Blood Lipids and Lipoproteins: Quantitation, Composition, and Metabolism

Blood Lipids and Lipoproteins: Quantitation, Composition, and Metabolism

EDITED BY

GARY J. NELSON

Ernest O. Lawrence Livermore Laboratory
Livermore, California

WILEY-INTERSCIENCE

a Division of John Wiley & Sons, Inc.

New York • London • Sydney • Toronto

Library of Congress Catalog Card Number: 76-178147

ISBN 0-471-63158-2

Printed in the United States of America.

10 9 8 7 6 5 4 3 2 1

Contributors

MARION BARCLAY, *Division of Experimental Chemotherapy, Sloan-Kettering Institute for Cancer Research, Walker Laboratory, Rye, New York*

VICTOR H. BLATON, *Simon Stevin Institute for Scientific Research, Bruges, Belgium*

DAVID CAPUZZI, *Department of Medicine, The Johns Hopkins University, Baltimore, Maryland*

NORMAN K. FREEMAN, *Donner Laboratory of Medical Physics and Biophysics, Ernest O. Lawrence Berkeley Laboratory, Berkeley, California*

JOHN A. GLOMSET, *Department of Medicine and Regional Primate Research Center, University of Washington, Seattle, Washington*

EUGENE L. GOTTFRIED, *Department of Medicine, Cornell University Medical College, New York, New York*

FREDERICK T. HATCH, *Bio-Medical Division, Ernest O. Lawrence Livermore Laboratory, Livermore, California*

LIN C. JENSEN, *Donner Laboratory of Medical Physics and Biophysics, Ernest O. Lawrence Berkeley Laboratory, Berkeley, California*

FRANK T. LINDGREN, *Donner Laboratory of Medical Physics and Biophysics, Ernest O. Lawrence Berkeley Laboratory, University of California, Berkeley, California*

AARON J. MARCUS, *Hematology Section, Veterans Administration Hospital, and Department of Medicine, New York Hospital-Cornell Medical Center, New York, New York*

SIMEON MARGOLIS, *Departments of Medicine and Physiological Chemistry, The Johns Hopkins University, Baltimore, Maryland*

GARY J. NELSON, *Bio-Medical Division, Ernest O. Lawrence Livermore Laboratory, Livermore, California*

HUBERT PEETERS, *Simon Stevin Institute for Scientific Research, Bruges, Belgium*

LENORE B. SAFIER, *Hematology Section, Veterans Administration Hospital, New York, New York*

BERNARD SHORE, *Bio-Medical Division, Ernest O. Lawrence Livermore Laboratory, Livermore, California*

VIRGIE G. SHORE, *Bio-Medical Division, Ernest O. Lawrence Livermore Laboratory, Livermore, California*

WILFRED J. SIMMONDS, *Department of Physiology, University of Western Australia, Nedlands, Australia*

VLADIMIR P. SKIPSKI, *Division of Experimental Chemotherapy, Sloan-Kettering Institute for Cancer Research, Walker Laboratory, Rye, New York*

HARRIS L. ULLMAN, *Hematology Section, Veterans Administration Hospital, New York, New York*

VIRGINIA S. WHITNER, *U.S. Department of Health, Education, and Welfare, Public Health Service, Lipid Standardization Laboratory, Atlanta, Georgia*

ROBERT F. WITTER, *U.S. Department of Health, Education, and Welfare, Public Health Service, Lipid Standardization Laboratory, Atlanta, Georgia*

Preface

The subject of blood lipids and lipoproteins covers a broad area of scientific knowledge that is not easily separated into the well-defined categories found in other scientific fields that are less interdisciplinary in character. The investigators interested in blood lipids are a heterogeneous group, ranging from theoretical biophysicists and structural organic chemists through biochemists and physiologists to practicing physicians. Consequently reports of original research in this field are scattered throughout the chemical and biomedical literature, making it difficult for even the specialist to retrieve significant information. And although there are a number of books on lipoproteins, as well as discussions of cellular lipids in several books on the erythrocyte, this problem is compounded by the lack of a modern, comprehensive treatise devoted exclusively to blood lipids and lipoproteins. This book attempts to fill this gap by providing in a single volume a reasonably complete summary of the field. Obviously it is not possible to cover thoroughly in a single volume all aspects of any scientific subject. Blood lipids and lipoproteins are certainly no exception. Yet I hope that the reader will find between the covers of this book adequate coverage of the overall subject without recourse to a full library, and at the same time adequate guidance to additional and more specialized information.

The authors were asked to treat their subject matter critically and objectively, but not to feel obligated to remove all signs of their own preferences and specialized interests. Thus each chapter reflects, more or less, the area of competence and specialization of its authors. No requirement was made to cite every publication or random hypothesis that has appeared in the last 50 years. Obviously, no matter how impartial an author tries to be, he brings a subjective bias to his subject matter. But this in itself can be useful. The reader can compare the chapters in this volume against those in past and future publications by others, thus obtaining a more balanced view of the subject than he can gain from the work of a single author.

Another reason for adding this book to the already prodigious number of scientific treatises currently available is my concern that an arbitrary segregation has occurred in the study of blood lipids, probably more through historical accident than through any deliberate actions on the part of the scientific community. Frequently the lipids and liproproteins of plasma and serum are treated separately from those of the cellular components of blood, and interactions between them are largely ignored. However, since it has been known for two decades that cholesterol is rapidly exchanged between erythrocytes and plasma, the justification for this type of treatment is questionable. More recently work on the plasma lecithin: cholesterol acyltransferase reaction has shown that lipids other than cholesterol also interact between cells and plasma. In addition, current studies on blood lipids in various diseases—such as acanthocytosis, hepatitis, and several anemias—have demonstrated that there is an intimate and vital relationship between the lipids of blood cells and plasma. Unquestionably, as we learn more about the structure and function of the lipids and lipoproteins of plasma and cells, their direct interrelationship with, and dependence on, one another will become even more manifest.

In any event the evidence is now overwhelming that lipids of both plasma and cells should be regarded as different facets of a single entity and that investigators should consider the possible consequences of lipid interactions between the two compartments regardless of their own specialized interests. My hope is that this volume will be a step in this direction.

I wish to acknowledge my gratitude to Dr. George Rouser for his assistance in the preliminary phases of the preparation of this volume and Dr. Valeska Evertsbusch for copy editing and reorganizing the tables in some of the chapters. To the authors of this volume I am grateful not only for their contributions but also for their understanding and patience during the preparation and production of this book. My thanks are also due to numerous publishers for permission to reproduce many of the figures and tables used in this volume.

GARY J. NELSON

Livermore, California
August 1971

Contents

PART III SOLUBLE LIPOPROTEINS

Blood Lipids and Lipoproteins: Quantitation, Composition, and Metabolism

Part I

ANALYTICAL METHODS

1. Handling, Extraction, and Storage of Blood Samples

GARY J. NELSON

Bio-Medical Division, Ernest O. Lawrence Livermore Laboratory, Livermore, California

I. INTRODUCTION

The withdrawal of blood for scientific purposes is as old as experimental biology. Early methods were crude and often involved simply cutting the skin or vein of the experimental subject (1). Blood sampling did not reach technical excellence until the advent of the centrifuge and anticoagulants in the early twentieth century (2). The phenomenon of clotting did not prevent some early studies on blood, particularly since serum can be recovered after blood has been allowed to clot for several hours (3). Early analyses of blood lipids were primarily qualitative (4, 5).

The pioneering work of Bloor (6, 7) marks the real beginning of the quantitative biochemistry of blood lipids. The difficulties encountered by early investigators are still major pitfalls today, and modern investigators should be cognizant of them. Briefly, they involve the coagulation of blood, contamination of serum with erythrocytes and/or platelets and leukocytes (and vice versa), and denaturation and autoxidation of lipids during isolation and storage. With due diligence and proper precautions, these problems can be avoided without inconvenience to the investigator. This chapter outlines procedures that, in the author's opinion, so facilitate the processing of blood samples that the experimental results are as accurate as the analytical procedures and are uninfluenced by sampling techniques. No attempt is made to present a historical development or to cite every technique reported in the literature.

II. DRAWING BLOOD SAMPLES

A. Preparation of Blood Containers

Small samples (approximately 1–25 ml) of blood can be drawn directly into evacuated centrifuge tubes. The tubes can be made of either glass or plastic and should be clean and sterile. Siliconizing, a useful technique in many procedures because it prevents the coagulation and cell fragmentation resulting from contact with glass surfaces (8), should be avoided when lipids are being analyzed, because silicone oil is soluble in organic solvents (9) and can be carried through the analytical procedures. A drop of heparin solution or a few crystals of heparin can be added to the tubes to prevent coagulation. The tubes should be shaken gently during the drawing of blood to distribute the anticoagulant uniformly throughout the sample. Without thorough mixing, coagulation may take place in the upper layers of the sample; this is particularly troublesome when large samples are drawn.

Samples of less than 20-ml total volume are often drawn directly into syringes (10), to which the anticoagulant can be added before the sample is drawn. Of course the sample must be transferred from the syringe to the centrifuge tube soon after sampling. Direct syringe sampling is also the method of choice for sampling the blood of small animals, since only small volumes can be obtained.

Blood bottles or plastic blood bags are the preferred containers for samples in the range of 50 to 500 ml. Within the last few years the plastic blood bag has almost entirely replaced the glass blood-storage bottle (11). However, hemolysis remains a problem with large-volume samples, even when plastic blood bags are used. The plastic blood bag need not be siliconized (11) and is unbreakable. However, it cannot be evacuated, and this may decrease the rate at which the sample can be drawn.

Methods for obtaining large samples of blood—for example, when a large animal is to be exsanguinated—cannot be standardized. Drawing the blood into large Erlenmeyer flasks is one method commonly used in the author's laboratory. Buckets and large beakers can also be used.

Anticoagulants are not always necessary (12). If only serum is needed, the blood is drawn and allowed to clot before the cells are separated from the serum. This simplifies the removal of the cells and, more important, removes the fibrinogen from the serum. This procedure has had noticeable success in studies of human-lipoprotein patterns (13) and in large-scale screening studies on the atherogenicity of lipoprotein levels (14) as well as in biophysical lipoprotein research (15). However, the procedure promotes the activity of plasma cholesterol acyltransesterase, which alters the serum-lipid patterns for cholesterol–cholesterol ester and lecithin–lysolecithin, as pointed out originally by Sperry (16) and more intensively studied by Glomset (17) (see Chapter 14).

Several anticoagulants are available to prevent clotting and the destruction of erythrocytes during blood sampling. Isotonic citrate dextrose solution, a good choice when whole blood must be preserved for metabolic studies or reused, as in infusion experiments (18, 19), has the disadvantages that it dilutes the blood and significantly increases the volume. This is particularly annoying when large amounts of blood are processed in the laboratory. The preferred anticoagulants are ethylenediaminetetraacetic acid (EDTA) and heparin (20–22). In the author's experience heparin in solution is a convenient anticoagulant, having little or no effect on the blood lipids. Ethylenediaminetetraacetic acid is also a reliable anticoagulant; moreover, it sequesters the divalent metallic ions that promote the autoxidation of unsaturated fatty acids in blood lipids (23).

The use of antioxidants is also recommended. Initially the best way of avoiding autoxidation, which may be promoted enzymatically in drawn whole blood, is to cool the blood immediately after, or even during, the sampling process. Centrifuge tubes can be prechilled in an ice bath and immediately returned to the bath after receiving the sample. Plastic blood bags can be immersed in an ice bath even as the sample is drawn. The addition of such antioxidants as butylated hydroxytoluene (BHT) or tocopherol to fresh blood is not necessary when blood is kept below 10°C until processing, provided that processing is not unduly delayed. This is particularly true if EDTA is present. Antioxidants should be added to blood-lipid samples during lipid extraction by addition to the extracting solvents.

B. Methods of Sampling Animal Blood

The choice of sampling method depends on the size of the experimental animal and on the size of the desired sample. Sampling from human subjects presents a special case and is usually handled in clinics or hospitals. Procedures for sampling the blood of animals fall into two categories: (a) those used for small animals (e.g., rats, guinea pigs, and mice) and (b) those used for any larger animals.

Blood is often obtained from small animals by sacrificing and exsanguinating them. Heart puncture recovers much of the total blood from a rat or mouse (24). Small samples can be drawn from rats or mice by slicing off the tip of the tail and collecting the blood (25), but this method yields total volumes of less than 1 ml; alternatively hypodermic needles can be inserted into the veins of small rodents (26–28). For specific techniques and information on blood volumes in small animals the reader is referred to more specialized treatises (29). Animals weighing a few hundred grams or less have small blood volumes (30). Samples from several animals are usually pooled for lipid analysis because the amount of lipids present in the circulation is small (31). Ten milliliters is frequently the minimum needed for the chromatographic techniques described in other sections of this volume.

Small samples can be drawn from large animals by syringes without anesthesia (32, 33). The location of the puncture is chosen at the convenience of the investigator. The ear is a good site because the veins are visible under the epithelial layer (34). Dogs are often sampled in the veins of the hindlegs (34). Several specialized techniques and locations for drawing blood from large experimental animals have been reported; the reader is referred to texts on experimental physiology or veterinary medicine for details (24, 34, 35).

Venipuncture is the normal procedure for large animals, and the jugular vein is a convenient site (36). Large animals must be restrained or anesthetized (37). If blood is drawn from a specific internal site, it is necessary to use a catheterization procedure (38), which always requires anesthesia.

It is sometimes necessary to draw blood postmortem. Immediately after death blood can be drawn from experimental animals with no problems. If the animal has been dead for several hours, blood coagulation, along with other postmortem changes, often complicates or prevents meaningful analysis of the data (39). Death causes the activation of hemolytic and lipolytic enzymes (40) that may degrade or release lipids into the blood. In general, therefore, blood should be drawn as soon as possible after death. If it is not drawn within 1 hr of the death of the animal, the sample is worthless for lipid analysis; the results are more likely to reflect post-mortem changes than natural composition *in vivo*.

III. SEPARATION OF BLOOD FRACTIONS

A. Separation of Plasma or Serum from Cells

Serum can be obtained from whole blood that has been allowed to clot, but this procedure has several disadvantages, as already noted. Although it eliminates the need for anticoagulants, it is not recommended for modern lipid analysis. Serum can be obtained from blood without clotting and without anticoagulants if the blood is carefully defibrinated (41).

Centrifugation is the standard method for separating cells from plasma. Samples of less than 15 ml can be processed in 15-ml centrifube tubes in a small clinical centrifuge. Larger volumes are handled in 40-ml plastic centrifuge tubes. A refrigerated centrifuge is preferable because the speed and duration of centrifugation otherwise heat the sample to undesirable temperatures.

The centrifugal force necessary to sediment the erythrocytes is relatively small. Adequate separations can be obtained at less than 1000 *g* (42); at this rate, however, long centrifuge runs are necessary for effective separations. At greater forces, such as 1600 *g*, cells are well separated from plasma in about 15 to 20 min. Greater centrifugal force yields cleaner separations and also provides more complete removal of platelets and platelet fragments from the plasma (43).

A disadvantage of high-speed centrifugation is that, since differences in red-cell density have more influence at greater centrifugal forces, there is a much more pronounced separation of young and old cells (44, 45). This may be desirable or undesirable, depending on the nature of the experiment. A disadvantage arises if the cells are being thoroughly washed to facilitate removal of residual plasma and leukocytes; younger cells are selectively removed from the sample. Because younger cells may differ from older cells in other ways (46), such centrifugation and washing could alter the results of the experiment. The effects of washing and recentrifugation are discussed further in Section III.B.

One centrifugation is enough to free the cells of plasma, provided that the centrifugal force and the centrifugation time are adequate. A low-speed centrifugation to remove most of the erythrocytes and leukocytes from the sample, followed by a high-speed centrifugation to remove the remaining cells and platelets, yields a cleaner plasma sample than a single high-speed run. In many experiments a trace of platelets in the plasma does not appreciably affect the analytical data. Hence the choice of sample-preparation technique is at the discretion of the investigator.

B. Isolation and Purification of Erythrocytes

Red cells must be washed thoroughly to remove residual plasma lipoproteins. Plasma contamination of erythrocytes has been a particularly vexing problem in the analysis of neutral lipids from erythrocytes (47). Some studies that report appreciable amounts of neutral lipids in erythrocytes may reflect inadequate removal of plasma from the cells. The cells must be washed at least three times with isotonic buffer before they can be considered to be free of plasma lipoproteins, and four washes are preferable (47).

Several buffer systems are available for washing red cells (48–51). The most common wash is isotonic saline. The isotonic saline solution supplied commercially is not buffered at physiological pH and may be unacceptable for many experiments. It can, however, be buffered with low concentrations of tris(hydroxymethyl)aminomethane (tris buffer) to physiological pH (49). Another wash medium that is frequently used is isotonic phosphate buffer, which has worked well for a wide variety of erythrocytes from a number of different species (52). Other washing media can be used, but they are largely variations of the above solutions and are often designed for specific problems (53–55).

The washes necessary to free the erythrocytes of plasma lipoproteins and leukocytes may cause some loss of lipid from the cell during the washing cycles. Some investigators (56, 57) have claimed that lipid is lost during the washing of intact cells with isotonic solutions, but this has not been true in my experience, particularly if the wash solution is buffered at physiological pH (52). There may be considerable loss of protein as well as lipid from the cell if the wash is not buffered adequately. Hemolysis of erythrocytes is associated with loss of cellular enzymes (58, 59), but loss of cellular lipids has not been proved.

Lipids bound to the outer surface of the plasma membrane can be removed by extensive washing. These lipids (e.g., lysolecithin and free fatty acids) are not considered to be integral components of the membrane but are reversibly attached to it in dynamic equilibrium with the plasma (60). Exchanges between membrane lipids and plasma lipoprotein occur in 1 : 1 ratios; hence no net loss of lipids is expected from such reactions (61–63).

Multiple washing is necessary to remove leukocytes and platelets from erythrocytes. Leukocytes particularly should be completely removed, because they contain some lipids (see Chapter 8) that are not present in erythrocytes. Furthermore, the presence of a few leukocytes can grossly affect the outcome of metabolic studies, because these cells are very active metabolically. The presence of leukocytes in the preparation can be determined by staining a smear of the cells with a nucleophilic dye (e.g., Giemsa stain). The washing technique is usually adequate if it reduces the leukocytes to less than one per 10^4 erythrocytes, a level considered acceptable for erythrocyte-lipid analyses or metabolic experiments (64). If the staining reveals larger numbers of leukocytes, the preparation should be subjected to additional washings. For details of the staining techniques one of the volumes on histochemical procedures should be consulted (65, 66).

The platelet content of erythrocyte preparations is difficult to estimate, but the leukocyte content is usually a good index of the platelet count, since platelets are easier to remove than leukocytes. A good way of removing platelets is to spin the whole blood for 10 min at 400 *g* and then to remove the plasma. This leaves the platelets in the plasma while most of the leukocytes and red cells are sedimented (67).

The erythrocyte preparation can then either be extracted directly or first freed of hemoglobin by lysis; however, lysing lengthens the time of the analysis. The end product of lysing is the erythrocyte "ghost," which is essentially the intact membrane of the erythrocyte, free of hemoglobin. The ghost has most of the properties of the intact membrane, except that some membrane proteins are lost (56). Extracts prepared from ghosts are free of heme pigments, which are undesirable because they promote the autoxidation of lipids (68). All extraction procedures extract some pigments from the intact erythrocyte.

Many hemolysis procedures have been reported in the literature (56, 69–73). In the simplest method the washed cells are added directly to a large volume of distilled water (69); this fragments the membrane, however, and does not yield ghosts that are completely free of hemoglobin (71). The ionic strength and the pH of the hypotonic medium are very important in the production of hemoglobin-free ghosts that still retain most, if not all, of the characteristics of the original cell membrane (58). Ghosts cannot be sedimented with low-speed clinical centrifuges; forces of 10,000 *g* or greater are necessary to sediment and pack the ghosts firmly enough to allow the removal of the supernatant without disturbing them.

In the older methods ghosts were prepared by the action of such chemical lysins as digitonin and saponin (72) or 0.1% sodium chloride saturated with carbon dioxide (74), or by successively freezing and thawing, as proposed by Jorpes (75). These techniques are either relatively inconvenient or fail to yield hemoglobin-free preparations; they also can fragment the cell membranes, lowering the yield of intact ghosts. A satisfactory but time-consuming procedure hemolyzes the cells by passing them through a series of successively more dilute solutions of saline, starting with 100 m*M*, followed by 60 and then 30 m*M* solutions (71). These solutions are buffered at pH 7.2. Weed, Reed, and Berg (55) found that the addition of 1 m*M* Na_2EDTA to the hypotonic solutions enhances the removal of hemoglobin from the cells.

Dodge, Mitchell, and Hanahan (58) have reported a method for producing ghosts from human red cells with only a single lysing medium. The solution consists of 20 milliosmolar phosphate buffer at a pH of 7.4, which controls both the ionic strength and the pH of the solution. Dodge and co-workers state that hemolysis in three washes of this hypotonic medium yields intact ghosts that are essentially free of hemoglobin, with no loss of membrane lipids and only minor loss of membrane proteins. This procedure would seem to be a convenient and simple way of preparing ghosts in large quantities.

Another point to be considered, besides loss of membrane lipids and lipoproteins during hemolysis, is whether the extra time *involved* is warranted by the advantages of a heme-free extract. Dodge and Phillips (68) showed that heme pigments do not cause deterioration if an antioxidant is added to the lipid extract. Hence hemolysis of the cells before extraction is at the discretion of the experimenter.

IV. EXTRACTION OF LIPIDS AND PURIFICATION OF EXTRACTS

A. Extraction of Plasma and Serum

Several solvent systems have been used to extract lipids from plasma (76–81). These systems include ethanol–acetone, ethanol–ether, isooctane–ether–ethanol, methanol–hexane, and other mixtures. Since the report by Sperry and Brand (82), based on work initiated by Folch and co-workers (83, 84), chloroform–methanol mixtures are the solvent systems of choice for the extraction of lipids from plasma and other tissues. Several variations of the Sperry and Brand method have appeared, but these are usually minor modifications of the original procedure. Some of these variations consist of adding first one solvent and then the other, shaking, heating, and varying the proportions of the chloroform–methanol mixture (85, 86).

Sperry and Brand initially recommended a solvent-to-sample ratio of 24 : 1 and used 2 : 1 chloroform–methanol (v/v). After adding the sample slowly to methanol, they added half the chloroform and brought the solution to a boil. After it had cooled to room temperature, the solution was brought up to volume with chloroform and filtered to remove the precipitated protein. This procedure does quantitatively extract the plasma, but to avoid autoxidation and degradation of the lipids, the heating step can be, and usually is, omitted. In the author's laboratory the solvent-to-sample ratio is 50 : 1, and BHT is added to all solvents used in the extraction. All extractions are performed at 0°C in an ice bath. After adding the sample dropwise to the methanol, half the chloroform is added, and the solution is stirred for 5 min. It is then brought up to volume with chloroform. After being allowed to stand for another 5 min, it is filtered through a sintered-glass filter or a fast filter paper previously washed with solvent to remove organic or water-soluble contaminants in the paper (87). Sintered-glass funnels are preferable because they can be cleaned thoroughly with acid and solvents, but they tend to clog easily and increase the filtration time. The residue in the funnel should be thoroughly washed with solvent. In the method of Sperry and Brand the residue was not washed. Sperry and Brand assumed that the volume of solvent lost in filtration contained lipids in direct proportion to those in the recovered solution. Their assumption cannot always be justified, but it is adequate in procedures for total-lipid determinations. For more sophisticated analyses, however, the residue must be thoroughly washed and then perhaps reextracted.

We find that by using a solvent-to-sample ratio of 50 : 1 and thoroughly washing the residue and the extraction flask with 2 : 1 chloroform–methanol we can recover 95 to 98% of the lipids. If the residue is reextracted with the same volume of 2 : 1 chloroform–methanol, the recovery is 97 to 100%. Acidification of the reextraction solvent helps recover all of the lipids in the sample; the free fatty acids are converted to the nonionized form, in which they are more soluble in the extraction solvent. There is no apparent advantage to using a basic solvent system containing ammonia or ammonium acetate in the extraction of plasma.

After the extraction steps listed above, the reextracted residue can be dried and then digested with 2 *N* KOH for several days (88). The digest is then neutralized and extracted once or twice with hexane and then with chloroform. Any lipids in the residue are recovered as free fatty acids or unsaponifiable matter (89, 90). If the first steps in the extraction are performed correctly, the saponification yields less than 0.5% of the mate-

Table I. Recovery of Lipids from Exhaustive Extraction of Sheep Plasma[a]

Step	Procedure	Before Sephadex mg	Before Sephadex %	After Sephadex[b] mg	After Sephadex[b] %
1	First extraction, 1000 ml of $CHCl_3$–MeOH, 2:1 (v/v) MeOH, 2:1 (v/v)	63.92	76.8	48.82	97.4
2	Second extraction (insoluble residue), 1000 ml of acidified $CHCl_3$–MeOH, 2:3(v/v)	5.84	7.0	0.75	1.5
3	Third extraction (insoluble residue), 500 ml of the solvent used in step 2	12.47	15.0	0.20	0.4
4	Hexane extraction of neutralized KOH digest of insoluble residue from step 3	0.35	0.4	0.30	0.6
5	Chloroform extraction of neutralized KOH digest following step 4	0.62	0.7	0.05	0.1
6	Total extracted	83.20		50.12	

[a] A 20-ml volume.
[b] Sephadex fraction I only.

rial recovered in steps 1 and 2 (see Table I). The only reason for an exhaustive digestion of the extracted residue is to check the efficiency of the initial extraction; recoveries of 1.0% or greater from the digestion indicate difficulties in the initial extraction.

B. Extraction of Erythrocytes

Chloroform–methanol mixtures are commonly used to extract lipids from erythrocytes (91–95), but acetone–ethanol and other solvent systems were used previously (96–98). Rose and Oklander (99) proposed the replacement of methanol by isopropanol to reduce the amount of heme pigments extracted. Several authors have used 1 : 1 methanol–chloroform and reextracted three or four times with this solvent (58, 100). A single extraction with 2 : 1 chloroform–methanol fails to recover all the lipids from erythrocytes. In the author's experience, however, the recovered proportions of lipids are the same, except perhaps for the gangliosides, but the amount is 5% less than that obtained by exhaustive reextraction of the cells. Hence the purpose of the experiment frequently determines the necessity for exhaustive reextraction. Reextraction increases the amount of nonlipids in the extract. If reextraction is necessary, the solvent system should be changed after the second extraction of the residue.

Table II lists the recovery of lipids from an exhaustive extraction of intact sheep erythrocytes. The amount of lipids recovered in the initial extract can be increased substantially by increasing the solvent-to-sample ratio and by thoroughly washing the filtrate with 2 : 1 chloroform–methanol. Extracting intact erythrocytes is complicated by the fact that denatured hemoglobin retains large amounts of solvent and lipids in a matrix that is difficult to flush adequately.

For extraction it is not necessary to grind or disrupt the cells if they are added slowly to methanol. Dropwise addition of the cells to a large volume of methanol, 10 : 1 solvent-to-sample ratio, results in a fine dispersion of the precipitated hemoglobin, provided that the solution is stirred. If they are added rapidly to 1 : 1 chloroform–methanol, the cells

Table II. Recovery of Lipids from Exhaustive Extraction of Packed Sheep Erythrocytes[a]

Step	Procedure	Before Sephadex		After Sephadex[b]	
		mg	%	mg	%
1	First extraction, 1000 ml of $CHCl_3$–MeOH[c]	85.02	55.7	78.23	95.9
2	Second extraction (insoluble residue), 1000 ml of $CHCl_3$–MeOH[c]	2.64	1.7	2.12	2.6
3	Third extraction (insoluble residue), 500 ml of $CHCl_3$–MeOH[c] saturated with 28% (w/w) acqeous ammonia	2.39	1.6	0.16	0.2
4	Fourth extraction (insoluble residue), 500 ml of $CHCl_3$–MeOH[c] acidified with 1% concentrated HCl	60.83	39.9	0.00[d]	0.0
5	Hexane extract of neutralized KOH digest of insoluble residue from step 4	0.77	0.5	0.75	0.9
6	Chloroform extraction of neutralized KOH digest following step 5	0.97	0.6	0.32	0.4
7	Total extracted	152.62		81.58	

[a] A 15-ml volume.

[b] Sephadex fractions I and II only.

[c] $CHCl_3$–MeOH 2:1 (v/v).

[d] Excluding heme pigments (48.0 mg).

tend to form large clumps that are difficult to disperse. Ghosts do not react in this way, presumably because they lack hemoglobin; hence smaller solvent-to-sample ratios can be used. These observations suggest that the extraction of lipids from red cells is complicated by the presence of hemoglobin but that the binding of lipids in membranes differs little from that encountered with serum lipoproteins.

The methanol–chloroform solution is filtered in the same way as the plasma extracts. The residue is larger, and hence a larger funnel may be needed for the same volume of solution. A sintered-glass funnel is convenient, but filter paper, if washed to remove organic residues, can be used. The sintered-glass funnel must be cleaned relatively soon after filtration, because the hemoglobin residue tends to polymerize in air and sets in the funnel to a hard, solid sheet that is very difficult to remove. The exhaustive-extraction technique should remove 99.0% of the lipids from the cells. The extraction can be checked if necessary by digestion of the residue at basic pH, but this step is neither necessary nor desirable; it is time consuming and inconvenient.

The Sephadex procedure (see Section IV.E) is used to remove the impurities from the red-cell extract. Aqueous washes should not be used to remove nonlipid impurities from the extract because gangliosides, phosphatidylinositol, and phosphatidic acid are all easily lost in the aqueous phase. For erythrocyte extracts we recommend either no purification or the Sephadex column procedure in preference to the aqueous wash.

C. Extraction of Leukocytes

Leukocytes are extracted by procedures similar to those used with erythrocytes. Fortunately, since leukocytes contain no hemoglobin, the removal of heme and heme pigments from the extract is not a problem. The other major consideration in extracting leukocytes is that these cells are fully functional and contain all of the enzymes and metabolites present in the solid organs of the body. Thus a leukocyte extract is a mixture of lipids from microsomes, vacuoles, and plasma, nuclear, and inner and outer mitochondrial membranes. If a particular subcellular fraction of the leukocyte is studied, fractionation of the cell must be undertaken; for details the reader is referred to works on the fractionation of subcellular particles (101).

D. Extraction of Platelets

Platelets are extracted by procedures similar to those described for red cells and leukocytes, without special modifications.

E. Purification of Lipid Extracts

A 2 : 1 (v/v) chloroform–methanol mixture extracts a considerable quantity of nonlipids, perhaps more than solvent systems consisting of ethanol–ether (102) or isopropanol–chloroform (99). Its advantage is its greater efficiency in extracting lipids. Some extra steps, however, are necessary to remove the nonlipid substances from the lipid extract, no matter which solvent system is used.

Until the development of the cellulose-column purification technique (103) for lipid extracts, impurities in the extract were removed by repeatedly dissolving the sample in dry organic solvents or, more commonly, by an aqueous wash of the chloroform–methanol extract (83, 84). Sperry and Brand presented two aqueous wash procedures in their 1955 paper (82). The first, which was essentially identical with the procedure of Folch et al. (84), used a large volume of water. The second used an aqueous wash containing 0.02% calcium chloride at only 20% the volume of the organic phase (82). The second method, because of its simplicity and rapidity, is widely used.

Bligh and Dyer were not specifically concerned with blood lipids, but published (104) a useful detailed report on the extraction and purification of lipid extracts with biphasic methanol–chloroform–water systems. This paper is strongly recommended to investigators who use aqueous washing procedures. This technique unfortunately does not yield a lipid extract that is totally free of nonlipid impurities (105), and lipids are frequently lost in the aqueous phase, particularly if the rigorous conditions proposed by Bligh and Dyer (104) are not followed exactly. These problems are not major ones in the extraction of plasma or serum, but nevertheless they should be considered, particularly for radiotracer studies (106).

Cellulose-column purification of lipid extracts was discovered almost accidentally in a study in which Lea and Rhodes (107) showed that cellulose columns did not separate phosphatidylethanolamine from lecithin (108); they suggested that cellulose could be used to remove nonlipids from lipid extracts. Others (109, 110) followed their suggestion, but their procedures were time consuming and often inadequate. Wells and Dittmer (111) described a method in which a dextran gel (Sephadex) is used and which is relatively simple and appears to provide good separation of lipids from nonlipids. However, Siakotos and Rouser (112) and Wuthier (113) found difficulties with the Wells–Dittmer procedure and modified it to give complete purification of lipid extracts regardless of the degree of contamination by nonlipid impurities. For details and variations of the Sephadex procedures the reader is referred to the original papers of

Siakotos and Rouser (112) or Wuthier (113). Details of the Sephadex procedure are given in Chapter 2 and are not discussed further here.

V. STORAGE OF BLOOD AND EXTRACTS

A. Storage of Whole Blood, Plasma, and Cells

Whole blood can be preserved for only a limited time. When it is frozen in the natural state and then thawed, the result is essentially total destruction of the cells and denaturation of plasma proteins (114). Hence it can only be stored above 0°C, but at these temperatures enzymatic reactions, though slowed, continue to occur and the cell continues to age. Furthermore, the life span of the erythrocyte is short, and any population of freshly drawn cells has a mixture of old and new cells. Some cells hemolyze soon after drawing, and in the absence of the *in vivo* clearing mechanism that removes the free hemoglobin and cell fragments, the preserved blood becomes contaminated with free hemoglobin, heme pigments, and lipids or lipoproteins (or both) in various states of denaturation (115). It is not practicable to preserve whole blood beyond a month (116); even then whole blood requires the addition of a preservative, such as isotonic citrate dextrose solution. A practical limit to the storage of anticoagulated whole blood without addition of an energy source like glucose is a few days.

Fortunately several alternatives are available for preserving blood samples. The best procedures require separation of cells from plasma immediately after the sample is drawn. Frozen plasma can be stored almost indefinitely provided that the plasma proteins need not be preserved in their natural state. Plasma is a good antioxidant and provides good protection to its component lipids (117). Hence at —20°C the lipid stored in plasma will not be degraded for several years or longer; the lipoproteins, however, will show discrete changes (118). The isolated lipoprotein fractions are labile and cannot be stored as long as whole plasma without severe denaturation (118). Antioxidants effectively preserve the lipids from deterioration, but the protein moieties are denatured by ice-crystal formation in the solid state (119).

Erythrocytes can be similarly preserved by freezing once they are freed of plasma and leukocytes. When thawed they hemolyze, but the lipids can be extracted as before without degradation. Leukocytes cannot be preserved in a viable condition by freezing (120).

The loss of lipids from intact erythrocytes stored under blood-bank conditions at 4°C has been studied (121, 122). According to Rimon, Brok, and Rimon (122), from 15 to 30% of the erythrocyte lipids is lost in 21 days; no further loss occurs up to 42 days, at which time their experiment was terminated.

Rimon and co-workers (122) postulated the existence of two pools of lipids in the erythrocyte membrane because of the rather peculiar characteristics of lipid loss from stored cells. The major loss of lipids seems to occur within 10 to 12 days of storage (other authors (121) report longer periods) and does not increase appreciably after this time until the cells undergo total destruction. Rimon et al. (122) thought that the 30% loss represented lipid that was not a structural part of the membrane, whereas the remaining lipid represented structural material that could not be removed without catastrophic destruction of the cell. Furthermore, the loss of lipids was apparently independent of the energy metabolism of the cell because it did not correlate well with either decrease in adenosine triphosphate or increase in intracellular sodium ions.

It is not yet clear whether the two-pool view is the correct one. The rather drastic conditions necessary for the complete hemolysis of the red cell apparently remove no lipids, except perhaps gangliosides, from the cell (58). Some authors have proposed that the loss of lecithin is a natural consequence of the aging of the red cell (123), but others have disputed this (124). This point is discussed further in Chapter 7.

Storage of whole blood prior to extraction of the lipids is not acceptable if rigorous lipid analysis is contemplated. Storage of the separated plasma (or serum) and cells is possible for long periods in the frozen state provided that only the lipid composition of the sample is to be analyzed; frozen stored samples are not recommended for metabolic studies or investigations of intact lipoproteins.

Whole blood can be stored frozen if preservatives like glycerol or dimethyl sulfoxide are added to the sample (125, 126). These additives keep the erythrocytes viable by preventing the formation of ice crystals; the blood can be used for transfusions after thawing and removing the additive. Unfortunately the lipids of such preparations have not been studied. Since changes may be induced by the presence of the preservative agent, these methods of preserving samples cannot be recommended at present to the lipid biochemist.

B. Storage of Lipid Extracts

The lipids extracted from blood are small molecules and not subject to conformational changes such as those that cause the denaturation of protein molecules. Under strictly defined conditions total lipid extracts and purified lipid fractions can be stored for long periods without significant deterioration, but they rapidly deteriorate if proper precautions are not observed (127–131). The storage of radioactive lipids presents a special problem, discussed at the end of this section.

Three basic precautions should be observed in the storage of all lipid samples:

1. They should be stored at as low a temperature as possible, but in any event at least —20°C.
2. Oxygen should be excluded from the sample during storage, and during handling if possible.
3. The sample should be stored in the dark.

If these rules are followed, samples can be stored for long periods.

Additional precautions that greatly increase the lifetime of stored samples are as follows:

1. The samples should be stored as solutions in organic solvents. For some reason solid, dry lipids have short half-lives; it has been suggested that glass surfaces may catalyze lipid deterioration (103).
2. Antioxidants should be added to the lipid solution. The antioxidant prevents autoxidation during storage and, perhaps more usefully, during subsequent processing. This is particularly helpful in the storage of a stock solution from which aliquots are taken at various times. Oxygen is difficult to exclude, and the effects of repeated exposure become cumulative so that the final analysis may no longer represent the original sample.

The storage container deserves to be chosen carefully. No cork or rubber stopper should ever be used with organic solvents. Ground-glass-stoppered vials and flasks are acceptable, provided that the stopper fits well. Commercial ground-glass-stoppered glassware is not ground fine enough to provide an adequate seal for organic solvents (103). The solvent evaporates from the vial or flask, and oxygen reaches the sample. The seal can be made tight enough by regrinding the commercial stopper with a glass-grinding compound (aluminum oxide, 800 grit size). A brief regrinding yields a stopper that seals well with all organic solvents except perhaps diethyl ether.

Samples can be stored in screw-cap vials when the caps have been thoroughly washed, cleaned, and lined with Teflon or polyethylene sealers. Caps with bonded paper liners or plastic liners should never be used. The bonding agents are soluble in organic solvents and can find their way into the sample, much to the chagrin of the experimenter. The threads of the cap and vial should be checked to ensure that an adequate seal can be made without breaking the vial or leaving an air gap between the liner and the lip of the vial; small irregularities in the lip of the vial can cause trouble. The fit can be improved by grinding the lips of the vials flat; only a few mils of glass need be removed to ensure a good seal.

There are commercial storage vials that are specifically designed for the storage of lipids in organic solvents. One is made by the Glass Engineering Company of Houston, Texas.[1] They can be purchased either graduated or ungraduated in 1- and 3-ml sizes. These vials have a Teflon stopper that is easy to insert and remove, yet forms a tight seal that allows neither evaporation of solvent nor passage of oxygen into the sample.

Total lipid extracts can be stored in a 19 : 1 chloroform–methanol (v/v) mixture saturated with water. However, a 9 : 1 chloroform–methanol (v/v) mixture saturated with water may be preferable for samples containing large amounts of glycosphingolipids and gangliosides. Purified lipids can be stored in the same solvents, but it is more convenient to store them in a single solvent like hexane or chloroform, because methanol is less easily removed. Neutral lipids like fatty acids, cholesterol, or triglycerides can be stored in pure hexane. Most phospholipids can be stored in chloroform; glycolipids can be stored in 9 : 1 chloroform–methanol (v/v).

As already mentioned, radioactive lipid samples present special problems, particularly if long-term storage is contemplated. Radioactively labeled organic compounds suffer radiation-induced decomposition (132), a problem that is not peculiar to lipids but is at times more pronounced because of the natural lability of many lipids. There are few reports on the specific susceptibility of lipids, but the general principles governing deterioration of radioactive organic compounds apply. Samples of high specific activity show greater deterioration. Phospholipids containing choline or nitrogenous bases can be considerably more susceptible to radioactively induced decomposition (133, 134). On the other hand, Mangold and Sand (135) reported that ^{14}C-labeled fatty acid methyl esters containing up to three double bonds with specific activities of approximately 100 μCi/mM were remarkably resistant to radiation-induced decomposition after storage at $-30°C$ as the solid for 10 years in sealed vials.

It is prudent for an investigator to ascertain the state of any radioactively labeled lipid that has been stored before proceeding to use it in any experimental procedure. Without such a check, the experiment may be ruined and the results suspect.

VI. CONCLUSIONS

The methods available for sampling, extracting, and storing blood samples are quantitative and reproducible for whole blood, plasma, or

[1]Reference to a product or company name does not imply approval or recommendation of the product by the U.S. Atomic Energy Commission or the University of California to the exclusion of others that may be suitable.

serum, erythrocytes, and other formed bodies of blood. Further research to provide better methods is not mandatory. Although by no means precluding future advances, we believe that new methods need not be developed before starting an experiment because the existing methods are adequate for most purposes.

Certain points deserve emphasis. It is best to extract samples as quickly as possible after drawing; storage of whole blood should be avoided unless absolutely necessary. It is safer to extract the sample and store the extract than to store cells or plasma, although frozen packed-cell preparations or plasma can be stored for long periods without extensive degradation of the lipids.

All extraction techniques yield extracts contaminated with nonlipid impurities. Heme pigments are extracted by organic solvents and cause difficulties in the lipid analysis of erythrocytes. Lipid extracts are better purified by partition chromatography than by aqueous washing. The removal of nonlipids from extracts is particularly important in radiotracer experiments, where inorganic and nonlipid precursors of high specific activity must be completely removed. Earlier reports in the literature that indicated incorporation of inorganic phosphate into erythrocyte lipids can be traced to failure to remove all inorganic phosphate from the extract.

Thorough washing of erythrocytes to remove both leukocytes and plasma lipoproteins is also worthy of emphasis. Metabolic studies of erythrocyte lipids could be seriously compromised by the presence of only a few leukocytes (136), and the presence of bound plasma lipoproteins was probably responsible for reports of neutral lipids other than cholesterol in erythrocytes (47). Usually three or more washes of the packed erythrocytes are necessary to remove plasma and leukocytes.

Cells need not be hemolyzed before extraction. Hemolysis can result in loss of lipid and certainly causes loss of membrane protein from intact erythrocytes. Although hemolysis has advantages in certain experiments, the choice is up to the investigator and depends on the particular experiment and on the results desired. It is not recommended for the quantitative analysis of erythrocyte lipids.

Finally, in storing lipid extracts and samples it is mandatory to use low temperatures and exclude oxygen. Samples in solution and in the presence of antioxidants can be stored almost indefinitely if the proper conditions are observed.

VII. ACKNOWLEDGMENTS

The work described in this chapter was supported in part by the U.S. Atomic Energy Commission. Technical assistance in experimental aspects was given by Mr. R. A. Booth.

REFERENCES

1. Dreyfus, C., *Some Milestones in the History of Hematology*, Grune and Stratton, New York, 1957, pp. 1–45.
2. Lewishon, R., *Surg. Gynecol. Obstet.* **21**, 37–47 (1915).
3. White, C. S., and J. J. Weinstein, *Blood Derivatives and Substitutes*, Williams and Wilkins, New York, 1947, pp. 290–297.
4. Lecanu, L. R., *Ann. Chim. Phys.* **67**, 54–70 (1838).
5. Letsche, E., *Physiol. Chem.* **53**, 31–112 (1907)
6. Bloor, W. R., *J. Biol. Chem.* **25**, 577–599 (1916).
7. Bloor, W. R., and A. Knudson, *J. Biol. Chem.* **29**, 7–13 (1917).
8. Strumia, M. M., L. S. Colwell, and A. Dugan, *J. Lab. Clin. Med.* **53**, 106–116 (1959).
9. Rouser, G., G. Kritchevsky, M. Whatley, and C. F. Baxter, *Lipids* **1**, 107–112 (1966).
10. Darmady, E. M., and S. G. T. Davenport, *Hematological Technique*, Grune and Stratton, New York, 1954, pp. 181–182.
11. Strumia, M. M., L. S. Colwell, and K. Ellenberger, *J. Lab. Clin. Med.* **46**, 225–233 (1955).
12. Nelson, G. J., and N. K. Freeman, *J. Biol. Chem.* **235**, 578–583 (1960).
13. De Lalla, O. F., and J. W. Gofman, in *Methods of Biochemical Analysis*, D. Glick, Ed., Interscience, New York, 1954, pp. 459–478.
14. Gofman, J. W., *Coronary Heart Disease*, Charles C. Thomas, Springfield, Ill., 1959.
15. Lindgren, F. T., H. A. Elliott, and J. W. Gofman, *J. Phys. Colloid Chem.* **55**, 80–93 (1951).
16. Sperry, W. M., *J. Biol. Chem.* **111**, 467–478 (1935).
17. Glomset, J. A., *J. Lipid Res.* **9**, 155–167 (1968).
18. Gibson, J. G., R. D. Evans, and W. A. Scheitlin, *Amer. J. Clin. Pathol.* **26**, 855–873 (1965).
19. Wintrobe, M. M., *Clinical Hematology*, Lea and Febiger, Philadelphia, 1967, p. 410.
20. Hadley, G. G., and S. P. Weiss, *Amer. J. Clin. Pathol.* **25**, 1090–1093 (1955).
21. Hellen, V. G., and H. Paul, *J. Lab. Clin. Med.* **19**, 777–782 (1934).
22. Schmidt, C. H., M. E. Hane, and D. C. Gomez, *U.S. Armed Forces Med. J.* **4**, 1556–1562 (1953).
23. Ray, B. R., E. O. Davisson, and H. L. Crespi, *J. Phys. Chem.* **58**, 841–846 (1954).
24. Stubbs, E. L., *J. Amer. Vet. Med. Assoc.* **122**, 226–227 (1953).
25. Leahy, J. R., and P. Borrow, *Restraint of Animals*, Cornell Campus Store, Ithaca, N.Y., 1953.
26. Hales, M. R., W. E. Bloomer, and W. A. Widman, *J. Appl. Physiol.* **21**, 1649–1652 (1966).
27. Vallejo-Freore, A., *Science* **114**, 524–525 (1951).
28. Nobunaga, T., K. Nakamura, and T. Imamichi, *Lab. Anim. Care* **16**, 40–49 (1966).
29. Grice, H. C., *Lab. Anim. Care* **14**, 483–493 (1964).
30. Schalm, O. W., *Veterinary Hematology*, 2nd ed., Lea and Febiger, Philadelphia, 1965, pp. 46–129.
31. O'Amour, F. E., and F. R. Blood, *A Manual for Laboratory Work in Mammalian Physiology*, University of Chicago Press, Chicago, 1954.

32. Schalm, O. W., *Veterinary Hematology,* 2nd ed., Lea and Febiger, Philadelphia, 1965, pp. 1–45.
33. Hillyard, L. A., C. Entenman, H. Feinberg, and I. L. Chaikoff, *J. Biol. Chem.* **214**, 79–90 (1955).
34. Farris, E. J., and P. Q. Griffith, *The Rat in Laboratory Investigations*, 2nd ed., Lippincott, Philadelphia, 1944.
35. Ambrus, P. L., C. M. Ambrus, P. W. E. Harrison, C. A. Leonard, C. E. Moster, and H. Cravitz, *Amer. J. Pharm.* **123**, 100–104 (1951).
36. Everett, J. W., and C. H. Sawyer, *Nature* **178**, 268–269 (1956).
37. Pearce, K. A., *Nature* **180**, 709 (1957).
38. Keishlay, G., *Lab. Anim. Care* **16**, 185–187 (1966).
39. Rouser, G., and G. Kritchevsky, in *Phenylketonuria and Allied Diseases,* J. A. Anderson and K. F. Swaiman, Eds., U.S. Government Printing Office, Washington, D.C., 1967, pp. 214–225.
40. Rouser, G., G. J. Nelson, S. Fleischer, and G. Simon, in *Biological Membranes,* D. Chapman, Ed., Academic Press, New York, 1968, pp. 5–69.
41. Dacie, J. V., and S. M. Lewis, *Practical Haematology*, Grune and Stratton, New York, 1963, pp. 2 and 3.
42. Hanahan, D. J., R. M. Watts, and D. Pappajohn, *J. Lipid Res.* **1**, 421–432 (1960).
43. Nelson, G. J., *Lipids* **2**, 64–71 (1967).
44. Westerman, M. P., L. E. Pierce, and W. N. Jensen, *J. Lab. Clin. Med.* **62**, 394–400 (1963).
45. Van Gastel, C., D. van den Berg, J. de Gier, and L. L. M. Van Deenan, *Brit. J. Haematol.* **11**, 193–199 (1965).
46. Hallinan, T., and E. Eden, *Blood* **20**, 557–565 (1962).
47. Nelson, G. J., *J. Lipid Res.* **8**, 374–379 (1967).
48. Chanutin, A., and R. R. Curnish, *Arch. Biochem. Biophys.* **113**, 114–121 (1966).
49. Dodge, J. T., and G. B. Phillips, *J. Lipid Res.* **8**, 667–675 (1967).
50. Farnsworth, P., D. Danon, and A. Gellhorn, *Brit. J. Haematol.* **11**, 200–205 (1965).
51. Neerhout, R. C., *J. Lab. Clin. Med.* **71**, 438–447 (1968).
52. Nelson, G. J., *Biochim. Biophys. Acta* **144**, 221–232 (1967).
53. Chafee, R. B. J., W. S. Platner, J. Patton, and C. Jenny, *Proc. Soc. Exp. Biol. Med.* **127**, 102–106 (1968).
54. Shohet, S. B., D. G. Nathan, and M. L. Karnovsky, *J. Clin. Invest.* **47**, 1096–1108 (1968).
55. Weed, R. I., C. F. Reed, and G. Berg, *J. Clin. Invest.* **42**, 581–588 (1963).
56. Anderson, H. M., and J. C. Turner, *J. Clin. Invest.* **39**, 1–7 (1960).
57. Lovelock, J. E., *Biochem. J.* **60**, 692–696 (1955).
58. Dodge, J. T., C. Mitchell, and D. J. Hanahan, *Arch. Biochem. Biophys.* **100**, 119–130 (1963).
59. Burger, S. P., T. Fujii, and D. J. Hanahan, *Biochemistry* **7**, 3682–3700 (1968).
60. Stein, Y., and O. Stein, *Biochim. Biophys. Acta* **116**, 95–107 (1966).
61. Rowe, C. E., *Biochem. J.* **76**, 471–475 (1960).
62. Sakagami, T., O. Minara, and T. Orii, *Biochim. Biophys. Acta* **98**, 356–364 (1965).
63. Reed, C. F., *J. Clin. Invest.* **47**, 749–760 (1968).
64. Donabedian, R. K., and A. Karmen, *J. Clin. Invest.* **46**, 1017–1027 (1967).

65. Emmel, V. M., and E. V. Cowdry, *Techniques in Biology and Medicine*, 4th ed., Williams and Wilkins, Baltimore, 1964.
66. Maile, J. B., *Laboratory Medicine: Hematology*, 2nd ed., C. V. Mosby, St. Louis, Mo., 1962, pp. 797–885.
67. Marcus, A. J., and T. H. Spaet, *J. Clin. Invest.* **37**, 1836–1847 (1958).
68. Dodge, J. T., and G. B. Phillips, *J. Lipid Res.* **7**, 387–395 (1966).
69. Berstein, S. S., R. L. Jones, B. N. Erickson, H. H. Williams, I. Avrin, and I. G. Macy, *J. Biol. Chem.* **122**, 507–514 (1938).
70. Ponder, E., *J. Exp. Biol.* **18**, 257–265 (1942).
71. Hillier, J., and J. F. Hoffman, *J. Cell. Comp. Physiol.* **42**, 203–247 (1953).
72. Ponder, E., *Protoplasmatologia: Handbuch der Protoplasmataforschung*, Vol. 10, Springer, Vienna, 1955, pp. 1–123.
73. Danon, D., A. Nevo, and Y. Marikovsky, *Bull. Res. Counc. Israel* **E6**, 36–39 (1956).
74. Ponder, E., *Hemolysis and Related Phenomena*, Grune and Stratton, New York, 1948.
75. Jorpes, E., *Biochem. J.* **26**, 1488–1503 (1932).
76. Gorter, E., and F. Grendal, *J. Exp. Med.* **41**, 439–443 (1925).
77. Erickson, B. N., H. H. Williams, S. S. Berstein, I. Avrin, R. L. Jones, and I. G. Macy, *J. Biol. Chem.* **122**, 515–528 (1938).
78. Mcfarlane, A. S., *Nature* **149**, 439 (1942).
79. Bloor, W. R., *The Biochemistry of Fatty Acids*, Reinhold, New York, 1943.
80. Lis, E. W., and R. Okey, *J. Nutr.* **73**, 117–125 (1961).
81. Smith, E., *The Lipids in Human Blood Fractions*, thesis, Oregon State University, 1965.
82. Sperry, W. M., and F. C. Brand, *J. Biol. Chem.* **213**, 69–76 (1955).
83. Folch, J., I. Ascoli, M. Lees, J. A. Meath, and F. N. Le Baron, *J. Biol. Chem.* **191**, 833–841 (1951).
84. Folch, J., M. Lees, and G. H. S. Stanley, *J. Biol. Chem.* **226**, 497–509 (1957).
85. Nelson, G. J., *J. Lipid Res.* **3**, 71–79 (1962).
86. Freeman, N. K., *Ann. N.Y. Acad. Sci.* **69**, 131–144 (1957).
87. Lindgren, F. T., A. V. Nichols, N. K. Freeman, and R. D. Wills, *J. Lipid Res.* **3**, 390–391 (1962).
88. Hilditch, T. P., and P. N. Williams, *The Chemical Constitution of Natural Fats*, Wiley, New York, 1964, pp. 678–680.
89. Gorbach, G., in *Analysen der Fette und Fettproduckte,* H. P. Kaufman, Ed., Vol. 1, Springer, Berlin, 1958, pp. 390–416.
90. Baltes, J., in *Oil, Fats and Fat Products,* H. A. Boekenoogen, Ed., Vol. 1, Interscience, New York, 1964, pp. 1–58.
91. Blomstrand, R., F. Nakayama, and I. M. Nilsson, *J. Lab. Clin. Med.* **59**, 771–778 (1962).
92. Dawson, R. M. C., N. Hemington, and D. B. Lindsay, *Biochem. J.* **77**, 226–230 (1960).
93. Farquhar, J. W., and E. H. Ahrens, Jr., *J. Clin. Invest.* **42**, 675–685 (1963).
94. Hill, J. G., A. Kuksis, and J. M. R. Beveridge, *J. Amer. Oil Chem. Soc.* **41**, 393–397 (1965).
95. Walker, B. L., and M. Yurkowski, *Biochem. J.* **103**, 218–224 (1967).
96. Brun, G. C., *Acta Med. Scand.* **99**, 13–237 (1939).
97. Munn, J. I., *Brit. J. Haematol.* **4**, 344–349 (1958).
98. Boyd, E. M., *J. Biol. Chem.* **115**, 37–45 (1936).

99. Rose, H. G., and M. Oklander, *J. Lipid Res.* **6**, 428–431 (1965).
100. Reed, C. F., S. N. Swisher, G. V. Marinetti, and E. G. Eden, *J. Lab. Clin. Med.* **56**, 281–289 (1960).
101. Bresnick, E., and A. Schwartz, *Functional Dynamics of the Cell,* Academic Press, New York, 1968, pp. 39–46.
102. Freeman, N. K., F. T. Lindgren, Y. Ng, and A. V. Nichols, *J. Biol. Chem.* **227**, 449–464 (1957).
103. Rouser, G., G. Kritchevsky, and A. Yamamoto, in *Lipid Chromatographic Analysis,* G. V. Marinetti, Ed., Vol. 1, Dekker, New York, 1967, pp. 99–162.
104. Bligh, E. G., and W. J. Dyer, *Can. J. Biochem. Physiol.* **37**, 911–917 (1959).
105. Nazir, D., and G. Rouser, *Lipids* **1**, 159 (1966).
106. Nelson, G. J., *Lipids* **3**, 267–274 (1968).
107. Lea, C. H., and D. N. Rhodes, *Biochem. J.* **54**, 467–469 (1953).
108. Bevan, T. H., T. Malkin, and A. G. Poole, *J. Chem. Soc.* (*London*), 841–842 (1951).
109. Rouser, G., G. Kritchevsky, C. Galli, and D. Heller, *J. Amer. Oil Chem. Soc.* **42**, 215–227 (1965).
110. Bernhard, K., and P. Lesch, *Helv. Chim. Acta* **46**, 1798–1801 (1963).
111. Wells, M. A., and J. C. Dittmer, *Biochemistry* **2**, 1259–1263 (1963).
112. Siakotos, A. N., and G. Rouser, *J. Amer. Oil Chem. Soc.* **42**, 913–919 (1965).
113. Wuthier, R. E., *J. Lipid Res.* **7**, 558–561 (1966).
114. Tullis, J. L., in *The Red Blood Cell,* C. Bishop and D. M. Surgenor, Eds., Academic Press, New York, 1964, p. 492.
115. Weed, R. I., and C. F. Reed, *Amer. J. Med.* **41**, 681–698 (1966).
116. Gibson, J. G., in *The Red Blood Cell,* C. Bishop and D. M. Surgenor, Eds., Academic Press, New York, 1964, pp. 477–489.
117. Robison, W. L., and G. J. Nelson, *Biochem. Biophys. Acta* **175**, 448–450 (1969).
118. Del Gatto, L., A. V. Nichols, and F. T. Lindgren, *Proc. Soc. Exp. Biol. Med.* **101**, 54–61 (1959).
119. Lovelock, J., *Biochim. Biophys. Acta* **11**, 28–36 (1953).
120. Tullis, J. L., *Blood* **8**, 563–575 (1953).
121. Reed, C. F., E. G. Eden, and S. N. Swisher, *Clin. Res.* **6**, 186–191 (1958).
122. Rimon, S., F. Brok, and A. Rimon, *Clin. Chim. Acta* **12**, 22–26 (1965).
123. Raderecht, H. J., E. Scholzel, and S. M. Rapport, *Klin. Wochenschr.* **38**, 824–825 (1960).
124. Reed, C. F., and S. N. Swisher, *J. Clin. Invest.* **45**, 777–781 (1966).
125. Tullis, J. L., and H. M. Pyle, *Vox Sang.* **5**, 70–71 (1960).
126. Huggins, C., *Science* **134**, 504–505 (1963).
127. Lea, C. H., *Rancidity in Edible Fats,* Chemical Publishing Co., New York, 1938.
128. Holman, R. T., in *Progress in the Chemistry of Fats and Other Lipids,* R. T. Holman, W. O. Lundberg, and T. Malkins, Eds., Vol. 2, Pergamon Press, London, 1954, pp. 51–58.
129. Bergstrom, S., and B. Samuelson, in *Autoxidation and Antioxidants,* W. O. Lundberg, Ed., Vol. 1, Interscience, New York, 1961, pp. 233–248.
130. Farquhar, J. W., *Biochim. Biophys. Acta* **60**, 80–89 (1962).
131. Wren, J. J., and A. D. Szczepanowska, *J. Chromatogr.* **14**, 405–410 (1964).
132. Tolbert, B. M., in *Advances in Tracer Methodology,* S. Rothchild, Ed., Plenum Press, New York, 1963, pp. 64–68.
133. Tolbert, B. M., and R. M. Lemmon, *Radiat. Res.* **3**, 52–67 (1955).
134. Kanfer, J. N., and M. Williams, *Chem. Phys. Lipids* **6**, 121–124 (1971).
135. Mangold, H. K., and D. M. Sand, *Biochim. Biophys. Acta* **164**, 124–126 (1968).
136. James, A. T., J. E. Lovelock, and J. P. Webb, *Biochem. J.* **73**, 106–115 (1959).

2. Quantitative Analysis of Blood Lipids

GARY J. NELSON

Bio-Medical Division, Ernest O. Lawrence Livermore Laboratory, Livermore, California

I. INTRODUCTION

This chapter presents quantitative methods for the analysis of blood lipids. It is not a survey of the current literature but rather a description of the techniques that have proved to be useful and reliable in the author's laboratories for the study of the lipid constituents of both red cells and plasma. In general many of the techniques described are applicable to the analysis of lipids from any source, often without modification. Nevertheless, care must be used in extending the methods described here to samples of different origins. Several reviews and articles covering the general aspects of lipid analysis have been recently published (1–4); the reader is referred to these for a more extended treatment of particular analyses.

The literature contains an enormous number of papers on specific analytical procedures for a particular blood lipid, often involving specialized instrumentation or procedures. Except for occasional citations, these methods are not discussed here. What is discussed here are methods that have been in use in the author's laboratories for several years. They have proved to be entirely satisfactory for the analysis of both plasma and red-cell lipids from a wide variety of sources and have been duplicated satisfactorily in other laboratories. One area of lipid analysis that is discussed only briefly here is the analysis of glycosphingolipids. For more details on the analysis of this class of blood lipids, the reader is referred to the work of Sweeley and co-workers (5–7) and others (8–13).

II. GENERAL LABORATORY PROCEDURES

A. Solvent Handling

All solvents used in the extraction and chromatography of lipids should be redistilled from reagent-grade solvents. Higher grade solvents from commercial sources can often be used directly without redistillation, but each solvent should be checked before use to ensure that its nonvolatile residues are not excessive. This is done conveniently by carefully evaporating 500 ml of solvent to dryness in a beaker protected from other sources of contamination, such as vacuum-pump oil vapor, atmospheric dust, and/

or silicic acid fines. The dry beaker is then washed down with a minimum volume of solvent, and the residue is transferred to a small vial. If the solvent is adequate, the weight of the residue should be essentially zero. Therefore a further and better check is to take the residue up in a minimum volume of hexane, about 5 μl, and inject it into a gas chromatograph. The recorder trace then gives a good description of the solvent residue. A visual inspection of the trace is usually enough to determine whether the solvent is acceptable for lipid analysis.

If redistilled solvents are used, chloroform should be stabilized with methanol (0.25% by volume). Chromatography-grade aqueous ammonia can be prepared by bubbling gaseous ammonia into distilled water in an ice bath. Ammonium acetate for ion-exchange cellulose-column chromatography can be prepared by mixing freshly prepared aqueous ammonia and redistilled glacial acetic acid. All solvents should be deaerated by bubbling nitrogen through them before use. In addition, butylated hydroxytoluene (BHT) (0.1 gm/l) can be added to all solvents to serve as an antioxidant during the various analytical procedures.

B. Glassware

All glassware should be scrupulously cleaned. If detergents are used during washing, very thorough rinsing with distilled water is necessary to ensure complete removal of all traces of the detergents. This is particularly necessary for glassware used in phosphorus determinations. Since most detergents contain inorganic phosphate, it is not uncommon to find a phosphate residue on glassware washed with them; the result is high blank readings and erroneous analytical data.

It is best not to send any glassware used in phosphate determinations to a common dishwashing facility. All reaction tubes, reagent vessels, and cuvettes should be thoroughly washed immediately after the analysis. Only dilute cleaning acid and distilled water should be employed. Under these conditions, reagent blanks with an absorbance of 0.005 versus distilled water can be obtained routinely. Reagent blanks whose absorbance exceeds 0.010 can be attributed to phosphate contamination.

Similarly glass plates for thin-layer chromatography should be treated with care to avoid contamination. Silica gel on used plates can be rapidly removed with a photographic squeegee. The plate is then rinsed in distilled water and soaked for 12 hr in dilute chromic acid–sulfuric acid cleaning solution. They are then rinsed very extensively in distilled water, dried in an automatic drying oven, and stored in a closed container until the next use. It is convenient to separate stacked glass plates from one another by a lint-free paper like Kimwipe.[1] This reduces the chances of chipping or breaking a plate during storage.

No stopcock grease should ever be used in procedures for lipid analysis. All glassware should have ground-glass tapered joints, and Teflon stopcocks and stoppers. Ground-glass joints fitted with O-rings are unacceptable in apparatus used for lipid analysis because the O-rings are susceptible to attack by organic solvents, which leach organic polymers into the sample. This is particularly true of buna-N rubber O-rings. If O-rings are used, they should be made of Teflon or Viton A. Thin Teflon sleeves inserted around ground-glass joints are acceptable, but in our experience, they leak more than the plain joint, although they do prevent freezing.

One place where a rubber or Viton O-ring is a useful accessory in lipid analysis is as a seal for desiccators. These desiccator rings eliminate the need for stopcock grease on the desiccator lid and also allow it to be opened more easily. Since no solvents contact the O-ring in the desiccator, there is no danger of any contamination of the samples by the O-rings.

C. Evaporation of Solvents

The evaporation of solvents from lipid extracts and column fractions should always be carried out with due care and under the proper conditions. Lipids may deteriorate if allowed to dry out completely as thin films on glass surfaces (14, 15), although this is not always true (16). Despite the use of antioxidants and pure nitrogen, all air cannot be rigidly excluded from the sample. Thus it is prudent not to dry a lipid sample completely. In any event the sample is usually transferred in solution to another container; hence it is convenient to leave some solvent in the evaporation flask. This is particularly necessary in handling phosphatidylethanolamine and phosphatidylserine, both of which rapidly undergo decomposition. Phosphatidylserine forms phosphatidic acid; phosphatidylethanolamine produces several artifacts, including one that is devoid of phosphorus and migrates like cerebroside in thin-layer-chromatography systems. Acidic lipids, such as cardiolipin, also form many artifacts under similar conditions.

These undesirable changes can be mostly avoided by performing all evaporations at reduced temperature and pressure. There are many commercial evaporators; any that require stopcock grease should be avoided. A type used successfully in the author's laboratory is constructed entirely of glass and Teflon (manufactured by Calab Industries, Oakland, Calif.).

[1] Reference to a company or product name does not imply approval or recommendation by the University of California or the U.S. Atomic Energy Commission to the exclusion of others that may be suitable.

A vacuum pump or aspirator can be attached to a vacuum line while pure nitrogen is bled into the evaporation flask at a low rate. Thus the rate of evaporation can be evenly controlled by a needle valve on the nitrogen line. Usually the evaporation flask is placed in a water bath. The temperature of the flask can then be maintained between 0 and 15°C. Hydrocarbon and chlorinated hydrocarbon solvents can be easily removed by these procedures. Other solvents, such as alcohols, acetic acid, or water, are best removed by repeated dilution and evaporation with chloroform. Column fractions containing glacial acetic acid must be treated with special care. After all the acetic acid is removed, it is usually desirable to convert the acidic lipids to their ammonium salts by the addition of a small amount of aqueous ammonia. The excess ammonia and water are then removed by the repeated addition and evaporation of chloroform.

After its volume has been reduced to an appropriate size, the sample is transferred to a storage vial. If it is a crude lipid extract, it is usually necessary to pass the sample through a medium fritted-glass filter to remove any inorganic salts present as well as any proteinaceous material in the initial extract. Glass-stoppered graduated cylinders are convenient for volumes of 5 ml or more. For volumes of 1 to 3 ml accurately graduated Teflon-stoppered tubes are excellent containers. These tubes can be obtained commercially from Glenco, Inc., Houston, Texas.

D. Sources of Contamination

There are many possible sources of contamination in the average laboratory, varying from dirty hands to oily aerosols produced by the air-conditioning system or by vacuum pumps. Obviously stopcock grease is a considerable hazard in a lipid laboratory. This substance should be avoided completely if possible. Teflon stopcocks and ground-glass joints have largely eliminated the need for its use. Similarly rubber or cork stoppers should never be used. The danger of detergents has already been mentioned in connection with the cleaning of glassware. However, even clean glassware will become contaminated with a thin film of hydrocarbon after standing in the average laboratory for any appreciable time. Two methods can be used to avoid contaminating the samples. One is to wash the glassware with chloroform before using; the second, and preferred, method is to seal the glassware into clean polyethylene bags after cleaning.

E. Miscellaneous Items

It is often convenient to obtain total weights on the crude lipid extract or isolated column fractions. Since the total sample is never dried, the simplest way of obtaining this is to weigh a small aliquot of the sample.

Because of the chance of error in handling small volumes (5–50 μl), which will produce a significant error in the total weight of the sample when multiplied by a factor of 100 or more, we always obtain the weight in triplicate aliquots. The weighings can be performed on any sensitive balance. Electrobalances are very good for this purpose (2). Larger samples can also be weighed on a substitution microbalance like the Mettler M5SA, which is accurate to ±2 μg but has a capacity of 20 g. Most electrobalances cannot weigh more than 1 g accurately. Small screw-cap vials (2-ml size), which weigh approximately 2 g, are convenient weighing vessels for the aliquots on substitution microbalances, and they are also convenient for storing the sample for further analysis, if desired.

Another useful datum is the percentage of phosphorus in the total lipid extract. After the weight of the aliquot has been obtained, the same sample can be used for the phosphorus analysis, provided it contains about 4 μg of phosphorus. Usually it is necessary to dilute the weighed sample so that a fraction containing this amount of phosphorus can be obtained. The sample is then transferred to a digestion tube and analyzed as described in Section V.D.2.

III. PURIFICATION OF LIPID EXTRACTS AND SEPARATION OF GANGLIOSIDES BY SEPHADEX COLUMN CHROMATOGRAPHY

A. Preliminary Steps

Nonlipids (usually aqueous soluble materials, such as sugars, amino acids, and inorganic salts) are always extracted from the tissue sample along with the lipids and in fact are actually solubilized by the lipids in the extract, particularly with the water present in the tissue. Lyophilization of tissue before extraction will reduce the amount of nonlipid extracted, but the extra time and manipulations necessary for the lyophilization are not usually warranted except under special circumstances.

Some salts, particularly magnesium and potassium acetates, are sufficiently hydrogen bonded with solvents to be soluble in chloroform and chloroform–methanol mixtures, even in the absence of lipids. The aqueous washing techniques of Folch et al. (17) and Bligh and Dyer (18) are frequently unsuitable for precise quantitative work. In the technique of Folch et al. (17) one salt is exchanged for another in the extract, and in the method of Bligh and Dyer lipids may be lost into the aqueous phase. Gangliosides may appear in both the upper and lower phases in both procedures. The presence of magnesium ions in the aqueous phase converts the acidic lipids to their magnesium salt forms, which do not undergo ion exchange with diethylaminoethyl (DEAE) or triethylaminoethyl (TEAE) cellulose. This means that acidic lipids must be reconverted to their potassium or sodium salts prior to ion-exchange cellulose-column chromatography.

In our experience nonlipid contaminants can be removed from lipid extracts most satisfactorily by column chromatography on cross-linked dextran gels like Sephadex (19–21). Sephadex is superior to ordinary cellulose (2) for partition chromatography because Sephadex beads can retain a large volume of water–methanol that is not retained on ordinary cellulose columns when chloroform is passed through the column. Thus Sephadex columns have a much greater capacity than cellulose columns of the same size.

B. Column Packing and Eluting Solvents

The Sephadex used in this procedure is the ordinary G-25 coarse Sephadex.[2] The Sephadex beads are placed in methanol–water, 1 : 1, and the fines are removed by repeated (triple) decantation. The beads equilibrate within 3 to 5 hr at room temperature. Dissolved gas can be removed from the gel by gentle suction from a water aspirator with swirling to prevent bumping. Also the equilibrated gel is usually degassed again just before packing the column.

The column is packed as a slurry of Sephadex in methanol–chloroform, 1 : 1. It is best to allow the excess solvent to drain from the column as it is being packed, so that the beads settle rapidly in the bed; otherwise they can be fractionated by size during settling. If fractionation does occur, the column can be made uniform by inverting it and mixing the packing after the desired amount of Sephadex has been added.

If an open column is used for Sephadex chromatography, the Sephadex beads must be weighted down with a layer of clean sand to prevent the gel from floating in solvent mixtures containing chloroform (3–8 cm of sand are sufficient for 10–30 cm of Sephadex). We prefer to use closed columns in which the packing is held firmly in place by bed supports on both the top and bottom of the column. For most of the samples columns containing 10 g of Sephadex are satisfactory. This amount of Sephadex packs conveniently into a column 1.2 cm in diameter and 35 cm long.

After the column is prepared, the packing is washed with the entire sequence of solvent mixtures used during the column purification of the lipid extract. When not in use, columns are maintained in standby condi-

[2] Do not use lipophilic Sephadex; it will not work in this system.

tion in methanol–water, 1 : 1. Columns can be used almost indefinitely, provided that they are not allowed to run dry.

The eluting solvents are all mixtures of solvents prepared as follows:

1. Chloroform–methanol, 19 : 1, saturated with water (approximately 5 ml/l).
2. Chloroform–methanol, 19 : 1, five parts plus one part glacial acetic acid, saturated with water (approximately 25 ml/l).
3. Chloroform–methanol, 9 : 1, five parts plus one part glacial acetic acid, saturated with water (approximately 42 ml/l).
4. Methanol–water, 1 : 1.

The first three mixtures should be prepared in separatory funnels, and any excess water should be removed. Mixture 4 should be cooled if it is used immediately, because of the heat of mixing of methanol with water.

C. Sample Application and Elution

The column that has been standing in 1 : 1 methanol–water is flushed with 400 to 500 ml of solvent 1 immediately before the sample is placed on the column. Although the column can be flushed at a somewhat faster flow rate than that at which the sample is eluted, it is generally convenient to use the same flow rate for both flushing and sample elution.

The sample is applied to the column in solvent 1 and rinsed onto the column with the same solvent. Elution then proceeds immediately. For 10g Sephadex columns the fraction volumes are 170, 350, 170, and 400 ml for fractions I, II, III, and IV, respectively. The normal flow rate is 2 ml/min. In practice fractions II and III are collected together. Table I lists the substances eluted in the various fractions. Fractions II and III from blood-plasma lipids contain very little material. The fractions from red-cell extracts, on the other hand, contain appreciable amounts of gangliosides.

Table I. Substances Eluted in Various Sephadex Fractions

Fraction	Substances Eluted
I	Hydrocarbons and all lipids except gangliosides and conjugated bile salts (when applied as salt forms)
II	Gangliosides and conjugated bile salts (when applied as salt forms), urea, and uncharacterized organic compounds
III	Traces of gangliosides and bile salts, less polar amino acids like phenylalanine and tyrosine, and uncharacterized organic compounds
IV	Inorganic salts, carbohydrates, taurocholic acid, and amino acids

The flow should be slow enough for equilibrium to be achieved between the interior of the beads and the mobile phase, but fast enough for the fractions to be collectable in a reasonable time. With a 1.2 × 35-cm column flow rates of 0.5 to 3.0 ml/min are satisfactory. Column fractions are handled essentially in the same way as the initial extract once they are collected from the column. Fraction IV is usually discarded without further examination after its dry weight is obtained.

D. Automatic Apparatus for Sephadex Chromatography

1. Construction. Sephadex purification of lipid extracts is a relatively simple and straightforward technique, but it does involve four solvent changes and three changes of the collecting vessels, as well as charging the column. In order to decrease the labor required by this procedure we have constructed an apparatus to perform the entire operation.

The apparatus automates the procedure described by Siakotos and Rouser (20). The four solvent mixtures are passed through the column in the usual sequence. Three or four fractions are collected automatically in volumes determined before the run is begun. The initial flow rate is also determined before the start of the run. It can be changed at any time during the run without disrupting the separations; however, it is usually more convenient to keep the flow rate constant during the run. At the beginning of the run the sample is loaded on the column, and the system is sealed from the atmosphere. A start button is then pressed to begin the automatic operation, which continues without manual intervention until the run is completed.

The apparatus was designed and constructed at the Lawrence Livermore Laboratory with commercially available components wherever possible. Columns, fluid valves, metering pump, and line fittings were obtained from Chromatronix, Inc. (Berkeley, Calif.). The control unit was designed and built by the Electronics Engineering Department of the Lawrence Livermore Laboratory. All materials in contact with the organic solvents and samples are made of either glass or inert plastics like Teflon or Kel-F. The solvent reservoirs are modified 2-liter, ground-glass-stoppered, borosilicate-glass bottles. The solvent-line valves are actuated by air pressure, which in turn is controlled by electrically operated solenoid valves located in the electronics chassis. The unit operates on 110-volt alternating current and on compressed air or nitrogen at 80 psi. It is packaged in a cabinet made of aluminum frame bar (Fig. 1).

Figure 2, a diagram of the solvent path, also shows the valve arrangement. The descending mode of operation is used during a sample run, and the ascending mode is used during flushing and column regeneration. (The

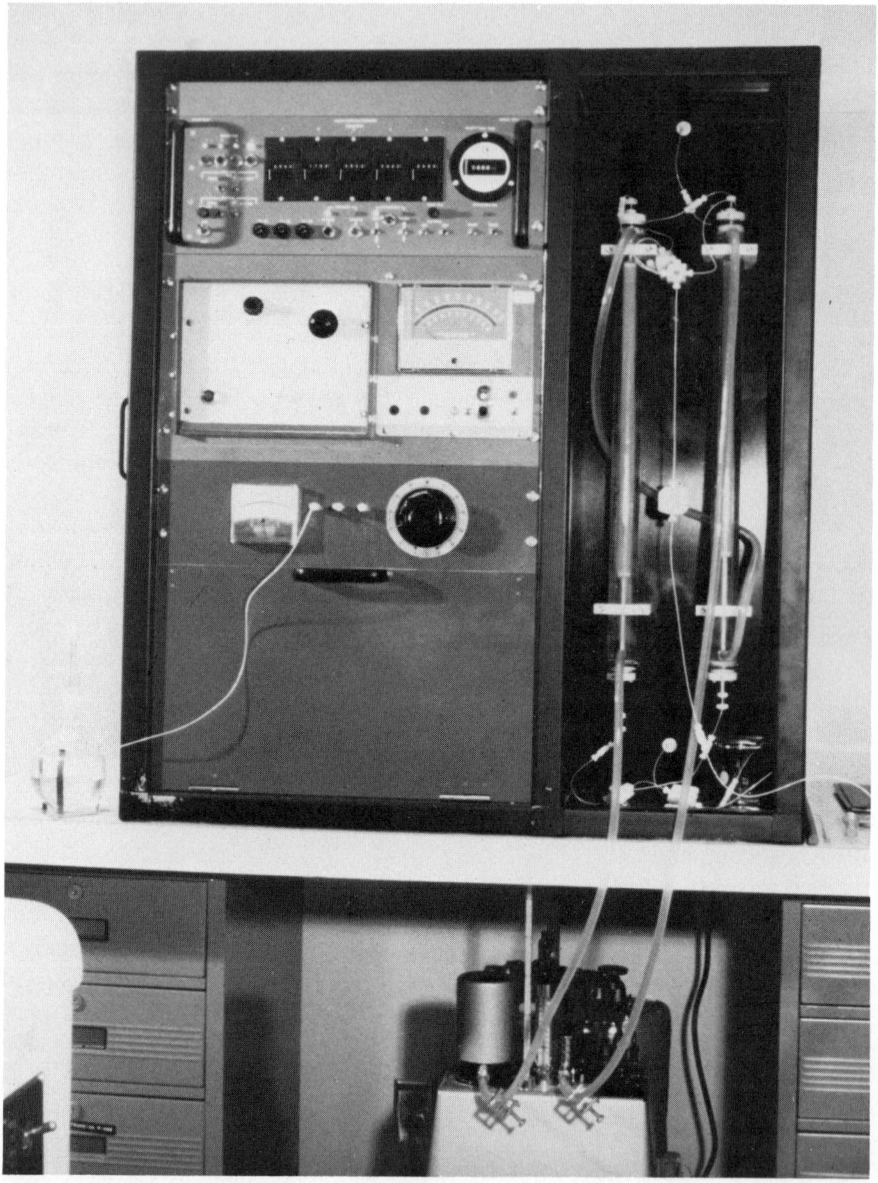

Fig. 1 A photograph of the automated column-chromatography apparatus for the purification of lipid extracts by gel filtration. Two columns are mounted on the right. Electronic controls and counters are in the upper left panel. The pump and the line-pressure gauge are immediately below the electronic panel, and below that are the thermocouple gauge and the temperature control for the solvent reservoirs. Under the cabinet is a circulating water bath that controls the column temperature. The fraction collector is not shown.

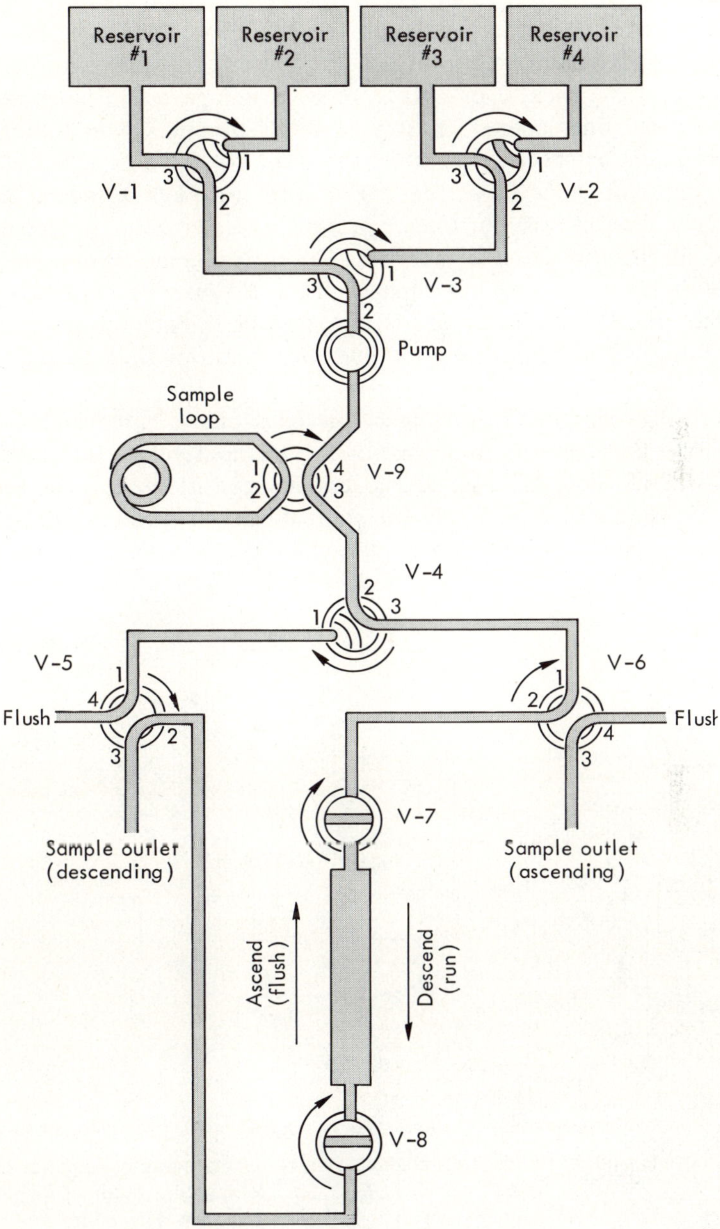

Fig. 2 Solvent flow diagram, showing valves, pump, and solvent reservoirs. Only one column is shown in the line. The automatic sampling valve is V-9. If a sample is placed on the column manually, the line is interrupted between valve 7 and the column.

reason for this is discussed further in the next section.) Two-liter solvent reservoirs are of convenient size, allowing three to five average runs before refilling. Larger volume reservoirs could be used, but since solvents should be made up fresh every 2 or 3 days, little advantage would be gained.

The solvent lines consist entirely of 0.024-in.-i.d. Teflon tubing. Since they are made as short as possible, the dead volume in the lines is quite small (approximately 0.003 ml/cm of tubing). The standard columns are 1.2-cm i.d. and 30 cm long. Larger or smaller columns can be substituted at the discretion of the user. These columns have a fixed bed volume that is not subject to change during a run. The fluid valves have essentially no dead volume; this is also true of the column connectors or other fittings. The compressed-air lines are made of 0.25-in.-o.d. copper tubing.

Figure 3, a simplified drawing of the electronic circuits in the control unit, shows the operating sequence of the solenoid valves that control the compressed-air flow. The electronic circuits consist entirely of switching relays operated either manually or automatically. The timing pulse to the counters is generated by a 1-rpm clock motor that turns a 10-notch cam,

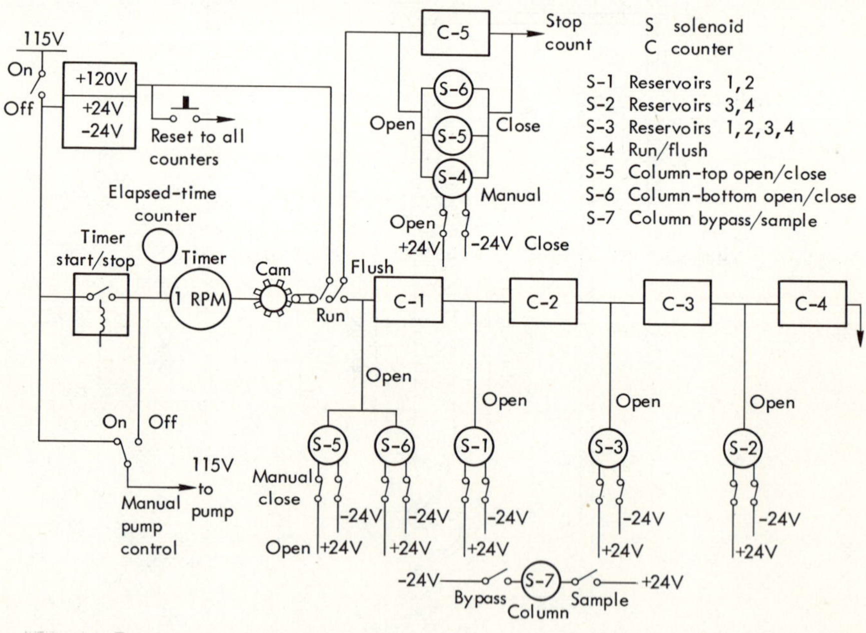

Fig. 3 Simplified block diagram of the electronic controls and solenoid valves in the electronic chassis of the automated column-chromatography apparatus. The unit is operated entirely by switching relays and counters.

which in turn actuates a microswitch. The pulse generated by the microswitch is sent to the counters. The operational sequence of the counters, electrical solenoids, and liquid-flow valves is shown in Fig. 4. The valves of the four solvent reservoirs are controlled by solenoids 1 through 3. The column and the direction of flow are controlled by solenoids 4 through 6 and valves 4 through 8. The sampling valve is operated only manually and is controlled by solenoid 7. When the system is operating automatically, each reservoir can be selected manually, the column can be opened or closed, and the pump can be turned on or off without disturbing the counting sequence.

The solvent reservoirs are mounted on a warm plate kept 5°C above ambient temperature; the columns are water jacketed and maintained at 15°C by a water bath. This combination effectively prevents the formation of gas bubbles in the columns and solvent lines during a run. A simple

Stand-by	Run sequence					Flush sequence	
	Counter #1 (Start)	Counter #2	Counter #3	Counter #4	Counter #5 (Stand-by)	Counter #5 (Start)	Counter out (Stand-by)
S-1 closed V-1 2-3		S-1 open V-1 1-2			S-1 closed V-1 2-3		
S-2 closed V-2 2-3				S-2 open V-2 1-2	S-2 closed V-2 2-3		
S-3 closed V-3 2-3			S-3 open V-3 1-2		S-3 closed V-3 2-3		
S-4 closed V-4 2-3						S-4 open V-4 1-2	S-4 closed V-4 2-3
S-4 closed V-5 [1-2, 3-4]						S-4 open V-5 [1-4, 3-2]	S-4 closed V-5 [1-2, 3-4]
S-4 closed V-6 [1-2, 3-4]						S-4 open V-6 [1-4, 3-2]	S-4 closed V-6 [1-2, 3-4]
S-5 closed V-7 closed	S-5 open V-7 open				S-5 closed V-7 closed	S-5 open V-7 open	S-5 closed V-7 closed
S-6 closed V-8 closed	S-6 open V-8 open				S-6 closed V-8 closed	S-6 open V-8 open	S-6 closed V-8 closed
S-7 closed V-9 [1-2, 3-4]	S-7 V-9 either position (manual)					S-7 } V-9 } either position (manual)	
Pump off	Pump on				Pump off	Pump on	Pump off

Fig. 4 Diagram showing the operational states of the seven compressed-air solenoid valves (S) and the nine liquid-flow valves (V) that they control during the run and flush sequences. The relationships of the valve-position numbers to flow in the system are shown graphically in Fig. 2. Solenoid 7 and valve 9 are controlled manually by a push button on the front panel, independently of the automatic operation.

resistance heater controlled by a variable transformer works well in a temperature-controlled room. In a location subject to large variations in ambient temperature it would be necessary to install a temperature regulator for the reservoir plate.

The pump (Chromatronix, Inc.) is a double-piston, constant-displacement unit constructed of glass, Kel-F, and Teflon. It operates over a pressure range of 0 to 500 psi without any change in flow rate. It also has a third piston to pressurize the inlet side to minimize pressure fluctuations that occur at back pressures above 50 psi. In this system all of the fittings and connector as well as the columns are rated at 500 psi. Other suitable pumps could undoubtedly be substituted for the Chromatronix unit provided they had adequate flow and pressure characteristics and were unaffected by the eluting solvents.

Since the pump can generate pressures higher than 500 psi (in testing pressures higher than 600 psi have been observed), a safety cutoff is necessary to avoid damage to the columns should the flow be inadvertently blocked. The system is therefore fitted with a pressure readout and a pressure-sensitive safety device. A pressure transducer (Statham Instruments) was incorporated into the solvent line next to the output side of the pump. The transducer is rated at 0 to 500 psi with an overrange to 750 psi and accuracy to 1% at full scale. The analog readout was modified by the incorporation of a pump-power-cutoff switch actuated by a relay. The relay can be tripped by any fluid pressure from 0 to 500 psi by setting a 10-turn potentiometer on the front panel. In routine operation the cutoff pressure is set between 450 and 475 psi. If the pressure limit is exceeded, the pump is turned off and remains off until a reset button is actuated, even though the pressure falls below the cutoff level.

In our instrument (Fig. 1) provision was made for mounting two columns on the rack for convenience; however, as indicated in Fig. 2, only one column can be operated at a time. The second column is on standby and can be alternated with the line column by manually actuated three-way valves (not shown on the flow diagram of Fig. 2).

Figure 5, a photograph of the main electronic control panel, shows the reservoir, column, run, and start buttons along with the counters and elapsed-time clock. Figure 6 shows the arrangement of the four reservoirs, liquid valves, and plumbing inside the cabinet.

2. Operational Sequence. The column is packed with 10 g of G-25 coarse Sephadex, conditioned as described in Section III.B. The column is then conditioned with at least 400 ml of solvent 4 (methanol–water, 1 : 1, v/v) and the resistance of the column is measured. The system can be operated in either the ascending or the descending mode. In dealing

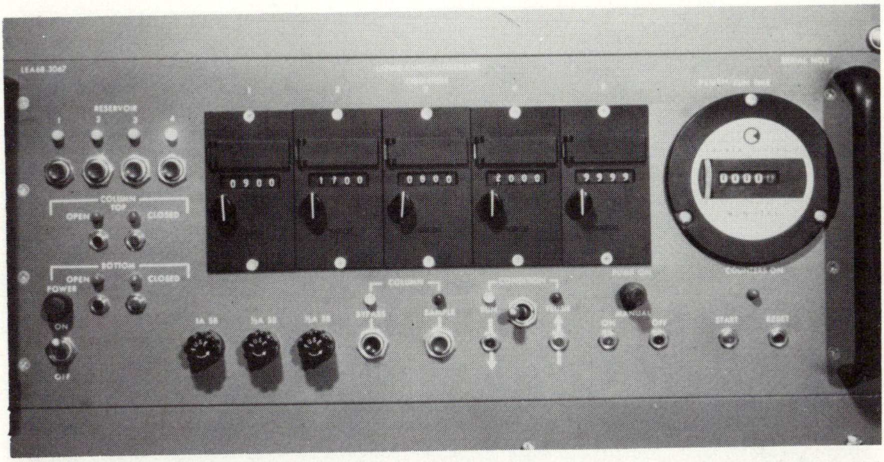

Fig. 5 Close-up view of the electronic panel and controls. Operating modes and positions of all valves are indicated continuously during a run by the pilot lights adjacent to each push button.

with immiscible solvents of differing densities, however, the direction of flow must be selected so that the denser solvent is always the lower phase. Thus solvent 4 must be flushed from the column by solvent 1 (chloroform–methanol, 19 : 1, v/v) in the ascending mode. Conversely the sample run must be performed in the descending mode, because the density of the solvents decreases in the order 1 to 4.

Before a sample is applied to the column, each of the four counters is set for the desired fraction volume. For routine runs the usual volumes are 170, 350, 170, and 400 ml for fractions I through IV, respectively. The counters can be set from 0 to 999.9 for each of the four fractions. Since the counters are actually timers, the volume collected depends both on the counter setting and on the flow rate. The available flow rates are 2.4, 6.0, 12.0, 24.0, 60.0, and 120.0 ml/hr; the last two are usually most convenient for a run. If 60 ml/hr is selected, the setting on the counters will correspond to the volume of each fraction.

After the column is conditioned, it is flushed with 500 ml of solvent 1 immediately before the sample is applied. The column is usually conditioned overnight so that the sample run can be started in the morning. The sample is dissolved in solvent 1 for application to the column. The automatic sampling valve (valve 9, Fig. 2) in this unit is useful for placing a known volume of sample on the column without opening the system to the atmosphere, particularly when excess sample is available. Alternatively, when the entire sample must be utilized, the sample can be placed on the column

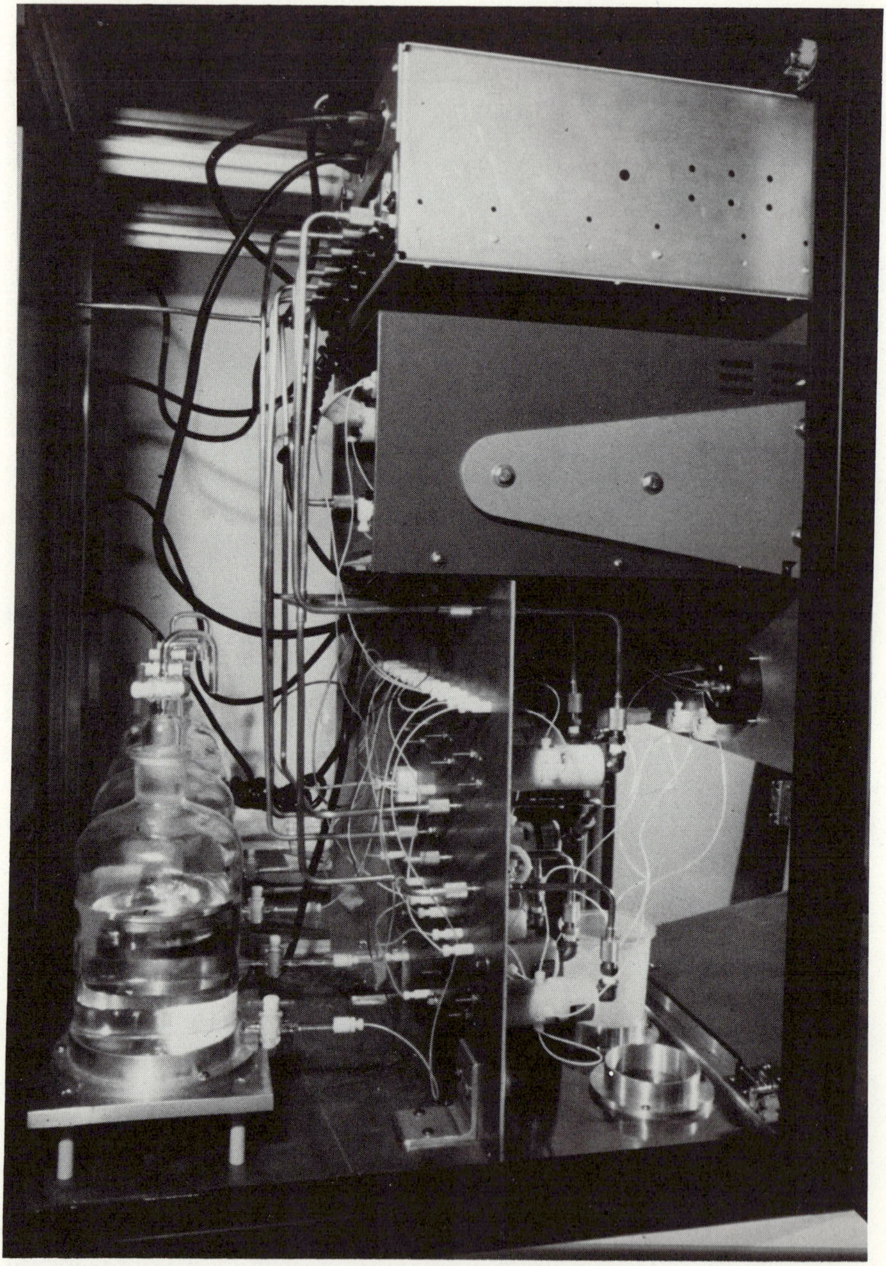

Fig. 6 Inside view of apparatus, showing the solvent reservoirs, valving, back of electronic chassis, pump, and plumbing. All compressed-air lines are made of copper, and all liquid lines are made of Teflon.

manually with a syringe, which is then flushed with excess solvent. The manual procedure is somewhat more time consuming and also opens the column to the atmosphere for a short period, but it is best for conserving small samples.

Once the column is charged and the system is sealed, the run is started by pressing first the reset button, to clear the counting circuits, and then the start button, to actuate the timers, counters, fraction collector, and pump. The solvent from reservoir 1 is pumped through the column until counter 1 is shut off by its timer mechanism. Then the second reservoir is immediately brought onstream and counter 2 is actuated. The sequence is repeated until counter 4 shuts off and the run ends; the pump is then shut off and the column is closed at valves 7 and 8. The fractions can be collected either in an automatic fraction collector or manually. The automatic fraction collector can be synchronized to change at the time the solvent reservoirs are switched or after a delay to compensate for the void volumes of the lines and the column.

To regenerate the column after a run, the flush-run switch on the front panel is placed in the flush position, and the volume of flushing solvent is selected on counter 5 with the appropriate flow rate. The flush sequence is begun by pressing the reset button and then the start button. When counter 5 stops, the pump turns off and the column is closed off at both ends by valves 7 and 8. The flush-run switch must be returned to the run position manually before the next sample run is begun.

3. Performance Characteristics. Tables II and III present some data on the performance of the instrument in processing total lipid extracts from sheep erythrocytes. Table II demonstrates that inorganic phosphate, free amino acids, and carbohydrates are effectively removed from the red-cell lipid extract (fraction I). Table III indicates that all of the lipids are recovered in fraction I and that the separation is highly reproducible. Essentially the data in Tables II and III confirm that the automated system is capable of duplicating the performance of the manual method as described originally by Siakotos and Rouser (20).

The packing of the Sephadex column has shown no evidence of deterioration after 6 months of continuous operation. In fact the columns function somewhat better after being used for several months than they do initially.

When a column is packed, it is essential not to compress the bed too tightly, because the flow could be impeded by a resistance change that occurs when solvent 4 replaces solvent 3 in the column. A column packed with 10 g of Sephadex should have an initial resistance of no more than 5 psi with solvent 1 and no more than 10 psi with solvent 4 at a flow rate

Table II. Performance of Sephadex Column During Automatic Operation

Sample	Weight (mg)	Total Activity (cpm)	Recovery (cpm) Fraction I	Fraction II	Fraction III	Total (%)
Sheep blood lipid extract + inorganic ^{32}P	105.3	4.91×10^6	0	5	4.73×10^6	96.3
Sheep blood lipid extract + radioactive amino acids and sugar (^{14}C-labeled)	98.7	1.72×10^6	10	1.03×10^5 [a]	1.60×10^6	99.0

[a] Phenylalanine labeled with ^{14}C.

Table III. Recovery and Reproducibility of Sephadex Column Performance in the Purification of Total Lipid Extract of Sheep Erythrocytes

Run	Sample	Weight (mg)	Fraction I (mg)	Fraction I (%)	Fraction II (mg)	Fraction II (%)	Fraction III (mg)	Fraction III (%)	Total Recovery (%)
1A	Initial chloroform–methanol extract	143.8	114.9	79.90	6.7	4.65	23.5	16.34	100.9
1B	Duplicate	143.8	115.3	80.18	6.4	4.45	22.1	15.36	100.0
2A	Rerun of fraction I on column	114.9	113.8	99.04	0.8	0.69	0.2	0.17	99.9
2B	Duplicate	115.3	114.0	98.87	0.9	0.78	0.4	0.34	100.0

of 120 ml/hr. Figure 7 is a plot of column-inlet pressure versus time during the change from solvent 3 to solvent 4. The column resistance is changed by the swelling of the Sephadex beads in methanol–water in a fixed bed volume. Why the beads contract after all of the third solvent has washed from the column is unclear. Some evidence suggests that the dissociation of acetic acid in solvent 4 causes a change in the ionic strength of the intrabead fluid and thus is the principal cause of the swelling. As the acetic acid is washed from the column, the beads contract again. In any event this phenomenon has no influence on the performance of the column other than to introduce the danger of column breakage from excess pressure, and this is prevented by the pressure-limit safety switch.

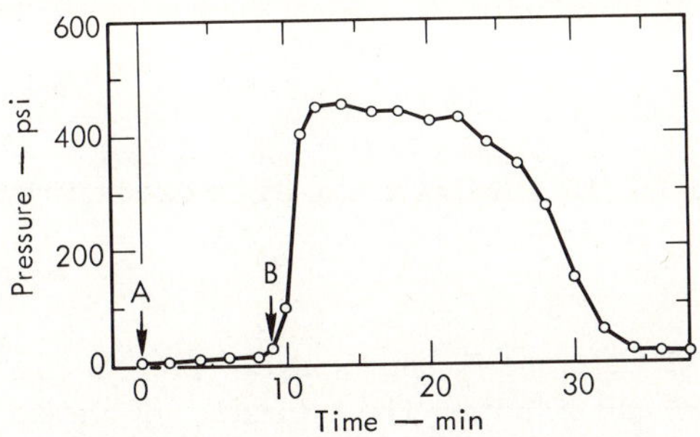

Fig. 7 Line pressure versus time, measured at the output side of the pump during a sample run at the time when solvent 4 displaces solvent 3 in the column. Arrow *A*, solvent 4 enters to top of the column; arrow *B*, solvent 4 begins to elute from the column. The flow rate was 60 ml/hr. The column pressure did not change after 40 min.

In over a year of continuous operation this instrument has proved to be reliable and very useful. It has relieved the technicians from many tedious hours of "column watching" and also has increased the productivity of the laboratory by its untended operation during nights and weekends.

E. Other Lipid-Purification Techniques

Several other methods for the purification of lipid extracts have been reported in the literature (17, 18, 22–25). In general the older procedures were probably less effective than they were thought to be, because of the inadequate methods used for lipid analysis at the time.

Maxwell and Williams (26) reported a Sephadex chromatographic procedure with lipophilic Sephadex, LH-20, for the purification of lipids from plant leaves. It is not clear, however, whether this method effectively separates gangliosides from other lipids in the extracts.

Another technique, using Sephadex G-25 coarse, was recently reported by Williams and Merrilees (27); it does not involve column chromatography. In this procedure dry Sephadex is added directly to the organic extract, in an approximate ratio of 1:1 by weight of water in the wet tissue to Sephadex. As the solvents are being removed by evaporation, the Sephadex absorbs all the water from the extract along with the nonlipid impurities. In preliminary studies we were able to duplicate these results; we found that the method is effective, except that gangliosides are retained in the Sephadex. However, the gangliosides can be recovered from the beads by washing with solvent 2 from the column-chromatography method. This procedure, because of its ease and time-saving features, should be explored intensively. It may well be the method of choice for the purification of lipid extracts.

IV. SEPARATION OF LIPIDS BY COLUMN CHROMATOGRAPHY

A. Neutral Lipids

1. Silicic Acid Columns. The neutral lipids in blood plasma can be resolved on silicic acid columns. The procedure of Hirsch and Ahrens (28) is satisfactory but rather time consuming by modern standards. The large columns used require relatively large samples. Of course the entire operation can be scaled down for small samples.

Another silicic-acid-column procedure that works well for small plasma

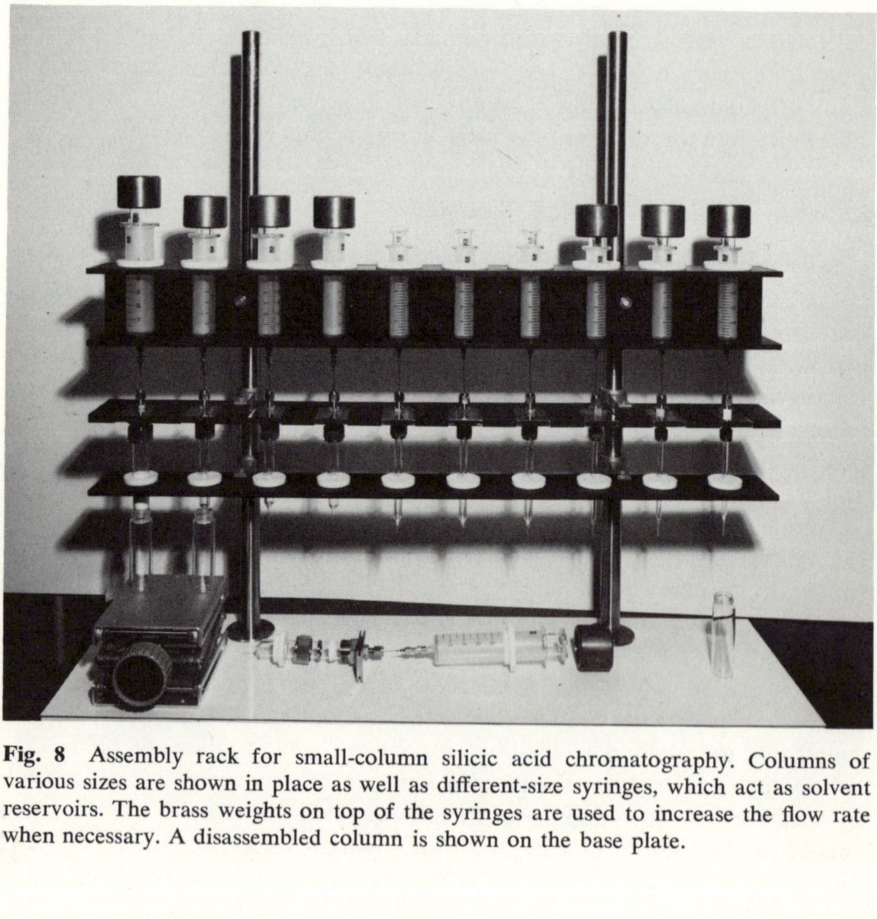

Fig. 8 Assembly rack for small-column silicic acid chromatography. Columns of various sizes are shown in place as well as different-size syringes, which act as solvent reservoirs. The brass weights on top of the syringes are used to increase the flow rate when necessary. A disassembled column is shown on the base plate.

or serum lipid samples was described by Freeman et al. (29). It combines chromatography with infrared spectrophotometry (see Chapter 4).

In the author's laboratory a number of small silicic acid columns (i.d. varying from 3 to 18 mm) have been used for loads between 0.5 and 20 mg of total lipids. Figure 8, a photograph of the column rack assembly, shows the Swagelok fittings and syringes fitted on the columns. These columns are quite useful for such simple separations as removing cholesterol from methyl esters in transesterification reactions or the separation of small samples into major lipid classes, such as neutral lipids, glycosphingolipids, and phospholipids.

2. Lipophilic Sephadex. Sephadex LH-20 has been used by several investigators to fractionate lipid mixtures (30–37). We have not used these systems, but they appear to be applicable to special problems in lipid analysis. The separation obtained on lipophilic Sephadex depends on a number of factors other than the adsorptivity of the lipids to the gel (32). Indeed it would seem that simple adsorptivity is the least important factor effecting the migration on the column. The primary factor controlling migration in LH-20, if a single solvent is used to elute the lipids, would still appear to be the shape and size of the molecule; that is, in essence it is gel-permeation chromatography with some polar and van der Waals interaction also (32). If multiple-solvent systems are used, then liquid–liquid partition-chromatography effects appear to dominate the results (32, 35).

Polar lipids, particularly phospholipids, do not fractionate appreciably on lipophilic Sephadex; however, they can be isolated free of neutral lipid on this material (31, 33, 36).

B. Phospholipids

Phospholipids can be fractionated on silicic acid columns, but with varying success (38–42). However, there are no reports of a single-column procedure that will successfully separate all of the common phospholipids. For this reason thin-layer chromatography has largely superseded silicic-acid-column chromatography of phospholipids, which nonetheless is often still useful for special purposes. For instance, acidic phospholipids can be separated from neutral phospholipids, such as lecithin and sphingomyelin, on silicic acid columns by using chloroform–methanol, 3:1, for acidic phospholipids and methanol for neutral phospholipids.

Another useful procedure on silicic acid columns was described by Rouser and co-workers (43) for the fractionation of total lipid extracts into neutral lipid, glycosphingolipid, and phospholipid fractions. The neutral lipids are removed from the column with chloroform. Glycosphingolipids can be removed with acetone and/or mixtures of ethyl acetate and acetone. Phospholipids are then removed from the column with methanol. This method is useful in preparing samples for further analysis by thin-layer chromatography.

At present thin-layer chromatography, particularly two-dimensional thin-layer chromatography, has proved to be the most useful procedure for the quantitative analysis of phospholipids, but it presents difficulties in handling trace components. Thus some form of column chromatography is very useful as a concentrating technique before quantitative analysis with thin-layer chromatography.

A very useful procedure for concentrating trace phospholipids is the ion-exchange chromatography on TEAE-cellulose, and DEAE-cellulose, developed by Rouser and co-workers (44, 45). The elution characteristics from an ion-exchange cellulose column place ionic lipids clearly into one of five groups. In order of elution these are the following:

1. Neutral (zwitterion) phospholipids, such as lecithin, lysolecithin, and sphingomyelin.
2. Very weakly acidic phospholipids, such as phosphatidylethanolamine, its lyso form, and the *N*-methyl derivatives of phosphatidylethanolamine.
3. Weakly acidic free fatty acids.
4. More polar, weakly acidic fatty acids, such as phosphatidylserine and its lyso form.
5. Strongly acidic compounds, such as phosphatidic acid.

Various solvent systems can be employed for elution of ion-exchange cellulose, providing a wide choice of procedures for special purposes.

Both DEAE and TEAE celluloses are useful packings for the separation of polar lipids. The DEAE form has an exchangeable proton, TEAE does not; this causes some differences in their retention characteristics. The former is more easily overloaded by weakly acidic lipids. Phosphatidylethanolamine is eluted from TEAE only by ionic solvents, but from DEAE it is eluted by chloroform–methanol mixtures. This is useful in the chromatography of erythrocyte lipids on TEAE, since the ceramide polyhexosides can be eluted with chloroform–methanol, 2:1, but phosphatidylethanolamine is retained on the column. Also, DEAE is used in the acetate form, and TEAE should be in the hydroxyl form. The relatively poor exchange capacity of the acetate form of TEAE causes strongly acidic phospholipids to be eluted with glacial acetic acid in contrast to DEAE, on which these phospholipids are firmly bound and are eluted only with ionic solvents. This is not a problem with the hydroxyl form of TEAE. With both DEAE and TEAE celluloses the best results are obtained with the standard grade rather than a fine grade.

When these materials are being packed into a column, the technician should be careful not to grind the fibers so that they are made into fines, because this could cause the resistance of the column to increase to the point where no solvent flow could be obtained at reasonable pressures. Properly packed TEAE columns can be reused many times provided the column is not allowed to run dry. Since TEAE columns appear to be the most useful for the separation of blood phospholipids, only the procedure for TEAE chromatography is presented here.

1. Washing TEAE-Cellulose. Prior to column chromatography, undesirable impurities are removed by washing the adsorbent with 1 *N* aqueous hydrochloric acid followed by water and then with 0.1 *N* aqueous potassium hydroxide followed by washing with water to neutrality. Three cycles of acid and base are used. Exposure to acid and base should be as brief as possible, and no more than 3 bed-volumes (i.e., the volume of solvent equal to the height of the absorbent layer) are required for either acid or base per cycle. The washing can be done in a Buchner or sintered-glass filter with gentle suction from a water aspirator. A piece of filter paper or several layers of cheese cloth are used to retain the cellulose and prevent clogging at the filter. After washing, the ion-exchange cellulose is first air dried and then dried to constant weight in a desiccator over potassium hydroxide pellets.

2. Packing TEAE-Cellulose Columns. Columns of 2.5-cm-i.d. and 20 cm long are generally useful for erythrocyte and plasma lipids applied in 100- to 200-mg amounts; directions are given therefore for columns of this size. The TEAE-cellulose (20 g of thoroughly dried ion-exchange cellulose) is treated overnight with glacial acetic acid to aid in breaking up aggregates and to facilitate uniform packing into the chromatographic tubes. Any visible aggregates still remaining after standing overnight are usually broken up with a glass rod before the slurry is transferred to the chromatographic tube. The chromatographic tube can be of double-walled Pyrex glass tubing (about 30 cm long) fitted with a Teflon stopcock and a solvent reservoir of about 1-liter capacity.

For packing, a clean glass-wool plug moistened with acetic acid is placed in the tube and a small volume of acetic acid is added. The plug is held in place by a glass rod while the first portion of the slurry of ion-exchange cellulose in acetic acid is poured into the chromatographic tube; then the rod is withdrawn and packing is continued. Approximately five equal portions can be packed to give a satisfactory column. After each addition, the excess acid is forced out under nitrogen pressure and the bed is pressed lightly and uniformly with a large-bore glass rod. After application of pressure the uppermost portion of the bed is gently stirred to free it of very tightly packed adsorbent before the next addition of slurry. The procedure is repeated until all the slurry has been transferred quantitatively into the tube to give a bed height of 20 ± 2 cm.

A common mistake in packing columns is uneven and excessive manual pressure. It introduces irregularities in the column, and these can lead to poor separations.

The bed should not be allowed to run dry at any stage of column preparation. The glacial acetic acid is allowed to run just to the top of the column, and the reservoir on top of the bed is freed of acid by several small additions of methanol, each of which is used to wash the solvent reservoir and then allowed to fall to the top of the bed. The bed is freed of acid by washing with 6 bed-volumes of methanol. The ion-exchange cellulose is then converted to the hydroxyl form by washing with 3 bed-volumes of 0.1 *N* potassium hydroxide in methanol, followed by 6 bed-volumes of methanol to remove excess base; it is then washed successively with 6 bed-volumes of chloroform–methanol, 2:1, and with chloroform. The column is then ready for testing.

The ion-exchange cellulose column is tested before sample application by passing through it a solution of 1 mg of the brightly colored hydrocarbon azulene applied in chloroform and eluted with the same solvent; the effluent is collected in a graduated cylinder. Imperfections in the column are easily seen as the blue hydrocarbon passes through the bed; the first appearance of the color in the column effluent gives an accurate measure of 1 column-volume (the volume occupied by the solvent). Columns are judged to be completely satisfactory if no mechanical imperfections are observed and when azulene appears after the collection of about 75 ml of solvent. If the column has been packed more tightly—for example, to 18 rather than 20 cm—azulene could appear after the collection of about 65 ml, whereas if the packing has been somewhat looser—for example, to a height of 22 cm—azulene could first be noted after the collection of 85 ml of the solvent. If the hydrocarbon appears before 60 ml of solvent has been collected, imperfections probably will be noted in the bed; if so, the column should be repacked. The test should be done just before applying the sample. If the test shows the column to be satisfactory, azulene is eluted quantitatively and quickly with chloroform, after which the sample can be applied. If the column must be repacked, the ion-exchange cellulose is gently extruded and repacked as a slurry in chloroform following the procedure described above. The flow rate during testing should be about 2.5 to 3 ml/min.

3. Application of Sample and Elution of Lipids from TEAE-Cellulose. The sample (100–200 mg) is applied in 5 to 10 ml of chloroform and quantitatively washed with the same solvent. There are many different ways to elute ion-exchange cellulose columns (2, 14, 43–45). The eluting solvents, the number of column-volumes required for total elution of a fraction, and the lipids eluted with the solvent are, for erythrocytes, as follows:

1. Chloroform: 5 column-volumes; elutes sterols, sterol esters, triglycerides, and ceramides.
2. Chloroform–methanol, 9:1: 8 column-volumes; elutes choline phospholipids (lecithin, lysolecithin, and sphingomyelin).
3. Chloroform–methanol, 2:1: 8 column-volumes; elutes ceramide polyhexosides.
4. Chloroform–methanol, 2:1, containing 1% glacial acetic acid: 8 column-volumes; elutes phosphatidylethanolamine, lysophosphatidylethanolamine, and free fatty acids, as well as dimethylphosphatidylethanolamine detectable in trace amounts in erythrocyte lipids.
5. Glacial acetic acid: 8 column-volumes; elutes phosphatidylserine.
6. Methanol wash: 3 column-volumes; elutes no lipid but is used for the removal of excess acetic acid.
7. Chloroform–methanol, 4:1, made 0.1 *M* in potassium acetate and with 20 ml/liter 28% aqueous ammonia added: 10 column-volumes, followed by methanol, 6 column-volumes; elutes the acidic phospholipids; the two solvents are pooled for evaporation.

The last three solvents are passed directly into a column (2.5-cm-i.d. and 10 cm long) of DEAE-cellulose in the acetate form in order to obtain complete separation of the strongly acidic phospholipids from phosphatidylserine.

Before reuse the TEAE-cellulose column is converted back to the hydroxyl form by treatment with 0.1 *N* potassium hydroxide in methanol and other washes as described in the preceding subsection for the initial preparation of the column.

Use of the above eluting sequence for plasma lipids results in the appearance of strongly acidic phospholipids in several fractions, probably because the acidic phospholipids are present as calcium and magnesium salts, which are not readily ion exchanged. The elution scheme for plasma therefore can be conveniently simplified, using only solvents 1, 2, and 7 to provide three useful fractions that contain respectively all the neutral lipids, all the choline lipids, and all phospholipids other than those containing choline.

A combination of ion-exchange cellulose-column techniques is necessary for the quantitative separation of erythrocyte-lipid classes. When phosphatidylserine is eluted with acetic acid, small amounts of other acidic phospholipids appear in the fraction. These are quantitatively separated from phosphatidylserine by passage of the acetic acid eluate from TEAE-cellulose through DEAE-cellulose (acetate form) in a 2.5-cm-i.d. by 10-cm column. All lipids other than phosphatidylserine are retained and can be eluted by passage of the final TEAE fraction through the DEAE column. Ion-exchange cellulose columns are eluted with glacial acetic acid or acidified solvents (in addition to chloroform and chloroform–methanol mixtures) that do not contain water; thus hydrolysis of plasmalogens is not encountered. Great care must be taken, however, to avoid evaporation to dryness of mixtures containing acetic acid, since acidic lipids are rapidly altered, with the production of artifacts that can suggest hydrolysis. After acetic acid is removed by the solvent-replacement procedure, it is advisable to add a few drops of aqueous ammonia to convert the acidic lipids to the more stable ammonium salt form.

C. Glycosphingolipids

Glycosphingolipids can be separated from other polar lipids by the silicic-acid-column chromatographic technique developed by Rouser and coworkers (43) and discussed in part B of this section. Gangliosides are best removed from a total lipid extract by the Sephadex procedure described in Section III.

If glycosphingolipids are to be separated from other polar lipids by the silicic-acid-column technique, very dry solvents should be used. Small amounts of water cause phospholipids to elute before all of the glycosphingolipids have been removed from the column. A typical separation of glycosphingolipids by this technique is as follows:

The sample (300 mg or less) is applied in chloroform, and the column is eluted at a flow rate of 3 ml/min with (a) chloroform (10 column-volumes, 350 ml); (b) hexane, 2 column-volumes (70 ml) to remove chloroform; (c) 3 column-volumes (105 ml) of ethyl acetate to ensure complete removal of cholesterol and other neutral lipids; (d) ethyl acetate–acetone, 1:3, 40 column-volumes (1400 ml) for the elution of glycosphingolipids; and (e) methanol, 10 column-volumes (350 ml) for the elution of phospholipids. The first three solvents are pooled as the neutral lipid fraction (sterols, sterol esters, triglycerides, free fatty acids, and ceramides). The ethyl acetate–acetone fraction contains any cerebroside and ceramide polyhexosides, including globoside. Gangliosides are not eluted, and only traces of phospholipids are found in the fractions. The phospholipid fraction eluted with methanol undergoes some slight decomposition as the result of adsorption onto silicic acid and is therefore less useful for quantitative analysis than that from direct two-dimensional thin-layer chromatography or ion-exchange cellulose-column chromatography followed by thin-layer-chromatography separation.

Once the glycosphingolipids are free of neutral lipids and phospholipids, they can be analyzed by any of several thin-layer procedures (46–49) or by the gas–liquid-chromatography techniques of Sweeley and co-workers (5–7). Gangliosides are also amenable to thin-layer-chromatography analysis (50–52). Structural distinctions and sugar linkages, however, are best determined by combinations of various chemical procedures (53–55).

V. QUANTITATIVE ANALYSIS BY THIN-LAYER CHROMATOGRAPHY

Despite many current developments in gas–liquid, liquid–liquid, and liquid–solid chromatography—developments that show considerable promise of future breakthroughs—thin-layer chromatography (TLC) on silica gel is still the method of choice for the analysis of intact lipids. Both one- and two-dimensional thin-layer procedures are useful for the nonpolar lipids. Gangliosides are preferably analyzed by one-dimensional thin-layer chromatography. Phospholipids and glycosphingolipids other than gangliosides are best handled by two-dimensional systems. The only major drawback to thin-layer chromatography for the analysis of complex lipid mixtures is the limited capacity of the technique, which prevents the accurate analysis of trace components without prior concentration by another procedure, usually column chromatography.

A. Preparation of Thin-Layer Plates

Borosilicate-glass plates (20 × 20 cm) are cleaned in a suitable detergent and then rinsed in dilute cleaning solution. The adsorbent is prepared as a slurry. We routinely use silica gel HR, which has no binder. Silica gel G contains a calcium sulfate binder and gives less satisfactory separation, less reproducibility, and also higher blank readings when used in the phosphate determination. Silica gel H is also acceptable and less expensive.

1. Preparation of Slurry. The dry silica gel HR is mixed with a solution of magnesium acetate, either 0.5 or 1.5 g to 20 g of absorbent. The optimum amount of magnesium silicate differs for various solvent systems. For most analytical thin-layer chromatography a layer of 250 microns is satisfactory. With the solvent most often used, 0.5 g of magnesium silicate to 20 g of silica gel HR provides the best resolution. For spreading plates it is preferable to use a spreading assembly that levels the upper, rather than the lower, surface of the plate, so that variations in plate thickness will not interfere with the spreading operation.

The slurry is prepared by weighing 30 g of silica gel HR into a 250-ml beaker, adding 10 ml of a solution of 7.5 wt % magnesium acetate, and then adding redistilled water to bring the total weight to 114.0 to 114.5 g. The slurry is mixed thoroughly with a Teflon stirring rod. It is also helpful to tap the beaker gently to remove any trapped air bubbles. The slurry is then poured into the reservoir of the spreader, and the plates are spread with a smooth, even pull. Abrupt stops or changes in speed produce nonuniform layers. Immediately after spreading and while the adsorbent is still wet, the spreading assembly is shaken or vibrated manually to eliminate small striations or unevenness in the layers. The plates are then air dried for 10 to 15 min at room temperature and then placed in an oven for 20 min at 110 to 120°C. After being removed from the oven, they can be stored in a desiccator until needed.

2. Sample Application. Before the sample is applied to the plate, it is subjected to several minor operations. All plates, whether used in one- or two-dimensional chromatography, first have the absorbent removed from the edges of the plate to a depth of 2 mm. Also, the position of the solvent front is indicated as well as reference marks for the origin. At this time the plate is activated by heating at 120°C for 10 min. When the plate is removed from the oven, it is immediately placed on a thermostated aluminum block maintained at 26°C and covered with a shield to prevent room air from circulating over the plate. After 3 min the plate, now at 26°C, is transferred to a nitrogen chamber for spotting.

Lang–Levy micropipettes or microliter syringes are used routinely for spotting. The micropipettes are more accurate than the microsyringes, but the latter are considerably easier to manipulate. Generally the sample is applied in chloroform–methanol, 19:1, at a concentration of 25 mg/ml. Water in the solution often affects the migration of components in the sample. If the applicating solvent is suspected of containing excess water, a stream of nitrogen can be directed at the spot for 5 min to ensure the removal of any water present. When large volumes are applied to a plate, repeated application with complete drying between applications is necessary to prevent excessive spreading of the sample. In two-dimensional thin-layer chromatography a second application of the sample is usually spotted in the corner opposite from the first. This spot is not chromatographed but is recovered after the spots are visualized and used to check the recovery of the sample.

The spotted plate is returned to the constant-temperature block for 2 min and then transferred to a humidity chamber for 7.5 min. The water content of the plate must be carefully controlled to obtain reproducible migration of the sample spots. It is best to have a humidity chamber in which nitrogen of known humidity flows around the plate. A chamber saturated with water vapor can also be used, provided that the degree of saturation is not unduly disturbed when the chamber is opened or closed. After being removed from the humidity chamber, the plates are immediately placed in the developing tank.

3. Development of Chromatograms. The chromatography jars must be prepared well in advance of the procedure, so that the solvent systems can equilibrate with the atmosphere in the jar. For reproducibility between runs and for uniform spot migration and straight solvent fronts, the jars should be lined with filter paper. If the glass-brick type of chromatograph jar is used, an 8.25 × 12.5-in. sheet of Whatman No. 4 filter paper, previously washed with organic solvents to remove impurities, makes an excellent liner. Two sheets are used per jar. One inch of the narrow ends of the paper is folded 90 degrees to allow the paper to cover the ends of the jar. The solvent is added to the jar at least 30 min before the plate is introduced into the chamber. It is convenient to pour the solvent over the filter papers so that they are thoroughly wetted from the moment the solvent is placed in the jar. A 95- to 100-ml volume of solvent is adequate for glass-brick jars.

The spotted plate is placed in the jar quickly to minimize the time the equilibrated chamber is open to the atmosphere. When the solvent front has migrated the desired distance, the plate is removed from the chamber, the back of the wet edge of the plate is wiped dry, and for two-dimensional thin-layer chromatography the plate is transferred to a closed chamber that is being continuously purged with dry nitrogen for 6 min. After removal from the nitrogen chamber, the plate is placed on the thermostated block for 2 min to ensure that it is at the proper temperature and is then placed in the chromatograph jar for development in the second dimension.

B. Developing Solvents

1. Neutral Lipids. The neutral lipids can be developed by any of several nonpolar solvent systems (56–58). One system that gives good results in that it separates cholesterol esters, triglycerides, free fatty acids, and cholesterol uniformly on the plate is hexane–diethyl ether–acetic acid, 85:15:2 (58). The presence of acetic acid ensures that all of the free fatty acids will be in the un-ionized form during chromatography. Benzene is a useful solvent in separating butylated hydroxytoluene (used as an antioxidant) from methyl ester samples and cholesterol.

2. Phospholipids and Glycosphingolipids. For general separation of mixtures of phospholipids and glycosphingolipids by two-dimensional thin-layer chromatography a solvent system of wide applicability and resolving power is the following: for the first dimension, chloroform–methanol–aqueous ammonia, 65:35:5 (by volume); for the second dimension, chloroform–acetone–methanol–acetic acid–water, 5:2:1:1:0.5 (by volume). A typical resolution of erythrocyte lipids is shown in Fig. 9. This solvent system is used with plates spread with 0.5 g of magnesium acetate to 20 g of silica gel HR. Another system that appears to be of equal resolving power uses in the first dimension chloroform–methanol–aqueous ammonia, 65:25:5 (by volume), and in the second dimension chloroform–acetone–

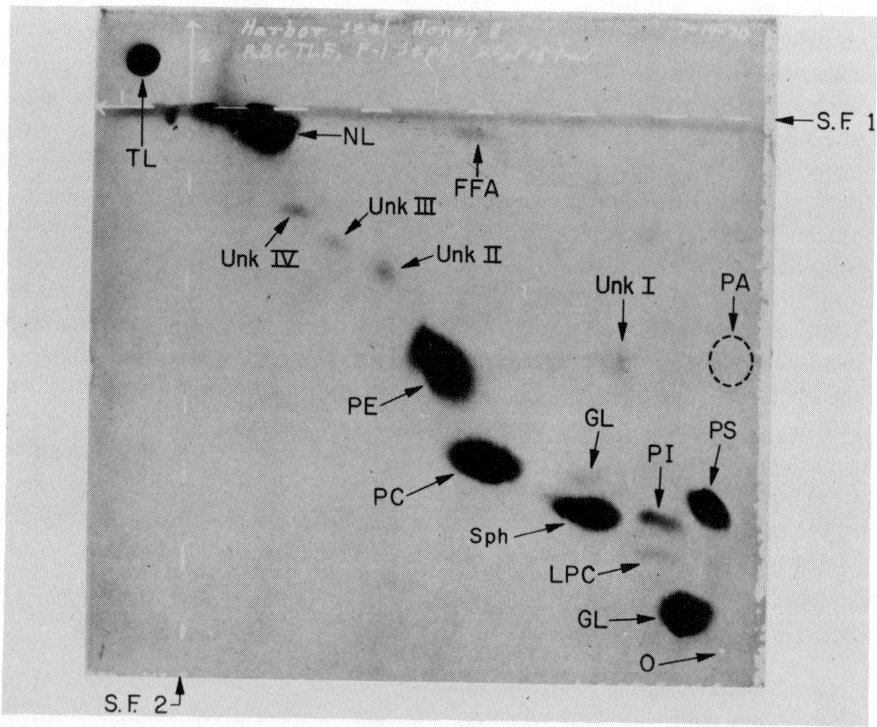

Fig. 9 A typical two-dimensional thin-layer chromatogram of seal-erythrocyte phospholipids. The sample was applied in the lower right-hand corner (600 μg of lipids). The solvent systems were as follows: in the first dimension, chloroform–methanol–aqueous ammonia, 65: 35: 5 (by volume); in the second dimension, chloroform–acetone–methanol–acetic acid–water, 5: 2: 1: 1: 0.5 (by volume). The plate was spread with silica gel HR containing 0.5 g of magnesium acetate per 20 g of silica gel. Abbreviations: O, origin; GL, glycosphingolipid; LPC, lysophosphatidylcholine; Sph, sphingomyelin; PI, phosphatidylinositol PS, phosphatidylserine; PC, phosphatidylcholine; PE, phosphatidylethanolamine; Unk, unidentified; PA, phosphatidic acid; FFA, free fatty acid; NL, neutral lipid; TL, total sample spot; S.F., solvent front. Spots were visualized by charring.

methanol–acetic acid–water, 3:4:1:1:0.5 (by volume). The plates spread for use with these solvents require 1.5 g of magnesium acetate for 20 g of silica gel HR. These pairs of solvent systems require about 35 min to develop in the first dimension and 45 to 50 min in the second.

Another useful solvent pair is (a) for the first dimension chloroform–methanol–water, 65:25:4 (v/v/v), and (b) for the second dimension butanol–acetic acid–water, 3:1:1 (v/v/v). No magnesium acetate should be incorporated into plates intended for use with these solvents. Because of the rather long development time in the second dimension, 2 to 3 hr, this system is generally used only to confirm results obtained with the other systems.

Because the phospholipids of mammalian plasma have a simple and consistent composition (59, 60), one-dimensional thin-layer chromatography can be used successfully for the quantitative analysis of the major phospholipids. The solvents for the first dimension in any of the above systems are satisfactory, but chloroform–methanol–aqueous ammonia, 65:25:5 (v/v/v), appears to be the best of the three used with the corresponding adsorbent. Figure 10 is an example of a plasma-phospholipid sample run in this manner.

3. Ceramides and Weakly Polar Lipids. Useful solvents in the first dimension are chloroform–methanol–ammonia, 95:5:0.5 (by volume), and in the second dimension chloroform–acetone–methanol–acetic acid–water, 8:1.5:0.5:0.5:0.5 (by volume). This pair of solvent mixtures is used with plain silica gel H.

4. Gangliosides. Gangliosides are separated in the one-dimensional system with plain silica gel H. The solvent should be propanol–water, 7:3 (v/v). Gangliosides should of course first be separated from other lipids by Sephadex column chromatography.

C. Detection Reagents

1. General Reagents. The most generally useful spray reagent for lipids on TLC plates is the char reagent. There are several variations of the basic char reagent, but they are mainly based on sulfuric acid (61–64) as the oxidizing agent. One is 50% sulfuric acid, which can be used, although saturated lipids do not char uniformly with it. A second, 0.6% potassium dichromate in 50% sulfuric acid, chars all lipids regardless of their degree of saturation (62). Another charring reagent that chars all lipids is composed of 3 volumes of 37% formaldehyde in 97 volumes of 98% sulfuric acid (64).

The plate should be sprayed with a fine mist of the reagent until the

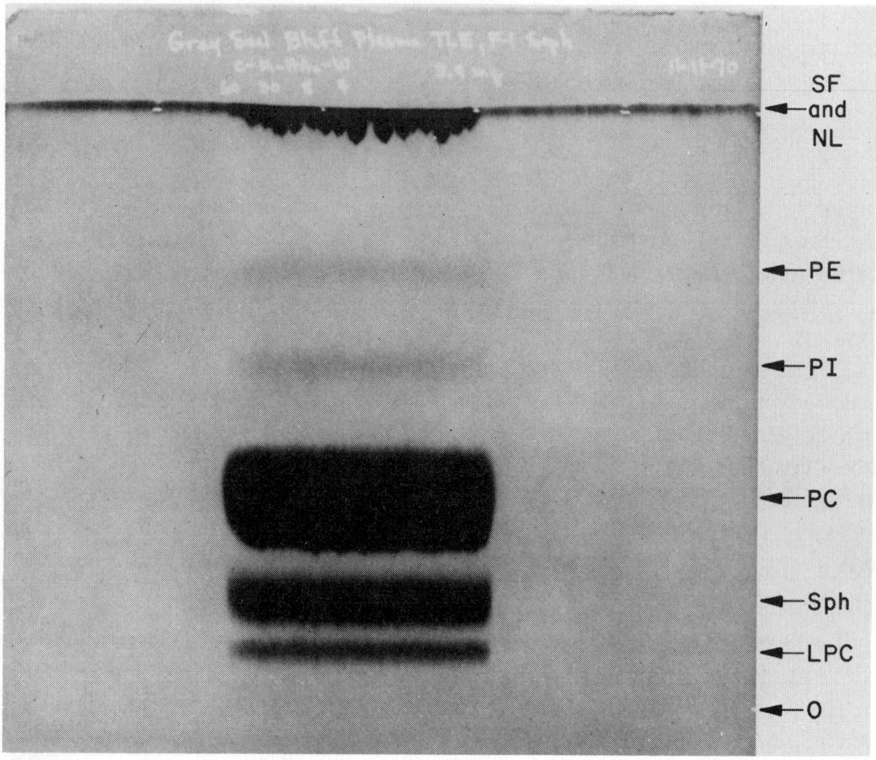

Fig. 10 A typical one-dimensional TLC separation of seal-plasma phospholipids. Sample was applied as a streak across the bottom of the plate (2000 μg of lipid, 20 μg P). The solvent was chloroform–methanol–aqueous ammonia, 65: 35: 5 (v/v/v). The adsorbent was silica gel HR containing 0.5 g of magnesium acetate per 20 g of silica gel. Abbreviations: O, origin; LPC, lysophosphatidylcholine; Sph, sphingomyelin; PC, phosphatidylcholine; PI, phosphatidylinositol; PE, phosphatidylethanolamine; NL, neutral lipid; SF, solvent front. Spots were visualized by charring.

layer is uniformly covered but does not appear moist. With the dichromate spray, the plate should be slightly and uniformly yellow. Underspraying with this reagent causes the layer to assume a dappled appearance. After spraying, the plate is immediately transferred to a forced-draft oven at 175 to 180°C for 20 min. If visible acid fumes are still being evolved from the plate after this time, the plate was oversprayed.

Nondestructive general spray reagents are water, rhodamine 6G (0.001% solution in water), and 2′,7′-dichlorofluorescein (0.03% in 0.01 *N* NaOH). With the latter two sprays the spots are visualized with shortwave ultraviolet light. Water is the mildest spray reagent but also the least sensitive, which limits its applications. With water-spraying the spots appear as opaque spots on a translucent background and are viewed best against a black background by reflected light. Since water and the fluorescent-dye sprays do not leave permanently visible marks on the plate, the location of the spots must be marked on the plate in some manner to provide a reference for further analysis.

Iodine vapor can also be used as a general detection reagent; it is considerably more sensitive for unsaturated lipids than for their fully saturated counterparts. Also, iodine vapors are unpleasant and potentially toxic, and hence the other spray reagents are preferable.

2. Specific Reagents. *Glycosphingolipids.* α-Naphthol 0.1% in 50:50 methanol–water is an excellent specific spray for glycosphingolipids. It has good sensitivity and high specificity. It yields a deep blue-purple color with all reducing sugars.

Phospholipids. The molybdenum reagent (65) gives a specific reaction with phosphorus-containing lipids, but it is not as sensitive as the general reagents. Phospholipids with amino groups (e.g., phosphatidylserine and phosphatidylethanolamine) can be located with ninhydrin spray.[3] The color is brought out by heating at 110 to 120°C for 7 min. Overheating reduces the color intensity, and the spots fade on standing after several hours. Choline-containing phospholipids can be located with the Dragendorff reagent, but our experience with this spray is not encouraging: its sensitivity is low and its specificity is poor.

Gangliosides. These compounds can be localized with an orcinol spray (66), which is specific for sialic acid. Gangliosides are the only lipids that contain this substance.

3. Photography of Plates After Visualization of Spots. It is useful to obtain photographic records of all plates after the spots are made visible. In the laboratory Polaroid film is the method of choice, because an immediately visible record of the sample is obtained. Also, it is possible to check the photograph to ensure that the spots on the plate are reproduced accurately. For charred plates back-lighting and photography with transmitted light appears to yield the best results. For most other color reagents front-lighting and photography with reflected light produce the best results. Polaroid film type 3000 or 155 is satisfactory for black-and-white reproductions. For color photographs it is best to use a 35mm camera equipped with type A Kodachrome film.

[3] An excellent commercial preparation of ninhydrin spray in an aerosol can is available from E. Merck and Co., through Brinkman Instruments, Inc.

D. Quantitative Analysis of Samples After Thin-Layer Chromatography

1. Recovery of Sample from Plate. Spots can be removed from the plates either by aspiration or by scraping the plate with a razor blade. Before a plate is scraped, it is useful, if the plates have been charred, to view the spots under long-wavelength ultraviolet light (3200 Å) (67). This facilitates the detection of trace components and allows the full extent of spot spreading to be determined. All spots to be scraped or aspirated are outlined on the plate with a sharp stainless-steel stylus.

We have found it useful also to rephotograph the plate with a grid overlay that determines an X-Y coordinate system for all spots on the plate, with $X = 0$, $Y = 0$ at the origin. Figure 11 is an example of a plate photographed with the overlay. This procedure helps to remove much of the subjective assignment of identity to the various spots.

Scraping the spots with a razor blade is an easy and straightforward method of removing the sample from the plate, but it is somewhat slower than the aspiration technique. Aspiration is very convenient and more rapid for the recovery of polar-lipid spots after two-dimensional thin-layer chromatography. It is conveniently done with a polyethylene-stoppered test tube into which two polyethylene tubes are inserted, one of them bent and drawn to a fine point to serve as the aspiration head and the other serving for attachment to a source of vacuum (a water pump is usually satisfactory).

Quantitative aspiration without loss of material into the vacuum side of the line is achieved by using an acid-washed, glass-fiber paper filter held in place by the vacuum. After aspiration of the spot, the filter is allowed to fall into the tube when the vacuum is withdrawn. Any adsorbent adhering to the plastic can be easily removed by gentle tapping. Glass-fiber paper can be cut reproducibly into suitable small circles with a paper punch; it should be washed first in redistilled (constant boiling) hydrochloric acid and then in distilled water to remove impurities that would otherwise add to blank values in some of the determinations.

2. Phosphorus Determinations on Charred TLC Samples. The coordinates of all sample spots are recorded in a notebook, and two blank areas are marked off on the plate. Since the adsorbent is not removed from the reaction tube during this procedure, reagent blanks containing adsorbent are carried through the entire sequence. Two adsorbent blanks are necessary because variations in spot area and the amount of phosphorus present in the spot are too great to be accurately measured in a single reaction volume.

Routinely two adsorbent blanks are prepared: one of 600 and one of

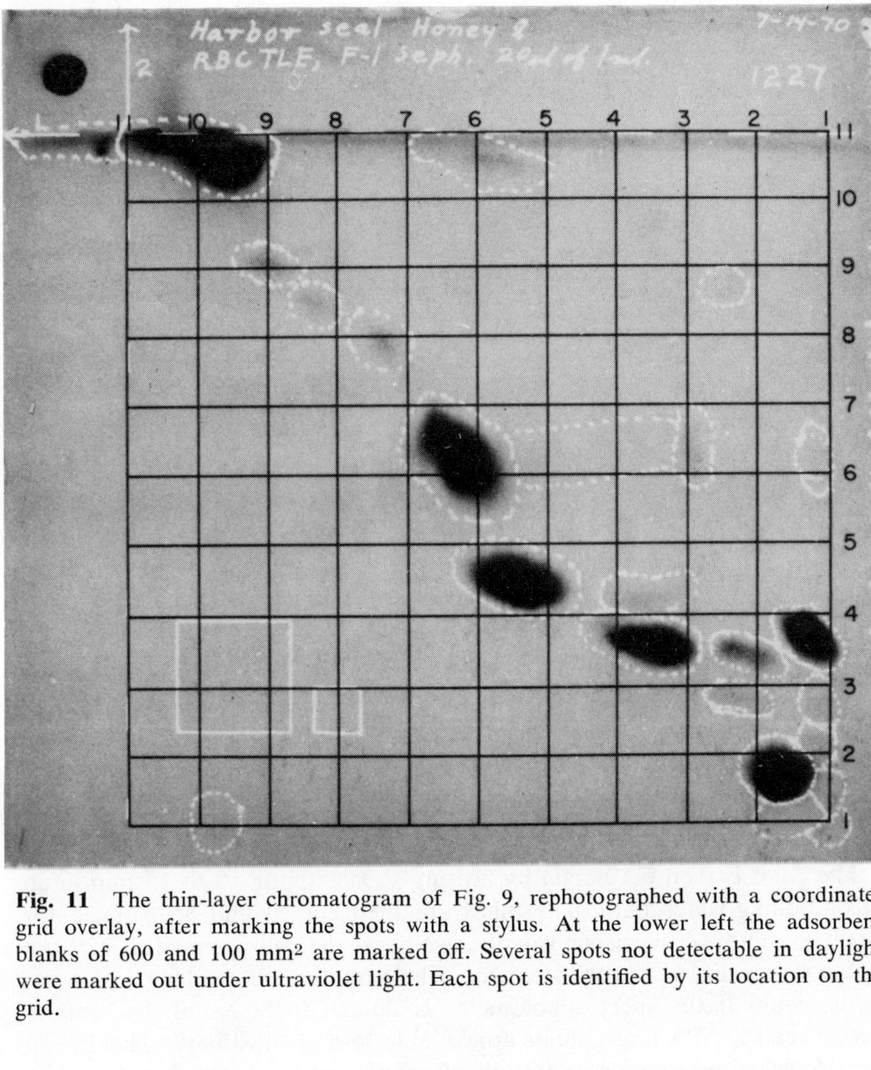

Fig. 11 The thin-layer chromatogram of Fig. 9, rephotographed with a coordinate-grid overlay, after marking the spots with a stylus. At the lower left the adsorbent blanks of 600 and 100 mm^2 are marked off. Several spots not detectable in daylight were marked out under ultraviolet light. Each spot is identified by its location on the grid.

100 mm^2. The 600-mm^2 blank is useful for spots containing 0.5 to 20 μg of phosphorus and is measured in a 5.0-ml reaction volume. The 100-mm^2 adsorbent blank can be used down to 0.01 μg of phosphorus but should not exceed 2 μg, and is measured in a 1.0-ml reaction volume. The area of each sample spot is estimated by comparison with a template on which are marked shapes of known area.

After the spots have been transferred to the reaction tubes, the samples are oxidized with a mixture of sulfuric and perchloric acids (2 volumes of

85% sulfuric acid to 1 volume of 72% perchloric acid.)[4] Then 0.5 ml of Oxidant is added to the 5-ml reaction tube and 0.1 ml to the 1-ml reaction tubes, and they are heated at 260°C for a minimum of 3 hr or until the solution is colorless. In practice it is convenient to place the tubes on the heating block at the end of the working day and allow them to digest overnight; they are then ready for analysis in the morning. Extended heating does not interfere with the determination, because the sulfuric acid is stable at 260°C; only the perchloric acid is removed.

The colored phosphomolybdate complex is developed essentially as described by Bartlett (68). The reducing agent is 1-amino-2-naphthol-4-sulfonic acid (ANSA) and is prepared 100 ml at a time by dissolving 2.72 g of $NaHSO_3$, 0.2 g of $NaSO_3$, and 0.1 g of ANSA in a 100-ml volumetric flask. Since ANSA dissolves rather slowly, it is useful to prepare the ANSA reagent the day before when the phosphate digestion tubes are placed on the heating block. Ammonium molybdate is prepared as a 2.5% solution in redistilled water. The ANSA reagent is stable for 2 weeks; the ammonium molybdate can be kept for a year in the dark.

All reagents are added to the reaction tubes with Repipettes (obtained from Lab Industries, Berkeley, Calif.). After the tubes are removed from the heating block, 1.61 ml of water is added to the 5-ml samples in such a manner as to wash down the sides of tube thoroughly; 0.64 ml of water is added to the 1.0-ml samples. For the 5.0-ml samples 0.5 ml of the ANSA reagent is added, followed by 1.0 ml of molybdate and 1.61 ml of water; for the 1.0-ml samples 0.1 ml of ANSA and 0.2 ml of molybdate are added. In adding reagents to the 1.0-ml sample care must be taken to keep them off the neck and sides of the tubes. The contents of the tubes are mixed with a vortex mixer after adding each reagent.

The color is then developed by heating at 100°C for 10 to 15 min in an oil or boiling-water bath. The tubes are then cooled and centrifuged for 5 min to remove any suspended silica gel, and the color is read at 820 nm in a good-quality spectrophotometer. The samples are read against a reagent blank. If the spectrophotometer is limited to 800 nm, the samples can be read at 795 nm without appreciable loss of sensitivity. The 1.0-ml sample yields approximately 0.9 ml of solution that can be transferred to a cuvette, so a semimicrocuvette must be used in the method as described. The Zeiss PMQ II spectrophotometer uses cuvettes of 1-cm path length and 0.25-ml total volume.

The adsorbent blanks are read against the reagent blank along with the sample spots. The absorbance of the adsorbent blank is subtracted from the absorbance of the samples in proportion to the area of the sample spots.

[4] This reagent can be obtained commercially from the G. Frederick Smith Chemical Co., Columbus, Ohio, and is known as Oxidant.

The amount of phosphorus is then determined from a standard curve prepared separately form a purified inorganic phosphate salt, such as potassium hydrogen phosphate. The results can be calculated with a computer. A small desk-top instrument like the Hewlett-Packard 9100 or Olivetti P-101 is satisfactory for these calculations, but larger computers can be used if available.

Computation of the results is simplified even further if the output of the spectrophotometer is converted to digital form and recorded on punched paper tape. The tape can then be fed directly to a computer, and all manual calculations are avoided. Figure 12 is an example of a printout

SAMPLE: 1230

SPOT NUMBER	MICROGM PHOS.	% OF TOTAL
1	0.0121	0.08
2	0.0613	0.38
3	0.0262	0.16
4	0.0078	0.05
5	0.0632	0.39
6	0.2908	1.81
7	0.0728	0.45
8	0.3082	1.92
9	2.4339	15.18
10	0.3781	2.36
11	2.6686	16.64
12	0.1808	1.13
13	4.7685	29.74
14	0.1341	0.84
15	0.1992	1.24
16	0.2204	1.37
17	3.7565	23.43
18	0.0763	0.48
19	0.0637	0.40
20	0.1181	0.74
21	0.1802	1.12
22	0.0066	0.04
23	0.0086	0.05

TOTAL: 16.0357

Fig. 12 A computer printout of the results of the phosphorus analyses of the spots from the two-dimensional TLC separation of seal-erythrocyte phospholipids shown in Figs. 9 and 11. The spots are numbered in the order in which they were read in the spectrophotometer; for identification they must be keyed back to the grid coordinates shown in Fig. 11. The second column gives the total amounts of phosphorus in each spot after subtraction of the adsorbent-blank values. The last column shows mole % phosphorus in each spot of the total recovered in all spots. The absorbance readout from the spectrophotometer is obtained on paper tape and fed directly to the computer. All of the calculations are performed by the computer, without any manual intervention.

of the calculations of a red-cell-phospholipid sample separated by two-dimensional thin-layer chromatography and analyzed by the phosphate method described above. Details of this conversion, which can be applied to any modern spectrophotometer, are available on request.

Other reducing agents, such as ascorbic acid and stannous chloride (69, 70), can be used in the phosphorus determinations. The choice of a particular reagent is at the discretion of the investigator. Ascorbic acid and stannous chloride can be used in the presence of perchloric acid, whereas ANSA cannot. Figure 13 shows a typical calibration curve for inorganic phosphate. The calibration is remarkably stable if all conditions are held constant. A standard curve should remain valid for years; the operator should be able to reproduce it at any time within the standard deviation of the method.

3. Determination of Glycosphingolipids by Hydrolysis and Reaction with Trinitrobenzenesulfonic Acid. The sample (14–140 μg of glycosphingolipid) is placed in a vial with a Teflon-lined screw cap. Any residual solvent is removed by evaporation under a stream of nitrogen,

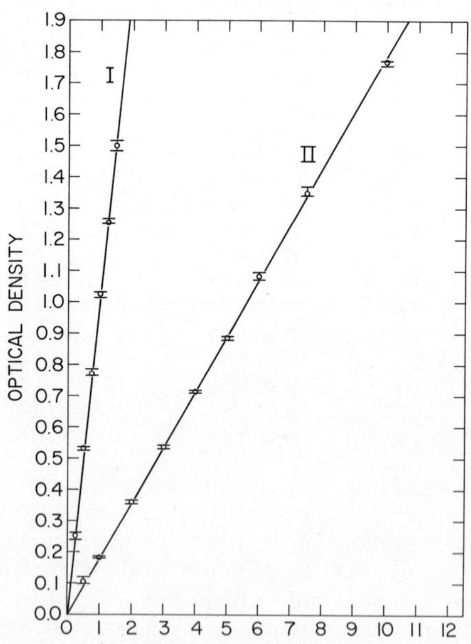

Fig. 13 A typical inorganic phosphate calibration curve prepared in the author's laboratory. Curve I is for a reagent volume of 1.0 ml and curve II is for a volume of 5.0 ml. Standard was NaH_2PO_4.

1.0 ml of boron trifluoride (14%) in methanol is added, the cap on the tube is tightened, and the tube is heated at 110°C for 1.5 hr. The tube is then cooled, 1.5 ml of water is added, and the mixture is extracted with three 2-ml portions of chloroform. The chloroform solution is transferred to glass-stoppered centrifuge tubes, the solvent is evaporated under a stream of nitrogen, and the residue is dissolved in methanol. Aqueous sodium bicarbonate (1 ml, 4% solution) and 1 ml of 0.1% aqueous trinitrobenzenesulfonic acid solution are added, and the solution is incubated for 1 hr at 40°C. Then 1 ml of 1 *N* hydrochloric acid in methanol is added, and the reaction product is extracted into *n*-hexane with 2-ml of solvent for each of three extractions; vigorous shaking is required, about 200 times manually or for 10 min with an automatic shaker. The solvent is evaporated under a stream of nitrogen. The solid is dissolved in 4 ml of 95% ethanol, and color intensity is read at 340 nm.

Commercially available pure preparations of cerebroside provide a convenient standard. A straight-line relationship is obtained when micrograms or micromoles of lipid are plotted against color intensity.

4. Determination of Cholesterol by the Acetyl Chloride–Zinc Chloride Method. In this procedure (71) a zinc chloride–acetic acid reagent is prepared from 40 g of anhydrous zinc chloride (sticks, analytical grade), which is crushed quickly, weighed in a dry 250-ml flask equipped with a glass stopper, and mixed with 150 ml of glacial acetic acid. The flask is stoppered and shaken, and then heated at 80°C for 2.5 hr with occasional shaking. The reagent is stored in a dark bottle and can be used until it becomes turbid when shaken with chloroform. Analytical grade acetyl chloride and redistilled chloroform are used.

After localization with a water or fluorescent-dye spray, the spots are allowed to dry in air, scraped into 12-ml screw-capped (Teflon-lined) centrifuge tubes, and dried over potassium hydroxide pellets in a desiccator. Chloroform (2 ml) is then added, followed by 1 ml of zinc chloride–acetic acid reagent and 1 ml of acetyl chloride, after which the screw cap is tightened and the tube contents are mixed thoroughly. The mixture is then heated at 65°C for 15 min, cooled in an ice bath for 15 min, diluted to 5 ml with chloroform, and centrifuged briefly to remove TLC adsorbent. The color intensity is read at 528 nm against a reagent blank. The amount of cholesterol is determined from a standard curve prepared from 5-, 10-, 25-, and 50-μg quantities of cholesterol.

5. Determination of Free Fatty Acids, Sterol Esters, and Triglycerides by Conversion to Fatty Acid Methyl Esters and Determination of Moles of Ester Group. The dry spots are aspirated or scraped from a TLC plate, 1.5 ml of boron trifluoride (14%) in methanol is added, and the screw-capped tube (Teflon-lined) is heated at 110°C for 5 min. The tube is cooled, 1.5 ml of water is added, and the fatty acid methyl esters are extracted into hexane with three 2-ml portions of solvent. The solvent is evaporated under a stream of nitrogen, and 3 ml of ether is added to the almost dry methyl esters. The tube is swirled, 0.1 ml of alkaline hydroxylamine solution is added and mixed by swirling, and the solvent is evaporated just to dryness in a water bath at 65°C with shaking to prevent bumping. Each tube is handled individually, and the operation requires about 1 min. The tube is then evacuated under reduced pressure from a water pump to remove the last traces of ethanol; 6 ml of acid ferric perchlorate solution is added with care to obtain thorough mixing and washing of the test-tube wall, and the color is determined after approximately 30 min at 530 nm against a 95% ethanol blank.

Reagent-grade absolute ether is used. A 3% solution of ethanolic hydroxylamine hydrochloride is prepared in 95% ethanol by dissolving 1.0 g of hydroxylamine hydrochloride in 1.7 ml of water followed by 32.3 ml of absolute ethanol (prepared fresh daily). Ethanolic sodium hydroxide is prepared as a 3% solution in 95% ethanol by dissolving 1.0 g of sodium hydroxide in 1.7 ml of water followed by addition of 32.3 ml of absolute ethanol. The alkaline hydroxylamine solution is prepared fresh daily by mixing equal volumes of ethanolic hydroxylamine hydrochloride and ethanolic sodium hydroxide; the precipitate of sodium chloride is removed by filtration. The reagent is stable for about 5 hr. The ethanolic acid–ferric perchlorate reagent is prepared by dissolving 0.50 g of ferric perchlorate (nonyellow, G. Frederick Smith Chemical Co., Columbus, Ohio) in a solution of 487 ml of 95% ethanol and 13 ml of 70% perchloric acid (double-distilled, G. Frederick Smith Chemical Co.). The pale-yellow solution should be stored in a brown bottle at 4 to 8°C; under such conditions it is stable for several weeks.

6. Determination of Plasmalogen Content by Reaction with p-Nitrophenylhydrazine. To the plasmalogen form of lipid (0.1–0.5 micromoles, about 80–400 μg) are added 4 ml of 95% ethanol, 0.5 ml of 0.02 *M* *p*-nitrophenylhydrazine in 95% ethanol, and 0.5 ml of 1 *N* sulfuric acid. After incubation at 70°C for 20 min, 2.5 ml of water is added, and the *p*-nitrophenylhydrazones are extracted into 5 ml of *n*-hexane. The hexane phase is washed twice with 5 ml of 0.05 *N* sulfuric acid in ethanol–water, 5 : 3; an aliquot of the solvent is evaporated under a stream of nitrogen, and the residue is dissolved in 95% ethanol. The color intensity is determined at 395 nm and compared with that of standards of palmitaldehyde.

7. Other Methods. Besides the methods described in detail above, several other colorimetric methods are directly applicable to thin-layer chromatography for specific reactions. A modified trinitrobenzenesulfonic acid reaction for free amino groups has been described by Siakotos (72). Direct charring in sulfuric acid solution has been used (73). If a nondestructive visualizing agent is used, the intact lipid can be eluted from the TLC plate and a direct weight can be obtained. Lipids recovered intact after chromatography (see Chapter 4) can also be analyzed by spectrophotometry.

E. Densitometry

Densitometry on TLC plates is a method of great potential usefulness because of its simplicity and rapidity. However, it has never realized its full potential for a number of reasons. The technique appears to be fraught with technological and methodological difficulties that have rendered it essentially useless for general application. Nevertheless, densitometric scanning of TLC plates could become the method of choice for routine quantitative analysis of samples by thin-layer chromatography. Some of the main difficulties with the method at present involve the nonuniformity of charring, lack of adequate standards, and poor control of migration and spot-spreading, among others. The reader is referred to articles by Privett and co-workers (60, 74–77) and others (63, 78, 79) for more details on the densitometric method. In any event its use is restricted at present to one-dimensional thin-layer chromatography.

VI. FATTY ACID ANALYSIS AFTER THIN-LAYER CHROMATOGRAPHY

The fatty acid composition of individual lipid classes can be determined after the sample has been purified by either one- or two-dimensional thin-layer chromatography. With trace components it is often necessary to concentrate the sample by column chromatography, as discussed in Section IV. However, to ensure that the sample is totally free of impurities or other trace components, it is often best to further purify the fractions obtained from the column procedures by thin-layer chromatography. The fatty acid composition of the major components can be analyzed directly after TLC separation.

A. Sample Handling

The lipid sample is handled up to visualization of the spots in the manner already described; however, the spots are visualized by spraying either with water or 2′,7′-dichlorofluorescein. The latter is preferable because of its greater sensitivity, but water is acceptable if only major components are being analyzed. The spots are then scraped directly into transmethylation tubes (screw-capped, 20 × 150-mm culture tubes obtained from Kimble Glass Co., Toledo, Ohio).

B. Transmethylation Procedure

1. Preparation of Reagent. Transmethylation can be done with either boron trifluoride in methanol or methanolic HCl. Either reagent should be absolutely free of water to prevent the formation of free fatty acids. These reagents can be purchased commercially or prepared in the laboratory. If they are prepared in the laboratory, it is best to prepare dry methanol rather than to use reagent-grade solvents, because the commercial reagent contains variable but significant amounts of water. Dry methanol can be conveniently prepared by the method of Vogel (80).

The reagent is then prepared from the dry methanol by bubbling the anhydrous HCl gas or boron trifluoride through methanol and measuring the weight of gas absorbed. Methanolic HCl should be at least 5% HCl by weight. The boron trifluoride reagent should contain at least 140 g of boron trifluoride per liter of methanol.

2. Transmethylation. Approximately 5 ml of the transmethylation reagent is added to each transmethylation tube containing sample and adsorbent. Several boiling chips previously washed with solvent and acid are added to each tube, and the tubes are capped with a reflux condenser and drying tube to prevent atmospheric moisture from reaching the sample. The boiling chips prevent the violent bumping that will occur in the presence of the adsorbent; no bumping occurs if the adsorbent is absent. The tubes are then heated for a minimum of 2 hr at 90 to 95°C.

The tubes are then cooled to room temperature, and 10 ml of ice-cold distilled water is added to each tube. The methyl esters are extracted with a minimum of three washes of 3 ml of hexane, containing 0.01% butylated hydroxytoluene. After the hexane is removed, the samples can be weighed to check the recovery of fatty acid methyl esters and to facilitate proper dilution for injection into the gas chromatograph.

3. Further Purification Steps. For samples containing material other than methyl esters the sample can be rechromatographed on a small silicic acid column as follows: fraction I, cut with 1% diethyl ether in hexane, will contain the methyl esters and butylated hydroxytoluene; fraction II, cut with methanol, contains the remaining material in the sample (e.g., cholesterol, sphingosine, and glycerol ethers). The dichlorofluorescein used to locate the spots is not extracted from the aqueous phase of the transmethylation procedure by hexane; hence it does not interfere with the subsequent analysis of the fatty acid methyl esters.

Butylated hydroxytoluene will chromatograph with the mobility of methyl myristate on polyester stationary phases, such as diethylene glycol succinate in packed columns. This may or may not interfere with the gas–liquid chromatography analysis, depending on the objective of the particular experiment.

If butylated hydroxytoluene is objectionable, it can be removed from the methyl ester sample by one-dimensional thin-layer chromatography. The TLC procedure can be used to replace the small silicic acid column, since it also allows removal of all other contaminants from the methyl ester sample. The procedure is as follows: The total hexane extract from the transmethylation is spotted on a plain silica gel H plate (several samples can be spotted on one plate) in bands 1 to 2 cm in length. The plate is then developed in pure benzene, and the bands are visualized with water. The sequence of bands is hydrocarbons, butylated hydroxytoluene, methyl esters, and cholesterol; more polar compounds remain at the origin. The methyl esters are widely separated from the other components in this system (see Fig. 14). The methyl ester band is scraped from the plate into a fine-grade sintered-glass funnel, and the methyl esters are eluted from the adsorbent with chloroform. They are now free of all impurities and can be prepared for injection into the gas chromatograph.

C. Quantitative Gas–Liquid Chromatography

Samples of fatty acid methyl esters for gas–lipid chromatography analysis are best handled in solution in hexane or pentane. The solubility of the longer chain saturated methyl ester is rather low in pentane; hence, if the sample contains appreciable quantities of these compounds, hexane is the preferred solvent. The sample should be prepared in a concentration of 10 to 20 μg/ml for most packed-column analyses. For capillary columns the dilution factor will vary with the split ratio of the particular instrument in use.

The vast number of commercial gas chromatographs available and the even greater number of books and monographs on the analysis of fatty acids by gas–liquid chromatography eliminate the need for extensive discussion of the mechanics of this technique. However, the reader should be warned that gas–liquid chromatography, as has been pointed out by Ackman (81, 82) is a much abused technique. It is not sufficient to make a single-column analysis of a sample containing unsaturated fatty acids on polyester columns and then immediately assume that all the components

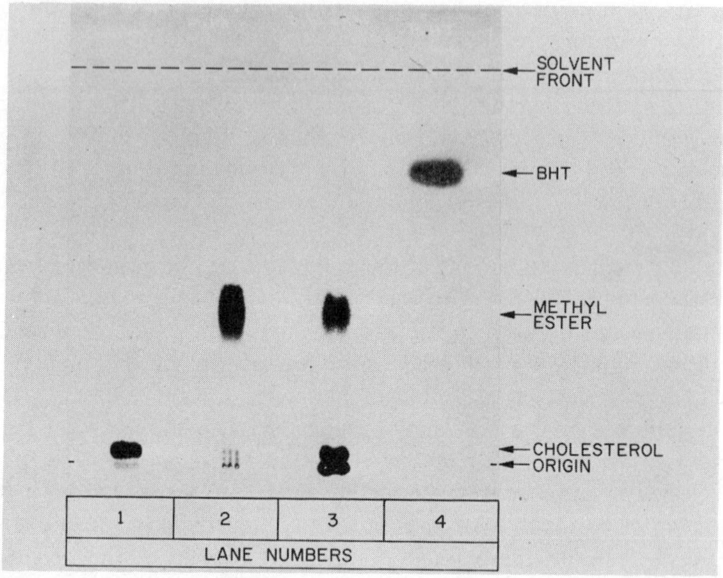

Fig. 14 A typical TLC separation of the products of a transmethylation reaction. The absorbent was plain silica gel HR; the solvent was benzene. Lane 1 contained a cholesterol standard; lane 2, a standard mixture of polyunsaturated fatty acid methyl esters; and lane 3, the hexane-soluble products of the transmethylation of a sample of dolphin-erythrocyte lipids. Sphingosine and other polar material remained at the origin. The butylated hydroxytoluene (BHT) is not visible (it chars very poorly), and a trace of hydrocarbon is above where the BHT should be. Lane 4 is pure BHT.

in the mixture have been either resolved or identified. Samples should be analyzed on two separate phases, such as polyethylene glycol succinate and Apiezon L. It is also wise to perform an analysis on a capillary column to resolve positional isomers and then to use both hydrogenation and ozonolysis to confirm the location of the double bonds. Only after this type of multiple analysis can the investigator be confident of the identity of the fatty acids in his samples.

It is also very helpful to use either argentation thin-layer chromatography (83, 84) or mercuric-adduct chromatography (85–87) to separate unsaturated fatty acids by the number of double bonds per molecule, thus simplifying the interpretation of the gas-chromatography data.

Besides the qualitative problems just listed, quantitation of gas-chromatography data also requires care. The response factors for each methyl ester in the sample should be checked, as well as losses of longer chain fatty acids on the column and the overall linearity of the system (81, 88). It is preferable to use an electronic integrator or digital computer to calculate the percentages in the reduction of gas-chromatography data. Manual methods like planimetry and triangulation are not only time consuming and tedious but also prone to both human and systemic errors. Of course electronic data reduction has its own set of problems, including expensive equipment, often extensive programming, calibration, and developmental difficulties. Nelson (89) has recently described a digital data station that takes the output from a gas chromatograph, converts it to digital form, and stores the results on magnetic tape so that they can be processed directly by a large digital computer. With this system no manual calculations are necessary to obtain the final results of the gas-chromatography analysis in a form useful to the investigator.

VII. CONCLUSIONS

No attempt has been made in this discussion to include all of the available procedures for the analysis of blood lipids, particularly all of the many analyses for specific lipids in the presence of the other lipid components of blood. These are of more interest in the clinical laboratory than in basic lipid research. For analyses of this kind the reader is referred to any of a number of texts on clinical biochemical methodology (90, 91).

Another area that has been neglected in this discussion and may be of interest to some readers is the analysis of glyceryl ethers, including both the alkyl-1-enyl and alkyl ethers; for specialized procedures, particularly the analysis of these compounds as derivatives by gas–liquid chromatography, the reader is urged to consult the recent works of Wood and co-workers (92–94). A new book by Litchfield (95) on the analysis of triglycerides also has many useful methods for the analysis of this interesting class of compounds, and mention has already been made of the work of Sweeley and co-workers on the analysis of glycosphingolipids in blood (5–7).

The analytical biochemistry of blood lipids is not at present an area of striking innovation and new developments. The techniques currently available allow complete quantitative analysis of practically all components. Newer developments will probably fall primarily in the area of computer-coupled instrumentation and automation of existing procedures, such as the automated Sephadex apparatus described here (96). Automation of the phosphorus procedure would obviously be a great boon to the investigator of phospholipid biochemistry. Fast liquid-column procedures with high pressures and very fine packings in narrow columns should also in the future provide new tools for the analysis of blood lipids.

Nevertheless, the methods described in this chapter will provide very good and fairly rapid analysis of blood lipids without the need for extensive modification or development by the investigator, particularly if he is unfamiliar with the field of lipid analysis. And in the absence of any new breakthroughs, these procedures should be useful for many years as they stand. This is particularly true of the two-dimensional thin-layer chromatography of phospholipid mixtures, which is an unsurpassed method for the analysis of this class of compounds when coupled with the colorimetric method for phosphorus. The recent reports by Turner and Rouser (97, 98) on the analysis of human red-cell and plasma lipids demonstrate well that these methods are capable of accurately quantitating blood lipids, including the most minor, and often unidentified, components.

VIII. ACKNOWLEDGMENTS

Mr. M. Hutton designed the electronics of the automatic Sephadex apparatus, and Mr. D. Hansen assembled and packaged the unit. Parts of this chapter were adapted, with permission, from publications of Dr. George Rouser. This work was supported in part by the U.S. Atomic Energy Commission.

REFERENCES

1. Renkonen, O., and P. Varo, in *Lipid Chromatographic Analysis*, G. V. Marinetti, Ed., Vol. 1, Dekker, New York, 1967, pp. 41–98.
2. Rouser, G., G. Kritchevsky, and A. Yamamoto, in *Lipid Chromatographic Analysis*, G. V. Marinetti, Ed., Vol. 1, Dekker, New York, 1967, pp. 99–162.
3. Rouser, G., G. Kritchevsky, D. Heller, and E. Leiber, *J. Amer. Oil Chem. Soc.* **40**, 425–454 (1963).
4. Lisboa, B. P., in *Lipid Chromatographic Analysis*, G. V. Marinetti, Ed., Vol. 2, Dekker, New York, 1969, pp. 57–147.
5. Sweeley, C. C., and D. E. Vance, in *Lipid Chromatographic Analysis*, G. V. Marinetti, Ed., Vol. 1. Dekker, New York, 1967, pp. 465–496.
6. Vance, D. E., and C. C. Sweeley, *J. Lipid Res.* **8**, 621–630 (1967).
7. Wells, W. W., C. C. Sweeley, and R. Bentley, in *Biomedical Applications of Gas Chromatography*, H. A. Szymanski, Ed., Plenum Press, New York, 1964, pp. 169–233.
8. Saifer, A., and S. Gerstenfeld, *J. Lab. Clin. Med.* **50**, 17–25 (1957).
9. Hess, H. H., and E. Rolde, *J. Biol. Chem.* **239**, 3215–3220 (1964).
10. Weiss, B., in *Lipid Chromatographic Analysis*, G. V. Marinetti, Ed., Vol. 1, Dekker, New York, 1967, pp. 429–446.
11. Eto, T., Y. Ichikawa, K. Nishimura, S. Ando, and T. Yamakawa, *J. Biochem. (Japan)* **64**, 205–213 (1968).
12. Klenk, E., in *Progress in the Chemistry of Fats and Other Lipids*, R. T. Holman, Ed., Vol. 10, Part 4, Pergamon Press, Oxford, 1969, pp. 411–431.

13. Coles, L., and G. M. Gray, *J. Lipid Res.* **11**, 164–166 (1970).
14. Rouser, G., G. Kritchevsky, C. Galli, A. Yamamoto, and A. G. Knudson, in *Inborn Disorders of Sphingolipid Metabolism*, S. M. Aronson and B. W. Volk, Eds., Pergamon Press, New York, 1967, pp. 303–316.
15. Rouser, G., and A. Yamamoto, in *Handbook of Neurochemistry*, A. Lajtha, Ed., Vol. 1, Plenum Press, New York, 1969, pp. 121–169.
16. Slawson, V., and R. A. Stein, *Lipids* **5**, 713–717 (1970).
17. Folch, J., M. Lees, and G. H. S. Stanley, *J. Biol. Chem.* **226**, 497–509 (1957).
18. Bligh, E. G., and W. J. Dyer, *Can. J. Biochem. Physiol.* **37**, 911–917 (1959).
19. Wells, M. A., and J. C. Dittmer, *Biochemistry* **2**, 1259–1263 (1963).
20. Siakotos, A. N., and G. Rouser, *J. Amer. Oil Chem. Soc.* **42**, 913–919 (1965).
21. Wuthier, R. E., *J. Lipid Res.* **7**, 558–561 (1966).
22. Lea, C. H., and D. N. Rhodes, *Biochem. J.* **54**, 467–469 (1953).
23. Westley, J., J. J. Wren, and H. K. Mitchell, *J. Biol. Chem.* **229**, 131–138 (1957).
24. Biezenski, J. J., *J. Lipid Res.* **3**, 120–125 (1962).
25. Lepage, M., *J. Chromatogr.* **13**, 99–103 (1964).
26. Maxwell, M. A. B., and J. P. Williams, *J. Chromatogr.* **31**, 62–68 (1967).
27. Williams, J. P., and P. A. Merrilees, *Lipids* **5**, 367–370 (1970).
28. Hirsch, J., and E. H. Ahrens, *J. Biol. Chem.* **233**, 311–320 (1958).
29. Freeman, N. K., F. Lindgren, Y. Ng., and A. V. Nichols, *J. Biol. Chem.* **227**, 449–464 (1957).
30. Soto, E. F., J. M. Pasquini, R. Placido, and J. L. La Torre, *J. Chromatogr.* **41**, 400–409 (1969).
31. Dittmer, J. C., *J. Chromatogr.* **43**, 512–514 (1969).
32. Brooks, C. J. W., and R. A. B. Keates, *J. Chromatogr.* **44**, 509–521 (1969).
33. Downey, W. K., R. F. Murphy, and M. K. Keogh, *J. Chromatogr.* **46**, 120–124 (1970).
34. Anggard, E., and H. Bergkuist, *J. Chromatogr.* **48**, 544–546 (1970).
35. Calderon, M., and W. J. Bauman, *J. Lipid Res.* **11**, 167–169 (1970).
36. Terner, C., E. I. Szabo, and N. L. Smith, *J. Chromatogr.* **47**, 15–19 (1970).
37. Ellingboe, J., E. Nystrom, and J. Sjovall, *J. Lipid Res.* **11**, 266–273 (1970).
38. Hanahan, D. J., J. C. Dittmer, and E. Warashina, *J. Biol. Chem.* **228**, 685–700 (1957).
39. Gjone, E., J. F. Berry, and D. A. Turner, *J. Lipid Res.* **1**, 66–71 (1959).
40. Nelson, G. J., and N. K. Freeman, *J. Biol. Chem.* **234**, 1375–1380 (1959).
41. Nelson, G. J., *J. Lipid Res.* **3**, 71–79 (1962).
42. Nelson, G. J., *Anal. Biochem.* **5**, 116–132 (1963).
43. Rouser, G., G. Kritchevsky, G. Simon, and G. J. Nelson, *Lipids* **2**, 37–40 (1967).
44. Rouser, G., C. Galli, E. Lieber, M. L. Blank, and O. S. Privett, *J. Amer. Oil Chem. Soc.* **41**, 836–840 (1964).
45. Feldman, G., L. S. Feldman, and G. Rouser, *Lipids* **1**, 27–30 (1966).
46. Young, O. M., and J. N. Kanfer, *J. Chromatogr.* **19**, 611–613 (1965).
47. Svennerholm, E., and L. Svennerholm, *Biochim. Biophys. Acta* **70**, 432–441 (1963).
48. Flowers, H. M., *Carbohydrate Res.* **2**, 371–379 (1966).
49. Panganamala, R. V., J. C. Geer, and D. G. Cornwell, *J. Lipid Res.* **10**, 445–455 (1969).
50. Kuhn, R., and H. Wiegandt, *Chem. Ber.* **96**, 866–880 (1963).
51. Wherret, J. R., and J. N. Cumings, *Biochem. J.* **86**, 378–383 (1963).
52. Ledeen, R., *J. Amer. Oil Chem. Soc.* **43**, 57–66 (1966).

53. Hakamori, S., *J. Lipid Res.* **7**, 789–792 (1966).
54. Ledeen, R., and K. Salsman, *Biochemistry* **4**, 2225–2232 (1965).
55. Wiegandt, H. *Angew. Chem.* **7**, 87–96 (1968).
56. Vogel, W. L., W. M. Doizaki, and L. Zieve, *J. Lipid Res.* **3**, 138–140 (1962).
57. Gloster, J., and R. F. Fletcher, *Clin. Chim. Acta* **13**, 235–240 (1966).
58. Mahadevan, V., in *Lipid Chromatographic Analysis*, G. V. Marinetti, Ed., Vol. 1, Dekker, New York, 1967, pp. 191–203.
59. Nelson, G. J., *Lipids* **2**, 323–328 (1967).
60. Vikrot, O., *Acta Med. Scand.* **175**, 443–453 (1964).
61. Privett, O. S., M. L. Blank, and W. O. Lundberg, *J. Amer. Oil Chem. Soc.* **38**, 312–316 (1961).
62. Privett, O. S., and M. L. Blank, *J. Amer. Oil Chem. Soc.* **39**, 520 (1962).
63. Downing, D. T., *J. Chromatogr.* **38**, 91–99 (1968).
64. Rouser, G., G. Simon, and G. Kritchevsky, *Lipids* **4**, 599–606 (1969).
65. Dittmer, J. C., and R. L. Lester, *J. Lipid Res.* **5**, 126–127 (1964).
66. Svennerholm, L., *Biochem. Biophys. Acta* **24**, 604–611 (1957).
67. Nelson, G. J., and R. A. Booth, *Anal. Biochem.* **20**, 198–199 (1967).
68. Bartlett, G. R., *J. Biol. Chem.* **234**, 466–468 (1959).
69. Rouser, G., S. Fleischer, and A. Yamamoto, *Lipids* **5**, 494–496 (1970).
70. Hesse, G., and K. Geller, *Mikrochim. Acta* **3**, 526–533 (1968).
71. Hanel, H. K., and H. Dam, *Acta Chem. Scand.* **9**, 677–682 (1955).
72. Siakotos, A. N., *Lipids* **2**, 87–88 (1967).
73. Marsh, J. B., and D. B. Weinstein, *J. Lipid Res.* **7**, 574–576 (1966).
74. Privett, O. S., and M. L. Blank, *J. Lipid Res.* **2**, 37–44 (1961).
75. Privett, O. S., and M. L. Blank, *J. Amer. Oil Chem. Soc.* **40**, 70–75 (1963).
76. Blank, M. L., J. A. Schmit, and O. S. Privett, *J. Amer. Oil Chem. Soc.* **41**, 371–376 (1964).
77. Privett, O. S., M. L. Blank, D. W. Codding, and E. C. Nickel, *J. Amer. Oil Chem. Soc.* **42**, 381–393 (1965).
78. Barrett, C. B., M. S. J. Dallas, and F. B. Padley, *J. Amer. Oil Chem. Soc.* **40**, 580–584 (1963).
79. Louis-Ferdinand, R. T., D. G. Therriault, W. F. Blatt, and M. Mager, *Clin. Chem.* **13**, 773–787 (1967).
80. Vogel, A., *Practical Organic Chemistry*, 3rd ed., Longmans, Green, New York, 1956, pp. 169–179.
81. Ackman, R. G., J. C. Sipos, and P. M. Jangaard, *Lipids* **2**, 251–257 (1967).
82. Ackman, R. G., *Lipids* **2**, 502–505 (1967).
83. De Vries, B., *Chem. Ind.* (*London*), 1049–1050 (1962).
84. Morris, L. J., *Chem. Ind.* (*London*), 1238–1240 (1962).
85. Wagner, H., and P. Pohl, *Biochem. Z.* **340**, 337–344 (1964).
86. White, H. B., *J. Chromatogr.* **21**, 213–222 (1966).
87. White, H. B., and S. S. Powell, *J. Chromatogr.* **32**, 451–457 (1968).
88. Ackman, R. G., and J. C. Sipos, *J. Amer. Oil Chem. Soc.* **41**, 377–378 (1964).
89. Nelson, G. J., *J. Amer. Oil Chem. Soc.*, **48**, 210–216 (1971).
90. Annino, J. S., *Clinical Chemistry, Principles and Procedures*, 3rd ed., Little, Brown and Co., Boston, 1964, pp. 269–289.
91. Henry, R. J., *Clinical Chemistry, Principles and Technics*, Harper and Row, New York, 1964, pp. 833–883.
92. Wood, R., and F. Snyder, *Lipids* **1**, 62–72 (1966).
93. Wood, R., and F. Snyder, *Lipids* **3**, 129–135 (1968).

94. Wood, R., and R. D. Harlow, *Lipids* **5**, 776–781 (1970).
95. Litchfield, C., *Analysis of Triglycerides,* in press, Academic Press, New York, 1972.
96. Nelson, G. J., *An Automatic Gel-Filtration Apparatus for the Purification of Lipid Extracts*, Lawrence Radiation Laboratory, Livermore, Report UCRL-50861, 1970.
97. Turner, J. D., and G. Rouser, *Anal. Biochem.,* **38**, 423–436 (1970).
98. Turner, J. D., and G. Rouser, *Anal. Biochem.,* **38**, 437–445 (1970).

3. Determination of Serum Triglycerides

ROBERT F. WITTER* and VIRGINIA S. WHITNER

U.S. Department of Health, Education, and Welfare, Public Health Service, Lipid Standardization Laboratory, Atlanta, Georgia

* Deceased.

I. INTRODUCTION

Interest in the determination of serum triglycerides has grown in the last decade because of the increasing evidence of the possible role of elevated levels of this lipid in the development of atherosclerosis and heart disease (1–7). Early procedures were based on the indirect determination of triglycerides as the difference between the total lipid content and the sum of the cholesterol, cholesterol esters, and phospholipid levels. More recently methods have been devised for the direct determination of triglycerides or neutral glycerides from the glycerol portion of the molecule or the ester groups.

The first direct procedure was published in 1957 by Van Handel and Zilversmit (8). In this manual method phospholipids are removed from the lipid extract by an adsorbent, and then the triglycerides are determined from the amount of glycerol released on saponification. This procedure has been widely adopted and subjected to modification by many investigators. In 1964 Lofland (9) devised an automated procedure for the determination of the glycerol and thus a semiautomated method for serum triglycerides. Two years later Kessler and Lederer (10) went one step further and automated saponification. These semiautomated methods have increased the number of determinations that can be carried out and are now being employed in both clinical and research laboratories. Recently methods for the specific enzymatic determination of glycerol have been incorporated into a method in which triglycerides are determined in the presence of phospholipids and in which the steps of saponification and extraction are combined (11).

In this chapter only the direct methods for the determination of triglycerides are reviewed. All of these procedures should be considered as methods for neutral glycerides since most of the partial glycerides, which make up from 2 (12) to 10% (13) of the total neutral glycerides, probably are determined along with the triglycerides.

Procedures based on thin-layer, gas–liquid, or column chromatography and infrared spectrophotometry are not discussed since they are covered in other chapters of this volume. However, column procedures used solely for the determination of triglycerides are considered. Indirect methods based on the calculation of triglycerides as the difference between total lipid content and the sum of cholesterol, cholesterol esters, and phospholipid levels are not discussed. These procedures are based on the assumption that the sphingomyelin content of serum phospholipids is constant and, in most cases, that the ratio between cholesterol and cholesterol esters is fixed. The analysis is subject to the errors of each of the individual determinations. These errors become more important as the triglyceride level approaches the normal range, in which the concentration of this class of lipid is about one-tenth to one-fifth that of the total lipid. Older methods for the determination of triglycerides by difference are reviewed by Carlson and Wadström (14) and Jacobs and Henry (15). More recent procedures based on the determination of glyceride ester groups have been presented by Reinhold, Yonan, and Gershman, (16), Eggstein (17), and Martinek (18).

A review of methods for the determination of glycerides has been published in the Soviet literature (19), and reviews of the semiautomated determination of blood lipids have appeared (20–22).

II. CLASSIFICATION OF DIRECT METHODS FOR THE DETERMINATION OF NEUTRAL GLYCERIDES

A. Principle of Methods

Methods for the direct determination of neutral glycerides can be divided into two groups: (a) procedures in which interfering phospholipids are removed before determination of the neutral glyceride and (b) methods in which neutral glycerides are not separated from phospholipids but are determined after saponification by a specific enzymatic procedure for glycerol. The procedures of type (a) include most of the manual and all of the semiautomated methods.

The steps in procedures of type (a) include the following:

1. Extraction of the lipids.
2. Adsorption of the phospholipids.
3. Saponification or transesterification of the phospholipid-free extract.

4a. Determination of glycerol released from the neutral glycerides.

4b. Alternatively, saponification of the phospholipid-free extract is omitted, and the ester groups in the neutral glycerides are determined.

In a number of methods that have been devised for the determination of triglycerides these basic steps are modified. A basic objective of many investigators has been to develop methods that are not only accurate and precise but also simple enough for adaptation to routine or clinical use. Hence, with only a few exceptions, phospholipids have been separated by a batch process rather than by column procedures. Furthermore, the solvents that have been used make it possible to carry out the extraction in the presence of the adsorbent, thus combining the steps of extraction and adsorption. Some recently published semiautomated (10, 20, 23–28) and manual (11, 29–33) procedures do not require the evaporation of the solvent, further simplifying the determination.

From 0.5 to 1.0 ml of serum is required for most procedures for the determination of serum triglycerides.

B. Classification of Methods

A classification of methods for the determination of serum neutral glycerides is presented in tabular form in Sections III through VI. The classification is based on the extracting solvent, the adsorbent, the solvent used for saponification, and the end reaction for the determination of glyceride glycerol or ester groups. The methods are grouped according to the end reaction. Each category or number does not necessarily represent a single method since several procedures may have common features that permit classification as one type of method. The following data are included:

1. Solvents that have been used for the extraction of triglycerides and the respective adsorbents.
2. References for experiments showing quantitative recovery of triglycerides (95–105%) and removal of phospholipids that have been carried out with the solvent–adsorbent systems.
3. Methods in which the extraction and adsorption steps are combined.
4. Conditions for the chromatographic separation of phospholipids in the few procedures in which small columns are used.

Batch methods for the removal of phospholipids are employed in the other procedures. In a batch process the serum sample itself plus the extracting solvent (adsorption and extraction steps combined) or a solution of the previously isolated serum lipids in a nonpolar solvent (extraction and adsorption steps separated) are shaken and/or allowed to stand in contact with the adsorbent. Under these conditions the quantitative extraction of the triglycerides and adsorption of the phospholipids depend on the sample-to-solvent and sample-to-adsorbent ratios, the degree of activation and particle size of the adsorbent, and the extent and duration of mixing.

An illustration of the conditions used for the extraction and adsorption steps with the chloroform–zeolite system is given in Table I. A similar

Table I. Conditions Used in the Chloroform–Zeolite System for the Extraction of Triglycerides and Adsorption of Phospholipids

Treatment of Zeolite Adsorbent	Ratio of Solvent to Sample (ml/ml)	Ratio of Adsorbent to Sample (g/ml)	Condition of Adsorption	Reference
Heated 4 hr at 125°C	12	4.0	Shake mixture vigorously for 10 min	8
Ground to 80–100 mesh, heated 4 hr at 125°C	12	4.0	Shake mixture, then allow to stand overnight	34
Ground to 80–100 mesh, heated 4 hr at 125°C	12	2.0	Allow mixture to stand 4 hr with occasional shaking or overnight	35
Heated 4 hr at 125°C	34	6.0	Shake at 1-min intervals for 5 min	36
Not activated	20	1.0	Shake mechanically at 270 oscillations per min for 10 min	37
20–80 mesh, heated 4 hr at 125°C	20	2.0	Allow mixture to stand 4 hr with occasional mixing or overnight	38
20–80 mesh, heated overnight at 170°C	25	5.0	Shake vigorously for 10 min	39

variety of conditions have been employed with other solvent–adsorbent systems in which batch processes are used. The original literature should be consulted for these data.

The species of animal from which the sample is taken has been shown to influence the conditions necessary for the quantitative extraction and complete adsorption in a batch process with the chloroform–zeolite (34) and isopropyl ether–silicic acid systems (22). More finely divided adsorbent is necessary with rat (34) or pig (22) plasma than with human plasma.

The conditions necessary for the quantitative extraction of neutral glycerides and adsorption of phospholipids are discussed in greater detail in Sections III through VI.

The saponification of triglycerides has been performed under various conditions. The most common procedure is saponification in ethanol containing potassium hydroxide. This process is carried out for 20 to 60 min at 60 to 70°C in 0.02 to 0.1 *M* (8, 34–36, 38, 40–51) or at 37 to 60°C in 0.22 to 1.7 *M* (11, 14, 31–33, 37, 39, 51–61) alkali. Automated saponification has taken place in isopropanol. Other solvents for the hydrolysis of neutral glycerides are discussed under individual methods and are listed in the tables.

Further steps in the analysis of glycerol, liberated after saponification, may include evaporation of the solvent employed in saponification, extraction of the glycerol into an aqueous phase and the cholesterol and liberated fatty acids into an organic phase, which is discarded. Which, if any, of these steps is required for a given method depends on the end reaction for the determination of glycerol. Hence these steps are discussed for each of the methods.

III. MANUAL PROCEDURES BASED ON THE DETERMINATION OF FORMALDEHYDE PRODUCED BY PERIODATE OXIDATION OF GLYCERIDE GLYCEROL

A. Periodate Oxidation of Glyceride Glycerol

Most of the procedures for the determination of neutral glycerides are based on the determination of formaldehyde produced by the periodate oxidation of glycerol liberated from the isolated neutral glycerides. Two moles of formaldehyde are produced per mole of glycerol.

$$\begin{array}{l} CH_2OH \\ | \\ CHOH + 2HIO_4 \rightarrow 2HCHO + HCOOH + H_2O + 2HIO_3 \\ | \\ CH_2OH \end{array} \qquad (1)$$

Oxidation is carried out in acid solution since formaldehyde can be oxidized under alkaline conditions (62). Periodic acid specifically oxidizes compounds that have two adjacent hydroxyl groups or a hydroxyl and amino group attached to adjacent carbon atoms (63). Hence common interfering compounds include glucose, serine, and sphingosine, or α-glycerol phosphate produced by the alkaline hydrolysis of phosphoglycerides.

B. Methods Based on Egriwe's Chromotropic Acid Reaction for Formaldehyde

Eegriwe's (64) chromotropic color reaction was adapted to spectrophotometry by MacFadyen (65). Formaldehyde is reacted with chromotropic acid (4,5-dihydroxy-2,7-naphthalenedisulfonic acid) in 9 to 10 *M* sulfuric acid for 30 min at 100°C to produce a violet-pink color (570 nm) that is stable in the dark for at least 3 days. According to Henry (66), the absorption peak is actually at 564 nm. Lambert and Neish (67) found that this reaction could be used to measure the formaldehyde produced by the periodate oxidation of glycerol if the interfering excess periodate was reduced with arsenite before formaldehyde was reacted with chromotropic acid. A tenfold excess of arsenite had to be used because of the reversibility of the reduction of periodate. Under these conditions an appreciable amount of chromogen was produced in the absence of formaldehyde. The blank could be reduced by lowering the concentration of periodate and arsenite. The blank also varies with different preparations of chromotropic (68) or sulfuric acid (69). Modifications in the color reaction that have been introduced by most investigators have been attempts to reduce the blank color.

Methods based on the Lambert and Neish (67) procedure for the determination of glycerol are outlined in Table II.[1] Experiments showing the quantitative recovery of triglycerides and removal of phospholipids have been carried out with most of the solvent–adsorbent systems used with the chromotropic acid reaction (Table II). Blankenhorn, Rouser, and Weimer (52) found up to 6% phospholipid left in eluates prepared with chloroform–zeolite according to the method of Van Handel and Zilversmit (8).

Chloroform–zeolite (8) and chloroform–silicic acid (72) extracts are relatively free of glucose and other formaldehydogenic compounds. The same thing is true of ethanol–ether extracts after treatment of the lipids in chloroform solution with silicic acid (46). Added glucose does not interfere in the chloroform–zeolite system (37), the chloroform–silicic acid system (72), or chloroform–methanol extracts prepared by the method of Folch (75). Blank glycerol (i.e., "glycerol" present in samples processed without saponification) was reduced in the chloroform–zeolite system by the use of a more finely divided adsorbent and a longer extraction time (35). Isopropyl ether–ethanol extracts of serum from diabetic patients gave the same blank as the reagent blank and hence are probably free of glucose (30).

Saponification is carried out in ethanolic potassium hydroxide with two exceptions. Methanol solutions are employed in the procedure of Chlouverakis, Hanley, and Butterfield (71), and 0.1 volume of 0.3 *M* potassium hydroxide is added to the phospholipid-free isopropyl ether–ethanol ex-

[1] Throughout this chapter the use of trade names is for identification only and does not constitute endorsement by the Public Health Service or by the U.S. Department of Health, Education, and Welfare.

Table II. Manual Procedures for Serum Neutral Glycerides Employing Periodate Oxidation of Glycerol and Egriwe's Reaction for Formaldehyde[a]

No.	Extractant	Adsorbent	Extraction and Adsorption Combined	References
1	Chloroform	Zeolite	Yes	8,[b,c] 34,[c] 35, 36,[b,c] 37,[b,c] 38,[c] 41, 42, 70
2	Chloroform	Zeolite	Yes	71[d]
3	Chloroform	Silicic acid	Yes	72[b,c]
4	Chloroform–methanol, 2:1 (v/v)[f]	Silicic acid	No	8,[e] 14,[b,c,e] 40,[b,c,e] 43, 55,[b,c] 56,[b,c] 72[b,c]
5	Chloroform–methanol, 2:1 (v/v)[f]	Florisil	No	37,[b,c,g] 73[b,c,g]
6	Ethanol–ethyl ether, 3:1 (v/v)[h]	Silicic acid	No	44–46[b,c]
7	Acetone–ethanol, 1:1 (v/v)	Florisil	No	52[b,c,i]
8	Isopropyl ether	Silicic acid	Yes	47[b,c]
9	Ethyl ether followed by isopropanol, 2:1 (v/v)	Florisil	Yes	74[b]
10	Isopropyl ether–ethanol, 95:5 (v/v)	Silicic acid	Yes	30[c,j]

[a] Saponification with ethanolic KOH unless otherwise noted.
[b] Triglycerides quantitatively recovered.
[c] Phospholipids quantitatively removed.
[d] Saponification with methanolic KOH.
[e] Lower phase after washing chloroform–methanol extracts as described in footnote f is applied to silicic acid Hyflo supercel column, and the neutral glycerides are eluted with chloroform.
[f] Chloroform–methanol extracts were washed with 1 volume of water (8); 1 volume of 0.15 *M* saline (40, 43); 0.4 volume of 0.15 *M* saline (14, 73); 0.25 volume of 0.04 *M* calcium chloride (37); 0.33 volume of 0.15 *M* saline (72); 0.2 volume of water (55); or 2 volumes of saturated saline solution (56). The chloroform phase is applied directly to the adsorbent except when 0.2 volume of water is used (55) or with the silicic acid column of Carlson and Wadström (14).
[g] Lower phase after washing chloroform extracts as described in footnote f is applied to a Florisil column, and the neutral glycerides are eluted with chloroform.
[h] Lipids from ethanol–ethyl ether extracts were redissolved in chloroform before treatment with silicic acid.
[i] Small column of Florisil containing 4% water. Lipids applied in petroleum ether–ethyl ether, 95:5 (v/v) and neutral glycerides eluted with chloroform–acetone–water 99:99:2 (v/v/v).
[j] Saponification with extractant plus 0.1 volume 0.3 *M* ethanolic KOH.

tract in order to carry out saponification by the method of Laurell (30). This method is based on the finding of Henriques (76) that saponification can take place in a solvent of low polarity after the addition of potassium hydroxide in ethanol.

In Laurell's procedure (30) fatty acids and cholesterol are removed. The addition of dilute sulfuric acid separates the saponified mixture into two phases. The upper, containing fatty acids and cholesterol, is completely removed; the liberated glycerol remains in the aqueous phase ready for periodate oxidation and the chromotropic acid reaction.

In regard to other methods conflicting reports have appeared as to what steps are necessary after saponification to prepare the glycerol solution for periodate oxidation and the chromotropic acid reaction. When methanol is the solvent for saponification, it must be removed (71) since it will react with chromotropic acid if the concentration of methanol is 10 or more times that of the formaldehyde produced from glycerol (64). Van Handel and Zilversmit (8) found turbidity in the color reaction to be associated with the presence of ethanol used for saponification. In contrast Moore (69) later claimed that ethanol caused a slight increase in the amount of chromogen formed in the chromotropic acid reaction and apparently an increase in the rate of reduction of periodate by arsenite. Thus some investigators recommend that after saponification the ethanol solution be evaporated to dryness (14, 36, 40, 44, 45, 47, 56, 73), although other workers do not consider this step to be necessary.

Conflicting evidence also exists as to whether cholesterol and fatty acids do (14, 41, 44, 69, 72) or do not (8, 45, 71) give increased color in the chromotropic acid reaction and hence must be removed by hexane extraction before periodate oxidation and color reaction. This step is included in the manual procedures devised by various investigators (14, 30, 36, 40–44, 46, 56, 69, 72, 73) but omitted by others (8, 34, 35, 37, 38, 45, 47, 52, 55, 70, 71, 74). If hexane extraction is included in the procedure, all traces of the solvent must be removed by heating at 60 to 70°C for 2 or 3 min since the chromogen produced in the chromotropic acid reaction is selectively extracted into any droplets that remain (69).

The glycerol that has been liberated by saponification and treated as described in the preceding section is now subjected to periodate oxidation. With the exception of Blankenhorn and co-workers (52), investigators have lowered the periodate concentration from the 0.02 *M* recommended by Lambert and Neish (67) to 0.009 *M* (8, 34, 40, 41, 69–71, 74), 0.005 *M* (14, 30, 35, 37, 43–45, 56, 72, 73), or lower (36, 42, 46, 47, 55) and extended the reaction time from 5 to 10 or 15 min in an attempt to reduce the blank and still obtain quantitative oxidation. At low periodate concentrations, iodine may be liberated (62).

Table III. Manual Procedures for Serum Neutral Glycerides Employing Various Color Reactions for Formaldehyde[a]

No.	Extractant	Adsorbent	Extraction and Adsorption Combined	References
	Methods Employing Schryver's Reaction (79)			
11	Hexane–isopropanol, 1:1 (v/v)[d]	Silicic acid	No	80–82[b,c]
12	Chloroform–methanol, 2:1 (v/v)[e]	Silicic acid	No	57,[b,c] 58
13	Isopropyl ether	Silicic acid	Yes	48
14	Isopropanol–heptane–sulfuric acid, 40:10:1 (v/v/v)[f]	Silicic acid	No	59[b,c]
	Methods Employing Nash's Modification (68) of the Hantzsch Reaction			
15	Chloroform	Silicic acid	Yes	49[b]
16	Isopropanol	Zeolite + Lloyds reagent + $Ca(OH)_2$ + $CuSO_4 \cdot 5H_2O$, 100:10:10:5 (w/w/w/w)	Yes	29[b,g]
17	Chloroform–methanol, 2:1 (v/v)[h]	Silicic acid	No	53[b]
	Method Employing Pays' Reaction (83)			
18	Isopropanol–dichloromethane, 8:10 (v/v)[j]	Zeolite	No	84[i]

[a] Saponification with ethanolic KOH unless otherwise noted.
[b] Quantitative recovery of triglycerides.
[c] Quantitative removal of phospholipids.
[d] Hexane–isopropanol is partitioned by the addition of 4 volumes of 0.15 *M* saline into a polar and nonpolar phase. The nonpolar phase is brought to the composition petroleum ether–ethyl ether, 9:1 (v/v), and treated with silicic acid.
[e] Chloroform–methanol extracts are washed with 0.2 volume of water. The nonpolar phase is diluted with 1 volume of chloroform before adsorption on silicic acid.
[f] Isopropanol–heptane–sulfuric acid extracts are diluted with sufficient water and heptane to bring the composition to isopropanol–heptane–aqueous phase 80:80:62

The reducing agent, arsenite, has been replaced by bisulfite (36, 55), hydroxylamine (46), and lead acetate (37) in attempts to lower the blank. Frisell and Mackenzie (77) claimed that arsenite interfered in the reaction of formaldehyde with chromotropic acid and suggested bisulfite as the reducing agent, but other investigators have continued to use arsenite. Reduction with bisulfite produces 8% less chromogen than does reduction with arsenite (72). In our opinion there seems to be little advantage in the use of hydroxylamine or lead acetate.

Most investigators have employed the conditions of MacFadyen (65) for the chromotropic acid reaction. However, Chlouverakis et al. (71) have claimed that more precise results were obtained if the reaction is carried out in 5 to 7 *M* rather than the 9 to 10 *M* sulfuric acid recommended by MacFadyen (65). Also, with bisulfite as the reducing agent, the addition of thiourea just prior to reading the optical density was found to reduce the blank (36, 55).

The methods of Van Handel and Zilversmit (8) and Carlson (43) have been found to give comparable results (78).

C. Methods Based on Schryver's Reaction for Formaldehyde

Schryver's reaction (79) for the determination of formaldehyde was adapted to the determination of glycerol from neutral glycerides by Randrup (80–82). In this method, after glycerol is converted to formaldehyde by oxidation with 0.005 *M* periodate for 10 min at room temperature, 0.03 *M* phenylhydrazine hydrochloride is added, followed 10 min later by 0.005 *M* ferricyanide. The solution is allowed to chill 4 to 5 min at 0°C. Then concentrated hydrochloric acid is added and after 10 to 12 min the color is read at 540 nm. The product of the reaction between formaldehyde, phenylhydrazine, and ferricyanide has been identified tentatively from infrared and visible spectra (48) as 1,5-diphenylformazan.

Extracting solvents, adsorbents, and other data are listed in Table III for methods (Nos. 11–14) in which Schryver's reaction is used. Nonpolar

---

(v/v/v). The nonpolar phase is evaporated, and the phospholipids are adsorbed with silicic acid from an ethyl ether solution.

[g] Saponification with isopropanol–water, 6:1 (v/v), containing 0.2 *M* KOH.

[h] Chloroform–methanol extracts are partitioned into polar and nonpolar phases with 1 volume of water. The nonpolar phase is passed through small silicic acid–HyFlo supercel columns as described by Van Handel and Zilversmit (8) (method 4).

[i] Saponification with isopropanol solution of KOH.

[j] Isopropanol–dichloromethane, 8:10 (v/v), extracts are diluted to isopropanol–dichloromethane, 8:17 (v/v), for the adsorption step.

phases produced by washing hexane–isopropanol and isopropanol–heptane–sulfuric acid extracts form the upper layer and can more readily be drawn off by pipette than can the nonpolar phase from chloroform–methanol. The nonpolar phase produced from isopropanol–heptane–sulfuric acid, after washing, is a poor extractant for phospholipids (85) since up to 1000 mg of lysolecithin did not interfere.

Cholesterol and fatty acids are extracted in all procedures (57–59, 80–82) except one (48) in which isopropanol is added before the absorbance is read in order to prevent turbidity. Oxidation is carried out in 0.005 *M* periodate (48, 58, 80–82) or at lower concentrations (57, 59). The color reaction is carried out essentially as outlined at the beginning of this section. Less variable results were found if the concentration of hydrochloric acid added to develop the color was increased 60% (81, 82). A fourfold increase in sensitivity was obtained by substituting a sulfuric acid–acetic acid reagent for the hydrochloric acid used for color development (48).

Each step in the Schryver color reaction must be carefully timed. The color fades rapidly, and the addition of the concentrated acid must be made at 0°C. On the other hand, there have been no reports of elevated blanks, which have been the reason for many investigations with the chromotropic acid reaction. Only 0.05 ml of serum is required for the method of Galletti (48).

The method of Lloyd and Goldrick (59), employing heptane–isopropanol–sulfuric acid extracts, gives results that are comparable to those obtained by the method of Carlson and Wadström (14).

D. Methods Based on the Hantzsch Reaction for Formaldehyde

Recently a number of triglyceride-determination procedures that are based on the Hantzsch reaction for the determination of formaldehyde have appeared. In this reaction formaldehyde reacts with ammonium acetate and acetylacetone to form 3,5-diacetyl-1,4-dihydrolutidine. The yellow product can be determined quantitatively from its absorbance at 412 nm (68) or its fluorescence (86). The fluorometric reaction has been applied to semiautomated methods and is discussed in Section VI.C. The colorimetric procedure developed by Nash (68) is carried out at a pH of 5.5 to 6.5 for 40 min at 37°C with 1 *M* ammonium acetate and 0.01 *M* acetylacetone. The yellow chromogen is stable overnight if left in the dark but fades in the light. A large excess of ammonium acetate must be present; however, the reaction rate is not as sensitive to decreased acetylacetone concentration. If present, periodate causes the color to fade (68).

Table III lists the extracting solvents, adsorbents, and other data for methods (Nos. 15–17) in which the Hantzsch reaction is used. Periodate oxidation is carried out with 0.005 (49, 53) or 0.0008 *M* solutions (29). Arsenite reduction is omitted at the lower concentration of periodate since under these conditions periodate did not interfere in the color reaction (29). Color development is carried out at 50 to 60°C for 10 to 30 min under conditions similar to those of Nash (68). However, in the procedure of Dunsbach (49) the chromogen is extracted into isoamyl alcohol. The method of Fletcher (29) is the only manual procedure in which all steps are carried out with the original phospholipid-free extract.

In none of these procedures were the solvents used for saponification evaporated, nor were the hydrolysates extracted to remove cholesterol or fatty acids. Dunsbach (49) found that ethanol, present in the saponification mixture, has no effect on the reaction; the effects of cholesterol and fatty acids have not been studied, however. In each procedure the blank (non-saponified sample) for most serum samples is negligible. None of the manual methods employing the Hantzsch procedure has been compared with other procedures.

The advantages of the methods employing this color reaction are (a) the color can be developed at a lower temperature than in methods employing chromotropic acid, (b) fewer reagents are required, and (c) none of the reagents is corrosive.

E. Methods Based on Pays' Reaction for Formaldehyde

A color reaction between formaldehyde, 3-methylbenzothiozolin-2-one, and ferric chloride to give a chromogen absorbing at 620 nm (83) is the basis of a recent method for triglycerides (84) outlined in Table III (No. 18).

IV. MANUAL PROCEDURES BASED ON THE DETERMINATION OF GLYCERIDE GLYCEROL

A. Methods Based on the Skraup Reaction for Glycerol

In the Skraup reaction (87) glycerol liberated from neutral glycerides is heated at 170°C with *o*-aminophenol to form 8-hydroxyquinoline in the presence of an oxidizing agent (arsenic acid) and sulfuric acid (88). The fluorescence produced by chelation with magnesium gives a quantitative measure of glycerol.

The procedure (88) is carried out as outlined in Table IV (No. 19). Phospholipids, cholesterol, and fatty acids interfere and are removed before

Table IV. Manual Procedures for the Determination of Glyceride Glycerol Employing Various Reactions for Glycerol[a]

No.	Extractant	Adsorbent	Extraction and Adsorption Combined	References
	Method Based on the Skraup Reaction (87)			
19	Isopropyl ether	Silicic acid	Yes	88[b–d]
	Glycerol Determined by the Modified Wieland Enzymatic Reaction (89)			
20	Chloroform–methanol, 2:1 (v/v)	Silicic acid	No	54[e]
	Glycerol Determined by the Modified Enzymatic Reaction of Garland and Randle (90)			
21	Chloroform	Zeolite	Yes	39
22	Chloroform–methanol, 2:1 (v/v)	—	—	33[b]
23	Isopropanol	Zeolite	Yes	51[b,c]
24	Ethanolic KOH, 0.5 *M*	—	—	11, 31, 32, 33,[b] 60, 61[f]

[a] Saponification with ethanolic KOH unless otherwise noted.
[b] Triglycerides quantitatively recovered. Lipids from chloroform–methanol were taken up in ethanolic KOH.
[c] Phospholipids quantitatively removed.
[d] Saponification with methonolic KOH.
[e] Small silicic acid column, method of Carlson and Wadström (14) (method 4).
[f] In all of these procedures saponification occurs during extraction with ethanolic KOH, 0.5 *M*, for 20 min at 70°C.

the fluorescent reaction is carried out. The *o*-aminophenol must be purified by sublimation at 170°C and recrystallization from isopropyl ether and then left under nitrogen. The levels of triglycerides obtained by this batch process on 15 samples agreed with those obtained with silicic-acid-column chromatography as described by Barron and Hanahan (91).

B. Methods Based on the Enzymatic Determination of Glycerol

Methods based on the enzymatic determination of glycerol liberated from neutral glycerides are outlined in Table IV (Nos. 20–24). In all of these methods cholesterol and fatty acids produced by saponification are removed before the enzymatic reactions are carried out. Two enzymatic methods have been employed for the determination of glycerol. The first method is a modification of the procedure of Wieland (89) and consists of the following coupled reactions:

$$\text{glycerol} + \text{ATP} \xrightarrow[\text{Mg}^{2+}]{\text{glycerokinase}} \alpha\text{-glycerolphosphate} + \text{ADP} \quad (2)$$

$$\text{NAD}^{+} + \alpha\text{-glycerolphosphate} \underset{\substack{\text{glycerol-}\\\text{phosphate}\\\text{dehydrogenase}}}{\rightleftarrows} \text{NADH} + \text{H}^{+} + \text{dihydroxyacetone phosphate} \quad (3)$$

Glycerol reacts at pH 9.4 in hydrazine buffer with ATP in the presence of glycerokinase, magnesium ion, and cysteine to form ADP. After 10 min at 30°C, α-glycerolphosphate dehydroxygenase is added with subsequent conversion of α-glycerolphosphate and NADH to dihydroxyacetone phosphate and $NADH_2$. The reaction is complete after 10 min at 30°C. The difference in optical densities at 340 nm before and after the addition of α-glycerolphosphate dehydrogenase is proportional to the amount of glycerol present.

Spinella and Mager (54) used this enzymatic method to determine glycerol released on the saponification of phospholipid-free extracts prepared according to the method of Carlson and Wadström (14). The enzymatic procedure and the original colorimetric method gave the same results on 17 samples ranging in concentration from 0.42 to 2.45 mM/l. These results indicate the specificity of the color reaction under these conditions (54).

The second enzymatic method employed for the determination of glycerol released from neutral glycerides is based on the procedure of Garland and Randle (90)

$$\text{glycerol} + \text{ATP} \xrightarrow[\text{glycerokinase}]{} \alpha\text{-glycerolphosphate} + \text{ADP} \quad (4)$$

$$\text{ADP} + \text{phosphoenolpyruvate} \xrightarrow[\substack{\text{pyruvate}\\\text{kinase}}]{} \text{ATP} + \text{pyruvate} \quad (5)$$

$$\text{H}^{+} + \text{pyruvate} + \text{NADH} \xrightarrow[\substack{\text{lactic}\\\text{dehydrogenase}}]{} \text{lactate} + \text{NAD}^{+} \quad (6)$$

The reaction takes place in the presence of the magnesium ion at pH 7.2. Glycerol and ATP react to form α-glycerolphosphate and ADP. However, unlike the method of Wieland (89), further reactions are carried out with ADP rather than with α-glycerolphosphate. The assay is started by the addition of glycerokinase to the otherwise complete reaction mixture. The change in absorbance at 340 or 366 nm is proportional to the concentration of glycerol. The method is specific for glycerol since the other substrates for glycerokinase, glyceraldehyde, or dihydroxyacetone, are not present in serum (11).

Garland and Randle's procedure (90) has been applied to the analysis of phospholipid-free extracts prepared with chloroform–zeolite (39) or isopropanol–zeolite (51), as outlined in Table IV (methods 21 and 23). Glycerol added to the serum or the level of the free glycerol in the serum did not influence triglyceride levels determined with the chloroform–zeolite system (39). Results with the two procedures correlate with those found on the same sera with the Van Handel and Zilversmit (8) (method 1) procedure (39, 51).

Garland and Randle's reaction (90) has also been applied to procedures (methods 22 and 24) in which phospholipids are not removed before saponification of the lipids. These procedures depend for accuracy on the specificity of the enzymatic reaction for glycerol.

In 1966 Eggstein and Kreutz (11) published a method for the determination of neutral glycerides in which the serum lipids were extracted and simultaneously hydrolyzed in ethanolic potassium hydroxide. After precipitation of protein, cholesterol, and fatty acids with perchloric acid, the enzymatic reaction is carried out. Magnesium sulfate has been substituted for perchloric acid since it is unnecessary to adjust the pH after addition of the salt (33). A "kit" of reagents incorporating this modification is available commercially (61). A semimicro adaptation of this procedure (32) requires only 0.04 ml of serum for a determination.

The glycerol determined in this manner is the sum of the neutral glyceride glycerol and the "free" glycerol. The latter is estimated on the unhydrolyzed serum by using the same enzymatic reaction. Neutral glyceride glycerol is calculated as the difference between "total glycerol" and "free glycerol." The latter is about 10% of the total glycerol (11, 33).

Lecithin, dipalmityl phosphatidylserine (33), and α-glycerolphosphate (32), the products of the hydrolysis of phosphoglycerides, do not react in the enzymatic method of Garland and Randle (90). Methanol cannot be substituted for ethanol in saponification since the enzymatic assay is inhibited by products formed from methanol (60). Quantitative recoveries of triolein added to serum were found by Schmidt and von Dahl (33). Results obtained by the method of Eggstein and Kreutz (11) agree with those obtained as the difference between total lipids and total cholesterol plus phospholipids (17) or by the application of Garland and Randle's enzymatic method (90) for glycerol to chloroform–methanol extracts containing phospholipids (32, 33) (method 22).

Impurities in the reagents used for the method of Eggstein and Kreutz (11) can lead to variable and inaccurate results. Some batches of potassium hydroxide contain sufficient glycerol to give triglyceride values that are 0.48 (31) to 0.74 (33) mM/l too high, since this reagent is not included in the determination of free glycerol. Some preparations of glycerokinase contain glycerol or hexokinase. In the presence of the latter glucose in the sample and ATP in the reagent yield ADP, which in turn fosters the oxidation of $NADH_2$. Thus the decrease in absorbance at 340 or 366 nm does not come to an abrupt halt but continues at a slower rate. Under these circumstances the fast initial rate due to the presence of glycerol must be corrected for the slow rate.

Usually the correction for hexokinase and glucose is made just for "free" glycerol since enzymatically active glucose is destroyed under the conditions used in saponification (11, 33). On the other hand, glucose active to glucose oxidase is not completely destroyed during saponification (51). In the procedure supplied with the "kit" of the Boehringer-Mannheim Corporation (61), an example of the correction of "total" glycerides for free glycerol is given. If reagents have been improperly stored, ATP may break down to ADP, which in turn can lead to the oxidation of sufficient $NADH_2$ to limit the amount of glycerol that can be determined (61).

V. MANUAL PROCEDURES BASED ON THE DETERMINATION OF GLYCERIDE ESTER GROUPS

Two methods based on the determination of neutral glyceride ester groups are outlined in Table V. In the first method neutral glycerides in phospholipid-free extracts are determined from the infrared absorption at 1745 cm^{-1} (92). The method is presented in more detail in Chapter 4.

Table V. Manual Procedures for Neutral Glycerides Based on the Determination of Ester Groups[a]

No.	Adsorbent	End Reaction	Reference
25	Silicic acid	Neutral glyceride ester carbonyl absorption at 1745 cm^{-1} in infrared	92[b,c]
26	Florisil	Hydroxamic acid reaction	93[d,e]

[a] In both methods the extractant is chloroform–methanol, 2:1 (v/v). Extraction and adsorption are not combined.
[b] After washing extract according to Folch et al. (75), the lipids are taken up in acetone–chloroform, 5:1 (v/v), for the adsorption step.
[c] Quantitative recovery of triglycerides and removal of phospholipids.
[d] Petroleum ether solution of lipids is adsorbed on Florisil. In a batch process cholesterol ester is eluted with petroleum ether–ethyl ether, 98:2 (v/v), followed by triglycerides and free cholesterol with 100% ethyl ether, and free fatty acids with ethyl ether–glacial acetic acid, 96:4 (v/v).
[e] Recovery of triglycerides in the triglyceride–cholesterol fraction is 95%.

In the second method the hydroxylamine–ferric chloride hydroxamic acid reaction is applied to the triglyceride and free-cholesterol fraction obtained in a batch process from Florisil. Small amounts of triglycerides remain in the cholesterol-ester and free-fatty-acids fraction (93).

VI. SEMIAUTOMATED PROCEDURES FOR THE DETERMINATION OF TRIGLYCERIDES

A. Principles of Semiautomated Methods

Phospholipid-free extracts for semiautomated procedures are prepared manually by batch processes, using solvents that make it possible to combine the steps of lipid extraction and phospholipid adsorption. Solvent–adsorbent systems, conditions for saponification or transesterification for release of glycerol, and other data are given in Table VI.

Automation of the steps of saponification or transesterification and the determination of glycerol in triglyceride determinations has been accomplished by using the Technicon AutoAnalyzer system. In this system, introduced by Skeggs in 1957 (94), the discrete step-by-step operations of a manual procedure are replaced by a continuously flowing, air-segmented stream in which the chemical reactions take place. Reactants are pumped at a constant speed through a system of tubing. Reagents and air bubbles are added continuously, but samples or standards are added intermittently at a preset rate, separated by a wash fluid that is preceded and followed by a segment of air. Under these circumstances, the amount of a given reactant added to the moving stream is governed by the diameter of the tubing through which the reactant is pumped, and the sequence in which it is added depends on the point beyond the pump at which the tubing is connected to the moving stream. The bubbles of air, which are removed before the stream enters the detection system, segment the moving stream into a consistent pattern of small portions and assist in the complete mixing of reactants in each portion and in separating samples.

The system of tubing, glass connectors, pressure-regulating chambers and tubes, and coils of glass tubing for mixing and permitting time for reactions to occur is called a manifold. The latter is connected to heating baths and a detector system through which the moving stream passes. The absorbance or emission is recorded automatically. Each method has an individual manifold, and the sequence of events that occur in the flowing stream of reactants is analogous to those of manual pipetting of known volumes of reactants, heating at controlled temperature for definite lengths of time, and recording the products of end reactions in appropriate detector systems.

Although the proportions of reactants and the time and temperature of reactions duplicate as nearly as possible the sequence of events in manual procedures, the chemical reactions do not necessarily reach the same degree of completion. Results are based on a comparison of unknown specimens with standard solutions, both of which have automatically received the same proportion of reagents and have been exposed for the same length of time to the same conditions.

B. Methods Based on Periodate Oxidation of Glycerol to Formaldehyde and Determination of the Latter with Eegriwe's Reaction

Solvents, adsorbents, and conditions of saponification for methods employing Lofland's (9, 50) automation of the determination of glycerol by the method of Lambert and Neish (67) are presented in Table VI (Nos. 27–31).

Isopropanol–zeolite extracts prepared with 1 g of zeolite per milliliter of serum (9, 50) were found to contain a formaldehydogenic substance (10, 22, 23, 51, 95), identified as glucose (51), that resulted in falsely elevated values for serum triglycerides (10, 22, 23, 51, 95). Phospholipids also were found to be present (74, 95), although other investigators did not detect this class of lipids (9, 10, 51). The interfering substances could be removed from a more dilute extract (i.e., a 1:20 rather than a 1:12 dilution of the sample) by increasing the amount of zeolite to 6 g/ml of serum (23) or by adding 4 g of a mixture of zeolite, copper sulfate, calcium hydroxide, and Lloyd's reagent per milliliter of serum (10, 22, 23, 51). Lloyd's reagent served to remove bilirubin and some phospholipids, but copper sulfate and calcium hydroxide were added to remove carbohydrates (10). However, serum blanks (i.e., unsaponified samples) still had to be run with the isopropanol extracts (23, 51), but not with chloroform–silicic acid (95) or isopropyl ether–silicic acid extracts (22).

Saponification takes place manually as described in Table VI in isopropanol–ethanol and ethanol. Ethanol may (22, 23, 50) or may not be evaporated (51, 95), but isopropanol is removed (9, 51) before the automated periodate oxidation and chromotropic acid color reaction. Chlouverakis et al. (71) had shown previously that as little as 3% isopropanol causes the chromogen of the chromotropic acid reaction to fade.

Cholesterol and fatty acids liberated during saponification do not interfere in the automated periodate oxidation and chromotropic acid reaction (22, 95), although these substances are removed in one procedure (51).

The automated procedure, first devised by Lofland (9, 50), for the periodate oxidation of glycerol and the chromotropic acid reaction for formaldehyde takes place as shown schematically in Fig. 1. The glycerol sample

Table VI. Semiautomated Triglyceride Methods Classified According to End Reaction[a]

No.	Extractant	Adsorbent	Saponification or Transesterification	References
		Eegriwe's (64) Chromotropic Acid Reaction for Formaldehyde		
27	Isopropanol	Zeolite	Ethanolic KOH added to isopropanol extract (manual)	9,[b,c] 23[b]
28	Isopropanol	Zeolite	Ethanolic KOH (manual)	50
29	Isopropanol	Zeolite + Lloyd's reagent + $CuSO_4 \cdot 5H_2O$ + $Ca(OH)_2$, 100:10:5:10 (w/w/w/w)	Ethanolic KOH (manual)	51[b,c]
30	Isopropyl ether–acetic acid, 1000:1 (v/v)	Silicic acid	Ethanolic KOH (manual)	22[b,c]
31	Chloroform	Silicic acid	Ethanolic KOH (manual)	95[b,c]
		Belman's (86) Modification of the Hantzsch Reaction for Formaldehyde		
32	Isopropanol	Zeolite + Lloyd's reagent + $CuSO_4 \cdot 5H_2O$ + $Ca(OH)_2$, 100:10:5:10 (w/w/w/w)	Isopropanolic KOH (semiautomated)	10,[b,c] 20,[b] 23,[b] 24,[b] 26, 27
33	Isopropanol	Silicic acid + $CuSO_4 \cdot 5H_2O$ + $Ca(OH)_2$, 100:5:10 (w/w/w)	Isopropanolic KOH (semiautomated)	25[b]
34	Isopropyl ether–acetic acid, 1000:1 (v/v)	Silicic acid	Isopropanolic KOH (semiautomated)	22[b,c]
35	Nonane–isopropanol–0.08 *N* H_2SO_4, 2:3.5:1 (v/v/v)	—	Sodium methylate in isopropanol (semiautomated)	28[b,c]

Table VI. Continued

No.	Extractant	Adsorbent	Saponification or Transesterification	References
	Glycerol Determined by Modified Enzymatic Reaction of Garland and Randle (90)			
36	Isopropyl ether–acetic acid, 1000:1 (v/v)	Silicic acid	Ethanolic KOH (manual)	22[b,c]

[a] The ratios of sample volume (ml) to extract (ml), to adsorbent (grams) employed by the investigators listed in Table VI are as follows: 1:12:1 (9, 50); 1:20:6 (23); 1:20:4 (10, 20, 24–27, 51, 95); and 1:25:4 (22). The ratio of nonane–isopropanol–sulfuric acid to serum is 13:1 (v/v). Adsorbent is not usually added, but if needed, 80 mg of Florisil is added per 1.5 ml of nonane phase (28).
[b] Triglycerides quantitatively recovered.
[c] Phospholipids quantitatively removed.

in 0.2 *N* sulfuric acid is added to the air-segmented stream of 0.2 *N* sulfuric acid and then reacted with periodic acid in a time-delay coil. Reduction of excess periodate with arsenite follows. Then the stream is mixed with the chromotropic acid reagent and heated at 95°C. After the air is removed by the debubbler, the reactants pass through the flow cell of the colorimeter, and absorbance at 570 nm is recorded. The system has been modified by Yert et al. (95) resulting in the elimination of a pumping tube and a mixing coil, and by Krehl et al. (23) and Antonis (22), who have adjusted pressures in the system, as indicated in the caption for Fig. 1.

Samples are taken at a rate of 40 per hour with 60 sec of sampling and 30 sec of wash cycle (9, 21–23, 50, 51). Precision of the analysis has been improved (95) by sampling at the rate of 30 per hour with sampling and washing cycles of 60 sec each.

C. Methods Based on Periodate Oxidation of Glycerol to Formaldehyde and Determination of the Latter with the Hantzsch Reaction

Solvents and adsorbents for the methods employing an automated saponification or transesterification of neutral glycerides and determination of the resulting glycerol by Belman's (86) fluorometric adaptation of the Hantzsch reaction for formaldehyde (10) are listed in Table VI (methods 32–35).

Isopropanol extracts after treatment with a mixture of zeolite, Lloyd's reagent, copper sulfate, and calcium hydroxide (10, 20, 23, 24, 26, 27)

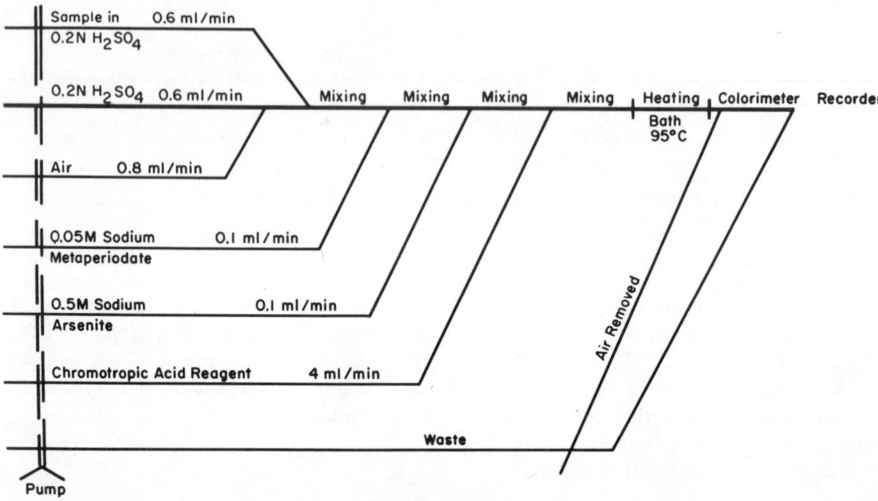

Fig. 1 Schematic diagram of manifold for semiautomated periodate oxidation and the chromotropic acid reaction (methods 27–31). The system has been modified by Yert, Mather, Whitner, and Witter (95) (method 31) in the following manner: The sample in 0.2 *N* sulfuric acid, pumped at 0.8 ml/min, is introduced into the air-segmented stream of periodate, which is pumped at 0.8 ml/min, thereby eliminating one pumping tube and mixing coil. The sodium arsenite concentration is raised to 0.1 *M*, but sodium arsenite is still pumped at 0.1 ml/min. The chromotropic acid reagent is made up of 2.5 g of disodium salt instead of 2 g of the free acid per liter of 10 *M* sulfuric acid as in the other semiautomated methods, and the volume pumped is increased to 5 ml/min.

Krehl and co-workers (23) (method 27) and Antonis (22) (method 30) have added pulse suppressors, and Antonis (22) also has debubbled the stream and repumped it and again added air to the reactants before entrance into the heating bath.

or silicic acid plus copper sulfate and calcium hydroxide (25) are introduced into the automated system for saponification with potassium hydroxide in isopropanol, whereas isopropyl ether extracts from silicic acid are evaporated and reconstituted in isopropanol (22) before automated saponification. Steps that occur in the automated system are illustrated in Fig. 2.

Saponification of neutral glycerides takes place as the sample, in a phospholipid- and glucose-free isopropanol solution, is introduced into an air-segmented stream of potassium hydroxide in isopropanol–water and passes through the 50°C heating bath. Simultaneously sodium periodate in acetic acid and acetylacetone in ammonium acetate, pH 6.0, are added to the stream, which again passes through the 50°C heating bath. Glycerol is oxidized to formaldehyde, which then is converted in the presence of am-

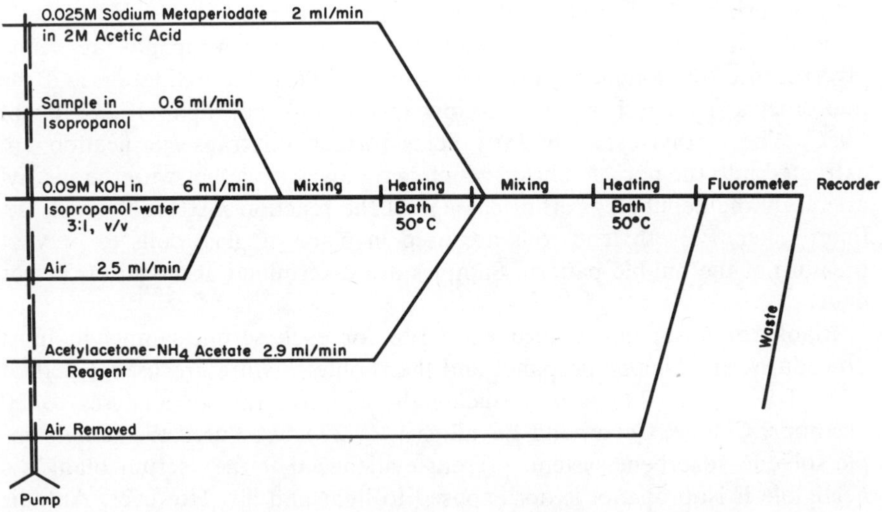

Fig. 2 Schematic diagram for semiautomated saponification, periodate oxidation, and fluorometric Hantzsch reaction of Kessler and Lederer (methods 32–34). Cramp and Robertson (25) have modified the system as follows: (a) sample is pumped at 0.7 ml/min; (b) air at 2.0 ml/min; (c) potassium hydroxide, 0.18 *M* in isopropanol–water, 1:1 (v/v), is pumped at 2 ml/min; (d) sodium metaperiodate, 0.005 *M*, is pumped at 0.32 ml/min; (e) 0.14 *M* acetylacetone in 2 *M* ammonium acetate, pH 6.0, is pumped at 0.8 ml/min; and (f) the temperature of the heating bath is raised to 58°C.

monia and acetylacetone to 3,5-diacetyl-1,4-dihydrolutidine. After debubbling, the reaction mixture enters the fluorometer (primary wavelength, 405 nm; secondary wavelength, 485 nm). Although Belman (86) found that periodate caused the color to fade, the reduction of excess periodate is not necessary under the conditions of automation established by Kessler and Lederer (10).

The manifold has been modified by the introduction of pulse chambers and suppressors in order to regulate pressures in the system (24–27). Further modifications by Cramp and Robertson (25) include changes in concentrations and rates of flow of reagents and in the temperature of reaction (see caption for Fig. 2).

The samples are analyzed at a rate of 40 per hour with sample and wash cycles of 60 and 30 sec, respectively. However, the precision of the analyses has been improved (22) by sampling at a rate of 30 per hour.

In method 35 the nonane phase from the nonane–isopropanol–0.08 *M* sulfuric acid solvent (28), containing about 1% of the phospholipid originally present, is introduced into the automated system without treatment with adsorbent. The triglycerides in the nonane phase are automatically transesterified at 50°C with sodium methylate in isopropanol, releasing glycerol into the nonane–isopropanol solution. Periodate oxidation and the fluorometric Hantzsch reaction follow in aqueous isopropanol solution at 50°C. The methyl esters of fatty acids formed on transesterification are extracted into the nonane phase, which is removed, together with the methyl esters, by the debubbler before passage of the reaction mixture through the fluorometer. Polyethylene coils are used in place of glass coils to prevent breakup of the bubble pattern. Samples are determined at a rate of 50 per hour.

Blanks of unsaponified serum are run for each serum sample in most procedures in which isopropanol and the zeolite mixture are used (method 32) (10, 20, 23, 24), thus reducing the effective rate of analyses to 20 per hour. Claude, Corre, and Levallois (26, 27), who used the same sample solvent–adsorbent system, present evidence that the "serum blank" is negligible if isopropanol is not exposed to light and air. However, Antonis (22) has pointed out that isopropanol extracts treated with the zeolite mixture still contain glycerol and other metabolites that are not present in isopropyl ether–silicic acid (22) or chloroform–zeolite extracts (34). Cramp and Robertson (25) found that serum blanks are insignificant with the isopropanol–silicic acid–copper–lime system when the serum-extract mixture is allowed to stand for 24 hr before removal of the adsorbent unless serum free-glycerol levels are above 200 μM/l (four times those found in normals, or twice those in diabetics) (90).

Interference from glucose, glycerol, or serine added to the nonane–isopropanol–0.08 *M* sulfuric acid system, even in the absence of adsorbent, amounts to less than 0.2% of the amount possible at the level of these substances in normal serum (28). Serum blanks probably are not needed; however, levels of such blanks in abnormal samples have not been presented. Although unsaturated fatty acids have not been shown to interfere in the fluorometric Hantzsch reaction, the methyl esters of the fatty acids are automatically removed from the reaction mixture. The level of interfering compounds, including phospholipids, can be further reduced by treatment of the nonane phase with Florisil (28).

D. Methods Based on the Enzymatic Determination of Neutral Glyceride Gycerol

In this approach to automation (22) glycerol is estimated automatically by the method of Garland and Randle (90), with the decrease in $NADH_2$ being measured fluorometrically. Phospholipid-free lipids from isopropyl ether–acetic acid extracts are saponified manually in ethanol. In the automated system the glycerol solution in phosphate buffer, pH 7.0, joins the air-segmented phosphate buffer solution of enzymes and cofactors to react at 25°C. Air is removed, and the reaction mixture passes through the flow cell of the fluorometer, where the $NADH_2$ is activated with light at 365 nm, and the excited fluorescence is measured at 470 nm. Determinations can be carried out at a rate of 60 per hour.

E. Comparison of Semiautomated and Manual Procedures

The results of semiautomated methods have shown excellent agreement with those obtained by manual procedures. Some semiautomated procedures (9, 22, 25–27, 51) have been compared with the manual procedure of Van Handel and Zilversmit (8); two (·10, 24) with the manual method of Carlson and Wadström (14); one (23) with the method of Blankenhorn et al. (52); and another (51) with an enzymatic procedure (51). In addition, phospholipid-free isopropyl ether–acetic acid extracts gave similar triglyceride values (22) when analyzed by (a) the semiautomated procedure of Lofland (9) for periodate oxidation and the chromotropic acid reaction; (b) the semiautomated procedure of Kessler and Lederer (10) for saponification, periodate oxidation, and fluorometric Hantzsch reaction; and (c) a semiautomated enzymatic method for glycerol (22).

Similarly the results obtained by the semiautomated procedure of Lofland (50) and Kessler and Lederer (10) were found to agree if the interfering substances in the isopropanol–zeolite extracts of the former method were removed by increasing the amount of zeolite alone (23) or by using instead of zeolite the zeolite mixture (51) described by Kessler and Lederer (10). Agreement also was noted (28) between the values obtained with the semiautomated procedure of Royer and Ko (28) and an unpublished modification (28) of the semiautomated method of Lofland (9).

F. Determination of Triglycerides and Cholesterol in the Same Extract

In many laboratories in which semiautomated methods for triglycerides are carried out there also is interest in the determination of cholesterol. Cholesterol can be determined manually in the same chloroform–zeolite (34) or isopropyl ether–silicic acid extracts (47, 88) that are used for triglyceride determinations. The cholesterol levels found with such extracts agree with those found by the reference method of Abell and co-workers (96). However, Ryan and Rasho (74) found that isopropyl ether–silicic acid extracts yielded much lower triglyceride and cholesterol levels than did extracts prepared with ethyl ether and Florisil followed by isopropanol. Further studies are needed to confirm the extraction of (a) cholesterol with the chloroform or isopropyl ether systems or (b) cholesterol and triglycerides with the ethyl ether–Florisil–isopropanol solvent.

Chloroform–methanol, ethanol–ether, and ethanol–acetone are well-accepted polar solvents for the extraction of triglycerides and cholesterol. Methods have been developed for the determination of triglycerides (8, 14, 33, 37, 40, 43–46, 52–58, 72, 73, 92, 93) or cholesterol (97) in these solvents. None of the previously mentioned solvents can be used in present semiautomated methods for the determination of cholesterol and triglycerides with Technicon equipment. However, isopropanol extracts of serum can be used directly for semiautomated methods for cholesterol (21, 24) or, after the removal of phospholipids and carbohydrates, for the determination of triglycerides by the automated fluorometric method of Kessler and Lederer (10, 20, 21, 24, 26, 27).

Investigators who do not wish to purchase an expensive fluorometer can utilize a modification of the automated colorimetric method of Lofland (9, 50) for the determination of glycerol; but the isopropanol extracts, after treatment to remove phospholipids and interfering carbohydrates (23, 51), must be evaporated, and the lipids must be saponified before introducing glycerol into the automated system.

VII. SOURCES OF ERROR IN THE DETERMINATION OF TRIGLYCERIDES

A. Errors Due to Method

Solvents for the extraction of triglycerides should be of reagent grade or freshly redistilled. Aldehyde-free isopropanol and peroxide-free ethyl or isopropyl ether should be employed. Chloroform–methanol extracts should be washed with no less than 0.2 volume of saline if the nonpolar phase is to be used directly for the adsorption step (14, 55). With methods in which the extraction and adsorption steps are combined, the limiting ratios of sample to extractant that yield sufficient water to permit quantitative extraction of triglycerides and removal of phospholipids should be determined. Thus Kessler and Lederer (10) found complete recovery of triglycerides and removal of phospholipids from the zeolite mixture within the limits of a 1:10 or a 1:25 dilution of the sample with isopropanol. The particle size and means of activation of the adsorbent also should be specified. The recovery of triglycerides and the removal of phospholipids should be checked in order to find the limiting ratio of sample to solvent and the proper ratio of sample to adsorbent.

Once conditions have been established for quantitative recovery and removal, the procedure should not be changed. The extraction and adsorption steps should be reinvestigated with each new lot of adsorbent. Extracts to be used in methods employing periodate oxidation of glycerol to formaldehyde must be free of glucose since the presence of this carbohydrate can lead not only to falsely high results but also, if small amounts remain, to highly variable results, as the oxidation of glucose may not take place at the same rate in replicate extracts (51). The removal of glucose and interfering pigments has been discussed under the individual methods.

Saponification has been carried out under a number of conditions with potassium hydroxide in ethanol, methanol, or isopropanol. These solvents should be free of aldehyde. Some lots of potassium hydroxide are contaminated with glycerol (31, 33, 59), which could increase the reagent blank or give erroneous values. Investigators do not agree as to the conditions under which aqueous ethanol (8, 14, 35, 36, 43, 47, 69) or methanol (71, 88) solutions may be heated or evaporated to dryness in order to avoid loss of glycerol, which can distill from ethanol solutions (98). It seems reasonable to carry out manual saponification in glass tubes with well-fitted glass stoppers and to bring the temperature no higher than 70°C at any time prior to the color reaction, as suggested by Moore (69). Furthermore, if ethanol, methanol, or isopropanol saponification mixtures are to be evaporated to dryness, the solvent should be evaporated at room temperature under vacuum or under a gentle stream of nitrogen. However, this step appears to be unnecessary in many of the procedures outlined in this chapter. Isopropanol or methanol must be removed if the chromotropic acid reaction is to be used (71).

On the other hand, extraction of the liberated cholesterol and fatty acids after saponification does not appear to be necessary for the semiautomated or manual procedures based on the Hantzsch reaction. Turbidity caused by the presence of these substances in the Schryver reaction can be avoided by addition of isopropanol just before absorbance is determined (48). In the reviewers' experience the presence of cholesterol and fatty acids causes only a small increase in absorbance in the chromotropic acid reaction. However, since the factors that control the extent of the interference are unknown, the effects of the presence of cholesterol and fatty acids should be studied when methods that include the chromotropic acid reaction are to be employed. These lipids are removed in manual procedures in which enzymatic end reactions are used. Sources of errors associated with the various end reactions for glycerol have been mentioned in the discussion of the reactions.

B. Errors Due to Standards and Units

The compound employed as a primary standard and the manner in which it is handled in every step in the analysis of serum triglycerides can be important sources of error. In our opinion pure triglycerides should be used as the primary standard. Furthermore, the latter should be subjected to every step in the procedure, even to substituting saline or water for the serum aliquot as the standard solution is carried through the extraction and adsorption steps.

Glycerol and mannitol are not suitable primary standards. Since glycerol is hygroscopic, its concentration should be checked by means of refractive index or by iodometry, if used. In contrast, mannitol is not hygroscopic but is oxidized quantitatively to formaldehyde under the usual conditions of periodate oxidation (99). Moreover, glycerol and mannitol standards do not reveal variation in the steps of extraction, adsorption, and saponification. These steps have been shown (10, 60, 100) to make major contributions to the total variation in serum-triglyceride analyses. This observation is understandable when it is remembered that in most procedures the phospholipid-free extracts are not made up to a known volume. Therefore the proportion of these extracts taken as aliquots for saponification and the lipids present in such aliquots may vary with temperature, in the case of volatile solvents; with the ratio of serum aliquot to solvent and to adsorbent, since water may be retained by the latter; and with the proportion of aqueous solution used to produce the nonpolar phase with such extractants as chloroform–methanol, isopropanol–heptane–sulfuric acid, or hexane–isopropanol. Glycerol or mannitol standards, when introduced into the various procedures after the saponification step, may be useful in locating sources of error.

The triglyceride standard itself can be a source of error. Preparations of corn oil, the standard used by Van Handel and Zilversmit (8, 35), may vary in composition. This glyceride should be purified by shaking with zeolite, as corn oil may contain impurities that cause a high blank, increased variability, and deviation from Beer's law (35). Highly purified triglycerides are available from commercial sources. However, it is a good idea to check these standards for the presence of impurities by chromatography on thin layers of silicic acid with acetic acid–ethyl ether–light petroleum ether, 1:25:74 (v/v/v), (43). We have favored the use, with chloroform extracts, of a mixture of triolein and tripalmitin, 2:1 (w/w), since the degree of unsaturation is similar to that of serum triglycerides. However, tripalmitin is not soluble enough in isopropanol for the preparation of standards containing 2.5 mM/l; hence triolein has been advocated as a standard with this extractant (10).

The triglyceride standards employed by various investigators have varied in molecular weight from 639 (trilaurin) to 891 (tristearin). Many authors have given results as "mg %" without stating the molecular weight of the triglyceride reported. In theory a difference of 10% would exist between the results obtained on a sample analyzed by using a tripalmitin standard (molecular weight 807) and those obtained on the same sample with a triolein standard (molecular weight 885). It is evident that triglyceride levels should be reported in molar units.

C. Errors Due to Sample

The sample itself can introduce errors into the measurement of serum triglycerides. The content of monoglycerides or diglycerides in plasma or serum does not appear to lead to serious errors. Even in hyperlipemic sera the partial glycerides account for less than 2% of the total neutral lipids according to Hirsch and Ahrens (12). Previously Carlson and Wadström (13) had found less than 2 mole % of monoglycerides and 9 mole % of diglycerides in the total neutral glycerides of fasting persons. Only about half the added monoglycerides are recovered from the chloroform–zeolite (37, 52) and the chloroform–silicic acid systems (72), whereas under the same conditions diglycerides and triglycerides are recovered. Similar results were obtained by Jover (57) for chloroform–methanol extracts treated as described in Table III (method 12). The chromatographic systems of Blankenhorn et al. (52) and Carlson and Wadström (14) (methods 7 and 4, respectively) are the only procedures reviewed that give complete recovery of monoglycerides as well as diglycerides and triglycerides. Other solvent–adsorbent systems have not been tested for recovery of partial glycerides; hence present methods should be considered as procedures for neutral glycerides rather than for triglycerides.

The neutral glyceride content of serum samples appears to be relatively stable in storage. The glyceride level of heparinized plasma samples is stable when stored for 12 weeks at 4°C; hyperlipemic samples can be kept up to 8 weeks at the same temperature (59). The levels seemed to be stable at —20°C for as long as 12 weeks (59) and up to 2 years in our laboratory. Heparinized blood can be kept for as long as 2 hr at room temperature without change in triglyceride content as determined by the method of Lloyd and Goldrick (59). Serum glyceride values, when determined by the method of Carlson and Wadström (14), decline 10% after 6 days at 25°C (66). Thin-layer chromatography of serum stored at 4°C for several weeks or at —20°C for several months shows the formation of monoglycerides and diglycerides (101). Whether these changes result in a decrease in triglycerides that is large enough to be detected by methods specific for triglycerides is unknown.

VIII. PRECISION OF METHODS FOR SERUM TRIGLYCERIDES

Although many investigators have measured the precision of manual (11, 14, 29, 30, 33–35, 37, 38, 40, 41, 44–49, 52, 54, 55, 57, 58, 71, 80, 81, 88, 93) or semiautomated procedures (10, 22–28, 51), the methods by which precision was determined and the statistics calculated have varied so much from one investigator to another that it is not possible to draw conclusions from these data as to the relative precision of methods except for those compared in the same laboratory. Four (22–24, 27) out of five (22–24, 27, 51) groups of investigators have reported improved precision with semiautomated procedures as compared with manual methods. The semiautomated method of Kessler and Lederer (10) gave more precise results (23) than those obtained with Lofland's procedure (50). Similarly, when the semiautomated method of Kessler and Lederer (10) and the procedure of Lofland (50) were applied to phospholipid-free isopropyl ether extracts, more precise results were obtained with the fluorometric procedure of Kessler and Lederer (10). With few exceptions (10, 24), the component of day-to-day variation has not been included in studies of the precision of methods.

Recent studies in which the same frozen serum samples have been analyzed in 68 different laboratories have provided a measure of the precision that can be attained in triglyceride analyses over a period of 3 months under routine operating conditions (102). The precision was calculated as the standard deviation of a single determination repeated on different days. In this study 20 replicate analyses were run in each laboratory over a period of 10 analytical runs on each of two serum pools with concentrations of 1.11 and 1.74 mM/l, respectively. Thirty-six of the sixty-eight participants attained a standard deviation ranging from 0.03 to 0.10 mM/l for the 1.11-mM pool and from 0.04 to 0.14 mM/l for the 1.74-mM pool. Seventeen of the thirty-six investigators obtained mean values ranging within $\pm$ 0.1 mM/l of the concentration of each of the two pools and were thus considered to be comparable.

These laboratories are grouped in Table VII according to the type of method used. The standard deviation for a single analysis and the mean concentration of triglycerides obtained for each pool are listed for each laboratory.

Table VII. Precision of Triglyceride Analyses in Laboratories in Which Comparable Results Were Obtained

End Reaction	Method No.[c]	Mean Triglyceride Concentration[a] (mM/l)		Standard Deviation[b] (mM/l)		Reference
		1.11-mM Pool	1.74-mM Pool	1.11-mM Pool	1.74-mM Pool	
Manual Methods						
Eegriwe	1	1.10	1.73	0.07	0.06	36
Eegriwe	4	1.13	1.73	0.10	0.14	43
Eegriwe	—	1.17	1.83	0.04	0.06	14,52,80
Eegriwe	—	1.21	1.83	0.06	0.06	8,36,37
Eegriwe	—	1.12	1.73	0.06	0.09	35,38
Enzymatic	24	1.08	1.71	0.04	0.07	33
Infrared spectrophotometry	25	1.10	1.74	0.06	0.09	92
Gas–liquid chromotography	—	1.03	1.66	0.04	0.05	103
Semiautomated Methods						
Eegriwe	31	1.14	1.83	0.08	0.10	95
Eegriwe	31	1.13	1.71	0.07	0.06	95
Eegriwe	31	1.12	1.75	0.05	0.06	95
Hantzsch[d]	32	1.17	1.83	0.10	0.13	10
Hantzsch[d]	32	1.12	1.74	0.05	0.05	10
Hantzsch[d]	32	1.06	1.76	0.09	0.12	10
Hantzsch[d]	32	1.12	1.83	0.05	0.08	10
Hantzsch[d]	32	1.09	1.70	0.07	0.08	10
Hantzsch[d]	32	1.12	1.79	0.03	0.04	10
Hantzsch[d]	32	1.10	1.74	0.09	0.12	24

[a] The arithmetic mean, calculated for each laboratory from 20 analyses from each serum pool, was used as a basis for the comparison of triglyceride values among laboratories. The designated values, 1.11 and 1.74 mM/l, were established from 88 analyses per pool performed in our laboratory by the method of Yert et al. (95).

[b] The standard deviation represents the variability of a single analysis repeated on different days.

[c] See Tables II, IV, V, and VI.

[d] Fluorometric method.

IX. NORMAL LEVELS OF SERUM TRIGLYCERIDES

Triglyceride levels of plasma or serum have been reported to change with food intake and to show a diurnal variation (3, 104–107). Hence measurements of the concentration of this class of lipid usually are made after the subject has fasted overnight. The level of neutral lipids has been found to increase with age (29, 58, 60, 105, 108, 109). However, Brown, Heslin, and Doyle (104) found an increase for a few months after birth, but none in individuals up to their thirtieth year. Men have been reported to have higher triglyceride levels than women (29, 58, 60, 105, 108). Schaefer (110) observed this difference up to age 58 and comparable values for both sexes from 58 to 67 years of age. On the other hand, Brown et al. (104) found no sex differences in triglyceride levels.

Normal levels for fasting serum triglycerides, taken from studies published in the last decade, are presented in Table VIII. These data were

Table VIII. Normal Fasting Levels for Serum Neutral Glycerides

Number of Subjects	Age	Mean Levels ± S.D.[a] (mM/l)	Method No.[b]	Reference	Year
53	19–84	0.91 ± 0.27	4	55	1962
68	18–30	1.23 ± 0.30	1[c]	104	1963
56	20–40	1.39 ± 0.55	24	60	1966
57	—	0.96 ± 0.36	21	39	1967
52	18–49	0.98 ± 0.31	16	29	1968
77	20–65	1.32 ± 0.62	1[c]	105	1968

[a] Standard deviation.
[b] See Tables II, III, and IV.
[c] Method 1, Van Handel and Zilversmit (8).

selected on the following basis: both sexes were included in the study, and at least 50 subjects were investigated; triglyceride levels were determined by direct methods, and sufficient information was given to permit calculation of the results on a molar basis. Changes in triglyceride levels under pathological conditions are presented in Chapter 11.

X. QUALITY CONTROL SYSTEMS FOR TRIGLYCERIDE ANALYSIS

Quality control programs for systematically monitoring all steps in a chemical assay by means of a control material are widely employed in clinical chemistry laboratories. The establishment, maintenance, and usefulness of such programs have been discussed by Whitby, Mitchell, and Moss (111) and Cooper (112). We recommend that a quality control system be installed in laboratories in which serum triglyceride analyses are performed.

Control samples of lyophilized or frozen serum are available from commercial sources and are widely used in clinical laboratories. A few suppliers do offer samples for triglyceride analyses, but in our experience (113), the triglyceride levels of such samples are too low, being in the lower portion of the normal range. Pooled human serum that has been filtered through clarifying membrane filters retaining particles larger than 5 microns is suitable control material. The neutral-glyceride content of such preparations does not change over a period of at least 2 years at —20°C, although a small amount of monoglycerides and diglycerides will appear after several months of storage (101).

XI. SUMMARY AND CONCLUSIONS

Over the last decade a number of methods for the direct determination of serum triglycerides or, more properly, neutral glycerides have been developed. These methods are based on the determination of glyceride esters or, more commonly, glyceride glycerol in phospholipid-free lipid extracts. In some methods phospholipids are adsorbed after extraction of the lipids and replacement of the polar extracting solvent with a nonpolar one. However, in most procedures the steps of lipid extraction and phospholipid adsorption are combined. After either type of extraction and adsorption, glyceride glycerol is determined enzymatically or by the Skraup reaction, or, more generally, by periodate oxidation to formaldehyde and subsequent determination of the latter by the Eegriwe, Schryver, or Hantzsch reactions.

Semiautomated procedures include a manual step for the combined extraction of lipids and removal of phospholipids and other interfering compounds. Glyceride glycerol is determined automatically with Technicon equipment by means of an enzymatic reaction or, more frequently, by periodate oxidation to formaldehyde followed by Eegriwe's colorimetric or Hantzsch's fluorometric reaction. Automated saponification or transesterification is included only in those procedures in which the fluorometric Hantzsch reaction is used.

Inadequate recovery of triglycerides and removal of phospholipids, carbohydrates, or other interfering compounds from the lipid extract and failure to give results in molar units are major sources of error. Recent studies indicate that precise and comparable results can be obtained under routine operating conditions with both manual and semiautomated methods.

XII. ACKNOWLEDGMENT

This work was performed as a cooperative effort with the Heart Disease and Stroke Control Program, Regional Medical Programs, Health Services and Mental Health Administration, U.S. Department of Health, Education, and Welfare, Arlington, Virginia.

REFERENCES

1. Albrink, M. J., and E. B. Man, *Arch. Intern. Med.* **103**, 4–8 (1959).
2. Albrink, M. J., *Arch. Intern. Med.* **109**, 345–359 (1962).
3. Antonis, A., and I. Bersohn, *Lancet* **1**, 998–1002 (1960).
4. Carlson, L. A., *Acta Med. Scand.* **167**, 399–413 (1960).
5. Hayes, D., and D. W. Neill, *Clin. Sci.* **26**, 185–192 (1964).
6. Nicolaysen, R., and K. Westlund, *Scand. J. Clin. Lab. Invest.* **15**, 291–298 (1963).
7. Brown, D. F., S. H. Kinch, and J. T. Doyle, *New Eng. J. Med.* **273**, 947–952 (1965).
8. Van Handel, E., and D. B. Zilversmit, *J. Lab. Clin. Med.* **50**, 152–157 (1957).
9. Lofland, H. B., Jr., *Anal. Biochem.* **9**, 393–400 (1964).
10. Kessler, G., and H. Lederer, in *Automation in Analytical Chemistry*, L. Skeggs, Ed., Mediad, New York, 1966, pp. 341–344.
11. Eggstein, M., and F. H. Kreutz, *Klin. Wochenschr.* **44**, 262–267 (1966).
12. Hirsch, J., and E. H. Ahrens, Jr., *J. Biol. Chem.* **233**, 311–320 (1958).
13. Carlson, L. A., and L. B. Wadström, in *3rd Intern. Conf. Biochem. Problems of Lipids*, R. Ruyssen, Ed., Palais des Academien, Brussels, 1956, p. 123.
14. Carlson, L. A., and L. B. Wadström, *Clin. Chim. Acta* **4**, 197–205 (1959).
15. Jacobs, S. L., and R. J. Henry, *Clin. Chim. Acta* **7**, 270–276 (1962).
16. Reinhold, J. G., V. L. Yonan, and E. R. Gershman, in *Standard Methods of Clinical Chemistry*, D. Seligson, Ed., Vol. 4, Academic Press, New York, 1963, pp. 85–99.
17. Eggstein, M., *Klin. Wochenschr.* **43**, 1031–1038 (1965).
18. Martinek, R. G., *J. Amer. Med. Technol.* **30**, 274–278 (1968).
19. Pokrovskii, E. A., *Vopr. Med. Khim.* **11**, 78–82 (1965); through *Chem. Abstr.* **63**, 13679*c* (1965).
20. Kessler, G., in *Advances in Clinical Chemistry*, O. Bodansky and C. P. Stewart, Eds., Vol. 10, Academic Press, New York, 1967, pp. 45–64.
21. Levine, J. B., *J. Amer. Oil Chem. Soc.* **44**, 95–98 (1967).
22. Antonis, A., *J. Amer. Oil Chem. Soc.* **44**, 333–340 (1967).
23. Krehl, W. A., A. Lopez-S., and E. I. Good, *Amer. J. Clin. Nutr.* **20**, 968–977 (1967).
24. Block, W. D., and K. J. Jarrett, Jr., *Amer. J. Med. Technol.* **35**, 93–102 (1969).
25. Cramp, D. G., and G. Robertson, *Anal. Biochem.* **25**, 246–251 (1968).
26. Claude, J. R., and F. Corre, *Ann. Biol. Clin.* **26**, 451–464 (1968).
27. Claude, J. R., F. Corre, and C. Levallois, *Clin. Chim. Acta* **19**, 231–234 (1968).
28. Royer, M. E., and H. Ko, *Anal. Biochem.* **29**, 405–416 (1969).

29. Fletcher, M. J., *Clin. Chim. Acta* **22**, 393–397 (1968).
30. Laurell, S., *Scand. J. Clin. Lab. Invest.* **18**, 668–672 (1966).
31. Willms, B., and H. D. Söling, *Z. Klin. Chem. Klin. Biochem.* **5**, 276–277 (1967).
32. Wolf, H., M. Kochsiek-Schuster, and H. Löhr, *Z. Klin. Chem. Klin. Biochem.* **5**, 205–209 (1967).
33. Schmidt, F. H., and K. von Dahl, *Z. Klin. Chem. Klin. Biochem.* **6**, 156–159 (1968).
34. Cheng, A. L. S., and D. B. Zilversmit, *J. Lipid Res.* **1**, 190–191 (1960).
35. Van Handel, E., *Clin. Chem.* **7**, 249–251 (1961).
36. Jagannathan, S. N., *Can. J. Biochem.* **42**, 566–570 (1964).
37. Vanzetti, G., and G. Denegri, *G. Biochim.* **13**, 391–400 (1964).
38. Kaplan, A., and V. F. Lee, *Proc. Soc. Exp. Biol. Med.* **118**, 296–297 (1965).
39. Altmann, A., A. Bach, and P. Metais, *Ann. Biol. Clin.* **25**, 439–452 (1967).
40. Ignatowska, H., *Pol. Arch. Med. Wewn.* **34**, 273–278 (1964).
41. Leveille, G. A., J. W. Shockley, and H. E. Sauberlich, *Poultry Sci.* **40**, 1361–1362 (1961).
42. Sordi, A., *Arch. Studio Fisiopatol. Clin. Ricambio.* **24**, 448–474 (1960); through *Chem. Abstr.* **57**, 11473c (1962).
43. Carlson, L. A., *J. Atheroscler. Res.* **3**, 334–336 (1963).
44. de Mets, M., *Bull. Soc. Chim. Belg.* **72**, 508–512 (1963).
45. Young, G., and R. Eastman, *South African J. Lab. Clin. Med.* **9**, 28–31 (1963).
46. Christophe, A., and F. Matthijs, *Bull. Soc. Chim. Belg.* **73**, 592–596 (1964).
47. Azarnoff, D. L., M. M. Esker, and F. E. Brock, *J. Lab. Clin. Med.* **60**, 331–338 (1962).
48. Galletti, F., *Clin. Chim. Acta* **15**, 184–186 (1967).
49. Dunsbach, F., *Z. Klin. Chem.* **4**, 262–264 (1966).
50. Lofland, H. B., Jr., *Anal. Biochem.* **10**, 178 (1965).
51. Timms, A. R., L. A. Kelly, J. A. Spirito, and R. G. Engstrom, *J. Lipid Res.* **9**, 675–680 (1968).
52. Blankenhorn, D. H., G. Rouser, and T. J. Weimer, *J. Lipid Res.* **2**, 281–283 (1961).
53. Sardesia, V. R., and J. A. Manning, *Clin. Chem.* **14**, 156–161 (1968).
54. Spinella, C. J., and M. Mager, *J. Lipid Res.* **7**, 167–169 (1966).
55. Kawade, M., *Mie. Med.* **11**, 399–407 (1962).
56. Nicolaysen, R., and A. P. Nygaard, *Scand. J. Clin. Lab. Invest.* **15**, 79–82 (1963).
57. Jover, A., *J. Lipid Res.* **4**, 228–230 (1963).
58. Buckley, G. C., J. M. Cutler, and J. A. Little, *Can. Med. Assoc. J.* **94**, 886–888 (1966).
59. Lloyd, M. R., and R. B. Goldrick, *Med. J. Aust.* **2**, 493–496 (1968).
60. Eggstein, M., *Klin. Wochenschr.* **44**, 267–273 (1966).
61. Boehringer-Mannheim Corp., *Determination of Glycerol and Triglycerides (Neutral Fat) in Serum*, New York, 1968.
62. Dyer, J. R., in *Methods of Biochemical Analysis*, D. Glick, Ed., Vol. 3, Interscience, New York, 1956, pp. 111–152.
63. Jackson, E. L., in *Organic Reactions*, R. Adams, Ed., Vol. 2, Wiley, New York, 1944, pp. 341–375.
64. Eegriwe, E., *Z. Anal. Chem.* **110**, 22 (1937).
65. MacFadyen, D. A., *J. Biol. Chem.* **158**, 107–133 (1945).
66. Henry, R. J., *Clinical Chemistry, Principles and Techniques*, Harper and Row, New York, 1964, pp. 864–870.

67. Lambert, M., and A. C. Neish, *Can. J. Res.* **28B**, 83–89 (1950).
68. Nash, T., *Biochem. J.* **55**, 416–421 (1953).
69. Moore, J. H., *J. Dairy Res.* **29**, 141–147 (1962).
70. Pokrovskii, E. A., *Vopr. Med. Khim.* **11**, 74–77 (1965); through *Chem. Abstr.* **63**, 6092 (1965).
71. Chlouverakis, C., T. Hanley, and W. J. H. Butterfield, *Guy's Hosp. Rept.* **112**, 193–198 (1963).
72. Whitner, V. S., A. N. Mann, and R. F. Witter, unpublished results (1965).
73. Suehiro, M., *Seikagaku* **33**, 387–390 (1961); through *Chem. Abstr.* **55**, 23644*f* (1961).
74. Ryan, W. G., and O. M. Rasho, *Clin. Chem.* **13**, 769–772 (1967).
75. Folch, J., M. Lees, and G. H. Sloane Stanley, *J. Biol. Chem.* **226**, 497–509 (1957).
76. Henriques, R., *Z. Angew. Chem.* **24**, 721 (1895).
77. Frisell, W. R., and C. G. Mackenzie, in *Methods of Biochemical Analysis*, D. Glick, Ed., Vol. 6, Interscience, New York, 1958, p. 63.
78. Szostak, W. B., *Pol. Med. Sci. Hist. Bull.* **11**, 58–59 (1968); through *Chem. Abstr.* **69**, 41647*j* (1968).
79. Schryver, S. B., *Proc. Roy. Soc.* (*London*) **82B**, 226 (1910).
80. Randrup, A., *Scand. J. Clin. Lab. Invest.* **12**, 1–9 (1960).
81. Randrup, A., *Scand. J. Clin. Lab. Invest.* **14**, 578–580 (1962).
82. Randrup, A., *J. Atheroscler. Res.* **2**, 373–381 (1962).
83. Pays, M., *Ann. Pharm. Franc.* **12**, 763 (1966).
84. Malangeau, P., and M. Pays, *Ann. Biol. Clin.* **25**, 845–851 (1967).
85. Dole, V. P., and H. Meinertz, *J. Biol. Chem.* **235**, 2595–2599 (1960).
86. Belman, S., *Anal. Chim. Acta* **29**, 120–126 (1963).
87. Skraup, H., *Mo* **2**, 139 (1881).
88. Mendelsohn, D., and A. Antonis, *J. Lipid Res.* **2**, 45–50 (1961).
89. Wieland, O., *Biochem. Z.* **329**, 313 (1957).
90. Garland, P. B., and P. J. Randle, *Nature* **196**, 987 (1962).
91. Barron, E. J., and D. J. Hanahan, *J. Biol. Chem.* **231**, 493 (1958).
92. Freeman, N. K., *J. Lipid Res.* **5**, 236–241 (1964).
93. Michaels, G., *Metabolism* **11**, 833–839 (1962).
94. Skeggs, L. T., Jr., *Amer. J. Clin. Pathol.* **28**, 311–322 (1957).
95. Yert, A. L., A. Mather, V. S. Whitner, and R. F. Witter, unpublished results (1966).
96. Abell, L. L., B. B. Levy, B. B. Brodie, and F. E. Kendall, *J. Biol. Chem.* **195**, 357–366 (1952).
97. Tonks, D. B., *Clin. Biochem.* **1**, 12–29 (1967).
98. Hehner, O., *Analyst* **12**, 65 (1887).
99. Kanter, S. L., *Clin. Chim. Acta* **16**, 177–178 (1967).
100. Fleischman, A. I., T. Hayton, M. L. Bierenbaum, and E. Wildrick, *Technicon Symposia*, Mediad, New York, 1968, pp. 21–24.
101. Whitner, V. S., O. T. Grier, A. N. Mann, and R. F. Witter, 56th Annual Meeting American Oil Chemists' Society 1965 abst. 133 *J. Amer. Oil Chem. Soc.* **42**, 146A (1965).
102. Whitner, V. S., C. L. Winn, R. F. Witter, E. C. Hall, and G. R. Cooper, 22nd National Meeting American Association of Clinical Chemists 1970 abst. 89, *Clin. Chem.* **16**, 534 (1970).
103. Kuksis, A. L., L. Marai, and D. A. Gornall, *J. Lipid Res.* **8**, 352–358 (1967).

104. Brown, D. F., A. S. Heslin, and J. T. Doyle, *Amer. J. Clin. Nutr.* **13**, 1–7 (1963).
105. Zweers, A., E. Yaron, and J. J. Groen, *Clin. Chim. Acta* **19**, 267–275 (1968).
106. Stormont, J. M., and C. Waterhouse, *J. Lab. Clin. Med.* **61**, 826–831 (1963).
107. Hollister, L. E., and A. Wright, *J. Atheroscler. Res.* **5**, 445–450 (1965).
108. Fredrickson, D. S., R. I. Levy, and R. S. Lees, *New Eng. J. Med.* **276**, 148–156 (1967).
109. Carlson, L. A., *Acta Med. Scand.* **167**, 377–398 (1960).
110. Schaefer, L. E., *Amer. J. Med.* **36**, 262–268 (1964).
111. Whitby, L. G., F. L. Mitchell, and D. W. Moss, in *Advances in Clinical Chemistry,* O. Bodansky and C. P. Stewart, Eds., Vol. 10, Academic Press, New York, 1967, pp. 65–156.
112. Cooper, G. R., in *Progress in Clinical Pathology,* M. Stefanini, Ed., Vol. 3, Grune & Stratton, New York, 1969, pp. 1–71.
113. Witter, R. F., M. Kuchmak, J. H. Williams, V. S. Whitner, and C. L. Winn, *Clin. Chem.* **16**, 743–748 (1970).

4. Analysis of Blood Lipids by Infrared Spectrometry

NORMAN K. FREEMAN

Donner Laboratory of Medical Physics and Biophysics, Ernest O. Lawrence Berkeley Laboratory, Berkeley, California

I. INTRODUCTION

Among the various physical and spectroscopic tools that have been adopted by chemists in the last two decades, one of the most widely useful is infrared spectrometry. It has a number of favorable attributes that have led to its introduction into almost all branches of chemistry, both theoretical and applied. Perhaps the most fundamental of these attributes is the high content of information about molecular structure that is inherent in the infrared spectrum of a substance. The spectrum is a display of the frequencies of radiation that are absorbed, and in the infrared these correspond to the frequencies of the internal vibration of molecules. From a theoretical point of view, mathematical analysis of the vibrational spectrum leads to a description of the modes of vibration and permits the establishment or verification of certain architectural features of individual molecules.

In most applied or analytical usage, however, the infrared spectrum is used empirically. That is to say it is one of the observable properties of a substance that can be compared with the corresponding established properties of known substances as an identification procedure. (Alternatively the measurement of absorption intensity at some selected spectral position can be made the basis of a quantitative analysis.) In the so-called fingerprint technique one searches a collection of spectra of known compounds to find a spectrum matching that of the unknown compound. No knowledge or interpretation of the spectral content may be required in this case, and the matching process is often the task of a machine or computer.

Although the fingerprint technique is quite general in principle, its successful application depends somewhat on the richness and variability of spectral detail. These qualities do not characterize the spectra of the long-chain fatty acids and their derivatives, since the differences resulting from additional methylene groups or double bonds may not be easily perceptible. Furthermore, in dealing with a limited group of well-known lipid classes, it soon becomes possible to recognize the spectral features of each class without searching through a large file of reference curves. For the present purpose then we shall have no further concern with either the purely theoretical (mathematical) analysis of spectra or the purely empirical approach based on a reference catalog. General reference works on infrared spectroscopy may be consulted for background information in these areas (1–5).

Most of the spectra that are presented and discussed in this chapter are those of representative types of blood lipids. They are illustrative of the spectral patterns that are encountered, and in a limited sense they can be regarded as a reference collection. However, it is equally important to consider the significant spectral features that can be interpreted from group correlations. Group correlations are the established characteristic frequencies of absorption associated with various bond types, functional groups (hydroxyl, carbonyl, ether, etc.) or structural features (*cis* and *trans* isomers, rings, etc.). Knowledge of the characteristic frequencies of such groups enables one to recognize the spectral indications of them and thus to make valuable inferences about the chemical structure of a substance, even if a complete identification is not possible from the spectrum alone. Condensed summaries of group correlations are available in the form of tables or charts, the most widely distributed being those of Colthup (6). Copies are obtainable from instrument manufacturers. Such charts should be used with some caution, with due regard for the complexity of the spectrum and for alternative assignments of a given absorption band. A complete and detailed discussion of group frequencies has been presented by Bellamy (7, 8).

From the point of view of structural investigation, Chapman's treatise on the structure of lipids (9) includes a thorough discussion of infrared spectrometry as well as a number of other physical and spectroscopic tools. This valuable reference work deals extensively with basic physical properties—modes of vibration, molecular configuration, crystal forms, and thermal effects—and their relationships to spectroscopic observations. Other reviews of the infrared spectroscopy of lipids have been published by O'Connor (10), Schwarz and co-workers (11, 12), and Freeman (13, 14). O'Connor's review contains an extensive table of group frequencies that are pertinent to lipid spectra. This table has also been reproduced by Chapman (9).

In addition to the qualitative aspects of lipid spectra, this chapter covers their application to quantitative analysis. Basically the spectrophotometric principles are the same for measurements in the infrared, visible, and ultraviolet regions. However, differences in sampling considerations and techniques need to be pointed out. The specific types of blood-lipid analyses that have been done and can be done are reviewed.

The methodology of infrared spectrometry is fairly well established. After about three decades it has reached a plateau of development where further innovations are infrequent. Commercial spectrophotometers and accessories are available in some variety, and our discussions of these instruments are limited. Factors bearing on applications are indicated, with very little reference to optical principles or mechanical design details. Modes of sample handling need more emphasis, however. These techniques are quite general, and most of them are potentially useful in lipid work. Some—such as gas sampling—may be used very little if at all; others are considered according to their importance in lipid work.

Much of the information derived for lipids in general is relevant to blood lipids in particular. The latter are in fact limited to a fairly small number of compound types. Cholesterol, cholesteryl esters, glyceryl esters, and three principal kinds of phospholipid ordinarily comprise more than 95% of the lipids in blood. These major lipids, together with the minor lipid constituents of blood and a few significant related compounds, are the focus of attention in this chapter. The intent is to provide a concise package of information that is of practical interest to the lipid chemist whose work involves these classes of compounds.

II. METHODS OF OBTAINING SPECTRA

A. Instruments

The infrared spectrum of a substance is represented as the graph of its transmittance (of radiation) versus wavelength over some defined interval. Although the word "infrared" might imply any wavelength beyond the red end of the visible spectrum, the range of most common interest extends from about 2.5 to about 16 μm.[1] In frequency (reciprocal-wavelength) units[2] these limits correspond to 4000 and 625 cm^{-1}. This range includes most of the fundamental modes of molecular vibration in organic molecules. It is the most thoroughly studied and documented, and except where otherwise specified, it is the range denoted by the term "infrared spectrum" throughout this chapter.

The spectral region between the visible limit and 2.5 μm is usually called near infrared. Absorption bands observed in this region are much weaker, since for the most part they are overtones (harmonics) or combinations of fundamental frequencies. Experimentally near-infrared spectra are obtained by apparatus and techniques that are more nearly akin to those used in visible-range spectrometry. Although they are generally less useful than infrared spectra of the fundamental region, some potential applications in the lipid field have been discussed by Holman and coworkers (15, 16).

There are instruments that are capable of measuring spectra beyond 16 μm and some distance into the far infrared, but at present very little of such data is pertinent to lipids, and no further mention is made of it.

For the spectral range that has been designated as infrared a variety of commercial spectrophotometers are available. Although they can be categorized according to their complexity, versatility, performance, or price, they have some common basic elements:

1. A source of radiation.
2. A monochromator.
3. A radiation detector.
4. A measuring system (which almost always implies recording of the spectrum during a continuous scan).

Another common feature is the use of reflecting optics—front-surface

[1] 1 μm = 1 micrometer = 10^{-6} meter = 10^{-3} mm (formerly μ, micron).

[2] 1 cm^{-1} = 1 wave per centimeter (1 μm = 10,000 cm^{-1}). This is a more convenient unit than frequency in time (sec^{-1}), to which it is related by the velocity of light, i.e., $cm^{-1} = sec^{-1}/c$.

mirrors—throughout (except for sample cells, detector window, certain filters, and of course a prism if one is used). Radiation sources are thermal, usually a nichrome wire or nonmetallic rod heated by an electric current. The energy distribution has the approximate shape of a blackbody curve, with its maximum somewhere near the short-wavelength (2 μm) end of the infrared range. As the wavelength is increased, the energy falls continuously, and it is down by a factor of about 100 at the long-wavelength end. To compensate for this decrease the spectrometer slits must be correspondingly widened so that the available energy remains adequate for measurement.

In the monochromator the focused radiation from the source enters through a slit, is collimated, and is then dispersed in space by a prism or a diffraction grating. The spectrum thus formed is refocused in the plane of an exit slit, which allows the passage of only a narrow wavelength interval. The location of the emerging spectral band is determined by the geometry of the system and can be varied over the whole range by changing the angular relationship of the prism or grating in the monochromator. The width of the interval, which is basically related to the resolution to be achieved, is determined by the dispersing power of the prism or grating and by the actual slit width.

The output radiation from the monochromator may be on the order of microwatts or less, and a very sensitive thermal detector is required to measure it. In most commercial spectrophotometers a radiation thermocouple is used. Some less common detectors are bolometers, pneumatic detectors, and semiconductor devices, the latter being largely limited to special purpose instruments. In the detector the incident energy is converted to an electrical signal, which is amplified and used to drive the recording system.

In order to facilitate continuous and automatic recording of spectra, some additional features are embodied in most infrared spectrophotometers. A double-beam system is usually employed, in which the source radiation is directed along two paths. The sample is placed in one path and an appropriate reference or blank in the other. The two beams are pulsed alternately into the monochromator at a suitable frequency, and the intensity in each beam generates its own signal. If they are equal, the transmittance is recorded as 100% (ratio of sample-beam energy to reference-beam energy is unity). If there is excess absorption in the sample beam, the difference in intensities gives rise to an alternating signal in the detector, which (when amplified) causes a servosystem to adjust an attenuator in the reference beam to restore intensity balance. Motion of the attenuator drives the recorder pen to a position on the scale corresponding to the absorption in the sample beam. If all other losses in the sample beam (such as cell absorption, solvent absorption, surface reflections, and scattering) are suitably balanced out, the value indicated by the pen is sample transmittance.

In recording a spectrum over the specified range, then, the wavelength is changed continuously by rotation of the grating (or Littrow mirror in a prism instrument). At the same time the slits are being opened to maintain a constant order of background energy, and the recorder chart is being synchronously driven so that the abscissa corresponds to the wavelength (or frequency) being passed by the monochromator. The transmission is measured continuously during the scan and recorded as the ordinate value on the chart. It should be pointed out that the scanning speed may affect the resulting curve, and in general it should be slow enough for the recording system to have time to respond.

The rudimentary outline just given for an infrared spectrophotometer applies to both simple and complex instruments. In the simplest types the operating parameters (scanning speed, slit-width schedule, amplifier controls, etc.) are preset for some suitable average set of conditions for obtaining spectra, and this may be adequate in ordinary circumstances. In such an instrument operational control is reduced to two or three switches. More versatile (and expensive) instruments, on the other hand, provide for considerable variability in all operating factors, so that performance can be optimized for any given situation. Energy, resolution, scan speed, and noise level are all subject to some degree of control. In addition, such instruments are expected to be better engineered and to be capable of more accuracy and precision in both wavelength and intensity measurements.

It is an interesting coincidence that the most important part of the fundamental vibration region of the spectrum is nicely encompassed by the effective working range of a sodium chloride prism. The earliest spectrometers employed prisms cut from natural crystals, and this spectral interval became known as the rock-salt range. Development of the technology for making high-quality synthetic crystals large enough for prisms was one of the factors that made commercial infrared spectrometers feasible.

For a long time prism instruments were prevalent, but in recent years the trend has been toward the use of diffraction gratings—once again the result of technological advance. The most obvious advantage of gratings is higher resolving power. This is especially apparent at shorter wavelengths, where sodium chloride resolution is relatively poor. The adoption of gratings has been to some extent accompanied by a tendency to record spectra on a scale that is linear in frequency (cm^{-1}) rather than wavelength (μm). In comparison with the linear wavelength scale, the linear frequency scale expands the high-frequency region and compresses the low-frequency region. It is thus more appropriate for the resolving power of the grating.

The instrumental requirements for applications in lipid chemistry are probably intermediate in both complexity and cost. Simple instruments may be adequate for simple qualitative identification work, but some degree of flexibility is desirable to meet unusual sampling situations and for quantitative analysis. The resolving power of the grating can be of significant advantage for certain purposes, which are discussed later.

B. Sampling

The general methods of sample handling are applicable to lipids, except that gas-phase techniques can be safely ignored. Solutions can be used for either solids or liquids, but the number of useful solvents is extremely limited. Reagent-grade solvents are adequate for most purposes, except that the small amount of ethanol normally present in chloroform as a preservative should be removed by passage through a silica-gel or alumina column.

The spectra of carbon tetrachloride, carbon disulfide, and chloroform are shown in Fig. 1. It is evident that in each of the solvents there is at least one region of the spectrum that is obscured by strong solvent absorption. Nevertheless, by taking part of the spectrum in carbon tetrachloride and part in carbon disulfide the entire range can be covered except for a short interval between 6 and 7 μm in which both solvents absorb. Bromoform has been suggested as a solvent with which to bridge that gap (17). Solvents whose molecules are more complex or more polar have correspondingly complex spectra and stronger absorption bands and are of little utility.[3]

In spite of these limitations, solutions are generally preferable for quantitative analysis, and absorption bands to be measured can usually be found elsewhere than in regions of strong solvent absorption. Most lipids, except some of the more polar ones, are sufficiently soluble in the acceptable solvents. Since for qualitative purposes it may often be desirable to avoid the use of solvents, the techniques for liquid and solid samples are outlined in this section. These procedures are less convenient for quantitative work but can be so used for substances that are not sufficiently soluble.

[3] Water, although a simple molecule, is highly polar and absorbs intensely in the infrared. There are, however, some limited regions where it is sufficiently transparent in very thin layers for partial spectra to be obtained of substances in water solution. This point is not especially significant in connection with lipids but may be pertinent to lipoproteins.

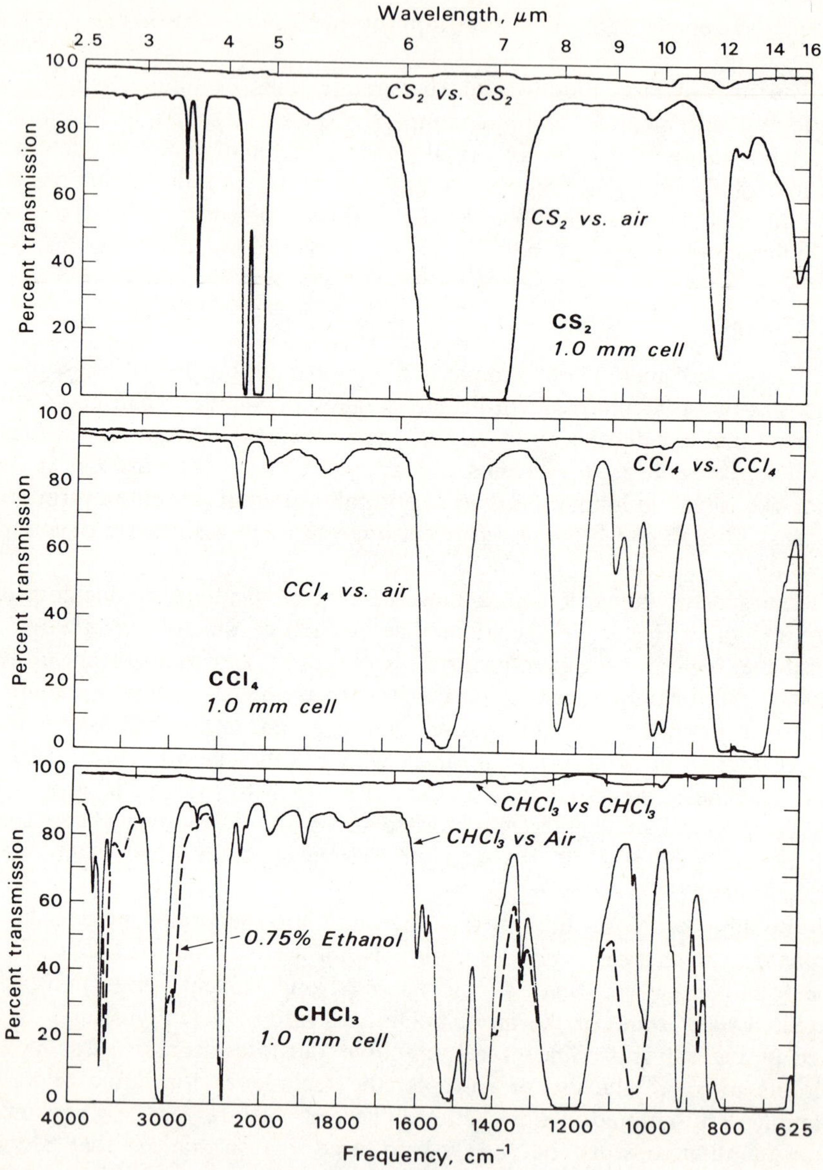

Fig. 1 Infrared spectra of reagent-grade carbon disulfide, carbon tetrachloride, and chloroform in 1.0-mm cells. Broken lines in the spectrum of chloroform indicate absorption bands of ethanol (normally present in chloroform as a preservative).

1. Liquids. Two types of absorption cells are used for liquids. The first type—called demountable—is assembled and disassembled for each sample. The technique is nevertheless extremely simple. A few drops of liquid are placed on a polished salt (NaCl) plate; a similar plate is set on top to form a "sandwich"; and the assembly is clamped lightly in a suitable frame to be placed in the spectrophotometer. In this instance the thickness of the liquid film is unknown and is controlled only by the viscosity of the liquid and the tightness of clamping. It is sometimes called simply a capillary film. If a thicker film is needed, a spacer in the form of a thin metal washer can be put between the plates, with the sample in the open center. (For a mobile or volatile liquid a spacer also acts as a seal. It is usually cut from lead foil, but insoluble plastic is sometimes used.) The spacer determines the thickness of the liquid layer, but not precisely enough for good quantitative work. There are also demountable cells in which the sample thickness is approximately determined by the depth of a shallow depression in one or both windows. Depending on the absorption properties of the substance, the required thickness usually ranges from 0.01 to 0.05 mm.

The second type of liquid cell—also made with salt windows—is permanently assembled and has a fixed thickness. This type is strongly preferred for the quantitative analysis of either solutions or undiluted liquids. In the latter case the path length is usually 0.01 to 0.05 mm (as in the demountable cell), whereas for solutions the cells are usually thicker, ranging up to 1.0 mm or more. These cells have stoppered filling ports and can be filled from a syringe or a dropper.

Some lipids have the consistency of a soft wax or grease and can be squeezed into a thin film between salt plates. Others may be too firm for this procedure but will form a suitable film when a solution is evaporated to dryness on a salt plate. Still others tend to crystallize on evaporation and form layers that are particulate and transmit poorly because of scattering. These may be dealt with by one or the other of two general methods for handling solids.

2. Solids. In the potassium bromide pellet method a solid sample is finely ground and uniformly dispersed in dry potassium bromide. The mixture is then pressed in a suitable die in a hydraulic press to form a pellet. Grinding and mixing can be done with a mortar and pestle or in a mechanical device, such as a dental amalgamator. The die is usually evacuated, and the required pressure is 80,000 to 100,000 psi. Equipment is available from manufacturers of instruments and accessories. Pellets are commonly disk shaped, but dies are also available for making them rectangular.

Blank disks can be made optically transparent, and many types of samples can be incorporated without significantly reducing their quality. Numerous factors, however, can cause the prepared disks to exhibit some degree of fogginess. If moderate, it may not impair the usefulness of the disk, and the observed effect on the spectrum is a sloping background, with transmission falling as the short-wavelength limit is approached.[4] This background phenomenon is a result of scattering loss, which can be more severe as the disk is whiter or chalkier. In such a case the transmission may be too low to obtain a spectrum at all.

Some possible causes of poor disks are the following:

1. Unsuitable particle size (too large).
2. Nonuniform distribution of material.
3. Water in sample.
4. Chemical or physical alteration of the sample.
5. Insufficient force on die.
6. Impure potassium bromide.
7. Inadequate vacuum.

Prepared potassium bromide—pure, dry, and of suitable particle size—is obtainable from commercial suppliers. It should be protected from exposure to atmospheric moisture, and some pains may be taken to dry it more exhaustively. It is, however, very difficult to avoid traces of water in the final pellet, as evidenced by the appearance of two slight dips in the spectrum at about 3 and 6.1 μm.[5] Other than these a potassium bromide blank should be free of absorption bands. The pellet method has been discussed critically and in detail by Fridmann (18).

For some purposes freeze-drying is an attractive alternative procedure for preparing a KBr–sample mixture. Since it evidently yields a molecular dispersion that is essentially amorphous, it avoids such difficulties as particle-size effects and crystal polymorphism. The spectral characteristics of a freeze-dried compound are somewhat like those of the liquid state, whereas the spectra of crystals (as prepared by grinding) tend to have sharper, more numerous, and more discrete bands. This difference (as well as the possibility of polymorphism) should be borne in mind in connection with the qualitative spectral identification of solid samples. Their solid-state spectra should be compared only with those of reference compounds prepared in the same way. The freeze-drying method can be recommended for quantitative analysis by virtue of its reproducibility, and

[4] Some of the KBr pellet spectra of lipids in Section III.B illustrate this effect. An attenuator has been used in the reference beam instead of a blank.

[5] This is shown in the cholesterol spectrum in Section III.B (Fig. 9).

also because it is a feasible technique for handling microgram amounts of material. Such procedures have been described in detail by Schwartz (12) for tissue lipids, and by Mason (19), who recommends two stages of lyophilization for substances (i.e., lipids) that are not water soluble.

An older method of treating solids is to grind the sample to a fine powder in a mortar and disperse it as a paste or mull by further grinding in a few drops of white mineral oil. This mixture is then squeezed into a film between salt plates. Operationally this procedure is extremely simple, and for many qualitative purposes it is quite adequate. Oil obscures the regions of absorption by CH_2- and CH_3-groups, but substantial and significant portions of its spectrum are relatively transparent (see Fig. 2). As in the case of undiluted liquids, quantitative analysis can only be done with the use of an internal standard.

3. Sample Size. The amount of sample required when standard instrumentation and cells are used is ordinarily 1 to 10 mg. However, special cells and accessories are available for working with quantities as small as a few micrograms. The first requirement in microsampling is to reduce the cross-sectional area occupied by the sample, keeping the thickness and concentration the same. By bringing the sample as near as possible to the slit (or some other focal point), its area can be made comparable to the slit dimensions with little or no loss of energy. Samples well below 1 mg

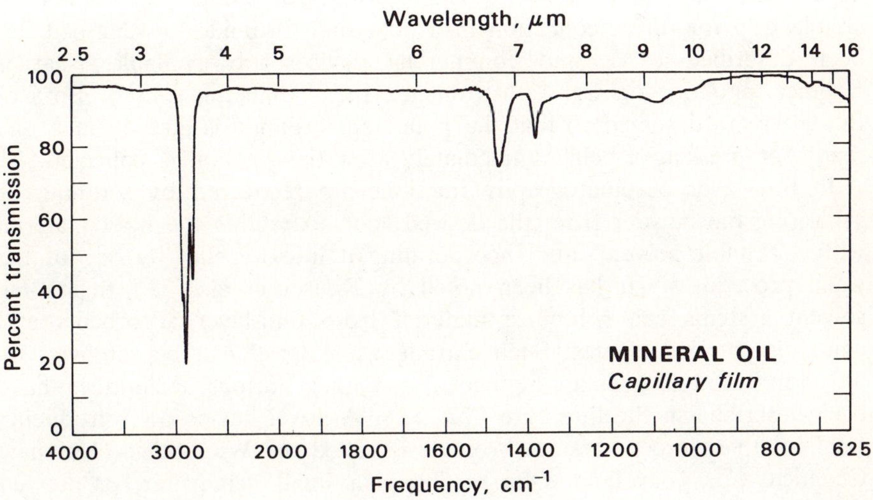

Fig. 2 Infrared spectrum of white mineral oil (Nujol). Capillary film between NaCl plates.

can be handled in this way with suitable microcells or small rectangular pellets.

Below about 100 μg the reduced sample area becomes substantially smaller than the minimum beam area, and a large fraction of the energy is lost or masked out. In this range it is therefore necessary to employ an auxiliary optical system, usually called a beam condenser. Such a device can be constructed with either transmitting or reflecting optics and provides in the sampling space an image of the source that is reduced in dimension by one-third to one-sixth. The beam energy is thereby concentrated in this smaller area, and still smaller cells or pellets can be used. Various auxiliary systems of this kind are provided by manufacturers of instruments and accessories. Pellets as small as 0.5 mm in diameter can be made. A microsampling technique of this sort is needed for the spectroscopic examination of fractions recovered from either gas–liquid or thin-layer chromatography.

4. Chromatography Fractions. If gas–liquid chromatography fractions are to be examined by infrared spectrometry, it is usually for the purpose of identification, since quantitation will have been already done. Depending on its amount and volatility, the material in the fraction may be collected in a simple solvent trap or cold trap as it emerges from the chromatograph and subsequently transferred to a suitable absorption cell. Direct collection of liquids in a microcell of 1-μl capacity is made possible by a special accessory (Barnes Engineering Co., Stamford, Conn.). A simple trap for direct collection in a potassium bromide powder bed has been described (20), and commercial devices are available (Barnes Engineering Co., and Carle Instruments, Inc., Anaheim, Calif.). Both of the latter are designed so that the potassium bromide is already in a die, ready for pressing a pellet immediately after the fraction is collected.

In thin-layer chromatography fractions are recovered by scraping or aspirating the powder from the desired spot, extracting the lipid material with a suitable solvent, and incorporating it into a pellet by one of the usual procedures. [It has been noted by Rouser et al. (21) that some solvent systems can solubilize material from thin-layer adsorbents and contaminate lipid eluates. Such extraneous material can be removed by filtration through a small Sephadex column.] Various techniques have been described in the literature (22, 23). A novel device for introducing small samples into potassium bromide is called the Wick-Stick (Harshaw Chemical Co., Cleveland, Ohio). This is a small, triangular, prepressed bed of potassium bromide that is placed upright in a small vessel together with a solution of the sample. On evaporation of the solvent the sample concentrates in the upper tip of the triangle, which is then broken off and made into a pellet.

III. QUALITATIVE APPLICATIONS

A. Interpretation of Infrared Spectra

Depending on the particular problem at hand, the lipid chemist may wish to use the infrared spectrum (a) to identify an isolated pure compound, either specifically or as to type; (b) to characterize mixtures with respect to probable constituents; or (c) to show the presence or absence of some particular chemical group or structural feature. Specific identification brings into play the catalog of reference spectra for direct comparison. Otherwise the background information consists basically of the group correlations mentioned in Section I.

Before describing the lipid spectra in these terms, it is perhaps worthwhile to discuss some general features of infrared spectra that guide the approach to their interpretation. The brief outline of these features here is tailored to the understanding of lipid spectra. For example, the spectral characteristics of aromatic compounds are not included. A more extensive and detailed discussion of characteristic group absorptions has been presented by Bellamy (7, 8).

For the purpose of "reading" an infrared spectrogram—in the sense of assigning structural groups to observed absorption bands—it is helpful at the outset to realize that the infrared range can be subdivided according to a broad classification of vibrational types. These subintervals are approximately as follows:

2.5 to 4.2 μm (4000–2400 cm^{-1}): hydrogen-stretching vibrations (O—H, N—H, C—H, S—H bonds).

4.2 to 6.5 μm (2400–1550 cm^{-1}): multiple-bond-stretching vibrations (C≡C, C≡N, C=C, C=N, C=O).

6 to 16 μm (1667–625 cm^{-1}): hydrogen-bending and single-bond (skeletal) stretching vibrations (C—C, C—O, etc.).

1. Hydrogen-Stretching Vibrations. The occurrence of the hydrogen-stretching vibrations at the high-frequency end of the spectrum is a logical consequence of considering a molecule as a system of coupled harmonic oscillators. As derived from Hooke's law, the frequency of a single oscillator is given by

$$\nu = \frac{1}{2\pi}\sqrt{f/M} \qquad (1)$$

where f is the restoring force per unit displacement and M is the reduced mass of the system. If the oscillator is a diatomic molecule, f is the force constant of the bond between the atoms and M is expressed as the product of the individual atomic masses divided by their sum. When one of the two atoms is hydrogen, the value of M is much smaller than that for a molecule composed of two heavier atoms; so for comparable force constants the vibration frequency is higher. Substantially all of the significant hydrogen-stretching frequencies fall within the range indicated; nearly all other vibrations are excluded, with the possible exception of weak overtones or combinations of lower frequencies.

Not all C—H bonds have the same single characteristic stretching frequency, represented in the absorption spectrum by a single peak. Rather there is in the spectrum of a (nonaromatic) hydrocarbon a pattern of absorption bands that is determined principally by methylene (CH_2), methyl (CH_3), and olefinic hydrogen (C=C—H) groups. In both CH_2- and CH_3-groups the stretching vibrations can be symmetric or antisymmetric. Thus each group has two frequencies, and four bands would be expected in the spectrum of a simple linear alkane. These are only partially resolvable, however, and in NaCl prism spectra two peaks are observed at about 3.4 and 3.5 μm (2920 and 2860 cm^{-1}). The first is a composite of the antisymmetric vibrations of both groups, and the second is the corresponding mixture of symmetric vibrations. In a branched alkane there is at least one tertiary hydrogen (R_3CH), whose absorption is relatively weak and also unresolvable. Stretching of a hydrogen on a double-bonded carbon atom has a slightly higher frequency, which is variable with double-bond type: 3.25 to 3.35 μm (3100–3000 cm^{-1}). The peak is observable but still poorly resolved in NaCl prism spectra of olefins. Grating spectra show fairly good resolution of this peak. Some other distinguishable types of C—H bond are acetylenic (C≡C—H; 3.05 μm, 3300 cm^{-1}) and aldehydic (O=C—H; 3.65 μm, 2730 cm^{-1}).

The hydroxyl (O—H) stretching frequency is strongly influenced by hydrogen bonding. For a very dilute solution in a nonpolar solvent, where little or no hydrogen bonding takes place, the absorption peak is sharp, at about 2.75 μm (3640 cm^{-1}). As the concentration (and hydrogen bonding) is increased, the peak broadens and intensifies, and its position moves to a longer wavelength. In the spectra of solid or undiluted liquid alcohols the band is quite broad, and its center is in the vicinity of 3.0 μm (3300–3400 cm^{-1}). It is in fact similar to the O—H stretching band of liquid water. An extreme case of hydrogen bonding is found in carboxyl groups, which associate pairwise to form cyclic dimers. In these structures the hydroxyl group of each mating molecule is hydrogen bonded to the carbonyl group of the other. The strength of these hydrogen bonds is such as to shift and broaden the absorption peak even more than in alcohols. The O—H stretching band of carboxyl extends from about 3 to 4 μm (3300–2500 cm^{-1}) and is seen in the spectra of fatty acids as broad shoulders on both sides of the C—H stretching bands.

The N—H stretching frequencies are very close to the O—H frequencies, and they are similarly affected by hydrogen bonding, although not as strongly. Unassociated NH-groups absorb at 2.85 to 3.05 μm (3500–3300 cm^{-1}). When involved in hydrogen bonding, they absorb between 2.95 and 3.2 μm (3400–3100 cm^{-1}). In the NH_2-groups of primary amines and amides there are also symmetric and antisymmetric stretching modes (just as in CH_2), giving rise to two distinct frequencies in these ranges. The presence of a positive charge on the nitrogen atom, as in amine salts or amino acids, usually has a further complicating effect on the spectrum, depending on the type of compound. Quite commonly new bands are observed at longer wavelengths, between 3.6 and 5 μm (2800–2000 cm^{-1}), but the possible effects are too varied to be discussed in detail here.

2. Multiple-Bond-Stretching Vibrations. The types of multiple bonds that are of some significance in relation to blood lipids are C=C and C=O. Triple bonds probably do not occur in mammalian lipids, and their absorptions are well segregated in the spectrum below 5 μm. The C=N double bond is also unlikely to be encountered and can for the most part be disregarded. Its stretching frequency falls in approximately the same narrow range as that of the C=C double bond: 5.95 to 6.15 μm (1680–1625 cm^{-1}).

The C=C stretching absorption is in fact relatively weak; for example, in methyl oleate it appears to be about two orders of magnitude weaker than the C=O band at 5.75 μm (1740 cm^{-1}).[6] This comparison illustrates the dependence of absorption intensity on the magnitude of the dipole-moment fluctuation that is associated with the vibrational motion of the atoms. The C=O bond is strongly polarized, whereas the C=C bond has a symmetrical charge distribution. If the C=C bond has a *cis* configuration, a small dipole can be generated by stretching. If it is *trans*, the electrical symmetry is maintained during the vibration and there is no absorption band at all.[7] If the C=C double bond is part of a conjugated system, the frequency is lowered and the intensity of absorption is increased.

The carbonyl absorption band is an important feature of infrared spectra generally and of lipid spectra as a class. Because it is relatively free from interference by other absorptions, it has been thoroughly studied, and its

[6] The spectrum of methyl oleate is shown in part B of this section (Fig. 5).
[7] See the spectrum of methyl elaidate in part B of this section (Fig. 4).

frequency ranges have been established for the various classes of carbonyl-containing compounds. Such other spectroscopic aspects as absolute intensities, solvent effects, and differences between the liquid and the solid states have also been investigated. All C=O absorptions occur within the limited range of 5.4 to 6.5 μm (1850–1540 cm^{-1}). Since virtually no other groups absorb between 5.4 and 5.95 μm, this is exclusively a carbonyl region. It includes most simple (or unconjugated) fatty acids, esters, ketones, aldehydes, anhydrides, and acid chlorides. Between 5.95 and 6.5 μm are found the absorption bands of amides, some conjugated carbonyls, and the carboxyl ion. The most common noncarbonyl absorbers in this range are C=C (weak), conjugated C=C (including aromatic), primary amines (NH_2 bending), and organic nitrate.

3. Hydrogen-Bending and Single-Bond-Stretching Vibrations. Patterns of absorption in the third spectral region (6–16 μm, 1667–625 cm^{-1}) can be quite complex, and for many classes of molecules only a few of the bands observed there can be assigned to group vibrations. Those for which correlations are best established include hydrogen bending and certain single-bond-stretching modes.

Hydrogen-bending Vibrations. Hydrogen bending implies deformation of bond angles by motions of the hydrogen atoms perpendicular to the bond directions. For example, the NH_2-group has a bending-vibration frequency at about 1610 cm^{-1} (6.2 μm); its occurrence there is the principal reason that the bending range overlaps the double-bond region. The C—H bending modes, which are of primary importance in lipids, are distributed over a wide range. As in the case of the stretching vibrations, these are best described as motions of CH_2-, CH_3-, and C=C—H-groups.

If a CH_2-group existed as a detached molecule, it would have only one bending mode: the angle deformation. As part of a chain of CH_2-groups linked by C—C bonds, its hydrogen atoms can execute four distinct types of in-phase motion that can be designated as bending modes:

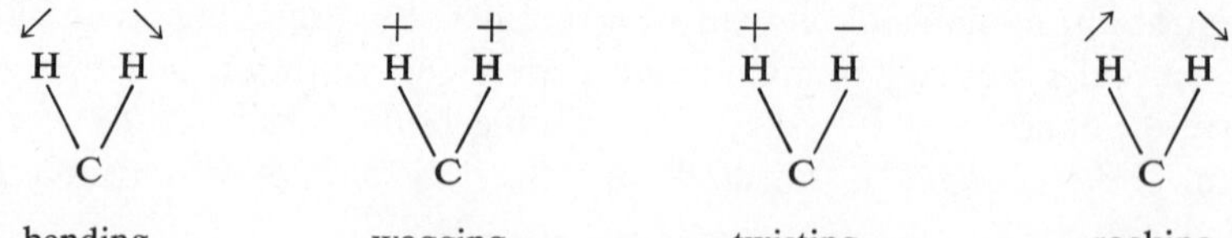

bending (deformation)	wagging	twisting	rocking
6.8 μm (1465 cm^{-1})	7.2–8.5 μm (1390–1180 cm^{-1})	7.7–8.55 μm (1300–1170 cm^{-1})	10–13.9 μm (1000–720 cm^{-1})

A half-cycle of each vibration is shown by the directions of motion of the hydrogen atoms, a plus sign indicating upward from the plane of the page and a minus sign indicating downward. The absorption band corresponding to the deformation mode appears at about 6.8 μm (1465 cm^{-1}) and is a prominent feature in the spectra of all long-chain compounds. The frequency of this vibration is lowered in a CH_2-group that is adjacent to a polar group or a double bond. If the polar group is a carbonyl (ester or fatty acid), the band is at 7.1 μm (1410 cm^{-1}). This is also the position of a weak carboxyl absorption. For a CH_2-group adjacent to a double bond the absorption is at 6.95 μm (1435 cm^{-1}) and tends to be overlapped by the main CH_2-band.

In theory, if a hydrocarbon chain is in the fully extended, planar zigzag form, the frequencies of the other bending vibrations occur as sequences distributed over a considerable spectral range. This is a result of interaction between the CH_2-groups and involves the phase relationships among the individual CH_2-group motions along the chain. The spectra of long-chain compounds in the crystalline state show such band sequences, whereas those of liquids do not. (It is presumed that in the liquid state, the chains are not constrained to the planar zigzag conformation, and the collective interaction among CH_2-groups is not definable.)

A prominent characteristic of the spectra of solid fatty acids and their esters is the "band progression" between about 7.2 and 8.5 μm (1390–1180 cm^{-1}). These band sequences in saturated straight-chain acids were analyzed by Jones, McKay, and Sinclair (24) and by Meiklejohn and co-workers (25), who minimized band interference by using fatty acid soaps. As n (the number of CH_2-groups) increases, the spacing between bands decreases, and there are approximately $n/2$ bands in the interval. The bands have been assigned as the CH_2-wagging modes, and in liquid or solution spectra they degenerate into a single weak band in the vicinity of 7.7 μm (1300 cm^{-1}). In lipids this band is often overlapped by stronger absorptions and is not readily discernible. The twisting modes are believed to occur in the same general frequency range as the wagging modes. They are evidently weaker; their identification and assignment have not been completely reliable; and they have little practical significance.

The rocking modes form a series whose long-wavelength limit is at 13.9 μm (720 cm^{-1}). In some instances other bands of the series can be identified, but usually it is only the 13.9-μm peak that is observed. For very short chains (less than four CH_2-groups) the band is shifted to shorter wavelengths: 13.5 μm (740 cm^{-1}) for propyl side chains and 12.9 μm (775 cm^{-1}) for ethyl side chains. Another very significant observation in connection with the CH_2-rocking frequency is its splitting into a doublet in certain crystalline forms. This has been attributed to interaction between CH_2-groups of adjacent chains, which is permitted only in a particular orientation.

A CH_3-group can have a bending vibration that is symmetric, in which all three hydrogens move inward and outward (with respect to the axis) in phase; or antisymmetric, in which one hydrogen moves inward while the other two move apart. The frequency of the latter mode is very close to that of the CH_2 deformation and usually appears as an unresolved shoulder (6.85 μm, 1460 cm^{-1}) on the long-wavelength side of the 6.8-μm (1465-cm^{-1}) peak. The symmetric vibration of a CH_3-group has a characteristic band at 7.25 μm (1375 cm^{-1}), nicely separated from the other alkane absorptions. Whenever two CH_3-groups are attached to the same carbon atom, their interaction results in a splitting of this band into a doublet. This is a useful diagnostic feature in relation to chain branching.

The bending vibrations of hydrogen on a double-bonded carbon atom can be classified as planar or nonplanar with respect to the C=CHR plane. Absorptions attributable to planar motions occur in the rather narrow range of 7.05 to 7.15 μm (1420–1400 cm^{-1}). The band is only strong when the structure is $R_2C{=}CH_2$, which occurs infrequently in the types of lipids with which we are concerned. For RHC=CHR (*cis*) the absorption is weak or moderate; for RHC=CHR (*trans*) it is zero (forbidden by symmetry). Since in fatty acids and their derivatives the α-methylene group absorbs at the same wavelength, these bands are not likely to be very useful.

The out-of-plane bending vibrations of olefinic hydrogen, on the other hand, are quite distinctive for each configuration. For unconjugated double bonds the structural correlation is as follows:

Group	Wavelength (μm)	Frequency (cm^{-1})
$RHC{=}CH_2$	10.1, 11.0	990, 910
$R_2C{=}CH_2$	11.25	890
RHC=CHR (*trans*)	10.35	965
RHC=CHR (*cis*)	~ 14.25	~700
$R_2C{=}CHR$	11.9–12.5	840–800

The first three types listed give strong, sharp, specific bands. The *cis* double-bond absorption is broader, less well defined, and overlaps the CH_2-rocking absorption at 720 cm^{-1}. The band for trialkylethylene is of only moderate intensity, also broad and more variable in position. Although these correlations do not apply to conjugated-double-bond systems, further distinctions of those structures can be made (26).

Single-Bond-Stretching Vibrations. In lipids the principal single-bond-stretching vibrations occur in the C—C and C—O bonds. The C—C bonds are mostly links in long alkyl chains and are subject to coupling interactions. This leads to a series of bands, just as for the coupled CH_2-group vibrations of long chains. Theoretically the C—C stretching sequence falls in the range between about 8.7 and 11.5 μm (1150–870 cm^{-1}). The number of vibrational modes is equal to the number of C—C bonds, but only some of these are active (allowed by symmetry) in the infrared. Because the dipole moments generated by these motions are very small, absorption is very weak and the bands are difficult to identify—especially in the longer chains. Since the C—C bands can also be easily obscured or confused with other absorptions in the spectra of nonhydrocarbons, they are of no practical utility in the interpretation of lipid spectra.

The ester group is a common feature of lipids, and its C—O stretching vibrations are responsible for prominent absorption bands in the range of 8 to 10 μm (1250–1000 cm^{-1}). Usually a strong band is observed between 8 and 8.7 μm (1250–1150 cm^{-1}) and a weaker one between 8.7 and 10 μm (1150–1000 cm^{-1}). In the spectra of acetates the strong band is characteristically near 8.05 μm (1245 cm^{-1}), and its position is relatively independent of the remainder of the molecule. This absorption is believed to be associated with the C—O bond nearest the carbonyl (although the two C—O bonds are coupled through the oxygen atom and the vibrations must interact). For large acyl groups (nonaromatic) this band moves to longer wavelengths, and in lipid spectra it is in the vicinity of 8.6 μm (1165 cm^{-1}). The weaker band appears in the spectra of acetates between 9.45 and 10 μm (1060–1000 cm^{-1}). It is poorly characterized, however, and its identification is uncertain in many ester spectra.

The C—O stretching vibration of alcohols has a wavelength range from about 8.5 to 10 μm (1175–1000 cm^{-1}). In simple noncyclic saturated alcohols a frequency correlation exists for primary, secondary, and tertiary structures. Their absorptions occur at about 9.5, 9.0, and 8.75 μm (1050, 1110, and 1140 cm^{-1}), respectively. Allylic alcohols have a band at about 9.9 μm (1010 cm^{-1}). Cholesterol is a cyclic secondary alcohol and does not conform to that correlation, having a C—O absorption at the primary alcohol position.

In simple saturated ethers the C—O—C group absorbs strongly in the vicinity of 9.0 μm (1110 cm^{-1}). This characteristic band position is shifted to about 8.35 μm (1200 cm^{-1}) in vinyl ethers and hence may be difficult to distinguish if ester groups are also present.

The various phospholipids are phosphate diesters. Strong absorptions of this structure are the P=O stretching band at about 8.1 to 8.3 μm (1235–1215 cm^{-1}) and bands attributable to P—O—C stretching between 9 and 9.5 μm (1100–1050 cm^{-1}). The P=O frequency falls outside the range designated for double bonds because the phosphorus atom has a larger mass than the carbon atom. The P—O—C bands are close to the C—O absorptions of alcohols and ethers, whose bands may be overlapped or obscured by the phosphate spectrum.

B. Lipid Spectra

Figures 3 through 12 are the spectra of lipid compounds that are of interest in the study of blood lipids. They have been chosen to be representative of the various lipid classes and to illustrate their spectral characteristics. Differences between solid-state and liquid or solution spectra are also exemplified.

1. Technical Data. Most of the compounds whose spectra are shown in this section were obtained from commercial suppliers, as designated. The phospholipids were stated to be 96 to 98% pure, other lipids at least 99% pure. Purities were not verified, but wherever possible the spectra were checked against known or previously published curves. Film thicknesses quoted are rough estimates on the basis of band intensities.

The spectra were recorded on a Perkin-Elmer Model 421 double-beam, filter-grating spectrophotometer. A scale-change mode was employed, in which the normal linear frequency scale is contracted by a factor of 2 between 4000 and 2000 cm^{-1} and expanded by a factor of 2 between 2000 and 625 cm^{-1}. The resulting curves resemble more closely the spectra recorded on a linear wavelength scale and are visually more nearly comparable with the prism spectra that appear in most of the earlier literature. Expansion of the low-frequency range can also be rationalized on the basis that this region contains the absorption patterns of principal qualitative significance. Relatively low resolution conditions (slit program = 1000 × 2) were used, but the observed resolution in the C—H stretching region (3.3–3.6 μm) is significantly better than that obtained with an NaCl prism. (This would be more clearly shown if the scale were not compressed in this region.)

Normally the recorded curve exhibits transient spikes at frequencies where the filter or grating is automatically changed (2500, 2000, 1580, 990 cm^{-1}). These spikes have been deleted, in some cases by raising the pen off the paper momentarily during recording, otherwise at the stage of photographing the original curves. This is noted only to explain an occasional irregularity in the curve at one of these frequencies. Such irregularities are of little consequence except at 990 cm^{-1}, where the recovery time from the transient is especially slow and the curve itself is apt to be changing more rapidly. In some spectra there may be a slight distortion of the curve at that point.

The curves were recorded directly on small charts (9 × 18.75 cm) for convenience in reproduction. Some accuracy is lost by this procedure, but the curves are believed to be correct within 5 cm^{-1} on the frequency scale between 2000 and 625 cm^{-1}, and within 20 cm^{-1} between 4000 and

2000 cm^{-1}. These limits are comparable to reading errors on the reduced scales and are probably adequate for most qualitative comparisons. Most of the wavelengths (frequencies) quoted in the text are approximate. Allowances must be made for the broadness of some bands, for variations in the calibration of different instruments, and for fluctuation in values taken from the literature. There may also be small differences between liquid and solid states, and in solvents of different polarity.

In the solution spectra regions of total absorption by the solvent have been omitted. Where there are other strong solvent bands (e.g., ~ 8 and ~ 10 μm in CCl_4) the reduced energy may cause slight blurring of the spectra.

2. Useful Features of Lipid Spectra. The most significant group correlations that are relevant to lipid spectra have been discussed in a general way in part A of this section. It may be profitable now to pinpoint some of the specific spectral characteristics that are most useful in the qualitative analysis of lipids. Aside from the identification of a lipid by simple recognition of its overall spectral pattern, various structural questions may be put regarding double bonds, chain length, branching, ester type, and the like. The spectrum provides answers of varying degrees of completeness, depending in part on whether the sample is an isolated pure compound, a mixture of homologs, or a mixture of classes. The basic information is to be found in the appropriate group correlations. Moreover, these correlations can be better defined for the limited set of lipid compounds if the reference spectra of pure lipids are examined against them as a background. There are some spectral features that distinguish various classes of lipids from one another. Other features persist through all or most of the classes because they are associated with the hydrocarbon-chain moieties.

The fatty acids have some unusual absorption bands that are attributable to their dimerized structure. One of these is the absorption of the strongly-hydrogen-bonded hydroxyl of the COOH-group. This is a broad band extending from about 3 to 4 μm (3300–2500 cm^{-1}) and appears in the spectrum (e.g., Fig. 3) as broad shoulders on both sides of the sharper C—H stretching bands. The hydroxyl hydrogens—because they are constrained in the ring structure formed by the dimer—can also oscillate in a direction perpendicular to the plane of the ring. This nonplanar bending mode is responsible for a characteristic fatty acid absorption at about 10.7 μm (935 cm^{-1}). The C=O stretching frequency for the dimerized form in solution is observed at about 5.85 μm (1710 cm^{-1}). At high dilution, however, a band of the monomer may also appear at a higher frequency (~ 1760 cm^{-1}). The spectrum of a soap is not shown here, but ionization of the carboxyl group shifts the carbonyl absorption into the range of 6.2 to 6.45 μm (1610–1550 cm^{-1}). This band is quite strong.

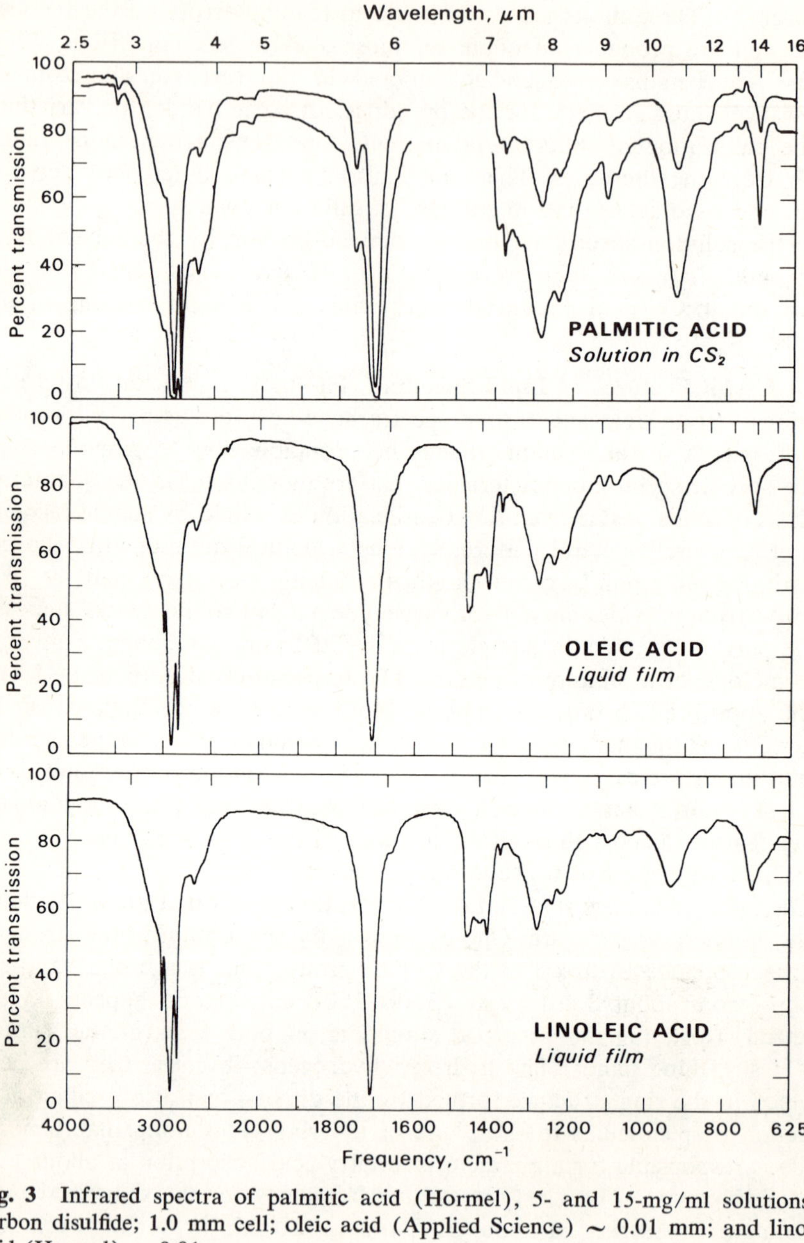

Fig. 3 Infrared spectra of palmitic acid (Hormel), 5- and 15-mg/ml solutions in carbon disulfide; 1.0 mm cell; oleic acid (Applied Science) ~ 0.01 mm; and linoleic acid (Hormel) ~ 0.01 mm.

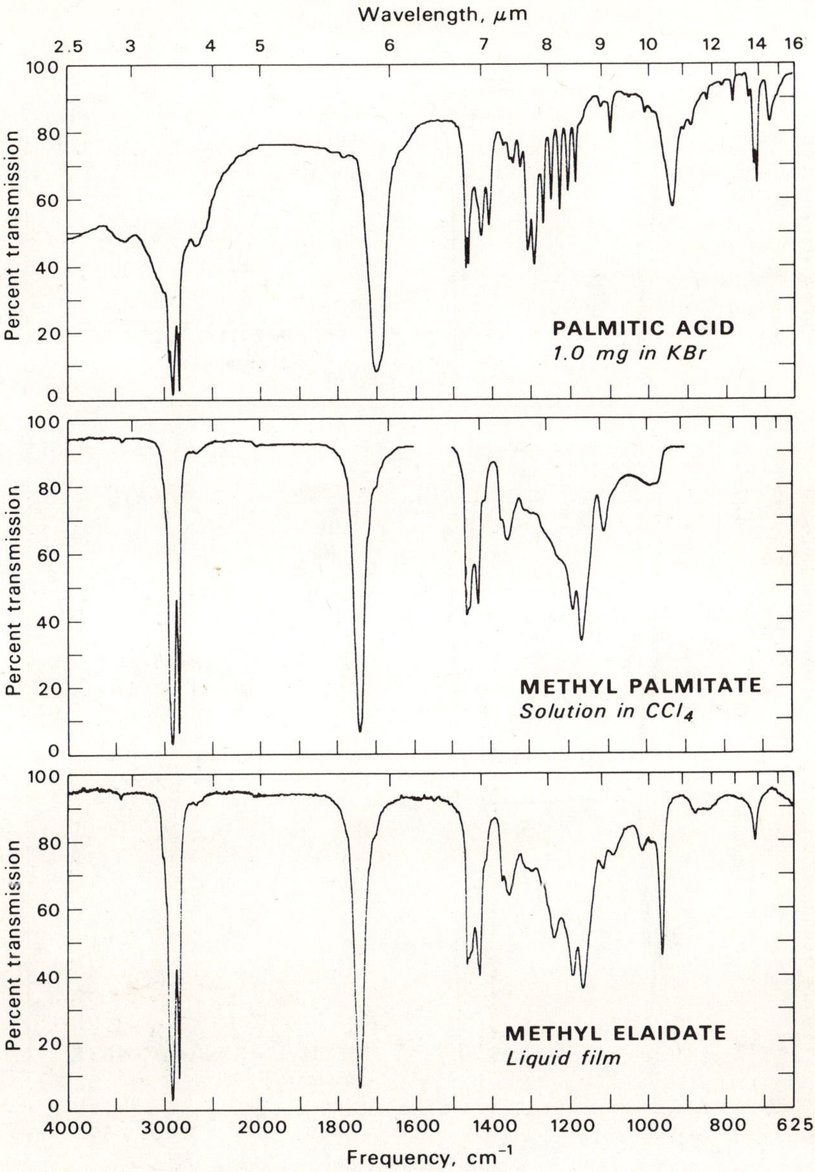

Fig. 4 Infrared spectra of palmitic acid (Hormel), solid; methyl palmitate (redistilled), 7-mg/ml solution in carbon tetrachloride, 1.0-mm cell; and methyl elaidate (Supelco) ~ 0.01 mm.

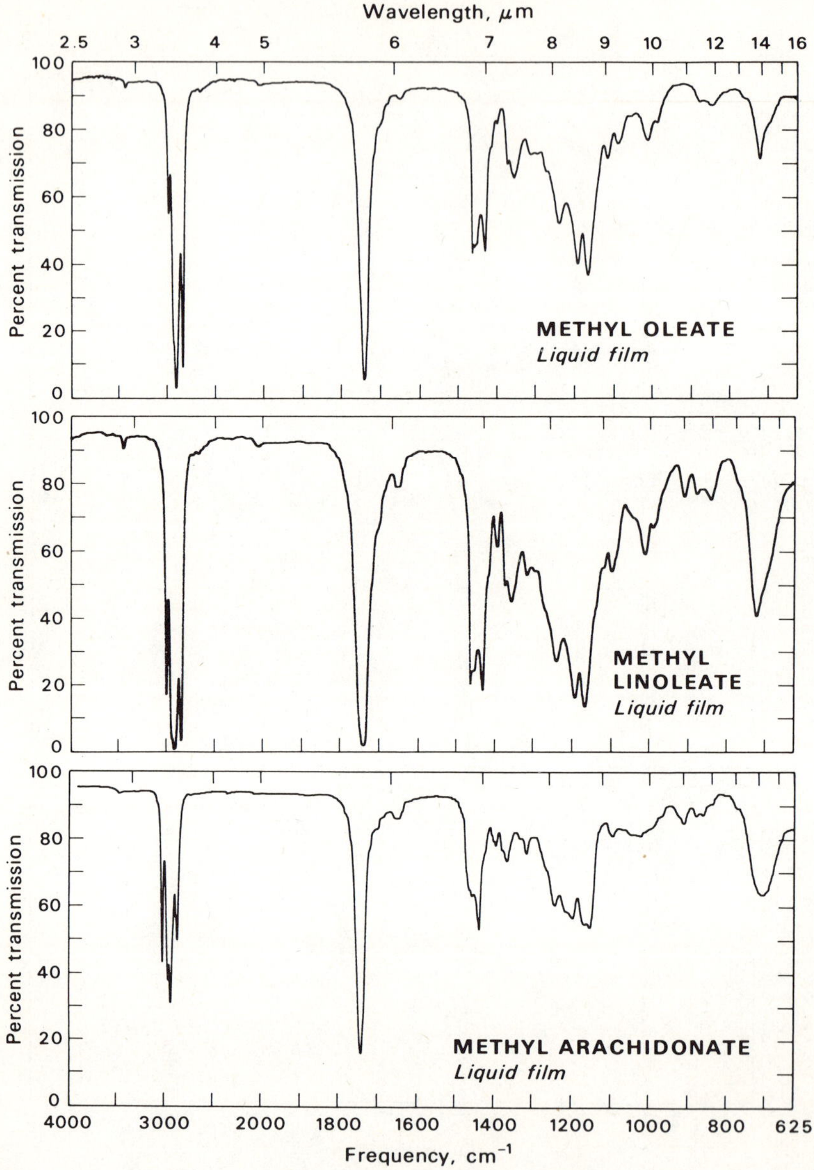

Fig. 5 Infrared spectra of methyl oleate (Hormel) ~ 0.01 mm; methyl linoleate (Hormel) ~ 0.02 mm; and methyl arachidonate (Hormel) ~ 0.01 mm.

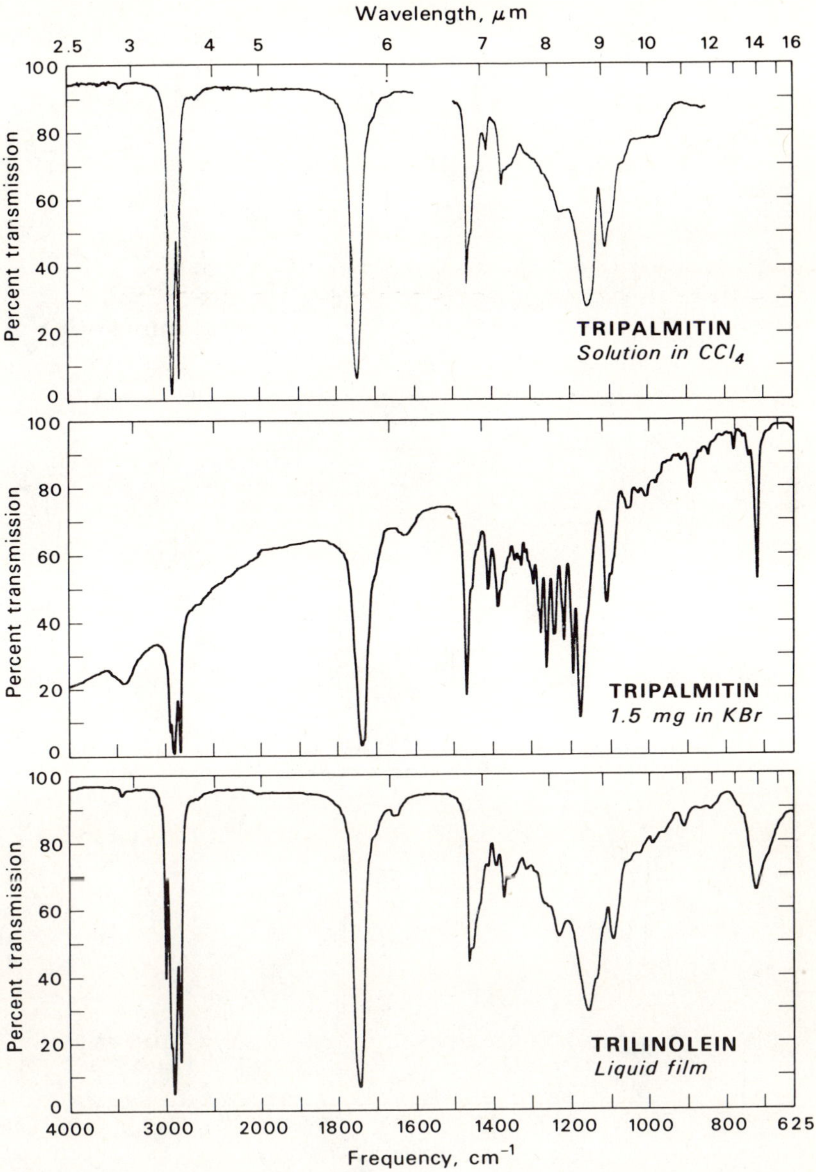

Fig. 6 Infrared spectra of tripalmitin (Hormel), 7-mg/ml solution in carbon tetrachloride, 1.0-mm cell; tripalmitin (Hormel), solid; and trilinolein (Hormel) ~ 0.01 mm.

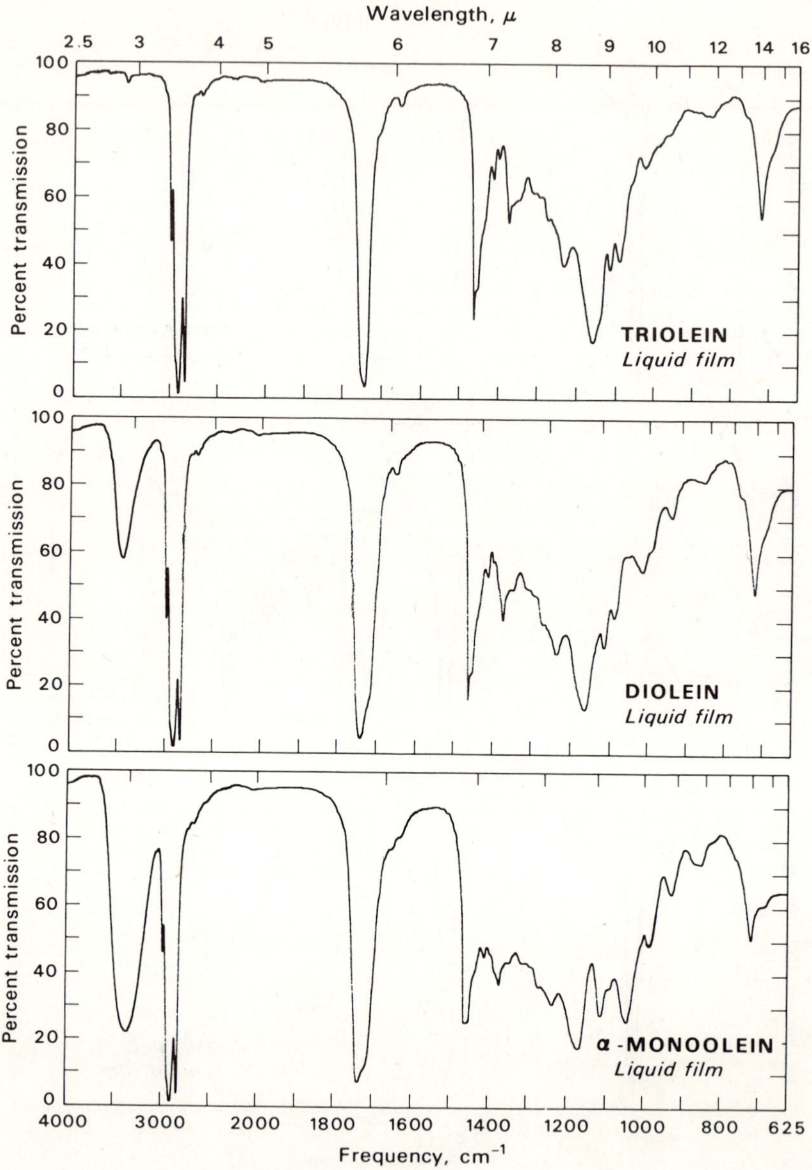

Fig. 7 Infrared spectra of triolein (Hormel) ~ 0.02 mm; diolein (Hormel) ~ 0.02 mm; and α-monoolein (Supelco) ~ 0.02 mm.

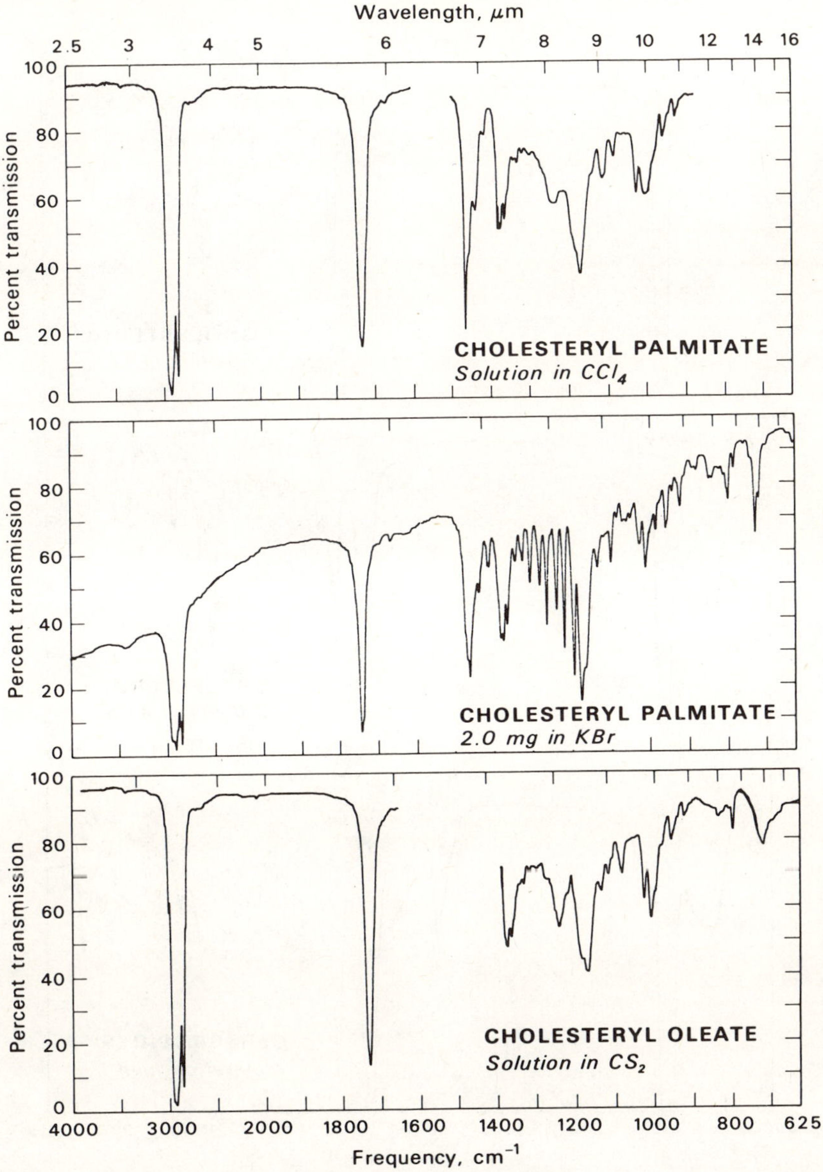

Fig. 8 Infrared spectra of cholesteryl palmitate (Supelco), 10-mg/ml solution in carbon tetrachloride, 1.0-mm cell; cholesteryl palmitate (Supelco), solid; and cholesteryl oleate (Supelco), 10-mg/ml solution in carbon disulfide, 1.0-mm cell.

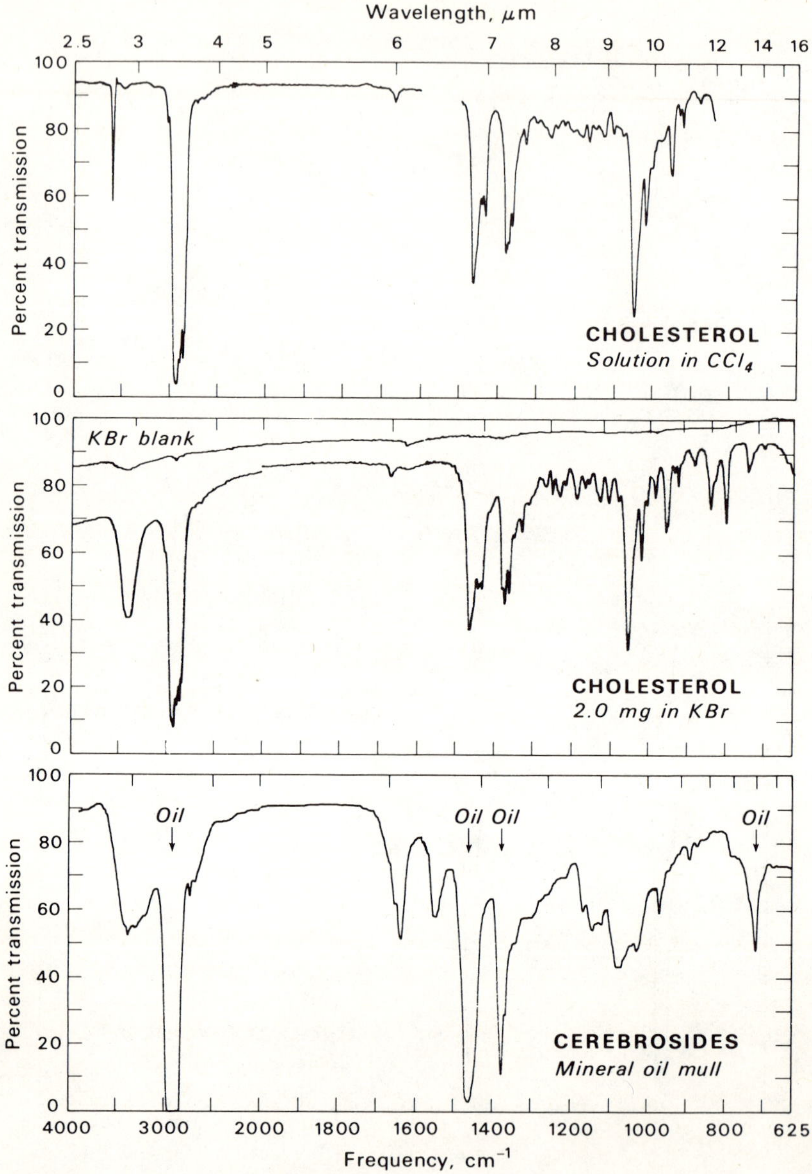

Fig. 9 Infrared spectra of cholesterol (Hormel), 10-mg/ml solution in carbon tetrachloride, 1.0-mm cell; cholesterol (Hormel), solid; and cerebrosides (bovine, Supelco), solid.

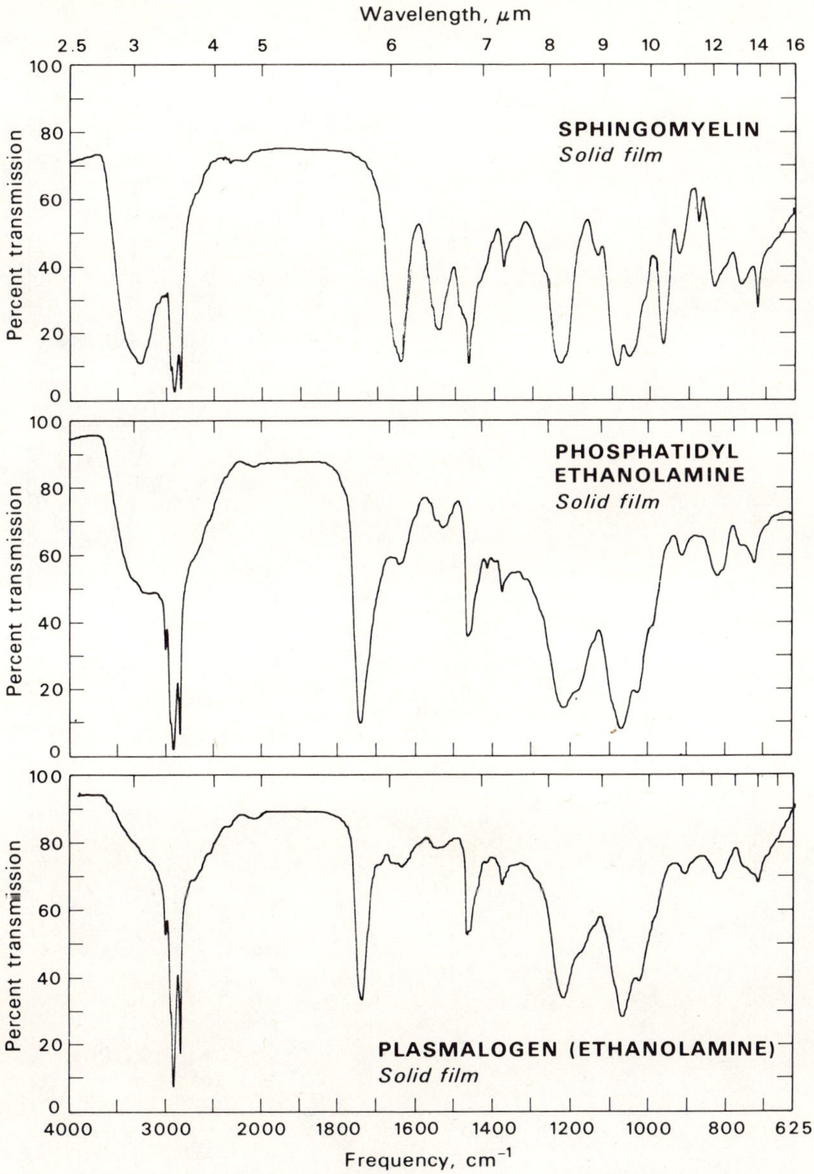

Fig. 10 Infrared spectra of sphingomyelin (bovine, Applied Science) ~ 0.02 mm; phosphatidylethanolamine (Applied Science) ~ 0.01 mm; and plasmalogen (ethanolamine) (white matter, Supelco) < 0.01 mm.

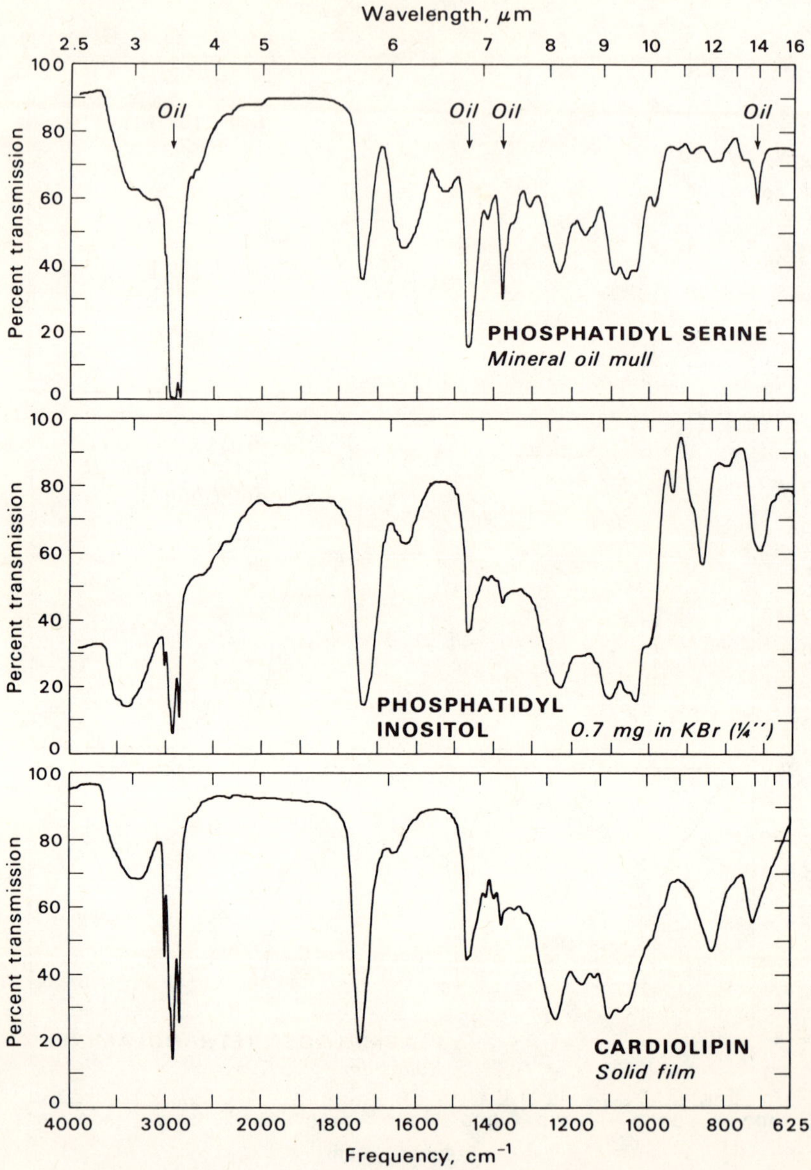

Fig. 11 Infrared spectra of phosphatidylserine (Supelco), solid; phosphatidylinositol (Supelco), solid; cardiolipin (Applied Science) ~ 0.01 mm.

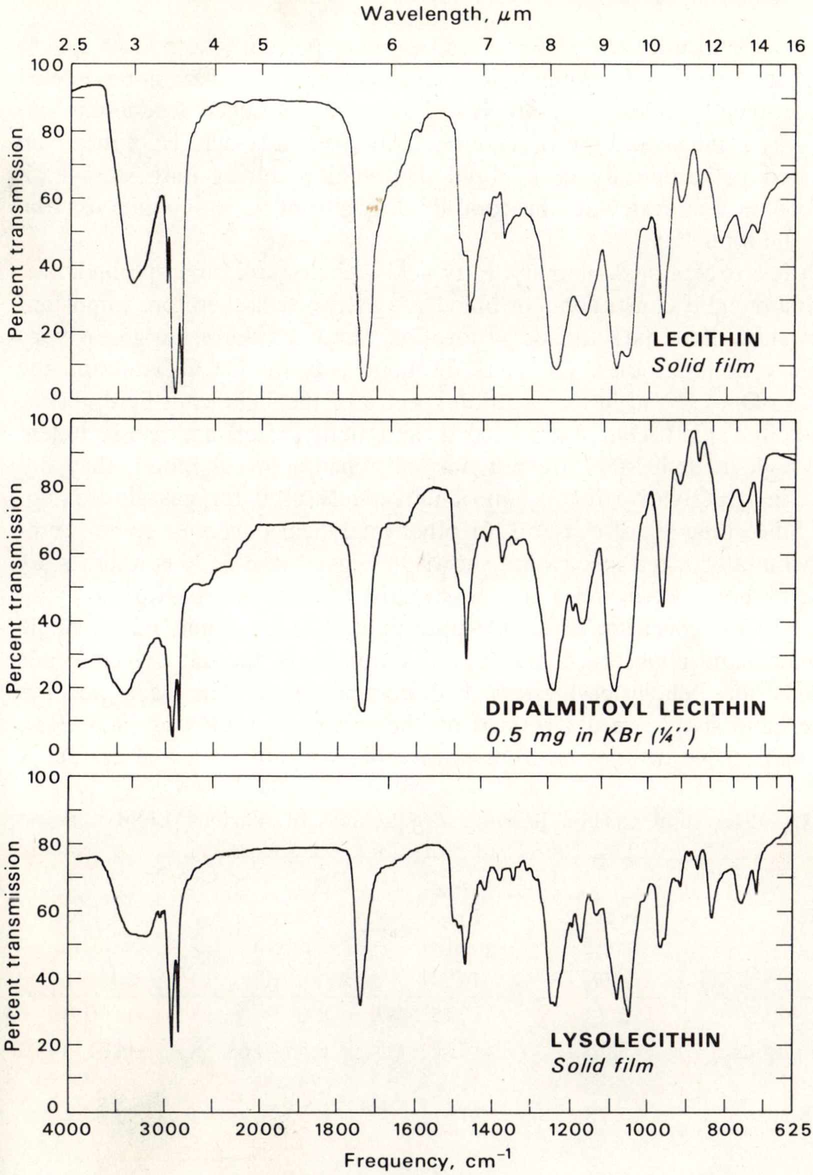

Fig. 12 Infrared spectra of lecithin (egg, Analabs) ~ 0.02 mm; dipalmitoyl lecithin (Supelco), solid; and lysolecithin (Supelco) ~ 0.01 mm.

Fatty acids in unesterified form are normally present in blood as a very small percentage of the total lipids. Consequently they are not detected spectroscopically unless they are isolated—or an enriched fraction is obtained—by some separation procedure. If the free-fatty-acid level in serum is elevated pathologically or by lipid degradation during long storage, it may become manifested in the total-lipid spectrum as a shoulder on the side of the ester band.

With few exceptions—namely, fatty acids, cholesterol, and sphingolipids—the major lipid constituents in blood are esters. It is therefore important to know how the characteristic absorption bands of the ester group vary from one type to another. The peak frequencies of the C=O band and the major C—O—C band in the solution spectra of the significant lipid classes are listed in Table I. Data for fatty acids and methyl esters are also included.

Although methyl esters are not normal constituents of blood, they are a convenient derivative form, almost universally used for gas chromatography. Since they are also useful for other analytical purposes, some representative methyl ester spectra are shown in Figs. 4 and 5. It is noteworthy that the carbonyl frequencies are measurably different for the various types of ester. In the spectrum of a total-lipid extract from serum only a single absorption band is observed, but it is a composite of the unresolved bands of triglycerides, cholesteryl esters, and phospholipids. The peak position and the band shape are determined by the relative amounts of each class. It is thus possible to infer on a qualitative basis whether a given extract is

Table I. Ester- and Carboxyl-Group Frequencies of Various Lipid Classes[a]

	C=O		C—O[b]	
Lipid Class	Wave-length (μm)	Fre-quency (cm^{-1})	Wave-length (μm)	Fre-quency (cm^{-1})
Triglycerides	5.73	1745	8.6	1160
Phospholipids (esters)	5.76	1737	8.55–8.6	1165–1170
Cholesteryl esters	5.78	1731	8.55	1170
Methyl esters	5.74	1741	8.55	1170
Fatty acids	5.85	1710	7.8	1280[c]

[a] In carbon tetrachloride solution.

[b] Only the principal band of the C—O—C group is given. The second is not well identified.

[c] In fatty acids the C—O vibration is coupled with O—H bending, giving rise to a second band at about 7.1 μm (1410 cm^{-1}).

high or low in triglycerides (usually the most variable component). The use of the carbonyl band for quantitative analysis is discussed in Section IV.B.

The C—O—C absorption bands of the esters are somewhat broader than the C=O bands and less definitive in terms of their peak positions. However, each lipid class has a characteristic pattern of absorption between 8 and 10 μm (1250–1000 cm^{-1}) that serves to identify it. In methyl ester spectra (e.g., Fig. 5) there are three overlapping bands of increasing intensity at about 8.05, 8.35, and 8.55 μm (1240, 1200, and 1170 cm^{-1}, respectively). In triglyceride spectra the strong band at 8.6 μm (1160 cm^{-1}) is flanked by weaker absorptions at about 8.1 and 8.9 to 9.1 μm (1235 and 1125–1100 cm^{-1}, respectively). The cholesteryl ester pattern in this range is very similar to that of triglycerides except that the principal peak is sharper and at a slightly shorter wavelength (8.55 μm, 1170 cm^{-1}). In addition the spectra of cholesteryl esters contain a distinctive band of moderate intensity at about 9.9 μm (1010 cm^{-1}).

The spectra of monoglycerides and diglycerides resemble that of triglycerides to which have been added the principal absorption bands of the hydroxyl group (see Figs. 6 and 7).

The C—O—C absorption band of the ester group appears in the spectra of the glycerophosphatides (e.g., lecithin and phosphatidylethanolamine), but it is less prominent because of the much stronger phosphate ester bands. As might be predicted, it is absent from the spectrum of sphingomyelin.

The spectra of a number of cholesteryl esters were studied by Labarrère, Chipault, and Lundberg (27). In solid-state spectra of the saturated fatty acid esters they observed the usual band progressions (see Fig. 8) that are correlated with chain length. It was also noted that in the solid-laurate spectrum the 13.9-μm CH_2-rocking band has a single peak, whereas in the spectra of compounds with longer chains this band is a doublet. Labarrère et al. concluded that two different crystal forms are indicated, possibly governed by chain length. The unsaturated fatty acid esters are differentiated from each other and from saturated esters by the pattern of weak bands in the vicinity of 9 μm (1100 cm^{-1}). Small bands at 8.8 and 9.04 μm (1135 and 1105 cm^{-1}) increase in intensity with the degree of unsaturation, whereas another band at 8.94 μm (1120 cm^{-1}) decreases. The 8.8-μm peak is absent from the spectra of saturated esters. Although these differences appear to be distinctive, the bands are probably too weak to be of use in evaluating mixtures on the basis of relative intensities. Sinclair and co-workers (28) concluded that similar bands in the spectra of fatty acids are not suitable for analytical purposes.

Cholesterol is unique among the blood lipids in having no carbonyl group. Its principal spectral features are associated with the OH-group, the relative preponderance of CH_3-groups, and its cyclic structure. An O—H stretching absorption appears in dilute-solution spectra (Fig. 9) as a sharp band at 2.75 μm (3640 cm^{-1}). In concentrated-solution or solid spectra the band becomes broad, with the maximum absorption at about 3.0 μm (3330 cm^{-1}). The C—O stretching band at 9.5 μm (1055 cm^{-1}) is the most prominent band in the long-wavelength region of the spectrum. The five CH_3-groups of cholesterol enhance the 7.25-μm (1380-cm^{-1}) absorption in comparison with straight-chain compounds. The intensity of this band can be judged in relation to the 6.85-μm (1465-cm^{-1}) band, which on a mass basis is about the same for the two types of compound (cf. triolein, Fig. 7, and cholesteryl palmitate, Fig. 8).

It may be noted that there is considerable detail in the "fingerprint" region (beyond 7.5 μ) of the cholesterol spectrum, and it is virtually the same for solid and solution. This is in contrast to the straight-chain compounds, whose solid spectra contain numerous sharp bands that are absent from their solution spectra. This difference can be explained on the basis of the rigidity imparted to the cholesterol molecule by its condensed-ring structure. Thus its configuration does not change appreciably on going into solution, and its relatively complex spectral pattern is retained. On the other hand, straight-chain compounds, which exist in the crystal as extended planar zigzag chains, undergo deformations in solution (or the liquid state) as a result of internal rotations, with a consequent loss of spectral detail.

The infrared spectra of numerous phospholipids appear in the work of Rouser et al. (29) in connection with brain-lipid studies. Nelson has presented the spectra of phospholipids isolated from the plasma and erythrocytes of various species (30, 31) and pointed out some of the characteristic spectral features (32). The phospholipids as a class have in common the phosphate ester group, which is characterized in their spectra by a strong P=O absorption band at 8.1 to 8.3 μm (1235–1215 cm^{-1}) and a P—O—C band of about equivalent intensity between 9 and 9.5 μm (1100–1050 cm^{-1}). These two absorptions are the dominant features that distinguish phospholipids from the other lipids. Cerebrosides absorb strongly between 9 and 10 μm (1100–1000 cm^{-1}) because of their C—O(H) groups, but they can be distinguished from phospholipids by the absence of a P=O band in their spectra.

Within the phospholipid class, those that contain the glyceryl ester moiety show a carbonyl absorption at about 5.76 μm (1737 cm^{-1}). The spectra of sphingolipids, which do not have carboxylic ester groups, are characterized instead by the distinctive bands of *N*-monosubstituted amides at about 6.1 and 6.45 μm (1640 and 1550 cm^{-1}) (Fig. 10). The presence of choline in the molecule is empirically associated with a sharp band of moderate intensity at 10.35 μm (965 cm^{-1}). The bond origin of this band is not known, but it may be a C—N vibration that has gained intensity from the charge on the nitrogen atom. There is no absorption band at this point in the spectra of phosphatidylethanolamine (Fig. 10), cardiolipin (Fig. 11), or phosphatidylserine (Fig. 11), and it has also been shown to be absent from the spectrum of *N, N*-dimethylphosphatidylethanolamine (32).

In phospholipid mixtures the 965-cm^{-1} band provides a positive means of detecting the presence of choline-containing species, but there is no corresponding band for the ethanolamine group. Indeed, except for indications of choline and the amide group, the spectra of phospholipids are so similar that minor components cannot be detected in mixtures. The curve of lysolecithin resembles that of lecithin except that the ester carbonyl band is somewhat weaker relative to the phosphate absorptions (Fig. 12). The ratio should be reduced by half, but this is not obvious in the film spectra shown. The same considerations apply to the spectra of plasmalogen and phosphatidylethanolamine (Fig. 10). A spectrum of lecithin plasmalogen (phosphatidal choline) has been published by Gottfried and Rapport (33). The curve shows a distinct, well-resolved C═C stretching absorption band at about 6.05 μm (1650 cm^{-1}), as would be expected for an alkenyl ether. Except for this band and diminished ester absorptions, the spectrum resembles that of lecithin. Absence of the C═C absorption in the spectrum of ethanolamine plasmalogen (Fig. 10) is not readily explicable, except possibly on the basis of impurity.

About 70% of the phospholipids in human plasma are lecithin and about 20% are sphingomyelin, the remaining 10% being composed mostly of phosphatidylethanolamine and lysolecithin. Both major components contain choline, and this is reflected in the spectrum of the total-phospholipid mixture by the presence of a prominent 965-cm^{-1} band. The relative proportions of lecithin and sphingomyelin can be judged from the intensities of the ester and amide carbonyl bands, bearing in mind that their absorptivities are not equal. As indicated above, the minor constituents cannot be identified without prior isolation. Although phosphatidylethanolamine is a more prominent constituent of erythrocyte phospholipids (31) and the plasma phospholipids of some species (30), this is only revealed indirectly by a relatively less intense 965-cm^{-1} band.

In the spectrum of phosphatidylserine (Fig. 11) there is a band of significant intensity at about 6.05 μm (1655 cm^{-1}) whose origin is not entirely clear. Kimura and Nagai (34) studied the spectra of this compound in various forms and observed that the band is absent from the spectrum of the metal-free form. They prepared monosodium and disodium salts, however, and found bands at 1645 and 1610 cm^{-1}, respectively. The latter band is quite broad and more nearly at the expected COO^- position. Thus, though the absorption appears to be related to the ionized carboxyl group, the frequency is shifted out of the normal range, possibly as a consequence of some complex interaction among ionized groups.

The presence of absorption bands at about 3 and 6.1 μm (3300 and 1640 cm^{-1}) in the spectrum of lecithin is best accounted for by bound water. These bands appear in the spectra of both natural and synthetic lecithins, but their intensities may vary with treatment.

The separation and identification of individual fatty acids by gas chromatography has largely preempted this area of lipid characterization. Nevertheless it is pertinent to indicate some of the spectral manifestations of fatty acid chain structure. Most of these persist through the spectra of the various lipid classes and are thus independent of lipid type. For example, the spectra of palmitic acid (Fig. 4) and its various esters in the solid state all exhibit the same characteristic band progressions between 7.2 and 8.5 μm (1390–1180 cm^{-1}). In an isolated species the chain length can be determined from these bands (25).

Some absorptions related to double-bond structures have been discussed in Section III.A. In blood lipids the double bonds are almost exclusively of the *cis* unconjugated type. The bands attributable to *cis* unsaturation can be seen most easily in the spectra of methyl esters (Figs. 4 and 5). Increasing in intensity with the number of double bonds, they are C=C—H stretch, 3.3 μm (3020 cm^{-1}); C=C stretch, 6.05 μm (1640 cm^{-1}); C=C—H planar bending, 7.1 μm (1410 cm^{-1}); C=C—H nonplanar bending, 14.2 μm (700 cm^{-1}). In addition, there is a change in the pattern of the CH_2-bending bands. The decrease in the number of CH_2-groups is reflected by a weaker 6.8-μm (1465-cm^{-1}) band, whereas the 6.95-μm (1435-cm^{-1}) band becomes stronger because more of the CH_2-groups are adjacent to double bonds. These effects are not very pronounced at low levels of unsaturation, but at higher levels they should be detectable in the spectra of any of the lipid classes.

Of the other double-bond configurations only the *trans* isomers are of significance in relation to blood lipids. They are present chiefly as a result of ingesting hydrogenated fats (or in ruminants by bacterial action in the rumen). Detection is by means of the 10.35-μm (965-cm^{-1}) band in all classes except phospholipids, which have an interfering band. For this class detection is made possible by conversion to methyl esters. Methanolysis is also helpful in fatty acids and cholesteryl esters when the level of *trans* isomers is very low.

Branching in fatty acid chains is of secondary interest in blood lipids, although some gas-chromatography investigations have suggested the presence of trace amounts. Spectral indications of branching have been described by Freeman (35), and more extensive and detailed studies of branched-chain acids were made by Fischmeister (36). Branching increases the proportion of methyl groups, which results in an increase in the intensity of the methyl band at 7.25 μm (1375 cm^{-1}). If the branching is such that there are two methyl groups on the same carbon atom, this band is split into a doublet. There are characteristic bands for ethyl groups (12.9 μm, 775 cm^{-1}) and propyl groups (13.5 μm, 740 cm^{-1}) at the distal end of the chain. Branching near the carboxyl group alters the pattern of the bands normally appearing at 7.8 and 8.1 μm (1285 and 1235 cm^{-1}).

C. Lipoprotein Spectra

There are two aspects to the study of lipoproteins by infrared spectrometry. One has to do with intact lipoproteins and the qualitative information that can be derived from their spectra. The other relates to the determination of their lipid compositions by the use of infrared analysis.

The spectra of serum lipoproteins as dried films on silver chloride plates have been published (37). Examples of high-density (HDL) and low-density (LDL) lipoproteins are shown in Fig. 13. The spectrum of egg lipoprotein [Fig. 14 *A(b)*] is virtually identical with that of very-low-density lipoproteins (VLDL) from serum.[8] The principal protein bands are those of the peptide (H—N(—)—C(—)=O) group. The N—H stretching absorption appears at about 3 μm (3300 cm^{-1}), the carbonyl-stretching band appears at about 6.05 μm (1650 cm^{-1}), and the 6.45-μm (1550-cm^{-1}) band arises from a complex vibrational mode of which N—H bending is a major component. The remaining bands are identifiable with lipid absorptions, and their chemical structure assignments are as shown in the spectrum of serum-lipid extract (see Fig. 18 in Section IV.B).

The 1650- and 1550-cm^{-1} protein bands have been commonly designated as Amide I and Amide II bands, respectively. Their use in the interpretation of protein structure goes back to the work of Ambrose and Elliott (38), who observed different band positions for folded-chain (α) and extended-chain (β) structures in the spectra of protein films. (The α-helix model had not yet been advanced.) Theoretical considerations of the manner in which the amide-group vibrations are affected by chain structure have been discussed by Miyazawa and Blout (39). More recently the frequency correlations have been examined for proteins in deuterium oxide solution by Susi, Timasheff, and Stevens (40, 41), who have given the following peak positions for the Amide I band in various structures: random

[8] These three major classes of lipoproteins are defined by their behavior in the ultracentrifuge under specified conditions (see Chapter 5).

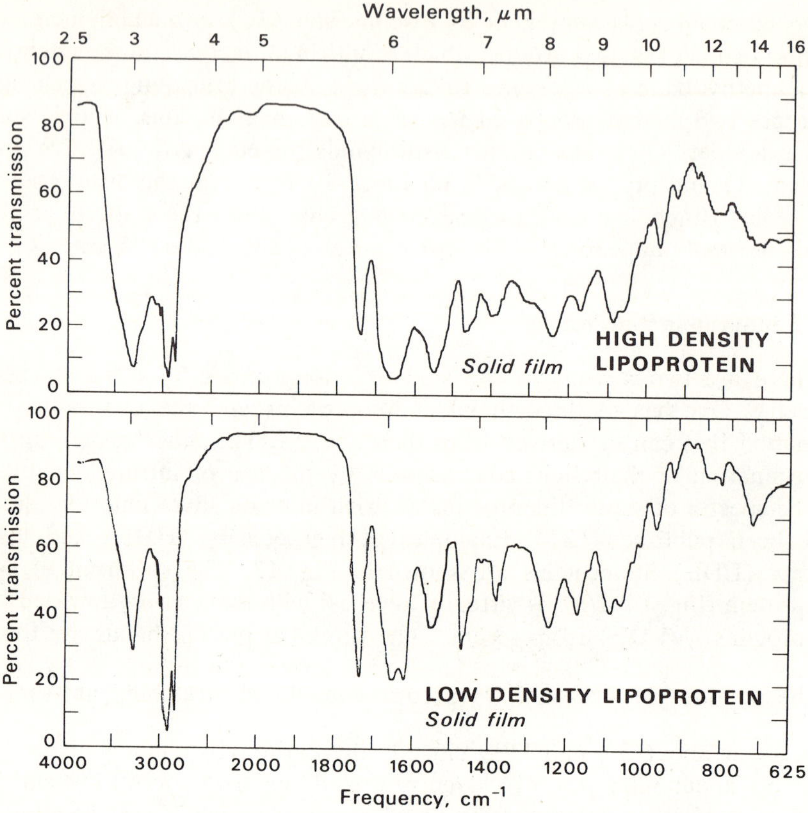

Fig. 13 Infrared spectra of serum lipoproteins; dried films on AgCl plates.

coil, 1640; α-helix, 1650; β (pleated sheet), 1625 cm^{-1}. In addition the antiparallel form of the β-structure has a weaker band at about 1680 cm^{-1} by which its presence can sometimes be recognized.

The spectrum of low-density serum lipoproteins in deuterium oxide solution has been studied by Gotto and co-workers (42), who observed a complex band with its principal maximum at 1625 to 1630 cm^{-1}, indicating a substantial proportion of β-structure. A distinct shoulder at 1640 cm^{-1} suggested the presence of some random coil, and another at 1680 to 1685 cm^{-1} implied that the β-structure is at least partly in the antiparallel form. A less well-defined shoulder was seen at 1650 cm^{-1}, indicating the possibility of some α-helix content. On addition of sodium decyl sulfate the β-peaks both disappeared, and the principal maximum shifted to 1650 cm^{-1}, the position characteristic of an α-helix. A shoulder at 1640 cm^{-1} (random coil) remained.

Dried-film spectra (Fig. 13) do not necessarily reflect the properties of lipoproteins in their native state. The low-density-lipoprotein spectrum appears to have two distinct peaks at about 1660 and 1625 cm^{-1}. The latter corresponds to the principal absorption maximum in deuterium oxide solution, attributed to β-structure. (Amide I frequencies are slightly higher in the solid state than in solution.) In the high-density-lipoprotein spectrum, however, only one absorption maximum is observed in the Amide I region at about 1650 to 1660 cm^{-1}. Thinner films do not reveal any other peaks, and 1650 cm^{-1} was reported for this frequency in a potassium bromide pellet preparation by Scanu and Granda (43). This broad band may be taken to indicate either an α-helix or a random-coil structure, or a mixture of the two. Scanu and Granda also concluded from circular-dichroism measurements that high-density lipoproteins contain a higher percentage ($\sim$ 70%) of α-helix than does the low-density class ($\sim$ 40%).

The infrared spectra of erythrocyte membranes in the form of dried films have been investigated by Maddy and Malcolm (44) and by Chapman, Kamat, and Levene (45). Except for relatively less intense lipid bands, these spectra bear considerable resemblance to the spectra of high-density lipoproteins from serum. Differences in lipid composition, and also the presence of a carbohydrate moiety, are responsible for small differences in the pattern beyond 8 μm (< 1250 cm^{-1}). The Amide I band appears at 1660 (44) or 1652 cm^{-1} (45), and no indications of β-structure are seen. Removal of the lipid by treatment with *n*-butanol does not alter the Amide I band, but heating with 50% ethanol at 70°C for 3 min results in the appearance of a second peak at about 1630 cm^{-1}. The spectrum in the amide region then resembles that of low-density lipoproteins (Fig. 13). The doublet peak, indicating partial transformation to the β-structure, was also observed by Chapman et al. in the spectra of erythrocyte membranes after treatment with various solvents. It did not, however, appear as a consequence of temperature change alone (−110 to +110°C).

In addition to the inferences regarding protein conformation in erythrocyte membranes, Chapman et al. (45) studied the 720-cm^{-1} CH_2-rocking absorption in the spectra of dried films. The fatty acid chains in the membranes are those of phospholipids, and the intensity of the CH_2-rocking band is taken as an indicator of the degree to which the CH_2-chains are extended in the all-*trans* zigzag configuration. In the membrane spectrum at room temperature the band is very weak, indicating very little of this structure. At lower temperatures the extended form is thermodynamically favored, and at −110°C the intensity of the 720-cm^{-1} band is significantly increased. In the spectra of lipid extracts from membranes the same relative intensity changes with temperature are seen, but at any given temperature the band is more prominent in the lipid spectrum than in the membrane spectrum. This observation seems to reflect a greater degree of disorder in the lipids when incorporated into the membrane structure. Some speculative interpretations of this difference were offered in terms of possible lipid–protein interactions.

With respect to the chemical composition of lipoproteins, the spectra of dried films provide little more than a qualitative indication of the lipid–protein ratio. This can be judged from the relative intensities of principal lipid bands (C—H, C—O) and protein bands (Amides I and II). These differences are apparent in the various lipoprotein spectra shown in Figs. 13 and 14. Although some tentative inferences about the major lipids are possible from the pattern beyond 8 μm, such spectra are not satisfactory for quantitative analysis. An early attempt to obtain quantitative information from them is exemplified by Fig. 14.

In this instance lipids were successively eluted from the lipoprotein film

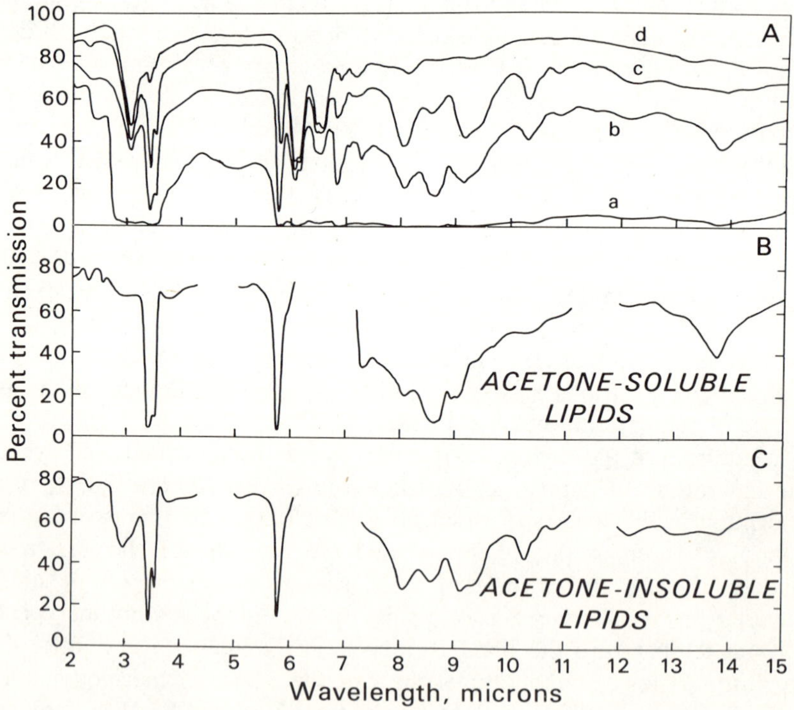

Fig. 14 Infrared spectra of egg lipoprotein and some of its components: (*A*) films (*a*, moist film; *b*, dried film; *c*, film after extraction with acetone; *d*, film after extraction with alcohol-chloroform, 1:1); (*B*) and (*C*) carbon disulfide solutions. (From Ref. 37. Reproduced by permission of the *Journal of Biological Chemistry*.)

by different solvents, taking advantage of the insolubility of phospholipids in acetone. Spectra of the lipid fractions in carbon disulfide solution are also shown. The spectrum of the acetone eluate of egg lipoprotein (or VLDL from serum) identifies it as principally triglyceride, whereas the corresponding eluates of low- and high-density lipoproteins have the spectral characteristics of cholesteryl esters. These eluates are nevertheless mixtures, which are not satisfactorily resolved by this method. Furthermore, solvent fractionation under these conditions is probably not reliable, so that this approach to quantitation is not very promising.

Lipoprotein lipids have been analyzed more successfully by extracting them from the isolated lipoprotein fractions and applying quantitative infrared methods, as described in Section IV. Results obtained by various combinations of these methods have been reported (46, 47). The compositions given by the most recent analyses (unpublished) are slightly revised from those previously found and are believed to be more reliable for the major components. Triglycerides and cholesteryl esters were determined by the two-component method (48) described in Section IV.B. In this procedure the adsorbed phospholipids were recovered and measured spectrometrically at the 9.15-μm (1090-cm^{-1}) peak (CCl_4 solution). This method does not yield a direct measurement of unesterified cholesterol, which is estimated either by difference or from cholesteryl esters, assuming that there is a constant ratio between free and esterified cholesterol. The latter assumption—although acceptable for total serum lipids—is not strictly true for the individual lipoprotein classes. Nevertheless the cholesterol results obtained by this method are more consistent than those obtained by difference. When calculated cholesterol values are added to the directly measured components, the average closures with total-lipid weight range from 96 to 102% in all classes except very-low-density lipoproteins (females). In this class the amount of material available was small (average 1.8 mg of lipid), and therefore the analytical accuracy was less than normal. Closures were more erratic, averaging about 90%. Although unesterified fatty acids may also be present in lipoproteins in very small amounts, they were not measured.

Composition data, determined for the three major lipoprotein classes from 16 normal males and 16 normal females (both nonfasting), are summarized in Table II. The standard deviations indicate that very-low-density lipoproteins exhibit greater variability in all components. This is consistent with the greater variability in density distribution within this class but may be due in part to lower analytical accuracy for the small amounts of lipid available. These data are cited here mainly as an illustration of infrared analysis and are not discussed further. They may be compared with the more extensive data on lipoprotein composition presented in Chapter 5 and in Part III of this volume.

Table II. Lipid Composition of Principal Serum-Lipoprotein Classes, by Infrared Analysis

Lipoprotein Class	Lipid Composition[a] (Average Percentage in Total-Lipid Extract ± S.D.)			
	Triglycerides	Cholesteryl Esters	Phospholipids	Unesterified Cholesterol[b]
VLDL:				
Males	60.4 ± 6.6	17.2 ± 3.7	19.0 ± 3.5	3.4 ± 0.7
Females	58.1 ± 4.5	20.6 ± 3.2	17.1 ± 5.0	4.2 ± 0.7
LDL:				
Males	9.4 ± 2.4	55.1 ± 1.5	24.4 ± 2.3	11.0 ± 0.3
Females	9.3 ± 2.3	53.4 ± 1.5	26.7 ± 1.8	10.6 ± 0.3
HDL:				
Males	8.8 ± 2.3	42.7 ± 2.2	40.1 ± 2.4	8.4 ± 0.4
Females	6.8 ± 2.1	41.8 ± 2.3	43.1 ± 1.7	8.3 ± 0.4

[a] Analyses of ultracentrifugal preparations from the sera of 16 normal males and 16 normal females (both nonfasting). Values have been adjusted proportionally to total 100% of extracted-lipid weight. (These data were obtained as part of an ultracentrifugal study discussed in some detail in Chapter 5 of this volume.)
[b] Not measured (calculated as cholesteryl esters × 0.198).

IV. QUANTITATIVE ANALYSIS

A. Measurements

The basic principles of spectrophotometry are applicable in the use of infrared absorption as a method of quantitative analysis (4, 49). The fundamental physical measurement is that of light intensity—or, more appropriately in the infrared, radiant power. The power is supplied by the radiation source; a narrow-wavelength interval is selected by the monochromator; and the emerging energy is measured by the thermocouple. The resultant electrical signal is proportional to the intensity I_0, which is to be compared with I_s, the corresponding energy measurement when an absorbing substance is placed in the radiation beam. The ratio of I_s to I_0 is the transmittance T of the sample. (In double-beam spectrophotometers, as described in Section II.A, I_s and I_0 are measured in separate sample and reference beams.)

Since transmittance is exponentially related to the concentration of the absorbing substance, a useful function is the absorbance A, which is equivalent to optical density and is defined as

$$A = -\log_{10} T = \log_{10} \frac{I_0}{I_s} \tag{2}$$

For a given substance at a given (monochromatic) wavelength λ the absorbance is determined by three factors:

1. The concentration C of the substance.
2. The path length b through the substance.
3. The absorptivity a_λ of the substance at wavelength λ.

The factors b and C define the number of molecules in the light path. Absorptivity (equivalent to the extinction coefficient) is equal to the absorbance at unit concentration and unit path length and is an intrinsic property of the substance. (The variation of absorptivity with wavelength is implicit in the spectral absorption curve.) The relationship of these factors is expressed as the well-known Beer–Lambert law:

$$A_\lambda = a_\lambda bC \tag{3}$$

For instrumental reasons it has not been generally possible in the infrared to establish absolute absorptivity values that can be used with confidence in all spectrophotometers. Furthermore, at the small path lengths used it is hazardous to rely on measured cell thicknesses. Rather it is common practice to carry out empirical calibrations with pure standard compounds in the same cell that is to be used subsequently for the analysis. If the working curve of absorbance versus concentration is a straight line, Equation 3 can be reduced to

$$A_\lambda = k_\lambda C \tag{4}$$

where k_λ, the empirically determined slope, represents a combination of a_λ and b for the particular cell.

A plot of A_λ versus C can be nonlinear for reasons that involve the relationship between band shape and spectral slit width. To avoid curvature from this cause, measurements should be made at band peaks rather than on steep sides of bands, and the spectral slit width should be kept narrower than the absorption-band width. The latter requirement may be in conflict with the necessity for a wide enough slit width to provide adequate energy for measurement, but in a grating instrument with slit control this does not usually present any difficulty.

Another possible cause of nonlinearity in the calibration of substances in solution is a change in band shape resulting from solute–solute interaction. Such interactions tend to increase with concentration and can be minimized by working in a low concentration range. This in turn may require the use of cells with relatively long path lengths. For most lipids that are soluble in carbon tetrachloride or carbon disulfide concentrations lower than 10 mg/ml in a 1.0-mm cell are satisfactory, and good approximations to linearity are usually obtained.

For quantitative measurements the use of dilute solutions has definite advantages over solid or undiluted liquid samples. If the amount of a lipid sample is about 2 mg or more, the technique is simple and straightforward and does not require accessory equipment. The minimum volume of solvent needed for a 1.0-mm cell is about 0.5 ml, which is large enough for solution volumes to be accurately measurable. Constancy of path length is ensured if all measurements are made in the same fixed-thickness cell. Furthermore, a duplicate cell filled with pure solvent in the reference beam is probably the most effective type of background cancellation. Pure solvent in *both* cells represents a zero concentration point, for which the instrument can be adjusted to read 100% T (or an appropriate correction can be made). Thin cells ($\leqslant$ 0.1 mm) are not very suitable for solution analysis because higher concentrations are necessary and the correspondingly smaller volumes are less accurately measurable. Moreover, the greater "dilution" of the solvent in the sample cell can cause a serious disparity with the amount of pure solvent in a matching reference cell. A variable-thickness reference cell is a possible means of correcting the solvent imbalance in that case.

Analysis in solution can be extended to the submilligram range by using microcells. Still longer path lengths (> 1 mm) are desirable to increase sensitivity and minimize volume-measurement problems. Solvent interference then becomes more likely, however.

If analysis in solution is precluded by insolubility, by solvent obscuration of the absorption band to be measured, or by a sample size that is too small, the potassium bromide pellet technique can be used. It is probably the only practicable technique for amounts smaller than about 100 μg. For a given pellet die the thickness of the pellet formed is proportional to the weight of potassium bromide. If the concentration is expressed on a weight-per-weight basis, Equation 3 becomes

$$A_\lambda = a_\lambda(kW)\left(\frac{w}{W}\right) \tag{5}$$

where k is a constant relating thickness to weight, W is the weight of the pellet, and w is the weight of sample in the pellet. The expression further reduces to

$$A_\lambda = k'w \tag{6}$$

where k' is the product of a_λ and k.

Thus the calibration can be established as absorbance versus sample weight, independent of pellet weight, provided all of the sample is in the pellet. If material is lost in preparing the pellet or only a portion of the total (sample–KBr) mixture is used, it is necessary to know both the weight of the pellet and the weight of the total mixture in order to account for the difference. Since the potassium bromide is usually weighed, and less than 1% of sample is added, the weight of the potassium bromide can be used as the total mixture weight.

The use of an internal standard in potassium bromide pellets was described by Wiberley, Sprague, and Campbell (50). In this procedure quantitation is based on the intensity ratio of an absorption band of the analyte and a band of a suitably chosen compound that is incorporated into the pellet in known amount. The requirements on the internal standard are that its spectrum be relatively simple, so as not to have too many interfering bands, and that it have a well-isolated band of sufficient intensity to be suitable as the reference band. Substances that have been used are potassium thiocyanate, lead thiocyanate, and potassium ferricyanide. In all of these the nitrile absorption is the reference band. If the amount of the internal standard is kept constant, we can write Beer's law expressions for the two independent bands and divide, obtaining

$$\frac{A_1}{A_2} = \frac{a_1 b C_1}{a_2 b C_2} = k C_1 \tag{7}$$

where the subscript "1" refers to the sample and subscript "2" to the standard. The ratio a_1/a_2 is constant, b/b is unity, and together with C_2 they can be combined into the constant k.

Oil mulls and films, either liquid or solid, are unfavorable sampling forms for quantitative analysis. They are neither accurate nor reproducible in thickness, and in the case of films deposited by evaporating solutions they are apt to be nonuniform as well. The internal standard method was proposed for mulls by Barnes et al. (51). In principle it is applicable to films, but its practical utility has evidently not been explored.

A method that is often useful for determining a minor component of a mixture is differential analysis. This is also applicable when the absorption band to be measured is overlapped by the band of another component. The procedure is essentially the solution procedure, except that as a reference pure solvent is replaced by a solution containing all the sample components other than the one to be determined. The absorption of the "other" components is thereby balanced out in the two beams. The band to be measured becomes more distinct, and the background is flattened out. The feasibility of this method will depend on the complexity of the mixture and needs to be evaluated for a particular problem. Robinson (52) has shown that optimum accuracy is attained when the concentration is adjusted to 37% transmittance without any compensation in the reference beam.

Whereas in solutions the transmittance of pure solvent establishes an I_0, or background level, potassium bromide blanks are not reproducible enough to be used as a reference for pelletized samples. The scattering background is much too variable from pellet to pellet, and especially from blank to sample. Under these circumstances it is necessary to estimate the I_0 value by somewhat arbitrary empirical methods.

One such approach is commonly called the base-line method, illustrated in Fig. 15. It consists of connecting two suitably chosen points, one on each side of the absorption band being measured, by a straight line. The

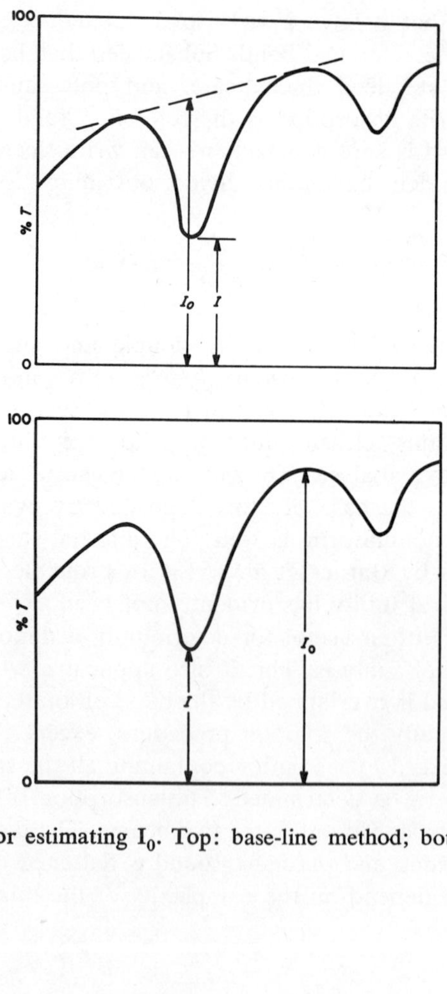

Fig. 15 Methods for estimating I_0. Top: base-line method; bottom: empirical ratio method.

ordinate value of this line at the wavelength of the band peak is taken as I_0. The case illustrated shows a well-separated absorption band, and the base line is drawn tangent to the curve near the adjacent transmission maxima. It is intended to be an objectively constructed representation of what the curve might be if the absorption band were not there.

An alternative method is the empirical ratio, also shown in Fig. 15. Here I_0 is taken as one of the transmission maxima adjacent to the absorption band.

In the simple cases illustrated the base-line method might seem to be the more rational choice. However, the true value of I_0 may lie somewhere between these two approximations, and only trial and error will show which is better. The choice may be even less obvious when the spectrum is more complex, with multiple or overlapping bands in the region of interest.

The contribution of instrumental measurement error to the overall analytical error can be estimated if it is assumed that the (transmittance) scale error is constant over the whole scale and applies equally to the 0%, 100%, and transmittance measurements. It was shown by Robinson (53) that a 1% scale-reading error leads to a minimum concentration error of about 3.5% at a transmittance value of 37%. The error increases at higher and lower transmittance values, becoming 4% at about 20 and 60% *T*, and 6% at about 10 and 75% *T*. At still higher and lower transmittances the error curve rises quite steeply, and it is generally recognized that these extremes should be avoided if possible. The better classes of modern spectrophotometers should be capable of precision well within 1%. If this measurement is the limiting error, and transmittances are kept between 20 and 70%, analytical precision of 3% or less should be possible. Background estimation in the spectra of solids is obviously subject to greater error than solution measurements. This reemphasizes the superiority of the solution mode.

The foregoing discussion has dealt mainly with the determination of a particular component by a single absorbance measurement. A simple example is the measurement of the amount of an isolated lipid or lipid class. In other cases, where more than one substance is present, the extraneous absorbances are considered as background and are accounted for by a suitably constructed base line or by a differential technique. For a mixture of only two components whose total amount is known one can establish a working curve for one component and determine the other by the difference.

To analyze for all *n* components of a mixture it is necessary (a) to know the components and (b) to be able to calibrate them independently with pure standards. Essentially the method consists of measuring *n* absorbances at n appropriately chosen spectral positions and inserting them in n linear equations:

$$\begin{aligned} C_1 &= k_{11}A_{\lambda_1} + k_{12}A_{\lambda_2} + \cdots + k_{1n}A_{\lambda_n} \\ C_2 &= k_{21}A_{\lambda_1} + k_{22}A_{\lambda_2} + \cdots + k_{2n}A_{\lambda_n} \\ &\vdots \\ C_n &= k_{n1}A_{\lambda_1} + k_{n2}A_{\lambda_2} + \cdots + k_{nn}A_{\lambda_n} \end{aligned} \tag{8}$$

where C_n is the concentration of the nth component, $A_{\lambda n}$ is the measured absorbance at λ_n, and each k_{ij} is a constant. The values of k_{ij} are derived by matrix inversion of the a terms in the set of equations:

$$\begin{aligned} A_{\lambda_1} &= a_{11}C_1 + a_{12}C_2 + \cdots + a_{1n}C_n \\ A_{\lambda_2} &= a_{21}C_1 + a_{22}C_2 + \cdots + a_{2n}C_n \\ &\vdots \\ A_{\lambda_n} &= a_{n1}C_1 + a_{n2}C_2 + \cdots + a_{nn}C_n \end{aligned} \tag{9}$$

where a_{ij} is the calibration coefficient of the jth component at λ_i. This formulation is based on the assumptions that (a) the individual calibration curves of all components at all wavelengths are linear; (b) the individual absorbances are independent and additive. Except in unusual cases of interaction between components, the latter assumption is generally valid. The first assumption (Beer's law) is tested in the course of calibration, and for most lipids in dilute solution the approximations to linearity are acceptable.

A further condition to be fulfilled is that for each component a wavelength (absorption band) can be chosen at which that component is the major absorber and all others absorb substantially less. Inability to meet this condition precludes the use of this multicomponent method for many complex mixtures, although in favorable cases as many as 10 components have been analyzed successfully. The problem of matrix inversion can now be handled easily by computers, although for just two components the arithmetic is very simple. Some useful two-component lipid analyses are cited in the next section.[9]

[9] A more extensive treatment of multicomponent analysis is given in Ref. 49, p. 403.

B. Analysis of Blood Lipids

Since infrared-absorption measurements are made almost exclusively in nonaqueous media, the analysis of blood lipids requires a preliminary extraction. Methods of extraction are discussed in Chapter 1 and are only touched on briefly here. In most instances a total-lipid extract is obtained and subsequent fractionation of some sort is carried out. Procedures that are adequate for extracting all of the lipids also carry along some nonlipid material, which should be removed as a first step of purification. For serum the method of Sperry and Brand (54) is generally satisfactory. The solvent used is chloroform–methanol (2 : 1, v/v), and the nonlipid material extracted is removed by a water wash. Nelson (31) has described a procedure for the extraction of red cells, in which chloroform–methanol is also used as the solvent. In this case the subsequent removal of nonlipid contaminants is accomplished by a gel-filtration technique, slightly modified from that of Siakotos and Rouser (55). Other extraction procedures may be adopted in special circumstances, and in consideration of the particular lipids to be determined and the type of fractionation to be employed.

The amount of a total-serum-lipid extract—purified as described above —can be determined with an accuracy and reproducibility of about $\pm 3\%$, as compared with weight measurement. This is done by measuring the absorbance in carbon tetrachloride solution at the CH_2-bending frequency, 6.8 μm (1465 cm^{-1}). Calibration of the various major components at this spectral position gives absorption coefficients that are all within a 10% range. Using an average value weighted according to a normal serum-lipid composition results in closer agreement. Wide variations in fatty acid chain length or degree of unsaturation would affect the intensity of this band and cause larger errors. Presumably the C—H stretching band near 3.45 μm (2900 cm^{-1}) could be used in a similar way, although the corresponding calibrations have not been carried out. These bands would be more suitable for microanalysis, since they are more intense and also more free from the solvent interference that may be encountered in cells with longer path lengths.

Any available separation method may be used to isolate lipid classes or to simplify the lipid mixture to be analyzed. In practice column or thin-layer chromatography is the most generally useful. These methods are also treated elsewhere in this volume and are described only minimally here as necessary. Better separations are usually possible by thin-layer chromatography, but the amounts are small enough to require micro-sampling techniques for infrared measurement, especially with the less abundant lipid species. Column chromatography can provide adequate sample sizes, but for some lipid classes the separation problem is formidable.

For an isolated lipid class the infrared analysis is straightforward. Taking account of possible spectral variations within the class, any absorption band—preferably a strong one—may be chosen for calibration and measurement. It should be noted, for example, that in an ester class (e.g., cholesteryl esters) containing several fatty acids the carbonyl absorption is proportional to the concentration of C=O groups. Calibration on a molar-concentration basis is therefore strictly valid, whereas for weight calibration an average molecular weight must be assumed. This is the same assumption that is commonly made in other methods of analysis, and it is not unreasonable for the fatty acid compositions normally encountered in blood lipids. It should be borne in mind, however, in unusual situations, such as the administration of high levels of medium-chain fatty acids in the diet.

A method for determining the major serum lipids by a combination of column chromatography and infrared measurement was devised by Freeman and co-workers (56). In view of the difficulty of isolating all of the lipid classes, they adopted a simplified, more manageable procedure in which only three fractions are obtained. Using small silicic acid columns (0.25 or 1.0 g), the total-lipid extract from 1.0 ml of serum is applied in hexane and eluted successively with hexane–chloroform (95 : 5), chloroform, and methanol. Each fraction is evaporated to dryness and redissolved in a known volume of carbon disulfide or carbon tetrachloride for infrared measurement.

Typical spectra are shown in Fig. 16. The first fraction contains only cholesteryl esters, which can be determined from the absorbance of the ester carbonyl band. The second fraction is a mixture of triglycerides, unesterified cholesterol, and unesterified fatty acids. Normally the amount of fatty acids is too small to be measured and its contribution to the spectrum (5.85 μm, 1710 cm^{-1}) can be ignored. In this case the concentration of triglycerides is found directly from the ester carbonyl band. (Cholesterol does not absorb in the carbonyl region.) The absorbance is then measured at the cholesterol peak at 9.5 μm (1050 cm^{-1}) and corrected for the contribution of the already calculated amount of triglycerides. The corrected absorbance value gives the cholesterol concentration. In cases where significant amounts of unesterified fatty acids are present, a two-component analysis based on the overlapping C=O bands is carried out, and a double correction is applied to the cholesterol-peak measurement. This method has been used in lipolysis experiments to follow the production of free fatty acids (57, 58).

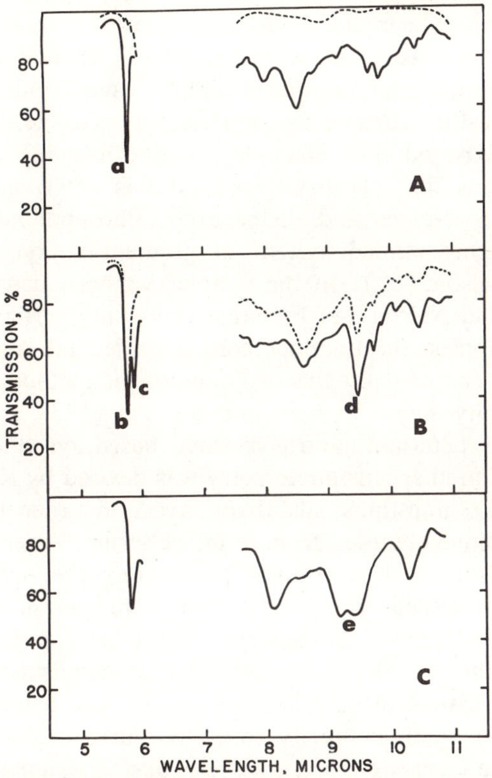

Fig. 16 Infrared spectra (carbon disulfide solutions) of serum-lipid fractions obtained by chromatography on silicic acid: (*A*) cholesteryl esters (broken curve is solvent background); (*B*) glycerides, fatty acids, cholesterol (two examples: broken curve, no fatty acids; solid curve, fatty acids present); (*C*) phospholipids. Lower case letters designate bands used for measurements. (From Ref. 56. Reproduced by permission of the *Journal of Biological Chemistry*.)

The fraction eluted by methanol consists of the total mixture of phospholipids. Its spectrum resembles that of lecithin, the only readily observable difference being a slightly lower relative intensity of the ester band due to the presence of 20% sphingomyelin. Among the stronger infrared bands, the best choice for absorbance measurement is one of the doublet peaks at about 9.1 and 9.4 μm (1100 and 1065 cm^{-1}). The absorptivities of the component phospholipids are nearly the same in this region, except that the absorptivity of phosphatidylethanolamine is slightly lower at the shorter wavelength peak. If this were a major constituent, the 9.4-μm peak would be preferable. The ester band at 5.76 μm (1737 cm^{-1}) can also be used, provided that the proportion of sphingomyelin is approximately constant in all samples. In the latter case the total-serum-phospholipid mixture is used as a calibration standard, whereas egg lecithin is a suitable reference material for the phosphate ester bands.

To the extent that further fractionation is possible, other individual lipids can be measured. For example, a more exacting chromatographic procedure, such as that of Hirsch and Ahrens (59), might be used to determine monoglycerides and diglycerides. Phospholipids can be separated by the highly refined system of gradient-elution chromatography developed by Nelson (60). In the simpler versions described earlier by Freeman (13) and Nelson and Freeman (61) only partial separations are achieved. Nevertheless the fractions containing lecithin and sphingomyelin together can be analyzed by the two-component method, using the ester and amide carbonyl bands at 5.76 and 6.1 μm (1737 and 1640 cm^{-1}).

A method for determining triglycerides based on thin-layer chromatography and infrared spectrophotometry was devised by Krell and Hashim (62), who used 1-mm-thick adsorbent layers in order to accommodate the amounts of lipid obtained from 1 ml of serum. After development of the plate, the adsorbent was scraped from triglyceride spot areas and the triglycerides were eluted from it. Spectra were run in carbon disulfide solutions, and absorbance was measured at the ester carbonyl peak, using the base-line method. Under these conditions some curvature was noted in the absorbance-versus-concentration plot, and this could be taken into account either by reading directly from the curve or by a mathematical correction to the measured absorbance value. Presumably this method could be used for other components as well.

Triglycerides and cholesteryl esters in serum can be determined simultaneously by the two-component method (48). This analysis requires the removal of the phospholipids from the total-lipid extract and infrared measurements of the remaining mixture. Such a separation is also required in the currently used chemical methods for determining triglycerides (63). It may be accomplished by batch adsorption on silicic acid from chloroform or chloroform–acetone solution, or by adsorption on a column. Another alternative procedure is to combine the extraction and adsorption in a single step, as described by Mendelsohn and Antonis (64). The latter yields comparable results for triglycerides and only slightly less reliable results for cholesterol esters. However achieved, the mixture after phospholipid removal contains cholesteryl esters and triglycerides as the major components, with lesser amounts of cholesterol and unesterified fatty acids. Cholesterol has negligible absorption in the carbonyl region, and with few exceptions fatty acids are present in serum in small enough concentrations for their contribution to the ester peak absorbances to be ignored.

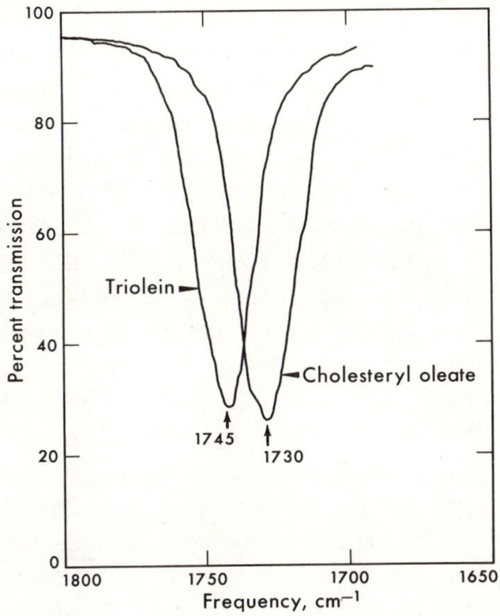

Fig. 17 Carbonyl absorption bands of triolein and cholesteryl oleate. Solutions in carbon tetrachloride: triolein, 3.11 mg/ml; cholesteryl oleate, 7.16 mg/ml. Cell thickness, 1.0 mm. Frequency scale expanded to five times normal. (From Ref. 48. Reproduced by permission of the *Journal of Lipid Research.*)

The overlapping carbonyl bands of cholesteryl esters and triglycerides are shown in Fig. 17. Measurements are made at the two peak positions. Where one component is the major absorber, there is a contribution to the absorbance from the side of the band of the other component. Thus not only good resolving power but also good reproducibility of frequency settings are needed. A grating instrument is preferred, but if other requirements are met, it may be possible to use a sodium chloride prism and very narrow slits. Absorbances are not measured on a recorded scan but at stationary points set manually. Calculations are made by a two-component matrix as already described. The prime virtue of this method is operational simplicity, and it is also nondestructive. By using a microcell it can be adapted to smaller quantities of serum, down to 0.1 ml.

A prototype instrument has been described for carrying out the triglyceride–cholesteryl ester analysis in a semiautomatic manner (65). This device incorporates a small single-beam grating spectrophotometer, which must be purged with dry air to minimize water-vapor absorption. It is equipped with a motor-actuated grating positioner, programmed to be set alternately at the two measurement frequencies. The transmittance measurements, represented by voltages, are first converted electronically to absorbances. These are multiplied by the predetermined constants of the matrix equations, and the appropriate terms are combined. Calculated results are displayed on a digital voltmeter and also printed on tape.

Infrared spectrometric analysis of total-unfractionated-lipid extract from serum has been undertaken (13), but with limited success. Examination of the spectrum of the total lipids (Fig. 18) with reference to the component spectra leads to the conclusion that the characteristic absorption bands for the various lipid classes are not sufficiently distinctive to permit a multicomponent analysis of the mixture in lipid-class terms. For example, the differentiation of triglycerides and cholesteryl esters in the presence of phospholipids is difficult if not impossible.

However, instead of the actual classes, components can be defined on the basis of significant absorption bands related to chemical groups. Thus the carbonyl band might be used for measuring total esterified fatty acids (TEFA), one of the phosphate ester bands might be used for the phospholipids (PL), and the CH_3-group band might be used for total cholesterol (TC). Since phospholipids contain esterified fatty acids, these three arbitrary components are not independent. It is necessary to define an artificial phospholipid as the residue obtained from the total phospholipids by removal of the esterified fatty acids (EFA). If it is assumed that the residue is a constant fraction of the total, the conversion can be made by a simple numerical factor. Calling this defined component residual phospholipid

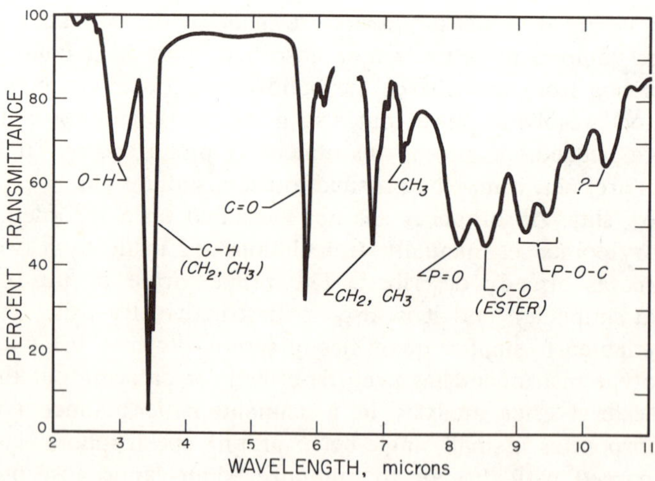

Fig. 18 Infrared spectrum of a total-lipid extract from serum (10 mg/ml in carbon tetrachloride). Cell thickness, 0.9 mm. (From Ref. 13. Reproduced by permission of the *Annals of the New York Academy of Sciences.*)

(RPL) and ignoring glycerol and free fatty acids, we have three things that add up to the total lipid (TL):

$$\mathrm{TL} = \mathrm{TEFA} + \mathrm{TC} + \mathrm{RPL}$$

Since each is associated with a different characteristic absorption band, it should be possible to set up a three-component analysis based on the usual equations:

$$\begin{aligned} A_{\lambda_1} &= a_{11}C_{\mathrm{TEFA}} + a_{12}C_{\mathrm{RPL}} + a_{13}C_{\mathrm{TC}} \\ A_{\lambda_2} &= a_{21}C_{\mathrm{TEFA}} + a_{22}C_{\mathrm{RPL}} + a_{23}C_{\mathrm{TC}} \\ A_{\lambda_3} &= a_{31}C_{\mathrm{TEFA}} + a_{32}C_{\mathrm{RPL}} + a_{33}C_{\mathrm{TC}} \end{aligned} \qquad (10)$$

where A is absorbance, C is concentration, λ_1 is 5.76 μm (carbonyl), λ_2 is 9.1 μm (phosphate ester), λ_3 is 7.25 μm (methyl), and a_{ij} is the calibration coefficient of component j at wavelength i.

To proceed according to this formulation it is necessary to evaluate the quantities a_{ij}, and here some difficulties are encountered. Whereas normally these would be calibration coefficients determined for specific compounds, in this instance, this is true only for cholesterol, and all others are derived. For example, a coefficient for total esterified fatty acids at λ_3 can be determined from separate calibrations of cholesteryl ester (CE) and unesterified cholesterol (UC). The assumption is made that the ester absorptivity is the weighted sum of its component absorptivities:

$$a_{\mathrm{CE}} = a_{\mathrm{EFA}}W_{\mathrm{EFA}} + a_{\mathrm{UC}}W_{\mathrm{UC}} \qquad (11)$$

where W is weight fraction.

The value of a_{EFA} (a_{31}) so obtained is in good agreement with the value derived from triglyceride calibration. For some of the other coefficients obtained in a similar way, however, there is greater variability, so that the use of average values leads to errors at extremes of sample composition.

At λ_1 only the ester groups absorb. For the various esters the absorbance per fatty acid (concentration) can be determined simply from the molecular-weight ratio of ester to fatty acid. Since the carbonyl-peak positions of cholesteryl esters, triglycerides, and phospholipids are not precisely the same, λ_1 has to be carefully selected so that a_{11} is as nearly equal as possible in all three classes. This point corresponds approximately to the phospholipid peak.[10] Since cholesterol does not absorb in the carbonyl region, and residual phospholipid has been defined to exclude fatty ester groups, both a_{12} and a_{13} can be set equal to zero. The first equation is thereby reduced to a single term, and the total esterified fatty acids can be

[10] This can be seen in Fig. 22 in the next section.

calculated independently from a single absorbance measurement. This can then be substituted in the other two equations, reducing each of them by one term. There remains then a 2×2 matrix, but the absorptivity of cholesterol at λ_2 is very small and can be neglected. This eliminates another term from the second equation. The concentration of residual phospholipids can be calculated from the remaining term and substituted in the third equation, which is then simply solved for cholesterol concentration. Thus the zero-absorptivity values permit the matrix calculation to be avoided altogether.

Operationally this method is extremely simple. Spectrophotometry is carried out directly on the purified serum-lipid extract dissolved in a measured volume of carbon tetrachloride. The information obtained is essentially that from separate chemical determinations of total cholesterol, total esterified fatty acids, and lipid phosphorus. (A total-lipid measurement can also be made at the same time.) The method has good precision and is accurate to about 5 to 10% in the normal range of serum-lipid compositions, for which its inherent assumptions and empirical averages are acceptable. However, it cannot be regarded as generally useful for a wide range of lipid compositions. Furthermore, it does not provide a good determination of triglycerides, since it would depend on calculations of difference between total fatty acids and the fatty acids of cholesteryl esters and phospholipids, just as in the older indirect chemical methods.

An infrared method has been used in conjunction with ultracentrifugal fractionation to measure serum chylomicrons at the microgram level (66). The isolation of the chylomicron-containing fraction is carried out by flotation in a sodium chloride density-gradient solution, using a swinging-bucket rotor. After centrifugation the top milliliter in the tube contains the serum lipoproteins whose Svedberg flotation constant (S_f) is greater than 400 and which are made up principally of the chylomicrons. Since the solution contains a known concentration of sodium chloride, it is possible to lyophilize an aliquot and prepare a pellet of sodium chloride in the manner described for potassium bromide. A microdie is used, forming a pellet 1.5 mm in diameter and containing about 5 mg of sodium chloride. For this size of pellet a beam condenser is used. The amount of chylomicrons that can be measured (without dilution) is 1 to 40 μg. Some curvature of the calibration curve is indicated above about 25 μg. Absorbance is measured at the triglyceride peak, using a base-line method, as shown in Fig. 19. Calibration is carried out with dilutions of a concentrated chylomicron preparation, in which the triglyceride content is known from independent analysis.

In addition to the determination of the lipid classes, there are some infrared analyses related to fatty acid characteristics. Since quantitation

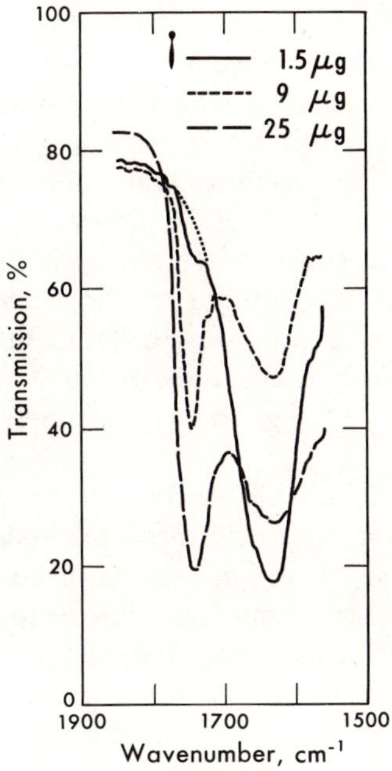

Fig. 19 Infrared-absorption bands of triglycerides (1745 cm^{-1}) and residual water (1640 cm^{-1}) in NaCl pellets (1.5-mm diameter) made from lyophilized chylomicron preparations. A base line for the solid curve has been sketched in (dotted curve). (From Ref. 66. Reproduced by permission of *Lipids*.)

of individual fatty acids is done largely by gas chromatography, the infrared methods are supplementary, or they are applied to mixed lipids or lipid classes for special purposes. Perhaps most significant are those related to unsaturation.

On the assumption that all of the double bonds in the fatty acids of blood lipids are of the *cis* unconjugated type, total unsaturation can be measured at either of two absorption bands. One of these bands is the (C=)C—H stretching absorption at 3.3 μm (3020 cm^{-1}). Sinclair et al. (28) proposed a method for the fatty acids, suitable also for triglycerides, methyl esters, and presumably other classes as well. In this method the ratio of the intensity of the 3020-cm^{-1} band to the difference between it and the CH_2-stretching intensity at 3.4 μm (2920 cm^{-1}) is plotted as a linear function of the number of double bonds per molecule. Since a ratio is used, the total concentration need not be known. An alternative is to plot the intensity of the 3020-cm^{-1} band against the degree of unsaturation, using a fixed ester concentration. With a sodium chloride prism instrument this band is not well enough resolved for good measurement, but any higher degree of resolution is satisfactory. A fluorite prism was used by Sinclair et al., and a grating is clearly adequate.

The other absorption band at which *cis* unsaturation can be measured is at 14.2 μm (700 cm^{-1}). Here resolution is not a problem. This band is overlapped by the CH_2-chain-rocking absorption at 13.9 μm (720 cm^{-1}), but it can be calibrated either directly or by a differential method (14). In the latter procedure triglycerides were used, with the sample being measured against tripalmitin (both in carbon disulfide at the same concentration: 40 mg/ml in a 0.9-mm cell). Calibration spectra are shown in Fig. 20. At low degrees of unsaturation this band (as well as the 3020-cm^{-1} band) is not very strong, so that relatively high concentrations are needed.

The determination of unconjugated *trans* isomers of unsaturated fatty acids is perhaps the best known infrared method in the chemistry of fats and oils, mainly because of its importance in connection with the hydrogenation process, but also because gas-chromatography separation of the isomers is difficult. The method was first described by Shreve et al. (67), and numerous variations of it have been published. One procedure has been adopted as Standard Method Cd 14–61 of the American Oil Chemists' Society.

The levels of *trans* isomer are low in blood lipids, and they are believed

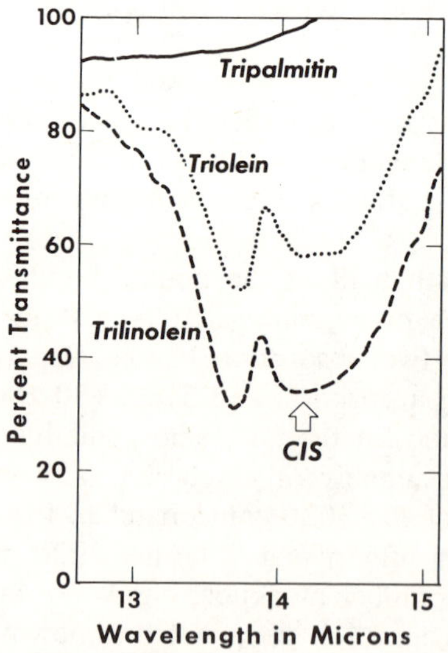

Fig. 20 The *cis*-double-bond absorption in triglycerides. Solutions in carbon disulfide, 40 mg/ml, 0.9-mm cells. Differential spectra, tripalmitin solution in reference cell. (From Ref. 14. Reproduced by permission of the *Journal of the American Oil Chemists' Society*.)

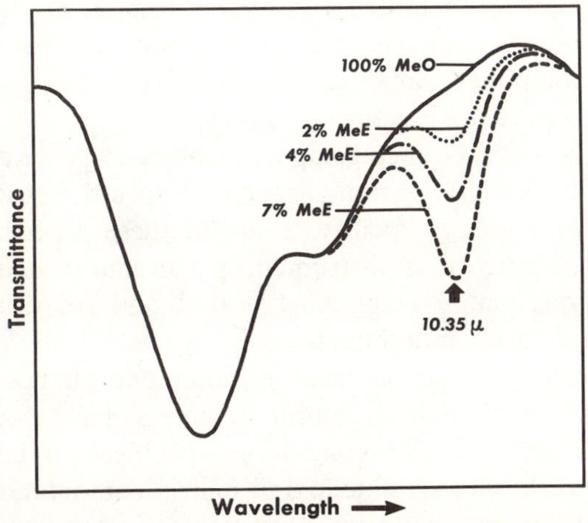

Fig. 21 Infrared spectra (9.5–10.5 μm) of mixtures of methyl oleate (MeO) and methyl elaidate (MeE) in carbon disulfide solutions, 15 mg/ml, 3.5-mm microcell. (From Ref. 14. Reproduced by permission of the *Journal of the American Oil Chemists' Society*.)

to be of exclusively dietary origin. No definitive study of them has been made, although an adaptation of the method and a few measurements have been reported (68). In this procedure the serum lipids are methanolyzed to obtain methyl esters. The ester spectra are recorded in carbon disulfide solution at a concentration of 15 mg/ml in a 3.5-mm microcell. Curves in the spectral interval between 9.5 and 10.5 μm (1050–950 cm^{-1}) are shown in Fig. 21 for various percentages of methyl elaidate in methyl oleate. Band intensities are measured by the base-line method, in which the 100% oleate curve approximates the background. By using the same solution for spectral measurement at 14.2 μm (700 cm^{-1}), the *cis* double bonds are determined in the same sample, thus giving total unsaturation.

It is possible to estimate the average chain length in mixed saturated fatty acids from the ratio of C—H to C=O absorptions (69), but this method is of little utility in the blood-lipid system. Also the estimation of the degree of branching from the CH_3-symmetrical-bending band (34) is not likely to be applicable, since branched acids—if they occur in blood lipids—are at most trace components.

C. Use of Computers

Specialized computing devices have been used for a long time in conjunction with infrared spectrometry. A particular application has been in connection with multicomponent analyses, in which large matrices are required. These can be handled by analog computers designed for this purpose, using absorbances measured in the usual way as input data. The automatic two-component analyzer mentioned in the preceding section contains simple computing circuitry of this type.

In recent years, with the increasing availability of general-purpose large-memory digital computers, various aspects of spectrometric data handling can be treated with greater facility. Some of these aspects are related to the techniques of correcting instrument performance, refining data and improving spectral quality (e.g., background and frequency corrections, peak location, and curve smoothing).

Applications of this type, as well as computer methods for spectrum identification and qualitative structural diagnosis, have been reviewed by Crisler (70). Other applications are more specifically related to analysis, and in addition to straight arithmetic and matrix computation these include the determination of integrated band intensities, resolution of overlapping bands, and component band summation.

For use by the computer the output of the spectrometer is first converted to digital form and stored on punched cards, magnetic tape, or punched paper tape. The spectrum is thereby represented as a sequence of transmittance or absorbance values measured at closely spaced intervals over the whole range. A limited spectral range may be selected for a specific purpose, and all or part of the spectrum can be plotted on any desired scale from the stored data.

Computer methods have been explored in connection with some infrared analyses of blood lipids (14). One approach is to use integrated band intensities, which are often more reliable than peak absorbances. A determination for which this method can be used is that of total esterified fatty acids, based on measurement of the ester carbonyl band. Although in the spectrum of a serum-lipid extract this band has a single peak, it is a composite of the absorptions of cholesteryl esters, triglycerides, and phospholipids.

The individual bands of these ester classes are shown on an expanded scale in Fig. 22. Concentrations have been adjusted to equivalent fatty acid concentration for all types. Although a curve is included for unesterified fatty acids at the same level, the amount of this component in serum is normally less than 10% of the total fatty acids. In the method described in the preceding section total esterified fatty acids are estimated from an absorbance measured at approximately the lecithin-peak position. At that point the absorbance per fatty acid is nearly the same for all three components. However, the measurement is off the peaks of both triglyceride and cholesteryl ester, and therefore highly dependent on the reproducibility of the frequency setting. It is particularly subject to errors at very high

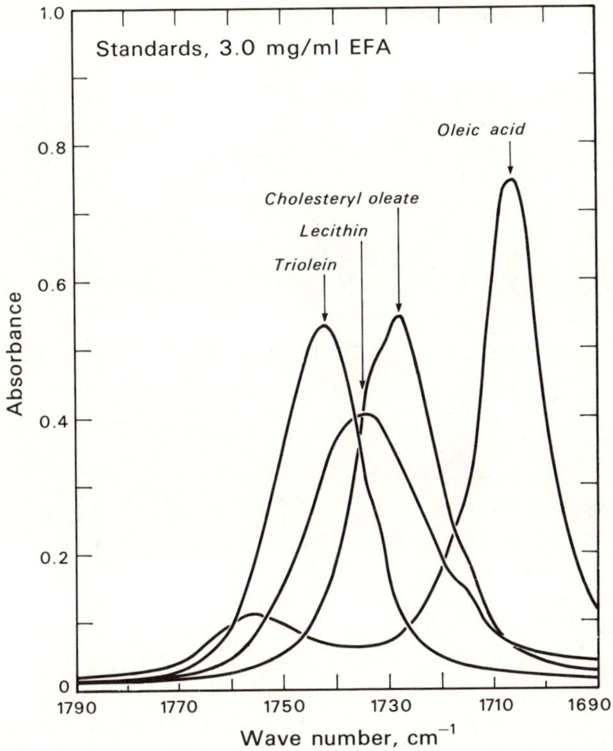

Fig. 22 Carbonyl absorption bands of representative serum-lipid types. The concentration of each has been adjusted to a fatty acid content of 3.0 mg/ml. Carbon tetrachloride solutions, 1.0-mm cell. (From Ref. 14. Reproduced by permission of the *Journal of the American Oil Chemists' Society*.)

or very low triglyceride content. The use of integrated band intensities avoids this difficulty and should be more reliable.

The integrated intensities used here are not absolute but are empirically measured band areas. Over the interval from 1690 to 1790 cm^{-1} a transmittance value is recorded every 0.5 cm^{-1}. These values are converted to absorbances, which are then summed and multiplied by 0.5 to obtain the area. This calculation is expressed as:

$$\text{band area} = B = \int_{\nu_1}^{\nu_2} A\,d\nu = \sum_{1690}^{1790} A\,\Delta\nu = 0.5 \sum_{1690}^{1790} A \qquad (12)$$

The band-area data for absorption by various lipids in this spectral interval are summarized in Table III. In this table the ranges of values

Table III. Carbonyl-Band Areas for Representative Lipids (1690–1790 cm^{-1}) (14)

Compound	C (mg/ml)	Band Area B[a]	B/C	B/C_{FA}[b]
Triolein	0.89–3.54	3.72–14.51	4.16 –4.09	4.35–4.28
Cholesteryl oleate	1.94–7.75	3.70–14.61	1.91 –1.83	4.42–4.22
Lecithin (egg)	2.38–5.96	7.71–19.16	3.24 –3.18	4.44–4.38
Methyl oleate	0.78–5.29	3.20–21.50	4.16 –4.06	4.37–4.26
Oleic acid	0.75–3.04	4.23–17.28	5.71 –5.63	5.71–5.63
Cholesterol	2.02–9.09	0.13– 0.48	0.063–0.053	—

[a] See Equation 12.
[b] C_{FA} = concentration of fatty acids (mg/ml).

correspond to indicated ranges of concentration. The value B/C does not vary appreciably in these ranges, indicating adherence to Beer's law. The constancy of B/C_{FA} over all four ester classes verifies that the band area per ester group is the same for all of the ester types and is therefore valid for their mixtures. In known mixtures that do not include unesterified fatty acids the accuracy of the determination has been estimated to be about ±2%. When free fatty acids are present, the error increases with their amount and reaches about 10% when the fatty acids comprise 10% of the total. This error can be reduced to less than 5% by choosing a narrower spectral interval (1770–1710 cm^{-1}), which excludes a large part of the fatty acid absorption band without seriously affecting the constancy of the ester-band area.

This procedure has also been applied to the measurement of total lipids, using the CH_2-bending band. It has been noted in the preceding section that the 6.8-μm (1465-cm^{-1}) peak can be used successfully for this determination in serum lipids. By the use of band areas it appears that the measurement is valid over a wider range of sample compositions. Figure 23 shows the band patterns for representative lipids, and two possible integration intervals are indicated.

In Table IV the areas are compared with peak absorbances for various lipid classes, some of which include fatty acids of differing unsaturation. The effect of unsaturation is clearly revealed in these data. The overall constancy with respect to both lipid classes and unsaturation is greatest in

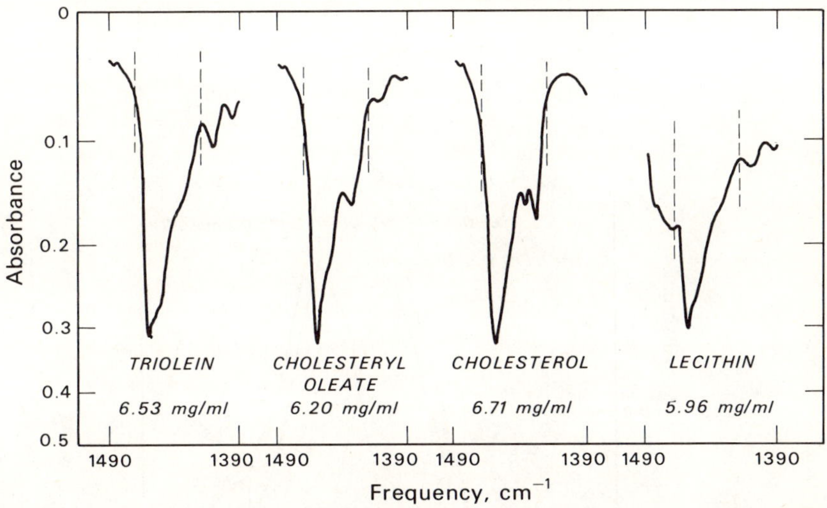

Fig. 23 Infrared spectra of representative serum-lipid types in the region of the CH_2-bending absorption. Roughly comparable concentrations in carbon tetrachloride, 1.0-mm cell. (From Ref. 14. Reproduced by permission of the *Journal of the American Oil Chemists' Society*.)

the integrated absorptivities of the narrower interval (1470–1420 cm^{-1}). This area therefore should be least affected by sample composition.

Another way of using the computer is to match the absorption curve of a mixture to the summation of the individual component curves, as

Table IV. Absorptivities of Various Lipids in the CH_2-Bending Band (14)

Compound	α, Peak[a]	β,[b] 1490–1390 cm^{-1}	β,[b] 1470–1420 cm^{-1}
Tripalmitin	0.0515	1.68	1.31
Triolein	0.0443	1.64	1.27
Trilinolein	0.0380	1.61	1.19
Cholesteryl palmitate	0.0509	1.49	1.25
Cholesteryl oleate	0.0476	1.50	1.24
Cholesteryl linoleate	0.0450	1.46	1.19
Cholesterol	0.0446	1.38	1.19
Lecithin (egg)	0.0424	2.08	1.31
Diolein	0.0428	1.77	1.30
Monoolein	0.0404	1.85	1.26

[a] α = absorbance per mg/ml.
[b] β = band area per mg/ml.

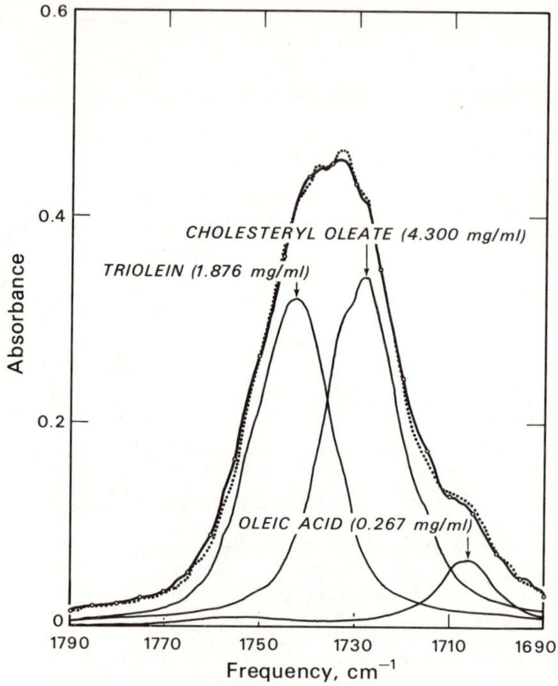

Fig. 24 Dotted curve is a computer plot of the recorded spectrum (1790–1690 cm^{-1}) of the mixture of the three lipid components indicated. The approximately superimposed solid curve is the summation of individual pure component (lower) curves, calculated as a least-squares fit. (From Ref. 14. Reproduced by permission of the *Journal of the American Oil Chemists' Society*.)

illustrated in Fig. 24. Here the dotted curve was regenerated from the spectrum recorded for a known mixture of triolein, cholesteryl oleate, and oleic acid. These represent the nonphospholipid serum components that can be measured in this spectral interval. The upper solid curve is the sum at every abscissa point of the ordinates of the three lower curves, which are the spectra of the standards. Component concentrations indicated for the standards are those determined by the computer by a least-squares curve-fitting method, such that the summation curve is the best possible fit to the recorded curve. The average error for triglycerides and cholesteryl esters in a series of such mixtures was about 3%. Since the amount of fatty acids is very small, the relative error for this component is high—about 20% at the level in the example used here. Although an accurate determination of free fatty acids is not to be expected under these conditions, a useful analysis for them should be possible by careful refinement of this method.

Two possibilities may be suggested for using a computer to assist in the analysis of total unfractionated serum lipids. One is an elaboration of the method outlined in the preceding section, wherein total lipids, total cholesterol, esterified fatty acids, and total phospholipids are determined. Modifications to that procedure might include replacement of peak absorbances by band-area measurements and the use of an iterative calculation with adjustable constants. The second approach is to analyze the carbonyl band for the three major ester components by the least-squares curve-fitting procedure mentioned above. A preliminary investigation of this method has been reported (14), but more development work is needed in these areas. Since neither method determines all components, some combination of them may be necessary for a total analysis.

There is a clear trend toward the use of computers in conjunction with several aspects of infrared spectroscopy, as there is indeed with nearly all analytical systems. Although the automation of relatively simple analyses is a worthwhile function, it is often the capability of performing more sophisticated or complex analyses that makes the computer attractive. In this respect blood lipids are still a challenge. As instrumentation develops, infrared spectrophotometers will become more adaptable to direct interfacing with computers, thereby eliminating the intermediate stage of recording data on tape. It seems probable that in the future most infrared analyses—possibly including blood-lipid analyses—will be "on line" with the computer.

V. ACKNOWLEDGMENTS

This work has been done under the auspices of the U.S. Atomic Energy Commission. The invaluable assistance of Mrs. Dorothy Sprague in preparing the manuscript is gratefully acknowledged.

REFERENCES

1. Potts, W. J., Jr., *Chemical Infrared Spectroscopy*, Vol. 1, *Techniques*, Wiley, New York, 1963.
2. Rao, C. N. R., *Chemical Applications of Infrared Spectroscopy,* Academic Press, New York, 1964.
3. Meloan, C. E., *Elementary Infrared Spectroscopy*, Macmillan, New York, 1963.
4. Szymanski, H. A., *Theory and Practice of Infrared Spectroscopy,* Plenum Press, New York, 1964.
5. Colthup, N. B., L. H. Daly, and S. E. Wiberley. *Introduction to Infrared and Raman Spectroscopy,* Academic Press, New York, 1964.
6. Colthup, N. B., *J. Opt. Soc. Amer.* **40**, 397–400 (1950).

7. Bellamy, L. J., *The Infrared Spectra of Complex Molecules*, Wiley, New York, **1958.**
8. Bellamy, L. J., *Advances in Group Frequencies*, Methuen, London, 1968.
9. Chapman, D., *The Structure of Lipids,* Wiley, New York, 1965, pp. 52–132.
10. O'Connor, R. T., *J. Amer. Oil Chem. Soc.* **33**, 1–15 (1956).
11. Schwarz, H. P., L. Dreisbach, R. Childs, and S. V. Mastrangelo, *Ann. N.Y. Acad. Sci.* **69**, 116–130 (1957).
12. Schwarz, H. P., in *Advances in Clinical Chemistry,* H. Sobotka and C. P. Stewart, Eds., Vol. 3, Academic Press, New York, 1960, pp. 1–34.
13. Freeman, N. K., *Ann. N.Y. Acad. Sci.* **69**, 131–144 (1957).
14. Freeman, N. K., *J. Amer. Oil Chem. Soc.* **45**, 798–809 (1968).
15. Holman, R. T., and P. R. Edmondson, *Anal. Chem.* **28**, 1533–1538 (1956).
16. Holman, R. T., S. Ener, and P. R. Edmondson, *Arch. Biochem. Biophys.* **80**, 72–79 (1959).
17. Tarpley, W., and C. Vitiello, *Anal. Chem.* **24**, 315–318 (1952).
18. Fridmann, S. A., in *Progress in Infrared Spectroscopy,* H. A. Szymanski, Ed., Vol. 3, Plenum Press, New York, 1967, pp. 1–23.
19. Mason, W. B., *Microchem. J., Symp. Ser.* **1**, 293–310 (1961); also Sparagana, M., and W. B. Mason, *Steroids* **2**, 245–252 (1963).
20. Leggon, H. W., *Anal. Chem.* **33**, 1295–1296 (1961).
21. Rouser, G., G. Kritchevsky, M. Whatley, and C. F. Baxter, *Lipids* **1**, 107–112 (1966).
22. McCoy, R. N., and E. C. Fiebig, *Anal. Chem.* **37**, 593–595 (1965).
23. Goldrick, B., and J. Hirsch, *J. Lipid Res.* **4**, 482–483 (1963).
24. Jones, R. N., A. F. McKay, and R. G. Sinclair, *J. Amer. Chem. Soc.* **74**, 2575–2578 (1952).
25. Meiklejohn, R. A., R. J. Meyer, S. M. Aronovic, H. A. Schuette, and V. W. Meloch, *Anal. Chem.* **29**, 329–334 (1957).
26. Wolff, I. A., and T. K. Miwa, *J. Amer. Oil Chem. Soc.* **42**, 208–215 (1965).
27. Labarrère, J. A., J. R. Chipault, and W. O. Lundberg, *Anal. Chem.* **30**, 1466–1470 (1958).
28. Sinclair, R. G., A. F. McKay, G. S. Myers, and R. N. Jones, *J. Amer. Chem. Soc.* **74**, 2578–2585 (1952).
29. Rouser, G., G. Kritchevsky, D. Heller, and E. Lieber, *J. Amer. Oil Chem. Soc.* **40**, 425–454 (1963).
30. Nelson, G. J., *Lipids* **2**, 323–328 (1967).
31. Nelson, G. J., *Biochem. Biophys. Acta,* **144**, 221–232 (1967).
32. Nelson, G. J., *Lipids* **3**, 104 (1968).
33. Gottfried, E. L., and M. M. Rapport, *J. Biol. Chem.* **237**, 329–333 (1962).
34. Kimura, Y., and Y. Nagai, *Biochem. J.* **77**, 3–4 (1960).
35. Freeman, N. K., *J. Amer. Chem. Soc.* **74**, 2523–2528 (1952).
36. Fischmeister, I., *Ark. Kemi* **20**, 353–367 (1962); *ibid.*, 385–397 (1962).
37. Freeman, N. K., F. T. Lindgren, Y. C. Ng, and A. V. Nichols, *J. Biol. Chem.* **203**, 293–304 (1953).
38. Ambrose, E. J., and A. Elliott, *Proc. Roy. Soc.* (*London*) **A208**, 75–90 (1951).
39. Miyazawa, T., and E. R. Blout, *J. Amer. Chem. Soc.* **83**, 712–719 (1961).
40. Susi, H., S. N. Timasheff, and L. Stevens, *J. Biol. Chem.* **242**, 5460–5466 (1967).
41. Timasheff, S. N., H. Susi, and L. Stevens, *J. Biol. Chem.* **242**, 5467–5473 (1967).
42. Gotto, A. M., R. I. Levy, A. S. Rosenthal, M. E. Birnbaumer, and D. S. Fredrickson, *Biochem. Biophys. Res. Commun.* **31**, 699–705 (1968).

43. Scanu, A., and J. L. Granda, in *Progress in Biochemical Pharmacology,* C. J. Miras, A. N. Howard, and R. Paoletti, Eds., Vol. 4, Karger, Basel, 1968, pp. 153–158.
44. Maddy, A. H., and B. R. Malcolm, *Science* **150**, 1616–1618 (1965).
45. Chapman, D., V. B. Kamat, and R. J. Levene, *Science* **160**, 314–316 (1968).
46. Freeman, N. K., F. T. Lindgren, and A. V. Nichols, in *Progress in the Chemistry of Fats and Other Lipids,* R. T. Holman, W. O. Lundberg, and T. Malkin, Eds., Vol. 6, Pergamon, London, 1963, pp. 228–233.
47. Ewing, A. M., N. K. Freeman, and F. T. Lindgren, in *Advances in Lipid Research,* R. Paoletti and D. Kritchevsky, Eds., Vol. 3, Academic Press, New York, 1965, pp. 50–51.
48. Freeman, N. K., *J. Lipid Res.* **5**, 236–241 (1964).
49. Bauman, R. P., *Absorption Spectroscopy,* Wiley, New York, 1962, pp. 364–433.
50. Wiberley, S. E., J. W. Sprague, and J. E. Campbell, *Anal. Chem.* **29**, 210–213 (1957).
51. Barnes, R. B., R. C. Gore, E. F. Williams, S. G. Linsley, and E. M. Peterson, *Ind. Eng. Chem., Anal. Ed.* **19**, 620–627 (1947).
52. Robinson, D. Z., *Anal. Chem.* **24**, 619–622 (1952).
53. Robinson, D. Z., *Anal. Chem.* **23**, 273–277 (1951).
54. Sperry, W. M., and F. C. Brand, *J. Biol. Chem.* **213**, 69–76 (1955).
55. Siakotos, A. N., and G. Rouser, *J. Amer. Oil Chem. Soc.* **42**, 913–919 (1965).
56. Freeman, N. K., F. T. Lindgren, Y. C. Ng, and A. V. Nichols, *J. Biol. Chem.* **227**, 449–464 (1957).
57. Shore, B., A. V. Nichols, and N. K. Freeman, *Proc. Soc. Exp. Biol. Med.* **83**, 216–220 (1953).
58. Young, W., and N. K. Freeman, *Proc. Soc. Exp. Biol. Med.* **90**, 463–466 (1955).
59. Hirsch, J., and E. H. Ahrens, Jr., *J. Biol. Chem.* **233**, 311–320 (1958).
60. Nelson, G. J., *J. Amer. Oil Chem. Soc.* **44**, 86–94 (1967).
61. Nelson, G. J., and N. K. Freeman, *J. Biol. Chem.* **234**, 1375–1380 (1959).
62. Krell, K., and S. A. Hashim, *J. Lipid Res.* **4**, 407–412 (1963).
63. Van Handel, E., and D. B. Zilversmit, *J. Lab. Clin. Med.* **50**, 152–157 (1957).
64. Mendelsohn, D., and A. Antonis, *J. Lipid Res.* **2**, 45–50 (1961).
65. Freeman, N. K., E. Lampo, and A. A. Windsor, *J. Amer. Oil Chem. Soc.* **44**, 1–4 (1967).
66. Hatch, F. T., N. K. Freeman, L. C. Jensen, G. R. Stevens, and F. T. Lindgren, *Lipids* **2**, 183–191 (1967).
67. Shreve, O. D., M. R. Heether, H. B. Knight, and D. Swern, *Anal. Chem.* **22**, 1261–1264 (1950).
68. Freeman, N. K., in *Semiannual Report,* Donner Laboratory, Lawrence Radiation Laboratory, UCRL-9897, 1961, pp. 96–102.
69. Keeney, P. G., *J. Amer. Oil Chem. Soc.* **39**, 304–305 (1962).
70. Crisler, R. O., *J. Amer. Oil Chem. Soc.* **45**, 818–822 (1968).

5. The Isolation and Quantitative Analysis of Serum Lipoproteins

FRANK T. LINDGREN and LIN C. JENSEN

Donner Laboratory of Medical Physics and Biophysics, Ernest O. Lawrence Berkeley Laboratory, University of California, Berkeley, California

FREDERICK T. HATCH

Bio-Medical Division, Ernest O. Lawrence Livermore Laboratory, Livermore, California

I. INTRODUCTION

During the last two decades there has developed a steadily increasing interest in, and literature on, human-serum lipoproteins and their relationship to health and disease. This followed the early pioneering work of Macheboeuf (1), McFarlane (2), the Cohn group (3), Pedersen (4), Gofman et al. (5), and others. In addition to a great variety of experimental studies with humans and animals, there has simultaneously developed a very substantial technology involving lipid and lipoprotein analysis. Because of the limitations of space we do not attempt to thoroughly review all this technology and its applications, since several comprehensive reviews are available (6–9).

Our main purpose is therefore to detail the present state of ultracentrifugal lipoprotein methodology as practiced at the Donner Laboratory. With the recent availability of high-speed, large-capacity computers, this technology has rapidly developed over the last few years. Essentially all procedures now involve at least one or more computer programs, many of which are constantly in a state of revision and improvement. In addition, computer programs are also used with each instrument involved in lipoprotein fractionation and analysis. For example, it would have been difficult to develop lipoprotein-subfractionation techniques on nonlinear density gradients without the aid of computer programs. Similarly the analysis of these subfractions by CHN elemental analysis is greatly facilitated by several computer programs.

After presenting the preparative and analytical ultracentrifugal methodology we consider some normal and clinical data illustrating the ultracentrifugal features of lipid and lipoprotein abnormalities. Then we discuss density-gradient procedures for the isolation of chylomicron-containing fractions and for the subfractionation of all major lipoprotein classes. Finally we consider the more widely used and latest techniques of paper and agarose electrophoresis and compare their results with those obtained by ultracentrifugal methods.

II. PREPARATIVE-ULTRACENTRIFUGATION TECHNIQUES FOR ISOLATION OF THE MAJOR LIPOPROTEIN CLASSES

Early lipoprotein-isolation procedures (10), particularly those of DeLalla and Gofman (11), were designed to obtain serum (or plasma) lipoprotein fractions for use in the analytical ultracentrifuge. However, with minor modifications (12–14), they are widely used for other purposes. Many laboratories interested in lipoprotein metabolism now have a growing need to study the physical and chemical properties of certain lipoprotein classes in normal and clinically abnormal states. The most important requirement in the preparative isolation of lipoproteins is the control and monitoring of density. This is most conveniently achieved by precision refractometry (15) with absolute calibration by pycnometry (16).

A. Density Monitoring, Manipulation, and Calculation

Although deuterium oxide and several salts are frequently employed for lipoprotein isolation, we consider here only two monovalent salt systems:

NaCl for low-density applications and NaCl-NaBr for high-density-lipoprotein work. With the exception of deuterium oxide (whose refractive index, $n_D^{26} = 1.32782$, differs little from that of water, $n_D^{26} = 1.33240$), the techniques for refractometry would of course apply to the other salt systems. For the preparation of accurate and reproducible salt solutions, it is recommended that only dry salts be used. For this purpose a large batch of salt should be calcined at 550°C overnight and stored in a Teflon-sealed jar in a desiccator.

If very limited applications are involved, manual calculations with data from the *International Critical Tables* (17) or the Chemical Rubber *Handbook* (18) are adequate. However, if lipoprotein fractionation involves several steps, density-gradient work, or analytical-ultracentrifugation analysis, computer-derived tables are recommended. These ideally should include values for the following parameters: ρ_{20}, η_{20}, ρ_{26}, η_{26}, g salt/l 20°C, g H_2O/l 20°C, g salt/g H_2O, molality, molarity, and wt %. In addition, at various calibration points n_D^{26} and refractometer ΔS values (characteristic of the instrument used) should be included. A complete table quadratically interpolated between each set of data points taken three at a time is easily constructed with a computer. The most convenient interpolation is to increment ρ_{20} one part in the fourth place for the complete range of salt parameters. Since preparation of salt solutions and density manipulations may be made over a temperature range, all solutions here are expressed in molal (m) concentrations (moles/1000 g H_2O) so as to avoid temperature dependence.

Although a salt solution of a given density (and volume) is easily prepared and monitored from the computer-derived tables discussed above, density manipulation is a somewhat different consideration. For example, one complication is that adding large amounts of salt significantly changes the initial solution volume. The simplest procedure, where precise density manipulations are needed, is to utilize the interpolated ratio of mass of salt to mass of water. Since this ratio is available for the initial and final density (and the initial masses of salt and water are known), the exact increment of salt needed to bring the initial solution to the final density can be calculated. Also, given the initial masses of water and salt, the added mass of salt and the final density of the solution, the volume of the final solution (and hence the volume change) is obtainable. Where a dual salt system is used, such as a low but constant 0.195 m NaCl content and a varying NaBr content, the 11.42 g/l NaCl content can be considered equivalent to 10.46 g/l NaBr, and the interpolated tables for NaBr alone can be used. Of course, for a given solution density, refractometer values would be different and somewhat lower for the pure NaBr system than those for the NaCl–NaBr system. Maintaining a constant 0.195 m NaCl content (approximately equivalent to the small-molecule serum background) simplifies the calculation and the monitoring of densities in the NaCl–NaBr system.

B. Preparation of Total-Lipoprotein Fractions

Exact manipulation of plasma or serum density is difficult because of variations in the amount of total macromolecules and in the composition of the small-molecule background. For most purposes, however, serum may be considered to be 94% by volume a solution with a density ρ of 1.0063 g/ml (0.195 *m* NaCl).[1] The examples presented here are based on this simplifying assumption.

The usual fractions prepared for use in the analytical ultracentrifuge are total-lipoprotein fractions with densities lower than 1.006, 1.063, and 1.203 g/ml (after preparative centrifugation). Each of these is conveniently prepared by mixing 2-ml serum aliquots with 4 ml of the following solutions:

1. 0.195 *m* NaCl ($\rho = 1.0063$ g/ml, $n_D^{26} = 1.33435$).
2. 2.505 *m* NaCl ($\rho = 1.0915$ g/ml, $n_D^{26} = 1.35451$).
3. 0.195 *m* NaCl and 4.507 *m* NaBr ($\rho = 1.3104$ g/ml, $n_D^{26} = 1.38596$).

All these solutions contain disodium ethylenediaminetetraacetate (EDTA) at a concentration of 10 mg/100 ml. The 6-ml serum mixtures are put into specially soaked and washed 0.5 × 2.5-in. heavy walled (0.014 in.) cellulose nitrate tubes and capped with an assembly having a stainless-steel stem. Preparative tubes should be carefully sized with a gauge for proper length and diameter. Oversized tubes may be shrunk by immersing in hot water for several days. All tubes should be soaked thoroughly in warm water overnight, rinsed 10 times, and then soaked overnight in distilled water. After being rinsed three times with distilled water, the tubes are placed in a basket to drain and are dried for 2 days at 37°C in an explosion-proof dust-free oven.

Depending on the desired rotor speed, preparative centrifugation is done in a 40.3 or a 50.3 rotor. For the two lower density fractions 18°C runs at 40,000 rpm for 18 hr are recommended. For the total high-density-lipoprotein (HDL) fraction 24 to 26 hr is needed at the same temperature and rotor speed. Although rotor speeds above 40,000 rpm may be desirable to reduce running time, this factor should be balanced against the increased hazard of occasional tube collapse, with sample loss. Nearly filling the preparative tube with additional background solutions will tend to minimize this loss, but it will make the quantitative removal of lipoproteins

[1] Unless otherwise indicated, all densities are given at 20°C.

much more difficult. Unless unusual circumstances require higher speeds, adding exactly 6.0 ml of the solution to each tube and running at 40,000 rpm is recommended.

C. Sequential Preparation of Serum Very-Low-Density, Low-Density, and High-Density Lipoproteins

It is frequently necessary to isolate the very-low-density, low-density, and high-density lipoprotein (VLDL, LDL, and HDL, respectively) fractions from plasma or serum. However, one difficulty involves the separation of exogenous chylomicrons and, for the most part endogenous, very-low-density lipoproteins. Perhaps at the present time the best approach to the problem is by an operational definition (19): lipoproteins whose svedberg flotation (S_f) rate exceeds 400 are classed as chylomicrons, and lipoproteins with S_f rates of 20 to 400 are defined as very-low-density lipoproteins. It should be understood that a given serum may contain exogenous lipoproteins whose S_f value is below 400 and endogenous lipoproteins whose S_f value exceeds 400 ($\sim$ 757-Å diameter). Indeed there is evidence that these two classes may have substantially overlapping distributions (20, 21).

Isolation of contamination-free total $S_f > 400$ lipoprotein fractions requires a special density-gradient procedure, which is described in Sections VI and VII. However, if they are present in serum in large amounts, $S_f > 400$ lipoproteins can be conveniently and quantitatively removed. By using a swinging-bucket rotor, such as the SW 25.3 (or SW 27) fitted with buckets to handle 0.5 $\times$ 2.5-in. preparative tubes, the procedure is simply to ultracentrifuge 7 ml of whole serum in each bucket for an appropriate time. This contrifugation is that calculated to quantitatively float S_f 400 molecules from the bottom of the preparative tube into the top 0.5-ml fraction. With serum values of $\eta = 1.755$ and $\rho = 1.0259$ g/ml at 23°C (22), the needed centrifugation is 5.74×10^6 *g*-min.[2] This requires a total of 79.9 min of full-speed centrifugation at 25,000 rpm (including one-third of the acceleration and deceleration times) with the SW 25.3 rotor (mean $r = 10.26$ cm).

After centrifugation the preparative tubes are carefully removed from each bucket and firmly held at a 45-degree angle. The $S_f < 400$ fraction is collected by puncturing the bottom of each tube at the lowest point with

[2] If very high serum concentrations of chylomicrons are present, a similar centrifugation of 7 ml of whole serum at 2.27×10^6 *g*-min (23°C) quantitatively removes $S_f > 1000$ lipoproteins into the top 0.5 ml. The 6.5 ml subnatant may be easily used for preparing fractions for analytical ultracentrifugation (Section II.B), with appropriate corrections for partial removal of S_f 0–400 lipoproteins (Section IV.E).

a sharp No. 22 needle and collecting the 6.5 ml subnatant. Before puncturing the preparative tube, the bottom is wiped with clean gauze dampened with distilled water and then dried with a lint-free wiper (e.g., Kimwipe).[3]

Although $S_f > 400$ molecules are removed from the subnatant fraction, this procedure also partially removes some S_f 20–400 very-low-density lipoproteins. Thus the $S_f < 400$ subnatant contains a somewhat *distorted* and reduced VLDL distribution compared with that present in the original serum sample (see Section VI.E). In preparing VLDL fractions the advantage of removing $S_f > 400$ lipoproteins as well as the disadvantage of recovering a distorted VLDL distribution should be considered. Generally, when $S_f > 400$ lipoproteins are present in relatively large amounts, the above procedure is recommended.

After collecting the $S_f < 400$ serum subnatant, sequential isolation of the VLDL, LDL, and HDL fractions utilizes 0.5 × 2.5-in. cellulose nitrate tubes and either 40.3 or 50.3 Beckman rotors (Beckman Instruments, Palo Alto, Calif.). All runs are made at approximately 18°C in a Beckman preparative ultracentrifuge equipped with a diffusion pump. A 6-ml volume of a serum solution containing 2 to 6 ml of serum $S_f < 400$ subnatant (the balance supplied by 0.195 *m* NaCl, $p = 1.0063$ g/ml $n_D^{26} = 1.33435$) is ultracentrifuged for 18 hr at 40,000 rpm. All solutions used contain EDTA at a concentration of 10 mg/100 ml. The S_f 20–400 VLDL fraction is quantitatively removed in the first 1 ml, and a second 1 ml is taken as a reference. Then the 4-ml bottom fraction is mixed with 2 ml of a 0.195 *m* NaCl and 2.434 *m* NaBr solution ($n_D^{26} = 1.36446$, $\rho = 1.1816$ g/ml), giving a resultant density before centrifugation of 1.065 g/ml.

After again centrifuging for 18 hr (in new preparative tubes), the S_f 0–20 LDL fraction is quantitatively recovered in the top of 1 ml of background density $\rho = 1.063$ g/ml, and a second 1 ml is taken as a reference. The 4-ml bottom fraction is mixed with 2 ml of a solution consisting of 0.195 *m* NaCl and 7.570 *m* NaBr ($n_D^{26} = 1.41205$, $\rho = 1.4744$ g/ml), this time resulting in a solution whose density before centrifugation is 1.216 g/ml. After a final centrifugation for 24 to 26 hr, the total HDL fraction is collected in the top 1 ml of background density $\rho = 1.203$ g/ml, and a second 0.5 ml is taken as a reference.

It is recommended that each fraction, particularly the reference fractions, be measured by refractometry to verify background densities. If salt redistribution is considered, the second 1-ml (or 0.5-ml) fraction can be extrapolated to give the appropriate background refractive index and den-

[3] Throughout this chapter, reference to a company or product name does not imply approval or recommendation of the product by the University of California or the U.S. Atomic Energy Commission to the exclusion of others that may be suitable.

sity of the lipoprotein fraction. Precision refractometry, as described in Section III, can provide convenient quantification of each lipoprotein fraction.

D. Quantitative Removal of Preparative Lipoprotein Fractions

Although the use of a tube-slicing device may have advantages in special applications, it is not recommended for lipoprotein work. Pipetting provides the best quantitative removal of lipoprotein fractions, with visual evaluation of completeness and with minimal disturbance to the remainder of the preparative tube. A special thin-walled Pasteur pipette with an inside bore of 0.4 to 0.6 mm is available commercially (Microchemical Specialties, Berkeley, Calif.). Pipetting is done in a darkened room on a fixture equipped with a focused light beam, allowing visualization of the lipoproteins by their Tyndall scattering.

After the rotor has stopped, great care should be exercised to avoid any abrupt movement of the rotor or of each individual preparative tube during manipulation prior to pipetting. Normally, for each lipoprotein-containing sample, two fractions are pipetted in depth, the top 1 ml containing quantitatively the lipoprotein fraction and the second 1 ml (or 0.5 ml in the 1.20 g/ml HDL run) providing (for refractometry) a reference salt background for that sample. Where the presence of unexpectedly large amounts of lipoproteins prevents quantitative removal in 1 ml, the fractions may be removed in 2 ml (or 1.5 ml in the HDL run), with a third 1 ml taken as a salt reference for the 1.006 g/ml and 1.063 g/ml runs.

The fractions collected in calibrated 1-, 2-, or 0.5-ml volumetric vials are transferred for storage into 9-ml airtight screw-cap vials (No. 60910, Owens-Illinois Co., Toledo, Ohio) fitted with washed plain pulp liners and Teflon gaskets. On the same day when pipetting is done and before storage at 4°C, refractive-index measurements are made with a Bausch & Lomb precision Abbe refractometer (23) with an n_D range of 1.203 to 1.508. Ideally room temperature should be approximately 23°C, and the refractometer should be thermostated to 26 ± 0.03°C with a temperature controller (Precision Scientific Co., Chicago, Ill.).

E. Ultracentrifugal Redistribution of Salts and Background Density Calculation

During the preparative-ultracentrifugation runs described here for isolating all lipoprotein fractions, appreciable salt redistribution occurs from the top to the bottom of the preparative tube. The extent of this redistribution is dependent on the nature and concentration of the salt as well as the time

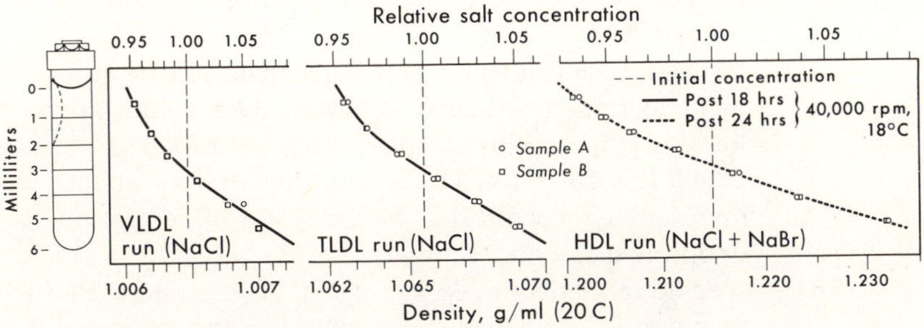

Fig. 1 Salt redistribution after typical runs (40.3 rotor): 1.006-g/ml NaCl, 1.065-g/ml NaCl [total low-density lipoproteins (TLDL)], and 1.216-g/ml NaBr. (From Ref. 23; reproduced by permission from the *Journal of Lipid Research.*)

and conditions of ultracentrifugation. Evaluation of this salt redistribution and its reproducibility for each type of run are easily achieved by running appropriate salt background solutions and measuring each fraction in depth by refractometry. Figure 1 shows the salt redistribution for typical 1.006 g/ml and 1.065 g/ml NaCl runs as well as for the 1.216 g/ml NaBr run. The differences between the second fraction and the first fraction in precision Abbe ΔS units and corresponding $\Delta\rho$ values are reproducible and known; therefore the background for each lipoprotein fraction can be determined from the second 1-ml fraction (or the second 0.5-ml fraction in the HDL run). These differences are as follows: $\Delta S = 0.005$ and $\Delta\rho = 0.0001$ g/ml for the 1.0063 g/ml run; $\Delta S = 0.043$ and $\Delta\rho = 0.0011$ g/ml for the 1.065 g/ml run; and $\Delta S = 0.115$ and $\Delta\rho = 0.0035$ g/ml for the 1.216 g/ml NaBr run.

III. EVALUATION OF LIPOPROTEIN CONCENTRATIONS BY REFRACTOMETRY

A. Determination of Lipoprotein Concentration

By measuring the refractive index of both the lipoprotein top fraction and the subnatant background, and correcting the latter to the first 1-ml fraction, lipoprotein concentrations are determined by using the following relationships:

$$\text{lipoprotein concentration, mg \%} = (\Delta S_{\text{TF}} - \Delta S_{\text{BG}}) \frac{k \times 10^3}{c_o \times \text{SRI}} \qquad (1)$$

where ΔS_{TF} = Abbe scale increment of lipoprotein top-fraction.

ΔS_{BG} = calculated Abbe scale increment of top-fraction salt background above water reference.

k = instrument-dependent factor for conversion of scale increment to refractive-index increment. Our values are as follows: $k_{TLDL} = 5.30 \times 10^{-3}$, $k_{VLDL} = 5.48 \times 10^{-3}$, $k_{HDL} = 4.97 \times 10^{-3}$ (TLDL = total low-density lipoproteins).

c_0 = lipoprotein-concentration factor (ratio of serum volume to lipoprotein-fraction volume).

SRI = specific refractive-index increment. As used here, SRI is the increase in refractive index n_D^{26} (of the indicated background salt solutions) resulting from the presence of 1 g of anhydrous lipoprotein per 100 ml of solution. Values used are 0.00158 for VLDL, 0.00154 for TLDL, and 0.00149 for HDL in 1.006 g/ml NaCl, 1.063 g/ml NaCl, and 1.203 g/ml NaBr, respectively (24).

Low-density-lipoprotein measurements by refractometry are useful for several purposes. Such measurements on a minimum of material provide an invariant physical method for VLDL and LDL measurement (by difference), without an analytical ultracentrifuge. If analytical centrifugation is performed, refractometry can easily be employed to monitor lipoprotein concentrations and ensure that only optimal concentrations of lipoproteins are run. First, if the LDL concentration in the isolated fraction is over 1300 mg/100 ml, the sample should be appropriately diluted, to avoid unnecessary and expensive reruns. Second, evaluation of lipoprotein background density in both the low- and high-density runs as well as in subfractionation work is essential for the complete ultracentrifugal analysis described later. Third, if refractometry of whole serum is performed and the total-lipoprotein content of serum is known, an accurate and reproducible value for the total serum proteins can be calculated (24).

B. Details of Refractometry Measurement

The most convenient and accurate refractometric analyses of small quantities of solution, equilibrated to room temperature, are made with the precision Abbe refractometer, temperature controlled to at least 0.1°C. Readings should be made above room temperature (in this procedure at 26°C) with scale readings estimated to within ± 0.005 unit. Over the range of measurements this accuracy corresponds to approximately ± 0.00003 in Δn (one to two parts in the fourth place for density measurements). An ordinary Abbe refractometer, though useful in monitoring densities, is not sufficiently accurate (± 0.0002 in Δn) to give satisfactory lipoprotein results by this method.

Refractometry is done with only one drop of the lipoprotein fraction (or salt solution) by taking the "reflection" reading. Thus nearly all the fraction is available for analytical ultracentrifugation or for lipid and protein analysis. The drop of lipoprotein solution should be placed slightly above the center of the outer ground-glass prism, and the prism should be closed immediately. Thereafter a delay of exactly 1 min between the application of the sample and the refractometric reading is recommended. This is sufficient for approximate temperature equilibration but insufficient for any significant evaporation. After each reading the surface of the opposing prisms is thoroughly washed by directing against each prism a stream of about 25 ml of distilled water from a polyethylene wash bottle. The prism surfaces are then wiped (unidirectionally) with a nonabrasive wiper (Kimberly Clark type 900-S). To ensure a dry prism surface, an unheated air stream is directed for 5 sec onto each prism surface from a hair dryer (Oster, Model 202).

IV. ANALYTICAL-ULTRACENTRIFUGATION ANALYSIS OF SERUM-LIPOPROTEIN FRACTIONS

Because ultracentrifugal studies of lipoproteins usually involve flotation analysis in salt solutions and because stability of preparations may be essential, special precautions are needed. For example, whenever salt solutions of greater than a few tenths molal concentration are used at a high rotor speed, significant and changing redistribution of salt occurs during the run. This requires that double-sectored cells be employed to allow accurate baseline evaluation in any frame. Since such base lines are a function of fluid-column height, the base-line and lipoprotein-fraction menisci should be as closely matched to one another as possible. Thus each sector is filled with 0.415 ml by using calibrated syringes. Also, it is highly desirable to use inert aluminum-filled epoxy centerpieces. Such cells in our hands are routinely capable of sustained operation at 52,640 rpm. Centerpieces are washed first with water, using a folded pipe cleaner, and then in an ultrasonic cleaning bath; they are thoroughly rinsed with distilled water and dried under a warm-air blower. No detergents or solvents are used.

A. Special Features of Cell Construction and Alignment

We have found that with slight modifications in design, the usual 2.5-degree double-sectored cells with 12-mm-thick centerpieces are desirable for lipoprotein analysis. These modifications include fabrication of both a standard and a 0.020 in. offset centerpiece (25), which allows accurate

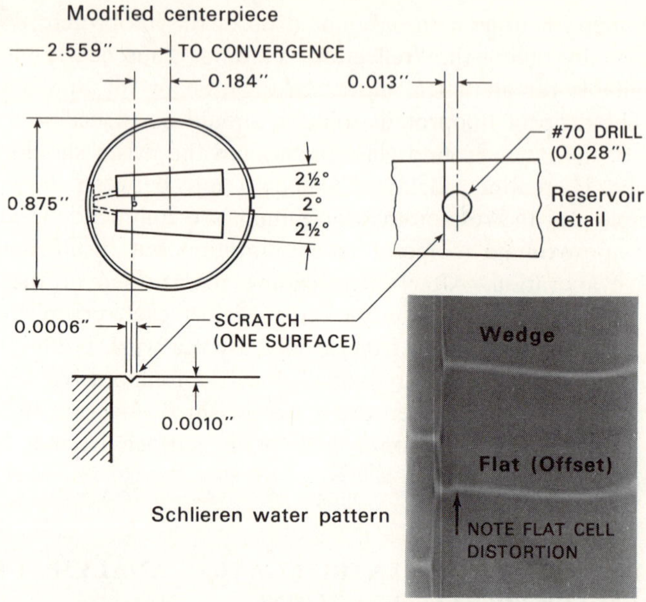

Fig. 2 Modified centerpiece with special reservoir. Note precise meniscus equalization in the schlieren water patterns obtained with flat (offset) and wedge cells.

base-of-cell identification when two samples are run simultaneously, such as in the standard low- and high-density run. Normally the offset centerpiece is run in a cell with a positive-wedge (48′30″) quartz disk, allowing clearer base-line resolution near the base of cell in the high-density run. We have found this arrangement superior to that shown in Section IV.E.

Another modification, shown in Fig. 2, is a reservoir in each centerpiece to equalize the meniscus in both the base-line and sample sectors. The dimensions of the scratch are important to allow meniscus equalization without exchange of fluid from one sector to another. Since under repeated stress the epoxy flows somewhat, after about 30 runs a centerpiece should be carefully rescribed with a sharp No. 22 gauge needle.

Precise cell alignment is very important in lipoprotein flotation analysis. Although scribe-line alignment of the cell in a rotor checked with an optical device (such as the Beckman microscope cell aligner) is usually adequate, occasionally cells may rotate slightly after proper alignment, giving striations in the schlieren pattern. This may be minimized by using a small amount of heavy silicone grease, which, however, prevents accurate weighing of the analytical cells.

Our procedure for achieving reproducible cell alignment is to use pinned rotors and notched cell housings, as shown in Fig. 3. Each cell housing must be matched with an appropriate centerpiece, so that the combined fully torqued assembly positioned in the rotor results in proper radial alignment. Our tolerance is that the top or bottom of the cell wall should be within ± 0.002 in. of perfect radial alignment, as checked on a special optical fixture. Whenever striations suddenly appear in a pattern, the cell alignment should be checked with the optical device.

Another useful design modification of the cell housing, shown in Fig. 3, involves relieving the diameter 0.001 in. for a distance of 0.310 in. from the screw-ring end. This minimizes scratch and wear within rotor holes and on the periphery of this specially stressed region of the cell housing.

Using filled-epoxy double-sectored centerpieces at high speed involves not only the risk of occasional gross cell leakage but also of subtle micro-leakage. Because the seal between the epoxy centerpiece and the quartz windows is not perfect, there is nearly always some slight leakage. Our cells routinely leak approximately 0.5 to 2.5 μl from one or both sectors during a standard low- and high-density run. Although this amount of leakage in-

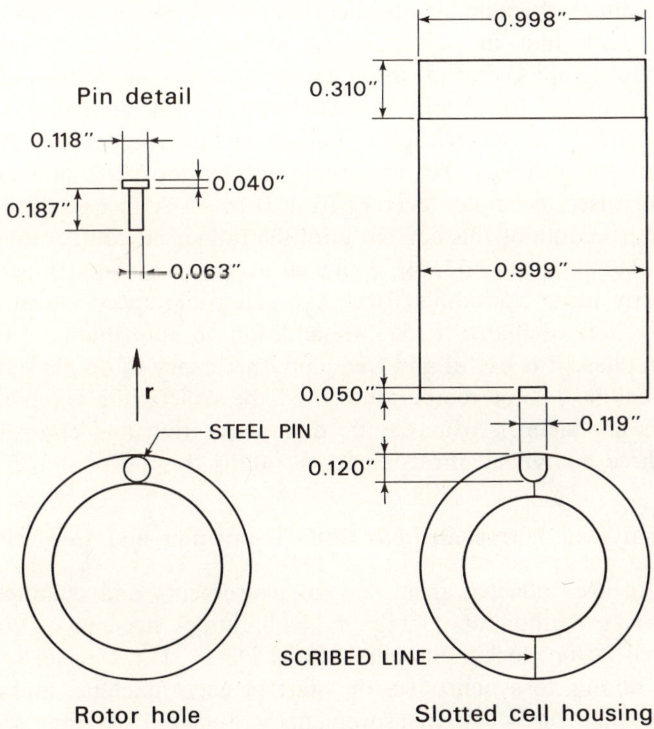

Fig. 3 Details of pinned rotor holes and special slotted cell housings.

volves only an imperceptible change in meniscus position, large losses can introduce appreciable and unacceptable inaccuracies, particularly when precision moving-boundary S_f rates are needed. Thus it is important to weigh each cell to $\pm$ 0.2 mg before and after each run. A new cell or a cell that has had one or more parts replaced should be run first with distilled water to identify any unusual cell distortion and to minimize lipoprotein-sample loss (see Fig. 2).

A critical manipulation to minimize cell leakage and avoid breakage is the proper torquing of the cells. Using only a dry lubricant, MS-122 Fluorocarbon (Miller-Stephenson Chemical Co., Chicago, Ill.), cells are torqued 50 to 70 in.-lb, depending on their age and history. Despite precautions cell leaks (greater than 5 mg) occur approximately once in 60 runs.

B. Some Useful Modifications of the Analytical Ultracentrifuge for Lipoprotein Work

Since lipoprotein analysis frequently involves macromolecules that migrate significantly during rotor acceleration to full speed (FS), it is important to define reproducibly the acceleration phase of the run. This is particularly important in our standard procedure, where we take two schlieren photographs during this period; ideally the value of $\omega_{FS}^{-2} \int \omega^2(t)\, dt$ is needed for appropriate analysis. Several modifications of the Beckman Model E ultracentrifuge and additional instrumentation fulfill this and other useful purposes. An automatic accelerator (26) actuated by a push button raises the motor current from 0 to 14 A in exactly 0.50 min and thereafter maintains this current until the full-speed control loop comes into range. At full speed (52,640 rpm) an accuracy of 2 parts per million is achieved by using a modified Beckman electronic speed control with a crystal-controlled oscillator (26). In addition to information about the acceleration phase it is useful and frequently necessary to obtain data about full-speed stability, rotor temperature, and the exact time when schlieren photographs are taken. An automatic data-acquisition and control system for up to three analytical ultracentrifuges fulfills this purpose (27).

C. An Analytical Ultracentrifuge Data-Acquisition and Control System

When data are collected from several instruments and channeled into one recorder, a method of coding and collating is necessary. We use a master digital 24-hr clock (Parabam Model DA24, Hawthorne, Calif.) to control the timing, to synchronize the start of each machine, and to code the data by time at which measurements are taken. A time sequencer switches from machine to machine, collecting data in a one-two-three sequence. An interface coupler (Dymec Model 2526, Hewlett-Packard, Palo Alto, Calif.) operates with an IBM 526 summary punch machine to store and record the data. Mercury reed relays select signals from gear-tooth counters (Electro Model 3010-A, Chicago, Ill.) for rotor-speed information and from radiometers for rotor-temperature information. The radiometer (Beckman Instruments, Palo Alto, Calif.) is the total-radiation heat-balance type used in the Model L2-65B preparative ultracentrifuge. The bottom of each analytical rotor is recessed 0.040 in. and painted flat black to optimize radiation exchange between the rotor and the radiometer; the latter is offset 0.75 in. from the rotor axis and spaced 0.25 in. from the rotor bottom. Reed relays select radiometer outputs to channel the corresponding ultracentrifuge temperature analog voltage to a digital voltmeter (Model 3460B, Hewlett-Packard). The overall block diagram of this system is shown in Fig. 4.

Each ultracentrifuge is designed to operate independently of the system (if desired) when the connector to the central system is replaced by an appropriate jumper plug. A timed cycle of rotor acceleration and photography is determined by a program card in each centrifuge; the cycle is

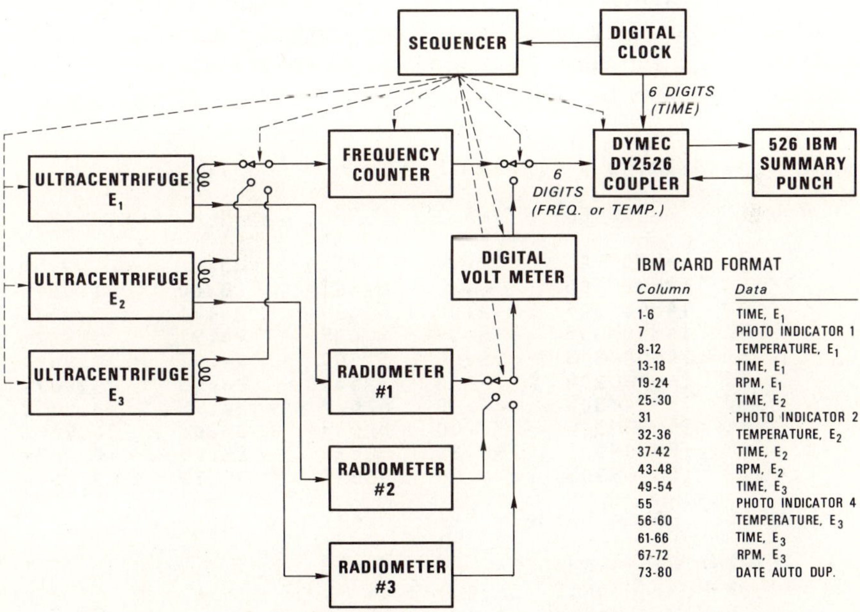

Fig. 4 Overall block diagram of an analytical ultracentrifuge data-acquisition and control system. (From Ref. 27; reproduced by permission from the *Review of Scientific Instruments*.)

initiated by a push button on each centrifuge. The Beckman commutator timer is replaced by an integrated circuit, giving flexibility of 99 possible photograph times taken at 2-min intervals over a period of 200 min.

A Fortran IV computer program processes the punched-card data, yielding graphs of rotor speed and temperature as functions of time as well as giving the cumulative value of $\omega_{FS}^{-2} \int \omega^2(t)\, dt$ for the mean time of each schlieren photograph. A typical computer output of a successful ultracentrifugal run is shown in Fig. 5. Had there been any error or failure, an error message (or messages) would describe the difficulty. An additional feature of the computer analysis, if desired, is shown in Fig. 6. Here a cathode-ray-tube plot gives the visual profile of acceleration and rotor temperature as well as the times at which photographs were taken.

We have chosen to obtain data directly in the form of IBM punched cards, which allow convenient and direct submission of data for computer analysis. Such data permit quick evaluation of each day's runs, machine performance, and error-detection capability. The equivalent up-to-speed (UTS) centrifugation of all the pictures is available with great accuracy; these data, particularly the zero-time up-to-speed value, are essential for accurate VLDL analysis where significant migration of molecules occurs during the acceleration phase of the run. Also, this data-acquisition system permits great flexibility in the actual run itself, for example, nonlinear acceleration or a run consisting entirely of programmed acceleration. The latter capability may be useful in minimizing the effects of adiabatic tem-

```
MACHINE 3, STARTED AT 14H37M 0S                  02/11/69

FRAME         CLOCK      TIME        RPM         TEMP   EQV. UTS

    1      14H40M30S     -2.00      34731        25.41        .4951
    2      14H42M30S      0.        52687        25.00       1.9670
    3      14H44M30S      2.00      52639        24.91       3.9674
    4      14H48M30S      6.00      52639        24.91       7.9673
    5      14H50M30S      8.00      52640        24.93       9.9672
    6      14H56M30S     14.00      52640        24.95      15.9671
    7      15H 4M30S     22.00      52639        24.99      23.9667
    8      15H12M30S     30.00      52639        25.02      31.9664
    9      15H30M30S     48.00      52639        25.06      49.9655
   10      15H46M30S     64.00      52639        25.13      65.9648

UP-TO-SPEED RPM = 52638.9 (+-     .63) N = 32

M-C TEMPERATURE AVERAGES..
         D-RUN, FRAMES  5-10   25.04
         G-RUN, FRAMES  2- 7   24.95
```

Fig. 5 Typical output showing computer evaluation of a successful ultracentrifuge run. (From Ref. 27; reproduced by permission from the *Review of Scientific Instruments.*)

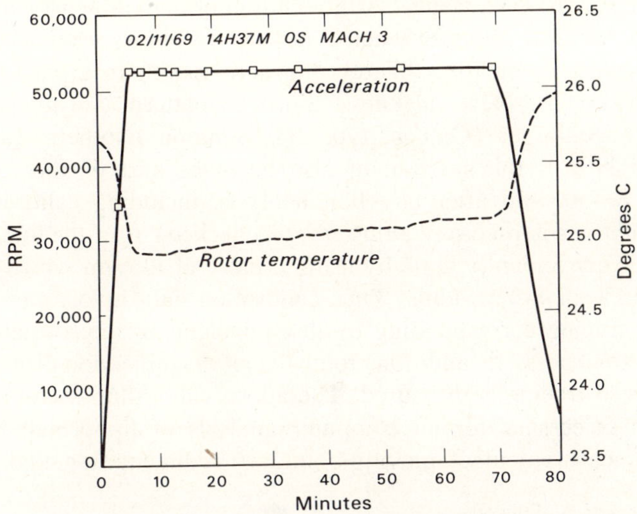

Fig. 6 Cathode-ray-tube plot (retraced) of rotor speed and temperature in the run evaluated in Fig. 5. Squares indicate times at which photographs were taken. (From Ref. 27; reproduced by permission from the *Review of Scientific Instruments.*)

perature changes during acceleration to full speed. Moreover, such a system should increase the accuracy of measured sedimentation and flotation rates, particularly at low rotor speeds.

Other modifications include a camera system using 4-in. roll film (25) of high dimensional stability (Tri-X Ortho Film Estar Thick Base, Eastman Kodak Co., Rochester, N.Y.). This capability permits recording of greater vertical schlieren deflections and is particularly advantageous when two patterns are routinely recorded. Furthermore, manipulation of films presents no hazard of potential breakage, and film storage is greatly simplified. Another useful device is a vacuum sentinel (28), which automatically shuts off the drive mechanism and applies the full brake in the event of a cell leak and subsequent vacuum loss. This device provides the capability of significantly decreasing the breakage of analytical cells and also provides automatic monitoring throughout each run.

D. Calibration of the Analytical Ultracentrifuge for Lipoprotein Analysis

Calibration of the analytical ultracentrifuge is conveniently done with an appropriate Beckman calibration cell. We routinely calibrate at approximately 4-month intervals, immediately after any manipulation of the optical system or after a drive exchange. Although film of high dimensional stability is employed, we also calibrate when a new lot of film is used. For a given calibration cell, area on the schlieren film corresponds to a particular total Δn for a given centerpiece thickness. Since all patterns are analyzed with the use of an enlarger (Omega, type B4, Simmon Brothers, Inc., Long Island City, N.Y.), this instrument also becomes part of the calibration procedure. Before and after any film analysis, including calibration patterns, the enlarger is precisely adjusted (or checked) to a fivefold enlargement. This is conveniently done by using a piece of film on which is lightly scribed a circle of 2-cm radius. Thus calibration data involve an enlarged area on the tracing corresponding to an equivalent Δn appropriate for the centerpiece thickness. In addition, total linear magnification from the cell to the enlarged tracing is measured. The above calibration factors for each machine are necessary for all computer analysis of lipoprotein fractions and in the measurement of moving-boundary sedimentation and flotation rates.

Although lipoprotein concentrations may be given in the invariant physical measurement of total refractive-index increment, lipoprotein concentrations are routinely expressed in mass per unit volume. Our ultracentrifugal data are calculated by assuming a constant specific refractive-index increment (SRI) of 0.00154 Δn/g/100 ml for the S_f 0–400 TLDL class, measured in 1.063 g/ml NaCl. High-density-lipoprotein concentrations are calculated by assuming an SRI of 0.00149 Δn/g/100 ml, measured in 1.203 g/ml NaBr. All schlieren runs are made between 25 and 26°C, using a phaseplate-wire combination (set at approximately 53 degrees) and a Wratten No. 16 filter so that the total lipoprotein Δn is obtained primarily with the green line of the mercury arc (5461 Å). Since dispersion effects are probably smaller than the SRI errors, these values are also used for refractometry at 5893 Å. It is anticipated that more accurate SRI data will be available soon on subfractions of the VLDL, LDL, and HDL classes.

E. Computer Analysis of Schlieren Lipoprotein Distributions

Computer analysis of the analytical low-density run (which includes the VLDL and LDL classes) and the HDL spectra is essentially as described in detail by Ewing, Freeman, and Lindgren (6). A total of 10 schlieren photographs are taken: one during acceleration and nine during the 64-min up-to-speed run at 52,640 rpm. Figure 7 shows selected schlieren photographs of a typical low- and high-density run. Note the use of the 0.020-in.-offset centerpiece in the flat cell, providing positive identification of the base-of-cell position in each run. Normally the zero-time, 6-min, and 30-min photographs are used for the low-density analysis of the S_f 100–400,

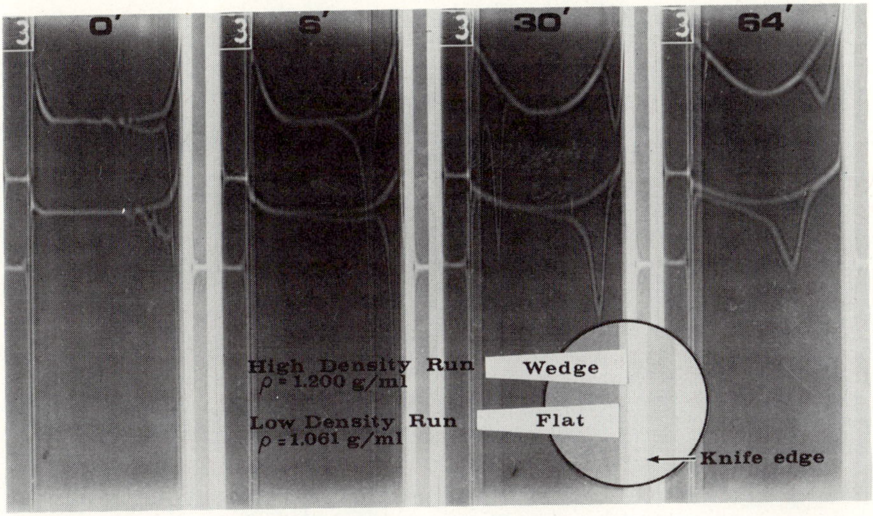

Fig. 7 Selected schlieren photographs from a typical standard low- and high-density lipoprotein run (case 710). (From Ref. 50; reproduced by permission from the American Oil Chemists' Society.)

S_f 20–100, and S_f 0–20 lipoproteins, respectively, and the 64-min frame for high-density analysis. However, when serum concentrations of S_f 20–400 lipoproteins are below 150 mg/100 ml, it is recommended that the S_f 20–100 lipoproteins be measured on the 2-min up-to-speed frame. A close estimate of this lipoprotein concentration is obtained by refractometry of the total VLDL fraction (Section III). Using a 5× enlarger in a darkroom, the appropriate frames are traced on precision photo-offset templates of proper linear magnification for each ultracentrifuge. Tick marks at selected S_f- and F-rate intervals on the template are connected with a sharp 7H pencil and a drafting machine, after which each ordinate height is manually measured. A total of 29 and 15 ordinate heights are measured in the standard low- and high-density patterns, respectively. All such data for each run are transcribed onto special keypunch forms, giving also the density of each fraction, concentration relative to serum, and the conditions of the analytical run (e.g., temperature, the up-to-speed equivalent of the zero-time up-to-speed picture, machine-calibration data, and useful alphanumeric coding information about the lipoprotein fraction).

Our Fortran IV program of 27,000-word field length, runs on a Control Data Corporation 6600 computer; however, with minor modifications it can be used with most high-speed, large-capacity computers. Figure 8 shows schematically the operation of the program, including all needed

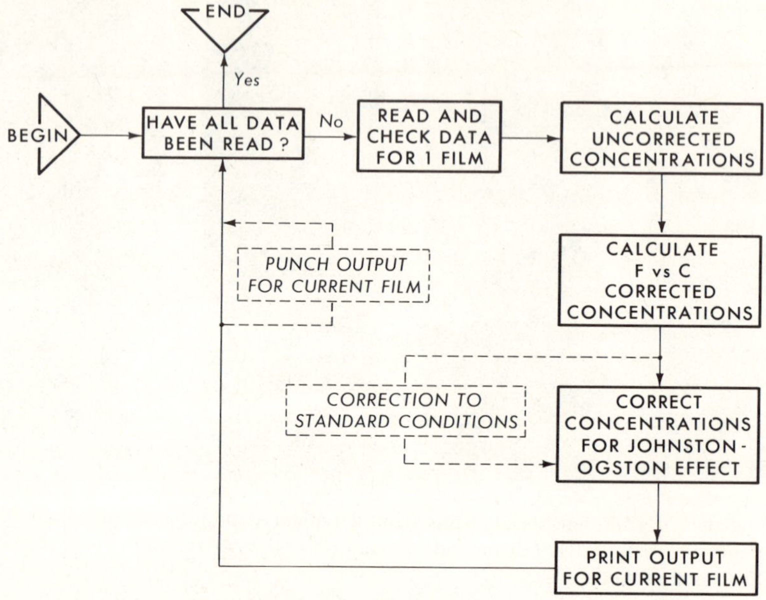

Fig. 8 Flow chart of program for analysis of ultracentrifuge schlieren patterns. Optional procedures are shown with dashed lines. (From Ref. 56; reproduced by permission from the American Oil Chemists' Society.)

corrections, such as flotation versus concentration dependence, Ogston–Johnston corrections, and corrections to standard conditions of density and temperature. Thus this computer program yields a numerical output that is fully corrected in terms of lipoprotein concentrations of the original sample, allowing valid comparisons to be made from sample to sample. It should be emphasized that the data-acquisition system described earlier provides the accumulated value of $\omega_{FS}^{-2} \int \omega^2(t)\, dt$ for all frames. Using these zero-time up-to-speed data, which can vary by as much as $\pm$ 10% from one run to the next, permits much more accurate schlieren analysis of the VLDL spectra. When unusually high concentrations of chylomicrons are present, $S_f > 1000$ lipoproteins are removed from the serum (Section II.C). An optional feature of this program uses the preparative recovery data and appropriately corrects the lipoprotein spectra for partial removal of S_f 0–400 lipoproteins.

F. Graphic Presentation of Schlieren Data

In order to extend and improve the computer analysis of lipoprotein distributions, another program presents these data in graphic form, allowing rapid visual evaluation, comparison of samples and population means, as well as providing for error detection (29). Although the program is used routinely for the graphical presentation of the low- and high-density spectra, other applications are available. For example, schlieren flotation (or sedimentation) patterns from any single frame, including an acceleration frame, can be analyzed at any time. The results from any frame can be plotted at any desired up-to-speed time value for ease in comparing data. This plotting program converts S_f° and $F_{1.20}^\circ$ rates (or *s* rates) into appropriate linear dimensions, and lipoprotein concentrations into areas equivalent to those of the corrected schlieren patterns, routinely presented at three times the concentration of serum.[4] It then calculates points along a best-fit curve through the resulting histogram from which the graph is plotted. We normally use a cathode-ray-tube plotter, but when greater dimensional accuracy is required, a California Computer Corporation plotter is used. Since the CalComp plotter is accurate to 0.01 in., it is also useful in drawing master templates for tracing schlieren patterns from any analytical ultracentrifuge, given the proper magnification factor and the conditions of the analytical run.

In addition to the actual plotting, the program sums lipoproteins of the total pattern and of the specified low-density subfractions (S_f° 0–12, S_f° 12–20, S_f° 20–100 and S_f° 100–400). The single-frame high-density analysis sums the $F_{1.20}^\circ$ 3.5–9 and $F_{1.20}^\circ$ 0–3.5 subfractions, which correspond roughly to the older HDL_2 and HDL_3 nomenclature (11). Final steps in the program are to draw a rectangle around each frame, with tick marks and frame boundaries that normally correspond to the templates on which the schlieren pattern was initially traced. The plots are labeled, and all standard-interval lipoprotein values are placed in the appropriate frames. The program is flexible, allowing one to plot several patterns on one frame for comparison or to plot the mean or standard deviation of a population (or both).

In the TLDL plots we normally use an S_f scale that is identical with that of the three-frame template used for tracing the enlarged schlieren patterns (see Fig. 9). However, the montage of three frames (taken at different times to include the total S_f° 0–400 lipoprotein distribution) results in a discontinuous curve (Fig. 9*a*), representing what is essentially a continuous spectrum. In Fig. 9*b* a logarithmic scale has been chosen to achieve con-

[4] The S_f rate is the uncorrected flotation rate, expressed in svedbergs (10^{-13} cm/sec/dyne/g), in an NaCl medium of 1.063 g/ml density. The F rate is the uncorrected flotation rate at any given density. The S_f° rate is the flotation rate fully corrected for effects of concentration dependence and to standard conditions of 1.744 *m* NaCl at 26°C ($\rho_{26} = 1.0630$ g/ml). Similarly the $F_{1.20}^\circ$ rate is the HDL flotation rate fully corrected for concentration dependence and to standard conditions of 0.195 *m* NaCl and 2.762 *m* NaBr at 26°C ($\rho_{26} = 1.2000$ g/ml).

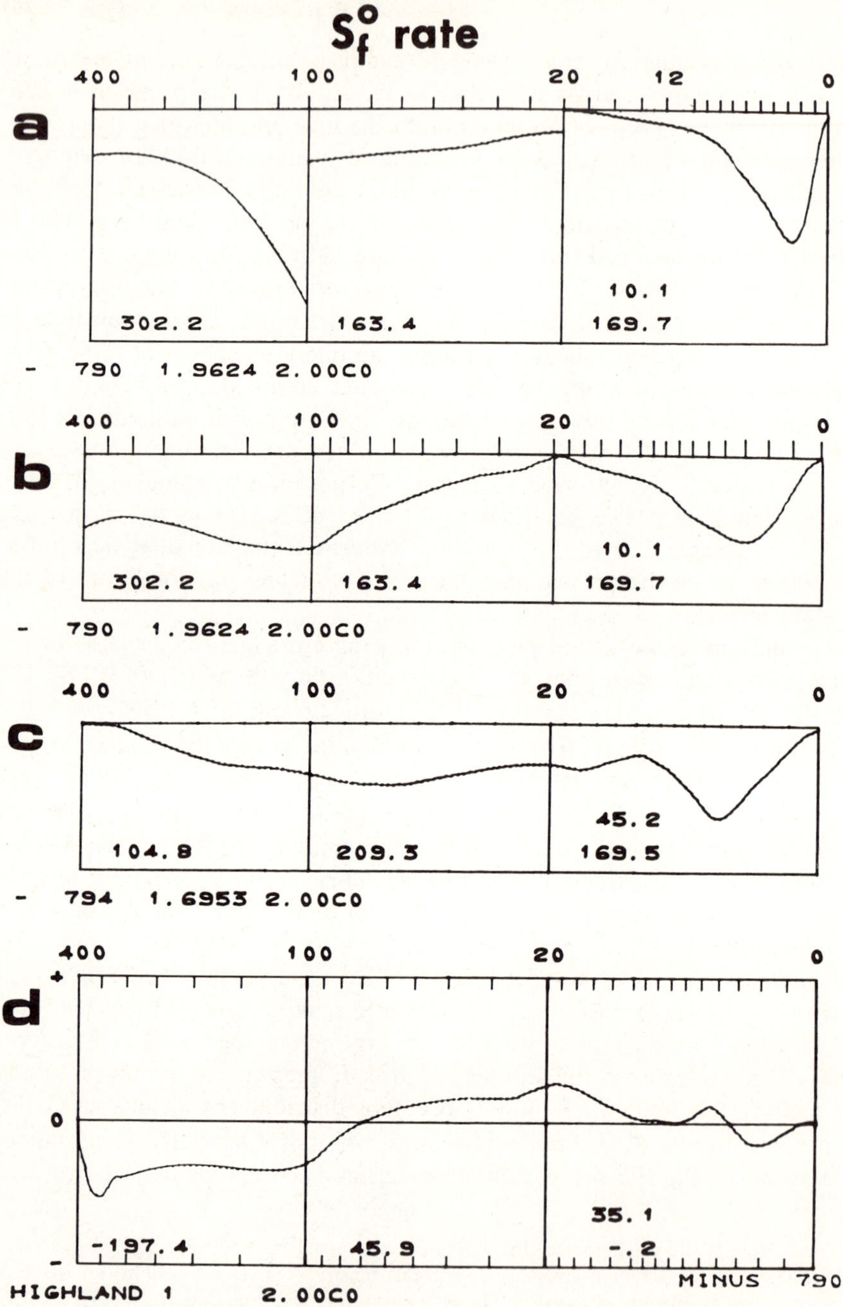

Fig. 9 Cathode-ray-tube plots of TLDL spectra: (*a*) traditional discontinuous plot and (*b*) continuous log plot for a fasting subject; (*c*) plot for the same subject 24 hr after a fat-tolerance test; (*d*) plot *b* subtracted from plot *c*. Although fully corrected, note significantly different up-to-speed equivalent (1.9624 and 1.6953 min) of the S_f 100–400 time frame for runs 790 and 794, respectively. (From Ref. 29; reproduced by permission from the American Oil Chemists' Society.)

tinuity while preserving the relative widths represented by the individual schlieren frames. To accomplish this a variable *k* log ($S_f^\circ + 5$) is used to avoid negative values. The usefulness of a similar logarithmic scale, particularly for the S_f 0–12 (LDL) spectra, has been discussed by Oncley (30). Another potentially useful scale, using the square root of the S_f rate, would yield a scale nearly linear in particle diameter.

Although patterns can be compared visually or by plotting them on a single graph, small but significant differences may still be hard to detect. Another version of the program subtracts the first pattern from one or more patterns, yielding difference plots at any specified magnification (see Fig. 9*d*).

For standard TLDL and HDL analysis the plotting program now runs as part of the same job, so that plots are routinely obtained, usually on an overnight basis. Since our data reduction from schlieren film to punch cards involves two technicians and two keypunch operators, occasional errors are made. However, nearly all such errors result in bumps or irregularities on an otherwise smooth and familiar schlieren curve and are now easily detected by visual examination of the cathode-ray-tube plots.

G. Normal and Abnormal Lipoprotein Spectra

Although it is not our purpose here to discuss in detail normal and abnormal lipoprotein spectra, it is nonetheless worthwhile to consider certain features of ultracentrifugal lipoprotein profiles. An extensive earlier study by Gofman et al. (31) defined many of the broad features in both normal and certain abnormal metabolic states. More recent detailed and comparative studies utilizing current methodology are presented elsewhere (32, 33).

Figures 10 and 11 show TLDL and HDL spectra for an adult normal male and female nonfasting population (Livermore G and H) as well as the main clinical types described by Fredrickson, Levy, and Lees (34). The latter profiles are from a previous study (32) and are from fasting plasma pools. The reason for presenting these data here is to familiarize the reader with the principal features of normal and abnormal patterns, using the new continuous logarithmic TLDL profiles. It is our opinion that in the future these profiles will replace the older discontinuous schlieren presentations.

Most abnormal lipoprotein patterns can be classified by paper (or agarose) electrophoresis or analytical ultracentrifugation (or both) as belonging to one of the types shown in Figs. 10 and 11. However, there are occasional patterns that seem to represent variations or combinations of the basic types. For example, certain type II hyperlipoproteinemia patients

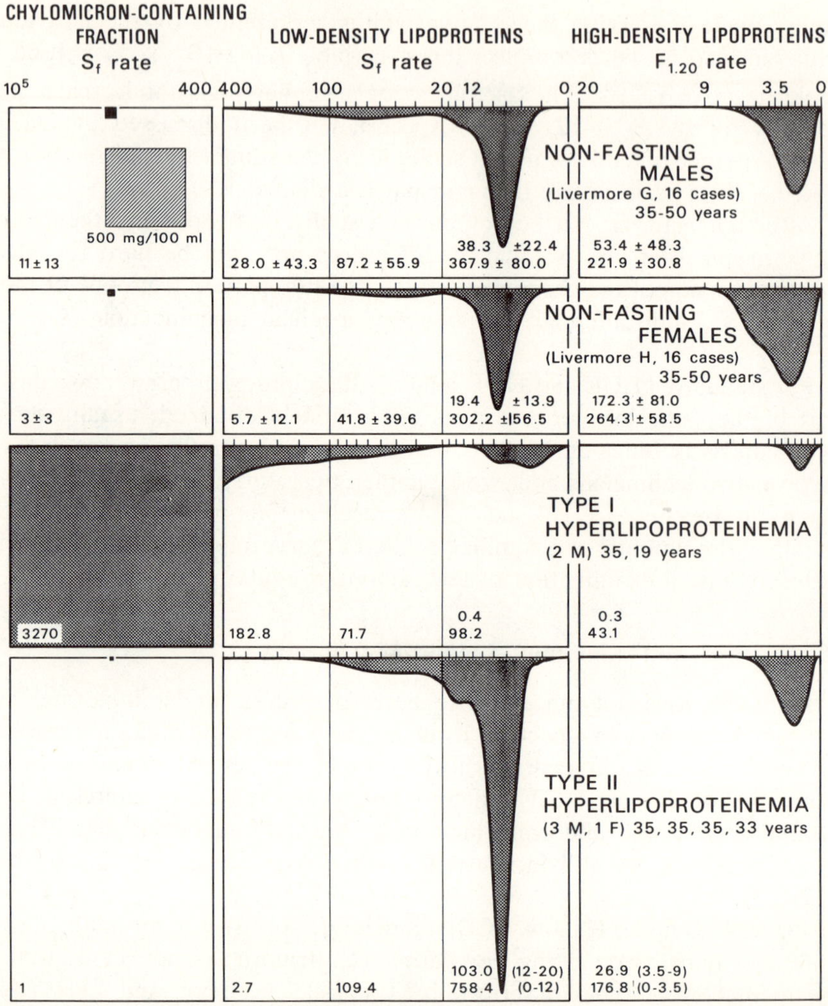

Fig. 10 Low- and high-density lipoprotein spectra for the indicated normal male and female populations, and for type I and II hyperlipoproteinemia fasting plasma pools. Where total S_f 20–400 concentrations are below 150 mg/100 ml (and in the type I hyperlipoproteinemia pool), the S_f 20–100 lipoproteins are measured in the 2-min up-to-speed schlieren photograph. Chylomicron quantification is as described in Sections VI.A and VI.B. For the two normal populations mean and standard-deviation lipoprotein values are given. (Data from Ref. 32.)

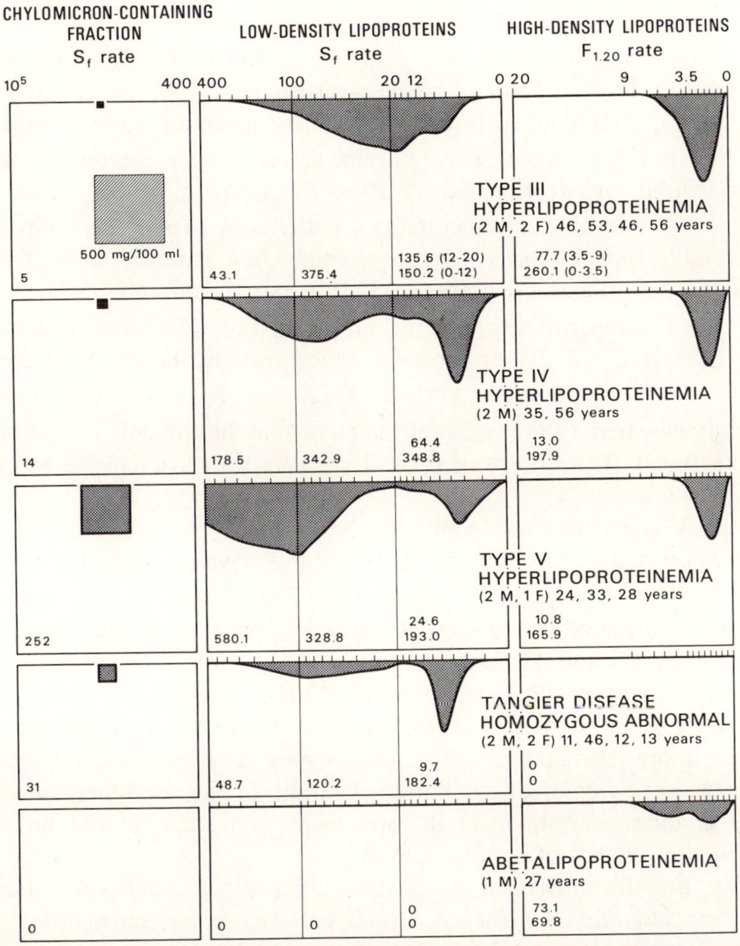

Fig. 11 Low- and high-density lipoprotein spectra of pooled plasma from fasting patients with type III, IV, and V hyperlipoproteinemias and Tangier disease, and plasma from one patient with abetalipoproteinemia. (Data from Ref. 32.)

(characterized by elevated S_f° 0–20 lipoprotein levels) may also exhibit elevated S_f° 20–400 lipoprotein levels (32), and this may reflect a sensitivity to carbohydrate ingestion (D. B. Blankenhorn, J. Jensen, L. C. Jensen, and F. T. Lindgren, unpublished observations). Also, type II hyperlipoproteinemia patients exhibit a wide range of S_f° 0–12 lipoprotein elevations, and those with concentrations above 700 mg/ml usually exhibit tendinous lesions (33).

Type III hyperlipoproteinemia is characterized by the presence of substantial amounts of lipoproteins that have the mobility of β-globulins in electrophoresis and float at 1.006 g/ml (34), and by S_f° 20–400 lipoproteins with an elevated ratio of cholesteryl esters to glycerides (35). Although the type III pool in Fig. 11 shows low levels of both S_f° 100–400 and $S_f > 400$ lipoproteins, when plasma glycerides are elevated, type III patients exhibit grossly elevated S_f° 20–400, and possibly $S_f > 400$, lipoprotein levels. Although ultracentrifugal patterns of these type III patients may resemble type IV or V hyperlipoproteinemia patterns, a relative increase in S_f° 12–30 and a decrease in S_f° 0–12 are usually observed.

The type IV hyperlipoproteinemia profile in Fig. 11 shows an approximately normal S_f° 0–20 lipoprotein concentration; however, there are instances where the levels of both S_f° 0–20 and S_f° 20–400 lipoproteins are grossly elevated (33), and such patterns may be difficult to distinguish ultracentrifugally from those of type II patients with a moderate glyceride elevation (32).

In type V hyperlipoproteinemia fasting patients characteristically have markedly elevated S_f° 20–400 VLDL levels and elevated $S_f > 400$ lipoprotein levels. However, there are patterns that indeed may be a combination of, or some intermediate gradation between, the type I and V patterns shown in Figs. 10 and 11. It becomes clear that some difficulty in placing all lipoprotein abnormalities in a limited primary category of types is to be expected. A given patient, for example, may exhibit a combination of metabolic lipoprotein abnormalities, one or more of which may be sensitive to such factors as caloric imbalance, alcoholic intake, or other acute nutritional changes, certain drug therapy, and even some of the unknown environmental factors of hospitalization.

Finally, Fig. 11 shows the two distinct lipoprotein deficiencies, Tangier disease and abetalipoproteinemia. Each pattern shows unusual features: the former an abnormal VLDL distribution, and the latter an unusually broad HDL pattern.

V. MEASUREMENT AND APPLICATION OF LIPOPROTEIN FLOTATION RATES

A. Moving-Boundary Peak Flotation Rates

The computer analysis of the TLDL and HDL spectra described in Section IV.E provides the S_f° or $F_{1.20}^\circ$ rate of the peak position. However, this determination is based on a single measurement of peak position and is sensitive to the correct base-of-cell position, which includes the problem of cell tilt. Therefore, wherever accurate flotation rates are needed, such as in the characterization of the major S_f 0–12 component, we use a computer program (24) to analyze peak flotation rates by the moving-boundary method (36, 37). In appropriate frames, using a fivefold projected enlargement, the distance of the maximum ordinate of the peak position is measured from the standard radial reference position of the inner knife edge. Using these measured distances and the times of the associated frame times t_i, the program computes the best-fit (least squares) straight line for the points ($\omega^2 t_i$ versus $\ln X_i$). Figure 12 shows the plot of this line, whose slope is the uncorrected flotation rate of the peak. In the low-density run the S_f rate of the major component of the S_f 0–12 class is normally measured in the 8-, 14-, 22-, 30-, 48- and 64-min up-to-speed frames. Such factors as increased lipoprotein concentration and salt redistribution with increasing time tend to change slightly the observed slope of the $\omega^2 t$ versus $\ln X_i$ plot. Since corrections for these changing conditions are not easily incorporated into the calculations, they are omitted from our current program. Other factors, such as the differential compressibility of the lipoprotein and its small-molecule background, present additional con-

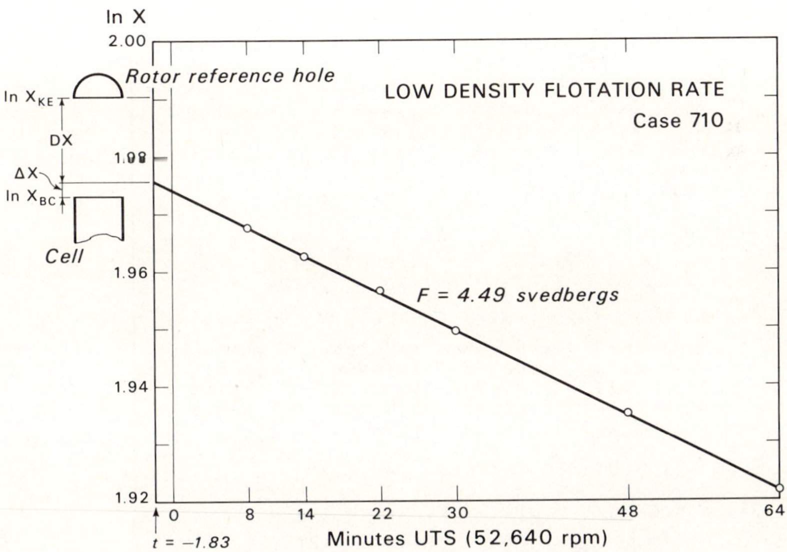

Fig. 12 Uncorrected flotation rate calculated from the 8-, 14-, 22-, 30-, 48-, and 64-min photographs after reaching full speed (52,640 rpm). The acceleration time of 5.2 min is approximately equivalent to 1.83 min of centrifugation at full speed.

siderations, although for the S_f 0–12 class these effects may be negligible (38).

Given the up-to-speed equivalent of the acceleration phase, the program can solve for the base-of-cell position (Fig. 13). This calculated base-of-cell position can be significantly displaced outward (by as much as 0.2 mm in the cell) from the observed base-of-cell position, especially in the late up-to-speed frames. A part of this displacement may be the result of cell tilt (39), estimated to be on the order of 0.1 mm. However, the presence of an inconspicuously small amount of sedimenting lipoprotein or protein can give rise to a false base of cell that moves out slightly as a function of time. As a consequence of these two factors, the more accurate uncorrected flotation rates computed by the best-fit moving-boundary method may be significantly faster than those computed by S_f rate measurement using the peak position and the base-of-cell position in the 30-min up-to-speed frame. It is obvious that small errors in the lipoprotein profile result from the above mentioned uncertainties in aligning the base-of-cell position on the photo-offset template with the assumed (or calculated) base-of-cell position of the schlieren projection.

The typical flotation-rate calculation shown in Fig. 13 utilizes data from

```
FILM      710D. E3 FACTOR = 11.51          JULY-20-67 YES-M    25 NOV 1969

TIME FRAME   DX(CM)     T*W**2      LN(X)       D LN(X)
      5       1.90     .001459     1.96766     -.00007
      6       2.32     .002552     1.96255     -.00027
      7       2.80     .004011     1.95667      .00041 <--
      8       3.37     .005470     1.94965     -.00005
      9       4.54     .008751     1.93507      .00013
     10       5.60     .011668     1.92169     -.00014       Calculation 1

   BEST FIT FLOTATION RATE =          -4.496

   BASE OF CELL/      UTS      DX(CM)      ABS R
                    1.733       1.23      7.2118
                    1.833       1.23      7.2124

TIME FRAME   DX(CM)     T*W**2      LN(X)       D LN(X)
      5       1.90     .001459     1.96766      .00006
      6       2.32     .002552     1.96255     -.00015
      8       3.37     .005470     1.94965      .00003
      9       4.54     .008751     1.93507      .00018
     10       5.60     .011668     1.92169     -.00013       Calculation 2

   BEST FIT FLOTATION RATE =          -4.485

   BASE OF CELL/      UTS      DX(CM)      ABS R
                    1.733       1.25      7.2107
                    1.833       1.24      7.2112
```

Fig. 13 Computer output for flotation-rate calculations (case 710), showing complete input data and best-fit flotation rate and base-of-cell output data.

three to six schlieren frames. The program also computes the deviation [D LN(X)] of each point from the best-fit straight line and then recalculates the slope by successively omitting the most deviant value until only two points remain or until no deviation is above 0.00030. Such presentation of the data allows detection of both reading errors and occasional but subtle cell leaks (if the cells are not weighed before and after the run). The program is flexible and allows measurement of flotation or sedimentation rates in any number of frames at any time, including frames taken during acceleration. In the latter case appropriate values of $\omega_{FS}^{-2} \int \omega^2(t)\,dt$ are obtained from the data-acquisition system. A special application of this technique to S_f 0–12 lipoprotein flotation rates in both low- and high-density media is discussed in the next section.

B. Low-Density-Lipoprotein S_f° Rates, Hydrated Densities, and Molecular Weights

Studies have indicated that the principal low-density S_f 0–12 lipoprotein class represents a distribution in molecular weight, hydrated density (σ), and chemical composition (40–42). The reported molecular weights of this class have ranged from 1.3×10^6 to 3×10^6 (10, 43–45) and depend, in part, on the techniques employed and the portion of the lipoprotein distribution studied. Protein content appears to be the major factor determining the hydrated densities of this class, which range from approximately 1.02 to 1.05 g/ml. Because of this distribution of values, for the specific physical characterization of a given LDL spectrum it is necessary to focus on the most abundant S_f 0–12 component as measured in the analytical ultracentrifuge. The flotation rate of this major low-density component varies from individual to individual, the range being about $S_f^\circ 4$ to $S_f^\circ 8$. The S_f° rates of normal females are approximately 1 S_f° unit faster than that of normal males (24, 46). Also, this component appears to have unusual flotation rates that are associated with specific lipid and lipoprotein abnormalities (32).

C. Utilization of the Standard TLDL and HDL Runs

In preceding sections we have considered computer methods for quantifying the TLDL and the HDL profiles as well as a flexible method for computer analysis of moving-boundary flotation (or sedimentation) rates —in particular, the flotation rate of the S_f 0–12 major component. Theoretically sufficient information is available from these standard low- and high-density runs to calculate more precise S_f° rates as well as hydrated densities (σ values) and molecular weights. Our next method utilizes the

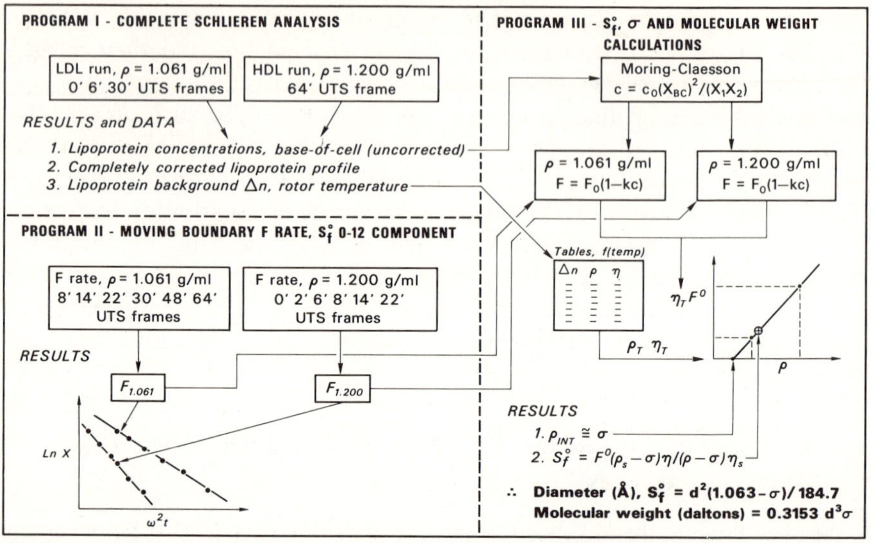

Fig. 14 Schematic diagram showing relationship and utilization of the results and data from three computer programs. Densities are for 26°C. (From Ref. 50; reproduced by permission from the American Oil Chemists' Society.)

results and data from these two programs as input to a third separate computer program, which calculates S_f° rates, σ values, and molecular weights. The relationships among these programs are shown in Fig. 14.

Program II calculates the classical moving-boundary flotation rates of the major S_f 0–12 component as measured in both 1.063 g/ml NaCl and 1.203 g/ml NaBr solutions. Measurements in 1.063 g/ml NaCl are as described in Section V. A, and measurements in 1.203 g/ml NaBr are usually measured in the 0-, 2-, 6-, 8-, 14-, and 22-min up-to-speed frames.

Program I, involving complete schlieren analysis, provides all needed lipoprotein concentrations and data (e.g., rotor temperature) that determine background density and viscosity. The background refractive indices of each lipoprotein subnatant are measured by precision refractometry. These values are extrapolated to the corresponding supernatant fraction. Thus the computer-generated salt tables described in Section II give η and ρ values corresponding to each measured flotation rate, corrected to the mean temperature of the analytical run.

A third program using the above data performs all the remaining calculations. Flotation rates are corrected for concentration dependence by the relationship $F = F^\circ\ (1 - kc)$ where $k = 0.89 \times 10^{-4}$ (mg/100 ml)$^{-1}$ and c is the lipoprotein concentration in the cell integrated up to the S_f

0–12 peak position, averaged over the time interval used in the moving-boundary flotation-rate measurement. This average is approximated by a Moring–Claesson type (47) correction:

$$c = \frac{c_o(X_{BC})^2}{(X_1X_2)} \tag{1}$$

where c_o is the initial base-of-cell concentration as determined in program I, X_{BC} is the base-of-cell radial distance, and X_1 and X_2 are the first and last radial peak positions measured. In the 1.203 g/ml run c is the sum of both the above LDL concentration and the total HDL concentration, similarly corrected. If the low- and high-density fractions are run at different concentrations, the program makes the appropriate corrections. From these data a plot of ηF° versus ρ is made and a ρ-intercept is calculated. The S_f° rates, corrected to standard conditions, are derived from the following relationship:

$$S_f^\circ = \frac{F^\circ(\rho_s - \sigma)\eta}{(\rho - \sigma)\eta_s} \tag{2}$$

where standard values at 26°C for 1.744 *m* NaCl are $\rho_s = 1.0630$ g/ml and $\eta_s = 1.0260$ cP.

Assuming Stokes' frictional factor for spheres, a molecular diameter may be calculated from the relationship:

$$S_f^\circ = \frac{d^2(\rho_s - \sigma)}{18\eta} = \frac{d^2(1.0630 - \sigma)}{184.7} \tag{3}$$

Here d is converted to angstroms in the final expression. Lastly a minimum hydrated molecular weight (MW) is calculated, assuming spheres, from the molecular volume, Avogadro's number N_0, and the hydrated density σ (the latter is closely approximated by the density of zero migration, or ρ-intercept:

$$\text{MW(daltons)} = \frac{\pi d^3}{6(10^{-8}\ \text{cm/Å})^3\ N_0\sigma} = 0.3153\ d^3\sigma \tag{4}$$

D. Use of ηF° versus ρ Techniques for Analysis of Isolated Lipoprotein Components

Classical ηF° versus ρ methodology involves the analysis of isolated homogeneous components at two or more densities. Since the three programs described in the preceding section are applicable to the analysis of single components, it is appropriate to consider their application to LDL subfractions. This application allows comparison and verification of the previous techniques; also this general method can be applied to any VLDL, LDL, and HDL subfractions, such as those obtained by the cumulative-flotation techniques described in Section VI.

Narrow-band low-density lipoproteins can be prepared on an approach-to-equilibrium NaBr density gradient (41). After ultracentrifugation at 50,000 rpm for 48 hr at 18°C, in a 50.3 rotor, fractions are isolated in the second, third, and fourth milliliters, corresponding to densities of approximately 1.031, 1.034, and 1.037 g/ml, respectively. The densities of the isolated lipoprotein fractions are manipulated to approximately 1.063 and 1.203 g/ml by adding solid NaBr, and the final fraction is monitored by precision refractometry. For precise density calculations the refractive-index increment of these lipoproteins was assumed to be 0.00154 and 0.00140 Δn/g/100 ml in the two media, respectively. Since the lipoprotein refractive-index increment is measured by the schlieren analysis program, the precise background refractive index, and hence the density of each fraction in each of the media, is known. As in the previous method, flotation rates are calculated and corrected to zero concentration. However, for this calculation the time-dependent total component concentration is used. Similarly ηF° versus ρ plots are made, and S_f° rates, hydrated densities, and molecular weights are calculated. In these studies with isolated components the problem of correcting for the concentration dependence of the LDL component in the presence of a time-dependent HDL concentration (which is different for each individual) is avoided. It is of interest that in this calculation ρ-intercept values are essentially independent of the concentration-dependent k-factor, although S_f° rates and molecular weights are affected.

E. Application of Techniques to Small Populations

A series of normal male and female subjects were clinically healthy employees of the Lawrence Radiation Laboratory at Livermore and Berkeley, California. Serum was prepared from midmorning nonfasting blood specimens. A complementary series of fasting male and female clinical referrals were obtained from the Kaiser Hospital, Oakland, California. Unless otherwise indicated, all serum or plasma samples studied contained 1/10,000 Merthiolate. Each population set was matched for age, and grossly overweight or underweight subjects were excluded.

In the normal nonfasting series studied the LDL fractions $1.006 < \sigma < 1.063$ g/ml (S_f 0–20) were isolated as described in Section II.C. Total lipids were extracted as previously described (6), and the cholesteryl ester, glyceride, and phospholipid contents were determined by infrared spectrometry (48).

Technical reproducibility was evaluated by using nine serum aliquots from a single nonfasting normal male subject. A measure of errors in our procedure employing TLDL and HDL fractions is the standard deviation of the results:

S_f° rate of major component $= 4.87 \pm 0.08$ (10^{-13} cm/sec/dyne/g)
Hydrated density $\sigma = \rho$-intercept $= 1.0360 \pm 0.0003$ g/ml (26°C)
Molecular weight $\approx (1.984 \pm 0.021) \times 10^6$ daltons

For appropriate comparison with nonfasting serum obtained earlier from the same male subject, ηF° versus ρ studies were made on isolated narrow-band LDL components, and the results were compared with those obtained by our standard low- and high-density technique. Figure 15 shows schlieren photographs of both the 1.063 g/ml NaBr and 1.203 g/ml NaBr runs of one of the narrow-band lipoprotein fractions prepared from the 1.034 g/ml density-gradient fraction (Merthiolate series). All density-gradient samples were analyzed at total component concentrations in the range of 261 to 704 mg/100 ml. Almost identical linear regression relationships between the S_f° rate and the ρ-intercept were obtained for the Merthiolate and non–Merthiolate fractions (Fig. 16). Also plotted are the results (from the same serum sample) of our procedure utilizing eight

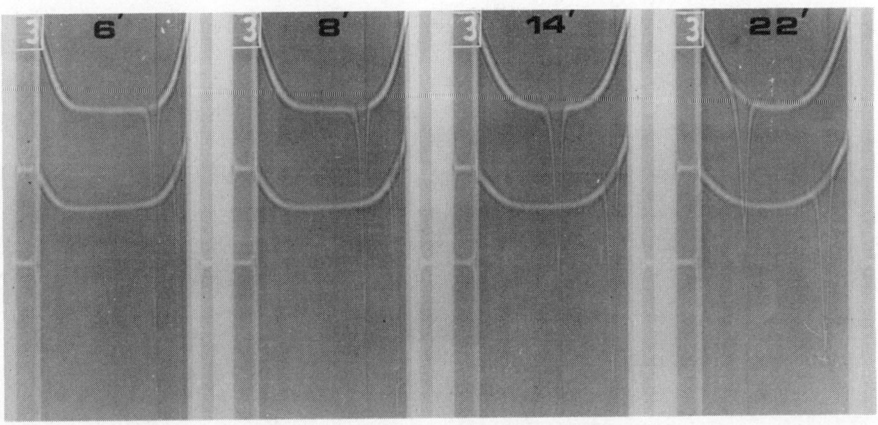

Fig. 15 Schlieren flotation photographs of isolated narrow-band S_f° 6.06 lipoproteins, Case 710. Conditions: 52,640 rpm, 26°C; upper wedge cell is $\rho_{26} = 1.200$ g/ml (2.762 *m* NaBr and 0.195 *m* NaCl), flat cell is $\rho_{26} = 1.061$ g/ml (0.744 *m* NaBr and 0.195 *m* NaCl). Lipoprotein concentration is 465 mg/100 ml. (From Ref. 50; reproduced by permission from the American Oil Chemists' Society.)

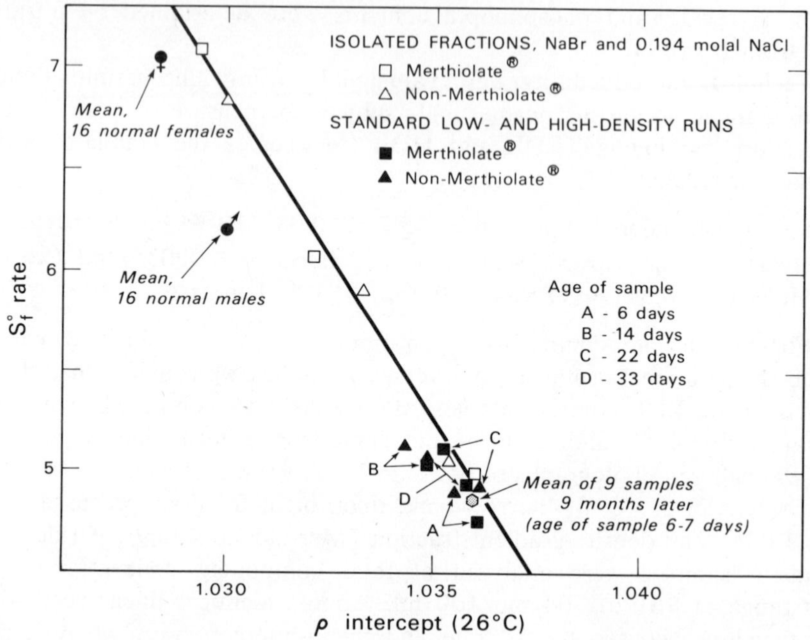

Fig. 16 Relationship between S_f°-rate and ρ-intercept obtained from isolated narrow-band LDL fractions and from the results of standard low- and high-density runs. (From Ref. 50; reproduced by permission from the American Oil Chemists' Society.)

standard TLDL and HDL analyses obtained over 33 days. Nine months later nine additional analyses by our method were performed on serum from the same nonfasting subject; a plot of the mean value suggested minimal biological variation in this person.

Figure 17 shows a similar linear-regression relationship between the S_f° rate and the molecular weight. Again, values obtained from simultaneous TLDL and HDL analyses indicate comparable results in the region of the major component compared with the same S_f° rate on the regression line obtained with isolated lipoprotein components. These results suggest that our TLDL and HDL analyses are closely similar to an ideal procedure. However, such a technically difficult method applied to each individual serum sample would require the identification and narrow-band isolation of the most abundant S_f 0–12 lipoprotein species, followed by a classical ηF° versus ρ analysis.

Preliminary application of this method involved nonfasting serum from a small population of normal adult males and females, 35 to 50 years old. Figures 18 and 19 show the relationship between the S_f° rate and the two

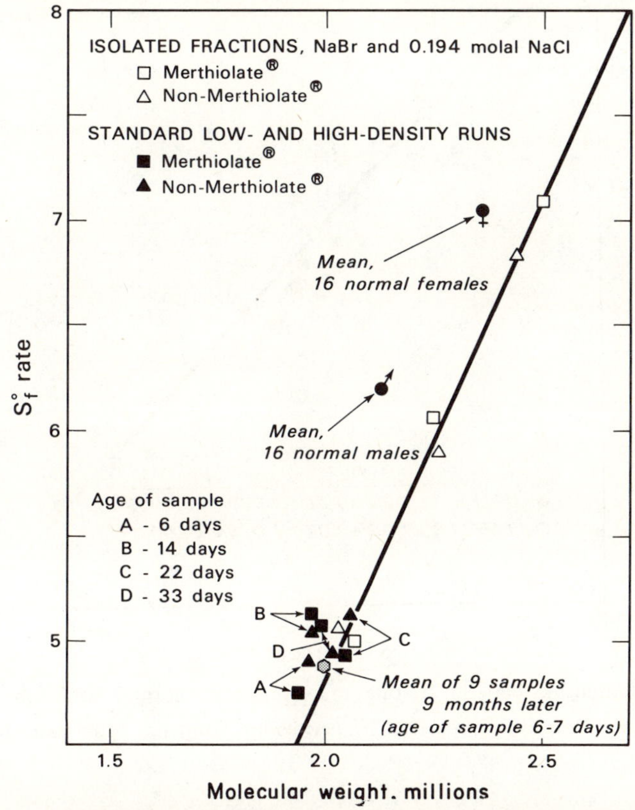

Fig. 17 Relationship between the S_f°-rate and molecular weight obtained from isolated narrow-band LDL fractions and from standard low- and high-density runs. (From Ref. 50; reproduced by permission from the American Oil Chemists' Society.)

calculated parameters, ρ-intercept and molecular weight, respectively. Similar regression is observed with this population as compared with the components isolated from a single normal male. For comparison with the isolated-component study the mean male and female values are also plotted in Figs. 16 and 17. Results indicate that at a given S_f° rate there is variability from person to person both in the ρ-intercept and in the molecular weight. Although the lipoproteins of females have significantly higher S_f° rates than those of males, there appear to be very similar regression relationships for each population. Table I presents the LDL results for this series of normal subjects, including the correlations among the four variables: S_f° rate, ρ-intercept, molecular weight of the major S_f° 0–12 component, and VLDL concentration. The lipoproteins of females

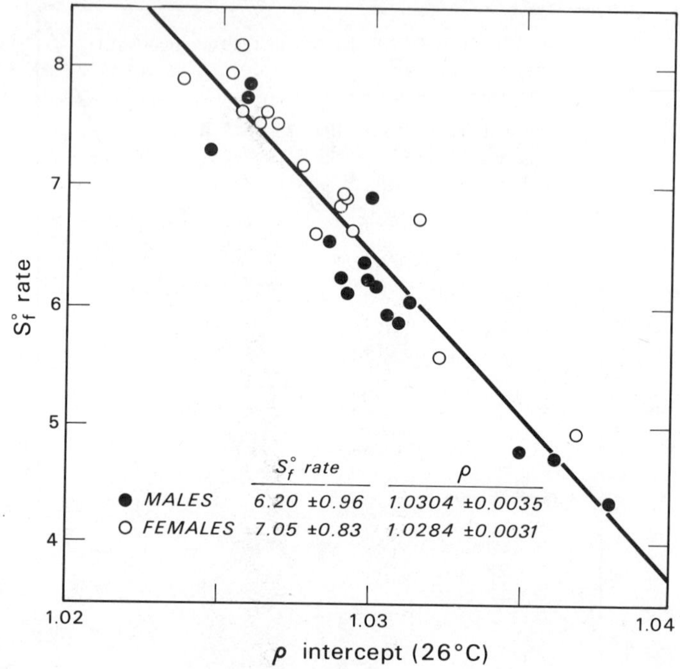

Fig. 18 Relationship between S_f°-rate and ρ-intercept; normal nonfasting males and females. (From Ref. 50; reproduced by permission from the American Oil Chemists' Society.)

(compared with those of males) have faster S_f° rates, as had been observed before (24, 46); they also have a mean molecular weight that is approximately 235,000 higher and a slightly lower mean hydrated density.

The lipoproteins of the S_f 0–20 class were isolated from each of the above normal nonfasting males and females. The cholesteryl ester, triglyceride, and phospholipid content of the total-lipid moiety is presented in Table II. The samples from females are higher in phospholipid, and lower in cholesteryl ester, content than those from males. However, the differences are small, and there is not much variability in lipid composition in these two populations. Although some relationships were observed in the females between these lipid values and the three physical parameters of the most abundant S_f 0–12 component (S_f° rate, σ, and molecular weight), no significant relationships were observed in the male population (see Table III). The calculated mean density of the lipid moieties of each population was almost identical. Although a high negative correlation between σ and phospholipid content was observed in

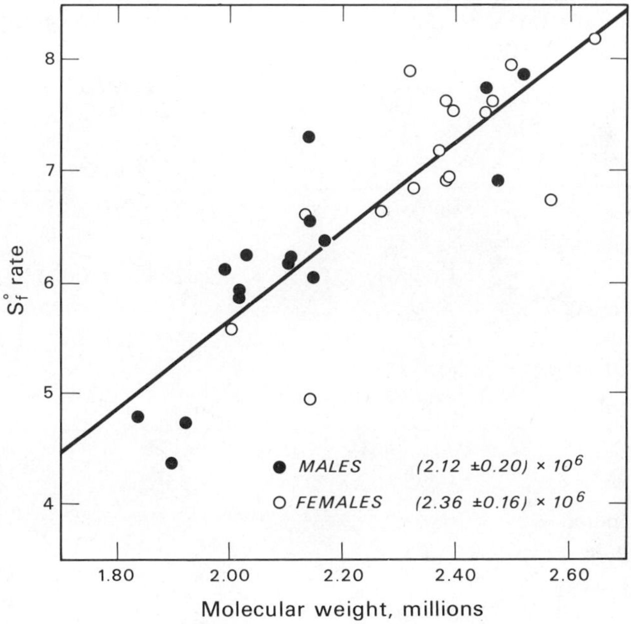

Fig. 19 Relationship between S_f°-rate and molecular weight; normal nonfasting males and females. (From Ref. 50; reproduced by permission from the American Oil Chemists' Society.)

the females, considering the small standard deviation of hydrated density σ (lipid) and phospholipid content, variations in the latter would not be expected to give the observed variations in hydrated density. Also, in the females there was a moderate positive correlation of glyceride content with σ (and a low-order positive correlation in the males).

These results suggest that the major factor contributing to changes in hydrated density within this class is not glyceride (wt %) content but the protein (wt %) content of the lipoprotein, as shown in Section VII.C. In a much earlier density-gradient study this relationship between protein content and lipoprotein density was also observed on subfractions of S_f° 3–10 from pooled human plasma (40). In a recent study (49), however, no significant correlation was found between the S_f° rate of the major LDL component and the protein content of the total-LDL fraction. Since the protein content increases with decreasing S_f° rate of LDL subfractions, the protein content of the total-LDL fraction is determined by the lipoprotein profile within intervals of the S_f 0–20 class and not by the S_f° rate of the major component (6).

Table I. Results for S_f 0–12 Major Component, Normal Nonfasting Subjects (Livermore G and H)[a]

Variable	Males ($n = 16$), 44 ± 3 Years	Females ($n = 16$), 43 ± 4 Years	Difference
S_f°-Rate	6.20 ± 0.96	7.05 ± 0.83	$p < .01$
Hydrated density σ (g/ml)[b]	1.0304 ± 0.0035	1.0284 ± 0.0031	N.S.
Molecular weight (10^6 daltons)	2.12 ± 0.20	2.36 ± 0.16	$p < .01$
S_f° 20–400 (VLDL) (mg/100 ml)	118 ± 105	36 ± 50	$p < .01$
Correlations:			
S_f° versus σ	−.95[c]	−.95[c]	
S_f° versus molecular weight	.87[c]	.76[c]	
σ versus molecular weight	−.69[c]	−.52[d]	
S_f° versus VLDL	−.72[c]	−.76[c]	

[a] Data from Ref. 50. All values are mean ± S.D.
[b] ρ-Intercept.
[c] $p < .01$.
[d] $p < .05$.

Table II. Lipid Composition and Lipid σ of S_f 0–20 Lipoproteins in Normal Males and Females[a]

Subjects	Component[b] PL	CE	TG	FC	Lipid σ (g/ml)[c]
Males ($n = 16$)	24.4 ± 2.3	55.1 ± 1.5	9.4 ± 2.4	11.0 ± 0.3	0.9803 ± 0.0016
Females ($n = 16$)	26.7 ± 1.8	53.4 ± 1.5	9.3 ± 2.3	10.6 ± 0.3	0.9798 ± 0.0015
Difference	$p < .01$	$p < .01$	N.S.	—	N.S.

[a] Data from Ref. 50. Values (mean ± S.D.) in weight percent of total lipids; free cholesterol is assumed to be 0.198 × cholesteryl ester. Lipoprotein lipid compositions of VLDL, LDL, and HDL (of this Livermore G and H series) are reported in Chapter 4.
[b] PL, CE, TG, and FC are abbreviations for phospholipids, cholesteryl esters, triglycerides, and free cholesterol, respectively.
[c] Calculated by assuming additivity of densities for PL, CE, TG, and FC; individual values used are 0.97, 0.99, 0.92, and 1.067 g/ml, respectively.

Table III. Correlations of S_f° Rate, σ, and Molecular Weight with S_f 0–20 Lipid Composition, Normal Subjects[a]

Parameter	Component[b] PL	CE	TG	Lipid σ
S_f°-Rate	.79[c] (.27)	−.02 (.07)	−.61[d] (−.30)	.47 (.26)
Hydrated density σ, (g/ml)	−.70[c] (−.29)	−.04 (.03)	.58[d] (.23)	−.47 (−.17)
Molecular weight	.70[c] (.23)	−.11 (.21)	−.46 (−.36)	.34 (.36)

[a] Data from Ref. 50; normal females and males (in parentheses).
[b] Abbreviations: PL, phospholipids; CE, cholesteryl esters; TG, triglycerides.
[c] $p < .01$.
[d] $p < .05$.

Another preliminary application of this method was to a small series of 16 male and 19 female clinical referrals from the Kaiser Hospital, Oakland, California. These patients were of a wider age range; many had high blood-lipid levels, and in contrast with the normals studied, they were fasting. Table IV presents the LDL results for these populations, including the statistical relationships. As in the normal populations, similar values, differences, and correlations were observed, although the somewhat lower S_f° rates observed probably reflect a clinical population with higher VLDL levels (see Tables I and IV). Lower S_f° rates would be expected, since in both normal male and female populations there was a significant negative correlation between the S_f° rate and VLDL concentration in this study and in a previous one (6).

From theoretical considerations molecular weights obtained by our technique might be expected to be low by as much as 10%, although differences between males and females as well as the observed relationships among S_f° rate, σ, and molecular weight would appear to be valid. These results, of course, apply to the small populations studied. However, it would seem unlikely, for example, that the shape factor for S_f° 4–8 lipoproteins would be different in males and females or would vary significantly from, say, $S_f^\circ 4$ to $S_f^\circ 8$. There are difficulties in applying corrections for concentration dependence in the flotation measurements, but there is no evidence that any of the observed relationships and relative differences are *k*-factor dependent. Recalculating all data by using *k*-factors of 0.44 or 1.78×10^{-4} (mg/100 ml)$^{-1}$ did not significantly alter any of the observed relationships. A 20% error in the *k*-factor used here, 0.89 $\times 10^{-4}$ (mg/100 ml)$^{-1}$, would involve approximately a 5% error in mo-

Table IV. Data for S_f 0–12 Major Component, Kaiser Clinical Referrals, Fasting[a]

Variable	Males ($n = 16$) 49 ± 11 Years	Females ($n = 19$) 51 ± 10 Years	Difference
S_f° Rate	5.85 ± 1.41	6.74 ± 0.97	$p < .05$
Hydrated density σ (g/ml)	1.0327 ± 0.0053	1.0293 ± 0.0037	$p < .05$
Molecular weight (10^6 daltons)	2.16 ± 0.28	2.29 ± 0.23	N.S.
S_f° 20–400 (VLDL) (mg/100 ml)	289 ± 285	108 ± 108	$p < .01$
Correlations:			
S_f° versus σ	−.96[b]	−.90[b]	
S_f° versus molecular weight	.89[b]	.72[b]	
σ versus molecular weight	−.73[b]	−.35	
S_f° versus VLDL	−.62[c]	−.74[b]	

[a] Data from Ref. 50. Values are mean ± S.D.
[b] $p < .01$.
[c] $p < .05$.

lecular weight. However, it is anticipated that as more data on concentration dependence and shape factors become available, more meaningful and accurate molecular-weight data may be obtained by this procedure. The main advantage of this technique is that all the needed information is derived from a single routine simultaneous TLDL and HDL analysis.

F. Comparison of Ultracentrifugal Techniques for Obtaining LDL Molecular Weight

Although our LDL molecular weights are compared with the results of others in some detail elsewhere (50), it is worthwhile to mention a few recent comparisons. For example, from somewhat similar ultracentrifugal data of the major LDL component (and assuming spheres) Oncley (44) obtained a molecular weight of 2.3×10^6 and a hydrated density of 1.032 g/ml. In their most recent hydrodynamic study Adams and Schumaker (51) obtained a mean and standard deviation for nine LDL samples (fasting males, ages 20–40) of $(2.38 \pm 0.13) \times 10^6$. These values assumed a shape factor of $f/f_0 = 1.05$ and 10% hydration. Had they assumed spheres and no hydration, the value would have been approximately $(2.16 \pm 0.13) \times 10^6$. From equilibrium data Scanu, Pollard, and Reader (52) have given a range of 2.2 to 2.3×10^6 for the major LDL component, $1.019 < \sigma < 1.063$ g/ml. Our data on both normals and clinical referrals are approximately of this magnitude.

VI. ISOLATION AND ANALYSIS OF SERUM-LIPOPROTEIN FRACTIONS WITH SWINGING-BUCKET ROTORS AND DENSITY GRADIENTS

A. Elemental Analysis of Lipoprotein Fractions

Although routine biochemical and physical methods are available for quantifying total lipoprotein lipids, constituent lipids (8, 53), and proteins (54, 55), these procedures have certain limitations and disadvantages. For example, if a limited lipoprotein sample is available and one is primarily interested in total lipoprotein mass, protein, and phospholipid content, a more convenient methodology is available, namely elemental CHN and P analysis. Since such data are presented in this section, which describes density-gradient preparation of lipoprotein fractions, it is appropriate to consider briefly these techniques now.

For elemental CHN analysis we use a modified CHN analyzer (Model 185, Hewlett-Packard, Palo Alto, Calif.). Aliquots of from 0.004 to 0.1 ml of lipoprotein solutions are pipetted into contamination-free aluminum boats (29–410M, Perkin-Elmer, Maywood, Ill.) and weighed on a semimicrobalance. Readings are taken 20 sec after pipetting, and corrections for evaporation may be made by adding the weight lost during an additional 20 sec period. Ideally, the total lipoprotein mass should be in the range of 200 to 400 μg. Triplicate samples are dried at 55°C overnight and at 110°C for 1 hr just before analysis. Other details of procedure, precautions against contamination, and absolute mass calibration of the instrument, including the computer program, are described in detail elsewhere (56, 57). The results of agreeing duplicates of the CHN analysis provide precise total CHN composition as well as N/CHN ratios for each lipoprotein fraction.

Since total lipoprotein N is derived almost exclusively from both proteins and phospholipids, the latter must also be determined.[5] The Bartlett method

[5] As summarized by Margolis in Ref. 9, pp. 388–389, defatted LDL and VLDL contain as much as 5 to 9% carbohydrate of which 1.5 to 3.5% is N-containing glucosamine and sialic acid; the remainder consists of neutral sugars. Delipidized HDL

(58) provides a precise semimicro phosphorus determination. As before, appropriate lipoprotein aliquots are accurately weighed so that the estimated phospholipid content will be in the approximate range of the standard sample, namely, 1 μg phosphorus. Contamination, especially from soaps and detergent residues on glassware and from smokers (igniting matches) should be scrupulously avoided. Cuvettes should be carefully matched, and absorbance readings should be obtained from a stable instrument, such as a Cary Model 14 recording spectrometer (Cary Instruments, Monrovia, Calif.). If no inorganic phosphorus is present in the lipoprotein fractions, we may assume that all elemental phosphorus is derived from lipoprotein phospholipids. Thus we can combine the results of the two elemental methods by using computer-derived tables. Knowing the total N + C + H and the approximate chemical composition of the lipoproteins, which yield an accurate ratio of N + C + H to the total mass, we obtain the total lipoprotein mass. From the N/CHN ratio corrected for the phospholipid N (assuming 1 atom of N per atom of P) we obtain a precise protein determination. In the calculations we assume a protein N/CHN ratio of 0.2000 for S_f 0–10^5 lipoproteins and 0.2056 for HDL lipoproteins; these values are derived from the amino acid composition of the LDL protein and HDL protein (7), respectively.

Under favorable operating conditions and optimum sample mass, this elemental analysis procedure routinely yields data with standard errors of measurement of approximately 0.5% for lipoprotein mass, 0.1 to 0.3% for weight percent of lipoprotein protein, and 0.5 to 1.0% for weight percent of phospholipids. In the future such data may be helpful in the detailed comparison of lipoprotein subfractions obtained from different patients exhibiting unusual lipoprotein abnormalities. Also, the accurate measurement of lipoprotein mass, independent of the presence of large amounts of inorganic salts, should permit very accurate evaluation of specific refractive-index increments for all LDL and HDL subfractions.

B. Isolation of total $S_f > 400$ Chylomicron-Containing Fractions

As already mentioned, a rigorous definition of the chylomicrons is difficult, particularly if fractions are isolated from plasma or serum instead of

contain approximately 3% carbohydrate of roughly similar composition (Scanu, in Ref. 9, pp. 435–438). The protein content reported here is uncorrected for the presence of this carbohydrate, although lipoprotein carbohydrate CHN is included in our analysis. Assuming 5% carbohydrate (2.5% galactose and 2.5% glucosamine) in all delipidized lipoprotein fractions, we have calculated approximate errors for lipoprotein mass and protein content. For $S_f > 400$, VLDL, LDL, and HDL, lipoprotein mass is underestimated by 0.07, 0.21, 0.5, and 1.3%, respectively; similarly protein content is overestimated by 0.04, 0.14, 0.4, and 0.9 wt %, respectively.

from chyle or lymph. Since their discovery by Gage (59) over 50 years ago, procedures for isolating and quantifying the chylomicrons have included the original method of dark-field counting of particles (60), turbidimetry (61, 62), flocculation by toluidine blue (63) or polyvinylpyrrolidone (64), and various combinations of ultracentrifugal isolation (65–68) and mass assay. Although these techniques are useful for specific experimental work, their limitation is the difficulty in reproducing and comparing the results from different laboratories. The two basic problems of chylomicron analysis are to define unambiguously the isolation procedure and to provide an accurate and reproducible mass assay. As recommended by Dole and Hamlin (67), the fractionation should be expressed in terms of the product of mean relative centrifugal force and time (*g*-min), and the conditions of preparative ultracentrifugation should be defined completely.

Our procedure defines a chylomicron-containing fraction isolated ultracentrifugally only in terms of its included S_f range of recovery. The method is essentially that described earlier (57), and the data given in Section IV.G were obtained by the original procedure. However, results obtained by our slightly modified and improved procedure would be very similar, except that the included S_f range is slightly larger, with less than 100% recovery, as defined below. With modifications only in the centrifugal conditions, larger samples may be used in the 12- and 17-ml buckets, and fractions may be obtained with any desired lower S_f range of recovery.

Since our overlayering procedure for preparing a nonlinear salt gradient is used for all our lipoprotein-subfractionation work, we present it in detail now. First, 84.6 mg of dry NaCl is weighed into a screw cap vial, and 1.00 ml of serum is added. The capped vial is swirled and allowed to stand for about 30 min. This bubble-free serum solution (background density 1.065 g/ml) is transferred to the bottom of a 0.5 × 2.5-in. cellulose nitrate tube. Before transferring, 10 drops of 1.065 g/ml NaCl solution is placed in the bottom, and a hemispherical epoxy insert is positioned, as shown in Fig. 20. This essentially eliminates the curvature in the lower boundary of the sample. The inserts for each tube size are made by casting plain epoxy or aluminum-filled epoxy in the bottom of appropriate preparative tubes. After hardening, the hemispheres are machined and lapped to final weights (which are within 20 mg for each type).

The plastic holder is now tilted to a position 25 degrees from horizontal, and during overlayering it is illuminated by a beam of light from the side in a darkened room (see Fig. 21). As shown in Fig. 20, precise volumes of the indicated NaCl solutions are added dropwise on the tube wall above the serum layer. All salt solutions used in the density-gradient procedures contain EDTA at a concentration of 3 mg/100 ml. This amount, rather than the usual 10 mg/100 ml, is necessary to minimize the CHN elemental

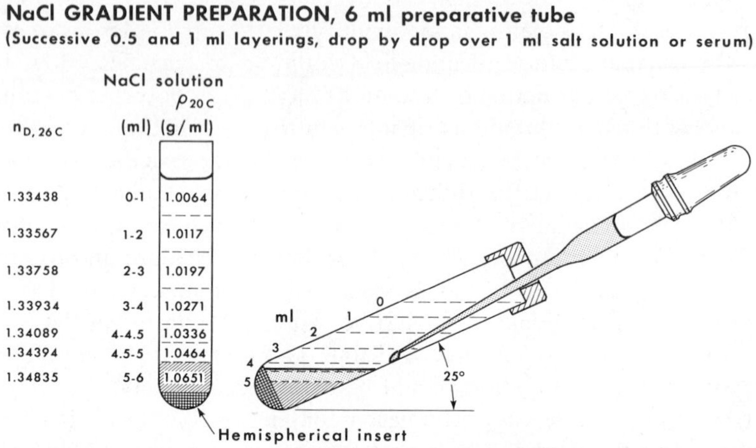

Fig. 20 Overlayering procedure for preparing nonlinear salt gradient for $S_f > 400$ fractionation. Each successive 0.5- and 1.0-ml layer is added drop by drop over the bottom 1 ml of salt solution or serum. (From Ref. 57; reproduced by permission from the American Oil Chemists' Society.)

background for both mass and protein determinations. After the gradient is finished, the holder is slowly rotated to the vertical position, and the layered preparative tube is carefully placed into the appropriate 6-ml bucket, which is then capped. Although we recommend a Beckman SW 25.3 rotor with special 6-ml buckets (mean $r = 10.44$ cm), a SW 25.1, SW 25.3, or SW 27 rotor equipped with 6-ml tube adapters may be used.

Temperature changes should be minimized in all lipoprotein density-gradient work. All our swinging-bucket centrifugations are carried out at room temperature (~ 23°C) in the Beckman L2-65 (or 65B) ultracentrifuge (modified to achieve temperature stability to ± 0.2°C, rotor-speed stability to ± 30 rpm, and equipped with a variable overspeed safety device). Precise lipoprotein recovery depends on the density and viscosity of all regions in the gradient; hence the initial rotor temperature (approximately equal to room temperature and the gradient temperature) of a particular run determines the equivalent up-to-speed centrifugation (full-speed time plus one-third of the sum of acceleration and deceleration). This value is obtained from computer tables (see Section VI.C) calculated for proper recovery over the range 22 to 26°C in 0.5°C increments. Although we recommend collection of the chylomicron-containing fraction in only 0.5-ml volumes, there may be circumstances when this is not possible. In these instances the initial serum solution may be diluted, or a full 1-ml fraction may be taken. In the latter case there will be a slightly different threshold

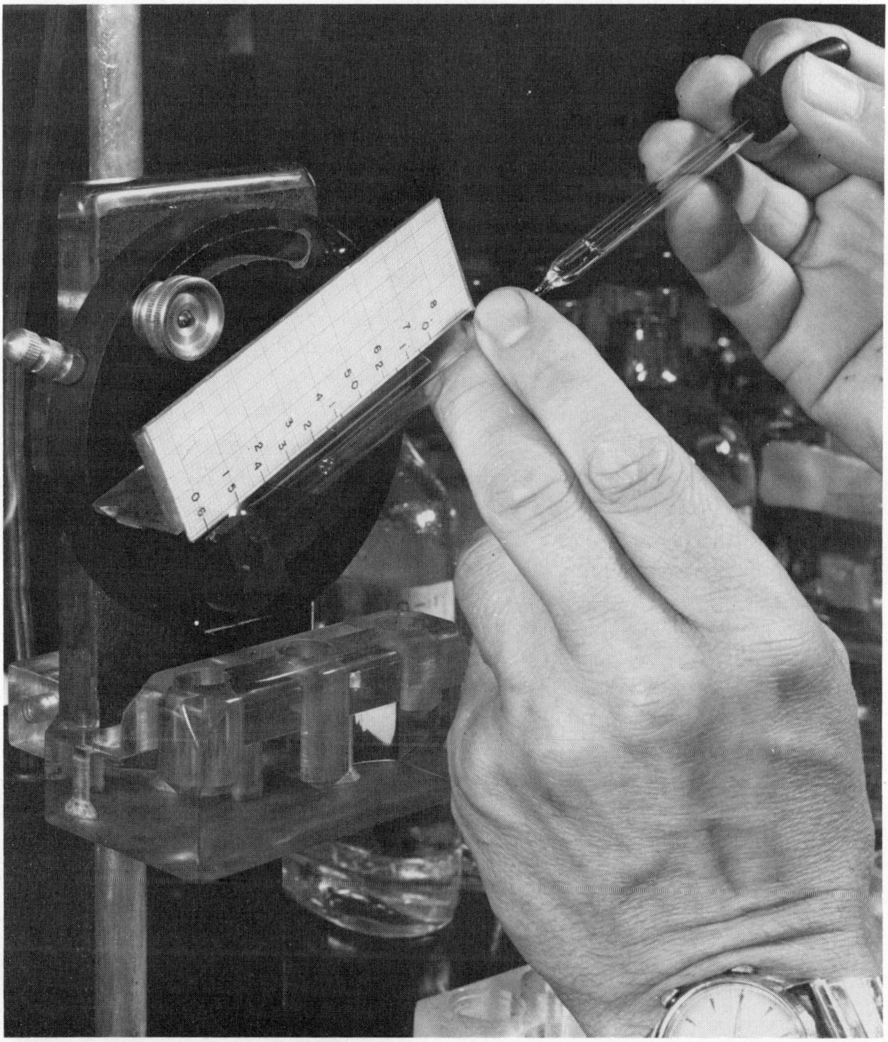

Fig. 21 Detail of lipoprotein-pipetting fixture, showing rotating preparative-tube holder and adjustable scale. Separate rotating tube holders with appropriate scales are substituted when using 12 ml and 17 ml preparative tubes. For pipetting lipoprotein fractions the holder is rotated to the vertical position and the upper region of the preparative tube is illuminated from above by a collimated light beam.

recovery. At 23°C the total *g*-min required for 100% recovery of $S_f > 400$ lipoproteins is 2.85×10^6 and 2.50×10^6 for 0.5- and 1.0-ml fractions, respectively.

Care should be exercised to start the centrifuge slowly; after reaching about 1000 rpm the speed control pot may be set at full speed. We do not use the brake. After centrifugation the 0.5-ml $S_f > 400$ fraction is quantitatively removed with a carefully selected capillary pipette (Section II.D), and two additional 0.5-ml fractions are taken as reference subnatants. Ideally the preparation of the gradient and the removal of the fractions, in this and all other density-gradient procedures, should be done as close to the centrifuge as laboratory conditions permit.

The stability of the salt gradient is shown in Fig. 22. Very little difference is observed between a gradient pipetted immediately and one allowed to stand at 1 *g* for 2.5 to 3.5 hr. More importantly, there is good reproducibility and very little difference between the static and dynamic gradients (61.0-min up-to-speed at 20,000 rpm). Accordingly, we use a mean of the dynamic gradient values for calculating lipoprotein recoveries in our chylomicron-containing fractions.

C. Calculation of Lipoprotein Recovery

Figure 23 shows a 6-ml preparative tube containing a dynamic salt gradient divided into 12 regions; to simplify the calculations each of the 12 regions can be considered a homogeneous region (j) of ρ_j *and* η_j, with a lower boundary at radial distance r_j determined by the rotor and rotor tube.

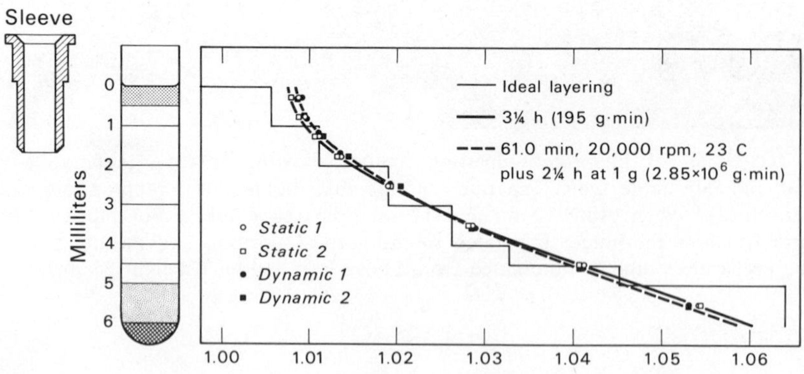

Fig.22 Stability of static and dynamic 6-ml NaCl gradients used for chylomicron isolation.

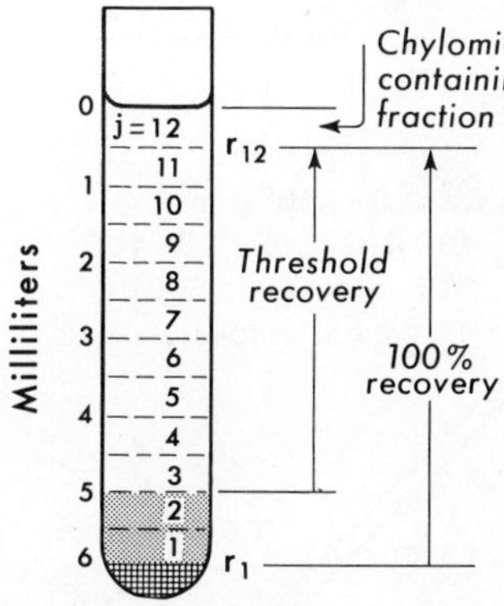

ρ_{23C} (g/ml)	η_{23C} (cp)
1.0088	0.9632
1.0097	0.9650
1.0113	0.9683
1.0141	0.9743
1.0184	0.9844
1.0213	0.9914
1.0265	1.0037
1.0309	1.0144
1.0375	1.0303
1.0434	1.0444
1.0701	1.8622
1.0765	1.8811

Fig. 23 Dynamic-gradient values of ρ and η used in calculating lipoprotein flotation recovery. (From Ref. 57; reproduced by permission from the American Oil Chemists' Society.)

Lipoprotein recovery for a specified top fraction may be defined in terms of 100% and threshold S_f rates. Migration up to the lower boundary of the fraction from the bottom and the top, respectively, of the layered sample is defined as 100% recovery and threshold recovery (0%). Ideally, all lipoproteins of S_f value greater than the 100% value should be recovered in the top fraction, but none lower than the threshold value should be included. By the use of a computer program written in Fortran IV, tables are constructed of centrifuge-run times for 100% recovery of specified S_f values at various temperature and rpm values. If a given S_f rate of hydrated density σ is to be recovered in fraction 12, the relation:

$$S_f = \frac{F_j(\rho_s - \sigma)\eta_j}{\eta_s(\rho_j - \sigma)} \tag{5}$$

yields the flotation rates F_j, which determine the times of migration Δt_j through each region:

$$F_j = \frac{\ln r_{j+1} - \ln r_j}{\omega^2 \ \Delta t_j} \tag{6}$$

Summing, we obtain

$$\omega^2 T = \Sigma_{j=1}^{11} \omega^2 \ \Delta t_j \tag{7}$$

where T is the total equivalent up-to-speed time. The program then converts this $\omega^2 T$ into shutoff times at specified rpm values, taking into account the acceleration and deceleration period. The conditions required to achieve 100% lipoprotein recovery with our 6-ml density gradient (23°C) are shown in Fig. 24. Times for a multistage run, such as the cumulative sub-

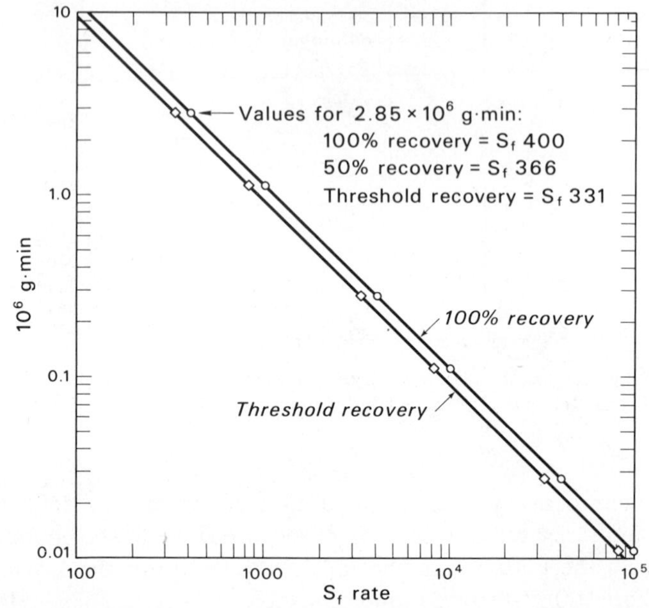

Fig. 24 Lipoprotein recovery (23°C, 6-ml gradient) over the range of 0.01×10^6 to 10×10^6 g-min. (From Ref. 57; reproduced by permission from the American Oil Chemists' Society.)

fractionation of lipoprotein classes, in which successive layers are removed, are also calculated from the increment of $\omega^2 T$ over the previous stage (for each successive run).

Calculating corresponding threshold recoveries, as well as 100% and threshold S_f values of a run that has been made under particular conditions of time, temperature, rpm, rotor, and gradient is accomplished by reversing the calculations. This involves iteration, because the hydrated density σ must be approximated for the unknown S_f value. For example, the 100% recovery calculation considers as a first approximation the flotation rate:

$$\mathrm{F} = \frac{\ln r_{12} - \ln r_1}{\omega^2 T} \tag{8}$$

Then assuming a mean ρ, η, and $\sigma_0 = 0.93$ g/ml, we obtain

$$\mathrm{S}_{f(1)} = \mathrm{F} \times 1.44 \quad \text{and} \quad \sigma_1 = f(\ln \mathrm{S}_{f(1)}) \tag{9}$$

from literature values (68, 69). An iterative calculation is started with $i = 1$, and F_j is calculated over each region j from

$$\mathrm{S}_{f(1)} \approx \frac{\mathrm{F}_j(\rho_s - \sigma_i)\eta_j}{\eta_s(\rho_j - \sigma_i)} \tag{10}$$

Then Δt_j and hence $(\Sigma_1^{11}\,\Delta t_j)_i$ can be calculated from

$$\mathrm{F}_j = \frac{\Delta \ln r_j}{\omega^2\,\Delta t_j} \tag{11}$$

A new approximation is now made, setting

$$\mathrm{S}_{f(i+1)} = \mathrm{S}_{f(i)}\,\frac{\Sigma_1^{11}\,\Delta t_j}{T} \tag{12}$$

and one continues to iterate for convergence until

$$\frac{|(\Sigma_1^{11}\,\Delta t_j)_n - T|}{T} < 0.001\,\cdot \tag{13}$$

D. Subfractionation of the $S_f > 400$ Lipoproteins

The following procedure scaled for subfractionating 3 to 18 ml of serum represents a modification and improvement of an earlier (69) cumulative-flotation procedure. Its application to the $S_f > 400$, VLDL, LDL, and HDL classes has been made possible by the development and availability of high-performance, long-radial path, swinging-bucket rotors. The subfractionation of each class involves overlayering serum or a serum-containing fraction with a particular nonlinear salt gradient, in a manner that resembles in many respects the procedure just described for total $S_f > 400$ lipoprotein fractionation.

In the first step of the procedure 254 mg of solid NaCl is added to 3 ml of plasma, raising the background density to 1.065 g/ml. Before the 3-ml sample is placed in a ⅝ × 4-in. heavy walled preparative tube, a few drops of 1.065 g/ml NaCl solution are added in the bottom. Then a solid epoxy hemispherical insert (which fits snugly) is positioned in the bottom of the tube, as shown in Fig. 25. A long Lucite sleeve is inserted in the top of the tube to avoid wall contamination, and the serum sample is carefully introduced into the bottom, avoiding any bubbles. Except for scaling up volumes, the gradient formation is similar to that of $S_f > 400$ fractionation. After rotating the tube to 25 degrees from the horizontal, the sample is overlayered with a 14-ml NaCl density gradient. Solutions are added (from highest to lowest density) in volumes of 1 ml each for the first two layers and 3 ml each for the remaining four layers. The densities are 1.0464, 1.0336, 1.0271, 1.0197, 1.0117, and 1.0064 g/ml, and the resulting gradient is as shown in Fig. 25. Corresponding n_{D}^{26} values are given in Fig. 20.

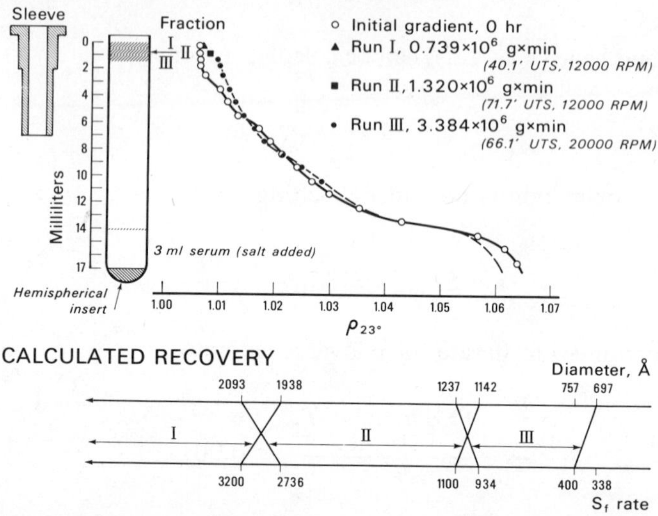

Fig. 25 Sodium chloride density gradient used for the subfractionation of the $S_f >$ 400 lipoproteins (17-ml gradient, SW 25.3 rotor, 23°C). The *g*-min values and needed equivalent full-speed centrifugation (including acceleration and deceleration) at the indicated conditions are given for each successive centrifugation. Diagrammed below the gradient are the calculated ranges of S_f-rates (and diameters, assuming spheres) for lipoproteins recovered under ideal conditions for each run. (From Ref. 70; reproduced by permission from the *Journal of Lipid Research.*)

The next steps consist of removing 0.5-ml layers from the tops of the tubes after three successive centrifugations at 0.739×10^6, 1.320×10^6, and 3.384×10^6 *g*-min. These runs are made in an SW 25.3 rotor (mean $r = 11.43$ cm) under such conditions that 100% recovery is achieved for $S_f > 3200$, $S_f > 1100$, and $S_f > 400$ fractions after the first, second, and third runs, respectively.

There are several reasons for fractionation in this manner rather than centrifuging once and removing several layers. Removal of thin layers at the top of the tubes concentrates each lipoprotein fraction, and the cumulative-flotation procedure minimizes the time lipoproteins are exposed to an aqueous–air interface. Also this procedure avoids the need to either isolate the total $S_f > 400$ lipoproteins free of contamination from other serum lipoproteins and proteins or to employ tedious washing procedures for each fraction. Furthermore, increasing the radial distance the lipoproteins in each fraction must travel by bringing them into a thin top 0.5-ml layer reduces the calculated differences in S_f rate between 100 and 0% (threshold) recovery. This also reduces overlap among the fractions collected.

Another factor favoring this procedure is that both small- and large-molecule contamination by diffusion and convection is essentially eliminated by collecting the fractions a maximum radial distance inward from the initially layered serum sample. Figure 25 shows the stability of this gradient as well as the centrifugal conditions required for each successive run. The calculated recovery, including overlap of the subfractions, is given in terms of both S_f rate and particle diameter. Although cuts at any desired S_f rate may be made, the suggested S_f rate intervals generally yield three $S_f > 400$ subfractions, concentrated approximately sixfold, that divide the total $S_f > 400$ lipoprotein mass into roughly equal parts. This consideration is useful in all lipoprotein-subfractionation studies in which detailed lipid and lipoprotein studies are involved.

E. Subfractionation of the S_f 20–400 Lipoproteins

The following procedure is scaled to permit VLDL subfractionation of from 2 to 12 ml of serum. As suggested in Section II.C, if $S_f > 400$ lipoproteins are present in significant amounts, they should be removed prior to VLDL subfractionation. After removal, 2 ml of $S_f < 400$ subnatant serum is added to 169 mg of solid NaCl, bringing the background density to 1.065 g/ml. Using hemispherical inserts and the same procedure of manipulation as in $S_f > 400$ lipoprotein subfractionation, the sample is placed in a heavy walled $\frac{9}{16} \times 3\frac{1}{2}$-in. cellulose nitrate preparative tube. The 2-ml serum sample is overlayered with a 10-ml NaCl salt gradient, using the same six solutions as in the $S_f > 400$ fractionation. The following volumes (from highest to lowest density) are 1 ml for the first two layers and 2 ml for the next four layers. The gradient and its stability are shown in Fig. 26. As before, 0.5-ml layers are removed after each of three successive centrifugations in an SW 41-Ti rotor calculated to bring up first the $S_f > 100$, $S_f > 60$, and finally $S_f > 20$ lipoproteins into each successive 0.5-ml top fraction. The necessary centrifugal conditions for each stage at 35,000 rpm and 23°C are listed in Fig. 26. At a mean radius of 10.76 cm the equivalent *g*-min values for these three centrifugations are 21.2×10^6, 15.0×10^6, and 164.7×10^6 *g*-min for the first, second, and third centrifugation, respectively. After collection of the third fraction an additional 0.5 ml is taken for measurement of the background salt density and evaluation of possible protein contamination.

F. Subfractionation of S_f 0–20 Lipoproteins

The following is a convenient subfractionation procedure (69a) scaled to permit the recovery of three LDL subfractions, each in 0.5- to 3-ml

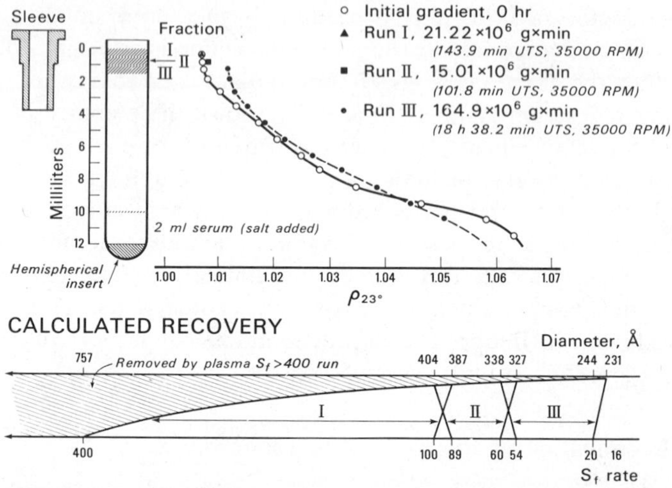

Fig. 26 Sodium chloride density gradient used for isolating three fractions of serum S_f 20–400 lipoproteins (12-ml gradient, SW 41 rotor, 23°C). Below is shown the partial removal of S_f 20–400 lipoproteins by the serum $S_f > 400$ run, as well as the calculated range of S_f-rates (and diameters) ideally recovered for each run. (From Ref. 70; reproduced by permission from the *Journal of Lipid Research.*)

volumes obtained from 2 to 12 ml of serum, respectively.[6] Before LDL subfractionation, $S_f > 20$ lipoproteins must first be removed from the serum. To achieve this, two-ml aliquots of serum are each mixed with 4 ml of 0.195 *m* NaCl, $p = 1.0063$ g/ml (containing EDTA at a concentration of 10 mg/100 ml). Normally six of these 6-ml serum mixtures are centrifuged at 40,000 rpm at 18°C for 18 hr in a 40.3 rotor. The $S_f > 20$ lipoproteins are removed in the top 1-ml; and three additional 1-ml fractions are removed.

After the top 1 in. of the preparative tube is cut off with a pair of surgical scissors, the bottom 2 ml of each preparative tube is mixed with a heavy

[6] This LDL gradient system may also be conveniently used to subfractionate all the major low density lipoprotein classes (69a). Using whole sera in the above gradient system and centrifuging in three steps, the $S_f > 400$, S_f 20–400, and S_f 4–20 fractions are successively removed as in the LDL fractionation. At 23°C the appropriate centrifugal conditions for each stage are 3.57×10^6, 56.5×10^6, and 164.2×10^6 g-min, respectively. A reasonable work cycle is achieved using 1 hr 14.2 min UTS equivalent at 20,000 rpm, 5 hr 43.1 min, and 16 hr 36.6 min UTS equivalent at 37,000 rpm, respectively. The advantage of this procedure is that the three major low density lipoprotein classes of metabolic interest are separated, without density manipulation, in an essentially contamination-free medium of defined small molecule composition.

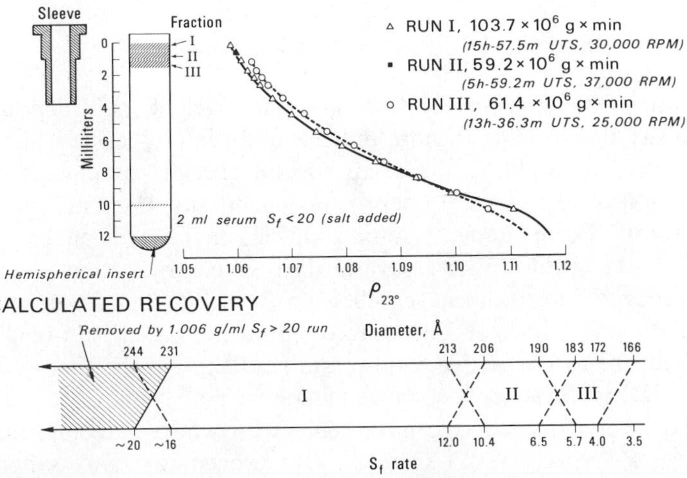

Fig. 27 Sodium chloride density gradient used for subfractionation of serum S_f 0–20 lipoproteins (12-ml gradient, SW 41 rotor, 23°C). The calculated recovery is shown at the bottom. (From Ref. 69a; reproduced by permission from the American Oil Chemists' Society.)

glass stirring rod (fire polished at each end) and all bottom fractions are pooled. The small-molecule salt background density is raised to 1.118 g/ml ($n_D^{26} = 1.36068$) by adding 2045 mg of dry NaCl to 12 ml of this $S_f <$ 20 serum fraction and thoroughly mixing. Two-ml aliquots of this bubble-free $S_f < 20$ fraction are overlayered, each with a 10-ml NaCl gradient in six $\frac{9}{16} \times 3\frac{1}{2}$-in. heavy walled preparative tubes. The solutions are added in volumes (from highest to lowest density) of 1 ml for the first two layers and 2 ml for the remainder. The densities are 1.0988, 1.0860, 1.0790, 1.0722, 1.0641, and 1.0588 g/ml. Corresponding n_D^{26} values are 1.35619, 1.35324, 1.35161, 1.35001, 1.34811, and 1.34686, respectively. Fractions containing 0.5-ml layers are removed from the top of the tubes after three successive centrifugations of 103.7×10^6, 59.2×10^6, and 61.4×10^6 g-min, respectively, at 23°C in an SW 41-Ti rotor (mean $r = 10.76$ cm).

Running times at the indicated rpms, as well as the gradient and its stability are shown in Fig. 27. Below the gradient is shown the anticipated recovery, both in terms of S_f rate and lipoprotein diameter (calculated as Stokes' spheres). As before, a fourth (and fifth) 0.5-ml fraction may be taken after the third centrifugation to evaluate possible contamination. The recommended rotor speeds are to allow a convenient work schedule and to minimize the risk of tube collapse, particularly during the second and third centrifugations.

G. Subfractionation of High-Density Lipoproteins

Because of their relatively low molecular weight, subfractionation of high-density lipoproteins is more difficult and requires a very high performance rotor. In addition there are several special complications in the fractionation of high-density lipoproteins on density gradients in swinging-bucket rotors. For example, a rotor with long-radial-path buckets, such as the SW 41-Ti, would involve several days of centrifugation at maximum rotor speeds. Of necessity an equilibrium-type salt gradient must be considered. However, since at a given rotor speed the radial path length determines both the extent of this equilibrium gradient and the time required to recover HDL subfractions, some reduction in path length and increase in performance is indicated. We have achieved a workable compromise with the use of a special SW 45-Ti rotor. Our procedure (69a) prepares two 1.0- to 3.0-ml HDL subfractions from approximately 4 to 12 ml of serum.

First, the total low-density lipoproteins ($\sigma < 1.063$ g/ml) must be removed. For this purpose and to achieve concentration of the high-density lipoproteins, three 4-ml aliquots of serum are mixed with 2 ml of a 0.195 *m* NaCl and 2.434 *m* NaBr solution ($p = 1.1816$ g/ml, $n_D^{26} = 1.36446$). After centrifugation for 24 hr at 18°C in a 40.3 rotor, the concentrated high-density lipoproteins are nearly quantitatively removed in the 3.5- to 5.5-ml layer. When remixed, this fraction has an approximately 5 to 8% serum protein background, desirable to stabilize the layering procedure and to provide the approximate viscosity and density increments of whole serum. If the serum protein background determined by refractometry is significantly different, two versions of our recovery program, one considering the bottom 1 ml fraction a salt solution only, permit appropriate (but minor) corrections in the centrifugal conditions needed for fractionation. To 6 ml of this HDL-containing fraction is added 3022 mg of solid NaBr, bringing the background density to approximately 1.395 g/ml, $n_D^{26} = 1.39973$. Aliquots of 1 ml of this fraction are placed in 0.5×2.5-in. heavy walled cellulose nitrate tubes and overlayered with an approximate equilibrium NaBr gradient. No hemispherical inserts are used, allowing a maximum radial path to be used. Two 0.5-ml solutions of 1.3622 and 1.3424 g/ml density are added first, then two 1-ml solutions of 1.3161 and 1.2856 g/ml density, and finally, two 1.5-ml solutions of 1.2521 and 1.1973 g/ml density complete the 7-ml density gradient. The corresponding n_D^{26} values are 1.39446, 1.39123, 1.38690, 1.38183, 1.37629, and 1.36711, respectively.

The details of this gradient, its stability and the anticipated recovery for two runs at 236.5×10^6 and 287.5×10^6 *g*-min are shown in Fig. 28.

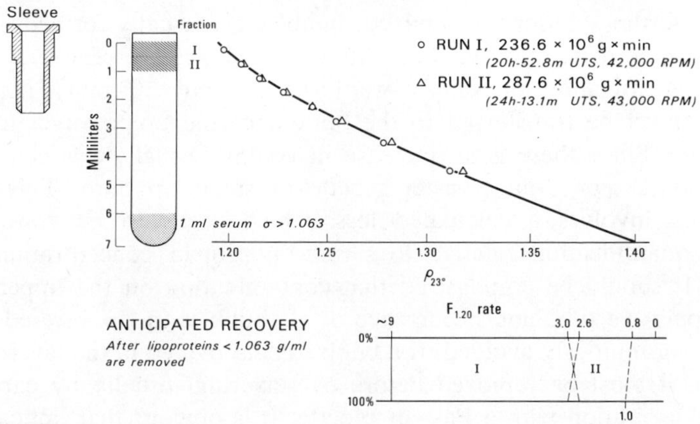

Fig. 28 Sodium bromide density gradient used for subfractionation of high-density lipoproteins (7-ml NaBr gradient, SW 45 rotor, 23°C). The calculated recovery is shown at the bottom. All NaBr solutions have a constant 0.195 *m* NaCl content. (From Ref. 69a; reproduced by permission from the American Oil Chemists' Society.)

Although the SW 45-Ti rotor (mean $r = 9.57$ cm) is rated to perform at 45,000 rpm, two factors require the lower rotor speeds. First, the gradient is of very high density and each tube is filled to the maximum (7 ml). Thus our first run at 42,000 rpm is actually close to the maximum safe speed, and after removal of 0.5 ml, the speed can safely be increased to 43,000 rpm. The other practical reason for limiting speed at this time is the strength and dimensional stability of the available preparative tubes. Above 43,000 rpm the tubes tend to collapse, and even if they do not, they expand and become increasingly difficult to remove from the buckets. Other suggested precautions in using this rotor include rigorous inspection and replacement (when necessary) of the bucket cap gaskets and the use of a vacuum sentinel (28) on the preparative centrifuge.

After each run, it still may be necessary to pipette the two 0.5-ml subfractions and one or more 0.5-ml reference fraction after the second run with the preparative tubes remaining in the buckets. This is recommended if the tubes cannot be easily and smoothly removed with a sterilized hemostat.

H. Special Considerations for All Density-Gradient Procedures

Before considering some preliminary results from these subfractionation techniques it is appropriate to make some general comments. First, all procedures involve addition of salt to serum or serum fractions with an approximate serum-protein content of 5 to 8%. When the salt is added to these serum solutions and mixed, bubbles are usually formed and there is an increase in solution volume. After the bubbles are removed (by low-speed centrifugation or simply waiting for about 30 min) appropriate aliquots must be transferred to the bottom of the preparative tubes with great care. Since there is an increase in volume, usually this can be done with a 1-, 2-, or 3-ml transfer pipette of small tip bore. This transfer procedure involves a calculated loss, which needs to be considered if precise quantification relative to serum-lipoprotein concentrations is required. It should be emphasized that contamination on the upper wall of the preparative tube and occurrence of air bubbles in the layered fraction must be scrupulously avoided. If a bubble is discovered in the layered serum solution, it must be removed before overlayering, usually by careful and minimal aspiration with a Pasteur pipette. It is obvious that optically clear cellulose nitrate (or polycarbonate) tubes must be used for these procedures.

In the preceding sections centrifugal conditions have all been given at 23°C; however, various laboratory conditions may require fractionation at temperatures from 20–26°C. Accordingly, a correction of the given total g-min and equivalent up-to-speed times in the amount of -2.1% per degree C (e.g., above 23°C) should be made.

Finally, because of the number of fractions and the length of fractionation time, it is not usually practical to subfractionate completely all lipoprotein classes from one single serum sample. If it is desirable to look at a patient's complete subfractions (e.g., in type V hyperlipoproteinemia), it would be advisable to take weekly samples from which one or at most two major classes are subfractionated in succession each week. It is for the above reasons that the examples presented in the next section are from different subjects or patients.

VII. RESULTS AND DISCUSSION OF DENSITY-GRADIENT LIPOPROTEIN SUBFRACTIONATIONS

A. $S_f > 400$ Lipoproteins

The examples of subfractionation of the $S_f > 400$ classes are taken from a previous study by Lossow and associates (70). In order to provide a sufficient quantity of $S_f > 400$ lipoproteins, two subjects were given 100 g of a safflower-oil preparation; one was a diabetic with normal blood lipids (sample 735), and the other was a type V hyperlipemic subject (sample 726). Plasma specimens were obtained 8 and 12 hr after the meal from the diabetic and type V patient, respectively. The results of the three-stage subfractionation were evaluated by electron microscopy, described in detail elsewhere (70).

Figure 29 compares the calculated recovery of sample 735 with the particle-size distribution determined by electron microscopy and elemental CHN total mass of each fraction. The measured recoveries, including overlap of fractions, agree well with the calculated recoveries of all fractions except fraction III. Although essentially all the mass of fraction III was recovered with measured diameters larger than those predicted for the lower boundary, approximately 45% of the mass included particles larger than 1175 Å. An almost identical histogram, including the discrepancy in fraction III, was obtained for sample 726. There appears to be no obvious explanation for this discrepancy.

A summary of the elemental CHN and P analysis is presented in Table V. The content (wt %) of both proteins and phospholipids increases with decreasing particle size, in general agreement with other data (68, 71). Also shown are the corrected serum concentrations of each lipopro-

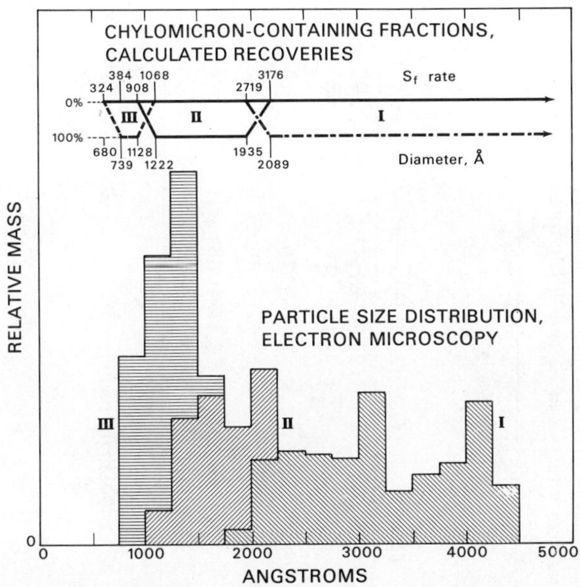

Fig. 29 Computer-constructed plot of lipoprotein mass versus particle diameter (sample 735) evaluated by electron microscopy. Each fraction is normalized to its total mass determined by elemental analysis. Above histogram is given the anticipated recovery for each of the three subfractions, calculated from the actual centrifugal conditions of each run. (From Ref. 70; reproduced by permission from the *Journal of Lipid Research.*)

Table V. Elemental Analysis of $S_f > 400$ Lipoprotein Subfractions[a]

						$S_f > 400$ Subfractions[b]	
Fraction	Case	Calculated Recovery	CHN Content (μg/0.1 ml)[d]	PL[c] (wt %)	Protein[d] (wt %)	Mass % of Total $S_f > 400$	mg/100 ml Serum
I	735	S_f 2719–10^5	390	2.8	1.17	43.3	75
	726	S_f 2694–10^5	941	3.0	1.02	29.1	182
II	735	S_f 908–3176	210	5.5	1.81	23.5	41
	726	S_f 902–3146	1192	2.1	1.98	36.9	230
III	735	S_f 324–1068	296	9.4	2.90	33.1	57
	726	S_f 324–1068	1100	7.7	2.81	34.0	213

[a] Data from Ref. 70.
[b] Mean mass of $S_f > 400$ lipoprotein $= 1.1287 \times (\Sigma N + C + H)$; fractions are concentrated $5.84c_0$ over serum.
[c] Phospholipids.
[d] Duplicate analysis.

tein subfraction, indicating the range of values that might be expected in such subjects after a fat-tolerance test.

B. S_f 20–400 Lipoproteins

The results of a typical VLDL subfractionation of the serum from a fasting patient with type IV hyperlipoproteinemia are shown in Fig. 30. The $S_f > 403$ lipoproteins were first removed by the procedure described in Section II.C, which also partially removes the S_f 20–400 very-low-density lipoproteins, as shown below the total VLDL schlieren pattern. As can be seen, the anticipated recovery and overlap agree very well with the schlieren patterns of the three subfractions. Details of these earlier data are given elsewhere (70).

Another, more complete, example of VLDL subfractionation and analysis of two sera from fasting patients with type III and IV hyperlipoproteinemia is shown in Fig. 31. As before, lipoprotein recovery in each

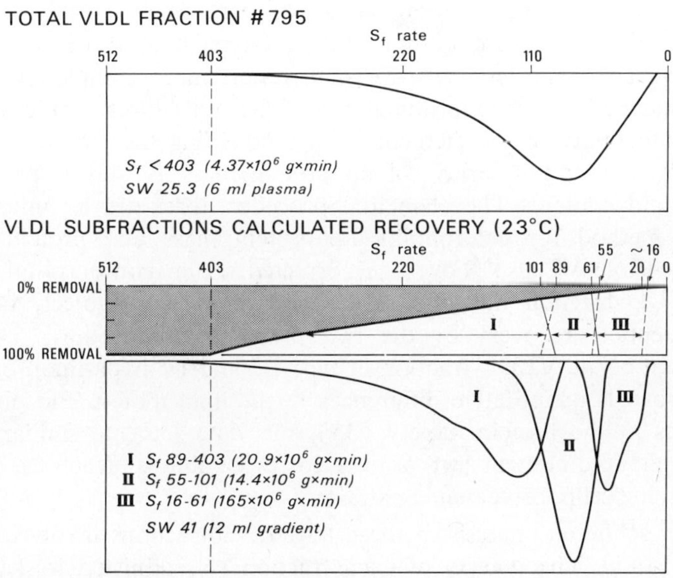

Fig. 30 Schlieren patterns for the three VLDL subfractions and the total VLDL fraction from sample 795. The VLDL distribution in all fractions has been distorted from that originally present in the serum by the continuously changing partial removal of the S_f 20–400 lipoproteins (shaded). The total VLDL fraction was isolated from a single-stage density-gradient run (200.4×10^6 *g*-min). Recoveries are calculated from the centrifugal conditions of each run. (From Ref. 70; reproduced by permission from the *Journal of Lipid Research*.)

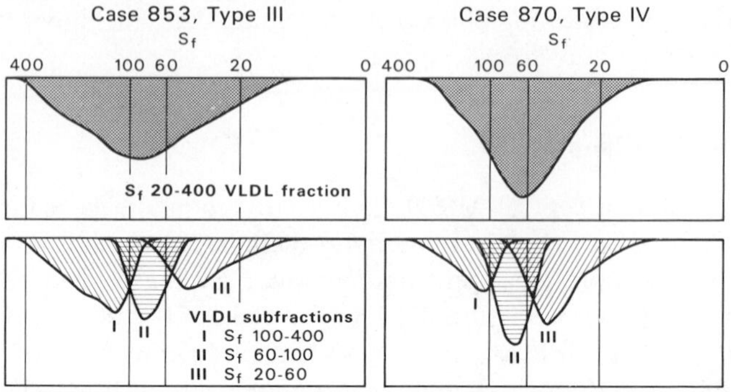

Fig. 31 Schlieren patterns, plotted logarithmically, of total VLDL and three VLDL subfractions from cases 853 and 870. (From Ref. 35; reproduced by permission from *Biophysica et Biochimica Acta.*)

subfraction is close to that predicted, and there is minimal overlap of adjacent fractions. Also, the sum of the three subfractions would yield a pattern very similar to the total VLDL pattern. Since the elemental data on these subfractions are both recent and typical of those obtained for all the fractions reported here, we shall report more completely the type of data obtained and the reproducibility of the procedures. Table VI shows the reproducibility of the elemental data, including the standard error of measurement (for this series) of lipoprotein mass as well as protein and phospholipid content. The elemental procedure provides an unusual and accurate method for determining lipoprotein mass and protein content (wt %). Table VI also shows the corrected serum concentrations of the total VLDL fraction and the subfractions for each subject, indicating almost identical recovery by the two preparative procedures. Although comparison of the VLDL fraction in type III and IV hyperlipoproteinemia patients reveals quantitative differences in the lipid moiety and qualitative differences in the protein moiety (35), our data indicate similar protein and phospholipid content (wt %) for corresponding subfractions obtained from each hyperlipoproteinemic patient.

Further schlieren analysis of these VLDL subfractions involved an ηF° versus ρ study. The density of each fraction was adjusted to 1.037 and 1.063 g/ml NaCl by appropriate addition of solid NaCl, and analytical runs were made at 34,000 rpm. The results are given in Table VII. These data on the S_f° rate, hydrated density σ, and molecular weight (see Figs. 32 and 33) are in general agreement with earlier data on subfractions of similar S_f ranges (68, 72, 73). For a given S_f rate there is approximately the same molecular weight for subfractions from both type III and IV hy-

Table VI. Reproducibility of Elemental CHN and P Analysis of VLDL Subfractions[a]

Subfraction	CHN Content (μg/0.1 g)	N/CHN	PL[b] (wt %)	Protein (wt %)	Lipoprotein Mass (μg/0.1 ml)		Mean Value at $1c_0$ (mg/100 ml)
Case 853 (Type III Hyperlipoproteinemia) Fasting							
S_f 100–400	1632	0.01221	12.6	5.46	1855		464
	1633	0.01244	12.4	5.60	1856		
S_f 60–100	1072	0.01799	18.2	7.84	1217		305
	1073	0.01814	19.2	7.92	1219		
S_f 20–60	1000	0.02529	22.7	11.94	1132		282
	996	0.02495	22.2	11.75	1127	Sum	1051
S_f 20–400[c]	1227	0.01817	17.0	8.24	1389		1044[c]
	1231	0.01766	20.2	7.95	1393		
Case 870 (Type IV Hyperlipoproteinemia) Fasting							
S_f 100–400	637	0.01417	16.4	6.21	724		181
	636	0.01437	15.6	6.32	723		
S_f 60–100	1006	0.01913	17.8	8.85	1143		285
	1000	0.01917	18.6	8.87	1136		
S_f 20–60	1178	0.02597	21.1	12.45	1333		331
	1161	0.02606	21.7	12.50	1314	Sum	797
S_f 20–400[c]	928	0.02114	18.8	10.10	1050		794[c]
	942	0.02128	18.0	10.10	1066		
Standard error of measurement			0.92%	0.10%	0.54%		

[a] Data from Ref. 35.
[b] Phospholipids.
[c] Recovery from a single-stage VLDL density-gradient run, 201×10^6 *g*-min at 23°C.

Table VII. Physical Data on VLDL Subfractions from Fasting Patients with Type III (Case 853) and Type IV (Case 870) Hyperlipoproteinemia

Fraction and Case	σ[a] (g/ml)	S_f° Rate[b]	Molecular Weight (10^6 daltons)
Fraction I, S_f 100–400:			
Case 853	0.9550	113.4	25.7
Case 853[c]	0.9551	115.2	26.4
Case 870	0.9502	103.6	20.9
Case 870[d]	0.9514	103.7	21.3
Fraction II, S_f 60–100:			
Case 853	0.9666	67.5	14.2
Case 870	0.9588	63.0	11.3
Fraction III, S_f 20–60:			
Case 853	0.9753	56.5[e]	12.6
Case 853	1.0013	24.3[f]	6.2
Case 870	0.9630	49.9	7.8

[a] Hydrated density (ρ-intercept).
[b] Component measured.
[c] Rerun.
[d] Reread.
[e] Fast.
[f] Slow.

perlipoproteinemia patients. However, at a given S_f rate there appears to be a somewhat higher hydrated density in all type III subfractions, which probably reflects the higher cholesteryl ester and lower glyceride content of all three fractions (35). A more complete analysis, including the clinical features of this study, is reported elsewhere (35).

C. S_f 0–20 Lipoproteins

Subfractionation of low-density lipoproteins was performed on plasma from two fasting patients, clinically characterized as type IV hyperlipoproteinemia. Figure 34 shows the corrected linear schlieren plots of each subfraction from each of the subjects. The observed recoveries agree reasonably well with that anticipated by calculation. The ηF° versus ρ studies were done at 52,640 rpm at densities of approximately 1.063 and

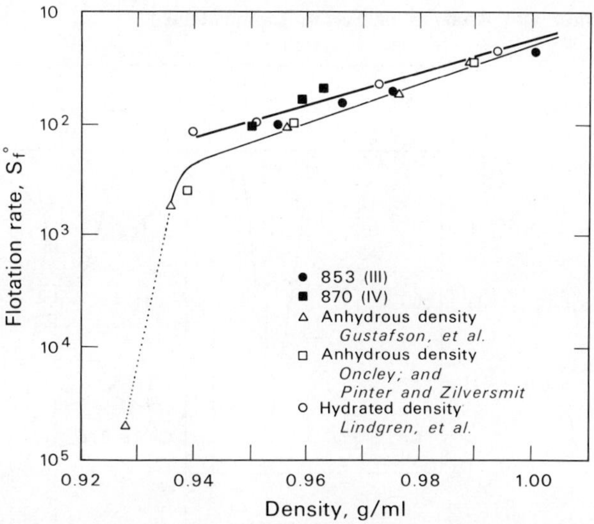

Fig. 32 Relationship between flotation rate and VLDL density: data on subfractions are from case 853 (type III hyperlipoproteinemia) and case 870 (type IV hyperlipoproteinemia); other literature data are from Gustafson et al. (68), Oncley (73), Pinter and Zilversmit (72), and Lindgren et al. (69).

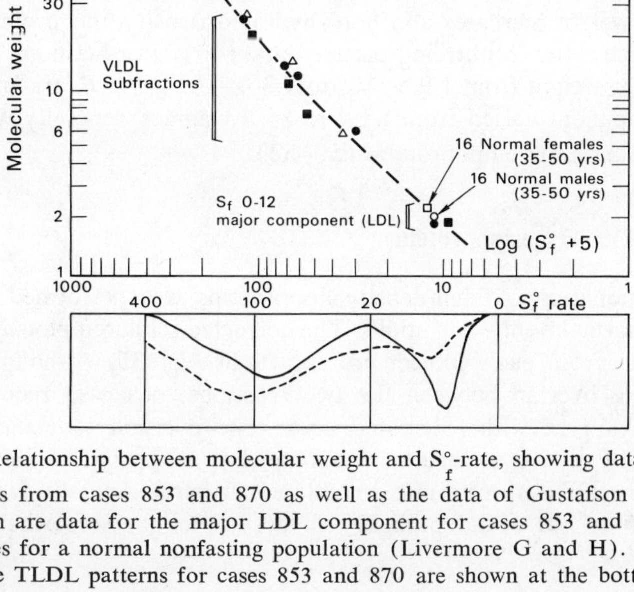

Fig. 33 Relationship between molecular weight and S_f°-rate, showing data for VLDL subfractions from cases 853 and 870 as well as the data of Gustafson et al. (68). Also shown are data for the major LDL component for cases 853 and 870 and the mean values for a normal nonfasting population (Livermore G and H). Logarithmic plots of the TLDL patterns for cases 853 and 870 are shown at the bottom.

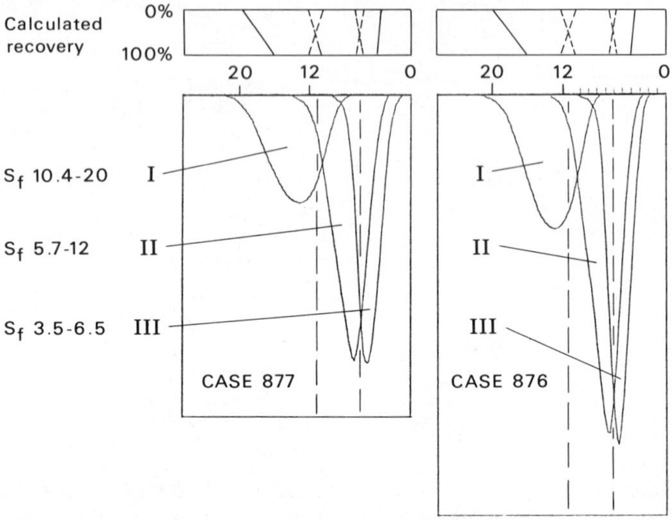

Fig. 34 Corrected schlieren patterns for LDL subfractions from patients with type IV hyperlipoproteinemia (cases 876 and 877). Calculated recovery is shown at the top.

1.097 g/ml NaCl (adjusted by appropriate solid NaCl addition), yielding S_f° rates, hydrated densities, and molecular weights of the major component of each subfraction. A summary of the physical and chemical data is presented in Table VIII. These results show that with increasing S_f° rate molecular weight increases and both hydrated density and protein content decrease, the latter confirming earlier data (40). Furthermore, the range of molecular weight from 1.9×10^6 to 3.3×10^6 for LDL fractions whose major component varied from S_f° 4 to S_f° 13 agrees generally with recent physical data on these lipoproteins (50–52).

D. High-Density Lipoproteins

Subfractionation of high-density lipoproteins was performed on serum from two normal nonfasting adults. The corrected schlieren plots for the two subfractions from each subject are shown in Fig. 35. Although there is considerable overlap between the two fractions, observed recoveries approximately agree with calculated ones. The decision to achieve 100% recovery of $F_{1.20}$ 3.0 molecules was somewhat arbitrary and was intended to divide the HDL spectra into roughly equal parts. Actually fractionation at $F_{1.20}$ 3.5 or 4.0 would probably yield subfractions somewhat closer in

Table VIII. Physical Data on LDL Subfractions from Fasting Patients with Type IV Hyperlipoproteinemia[e]

Fraction and Case	σ^a (g/ml)	Peak S_f°-Rate	MW[b] (10^6 daltons)	Protein (wt %)[d]	PL[c] (wt %)[d]
Fraction I, S_f 10.4–20.0:					
Case 876	1.0079	13.50	3.04	16.9	24.8
Case 877	1.0110	13.50	3.34	17.9	22.2
Fraction II, S_f 5.7–12.0:					
Case 876	1.0272	6.89	2.17	22.6	23.3
Case 877	1.0281	6.87	2.25	23.8	22.6
Fraction III, S_f 3.5–6.5:					
Case 876	1.0348	4.96	1.91	25.5	22.3
Case 877	1.0393	4.13	1.88	26.6	21.2

[a] Hydrated density (ρ-intercept).
[b] Molecular weight.
[c] Phospholipids.
[d] Duplicate CHN and P analysis.
[e] Data from Ref. 69a.

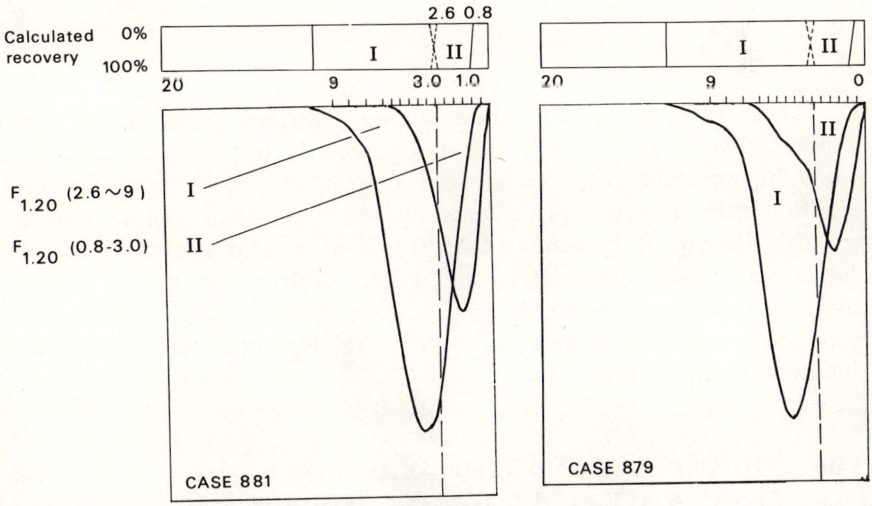

Fig. 35 Corrected schlieren patterns of HDL subfractions from normal subjects (cases 879 and 881). Calculated recovery is shown at the top.

identity to the earlier HDL_2 and HDL_3 components. It should be observed that the earlier techniques (11, 74) fractionate primarily on the basis of density, giving two fractions, HDL_2, ($1.063 < \sigma_2 < 1.125$ g/ml) and HDL_3 ($1.125 < \sigma_3 < 1.20$ g/ml). In contrast, our procedure fractionates essentially on the basis of particle size, and therefore the two procedures may be achieving a different type of fractionation within the HDL spectra.

Our ηF° versus ρ flotation studies were done at 52,640 rpm in media of approximately 1.203 and 1.290 g/ml density NaBr. Solid NaBr was added to aliquots of the two subfractions, raising their densities to the higher values. All the physical and chemical data are summarized in Table

Table IX. Physical Data on HDL Subfractions from Normal, Nonfasting Subjects[c]

Subfraction and Case	σ[a] (g/ml)	Peak $F^\circ_{1.20}$ Rate	Molecular Weight	Protein (wt %)	PL[b] (wt %)
$F_{1.20}$ 2.7–9.0:					
Case 879	1.0988	4.30	265,000	43.6	33.1
Case 881	1.0950	4.14	236,000	43.4	31.4
$F_{1.20}$ 0.8–3.0:					
Case 879	1.1437	1.73	170,000	53.9	27.0
Case 881	1.1346	1.84	148,000	55.0	25.7

[a] Hydrated density (ρ-intercept).
[b] Phospholipids.
[c] Data from Ref. 69a.

IX. These preliminary data show similar hydrated densities but lower molecular weights than earlier data, particularly for the less dense $F_{1.20}$ 3.0–9.0 component (74, 75). These discrepancies may be partly the result of different fractionation procedures. However, chemical composition, and in particular protein content (44–55%), is in general agreement with the data based on the older HDL_2 and HDL_3 subfractionation. In order to compare procedures rigorously in the future it will be necessary to determine the density heterogeneity of each subfraction acquired by cumulative-flotation-rate separations.

VIII. ADVANTAGES AND LIMITATIONS OF CUMULATIVE-FLOTATION PROCEDURES

It should be emphasized that the earlier preparative techniques continue to have certain advantages in that the use of angle-head rotors considerably simplifies methodology and at the same time permits fractionation on a much larger scale. However, there are uncertainties concerning lipoprotein structural stability during prolonged and repeated centrifugations in angle rotors, particularly with high-density lipoproteins (76–78). Many of these angle-rotor fractionations of necessity have involved serial centrifugations (75, 78) to avoid contamination from albumin and other nonlipoprotein protein. In addition, as a precaution against lipoprotein aggregation, especially for LDL in high salt media (79), the pH of solutions used for all lipoprotein fractionation should be maintained near neutrality (above pH 5.5).

On the other hand, our density-gradient procedures provide lipoprotein

Table X. Evaluation of Potential Contamination in Lipoprotein Subfractions[a]

Depth (ml)	LDL, 12 ml, Using 1.063 g/ml Bottom Fraction (μg/0.1 g)		HDL, 7 ml, Using 1.21 g/ml Bottom Fraction (μg/0.1 g)	
	Dynamic[b]	Static[c]	Dynamic[b]	Static[c]
0.0–0.5[d]	1.3	1.2	−1.0	−1.8
0.5–1.0[e]	−0.1	−0.9	1.4	−0.4
1.0–1.5[f]	−0.8	−0.5	1.8	0.4
1.5–2.0[g]	−1.4	−1.4	0.7	0.7
2.0–2.5	−0.5	−1.8	0.5	0.2
2.5–3.0	0.3	−1.2	2.2	2.2
3.0–4.0	−2.1	−2.8[h]	19.6	5.9[h]
4.0–5.0	−1.1	−2.2[h]	1083.0	160.0[h]
5.0–6.0	0.2	−0.7[h]	1585.0	1165.0[h]
6.0–7.0	6.5	2.6[h]	232.0	1822.0[h]
7.0–8.0	13.9	4.6[h]		
8.0–9.0	36.1	81.2[h]		
9.0–10.0	67.5	896.0[h]		
10.0–11.0	130.0	2823.0[h]		
11.0–12.0	6034.0	3461.0[h]		

[a] Matrix above catalyst (CAT), 7.8 μg/0.1 g; CAT above base line, 3.9 μg/0.1 g. Standard error of measurement of sample minus matrix, ±1.0 μg/0.1 g (calculated as methyl stearate, the standard).
[b] Standard isolation procedure.
[c] Control gradient allowed to stand at 1 *g* in a 23°C chamber.
[d] Fraction I.
[e] Fraction II.
[f] Fraction III.
[g] Fraction IV.
[h] Single determinations; all others are duplicate analyses.

fractions in a media of defined small-molecule composition, with minimal contamination from other plasma lipoproteins and proteins. There is also essentially no contamination from the plasma small-molecule components. The upper limits of such contamination can be evaluated, for example, by going through the cumulative-flotation procedure for LDL and HDL subfractionation, using 1.063 and 1.21 g/ml bottom fractions raised to the appropriate densities. These fractions should have essentially no LDL or HDL present, respectively, but would have all other serum components, which could potentially contaminate each lipoprotein subfraction. Table X shows the CHN elemental analysis of the LDL and HDL gradient fractions obtained by the standard isolation procedure (dynamic) and a control gradient allowed to stand at 1 *g* in a 23°C chamber (static). Considering the error of measurement of sample above matrix, there is no detectable contamination, as revealed by elemental analysis, in the fractions that would contain the lipoprotein subfractions. Where contamination is important, such as in lipoprotein immunological studies (78), such fractionation may help define more accurately the characteristics of the protein moiety within subfractions of all the plasma lipoproteins. In addition, the cumulative-flotation-rate procedure is flexible, allowing the collection of two, three, or more subfractions of any desired flotation-rate interval within each of the $S_f > 400$, VLDL, LDL, and HDL spectra. Where very large fractions from a single plasma sample are needed, this general technique might be used in a zonal-type rotor (80) with reduced resolution.

IX. ELECTROPHORESIS OF LIPOPROTEINS

A. Principles of Lipoprotein Electrophoresis

The surface electric charge of lipoproteins has become the basis of numerous electrophoretic methods, which rate second in importance after ultracentrifugation for lipoprotein analysis. The net charge on a lipoprotein molecule, which primarily determines its electrophoretic mobility, results from the balance of positive and negative charges on the terminal and side-chain amino acid residues. Additional charge contributions would be expected from adsorbed metal cations and fatty acid anions and to a small extent from those phospholipids that do not exist in the form of zwitterions at electrophoretic pH values (8).

The mobility of lipoproteins in free electrophoresis (i.e., where the lipoproteins are in buffered solution without supporting medium) is identical with that found in layers or blocks of potato starch granules. However, on paper, cellulose acetate, and various types of gels the migration of lipoproteins according to their net electric charge is modified by two types of interaction between the lipoproteins and the supporting media. First, all supporting media other than starch granules possess interstices of a range of sizes that offer resistance to the passage of chylomicrons and very-low-density lipoproteins. Second, chemical interactions between lipoproteins and supporting media probably make at least a small contribution to the electrophoretic pattern and to its variations in different media. Perhaps the most important such interaction occurs in paper electrophoresis. In barbital buffer, containing EDTA to minimize the effect of metal-ion contamination in the paper or reagents, the lipoprotein pattern shows a poorly defined α_1 (HDL) lipoprotein zone, fails to show resolution of the very-low-density lipoproteins from low-density lipoproteins, and exhibits considerable trailing of very-low-density lipoproteins between the β-region and the origin. The addition of human-serum albumin to the buffer solution sharpens the α_1-lipoprotein band, partially resolves pre-β-lipoproteins (VLDL) from β-lipoproteins (LDL), and limits trailing to samples containing large VLDL concentrations.

Our knowledge at present suggests that the electrophoretic mobilities of high-, low-, and very-low-density lipoproteins are largely determined by the presence of the apoproteins. The apoproteins consist of families of polypeptide subunits including a set A, found in high-density lipoproteins, a set B found in low-density lipoproteins, and a third set, found in very-low-density lipoproteins, which contains at least some members of sets A and B plus several additional polypeptides (81–85). The precise pattern obtained in a given electrophoretic medium is then modified by the mechanical and chemical interactions with the medium, as mentioned above. Figure 36 indicates the relationships between the patterns obtained in agarose-gel electrophoresis and the schlieren patterns obtained by analytical centrifugation. Figure 37 illustrates these relationships schematically in the four media principally used in lipoprotein electrophoresis.

B. Electrophoretic Mobility in Various Media

The correspondence between the electrophoretic zones and the standard ultracentrifugal fractions is summarized in Table XI. These relationships have been determined by the electrophoresis of fractions isolated with the preparative ultracentrifuge (87), and by indirect methods.

The electrophoretic mobility of high-density lipoproteins is between that of albumin and α_1-globulin. When this fraction is relatively abundant, partial resolution into two zones is often seen on paper and on other media. The minor zone (less uptake of fat stains) extends toward the

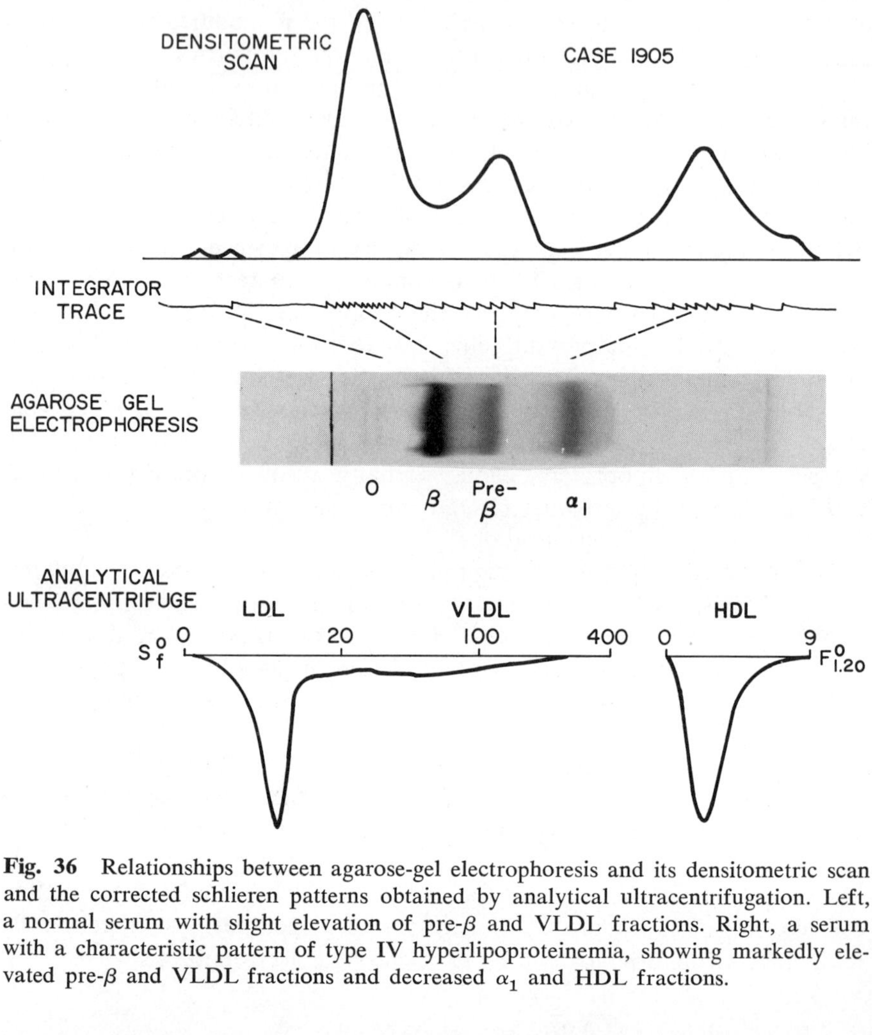

Fig. 36 Relationships between agarose-gel electrophoresis and its densitometric scan and the corrected schlieren patterns obtained by analytical ultracentrifugation. Left, a normal serum with slight elevation of pre-β and VLDL fractions. Right, a serum with a characteristic pattern of type IV hyperlipoproteinemia, showing markedly elevated pre-β and VLDL fractions and decreased α_1 and HDL fractions.

anode from the main zone and at least partially overlaps the albumin band. Some investigators have raised the question whether this minor anodal band of α_1-lipoproteins is really caused by staining of the free fatty acid–albumin complex rather than by a portion of high-density lipoproteins. We have recently shown after preparative electrophoresis of human serum in agarose (with G. J. Nelson and R. P. Noble, unpublished data) that this zone does contain all of the lipids expected in α_1-lipoproteins and is no more than slightly enriched in free fatty acids. It is still not clear, however, whether the resolution of α_1-lipoproteins on electrophoresis

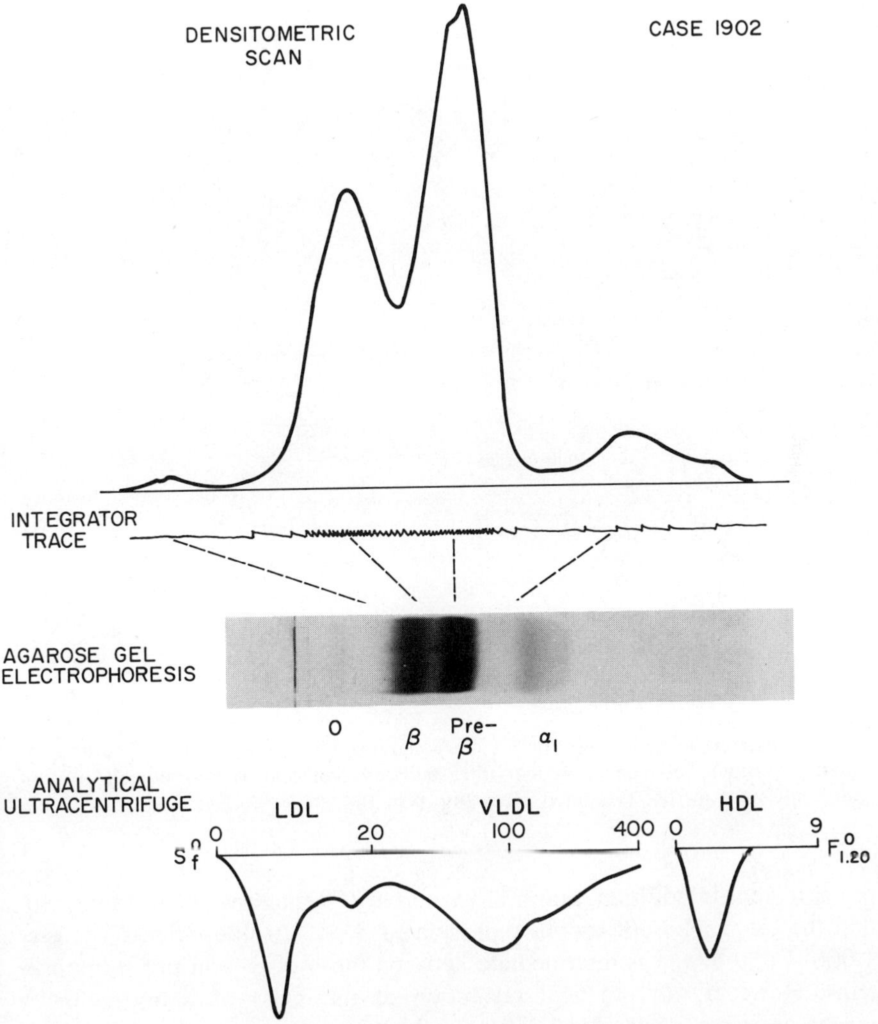

corresponds to the partial ultracentrifugal resolution of HDL_2 and HDL_3, but our evidence does not support such a relationship. M. Z. Nichaman and associates (personal communication) have noted progressive increases in the staining and degree of separation of the minor anodal component in certain sera during storage at 4°C.

The VLDL fraction moves in the region of the α_2-globulins in cellulose acetate and various gels. On paper, in barbital buffer containing albumin, these lipoproteins move slightly faster than the β-lipoproteins—in the

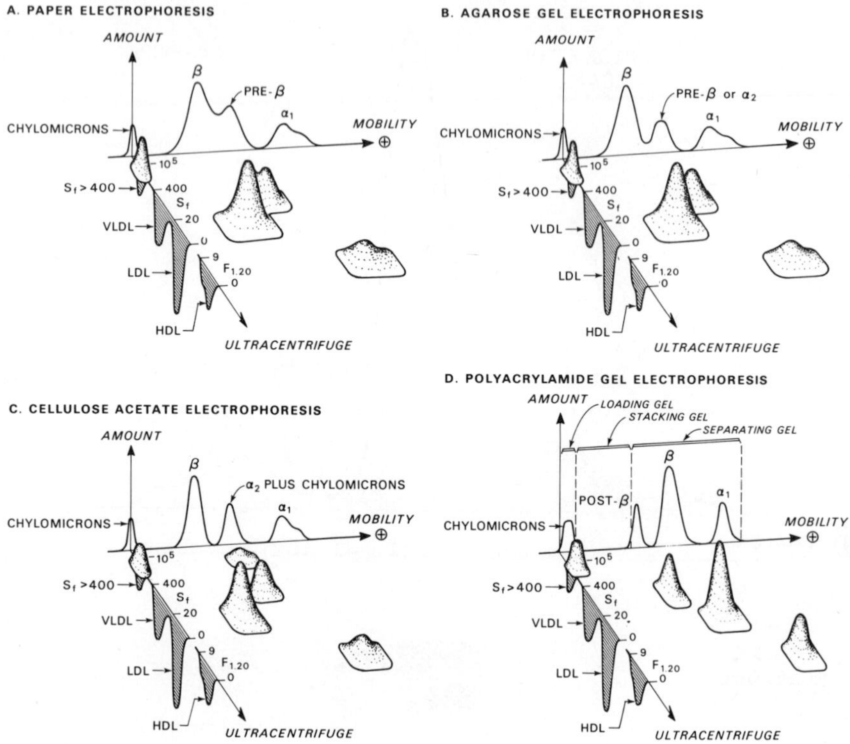

Fig. 37 Schematic representation of the relationships (in a typical hyperlipoproteinemic serum) between analytical ultracentrifugation and electrophoresis in four commonly used media. (Adapted from Fig. 9 in Ref. 86.)

pre-β-region. In addition, Smith has reported (88), and we have confirmed, that the electrophoretic mobility of isolated S_f 12–20 lipoproteins (density 1.006–1.019 g/ml) is intermediate between those of β- and pre-β-lipoproteins. However, no practical resolution of this class of lipoproteins by means of paper electrophoresis is possible. In agarose gel the mobility of the VLDL fraction in different human subjects varies from that of α_2-globulins into the pre-β-lipoprotein regions and occasionally is found to be resolved into two distinct bands (Fig. 38). The latter finding has most often been observed in subjects receiving either certain contraceptive drugs or clofibrate. In polyacrylamide gel, which has a smaller pore size than agarose, the VLDL molecules are trapped just after entering the separating gel from the stacking gel, thus migrating in a "post-β" position.

The low-density lipoproteins move in the β-globulin region. In media

Table XI. Correspondence of Paper and Agarose-Gel Electrophoresis and Ultracentrifugation

	Electrophoretic Zone	Ultracentrifugal Fraction
Origin	Chylomicrons	$S_f > 400$ (density gradient)
↓	Trail	S°_f 20–400 (when markedly elevated)
	β-Lipoproteins	S°_f 0–20
	Pre-β-lipoproteins	S°_f 20–400
	α_1-Lipoproteins	$F^\circ_{1.20}$ 0–9
Anode		

that are capable of resolving the β_1- and β_2-globulins of serum, the β-lipoproteins are found in the β_1 (faster) zone.

Chylomicrons, because of their large size, form a symmetrical band about the origin or point of application on paper. In the various gels they

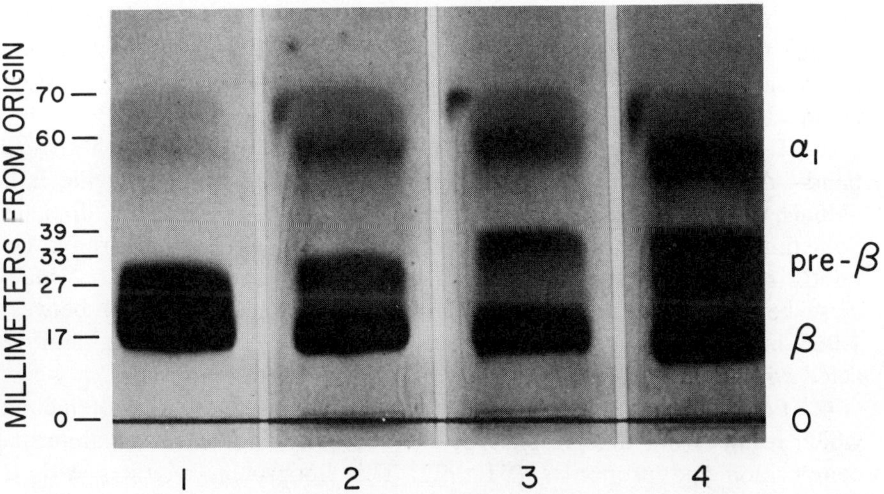

Fig. 38 Variations in the relative mobility of pre-β-lipoproteins in agarose-gel electrophoresis. Strip 4 illustrates the splitting of the pre-β-fraction that is observed occasionally in patients with uncontrolled diabetes and in subjects taking clofibrate or contraceptive drugs. Spots in the upper left of strips 2, 3, and 4 are bromphenol blue–albumin complex added before electrophoresis to mark the total migration distance. Relative mobilities of lipoprotein fractions can be determined in relation to the total migration. (Reprinted with permission of author and publisher from Ref. 97.)

remain in the origin well or in the starting gel. On cellulose acetate, however, it has been found that a part of the chylomicron fraction migrates to the α_2-region, thus producing ambiguity in the distinction between the VLDL fraction and chylomicrons.

C. Exceptional Electrophoretic Behavior of Lipoproteins

Recently four uncommon exceptions to the usual lipoprotein patterns have been observed:

1. In the type III hyperlipoproteinemia of Fredrickson et al. (34) a portion of the lipoproteins with a hydrated density of less than 1.006 g/ml exhibits β-globulin electrophoretic mobility ("floating β-lipoprotein"). Recent findings by Fisher suggest that lipoprotein of these characteristics is usually present in patients with elevated pre-β-lipoproteins (VLDL) (89). Thus the large amount of "floating β-lipoprotein" characteristic of type III hyperlipoproteinemia may indicate a quantitative, rather than qualitative, difference from type IV hyperlipoproteinemia. Quantitative limits may therefore have to be set for accurate differential diagnosis.
2. A new lipoprotein of pre-β mobility and the density of LDL ("sinking pre-β") has been found by Sodhi in a healthy 10-year-old boy (90); similar lipoproteins were observed in a considerable number of normal individuals in the Framingham study (W. B. Kannell and W. P. Castelli, personal communication).[7]
3. J. Davignon (personal communication) has observed a "retro-α_1" band—rarely in normal subjects and occasionally in hyperlipidemic individuals, usually in association with liver disease, obesity, or diabetes. Sometimes the band appeared in conjunction with clofibrate therapy. The faintly staining band was located between the β- and α_1-zones, usually close behind the main α_1-band. This lipoprotein had a density between 1.063 and 1.21 g/ml, was not precipitated by dextran sulfate, and reacted with α_1-lipoprotein antiserum in immunoelectrophoresis.
4. Patients with obstructive jaundice exhibit hyperlipoproteinemia, which results from the presence of a low-density lipoprotein of abnormal composition and properties (91, 92). This lipoprotein migrates with β-lipoproteins in agarose, but unexpectedly in a cathodal direction in agar gel (93).

One must therefore be aware that exceptional lipoprotein behavior will occasionally appear as total experience with electrophoretic methods in-

[7] It now appears that this type of lipoprotein is present in about 10% of normal populations and is identical with the previously known Lp antigen.

creases. For certain studies it may be important to carry out preparative ultracentrifugation at densities of 1.006 or 1.063 g/ml in conjunction with electrophoresis.

D. Qualitative Lipoprotein Electrophoresis

Zone electrophoresis in a supporting medium provides the only simple, direct evaluation of the main classes of serum lipoproteins that does not require the use of either an analytical or preparative ultracentrifuge. Qualitative interpretation of lipoprotein patterns has proved to be useful in clinical medicine and human genetics. A recent didactic classification of familial hyperlipoproteinemias and hypolipoproteinemias is based on this technique (34), and routine experience with this classification in other laboratories has been reported (94, 95). The typical patterns observed in paper and agarose-gel electrophoresis are presented in Figs. 39 and 40, respectively. Furthermore, numerous secondary hyperlipoproteinemias and hypolipoproteinemias have been observed in many other diseases (8, 34).

The paper-electrophoresis technique has been reviewed in detail by Hatch and Lees (8), and a recent modification has been presented by Moinuddin and Taylor (96). Various authors have described the techniques of agarose-gel (97–103), agar-gel (104), and polyacrylamide-gel (105–109) electrophoresis. The techniques of cellulose acetate electrophoresis have also been presented (110–113). Hence the technical details of these methods are not repeated here.

A comparison of several electrophoretic techniques has been presented in abstract form by Maskett, Levy, and Fredrickson (114). In type III hyperlipoproteinemia (34) correct diagnosis was obtained 50 to 55% of the time when only paper, agarose gel, or polyacrylamide gel was used; with a combination of paper and polyacrylamide gel correct diagnosis was obtained in over 90% of the cases (Maskett et al., Ref. 114 and personal communication).

Paper electrophoresis of lipoproteins has been widely applied in clinical laboratories and in some epidemiological studies. Lipoprotein electrophoresis in other media, with the possible exception of cellulose acetate, has so far been limited mostly to research laboratories. The advantages of agarose gel over paper—greater speed, resolution, and sensitivity—are offset by the need for daily preparation of the gel media and the need for more skillful technique. However, this situation is changing through the introduction of stable, ready made gels in package form by at least two companies: Analytical Chemists, Inc., Palo Alto, California, and Bio-Rad Laboratories, Inc., Richmond, California. Minor technical and packaging details are still being worked out. However, these products, and others

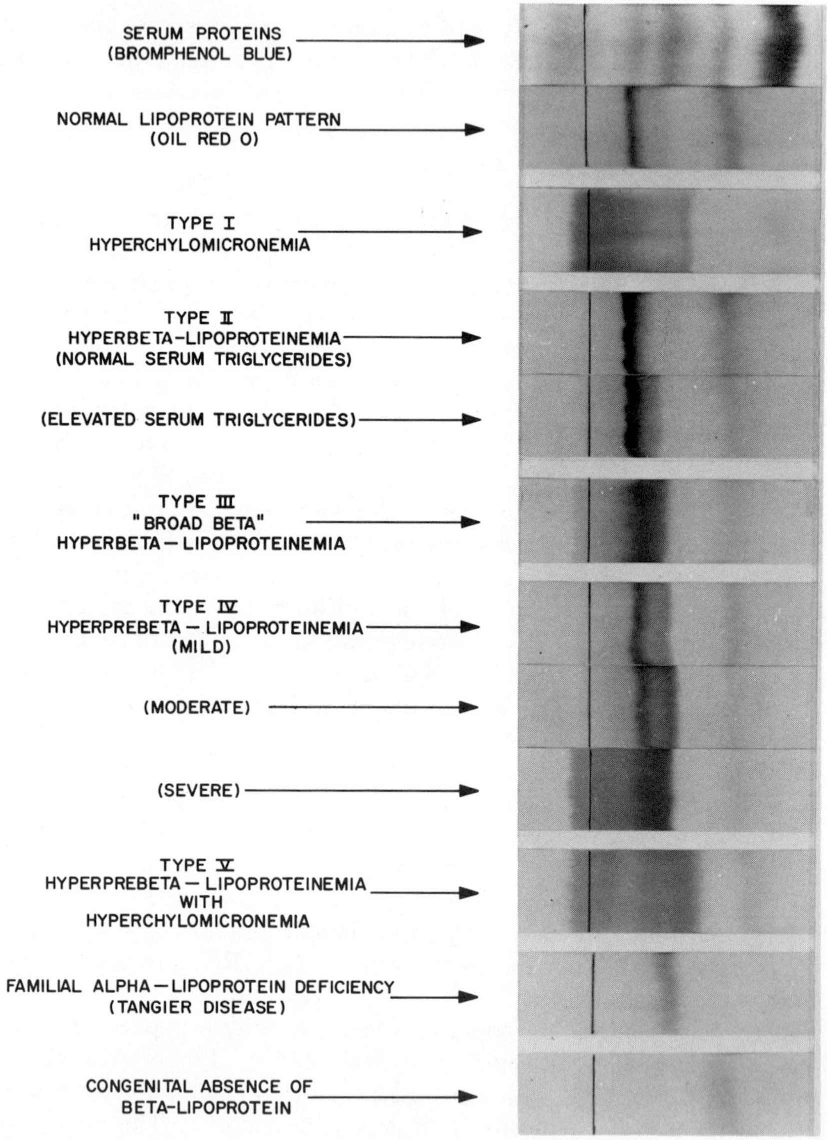

Fig. 39 Typical lipoprotein patterns observed in paper electrophoresis. (Reprinted with permission of the publisher from Ref. 8.)

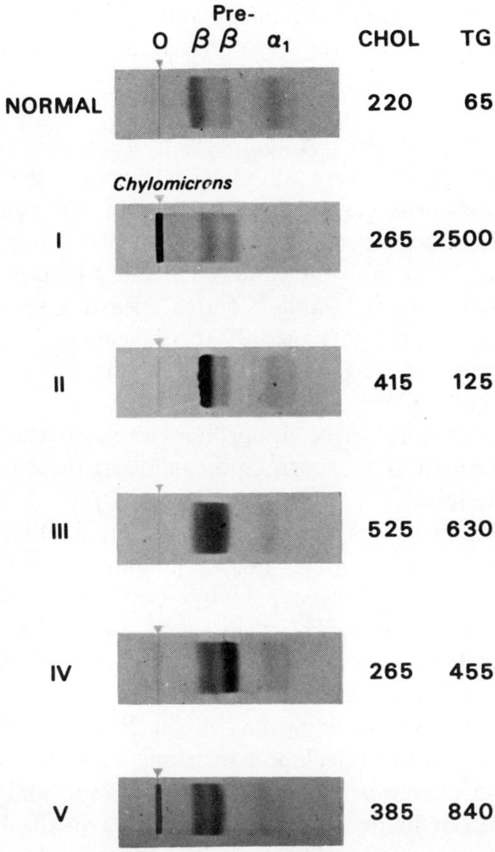

Fig. 40 Typical lipoprotein patterns observed in agarose-gel electrophoresis. Abbreviations: CHOL, serum total cholesterol (mg/dl); TG, serum triglycerides (mg/dl). The Roman numerals refer to the types of hyperlipoproteinemia as classified by Fredrickson, Levy, and Lees (34). (Courtesy of R. P. Noble.)

that may follow, should bring the gel technique within the capability of any clinical laboratory that employs paper electrophoresis. Results are obtained in about 1.5 hr (exclusive of scanning and interpretation), rather than the 10- to 24-hr period required for most of the methods available heretofore.

E. Semiquantitative Lipoprotein Electrophoresis and Comparison with Analytical Ultracentrifugation

Although qualitative interpretation of lipoprotein electrophoretic patterns has become widely accepted and is available in many clinical laboratories, the needs of epidemiologic teams and of clinical investigators using drug or diet therapy are served better by quantitative data presented in digital form.

1. Paper Electrophoresis. A comparison of quantitative measurements by paper electrophoresis and by analytical ultracentrifugation in 71 normal and abnormal cases was carried out in the authors' laboratories (115). Nonfasting morning serum samples were obtained from 15 healthy employed men aged 38 to 50 years and 16 healthy employed women aged 36 to 50 years (Livermore G and H series). Fasting serum samples were obtained from 20 male patients aged 29 to 66 years and 20 female patients aged 27 to 70 years. These patients exhibited miscellaneous hyperlipoproteinemias and were undergoing a variety of treatments. The three series of samples provided a range of lipoprotein levels in each major fraction that was adequate to test the correlation between the electrophoretic and ultracentrifugal methods.

Paper electrophoresis was performed in barbital buffer at pH 8.6 and ionic strength 0.1, containing 1% (w/v) human albumin, by the method of Lees and Hatch (116). For each sample duplicate electrophoretic strips were made on different days. The strips were stained for 6 hr at 37°C in Oil Red O (saturated solution in 60% ethanol). Details and discussion of this technique are presented elsewhere (8).

Scanning was performed with the Model RB Analytrol densitometer with automatic integration (Beckman Instruments, Inc., Palo Alto, Calif.). The standard B-5 cam was replaced by a B-2 cam, and a 520-nm filter was used in the front holder with a 500-nm filter in the rear holder. The slit width was 1.5 mm. The calibration set point was determined by interpolation in the table given in the instrument manual and was used without "color correction." The strip was located in the light path about 1 cm cathodal to the origin mark. The zero point was set, and the calibration set point was adjusted with the neutral density filter in the light path. The strip was scanned, and the scan was examined visually. If the base line of the scan was not close to the chart zero line behind the origin, between pre-β- and α_1-lipoproteins, and in front of α_1-lipoproteins, the zero point was reset, and the scan was repeated. Often the best setting for the base line was at the lowest point between the pre-β and α_1-lipoprotein zones.

Values obtained from the duplicate strips were averaged for statistical analysis. In a preliminary study on the 15 normal male subjects duplicate scans were made on each strip, duplicate strips were run in the same cell, and duplicate strips were run on different days in order to evaluate the sources of variation in the procedure.

The establishment of criteria for the boundaries of the electrophoretic zones is difficult. Our efforts were aided by data feedback from computer-plotted scatter diagrams that correlated the electrophoretic and ultracentrifugal data (117). The trail, and chylomicrons, if present, extended from slightly behind the point of application of the serum to the intersection with the base line of an extension of the linear portion of the rear of the β-peak. The β-peak was measured in two ways: by integrated area and by peak height; the latter method was easier and as accurate as the area method in this study. The most important, and the most difficult, demarcation was that of the boundary between β- and pre-β-lipoprotein zones. The best results were obtained at the midpoint between two lines perpendicular to the base line, located at the first and second perceptible deviations from the straight line describing the descending limb of the β-peak. This rule was inapplicable in those rare cases where the pre-β-component was higher than the β-component. The leading boundary of the pre-β-component was marked when the trace returned close to the base line. The boundaries for α_1-lipoproteins were usually easy to define.

Under magnification the boundaries were marked along the base line, and their vertical projections were located on the integrator trace. Integrator pips were counted and recorded in terms of integration units for each lipoprotein fraction. Peak height (mm) for β-lipoproteins could be approximately converted into integration units by multiplying the values by 0.63.

Correlation and regression relationships between the densitometric scans and the ultracentrifugal analyses were calculated with a CDC-6600 computer and graphs were prepared with a CalComp plotter.

Variation between scans of the same strip (mean deviation between duplicates) was much smaller (3–9%) than the other sources of variation (13–30%), so that duplicate scans were not made in the remainder of the study. Variation between strips run in the same cell was smaller than that between strips run on different days for the trail and pre-β-fractions, about equal for the β-fraction, and—unexpectedly—larger for the α_1-fraction. Thus for reliable results duplicate strips should be made for each serum sample, but it probably makes little difference whether these are made concurrently or on different days.

Our data relating the amounts of each major electrophoretic and ultracentrifugal fraction in the 71 serum samples are presented in Table XII; the last column shows the percentage of the 71 samples in which the actual ultracentrifugal value was within $\pm$ 30% of the value predicted by the regression line. We can thus imagine that if we had available only the electrophoretic measurements, we could have predicted the ultracentrifugal values of each major lipoprotein fraction within $\pm$ 30% from 83 to over 90% of the time. Although analytical ultracentrifugation is not entirely

Table XII. Semiquantitative Paper Electrophoresis of Serum Lipoproteins[a]

Electrophoretic Zone	Ultracentrifugal Fraction	Correlation Coefficient	Cases within ±30% of Regression Line (%)
β-Lipoproteins	S_f° 0–20	.76	87
Pre-β-lipoproteins	S_f° 20–400	.97	90[b]
β- + Pre-β-lipoproteins	S_f° 0–400	.90	96
α_1-Lipoproteins	$F^\circ_{1.20}$ 0–9	.75	83

[a] Three populations, 71 subjects. Data from Ref. 115.
[b] At very low levels scatter is greater than ± 30%, but not of practical significance.

error free, most of the deviations from a perfectly linear relationship undoubtedly came from the electrophoretic procedure.

In a more recent series we have found difficulty in measuring the β-lipoprotein zone in sera containing large amounts of very-low-density (pre-β) lipoproteins (118). Evidently a significant portion of these lipoproteins lies beneath the β-peak, resulting in erroneous increases in both peak height and area of the β-zone. For these occasional samples the best estimate of β-lipoproteins was obtained by subtracting the height of the chylomicron or trail fraction at the origin from the peak height of β-lipoproteins.

2. Agarose-Gel Electrophoresis. A collaborative comparison of both paper and agarose-gel electrophoresis with analytical ultracentrifugation has been published by Noble and associates (117). Recently a collaborative study (118) of a selected series of normal and abnormal subjects has been carried out by the authors in collaboration with S. Hulley, S. Cook, S. Wilson, and M. Z. Nichaman. The results of both paper and agarose-gel electrophoresis were compared with those obtained by analytical ultracentrifugation; the study covered 20 selected subjects, including 4 normal adults and 16 with hyperlipoproteinemias: six with type II, 5 with type IV, and five with type V, with marked elevations of VLDL and chylomicron levels. Since the electrophoretic techniques used in this study took advantage of the information gained from the other studies we have mentioned and appeared to give significantly better results for agarose electrophoresis, we wish to present the data as an example of the present state of the art of quantitative lipoprotein electrophoresis. An indication of the sensitivity and resolution of these electrophoretic data was their ability to point out a minor deficiency in the standard ultracentrifugal method for measuring low concentrations of S_f° 20–400 lipoproteins (below 150 mg/100 ml). For those samples an improved analysis of S_f° 20–100 lipoproteins was made by using the 2-min up-to-speed frame, as described in Section IV.E.

The methods of analytical ultracentrifugation employed in the collaborative study were those described in preceding sections of this chapter. Paper electrophoresis was carried out as described by Hatch and Lees (8). Only a single analysis was made on each sample. The agarose-electrophoresis technique was that of Noble (97) and was modified in three respects: (a) the strips were one-half the width employed previously, and the full width of the pattern was scanned, leading to better reproducibility of duplicate strips; (b) standardization of dye uptake by the electrophoretic strips on different days was improved by making daily dye-uptake controls with aliquots of a frozen, pooled serum and adjusting all values for test sera accordingly; and (c) duplicate analyses were performed and the data were averaged. The strips were stained with Oil Red O (prepared fresh every 2 months) at 40°C as described by Hatch and Lees (8); staining was carried out for 24 hr after preliminary studies showed that this time period provided reproducible and nearly maximal dye uptake by each lipoprotein fraction. The data were analyzed with a computer, as described by Noble et al. (117).

Table XIII. Correlations between Lipoprotein Electrophoresis and Analytical Ultracentrifugation[a]

Methods	β, or S_f 0–20[b]	Pre-β, or S_f 20–400	Chylomicrons, or $S_f > 400$	α_1, or HDL
Agarose versus ultracentrifugation	.978	.993	.854	.867
Paper versus ultracentrifugation	.691	.956	.888[c]	.786
Agarose versus paper	.685	.971	.942[c]	.708

[a] Data for agarose gel are the mean of duplicate determinations; for paper electrophoresis and ultracentrifugation single determinations were made. All correlations are $p < .01$.

[b] The comparisons are based on 20 cases, except for β-lipoproteins. Comparisons involving β-lipoproteins are based on 16 cases because agarose-gel data in four type V hyperlipoproteinemia cases had to be excluded, owing to obvious errors believed to result from partial trailing of pre-β-lipoproteins beneath the β-peak.

[c] In paper electrophoresis the chylomicron fraction includes material trailing between the origin and the β-zone.

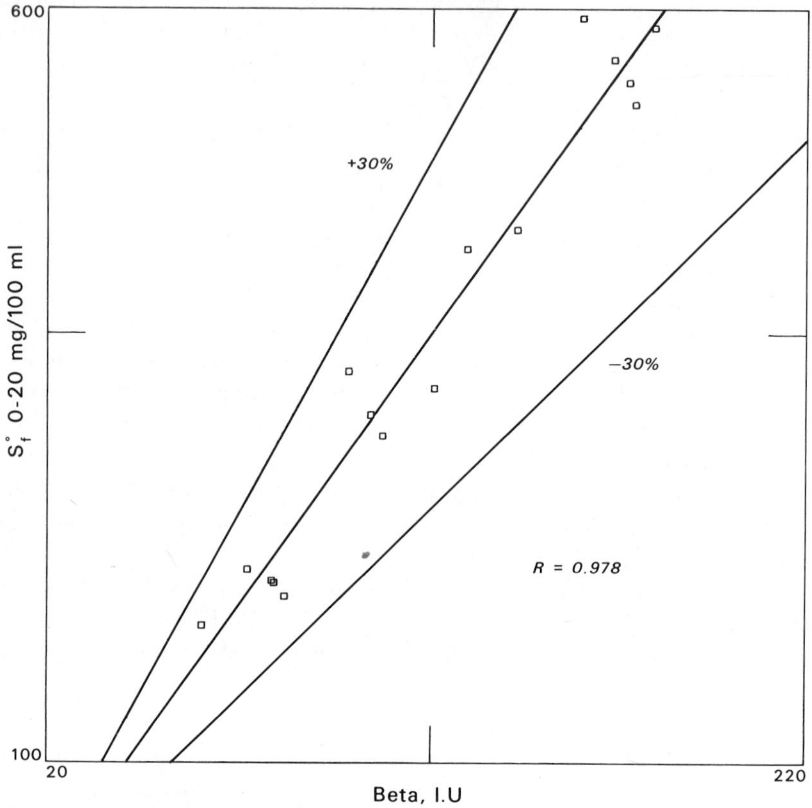

Fig. 41 Scatter diagrams relating data of agarose-gel electrophoresis to that of analytical ultracentrifugation by methods described in the text (see footnote b, Table XII). R = correlation coefficient; I. U. = integration units measured with the Beckman Analytrol densitometer and standardized as explained in the text. The central line is the regression line calculated by the method of least squares. The divergent lines are plotted 30% of the ultracentrifugal values above and below the regression line.

The correlation coefficients among lipoprotein separations in agarose gel and paper and the ultracentrifugal analyses are presented in Table XIII. Scatter diagrams are shown in Fig. 41. The results for agarose-gel electrophoresis were considerably better than those reported in the previous study, probably owing to the modified strips and more rigorous standardization of dye uptake.[8] The results for paper electrophoresis were substantially the same as those obtained previously (Table XII) (115, 117).

One useful indication of the accuracy of a method being tested by com-

[8] Recently the authors, with G. L. Adamson, have studied plasma from 23 patients

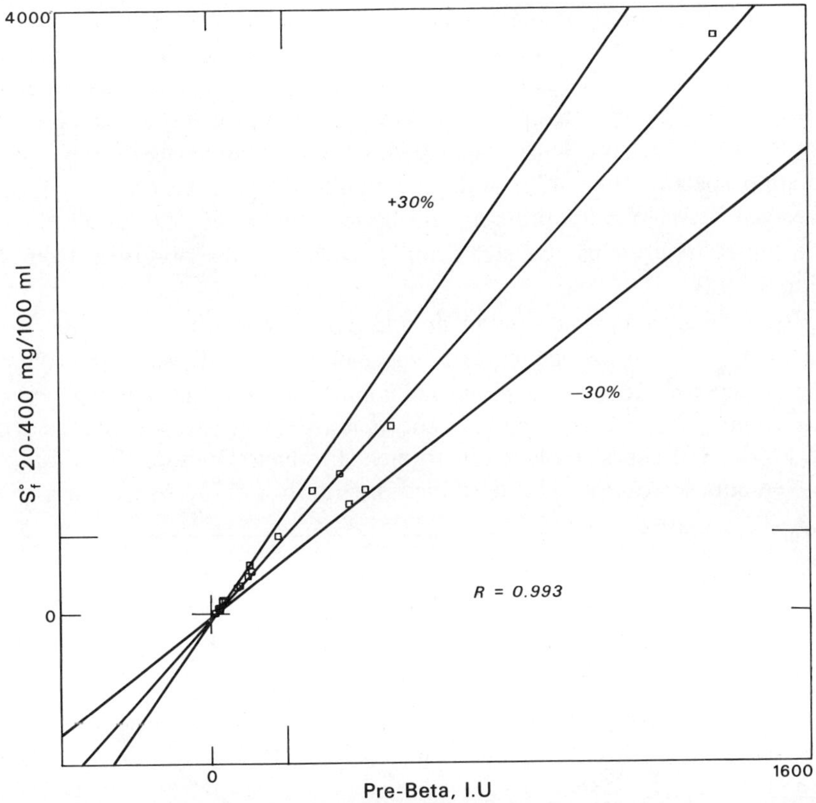

Fig. 41 *(continued)*

parison with an established method is the standard error of the estimate, $S_{y \cdot x}$. This is a measure of the statistical variation of the estimates of the "true" values obtained with the test method—that is, the variations about the least-squares regression line relating test-method values (x-variable) to standard-method values (y-variable) (119). Table XIV presents a comparison of $S_{y \cdot x}$ values obtained in a study by Hulley et al. (118) with those of previously published data. The results suggest that, after careful standardization, agarose-gel-electrophoresis data may be transformable into actual lipoprotein-concentration values (mg/100 ml) with an acceptable degree of accuracy.

with various lipoprotein levels, using one of the commercially available agarose-gel kits. With daily standardization against the β component of a frozen normal serum the following correlations were obtained: pre-β versus S° 20–400, $r = 0.98$; β versus S_f° 0–20, $r = 0.91$; and α_1 versus HDL, $r = 0.74$ (120). Total plasma glyceride and cholesterol data provide internal standardization, giving better results.

In order to relate the electrophoretic fractions observed in agarose gel to specific parts of the ultracentrifugal lipoprotein spectrum, correlation coefficients were calculated between the amounts of each electrophoretic fraction and the ultracentrifugally measured lipoproteins at small increments across the low-density (S_f° 0–400) and high-density ($F_{1.20}^\circ$ 0–9) flotation spectra (Fig. 42). A highly significant positive correlation was observed between β-lipoproteins and lipoproteins of S_f° 5 to about S_f° 12. For pre-β-lipoproteins the significant correlation was observed from S_f° 16 to S_f° 400.

For α_1-lipoproteins a significant correlation was observed from $F_{1.20}^\circ$ 1.5 to $F_{1.20}^\circ$ 7, which encompasses most of the high-density lipoproteins. The partial resolution of α_1-lipoproteins into a main band, denoted by α_x, and a minor faster anodal component, denoted by α_y, was evaluated with the Model 310 curve resolver (Instrument Products Division, E. I. duPont de Nemours & Co., Inc.), as described previously (117). As shown in Fig.

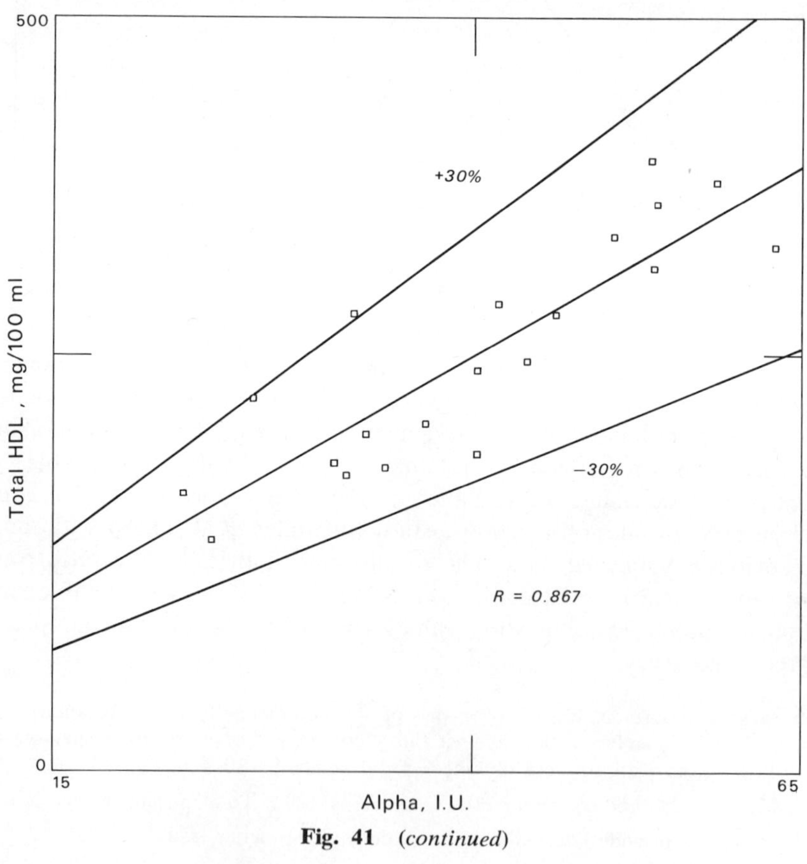

Fig. 41 (*continued*)

Table XIV. Means and Standard Errors of the Estimate ($S_{y.x}$) of Ultracentrifugal Values from Electrophoretic Data

Medium and Number of Cases n	Concentration (mg/100 ml)					
	β-Lipoproteins		Pre-β-lipoproteins		α_1-Lipoproteins	
	$\overline{y}$[a]	$S_{y.x}$[b]	$\overline{y}$[a]	$S_{y.x}$[b]	$\overline{y}$[a]	$S_{y.x}$[b]
Agarose gel:						
$n = 20$[c]	385[d]	32	520	104	276	38
$n = 28$[e]	535	73	125	50	344	70
Paper:						
$n = 20$[c]	385[d]	111	520	258	276	48
$n = 71$[f]	455	110	165	75	337	78

[a] Mean concentration (mg/100 ml) of the corresponding ultracentrifugal fraction.
[b] Standard error of the estimate derived by least-squares regression analysis of the relationship between electrophoresis (x-variable) and ultracentrifugation (y-variable).
[c] Data from S. B. Hulley et al. (118).
[d] Comparisons are based on 16 cases. Data for four type V hyperlipoproteinemia cases had to be excluded, owing to obvious errors believed to result from partial trailing of pre-β-lipoproteins beneath the β-lipoprotein peak.
[e] Data from Ref. 117.
[f] Data from Ref. 115.

42, the main α_x-component is well correlated with most of the HDL ultracentrifugal spectrum ($R = .89$), without any suggestion of preferential representation of HDL_2 ($F^\circ_{1.20}$ 3.5–9) or HDL_3 ($F^\circ_{1.20}$ 0–3.5). However, the minor α_y-component is not significantly correlated with any part of the HDL spectrum, despite the fact (mentioned earlier) that this zone contains lipids typical of high-density lipoproteins (R with total HDL $= .19$). In view of the equivocal nature of the α_y-zone, the semiquantitative estimation of α_1-lipoproteins by agarose-gel or paper electrophoresis should perhaps be limited to the main, or α_x, zone.

Finally, an approximate correspondence has been found between the chylomicron zone at the electrophoretic origin and $S_f > 400$ lipoproteins, determined by ultracentrifugation in a density gradient (see Section VI.E. and Table XIII). However, the number of sera containing chylomicrons and the range of chylomicron concentrations were still insufficient for a rigorous statistical analysis.

F. Evaluation of Lipoprotein Electrophoresis

Although a fair estimate of the amounts of β- and pre-β-lipoproteins can be inferred from chemical measurements of serum cholesterol and

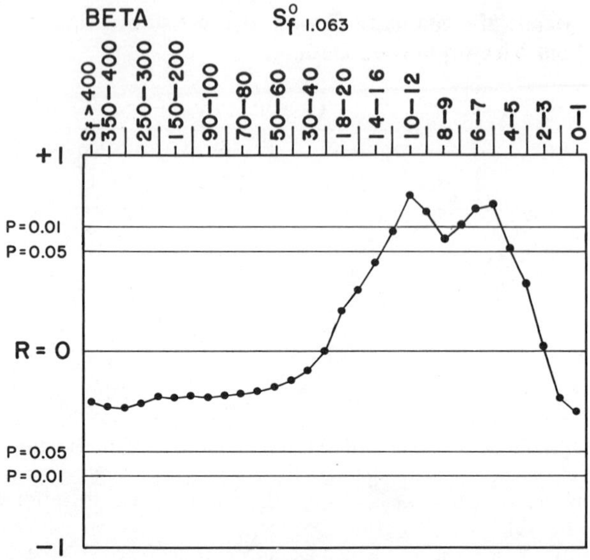

Fig. 42 Correlation profiles of the amounts of the electrophoretic fractions indicated at the upper left of each diagram across increments of the low-density ($S^\circ_{f\ 1.063}$) or high-density ($F^\circ_{1.20}$) ultracentrifugal schlieren patterns. The vertical axis ranges from correlation coefficients of −1 to +1. Transverse lines indicate the correlations required for probabilities of chance occurrence less than .05 to .01. Alpha$_x$ is the major band of α_1-lipoprotein; alpha$_y$ is the faster migrating minor component observed anodally to the major band (see text).

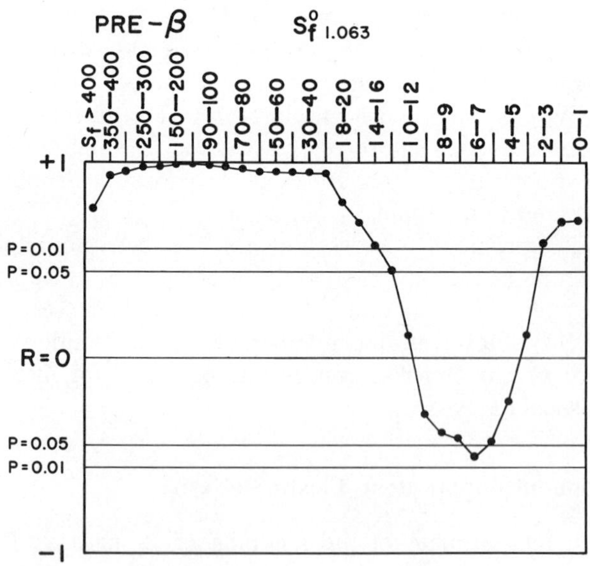

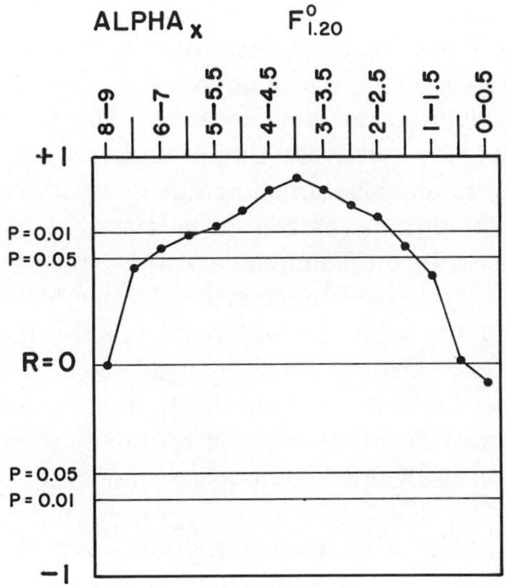

Fig. 42 (*continued*)

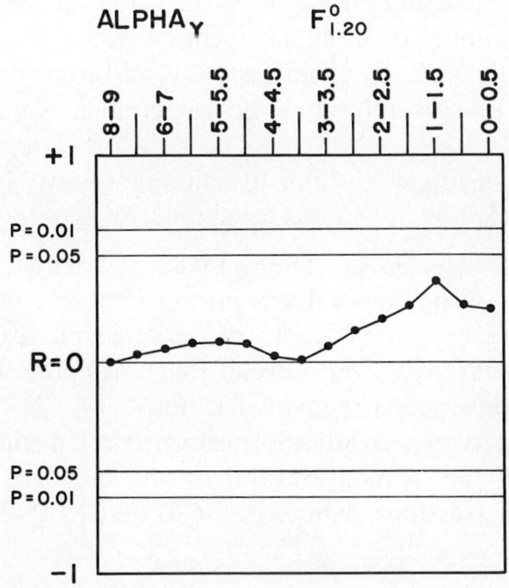

triglycerides, such inferences can be seriously in error in certain clinical disorders. The concentration of α_1-, or high-density, lipoproteins cannot be estimated directly from serum cholesterol and triglyceride levels. Thus a proper understanding of the distribution of the lipoproteins in plasma is best achieved by a direct method of assay. The semiquantitative correspondence between the relatively simple and inexpensive electrophoretic method and the more reliable, but elaborate, ultracentrifugal method means that plasma-lipoprotein patterns can be measured in clinical and epidemiological laboratories. In most individuals with either normal or abnormal plasma-lipoprotein levels the ultracentrifugal value for each major lipoprotein fraction could be estimated within $\pm$ 30% by paper electrophoresis and within somewhat narrower limits by agarose-gel electrophoresis. These electrophoretic methods can be considered to be semiquantitative. Since the significant clinical disorders and the results of successful therapy generally produce changes of much greater magnitude, this degree of accuracy is tolerable.

There are difficulties in achieving rigorous control over the complete sequence of operations in the semiquantitative electrophoretic technique. In our experience the features of the method that require particular attention are (a) careful addition of serum aliquots to the applicator and thence to the strips, (b) control of temperature and concentration of the dye solution, and (c) calibration of the scanning densitometer. Bush (121) and Winkelman and Wybenga (122) discuss certain features of the quantitative scanning technique.

Our semiquantitative electrophoretic data have been reported in terms of integration units, or millimeters of peak height in the case of β-lipoproteins. Within the limits of attained accuracy these data could be related to the values (mg/100 ml) obtained by ultracentrifugation; the latter method involves specific refractive-index-increment values that were standardized gravimetrically.

Laboratories wishing to establish semiquantitative lipoprotein electrophoresis have the following options for standardization:

1. Local assay of series of healthy males and females covering a range of ages, with establishment of local norms in terms of integration units.
2. Performance of a small series of direct comparisons with a reliable ultracentrifugal laboratory over a broad range of lipoprotein concentrations and subsequent conversion to gravimetric units.
3. If facilities for preparative ultracentrifugation and precision refractometry are available, standardization of the clinically important pre-β- and β-lipoprotein fractions with S_f 20–400 and S_f 0–20 lipoproteins, respectively, can be accomplished (23).[9]

[9] See Section III.

Of course, all of the usual admonitions about defining "normal" lipoprotein levels apply to these data. Our values were obtained from a healthy middle-aged population in which the males, especially, can be assumed to have a great deal of occult atherosclerosis. This limitation must be recognized by everyone who generates, or interprets clinically, semiquantitative data from lipoprotein electrophoresis.

X. CONCLUSIONS

We have considered in some detail the present state of the art of two widely used and important tools for lipoprotein research: ultracentrifugal fractionation and analysis, and lipoprotein characterization and semiquantification by the latest electrophoretic techniques. Throughout our presentation we have emphasized and illustrated the usefulness and frequent necessity of employing computer techniques in many aspects of instrumentation and data analysis. Scientists and students looking for a broader treatment of the subject of human plasma lipoproteins are referred to a review by Nichols (7), a book on clinical disorders by Sanbar (123) and a forthcoming *Scientific American* article by Lossow (124).

Currently there is an active ferment in the fields involving the study of serum lipoproteins and their metabolism. Many of these studies are concerned with such fundamental questions as the structure and physicochemical characterization of lipid–protein complexes. Other questions relate to the detailed characterization of the protein moieties, their substructure and conformation within each class of the serum lipoproteins. All such studies should increasingly contribute toward our understanding of how specific elevations and abnormalities of these important and complex molecules relate to states of health and disease.

The results we have presented show that the relatively simple and inexpensive electrophoretic methods correlate rather well with analytical ultracentrifugation. This means that semiquantitative measurement of the major lipoprotein fractions can be carried out in clinical and epidemiological laboratories, where there is great demand for these analyses for studies of human genetic disorders, cardiovascular-disease risk factors, secondary metabolic disorders, and evaluation of the results of drug and diet therapy.

In most scientific research the results of carefully planned experiments ultimately depend on the validity, reproducibility, and reliability of the methods employed to acquire and analyze the data. Therefore it is our hope that by emphasizing the unique capabilities, as well as the limitations, of ultracentrifugation and electrophoresis we shall assist the more biologically and metabolically oriented scientists working in lipoprotein research.

XI. ACKNOWLEDGMENTS

This work was supported in part by contract W-7405-eng-48, U.S. Atomic Energy Commission, and by Research Grant 5-RO1-HE-1882-15 from the National Heart Institute, U.S. Public Health Service.

We thank Drs. Robert I. Levy, Robert S. Lees, Edwin L. Bierman, William R. Hazzard, and Edward H. Strisower for kindly providing serum or plasma samples used to illustrate the lipoprotein characterization techniques. Also we especially thank Drs. Milton Z. Nichaman and Steven B. Hulley for making available agarose-gel-electrophoresis data from a collaborative study prior to normal publication. We particularly thank Mrs. Dorothy Sprague for help in preparing the manuscript.

For permission to use published data and to reproduce (in some cases with minor revisions) figures we thank the American Oil Chemists' Society, Academic Press, the *Review of Scientific Instruments,* the *Journal of Clinical Investigation,* the *Journal of Lipid Research,* and *Biophysica et Biochimica Acta.*

REFERENCES

1. Macheboeuf, M., *Bull. Soc. Chim. Biol.,* **11**, 268–293 (1929).
2. McFarlane, A. S., *Biochem. J.,* **29**, 660–693 (1935).
3. Cohn, E. J., F. R. N. Gurd, D. M. Surgenor, B. A. Barnes, R. K. Brown, G. Derouaux, J. M. Gillespie, F. W. Kahnt, W. F. Lever, C. H. Liu, D. Mittelman, R. F. Mouton, K. Schmid, and E. Uroma, *J. Amer. Chem. Soc.* **72**, 465–474 (1950).
4. Pedersen, K. O., *Ultracentrifugal Studies on Serum and Serum Fractions,* Almquist and Wiksells, Uppsala, 1945.
5. Gofman, J. W., F. T. Lindgren, and H. Elliott, *J. Biol. Chem.* **179**, 973–979 (1949).
6. Ewing, A. M., N. K. Freeman, and F. T. Lindgren, in *Advances in Lipid Research,* Vol. 3, R. Paoletti and D. Kritchevsky, Eds., Academic Press, New York, 1965, pp. 25–61.
7. Nichols, A. V., in *Advances in Biological and Medical Physics,* Vol. 11, J. Lawrence and J. Gofman, Eds., Academic Press, New York, 1967, pp. 110–158.
8. Hatch, F. T., and R. S. Lees, in *Advances in Lipid Research,* Vol. 6, R. Paoletti and D. Kritchevsky, Eds., Academic Press, New York, 1968, pp. 1–68.
9. Tria, E., and A. M. Scanu, Eds., *Structural and Functional Aspects of Lipoproteins in Living Systems,* Academic Press, New York, 1969.
10. Lindgren, F. T., H. A. Elliott, and J. W. Gofman, *J. Phys. Colloid Chem.* **55**, 80–93 (1951).
11. DeLalla, O., and J. Gofman, in *Methods of Biochemical Analysis,* Vol. 1, D. Glick, Ed., Interscience, New York, 1954, pp. 459–478.

12. Havel, R. J., H. A. Eder, and J. H. Bragdon, *J. Clin. Invest.* **34**, 1345–1353 (1955).
13. Hillyard, L. A., C. Entenman, H. Feinberg, and I. L. Chaikoff, *J. Biol. Chem.* **214**, 79–90 (1955).
14. Lindgren, F. T., A. V. Nichols, and N. K. Freeman, *J. Phys. Chem.* **59**, 930-938 (1955).
15. Bauer, N., and S. Z. Lewin, in *Physical Methods of Organic Chemistry,* 3rd ed., Vol. I, Part II, A. Weissberger, Ed., Interscience, New York, 1960, pp. 1239–1244.
16. Bauer, N., and S. Z. Lewin, in *Physical Methods of Organic Chemistry,* 3rd ed., Vol. I, Part I, A. Weissberger, Ed., Interscience, New York, 1960, pp. 131–190.
17. Washburn, E. W., Ed., *International Critical Tables of Numerical Data,* McGraw-Hill, New York, 1933.
18. Weast, R. C., Ed., *Handbook of Chemistry and Physics,* The Chemical Rubber Co., Cleveland, 1969.
19. *Proceedings of the Deuel Conference on Lipids, Carmel, Calif.,* U.S. Public Health Service, Washington, D.C., 1967, pp. 152–157.
20. Ockner, R. K., F. B. Hughes, and K. J. Isselbacher, *J. Clin. Invest.* **48**, 2079–2088 (1969).
21. Windmueller, H. G., F. T. Lindgren, W. J. Lossow, and R. I. Levy, *Biochim. Biophys. Acta* **202**, 506–516 (1970).
22. Dittmer, D., Ed., *Blood and Other Body Fluids,* Federation of American Societies for Experimental Biology, Washington, D.C., 1961, p. 13.
23. Lindgren, F. T., A. V. Nichols, N. K. Freeman, R. D. Wills, L. Wing, and J. E. Gullberg, *J. Lipid Res.* **5**, 68–74 (1964).
24. Lindgren, F. T., N. K. Freeman, A. M. Ewing, L. C. Jensen, *J. Amer. Oil Chem. Soc.* **43**, 281 285 (1966).
25. Lindgren, F. T., N. K. Freeman, and A. M. Ewing, in *Progress in Biochemical Pharmacology,* Vol. II, D. Kritchevsky, R. Paoletti and D. Steinberg, Eds., Karger, Basel, 1967, pp. 475–499.
26. Windsor, A. W., T. H. Rich, R. E. Doyle, and F. T. Lindgren, *Rev. Sci. Instr.* **38**, 949–952 (1967).
27. Windsor, A. W., L. C. Jensen, D. A. Hoopes, and F. T. Lindgren, *Rev. Sci. Instr.* **41**, 123–125 (1970).
28. Lindgren, F. T., and F. T. Upham, *Rev. Sci. Instr.* **33**, 1291–1292 (1962).
29. Jensen, L. C., T. H. Rich, and F. T. Lindgren, *Lipids* **5**, 491–493 (1970).
30. Oncley, J. L., *Biopolymers* **7**, 119–132 (1969).
31. Gofman, J. W., O. deLalla, F. Glazier, N. K. Freeman, F. T. Lindgren, A. V. Nichols, B. Strisower, and A. R. Tamplin, *Plasma* **2**, 413–484 (1954).
32. Fredrickson, D. S., R. I. Levy, and F. T. Lindgren, *J. Clin. Invest.* **47**, 2446–2457 (1968).
33. Strisower, E. H., G. L. Adamson, and B. Strisower, *Amer. J. Med.* **45**, 488–501 (1969).
34. Fredrickson, D. S., R. I. Levy, and R. S. Lees, *New Engl. J. Med.* **276**, 34–44, 94–103, 148–156, 215–225, 273–281 (1967).
35. Hazzard, W. R., F. T. Lindgren, and E. L. Bierman, *Biochim. Biophys. Acta* **202**, 517–525 (1970).
36. Svedberg, I., and K. O. Pedersen, *The Ultracentrifuge,* Oxford University Press, London and New York, 1940.
37. Schachman, H. K., *Ultracentrifugation in Biochemistry,* Academic Press, New York, 1959.

38. Adams, G. H., and V. N. Schumaker, *Biochim. Biophys. Acta,* **202**, 315–324 (1970).
39. Gropper, L., *Anal. Biochem.* **6**, 170–175 (1963).
40. Oncley, J. L., K. W. Walton, and D. G. Cornwell, *J. Amer. Chem. Soc.* **79**, 4666–4671 (1957).
41. Lindgren, F. T., A. V. Nichols, T. L. Hayes, N. K. Freeman, and J. W. Gofman, *Ann. N.Y. Acad. Sci.* **72**, 826–844 (1955).
42. Adams, G. H., and V. N. Schumaker, *Ann. N.Y. Acad. Sci.,* **164**, 130–146 (1969).
43. Oncley, J. L., G. Scatchard, and A. Brown, *J. Phys. Colloid Chem.* **51**, 184–198 (1947).
44. Oncley, J. L., *Vox Sang.* **5**, 91–92 (1960).
45. Bjorklund, R., and S. Katz, *J. Amer. Chem. Soc.* **78**, 2122–2126 (1956).
46. Mills, G. L., C. E. Taylaur, and P. A. Wilkinson, *Clin. Chim. Acta* **14**, 273–275 (1966).
47. Moring-Claesson, I., *Arkiv Kemi* **10**, 47–56 (1956).
48. Freeman, N. K., *J. Lipid Res.* **5**, 236–241 (1964).
49. Mills, G. L., *Biochim. Biophys. Acta,* **194**, 222–226 (1969).
50. Lindgren, F. T., L. C. Jensen, R. D. Wills, and N. K. Freeman, *Lipids* **4**, 337–344 (1969).
51. Adams, G. H., and V. N. Schumaker, *Anal. Biochem.* **29**, 117–129 (1969).
52. Scanu, A., H. Pollard, and W. Reader, *J. Lipid Res.* **9**, 243–349 (1968).
53. Freeman, N. K., in *Blood Lipids and Lipoproteins,* G. J. Nelson, Ed., Wiley-Interscience, New York, 1971, pp. 113–179.
54. Lowry, O. H., N. J. Rosebrough, A. L. Farr, and R. J. Randall, *J. Biol. Chem.* **193**, 265–275 (1951).
55. Lees, R. S., abstract, *Circulation* **40**, Suppl. III–15 (1969).
56. Jensen, L. C., A. M. Ewing, R. D. Wills, and F. T. Lindgren, *J. Amer. Oil Chem. Soc.* **44**, 5–10 (1967).
57. Hatch, F. T., N. K. Freeman, G. R. Stevens, and F. T. Lindgren, *Lipids* **2**, 183–191 (1967).
58. Bartlett, G. R., *J. Biol. Chem.* **234**, 466–468 (1959).
59. Gage, S. H., *Cornell Vet.* **10**, 154 (1920).
60. Gage, S. H., and P. A. Fish, *Amer. J. Anat.* **34**, 1–85 (1924).
61. Marder, L. G., H. Becker, B. Maizel, and H. Necheles, *Gastroenterology* **20**, 43–59 (1952).
62. Stone, M. C., and J. M. Thorp, *Clin. Chim. Acta* **14**, 812–830 (1966).
63. Laurell, C. B., *Scand. J. Clin. Lab. Invest.* **6**, 22–24 (1954).
64. Gordis, E., *Proc. Soc. Exp. Biol. Med.* **110**, 657–661 (1962).
65. Bragdon, J. H., R. J. Havel, and E. Boyle, *J. Lab. Clin. Med.* **48**, 36–42 (1956).
66. Cornwell, D. G., and F. A. Kruger, *J. Lipid Res.* **2**, 110–134 (1961).
67. Dole, V. P., and J. T. Hamlin, III, *Physiol. Rev.* **42**, 674–701 (1962).
68. Gustafson, A., P. Alaupovic, and R. H. Furman, *Biochemistry* 4, 596–605 (1965).
69. Lindgren, F. T., A. V. Nichols, F. T. Upham, and R. D. Wills, *J. Phys. Chem.* **66**, 2007–2011 (1962).
69a. Lindgren, F. T., L. C. Jensen, R. D. Wills, and G. R. Stevens, *Lipids,* in press (1972).
70. Lossow, W. J., F. T. Lindgren, J. C. Murchio, G. R. Stevens, and L. C. Jensen, *J. Lipid Res.* **10**, 68–76 (1969).
71. Yokoyama, A., and D. B. Zilversmit, *J. Lipid Res.* **6**, 241–246 (1965).

72. Pinter, G. G., and D. B. Zilversmit, *Biochim. Biophys. Acta* **59**, 116–127 (1962).
73. Oncley, J. L., *Brain Lipids and Lipoproteins, and the Leucodystrophies, Proc. Neurochemistry Symposium,* Rome, 1961, J. Folch-Pi and H. Bauer, Eds., Elsevier, New York, 1963, pp. 1–17.
74. Hazelwood, R. N., *J. Amer. Chem. Soc.* **80**, 2152–2156 (1958).
75. Scanu, A., and J. L. Granda, *Biochemistry* **5**, 446–455 (1966).
76. Scanu, A., and W. L. Hughes, *J. Biol. Chem.* **235**, 2876–2883 (1960).
77. Furman, R. H., S. S. Sanbar, P. Alaupovic, R. H. Bradford, and R. P. Howard, *J. Lab. Clin. Med.* **63**, 193–204 (1964).
78. Levy, R. I., and D. S. Fredrickson, *J. Clin. Invest.* **44**, 426–441 (1965).
79. Mauldin, J., and W. R. Fisher, *Biochemistry* **9**, 2015–2020 (1970).
80. Wilcox, H. G., D. C. Davis, and M. Heimberg, *J. Lipid Res.* **12**, 160–172 (1971).
81. Granda, J. L., and A. Scanu, *Biochemistry* **5**, 3301–3308 (1966).
82. Scanu, A., W. Reader, and C. Edelstein, *Biochim. Biophys. Acta* **160**, 32–45 (1968).
83. Alaupovic, P., R. H. Furman, W. H. Falor, M. L. Sullivan, S. L. Walraven, and A. C. Olson, *Ann. N.Y. Acad. Sci.* **149**, 791–807 (1968).
84. Shore, B., and V. Shore, *Biochemistry* **8**, 4510–4516 (1969).
85. Brown, W. V., R. I. Levy, and D. S. Fredrickson, *J. Biol. Chem.* **244**, 5687–5694 (1969).
86. Kunkel, H. G., and R. Trautman, *J. Clin. Invest.* **35**, 641 (1956).
87. Hatch, F. T., in *Serum Proteins and the Dysproteinemias,* F. W. Sunderman and F. W. Sunderman, Jr., Eds., Lippincott, Philadelphia, 1964, Fig. 5, p. 228.
88. Smith, E. B., *Lancet* **2**, 910–914 (1957).
89. Fisher, W. R., *J. Biol. Chem.* **245**, 877–884 (1970).
90. Sohdi, H. S., *Metabolism* **18**, 852–859 (1969).
91. Switzer, S., *J. Clin. Invest.* **46**, 1855–1866 (1967).
92. Mills, G. L., D. Seidel, and P. Alaupovic, *Clin. Chim. Acta* **26**, 239–244 (1969).
93. Seidel, D., P. Alaupovic, and R. H. Furman, *J. Clin. Invest.* **48**, 1211–1223 (1969).
94. Pries, C., C. M. Van Gent, H. Baes, M. K. Polano, H. A. M. Hulsman, and A. Querido, *Clin. Chim. Acta* **19**, 181–190 (1968).
95. Winkelman, J., and F. A. Ibbott, *Clin. Chim. Acta* **26**, 25–32 (1969).
96. Moinuddin, M., and L. Taylor, *Lipids* **4**, 186–189 (1969).
97. Noble, R. P., *J. Lipid Res.* **9**, 693–700 (1968).
98. Rapp, W., and W. Kahlke, *Clin. Chim. Acta* **19**, 493–498 (1968).
99. McGlashan, D. A. K., and T. R. E. Pilkington, *Clin. Chim. Acta* **22**, 646–647 (1968).
100. Papadopoulos, N. M., and J. A. Kintzios, *Anal. Biochem.* **30**, 421–462 (1969).
101. Irwin, W. C., Ph.D. thesis, University of Alberta, Edmonton, 1969.
102. Cawley, L. P., *Electrophoresis and Immunoelectrophoresis,* Little, Brown and Co., Boston, 1969, pp. 88–110, 264–266.
103. Houtsmuller, A. J., *Agarose-Gel-Electrophoresis of Lipoproteins,* Royal Vangorcum, The Netherlands, 1970.
104. Iammarino, R. M., M. Humphrey, and P. Antolik, *Clin. Chem.* **15**, 1218–1229 (1969).
105. Narayan, K. A., H. L. Creinin, and F. A. Kummerow, *J. Lipid Res.* **7**, 150–157 (1966).

106. Narayan, K. A., G. E. S. Mary, and H. P. Friedman, *Microchem. J.* **14**, 235–241 (1969).
107. Narayan, K. A., *Microchem. J.* **14**, 335–342 (1969).
108. Raymond, S., J. L. Miles, and J. C. J. Lee, *Science* **151**, 346–347 (1966).
109. Pratt, J. J., and W. G. Dangerfield, *Clin. Chim. Acta* **23**, 189–201 (1969).
110. Colfs, B., and J. Verheyden, *Clin. Chim. Acta* **18**, 325–334 (1967).
111. Chin, H. P., and D. H. Blankenhorn, *Clin. Chim. Acta* **20**, 305–314 (1968).
112. Farber, E. R., J. G. Batsakis, P. C. Giesen, and M. Thiessen, *Amer. J. Clin. Pathol.* **51**, 523–528 (1969).
113. Winkelman, J., F. A. Ibbott, C. Sobel, and D. R. Wybenga, *Clin. Chim. Acta* **26**, 33–39 (1969).
114. Maskett, B., R. I. Levy, and D. S. Fredrickson, abstract, *Circulation* **40**, Suppl. III–17 (1969).
115. Hatch, F. T., J. A. Mazrimas, J. L. Moore, F. T. Lindgren, L. C. Jensen, R. D. Wills, and G. L. Adamson, *Clin. Biochem.* **3**, 115–123 (1970).
116. Lees, R. S., and F. T. Hatch, *J. Lab. Clin. Med.* **61**, 518–528 (1963).
117. Noble, R. P., F. T. Hatch, J. A. Mazrimas, F. T. Lindgren, L. C. Jensen, and G. L. Adamson, *Lipids* **4**, 55–59 (1969).
118. Hulley, S. B., S. G. Cook, W. S. Wilson, M. Z. Nichaman, F. T. Hatch, and F. T. Lindgren, *J. Lipid Res.,* **12**, 420–433 (1971).
119. Dixon, W. J., and F. J. Massey, Jr., *Introduction to Statistical Analysis,* McGraw-Hill, 1951, p. 155.
120. Lindgren, F. T., G. L. Adamson, L. C. Jensen, and F. T. Hatch, *Circulation* **44**, Suppl. I, Abstract No. 191 (1971).
121. Bush, I. E., in *Methods of Biochemical Analysis,* Vol. 11, D. Glick, Ed., Interscience, New York, 1963, pp. 149–209.
122. Winkelman, J., and D. R. Wybenga, *Clin. Chem.* **15**, 708–711 (1969).
123. Sanbar, S. S., *Hyperlipidemia and Hyperlipoproteinemia,* Little, Brown and Co., Boston (1969).
124. Lossow, W. J., *Scientific American,* in press.

6. Integrated Approach to Plasma Lipid and Lipoprotein Analysis

VICTOR H. BLATON and HUBERT PEETERS

Simon Stevin Institute for Scientific Research, Bruges, Belgium

I. INTRODUCTION

The relationship between plasma lipids and atherosclerosis has been exhaustively studied for many decades, and a first integrated approach to the mechanism and disorders of fat transport in lipoproteins has been reviewed by Fredrickson, Levy, and Lees (1). Total cholesterol is the standard lipid determination recommended in cardiovascular epidemiology for the following reasons: it correlates as well or even better than other lipid fractions with the prevalence of ischemic heart disease and is known to be related to the risk of a future disease; it is the fraction about which there is the most information. However, we need clarification on how the serum cholesterol level is related to other arterial—cerebral and peripheral vascular—diseases and on its interrelations with other risk factors and other lipids. Several other lipid fractions, including phospholipids, have also received attention in the continuous attempt to delineate the pathogenic mechanisms in atherosclerosis.

Many older procedures did not resolve several of the blood lipid components but measured only groups or classes in toto. This is particularly true of phospholipids in whole-blood plasma and in erythrocytes. It is now obvious that specific changes occur within the specific lipid classes—changes that may go undetected by more general analytical procedures. Furthermore, blood lipids are manifestly important in diabetes, and they undergo changes in many hereditary anomalies.

The structure, definition, and interrelationship of plasma lipoproteins, and regulation of lipoprotein concentration, have become increasingly important topics because it is evident that abnormal lipoprotein concentrations accelerate the development of atherosclerosis. Therefore a rapid method for the separation and assessment of plasma lipoproteins is of importance. The development of new techniques constantly provides a stimulus for refinements in plasma lipid and lipoprotein analysis. In this chapter we attempt to show the necessity of a detailed analysis of the lipids and fatty acids in individual plasma lipoproteins.

Precise quantitative analysis of the lipid classes and their fatty acid composition in a complex mixture presents several analytical problems. The most precise procedures for quantitative analysis involve minimal handling of the lipid extract to avoid decomposing the sample or introducing contaminants. Most rapid procedures that are also accurate use electrochromatography and ultracentrifugation for lipoprotein separation, whereas lipids are analyzed by extraction thin-layer chromatography (TLC) and gas–liquid chromatography. Lipids are mixtures composed of many different classes of molecules, and the specific determination of each component is quite difficult. Characterization and analysis require the use of many procedures and extensive knowledge of the chemical characteristics of diverse types of organic compounds. Several components occur in trace amounts and are therefore more difficult to analyze. Because others are unknown or not fully identified and characterized, their determination cannot always be carried out with certainty. The polar lipids are complex molecules differing in the length and degree of saturation of their carbon chains. In addition, branched chains and various substitutions along the chain may be present. These different molecular species cannot be easily determined at this time. Some lipids are easily oxidized or otherwise altered. Nonlipid contaminants are extracted with lipids and must be removed.

All serum or plasma lipids are bound to proteins, and an accurate picture of them can only be obtained through an extensive separation and determination of the individual lipids in individual lipoproteins isolated on the basis of mobility, solubility, molecular weight, or density. We conclude that the analysis of separated α-lipoproteins [high-density lipoproteins (HDL), $1.083 < d < 1.20$] and β-lipoproteins [low-density lipoproteins (LDL), $1.019 < d < 1.063$] describes many differences that could not be seen in total plasma.

II. EXTRACTION OF LIPIDS

One major difficulty associated with any chemical or biochemical study of the simple and complex lipids is their isolation and separation into individual components and, concomitantly, definition of the proper purity criteria. The homogeneity, or uniformity, of a lipid fraction is often defined on the basis of the non-fatty-acid skeleton, but there is no doubt that the fatty acid composition significantly affects the physical and chemical properties of the fraction. Hence the term "pure lipid" is not rigorous. Closely related solubility properties, interassociative effects (the ability of one compound to solubilize another, etc.), and the influence of contaminants all contribute to the problem of lipid purification.

A second problem is the susceptibility of certain lipids and lipoproteins to oxidation. For this reason organic solvents should be treated to remove dissolved oxygen. Unsaturated fatty acids are susceptible to oxidation, and dienoic and polyenoic acids are more susceptible to oxidation than monoenoic acids. Furthermore, polyenoic acids of physiological origin are of the methylene-interrupted variety, which give rise to free radicals or peroxide free radicals.

In this section we describe some of these problems as well as ways of achieving a satisfactory fractionation.

A. Extraction Procedures for Plasma Lipids and Lipoproteins

1. Extraction of Plasma Lipids. Since many of the commonly occurring lipids are not entirely soluble in such solvents as ethanol, acetone, and methanol, it is always advisable to combine these with a less polar solvent like petroleum ether, chloroform, or diethyl ether. Depending on the extraction temperature, some or all of the plasma proteins may be denatured.

The various mixtures used for extracting lipids have been reviewed by Entenman (2). It is obvious from his paper that there are variations in the approaches used by different investigators; however, for most purposes an initial trial with a chloroform–methanol, 2:1 (v/v), or an ethanol–diethyl ether, 3:1 (v/v), mixture is highly recommended. For complete extraction most investigators use the Folch solvent, chloroform–methanol, 2:1. Important modifications of the procedure of Folch, Lees, and Sloane-Stanley (3) are the use of multiple, rather than single, extraction (4–6), the addition of an antioxidant (4), and extraction under nitrogen. Lipid extracts should be evaporated in the cold under nitrogen, taking care not to evaporate to complete dryness, to avoid decomposition of some lipids.

2. Delipidation of Plasma Lipoproteins. Plasma lipids are associated with specific proteins, often called apoproteins, with which they form lipid–protein complexes, whose structure and function are not yet clearly established. Available procedures for quantitative lipid separation and for the determination of lipid composition can establish the complete lipid patterns of plasma lipoproteins and follow lipid changes under pathological conditions.

It is more difficult to extract lipids from lipoproteins isolated by density centrifugation than to extract them from untreated plasma. The large amounts of salt added to adjust density during the fractionation of plasma may account for the change in the extractability of lipids. Table I shows

Table I. Composition of β-Lipoproteins

Preparation	Composition (%)		
	Phospholipids	Triglycerides	Cholesterol
Ultracentrifugation[a]	33	6	61
Heparin–Mn precipitation[a]	29	7	64
Sulfated dextran precipitation[b]	33	8	58
Electrochromatography[b]	33	8	58

[a] Data from Gotto, Levy, and Fredrickson (7).
[b] Data from Peeters (8).

the lipid composition of low-density lipoproteins ($1.019 < d < 1.063$) isolated on the basis of density, solubility, and mobility. No significant differences were found between the preparations of β-lipoproteins that were precipitated with heparin or sulfated dextran and those that were obtained by centrifugation or by electrochromatography. At the moment, however, we cannot explain how the lipoprotein-separation procedure affects the solubility of the protein moiety.

The lipoprotein complexes of blood plasma are so firmly bound that very little lipid is extracted by ethyl ether at room temperature. The addition of alcohol and the use of low temperatures and enzymes improve the extraction of lipids by ether. With this procedure cholesterol is more readily removed than phospholipids, indicating differences within the intramolecular binding forces (9). Alcohols promote the ether extraction of lipids from tissues or blood plasma, affecting the gross hydration of the protein moieties of the complex. The influence of alcohols on extractability by ether and chloroform indicates that the hydrophobic lipid moieties of lipoprotein complexes have weak internal lipid–lipid associations and are protected externally by ionization and hydration phenomena of the hydrophilic protein moieties. Alcohols are assumed to affect the permeability of the protective outer zone, allowing ether to reach the lipids and remove them.

Gustafson (10) performed *partial delipidation* and stressed the difficulty of removing all lipids from lipoproteins. The extraction of neutral lipids can be accelerated by the presence of starch, which increases the lyophilized lipoprotein's area of contact with the lipid solvent. By combining partial delipidation with thin-layer chromatography, Gustafson (10) found that in β-lipoproteins free cholesterol was more tightly bound than cholesteryl esters and triglycerides. The evidence for loosely bound cholesteryl esters is in agreement with earlier findings of cholesteryl ester loss in repeated ultracentrifugation. In α-lipoproteins the lipid-binding properties seem to be different (4). Cholesteryl esters are more tightly bound than free cholesterol, as judged by the sequence in lipid removal.

Extraction studies of *low-density lipoproteins* have rather distinct motivations. Most commonly the aim has been to understand the interactions between the lipid and the protein fractions and to gain insight into the lipid and fatty acid composition. In an analogous manner other investigators have attempted to show differences in the lipid composition of normal plasma and plasma from patients with some disease, such as atherosclerosis. Additional experiments have been directed toward the preparation of soluble, lipid-free apoproteins whose physical and chemical properties could be studied (11). The ease of extraction varies with the lipoprotein class: phospholipids are more readily extracted from very-low-density lipoproteins (VLDL) than from low- or high-density lipoproteins.

Lipid extractability can be increased by the addition of more polar solvents to ether, by adding detergents to the plasma or lipoprotein fraction, by physical or enzymatic modifications of the lipoproteins (7), or by using more vigorous extraction conditions. Macheboeuf (12) concluded that detergents take the place of lipids in the lipoproteins, enabling the displaced lipids to be extracted into the ether. More extensive extraction of lipids from low-density lipoproteins by lyophilization by ether prior to extraction with ether–ethanol yields a complete delipidation and a gellike material that is insoluble in water and urea. Exposure of a mixture of ether and human plasma or low-density lipoprotein to temperatures below −25°C substantially increases the amount of lipid extracted (13). Sonication of low-density lipoproteins also enhances lipid extraction by ether (14). The presence of albumin or γ-globulin during sonication of low density lipoproteins prevents cholesterol extraction. Digestion of low-density lipoproteins with trypsin or chymotrypsin increases the amount of lipids extracted by organic solvents.

The resistance of phospholipids to extraction may not necessarily be related to a specific affinity of these lipids for the protein, since aqueous dispersions of phospholipids are also resistant to extraction by diethyl ether or chloroform in the absence of protein. In general none of the discussed methods for total lipid extraction or delipidation of low-density lipoproteins is entirely satisfactory.

Delipidation of high-density lipoproteins with either 3:2 or 3:1 mixtures of ethanol–ethyl ether yields an apoprotein that is soluble in aqueous media (15). This mixture does not appear to be essential for lipid removal; other solvent combinations may prove to be useful as well. To date, however, the ethanol–ether technique of Scanu (16) has yielded the most reproducible and predictable results. During the preparation of a soluble apoprotein some hydrophobic compounds remain in the protein moiety. After ethanol–ether extraction, apo-HDL contains approximately 1% lipid, predominantly lecithin, and 3.3% carbohydrate as glucosamine, methylpentose, D-galactose, D-mannose, and sialic acid. Lipids, however, constitute the major and most thoroughly studied components of lipoproteins.

Table II shows the lipid compositions of the various lipoprotein classes. The LDL and VLDL fractions have some obvious similarities, as well as several important differences, in lipid composition. Both contain about 20% phopholipids and 8% free cholesterol. Whereas triglycerides constitute the main component of very-low-density lipoproteins, the principal lipids in low-density lipoproteins are cholesteryl esters, which account for about 37% of the LDL weight. In fact low-density lipoproteins carry 55 to 65% of the total cholesteryl esters found in the plasma of normal adults. The two subclasses HDL_2 and HDL_3 are quite similar in lipid composition except for the concentration of cholesteryl esters. The lipid-to-protein and phospholipid-to-protein ratios are highest in the VLDL class, intermediate in the LDL class, and lowest in the HDL class.

B. Contamination Problems

1. Contaminants. Lipids and other solvent-soluble contaminants may originate from greases, rubber and cork stoppers, pump oils, detergents, and from the solvents themselves. Since it is practically impossible to completely remove all sources of contamination, the lipid chemist needs rapid

Table II. Average Composition of Human-Plasma Lipoproteins

Lipoprotein Class and Density Range (g/ml)	Percentage of Total Weight[a]					
	PL	FC	CE	GL	FFA	PR
VLDL,[b] $0.95 < d < 1.018$, S_f 20–5000[c]	18	7	12	50	2	8
LDL,[b] $1.018 < d < 1.063$, S_f 0–20[c]	22	8	37	11	1	21
HDL_2,[d] $1.063 < d < 1.125$	24	2	20	4	—	50
HDL_3,[e] $1.125 < d < 1.21$	23.4	2.2	10.4	4.2	1.3	58.5
VHDL,[e] $d > 1.21$	28.0	0.3	3.2	4.6	0.6	62.4

[a] Abbreviations: PL, phospholipids; FC, free cholesterol; CE, cholesteryl esters; GL, glycerides; FFA, free fatty acids; PR, protein.
[b] Data from Ref. 17.
[c] Svedberg flotation rate.
[d] Data from Refs. 17 and 18.
[e] Data from Ref. 19.

methods for detecting contaminants and procedures that will minimize or prevent their introduction into preparations. In a review article Rouser and associates (20) have described both the detection of contaminants by thin-layer chromatography and infrared spectroscopy and the procedures that prevent, eliminate, or minimize contamination.

2. Alteration Products. Optimal conditions for extracting lipids vary with the nature of the sample, and the procedures that are used can significantly affect the results. Elevated temperatures can have detrimental effects on some lipids. Particularly pertinent is the activation of certain lipolytic enzymes by the solvents most commonly used in extraction; accompanied by an elevated temperature, this can have a deleterious effect on lipids, as noted by Hanahan and Chaikoff (21). Storage of lipid samples in polar solvents, evaporation to dryness, concentration of extracts under an air stream, and the type of column separation can modify the lipid composition and certainly the amount of unsaturated fatty acids.

It is clear that degrading influences of this type must be considered in any extraction procedure. The most satisfactory approach is perhaps the use of a number of extractions of brief duration at room temperature without further concentration of the sample and immediate determination of the lipid content.

3. Nonlipid Material. One of the most important steps in lipid analysis is the removal of nonlipid contaminants. During a study of the lipids of beef and human hearts Nazir and Rouser (22) discovered the presence of an unusually large amount of nonlipid contaminants in chloroform–methanol extracts. The phospholipids, more than the neutral lipids, show a remarkable ability to solubilize many nonlipid components, the most common ones being sugars, free amino acids, sterols and sterol esters, urea, and many inorganic substances. Though partly attributable to the solubility of these substances in the solvents used for lipid extraction, this effect is due mainly to the complexing ability of the various phospholipids.

On the other hand, low-density and very-low-density lipoproteins contain a certain number of carotenoids, which have not been detected in high-density lipoproteins and chylomicrons. The carotenoids have been studied by following the presence and intensity of their characteristic yellow color within lipoproteins and degradation products. Their extractability shows an interesting similarity to that of the phospholipids, as could be expected from earlier studies. Only a small amount is extracted by heptane, and most of the color apparently remains with the phospholipid-protein residue.

The most reproducible method for the removal of many of the impurities cited here is the special washing technique of Folch et al. (23). Unfortunately this widely used solvent-partition procedure for removing nonlipid contaminants causes some lipid to be lost into the aqueous phase. Other purification methods are also available, but not all of them are generally applicable. Dialysis of lipid emulsions against water is effective for some lipids, but Smith (24), working with rubber-latex phospholipids, found that certain nitrogen- and phosphorus-containing impurities still remained. Similarly a cellulose column has been effectively used to remove nitrogenous impurities (25).

The most satisfactory procedures for the quantitative removal of nonlipid products are ion-exchange chromatography on diethylaminoethyl (DEAE) cellulose and partition column chromatography with a cross-linked dextran gel (Sephadex), which quantitatively separates the water-soluble nonlipid contaminants from the lipids (25). Sephadex is preferable to cellulose because it permits more complete and reproducible separations and larger sample loads.

III. ISOLATION OF PURE LIPID CLASSES

Quantitative separation and analysis of lipid classes are usually based on chromatographic separations, which provide a high degree of specificity in the analysis. Separation is mostly performed by column or thin-layer chromatography or by a combination of these procedures (6, 25, 26). Since it is impossible to summarize all of the variations that have been used, the omission of a method does not necessarily imply that it is unsatisfactory.

A. General Procedures

Because of its versatility and improved separation, thin-layer chromatography has almost completely replaced paper chromatography, and, being more rapid, it is commonly preferred to column chromatography whenever possible. Most of the lipid classes, including their major and minor components, can be determined after extraction by one- or two-dimensional thin-layer chromatography, without column chromatography. Their speed, selectivity, and reproducibility make TLC procedures ideal for studies in which many samples are analyzed and compared, since it is only by comparison that specific changes can be detected. A combination of column and thin-layer chromatography is time consuming and relatively complicated, whereas the two-dimensional TLC procedure is relatively simple and rapid. The use of two-dimensional, rather than one-dimensional, thin-layer chromatography offers the advantages of improved resolution as well as the possibility of recognizing more components and identifying them more reliably (27).

On the other hand, the use of *column chromatography* prior to thin-layer chromatography provides several advantages. Larger amounts of lipids can be isolated in less time, and columns can be used to concentrate minor components that are not detectable by thin-layer chromatography alone. Chromatography on DEAE-cellulose columns has become one of the most commonly used chromatographic procedures for the separation of lipids from plasma and the nervous system (26, 28). Florisil, a synthetic magnesium silicate combined with silicic acid, has been used and developed for the separation of all glycolipids. More recently triethylaminoethyl (TEAE) cellulose has been shown to possess advantages for lipid-class separations. The advantages and limitations of the various procedures have been described in recent publications by Rouser and co-workers (25, 26).

B. Phospholipids

It is not always necessary to separate phospholipids from other lipids prior to a determination, nor to separate them one from another. A phosphorus determination on a washed total-lipid extract, when multiplied by the appropriate factor, will give the phospholipid content. There are, however, occasions when initial and further separations of phospholipids from other lipids are necessary. Techniques involving solvent fractionation and countercurrent distribution have been very useful in the separation of lipids but are of limited use in analysis because of the losses that occur and the large amount of starting material required. An ideal approach to combining the separation of nonpolar and polar lipids with phospholipid analysis would be reproducible chromatographic separation capable of reduction to microscale and involving only the determination of phosphorus. Sephadex G-25 and LH-20 are new tools for the further separation and characterization of plasma lipids.

The complexity and the enormous difficulties encountered during the separation and isolation of a pure native lipid component can be demonstrated by the isolation of phospholipids from egg yolk by column chromatography. This problem has been tackled in several laboratories, using silica (29, 30) and alumina (31) as adsorbents. In these procedures pure lecithin was isolated, but lysolecithin and degradation products were observed by Camejo (32) during separation on silica and by Renkonen (33) on alumina. Using a slight modification of the method of Singleton (31), we were able to separate pure lecithin, chemically characterized with respect to homogeneity and stability by gas–liquid, thin-layer, and ion-exchange (DEAE-cellulose) chromatography (28). The purity and stability of the isolated phospholipid fractions are very important.

The chromatographic homogeneity of the isolated lecithin remains unchanged if the sample is stored in solution. As shown in Table III, storage of dry lecithin for several days at room temperature results in the formation of degradation products (detectable by TLC) and in loss of linoleic, arachidonic, and all higher fatty acids. Contact of polar lipids with adsorbents must be reduced to a minimum to prevent the formation of methyl esters and artifacts.

Table III. Fatty Acid Distribution in Lecithin Kept in a Dry State

	Quantity (%)						
		One-Day Storage			Ten-Day Storage		
Fatty Acids[a]	Fresh Sample	−20°C	+4°C	+23°C	−20°C	+4°C	+23°C
16:0	28	30	29	29	31	28	40
18:0	14	12	14	12	14	15	18
18:1	30	30	31	28	29	30	34
18:2	17	18	15	16	16	17	4
20:4	4	4	4	5	4	4	[b]
Higher fatty acids	5	5	5	5	4	4	1

[a] Fatty acids are characterized by two quantities: number of carbon atoms and number of double bonds (e.g., 16:0).
[b] Trace.

IV. BIOCHEMICAL DETERMINATION OF LIPIDS

The chemical analyses and quantitative determinations of the lipid constituents of whole plasma and lipoproteins are an essential part of most studies concerning lipoprotein metabolism. Insight into the function and structure of plasma lipoproteins requires precise information on the physiological functions of the major classes of lipids and a complete quantitative picture of the constituent lipids, sugars, fatty acids, and proteins. The most important functions of the lipids can be summarized as follows (34):

1. Triglycerides are a source of fatty acids, which are oxidized by tissues to produce energy or stored as an energy reserve in triglyceride form. In response to energy needs the stored triglycerides are hydrolyzed, and the unesterified fatty acids are released into the circulation for transport to tissues.
2. Phospholipids are a major structural unit of many cellular membranes, which include plasma membranes as well as the membranes of cytoplasmic organelles like mitochondria and microsomes. These lipids concentrate at polar–polar interfaces and stabilize lipoprotein structures in aqueous media. Phospholipids have also a functional role in the living cell. Some evidence suggests that they are important for protein synthesis *in vivo* by binding ribosomes to membranes and may even indirectly control DNA replication through membrane-mediated structures.
3. Unesterified cholesterol is a component of many cell membranes and also serves as a precursor in the formation of bile acids and steroid hormones. Cholesteryl esters are present chiefly in the liver, adrenals, and plasma, and their functional role is still unclear.

On the basis of these functions, lipoproteins that are rich in triglycerides could be expected to participate in the transport function of sterol metabolism. One function of the phospholipids and proteins of lipoproteins could be the solubilization and transport of the highly nonpolar lipids (triglycerides, cholesterol, and cholesteryl esters) in plasma.

One of the most important steps in lipid-class analysis is the quantitative determination of each lipid either by weighing, turbidimetry, titration, absorption, or colorimetry.

A. Total-Lipid Determination

A simple measurement of the total lipid content of plasma is an efficient parameter for screening dyslipemic patients. Several useful methods are available (35). Some are relatively simple, such as those depending on turbidity; others, like the total-fatty-acid measurements of Stern and Shapiro (36), are more specific but also more complex. All of these procedures depend on lipid distribution, plasma viscosity, room temperature, and other physical environmental conditions and need careful standardization. The most widely accepted methods of measuring the total serum or plasma lipids by extraction and subsequent gravimetric analysis after chromatographic separation (37, 38) are not only tedious and time consuming but also prone to substantial errors.

In atherosclerosis research and in clinical work we do not need to know the exact amount of total plasma lipids to characterize a dyslipemia. On the other hand, there is a correlation between coronary heart disease and total lipid concentration; hence this value is still important.

A simple, rapid, and reliable method for the assay of plasma or serum lipids with the analytical integrity of the gravimetric method is still needed. Several basic approaches to this problem have been made. It is possible to perform cholesterol, phospholipid, and triglyceride assays, and then to calculate the total lipid concentration from the sum of values of the lipid fractions, as in the procedure of Cheek (39). This approach, however, is very time consuming, because three independent chemical determinations must be performed on purified samples. Moreover, it requires the use of the assumption, often incorrect, that 73% of the total cholesterol represents cholesteryl esters. The turbidimetric method for the assay of total lipids is rapid but has been shown to compare unfavorably with the gravimetric method. Frings and Dunn (40) described an improved colorimetric method for total plasma lipids based on the color reaction given by lipids with vanillin, using sulfophosphovanillin.

Table IV presents a comparison of the total lipid concentration in a series of samples evaluated by different methods. Turbidimetry (41) yields approximate, rather than quantitative, results, but when triglyceride values are normal, good results can be obtained. Its precision is sufficient for routine work if only a range of values is required. Only weighing lipid extracts can be recommended in quantitative lipid analyses, but the extracts are easily contaminated by solvent impurities, nonlipid material like urea and inorganic ions, or by partial oxidation.

The measurement of total lipids alone never provides a specific diagnosis, and occasionally abnormal but reciprocal changes in cholesterol and glyceride concentrations can occur without inducing abnormal values in the total-lipid data.

B. Combination of Lipid Analyses

An estimate of the distribution of lipoprotein fractions can be obtained indirectly from the plasma levels of cholesterol, triglycerides, and phospho-

Table IV. Evaluation of Total Plasma Lipids by Various Methods

	Total Lipid Concentration (mg/100 ml)		
Sample	Colorimetric	Turbidimetric	Gravimetric
1	552	540	570
2	360	380	415
3	665	680	665
4	640	630	650
5	569	540	565
6	569	520	665
7	1378	1390	1300
8	595	650	526
9	1442	1600	1395
10	641	650	669
11	659	640	714
12	561	540	583
13	720	710	721
14	680	640	764
15	573	520	612

lipids. Such data are based on the chemical composition of lipoproteins (Table I) and on a general knowledge of the types and patterns of pathological alterations of plasma lipoproteins. Plasma-lipid data define, within broad limits, the lipoprotein distribution in a given sample (42).

The following statements can be made:

1. High levels of cholesterol and phospholipids, but not triglycerides, denote increased LDL levels.
2. Simultaneous increase of the three lipid types denotes increased VLDL levels.
3. Increases predominantly in triglyceride levels indicate that the VLDL increase occurs chiefly in the largest particles, those with the highest flotation rate, or in the chylomicrons.
4. Pathological changes in HDL levels are in the direction of decreased concentration, except in biliary cirrhosis; the decrease is often accompanied by an increase in VLDL levels. The HDL concentration cannot be predicted from plasma-lipid levels in most cases.

Alterations of cholesterol concentration and distribution in various physiological and pathological conditions have been the subject of extensive studies by Roberts and Straus (43) and Gresham et al. (44). Methods for determining the total cholesterol concentration are widely available (45) and have been successfully automated. Recently a number of procedures for the direct determination of total plasma or serum cholesterol have been described—procedures that are claimed to be very rapid and sensitive. The precision and sensitivity of these various methods are questionable, because reagents and complexes are difficult to stabilize and the influence of high bilirubin concentrations on the reactions is difficult to eliminate.

In any simple scheme for screening hyperlipemia, or hyperlipoproteinemia, the cholesterol determination should be combined with other lipid tests, which should include the examination of plasma turbidity (a gross test for hyperglyceridemia) and the determination of either total-lipid or triglyceride levels. The best combination is the measurement of both cholesterol and glyceride concentrations (46). If both are clearly within normal limits, hyperlipoproteinemia can be ruled out with a degree of precision that is quite adequate for current use. Phenotyping of hyperlipemia, or hyperlipoproteinemia, according to Fredrickson, is important for routine clinical chemistry and for the choice of therapy; hence it requires a rapid lipid-screening technique.

We have developed and tested in our laboratory a basic set of lipid parameters for phenotyping the lipoprotein pattern in cellulose or paper electrophoresis (Table V).

Table V. Type of Hyperlipoproteinemia and Parameters for Their Classification

	Type of Hyperlipoproteinemia		
Parameter	II	III	IV[a]
Cholesterol content[b]	35	23–31	23
Triglyceride content[b]	20	20–35	35
Cholesterol-to-triglyceride ratio	1.9	0.7–1.5	0.3–0.7

[a] Data from Ref. 37.
[b] Percentage of total lipids.

Essential familial hypercholesterolemia is the severest of the congenital disorders of lipid metabolism. Numerically it is not as common as other predisposing illnesses, such as hypertension and diabetus mellitus, but the relative number of arteriosclerotics within this group is large. Table VI gives the data so far available on the correlation between essential familial hypercholesterolemia, xanthoma, and angina pectoris.

Complementary determination of the total phospholipid concentration (48) presents no special difficulty in interpretation. A high ratio of plasma cholesterol to phospholipids indicates a relative predominance of β-lipoproteins; this ratio is low when a great excess of α-lipoproteins is present,

Table VI. Essential Familial Hypercholesterolemia (EFH) and Prevalence of Coronary Sclerosis[a]

EFH[b]	Hypercholesterolemia	Xanthoma	Angina Pectoris
29	28	24	13
6	5	1	5
390	223	47	168
112	112	42	10
67	36	19	13
103	41	23	16
16	6	3	3
16	16	15	7
24	11	11	18
28	10	6	12
791	488	191	265

[a] Data from Ref. 47.
[b] Total number of cases exhibiting one or more of the symptoms.

as in obstructive liver disease. At the moment total-phospholipid determinations do not yield precise information about the type of hyperlipemia, but differential analyses of the individual phospholipid classes may be helpful in understanding the genesis of atherosclerosis.

V. INTEGRATED APPROACH TO LIPID AND LIPOPROTEIN ANALYSIS

Because plasma lipids are bound to proteins, their accurate description can only be obtained through a "fingerprint" of the individual lipids isolated from individual lipoproteins. Plasma-lipid values are relatively meaningless; for example, assay of total cholesterol shows neither the cholesterol distribution among the plasma lipoproteins nor the distribution changes induced by diet, disease, or drugs. This argument is also valid for the esterified lipids and fatty acids. In this section we discuss the methods that have been developed and combined in order to establish the state of the plasma in terms of the constituent lipids, lipoproteins, and fatty acids.

A. Procedure

The procedure is summarized in Fig. 1. Electrochromatography has been used for years in our laboratory as a rapid, efficient, and inexpensive means of separating lipoproteins into two groups on a paper curtain. In a

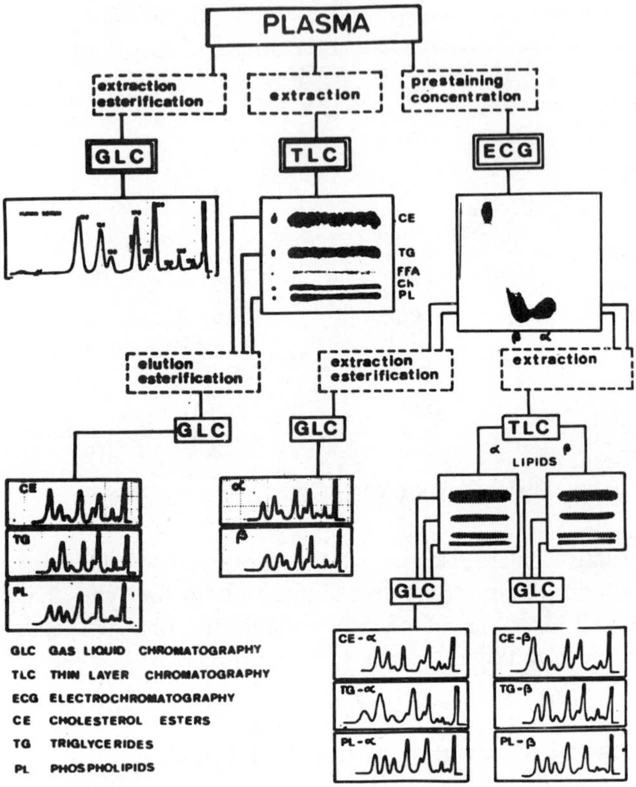

Fig. 1 Integrated lipid and lipoprotein analysis.

second stage the fractions are cut out and eluted, their lipids are extracted, and the polar and nonpolar lipid classes are separated by thin-layer chromatography. Gas-chromatography patterns are established for serum or plasma, the total α- and β-lipoproteins, and each of their lipid components. The amount of serum or plasma required for a complete analysis is about 20 ml. The total plasma or serum values are used as checks on the subsequent procedures and also have their own, though limited, significance.

Since there may be a correlation between increased plasma-lipid levels and coronary heart disease in man (49), plasma lipids have been investigated in detail in normal human subjects, in type II essential familial hyperlipemia, and in primates on atherogenic diets (experimental atherosclerosis).

The literature contains no systematic or complete comparative data on lipids, fatty acids, and lipoproteins in primates on a controlled and identical diet. Hence we initiated a comparative analysis of primate plasma lipids. All animals were kept at the zoo of Antwerpen (Belgium) on an identical diet and under the same hygienic conditions (8, 50). Such a comparison would be most valuable if uniform methods were used to collect the specimens and to evaluate the plasma and arterial lipid system.

Plasma lipids were extracted with chloroform–methanol 2 : 1 (v/v) for 10 min and with chloroform–methanol 1 : 1 (v/v) for 30 min (51). The lipid distribution in the plasma of normal male subjects and control primates is shown in Table VII. All the animals except the baboon and the

Table VII. Lipid Distribution in Primate Plasma

	Lipid Distribution (%)[a]			
Primate	FC	CE	TG	PL
Man	7	41	15	37
Chimpanzee	10	44	8	38
Mountain gorilla	12	42	8	38
Lowland gorilla	13	37	10	40
Baboon	8	34	10	48

[a] Abbreviations: FC, free cholesterol; CE, cholesteryl esters; TG, triglycerides; PL, phospholipids.

lowland gorilla have high total-lipid values, about three times the human value, but the relative amount of the phospholipids seems to increase with the phylogenetic distance from man and is related to a relative increase in high-density lipoproteins.

In our opinion a complete lipid analysis of primate plasma, including the lipid distribution in lipoproteins, is required to establish a valid base line or background for the study of the genesis of atherosclerosis in animals and its eventual extrapolation to the human disease.

1. Analysis of Lipids. The technique of electrochromatography (52) was developed specifically to obtain from plasma sufficient quantities of α- and β-lipoproteins for quantitative analyses, because a detailed analysis of these fractions is more useful than a study of plasma alone (51).

The quantitative determination of polar and nonpolar lipids has been discussed in Section IV. The same solvents are used for the elution of lipids from lipoproteins separated by electrochromatography. The last traces of phospholipids are extracted from the paper with chloroform–methanol–acetic acid. Silica gel G thin-layer plates are used to differentiate the lipids of plasma and of the α- and β-lipoproteins.

2. Analysis of Fatty Acids. Plasma or serum (0.2 ml) lipids are extracted by the multiextraction procedure with 4.8 ml of chloroform–methanol, 2 : 1 (v/v), for analysis and quantitation of the fatty acids. The fatty acid methyl esters are obtained by saponification of the lipids with potassium hydroxide–methanol and by esterification with boron trifluoride in dry methanol, followed by extraction with petroleum ether.

To obtain the fatty acid spectra of the lipoprotein fractions, 0.5 ml of prestained and concentrated plasma or serum is applied as a spot to the curtain. After a 3-hr migration, the α- and β-lipoprotein zones are cut out of the wet curtain. The lipids are then eluted with chloroform–methanol, 2 : 1 (v/v), and subjected to the saponification–esterification–extraction procedure described above.

To establish the fatty acid composition of the cholesteryl esters, triglycerides, and phospholipids 1 ml of plasma or serum was extracted and separated by thin-layer chromatography. The same treatment was applied to the cut out α- and β-lipoprotein fractions to determine the fatty acid spectrum of their lipid classes. To obtain sufficient lipid from α- and β-lipoproteins, fractions from 16 curtains were cut out and extracted.

3. Expression of Results. The fatty acid concentrations considered in our studies are expressed as percentages and as milligrams per 100 milliliters, but in the gas-chromatography spectrum the percentage of an individual fatty acid is a relative value. The establishment of fatty acid indices or ratios sometimes gives more comparable reference values.

With this procedure relative variations between lipids from different lipoprotein classes are obtained. Recently quantitative recovery of the curtain fractions gave quantitative results that are even more significant. The next section describes the techniques used and surveys results from human plasma and the plasma of primates under normal and atherogenic conditions (53, 54).

B. Separation of Lipoproteins by Electrochromatography

The separation of plasma lipoproteins has not advanced rapidly in clinical biochemistry. Some of the reasons are (a) the heterogeneity and relative instability of plasma lipoproteins, (b) the great variety of abnormal patterns that occur in disease, and (c) the relative lack of standards or standard techniques for evaluating new methods. With these objections in mind we compare and discuss the utilization of various lipoprotein properties as bases for separation and analysis.

For the isolation and characterization of plasma lipoproteins, solubilization methods have been useful, but salting-out methods have not been very helpful. Ion-exchange chromatography (55) and molecular sieving (56, 57) have also been applied to lipoprotein separation and purification with some success. Ultracentrifugation is very successful, but it is time consuming and too expensive in the clinical laboratory; moreover, the influence of changing the environment raises questions concerning the homogeneity of the lipid–protein complex.

Simple electrophoretic methods also allow the separation of several lipoprotein fractions from a complex mixture or from plasma. The one-dimensional paper-electrophoresis methods of Lees and Hatch (58) have been applied by Fredrickson et al. (1) to a classification system in which five types of pattern are distinguished. Starch granules or gel, cellulose acetate, and agarose gels have also been successfully used. Pure lipoprotein fractions are not obtained by electrophoresis alone. When, however, either zonal electrophoresis or electrochromatography is used to subfractionate plasma and applied as an analytical method in the study of lipoprotein homogeneity and composition, useful results are obtained.

The homogeneity of lipoproteins is very difficult to prove. Immunochemically the HDL and LDL classes appear to meet this test, but because they are multiple antigenic determinants that elicit heterogeneous antibodies, the test is probably not sufficiently stringent, at least with the existing antiserum systems. More detailed comparative analyses of their components—lipids, fatty acids, sugars, and especially peptides—may be a more rigorous procedure.

1. Method. In our studies electrochromatography has been selected as a rapid and inexpensive method of separating the plasma lipoproteins for the subsequent analysis of their lipids. The principle of the method is shown in Fig. 2. Electrophoresis combined with chromatography is a technique in which a horizontal electrical field and a vertical buffer flow are supported by a substrate like cellulose powder (59) or paper (60). Each particle migrates according to the resultant vector of the horizontal electrophoretic velocity and the vertical velocity of the buffer. Two problems had to be solved, one involving the electrodes or the supply of current to the curtain along the horizontal plane and the other the supply of buffer that ensures a vertical electrochromatographic dimension. These problems were solved by the combined use of washed cascade electrodes and of a trickle feeder for the buffer. The method can be used in two ways.

If the sample is applied continuously, the separated fractions can be collected in tubes at the bottom of the curtain. This method is called "continuous" electrophoresis. If the sample is applied as a spot, a two-dimensional pattern will be developed; this we called "star electrophoresis." An analogous method was described as free two-dimensional continuous

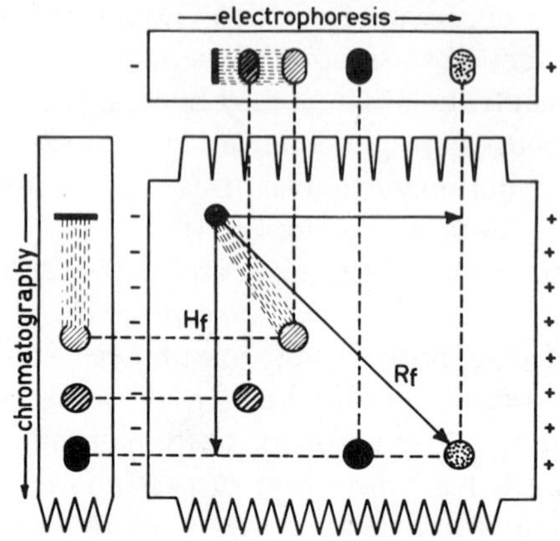

Fig. 2 Schematic diagram of the electrochromatographic procedure.

electrophoresis by Barrolier et al. (61) and also by Grassmann (60). The major advantage of electrochromatography is that each fraction migrates on its own pathway, avoiding contamination and yielding pure lipoproteins.

2. Lipoprotein Pattern. Plasma samples prestained with Sudan Black B are concentrated by ultrafiltration through a membrane filter LSG-60 (Membrane Filter Gesellschaft, Göttingen) under nitrogen pressure (10 kg/cm^2). The lipoproteins are then separated by electrochromatography on Whatman 3MM filter papers in a Veronal buffer (pH 8.6, ionic strength 0.033) for 3 hr (52, 62). Serum (0.5 ml) is prestained with 0.05 ml of purified Sudan Black B in 95% ethanol on a vibrating mixer, concentrated to one-third the initial volume by ultrafiltration (pore size < 5 mμ), and applied as a spot at the top of the curtain. Star electrophoresis is carried out at 27-mA constant current and 600-volts initial voltage. After 3 hr the voltage drops to 400 volts. Afterwards the paper is dried at 110°C in the oven; alternatively the prestained zones are cut out while wet and eluted. Staining procedures must take two variables into account: poststaining of a dried strip and prestaining of the serum. The materials used for staining lipoproteins in various electrophoretic methods have been well reviewed by Ribeiro (63), Schjeide (64), and their associates.

Specific chemical reactions that identify the lipid moieties of lipoproteins are not generally applicable when a supporting medium is present. Electrophoretic patterns of lipoproteins can be stained by the transfer of nonpolar dyes from aqueous or organic media to the lipoproteins. Locating lipoprotein zones is simple, but quantitative measurements by staining remain unsatisfactory. Heating the paper after electrophoresis to fix the proteins and prevent diffusion reduces the dye uptake, probably through partial oxidation of the lipid. On the other hand, nonpolar solvents dissolve the dyes and extract lipids from the denatured lipoprotein on the strip. De Keersgieter, Blaton, and Peeters (65) showed that individual lipids leach into the staining bath with a loss of 5 to 90%, depending on the type of lipid present. Lipoproteins show a preferential loss of phospholipids, cholesterol, and fatty acids. This behavior is partially predicted by experiments on isolated lipids. Unsaturated lipids also take up more dye than saturated lipids. Hence no simple correction factor is available. These observations indicate that quantitation of lipoprotein electrophoresis remains a problem.

Prestaining of plasma or serum before electrophoresis avoids staining of the background (which is particularly troublesome with supports like cellulose acetate) and also loss of lipids into the organic solvent containing the dye. Sudan Black B in various solvents has been widely used for prestaining serum; the end concentration of the solvent must remain low to avoid protein denaturation.

To obtain electrochromatographic lipoprotein patterns we used pure ultracentrifugal fractions from the plasma of normal subjects and the sera of patients with congenital and hyperlipemic dyslipoproteinemia. The plasma of control subjects yields four fractions: (a) chylomicrons ($d <$ 1.006 g/ml) at the starting point; (b) α_2-lipoproteins (VLDL, $1.006 < d < 1.019$); (c) β-lipoproteins (LDL, $1.019 < d < 1.063$); and (d) α-lipoproteins (HDL, $1.063 < d < 1.210$). In Fig. 3 the lipoprotein pattern obtained by electrochromatography is compared with those ob-

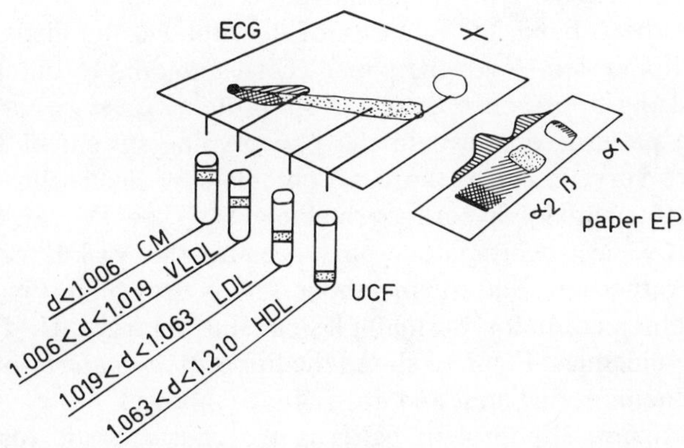

Fig. 3 Comparison of lipoproteins separated by electrochromatography (ECG), paper electrophoresis (EP), and ultracentrifugal fractions (UCF).

tained by electrophoretic and ultracentrifugal fractionation procedures. The normal pattern was confirmed by the use of pure ultracentrifugal fractions, by a case of congenital analphalipoproteinemia (Tangier disease) and abetalipoproteinemia, and by the immunological characteristics of both lipoprotein fractions.

3. Phenotyping of the Lipoprotein Pattern. The rationale for laboratory evaluation of the serum lipoproteins has been established. A method of lipoprotein analysis that depends on paper electrophoresis has become popular as the basis of a system for phenotyping patients with hyperlipoproteinemia. The classification of hyperlipoproteinemias suggested by Fredrickson et al. (1) provides a useful means of phenotyping hyperlipemic states and is a very selective method for clinical diagnosis, genetic investigations, and epidemiology. A nomogram was devised to facilitate classification of hyperlipoproteinemias when cholesterol and triglyceride values are available; it was found to be useful and generally accurate, but it does not replace electrophoresis. Lipoprotein electrophoresis and the nomogram have restrictions on their interpretation and both share some diagnostic ambiguities. The needs of epidemiologic teams and clinical investigators using drug or diet therapies are served better by quantitative data in digital form than by qualitative observations. The former reduce to some extent the bias and the day-to-day variations that are inherent in qualitative data. Quantitative data are also suitable for statistical analysis without artificial transformations, but densitometric evaluation of paper strips (18) is not satisfactory. Better results can be expected from densitometry and reflectometry of agarose plates (Fig. 4).

Electrochromatography reveals typical lipoprotein patterns in the various familial hyperlipemias. The quantitative variation of β-lipoproteins, the broadness of the β-band, the intensity of dye uptake, the dispersion of the low-density lipoproteins over the paper (corresponding to different density ranges), and the appearance of pre-β-lipoproteins must be carefully considered. The patterns obtained in the phenotyping system of Fredrickson et al. (1) are very similar to those we obtained by electrochromatography for type II, III, and IV hyperlipoproteinemias. Type IV can be detected more easily by electrochromatography, because the VLDL concentration in plasma is rather low, and the metabolic rate is very high. Figure 5 shows the lipoprotein picture for normal plasma and for type II, III, and IV hyperlipoproteinemias. Figure 6 shows the lipoprotein patterns of congenital dyslipoproteinemias, diabetes, and obstructive jaundice.

The hyperlipemic lipoprotein patterns are characteristic for given diseases and show the variability of β-lipoproteins that is known to be an important factor in pathological conditions.

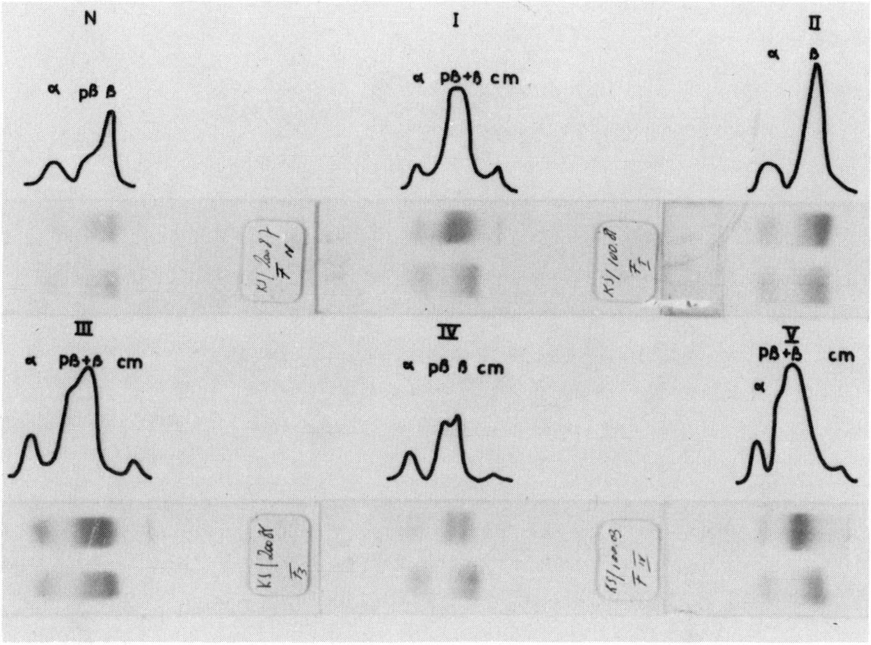

Fig. 4 Densitometric scanning of plasma-lipoprotein patterns on agarose.

As a whole electrochromatography is a rapid tool for lipoprotein evaluation, phenotyping, and separation.

4. Extraction of Lipoprotein Fragments from the Curtain. The fractions are localized by a standardized method based on the comparison between unstained, prestained, and poststained patterns. The fractions are cut out immediately from the wet curtain after separation, extracted with chloroform–methanol, 2 : 1 (v/v), and washed with aqueous calcium chloride solution for fatty acid analysis. Lipoproteins intended for lipid analysis are separated in the same manner but without prestaining.

Since elution of lipids from lipoproteins separated by electrochromatography with chloroform–methanol, 2 : 1 (v/v), results in the loss of 10% of the phospholipids, a new extraction procedure with chloroform–methanol and acetic acid was developed. The curtain fragments containing the α- and β-lipoprotein fractions from approximately 2 ml of plasma are lyophilized for 15 hr and then extracted with 100 ml chloroform–methanol, 1 : 1 (v/v), for 15 hr with constant stirring. After a second extraction for 2 hr with the same solvent, the last traces of phospholipids are extracted with methanol–acetic acid, 99 : 1 (v/v). Recovery of individual

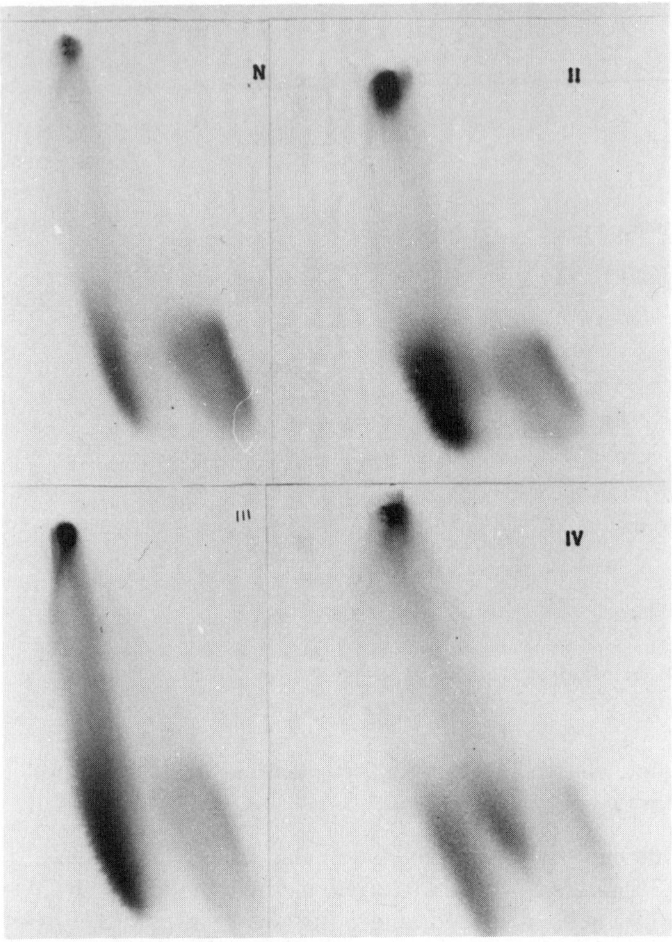

Fig. 5 Electrochromatographic patterns of plasma lipoproteins in various familial hyperlipoproteinemias.

lipids by elution from the paper was 99.2%. All extracts are combined and evaporated under nitrogen at 40°C. The dry extract is then dissolved in 15 ml of chloroform–methanol, 2 : 1 (v/v). The absolute concentrations are then calculated from the plasma-lipid values and from the ratios of the lipids in α- and β-lipoproteins.

C. Differentiation of Lipids in Plasma Lipoproteins

Thin-layer chromatography is a simple technique, requiring little equipment and minimal amounts of sample. Its advantages include sensitivity

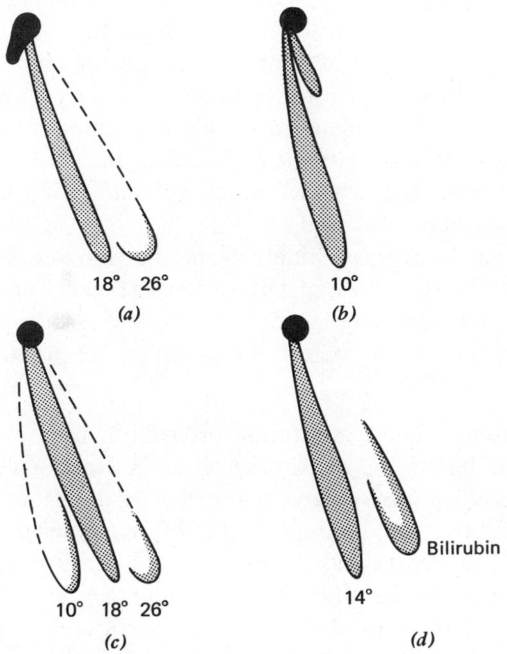

Fig. 6 Electrochromatographic patterns of plasma lipoproteins in (*a*) congenital α-β-lipoproteinemia, (*b*) congenital an-α_1-lipoproteinemia, (*c*) diabetes, and (*d*) obstructive jaundice.

and rapidity. Rouser, Siakotos, and Fleischer (66) and Renkonen and Varo (67) reviewed the basic TLC principles of thin-layer chromatography for the separation of apolar and polar lipids, but we wish to draw attention to some critical problems and potential difficulties.

1. Separation Problems. Many adsorbents are available for thin-layer chromatography, and these can be modified in several ways. Artifacts can be introduced by dirty silica-gel powder and contaminated solvents. The quality of both solvents and powder can be checked by two-dimensional TLC procedures, by using the same solvent in both directions. For spreading adsorbent over scrupulously clean glass plates we recommended the automatic Desaga No. 21,602 (Muttenz-Schweiz) equipment. It is also evident that along with the homogeneity of the layer, the moisture content influences the separation; therefore activation time and temperature must be standardized.

Autoxidation appears to be an important source of artifacts in lipid analysis. The danger of degradation is always present when lipids are manipulated in the laboratory and particularly when they are dispersed on a surface and exposed to air. Oxidation is a problem, particularly in multidevelopment, two-dimensional, or preparative thin-layer chromatography and in the analysis of lipids for fatty acids after TLC separation. Such questions as how to use antioxidants effectively, how to deliver unsaturated lipids onto TLC plates with minimal oxidative damage, how to handle the plates after development, whether the TLC tanks should be filled with inert gas, and whether silica gel and trace metal ions affect the oxidation are still unanswered.

Detection procedures vary widely from the universal qualitative spray to the more specific sprays (e.g., Dragendorff reagent for choline–containing lipids and ninhydrin for lipids with amino groups) and the more quantitative sprays mostly based on complete destruction of the lipid components by oxidation.

2. Quantitation. The quantitation procedures used in thin-layer chromatography are based on densitometry or reflectometry of colored or oxidized fractions, or on spectrophotometry of lipids removed from the plates. Dilute sulfuric acid containing 0.6% potassium dichromate is fairly specific for lipid detection and quantitation by densitometry or reflectometry. The formation of the molybdate blue complex with phospholipids on the layer itself and the phosphoric acid–copper acetate reaction may have possible applications in quantitative lipid analysis. Quantitative methods based on the removal of lipids from the TLC plates include extraction and recovery of intact lipids before the quantitative spectrophotometric analysis.

One-dimensional thin-layer chromatography is generally most convenient for the isolation of lipid classes and for fatty acid analysis. The problems in this type of work include localization of the spots, complete recovery of the intact lipid from the adsorbent, and avoidance of contamination, secondary reactions, and subsequent degradation. Rhodamine 6G (0.001% aqueous) can be used for spot localization, but most components can best be located under ultraviolet light after spraying with a fluorescent dye. In our laboratory the most precise lipid values are obtained by quantitation of the separated components, after removal of the support for nonpolar lipids and in the presence of the adsorbent for phospholipids.

3. Separation Procedure. Neutral lipids from electrochromatographic α- and β-lipoproteins are separated, in 20:1:80 (v/v/v) ether–acetic acid–petroleum ether (b.p. 40–60°C) (68), on silica gel G plates, activated, washed in chloroform–methanol–water, 80:35:5 (v/v/v), and reactivated at 110°C for 30 min. Chromatography is performed at room temperature in chambers lined with solvent-saturated Whatman 3MM paper. For fatty acid analysis the fractions are detected with a solution of 42 mg of Rhodamine B and 14 mg of 2,7-dichlorofluorescein in 100 ml ether-ethanol-water, 63:30:7 (v/v/v). The phospholipids are separated into classes by one-dimensional thin-layer chromatography, chloroform–methanol–water, 80:35:5, being used as the developing solvent. For phosphorus analysis silica gel HR is spread and heat activated for 30 min at 110°C, detection is performed with iodine, and the phosphorus content of the spots is analyzed in the presence of the adsorbent by a modification (69) of the method of Rouser et al. (27). Phospholipid separations for fatty acid analysis are done on silica gel G or F254. The detection is performed as for neutral lipids. The neutral solvent chloroform–methanol–water (80:35:5), however, only separates the four major components of plasma phospholipids. Further differentiations of the minor components can be obtained by using the same solvent system with chloroform–methanol–acetic acid–water, 50:25:8:4 (by volume), on basic plates or by two-dimensional thin-layer-chromatography in chloroform–methanol–acetone–acetic acid–water, 5:1:2:1:0.5 (by volume), and chloroform–methanol–ammonia, 65:35:5 (by volume), as described by Nelson (70) and Parsons (71).

4. Thin-Layer Patterns. It is valuable to investigate in detail the changes that occur in lipids and plasma lipoproteins in baboons and chimpanzees on atherogenic diets and to relate the changes to those seen in human type II hyperlipoproteinemia (51, 69).

In previous work Gresham and co-workers (44) demonstrated that experimental atherosclerosis can be induced in animals by feeding a high-

Table VIII. Lipid Content of α-Lipoproteins

		Concentration (mg/100 ml ± S.D.)[a]				
Primate	n[b]	PL	FC	CE	TG	C/PL[c]
Man:						
Normal	3	74 ± 4	12 ± 1	46 ± 3	14 ± 2	0.53 ± 0.03
Diseased[d]	3	85 ± 20	17 ± 4	73 ± 9	24 ± 4	0.74 ± 0.08
Chimpanzee:						
Controls	4	166 ± 10	26 ± 3	104 ± 14	19 ± 2	0.53 ± 0.01
Experimental[e]	6	163 ± 15	29 ± 2	110 ± 13	20 ± 2	0.58 ± 0.03
Baboon:						
Controls	3	82 ± 19	12 ± 2	81 ± 16	13 ± 2	0.76 ± 0.06
Experimental[e]	4	97 ± 7	17 ± 4	132 ± 17	11 ± 2	0.98 ± 0.07

[a] Abbreviations: PL, phospholipids; FC, free cholesterol; CE, cholesteryl esters; TG, triglycerides.
[b] Number of subjects.
[c] Cholesterol-to-phospholipid ratio.
[d] Type II hyperlipoproteinemia.
[e] Animals on high-fat atherogenic diets.

cholesterol diet of egg yolk and butter. There may be a correlation between plasma lipids and vascular disease in man.

Tables VIII and IX summarize our data on the lipid content of lipoproteins from human, chimpanzee, and baboon plasma under normal conditions and under atherogenic risk factors. The main effect of the atherogenic diet in these animals was an increase in β-lipoproteins and in their cholesterol and phospholipid, but not triglyceride, content, so that the lipoprotein pattern resembled that of type II hyperlipoproteinemia in man. The most marked changes occurred in β-lipoproteins. Similar trends were seen in α-lipoproteins, but the changes were quantitatively smaller and fell just below the level of statistical significance.

The most interesting differences between the α- and β-lipoproteins in baboons were in the cholesterol-to-phospholipid ratio (C/PL), which was decreased only in the β-fraction. It must be noted that the plasma C/PL ratio in baboons was unchanged because of the compensatory increase in the C/PL of the α-lipoproteins. This study was important because the C/PL ratio is generally believed to be an index of atherogenicity.

The animals on an atherogenic diet were found to have a 70% increase in plasma phospholipids (mg %). This can be attributed to a general increase in the phospholipid content of β-lipoproteins, although the greatest change occurred in the lecithin fraction (Table X). The phospholipid content of α-lipoproteins was unaffected (Table XI). Presumably the lecithin

Table IX. Lipid Content of β-Lipoproteins

		Concentration (mg/100 ml ± S.D.)				
Primate	n[b]	PL	FC	CE	TG	C/PL[c]
Man:						
Normal	3	88 ± 8	37 ± 4	117 ± 6	21 ± 2	1.24 ± 0.12
Diseased[d]	3	189 ± 23	83 ± 6	303 ± 54	51 ± 14	1.39 ± 0.08
Chimpanzee:						
Controls	4	129 ± 10	39 ± 7	222 ± 24	41 ± 9	1.33 ± 0.06
Experimental[e]	6	296 ± 42	136 ± 23	631 ± 86	45 ± 15	1.73 ± 0.11
Baboon:						
Controls	3	40 ± 6	9 ± 2	80 ± 11	25 ± 2	1.43 ± 0.07
Experimental[e]	4	105 ± 17	21 ± 3	145 ± 21	21 ± 2	1.03 ± 0.07

[a] Abbreviations: PL, phospholipids; FC, free cholesterol; CE, cholesteryl esters; TG, triglycerides.
[b] Number of subjects.
[c] Cholesterol-to-phospholipid ratio.
[d] Type II hyperlipoproteinemia.
[e] Animals on high-fat atherogenic diets.

Table X. Phospholipid Distribution in β-Lipoproteins

Primate	n[a]	Lecithin %	Lecithin mg/100 ml	Phosphatidyl-ethanolamine %	Phosphatidyl-ethanolamine mg/100 ml	Sphingomyelin %	Sphingomyelin mg/100 ml	Lysolecithin %	Lysolecithin mg/100 ml
Man:									
Normal	3	68.6	63	4.8	4	19.3	17	7.2	7
Diseased[b]	5	61.9	110	3.7	6	27.4	50	7.1	13
Chimpanzee:									
Controls[c]	4	69.8	90	5.6	7	21.1	27	3.5	4
Experimental[c,d]	6	66.5	197	5.6	17	24.7	73	3.2	9
Baboon:									
Controls	4	67.0	27	11.6	5	11.4	5	9.9	4
Experimental[d]	4	70.7	74	11.2	12	8.8	9	9.3	10

[a] Number of subjects.
[b] Type II hyperlipoproteinemia.
[c] Pooled samples.
[d] Animals on high-fat atherogenic diets.

Table XI. Phospholipid Distribution in α-Lipoproteins

Primate	n[a]	Lecithin %	Lecithin mg/100 ml	Phosphatidyl-ethanolamine %	Phosphatidyl-ethanolamine mg/100 ml	Sphingomyelin %	Sphingomyelin mg/100 ml	Lysolecithin %	Lysolecithin mg/100 ml
Man:									
Normal	3	66.5	51	5.4	4	19.1	15	9.1	7
Disease[b]	5	63.4	67	5.2	5	18.3	19	13.7	13
Chimpanzee:									
Controls[c]	4	68.2	113	6.5	11	12.8	21	12.5	20
Experimental[c,d]	6	73.0	119	6.6	11	12.0	19	8.4	13
Baboon:									
Controls	4	73.9	61	9.4	8	8.5	7	8.1	7
Experimental[d]	4	70.2	68	9.6	9	8.4	8	11.8	11

[a] Number of subjects.
[b] Type II hyperlipoproteinemia.
[c] Pooled samples.
[d] Animals on high-fat atherogenic diets.

content of β-lipoproteins is increased in an attempt to maintain the stability of the lipoprotein molecule by ensuring an adequate proportion of hydrophilic groups.

The integrated analysis of plasma lipids and lipoproteins indicates that the pathological effects of the atherogenic diet are due not only to an increased plasma level of β-lipoproteins but also to a change in composition, which decreases their stability while favoring the deposition of cholesteryl esters in the arterial wall.

D. Differentiation of Fatty Acids in Plasma Lipoproteins by Gas–Liquid Chromatography

The nature of the fatty acids in each lipid class is of particular interest, since the physical and chemical properties of lipid molecules depend on the length of the hydrocarbon chains and the number of double bonds. Thus the metabolic properties and physiological characteristics of lipoproteins may be correlated with variations in fatty acid composition.

The rapid development of gas chromatography has provided for the separation and quantitative determination of fatty acids in biological materials. Though the basic principles and methods are well known (72), the precision and accuracy vary significantly with the investigator. These variations may be due to instrument factors (apparatus, detection systems) and to such experimental factors as the selectivity and thermal stability of the column. Nonpolar phases, such as Apiezon and methyl silicones with a very low vapor pressure, have generally a higher thermal stability. Polyesters of succinic acid, adipic acid, and polyalcohols like ethylene glycol have greater selectivity. In our analyses the amount, selectivity, and thermal stability of the liquid phase were selected so that neither the column nor the detector was overloaded. Also temperatures must be selected so that all peaks can be measured accurately. Adsorptive properties of the solid supports can strongly influence the quantitative analysis of fatty acids, despite the fact that symmetrical peaks are obtained. Therefore adequate treatment of the support with acid and alkaline solutions or silylating reagents is necessary (73).

1. Preparation of Methyl Esters. The analytical procedure in preparing the sample for gas–liquid chromatography is of great interest. The separation of fatty acids as their methyl esters is the usual procedure. Quantitative analysis requires the complete conversion of fatty acids or their esters to methyl esters. Most of the methods that have been described used anhydrous methanol containing an acidic or basic catalyst and heating periods of up to 24 hr.

Metcalfe and Schmitz (74) completely converted *free fatty acids* into methyl esters by boiling them in an excess of boron trifluoride in methanol for 2 min. In a quantitative comparison of the four most commonly used reagents for methylation (diazomethane, methanol–hydrochloric acid with sublimation of the ester, methanol–hydrochloric acid on an ion-exchange resin, and methanol–boron trifluoride) Vorbeck et al. (75) concluded that the results are comparable when only higher-molecular-weight fatty acids are present. Fatty acids from plasma lipids can be prepared by direct transesterification or by esterification of the liberated fatty acids after saponification. Direct transesterification is sometimes incomplete because of the low solubility of some lipids in the reaction mixture. For quantitative transesterification of the various lipid classes with methanol–boron trifluoride, heating periods varying from 10 min for monoglycerides to 90 min for sphingomyelin are recommended.

Several authors have described the use of methanol–hydrochloric acid as reagent, but it was found to be unsuitable for the methylation of cholesteryl esters and sphingomyelin. When the method involves a saponification step, isomerization of highly unsaturated fatty acids may occur. By controlling the temperature, the reagent volumes, and the heating periods, however, isomerization can be prevented. A slight modification of the method of Ast (76) was selected for our analyses. The completeness of the methylation of the various lipids was checked by thin-layer chromatography, and no residual lipids were detected.

It has been demonstrated (77) that, in the determination of fatty acids in lipid fractions separated by thin-layer chromatography, elution of the lipid from the chromatographic plate is an unnecessary and time-consuming step. In our experience the refluxing time in the presence of boron trifluoride should be increased to 16 hr for sphingomyelin. Direct esterification of the adsorbed lipid eliminates the possibility of degradation during elution.

2. Analytical Procedure. As a first step, lipid samples are saponified with 3 ml of 3% potassium hydroxide in methanol for 30 min at 70°C. Then 2 ml of water is added, and the mixture is evaporated under nitrogen to about 2 ml to remove the methanol. This saponification cannot solve the problem of sphingomyelin esterification. Unsaponifiable matter is removed by extraction with 5 ml of petroleum ether. The aqueous phase is acidified with 4 *N* hydrochloric acid, and the fatty acids are extracted with 10 ml of petroleum ether. In a second step the dried extract is esterified with 2 ml of boron trifluoride–methanol (125 g/l) by heating for 30 min at 80°C in a sealed tube. The methyl esters are extracted with petroleum ether and concentrated, and 1 μl is used for injection.

The separation is performed on a gas chromatograph equipped with a 6-ft column (packed with 15% diethylene glycol succinate on Anakrom ABS, 110–120 mesh) and a flame ionization detector. The temperature is programmed to rise from 195 to 225°C at 2°C/min after an isothermal period of 5 min.

3. Results. The fatty acid compositions of serum lipoproteins from fasting normal human subjects and control primates have been compared. The fatty acid compositions of serum α- and β-lipoproteins separated by electrochromatography are shown in Table XII. The values obtained over an interval of several months indicate the constancy during this period; note that within the same plasma there are differences in the fatty acid compositions of α- and β-lipoproteins. In comparison with chimpanzees and baboons, human subjects demonstrated a greater content of unsaturated fatty acids in both α- and β-lipoproteins.

The information gained from the isolated lipoproteins differs greatly from the values obtained for total serum. The α_1- and β-lipoproteins are clearly characterized by different fatty acid indices, which reflect the specific lipid composition of these lipoproteins, so that it is more important to determine the internal fatty acid spectra of the separated α_1- and β-lipoprotein lipids than to give values for the total fraction. Moreover, the significance of the total serum values is still smaller, because the total ratios represent averages of the internal lipoprotein variations.

Since there appears to be a correlation between increased plasma lipids, fatty acids, and coronary heart disease in man, it is of value to investigate plasma fatty acids and lipids in animals on normal and atherogenic diets. The main aim of our procedure is to relate any changes in lipids and fatty acids to those seen in the very similar Fredrickson type II disease, hyperbetalipoproteinemia, in human patients.

Eighteen young baboons and twelve chimpanzees were divided into two equal groups and given either a control or an atherogenic diet. These animals were subjects in a long-term study on the effect of high-cholesterol diets on atherosclerosis and had been consuming the diets for 1.5 to 3 years. In Tables XIII and XIV we present as an example of the validity of our procedure the concentrations of the most important fatty acids in the α- and β-lipoproteins of normal human subjects, hypercholesterolemic patients with the type II hyperlipoproteinemia of Fredrickson et al., and chimpanzees and baboons on control and atherogenic diets.

Animals on both control and atherogenic diets demonstrated a greater content of saturated fatty acids in α_1- and β-lipoproteins than did human subjects (51). The diet, however, increased unsaturation in both α- and β-lipoproteins. In comparison with the control animals, baboons and chim-

Table XII. Fatty Acid Composition of Serum Lipoproteins

Fatty Acid[a]	Concentration (% ± S.D.)					
	Human Lipoproteins		Chimpanzee Lipoproteins		Baboon Lipoproteins	
	α	β	α	β	α	β
14:0	0.8 ± 0.1	0.7 ± 0.1	1.1 ± 0.1	0.8 ± 0.0	0.4 ± 0.2	0.8 ± 0.2
15:0	0.5 ± 0.1	0.6 ± 0.3	0.3 ± 0.0	0.3 ± 0.0	0.3 ± 0.2	0.1 ± 0.0
16:0	25.4 ± 0.7	19.7 ± 0.5	25.0 ± 0.5	20.9 ± 0.3	25.3 ± 0.3	21.9 ± 0.2
16:1	3.9 ± 0.5	3.6 ± 0.2	2.8 ± 0.3	2.7 ± 0.1	2.7 ± 0.1	2.2 ± 0.2
18:0	9.5 ± 0.5	5.6 ± 0.3	10.5 ± 0.6	7.9 ± 0.3	17.2 ± 0.2	12.7 ± 0.1
18:1	20.5 ± 0.3	23.4 ± 0.9	20.0 ± 1.4	21.0 ± 1.2	19.3 ± 0.1	20.1 ± 1.0
18:2	28.4 ± 1.4	37.0 ± 2.0	27.2 ± 1.0	33.5 ± 2.7	24.9 ± 0.1	33.7 ± 1.1
18:3	0.8 ± 0.1	0.5 ± 0.1	0.3 ± 0.1	0.4 ± 0.1	—	—
20:0	1.0 ± 0.1	0.9 ± 0.1	0.2 ± 0.0	0.2 ± 0.0	—	—
20:3	1.8 ± 0.2	1.5 ± 0.1	1.4 ± 0.1	1.8 ± 0.2	—	—
20:4	6.2 ± 0.7	5.5 ± 0.5	10.5 ± 0.7	9.6 ± 1.0	9.9 ± 0.8	8.6 ± 0.5
24:0	0.7 ± 0.1	0.5 ± 0.1	0.5 ± 0.1	0.7 ± 0.2	—	—
24:1	0.5 ± 0.1	0.5 ± 0.1	0.3 ± 0.1	0.3 ± 0.2	—	—

[a] Fatty acids are described by two quantities: the number of carbon atoms and the number of double bonds (e.g., 14:0).

Table XIII. Fatty Acid Composition of α-Lipoproteins

Primate[c]	Fatty Acid[a] (%, mean ± S.D.)[b] 16:0	16:1	18:0	18:1	18:2	20:4
Man:						
Normal ($n = 5$)	25.4 ± 0.7 (23)	3.9 ± 0.5 (4)	9.5 ± 0.5 (9)	20.5 ± 0.3 (19)	28.4 ± 1.4 (26)	6.2 ± 0.7 (6)
Diseased[d] ($n = 5$)	28.4 ± 0.7 (58)	4.8 ± 0.3 (10)	11.5 ± 0.8 (23)	25.5 ± 0.6 (52)	23.8 ± 1.3 (48)	3.5 ± 1.0 (7)
Chimpanzee:						
Controls ($n = 4$)	25.0 ± 1.6 (45)	2.8 ± 0.3 (5)	10.5 ± 0.6 (19)	20.0 ± 1.4 (37)	27.2 ± 1.0 (49)	10.5 ± 0.7 (19)
Experimental[e] ($n = 6$)	26.9 ± 0.7 (50)	3.3 ± 0.3 (6)	11.6 ± 0.6 (21)	22.4 ± 1.0 (41)	21.2 ± 1.1 (39)	10.6 ± 0.5 (19)
Baboon:						
Controls ($m = 2$)	25.3 ± 0.4 (27)	2.7 ± 0.1 (3)	17.2 ± 0.3 (18)	19.3 ± 0.1 (20)	24.9 ± 0.1 (26)	9.9 ± 0.8 (10)
Experimental[e] ($m = 2$)	21.4 ± 1.3 (29)	1.9 ± 0.1 (3)	15.4 ± 1.2 (22)	20.8 ± 0.5 (28)	22.8 ± 1.0 (31)	16.4 ± 1.0 (22)

[a] Fatty acids are described by two quantities: number of carbon atoms and number of double bonds (e.g., 16:0).
[b] Values in parentheses represent fatty acid concentration (mg/100 ml).
[c] n = Number of subjects; m = number of pools.
[d] Patients with type II hyperlipoproteinemia.
[e] Animals on high-cholesterol atherogenic diets.

Table XIV. Fatty Acid Composition of β-Lipoproteins

Primate[c]	Fatty Acid[a] (%, mean ± S.D.)[b]					
	16:0	16:1	18:0	18:1	18:2	20:4
Man:						
Normal						
($n = 5$)	19.7 ± 0.5 (27)	3.6 ± 0.2 (5)	5.6 ± 0.3 (8)	23.4 ± 0.9 (32)	37.0 ± 2.0 (51)	5.5 ± 0.5 (8)
Diseased[d]						
($n = 5$)	23.0 ± 0.3 (62)	4.3 ± 0.3 (12)	7.4 ± 0.5 (20)	24.8 ± 1.2 (67)	33.3 ± 1.1 (90)	5.3 ± 0.6 (14)
Chimpanzee:						
Controls						
($n = 4$)	20.9 ± 0.3 (47)	2.7 ± 0.1 (7)	7.9 ± 0.3 (18)	21.0 ± 1.2 (48)	33.5 ± 2.7 (74)	9.6 ± 1.0 (22)
Experimental[e]						
($n = 6$)	22.7 ± 0.6 (118)	2.4 ± 0.4 (10)	9.0 ± 0.5 (49)	23.4 ± 2.2 (118)	28.7 ± 1.6 (152)	9.7 ± 1.0 (54)
Baboon:						
Controls						
($m = 2$)	21.9 ± 0.2 (19)	2.2 ± 0.2 (2)	12.7 ± 0.1 (11)	20.1 ± 1.1 (18)	33.7 ± 1.1 (29)	8.6 ± 0.5 (8)
Experimental[e]						
($m = 2$)	16.7 ± 1.3 (27)	2.6 ± 0.0 (4)	12.8 ± 1.2 (20)	23.6 ± 0.4 (37)	29.7 ± 1.0 (47)	13.7 ± 1.1 (21)

[a] Fatty acids are described by two quantities: number of carbon atoms and number of double bonds (e.g., 16:0).
[b] Values in parentheses represent fatty acid concentration (mg/100 ml).
[c] n = Number of subjects; m = number of pools.
[d] Type II hyperlipoproteinemia.
[e] Animals on high-cholesterol atherogenic diets.

panzees on atherogenic diets had more oleic and arachidonic acids in their lipoproteins, expressed either as composition (%) or concentration (mg/100 ml). These increases were most pronounced in β-lipoproteins, in which the oleic acid content was doubled and the arachidonic acid content was 2.5 times the control concentration. The data obtained from control and atherogenic animals can be correlated with those from human subjects, who show similar trends in comparisons between control subjects and patients with type II hyperlipoproteinemia.

In view of these observations the proposed procedure consisting of electrochromatography separation, thin-layer-chromatography separation, and gas-chromatography determinations of the fatty acid spectra of individual lipids from isolated lipoproteins can be considered useful and valid for lipoprotein analysis and screening. The analysis of lipids from α- and β-lipoproteins after the rapid, precise, and convenient electrochromatographic separation shows up many details that are not observed in total plasma lipids.

VI. ACKNOWLEDGMENTS

We thank F. Soetewey for the data handling and W. De Keersgieter, B. Declercq, D. Vandamme, and the whole Simon Stevin Institute for their participation in the development of the methods. This work was supported by grants from the N.F.W.G.O. (Belgium), from the K.F.W.O. (Belgium), from the National Institutes of Health, Bethesda, Md. (P.H.S. grant No. HE-9969), and the World Health Organization.

REFERENCES

1. Fredrickson, D. S., R. I. Levy, and R. S. Lees, *N. Engl. J. Med.* **276**, 32–44, 94–103, 148–156, 215–226, 273–281 (1967).
2. Entenman, C., *Meth. Enzymol.* **3**, 299–317 (1957).
3. Folch, J., M. Lees, and G. H. Sloane-Stanley, *J. Biol. Chem.* **226**, 497–509 (1957).
4. Cook, W. H., and W. G. Martin, *Can. J. Biochem.* **40**, 1273–1285 (1962).
5. Rouser, G., A. J. Bauman, G. Kritchevsky, D. Heller, and J. O'Brien, *J. Amer. Oil Chem. Soc.* **38**, 544–555 (1961).
6. Rouser, G., G. Kritchevsky, C. Galli, A. Yamamoto, and A. Knudson, in *Inborn Disorders of Sphingolipid Metabolism,* S. M. Aronson and B. W. Volk, Eds., Pergamon Press, New York, 1967, pp. 303–316.
7. Gotto, A. M., R. I. Levy, and D. S. Fredrickson, *Lipids* **3**, 463–470 (1968).
8. Peeters, H., in *Protides of Biological Fluids, Proceedings of the 18th Colloquium,* H. Peeters, Ed., Pergamon Press, Oxford, 1971, pp. 3–26.

9. Waters, L. L., *Yale J. Biol. Med.* **37**, 204–210 (1964).
10. Gustafson, A., *J. Lipid Res.* **6**, 512–517 (1965).
11. Margolis, S., in *Structural and Functional Aspects of Lipoproteins in Living Systems,* E. Tria and A. Scanu, Eds., Academic Press, New York, 1969, pp. 369–424.
12. Macheboeuf, M. A., in *Blood Cells and Plasma Proteins, Their State in Nature,* J. L. Tullis, Ed., Academic Press, New York, 1953, pp. 358–377.
13. Oncley, J. L., F. R. N. Gurd, and M. Melin, *J. Amer. Chem. Soc.* **72**, 458–464 (1950).
14. Searcy, R. L., and L. M. Bergquist, *Biochim. Biophys. Acta* **106**, 603–615 (1965).
15. Scanu, A., L. A. Lewis, and F. M. Bumpus, *Arch. Biochem. Biophys.* **74**, 390–397 (1958).
16. Scanu, A., *J. Lipid Res.* **7**, 296–306 (1966).
17. Oncley, J. L., in *Brain Lipids and Lipoproteins and the Leucodystrophies,* J. Folch-Pi and H. J. Bauer, Eds., Elsevier, Amsterdam, 1963, pp. 1–17.
18. Hatch, F. K., and R. S. Lees, *Adv. Lipid Res.* **6**, 1–68 (1968).
19. Alaupovic, P., S. S. Senlar, R. H. Furman, M. L. Sullivan, and S. L. Walraven, *Biochemistry* **5**, 4044–4053 (1966).
20. Rouser, G., G. Kritchevsky, M. Whatley, and C. F. Baxter, *Lipids* **1**, 107–112 (1966).
21. Hanahan, D. J., and I. L. Chaikoff, *J. Biol. Chem.* **168**, 233–240 and **169**, 699–705 (1947).
22. Nazir, D., and G. Rouser, *Lipids* **1**, 159 (1966).
23. Folch, J., I. Ascoli, M. Lees, J. A. Meath, and F. N. Le Baron, *J. Biol. Chem.* **191**, 833–841 (1951).
24. Smith, R. H., *Biochem. J.* **57**, 130–139 (1954).
25. Rouser, G., G. Kritchevsky, and A. Yamamoto, in *Lipid Chromatographic Analysis,* Vol. 1, G. V. Marinetti, Ed., Dekker, New York, 1967, pp. 99–162.
26. Rouser, G., G. Kritchevsky, A. N. Siakotos, and A. Yamamoto, in *Neuropathology: Method and Diagnosis,* C. G. Tedeschi, Ed., Little Brown, Boston, 1970, pp. 691–753.
27. Rouser, G., G. Kritchevsky, C. Galli, and D. Heller, *J. Amer. Oil Chem. Soc.* **42**, 215–227 (1965).
28. Vandamme, D., V. Blaton, and H. Peeters, in *Fifth International Symposium on Chromatography and Electrophoresis,* Presses Academiques Europeennes, Brussels, 1968, pp. 268–272.
29. Lea, C. H., D. N. Rhodes, and R. D. Stoll, *Biochem. J.* **60**, 353–363 (1955).
30. McFarlane, A. S., *Nature* **149**, 439 (1942).
31. Singleton, W. S., M. S. Gray, M. L. Brown, and J. L. White, *J. Amer. Oil Chem. Soc.* **42**, 53–56 (1965).
32. Camejo, G., *J. Chromatogr.* **21**, 6–12 (1966).
33. Renkonen, O., *J. Lipid Res.* **3**, 181–183 (1962).
34. Nichols, A. V., *Proc. Natl. Acad. Sci. U.S.* **64**, 1128–1137 (1969).
35. Sunderman, F. W., and F. W. Sunderman, Jr., Eds., *Lipids and the Steroid Hormones in Clinical Medicine,* Part I, Lippincott, Philadelphia, 1960, pp. 3–85.
36. Stern, I., and B. Shapiro, *J. Clin. Pathol. (London)* **6**, 158–160 (1953).
37. Postma, T., and J. Stroes, *Clin. Chim. Acta* **22**, 569–578 (1968).
38. Sperry, W. M., in *Standard Methods of Clinical Chemistry,* Vol. 4, D. Seligson, Ed., Academic Press, New York, 1963, pp. 173–182.
39. Cheek, C. S., *Clin. Chem.* **15**, 102–107 (1969).
40. Frings, C. S., and R. T. Dunn, *Amer. J. Clin. Pathol.* **53**, 89–91 (1970).

41. De La Huerga, J., C. Yesinick, and H. Popper, *Amer. J. Clin. Pathol.* **23**, 1163–1167 (1953).
42. Albrink, M. J., *J. Clin. Invest.* **40**, 536–544 (1961).
43. Roberts, J. C., and R. Straus, in *Comparative Atherosclerosis,* Harper and Row, Hoeber Medical Division, New York, 1965, pp. 211–252.
44. Gresham, G. A., A. N. Howard, J. McQueen, and D. E. Bowyer, *Brit. J. Exp. Pathol.* **46**, 94–103 (1965).
45. Kabara, J. J., *Meth. Biochem. Anal.* **10**, 263–318 (1962).
46. Van Handel, E., and D. B. Zilversmit, *J. Lab. Clin. Med.* **50**, 152–157 (1957).
47. Boyd, G. S., F. P. Nobbe, and F. G. Schettler, in *Atherosclerosis,* F. G. Schettler and G. S. Boyd, Eds., Elsevier, Amsterdam, 1969, pp. 531–564.
48. Rouser, G., G. Kritchevsky, D. Heller, and E. Lieber, *J. Amer. Oil Chem. Soc.* **40**, 425–454 (1963).
49. Kannel, W. B., T. R. Dawber, A. Kagan, N. Revotskie, and J. Stokes, *Ann. Intern. Med.* **55**, 33–50 (1961).
50. Peeters, H., and V. Blaton, *Acta Zool. Pathol. Antverpiensia* **48**, 221–231 (1969).
51. Blaton, V., A. N. Howard, G. A. Gresham, D. Vandamme, and H. Peeters, *J. Atheroscler. Res.* **11**, 497–507 (1970).
52. Peeters, H., and E. Laga, in *Protides of the Biological Fluids, Proceedings of the 10th Colloquium,* H. Peeters, Ed., Elsevier, Amsterdam, 1962, pp. 134–139.
53. Peeters, H., and V. Blaton, *Progr. Biochem. Pharmacol.* **4**, 144–152 (1968).
54. Blaton, V., H. Peeters, G. A. Gresham, and A. N. Howard, *Progr. Biochem. Pharmacol.* **4**, 122–125 (1968).
55. Blaton, V., and H. Peeters, in *Protides of the Biological Fluids, Proccedings of the 14th Colloquium,* H. Peeters, Ed., Elsevier, Amsterdam, 1966, pp. 659–665.
56. Werner, M., *J. Chromatogr.* **25**, 63–70 (1966).
57. Blaton, V., and H. Peeters, in *Protides of the Biological Fluids, Proceedings of the 15th Colloquium,* H. Peeters, Ed., Elsevier, Amsterdam, 1967, pp. 585–589.
58. Lees, R. S., and F. T. Hatch, *J. Lab. Clin. Med.* **61**, 518–528 (1963).
59. Dicastro, G., *Bull. Soc. Chim. Belg.* **65**, 97–102 (1956).
60. Grassmann, W., discussion in *Protides of the Biological Fluids, Proceedings of the 8th Colloquium,* H. Peeters, Ed., Elsevier, Amsterdam, 1960, p. 344.
61. Barrollier, J., E. Watzke, and H. Gibian, *Z. Naturforsch.* **13**, 754–755 (1958).
62. Peeters, H., W. De Keersgieter, and E. Lamonte, in *Second International Symposium on Chromatography,* Belgisch Genootschap voor Pharmaceutische Wetenschappen, Brussels, 1962, pp. 113–123.
63. Ribeiro, L. P., E. Mitideri, and O. R. Affonso, *Paper Electrophoresis,* Elsevier, Amsterdam, 1961.
64. Schjeide, O. A., A. U. Rivin, and J. Yoshino, *Amer. J. Clin. Pathol.* **39**, 329–341 (1963).
65. De Keersgieter, W., V. Blaton, and H. Peeters, in *Fourth International Symposium on Chromatography and Electrophoresis,* Presses Academiques Europeennes, Brussels, 1964, pp. 604–611.
66. Rouser, G., A. N. Siakotos, and S. Fleischer, *Lipids* **1**, 85–86 (1966).
67. Renkonen, O., and P. Varo, in *Lipid Chromatography Analysis,* Vol. 1, G. V. Marinetti, Ed., Dekker, New York, 1967, pp. 41–98.
68. Wood, R., K. Imaichi, J. Knowles, and G. Michaels, *J. Lipid Res.* **5**, 225–231 (1964).
69. Peeters, H., V. Blaton, A. Howard, and G. Gresham, *Atherosclerosis* **12**, 283–290 (1970).

70. Nelson, G. J., in *Drugs Affecting Lipid Metabolism,* W. L. Holmes, L. A. Carlson, and R. Paoletti, Eds., Plenum, New York, 1969, pp. 583–596.
71. Parsons, J. G., *J. Lipid Res.* **8**, 696–698 (1967).
72. James, A. T., and A. J. P. Martin, *Biochem. J.* **50**, 679–690 (1952).
73. Buhring, H., *J. Chromatogr.* **11**, 452–458 (1963).
74. Metcalf, L. D., and A. A. Schmitz, *Anal. Chem.* **33**, 363–364 (1961).
75. Vorbeck, M. L., L. R. Mattick, F. A. Lee, and C. S. Pederson, *Anal. Chem.* **33**, 1512–1514 (1961).
76. Ast, H. J., *Anal. Chem.* **35**, 1539–1540 (1963).
77. Bowyer, D. E., W. M. F. Leat, A. N. Howard, and G. A. Gresham, *Biochim. Biophys. Acta* **70**, 423–431 (1963).

Part II

FORMED ELEMENTS OF BLOOD

7. Lipid Composition and Metabolism of Erythrocytes

GARY J. NELSON

Bio-Medical Division, Ernest O. Lawrence Livermore Laboratory, Livermore, California

I. INTRODUCTION

A. Historical Perspective

Interest in the lipid composition of erythrocytes dates back for several decades, but only in the last 10 years has accurate quantitative data on lipid distribution in the erythrocytes of man, and a limited number of other species, become available. Although early studies, particularly those on cellular membranes, contributed valuable knowledge, little was known about the distribution of the various lipid classes in the membrane. Gorter and Grendal (1) were the first to suggest that the erythrocyte was surrounded by a bilayer of lipid molecules. Later Danielli and Davson (2), without knowledge of the work of Gorter and Grendal, proposed a cell-membrane structure that was based on permeability considerations. The bilayer theory and/or unit membrane hypothesis (3) has recently come under increasing criticism (4, 5), but nonetheless it has proved to be a durable model and a valuable stimulus to membrane research.

Only recently Bar, Deamer, and Cornwall (6) repeated the work of Gorter and Grendal (1) and confirmed the essence of the results after over 40 years. They pointed out some errors in the original work—errors that fortuitously tended to cancel one another, so that the results were essentially correct. Whether the amount of lipid and its surface area are actually relevant to molecular architecture of the membrane is not at all clear. These experiments are considered further in Section V.

A remarkable feature of the early work on the lipids of the erythrocyte membrane was the lack of knowledge of the distribution of the lipid classes (1, 2). Cholesterol and phospholipids were known to be important lipids in the red cell (7), but there was no agreement as to the relative proportions and the major phospholipid classes. Hence most models of the cell membrane consisted of "black boxes" for the lipid region, which ignored differences in the types of lipids in the membrane. This is still true today more often than not.

Recent studies (8–10) suggest that individual lipids may be asymmetrically distributed in the membrane. Glycosphingolipids, particularly, may be distributed only on the surface of the cell (11, 12). Thus one reason for the failure of the classic bilayer theory may well be its failure to recognize differences in individual lipids and variation in lipid composition in various regions of the membrane. A uniform hydrocarbon region surrounded by proteins on both sides appears to be a highly oversimplified view of the cell membrane. Of course without sufficient data a more elaborate theory could not be formulated.

B. Scope of Presentation

This chapter reviews current data on the composition of erythrocytes in man and other animals. The emphasis is on the mammalian erythrocyte simply because data on the lipids of nonmammalian species are sparse or nonexistent. The review concentrates on recent values; the older work is discussed only where it is of particular interest or covers data not available in recent studies (or both). For references and review of the older literature the reader is referred to several excellent reviews (13–18).

The scheme of this work is to present the data on the normal composition of erythrocytes in man and other animals, including total lipids, individual lipid classes, and the fatty acid composition of each group, followed by a discussion of the lipid metabolism of erythrocytes and the effects of various diseases and diets on the lipids of the cell. The chapter concludes with a brief review of some current experiments and ideas on the structure of the red-cell membrane.

II. LIPID COMPOSITION OF ERYTHROCYTES

A. Nature of the Erythrocyte

The mammalian erythrocyte consists primarily of hemoglobin, water, and inorganic electrolytes: approximately 63% water, 3.5% potassium, 0.1% sodium, and 33% hemoglobin (19, 20). These values for wet cells are subject to error from liquid trapped in intercellular space when the cells are packed by centrifugation, but they are probably close to the normal *in vivo* values for healthy adults. Thus the dry mass of the cell is more than 90% hemoglobin.

When erythrocytes are lysed, the membrane, or stroma, can be isolated by centrifugation. Dodge, Mitchell, and Hanahan (21) estimated that the stroma obtained by lysing contains 1.3% of the dry mass of the cell. This may be somewhat less than the true mass of the membrane *in vivo* because some material may be lost from the membrane during the preparation of the stroma (22). Dodge et al. (21) report that 40% of the stroma consists of lipids; the rest is mainly protein with a small amount of carbohydrates (23).

The membranes contain many enzymes (19), some of which may be lipoproteins. The remaining protein may be "structural protein." Since the proteins of the erythrocyte are covered in Chapter 10 of this book, they are not discussed here.

Table I. Total Lipid, Total Cholesterol, and Total Phospholipid Content of Human Erythrocytes

Year	Total Lipids[a] mg/ml	Total Lipids[a] g/cell ($\times 10^{-13}$)	Total Cholesterol[b] mg/ml	Total Cholesterol[b] g/cell ($\times 10^{-13}$)	Total Phospholipids[c] mg/ml	Total Phospholipids[c] g/cell ($\times 10^{-13}$)	Ref.
1963		5.76		1.57		3.25	21
1963	5.30	4.79	1.24	1.12	3.32	3.00	27
1964		4.88		1.26		3.17	28
1964		4.83		1.18		2.90	29
1964			1.36				30
1965					3.22		31
1965	4.88	4.88	1.26	1.26	3.18	3.18	32
1965			1.49		4.46		33
1965			1.35		3.10		34
1965			1.46		3.33		35
1966				1.39		3.15	6
1966		5.90					36
1966		4.95		1.13		2.88	37
1966					2.63		38
1967		5.00		1.22		2.75	39
1967			1.22	1.25	3.03	3.10	40
1967					2.08		41
1967					3.13		42
1968				1.11		2.50	43
1968				1.22		2.87	44
1968	5.67	4.98	1.51	1.33	3.21	2.82	45
1968		5.05		1.07		3.20	46
1968			1.21				47
1968	5.07	5.07	1.33	1.33	3.05	3.05	48
1968					2.85		49
1968				1.10	3.74		50
1968				1.15	3.02		51
1968					3.25		52
1969				1.16		3.77	53
1969					3.95		54
1969				1.34		3.15	55
1969			1.27	1.16	4.13	3.77	56

[a] Average total-lipid values: 5.20 ± 0.27 mg/ml, $(5.09 \pm 0.36) \times 10^{-13}$ g/cell.

[b] Average total-cholesterol values: 1.31 ± 0.11 mg/ml, $(1.23 \pm 0.12) \times 10^{-13}$ g/cell. Average percentages: 25.2% of total lipids measured in milligrams per milliliter; 24.2% in grams per cell.

[c] Average total-phospholipid values: 3.26 ± 0.61 mg/ml, $(3.11 \pm 0.31) \times 10^{-13}$ g/cell. Average percentages: 62.7% of total lipids measured in milligrams per milliliter; 61.1% in grams per cell.

B. Total Lipid Composition

Table I lists some modern values for the total lipid content of human erythrocytes; some date back to 1963, but most have been reported since 1965. Some controversy has occurred over the loss of lipid when cells are repeatedly washed to remove plasma lipoproteins and leukocytes (24, 25), but more modern data (21) suggest that under proper conditions (pH, osmotic strength) little or no lipid is removed from the membrane. As the human red cell has an average volume of 100 cubic microns (26), the same quantity is obtained for the total lipid content in terms of both milligrams per milliliter and grams per cell ($\times 10^{-13}$) are given by the same number. Any variation is caused by differences in the technique of measuring the mean cell volume. The average value for the total lipid content is 5.20 ± 0.27 mg/ml for packed-cell preparations, or $(5.09 \pm 0.36) \times 10^{-13}$ g/cell. Similar agreement is noted for the cholesterol and total-phospholipid values.

The main types of lipids found in erythrocytes are cholesterol, glycosphingolipids, and phospholipids. In Table I it is apparent that the sum of the cholesterol and total-phospholipid values does not give the value for the total lipids in the cell.[1] The difference between that sum and the measured total lipids in the cell is the glycosphingolipid content of the cell. The value for the total glycosphingolipid content of human erythrocytes falls between 12 and 15% of the total-lipid value. The composition of the glycosphingolipid fraction is discussed further in Section II.D.

Table II lists the total lipid, total phospholipid, and cholesterol contents of the erythrocytes of various animal species. Since the size of the erythrocyte varies widely among different species (26), the values in milligrams per milliliter and grams per cell are not the same. On the other hand, the total-lipid values in milligrams per milliliter of packed cells are remarkably alike for all species, varying only from 4 to 6. Also, the relative amounts of cholesterol and phospholipids (as percentages of the total lipids) are similar for all species. The variation in total phospholipid content is somewhat greater than that in cholesterol. If this is not due to experimental error, it reflects variations in total glycosphingolipids or the substitution of glycosphingolipids for phospholipids in the membrane (or both). The latter assumption is unlikely, however, because there is no reason to assume that glycosphingolipids and phospholipids have equivalent roles in the bio-

[1] Most of the values for the total phospholipid content were obtained by multiplying the measured phosphorus content (mg) by 25; this is a good approximation for human-red-cell phospholipids.

Table II. Total Lipid, Total Cholesterol, and Total Phospholipid Contents of the Erythrocytes of Various Species

	Total Lipids		Total Cholesterol		Total Phospholipids		
Species	mg/ml	g/cell ($\times 10^{-13}$)	mg/ml	g/cell ($\times 10^{-13}$)	mg/ml	g/cell ($\times 10^{-13}$)	Ref.
Cow		3.00				1.63	57
	4.21	2.58	1.23	0.71		1.63	58
				0.82			59
				1.48	2.87	1.67	60
Rat	4.86	3.15	1.27		3.40		58
				0.89		2.03	59
			1.51		4.27		61
	5.26		1.11		3.39		62
			1.80		4.50		63
			1.45				64
Sheep	4.42	1.62	1.24	0.63		1.02	58
				0.56[a]			59
Dog	5.08	4.84	1.43	1.20	3.03	2.54	58
		3.60					65
		9.30[b]					65
	4.47				2.29		66
Rabbit	4.42	4.15	1.32	1.19	3.01	2.73	58
							67
							68
Chicken	5.00				3.56		69
	7.25		1.47		4.45		70
Guinea pig	5.72	4.41	1.54	1.19	3.50	2.45	71
			1.36		2.56		72
Goat	5.79	1.23	1.02	0.32	3.08	0.61	73
Horse	4.76	2.56	1.38	0.63	2.79	1.34	73
Pig	4.19	2.52	1.15	0.68	2.58	1.51	73
Cat	6.04	3.45	1.62	0.92	3.70	2.11	73
Seal:							
Elephant	4.07		1.05		2.42		74
Harp	4.03		1.07		2.63		74
Monkey					3.15		75

[a] Using a different extraction procedure, the same authors obtained a value of 0.64.
[b] Hyperlipemic.

chemistry of the membrane. Variations in cellular glycosphingolipid and phospholipid contents probably result from independent phenomena.

C. Neutral Lipids

The neutral lipids of erythrocytes consist almost exclusively of a single compound, cholesterol. The older data (76–79) reporting appreciable amounts of triglycerides and cholesteryl esters in red cells are not supported by later reports (32, 57, 58, 80, 81). The amount of triglycerides in mammalian red cells is negligible. Nelson (58) found no evidence of any neutral lipids other than cholesterol in red cells from a number of species. Payne and Masters (81) found that less than 1% of the neutral lipids of bovine red cells was not free cholesterol and that essentially no triglycerides or free fatty acids were present in well-washed cell preparations.

Figure 1 shows examples of separation by thin-layer chromatography of the neutral lipids from the total-lipid extracts of cow, sheep, and rat erythrocytes. Under visible light no spots for any neutral lipids other than cholesterol were visible; any lipid present to the extent of 0.5% of the total extract should have been visible. Under ultraviolet illumination faint spots for cholesteryl esters, triglycerides, and free fatty acids were detected; in these samples they could not have accounted for more than 0.3% of the total lipids applied to the plate.

The free-fatty-acid content of erythrocytes is difficult to measure, because the membrane can reversibly bind a large number of free-fatty-acid

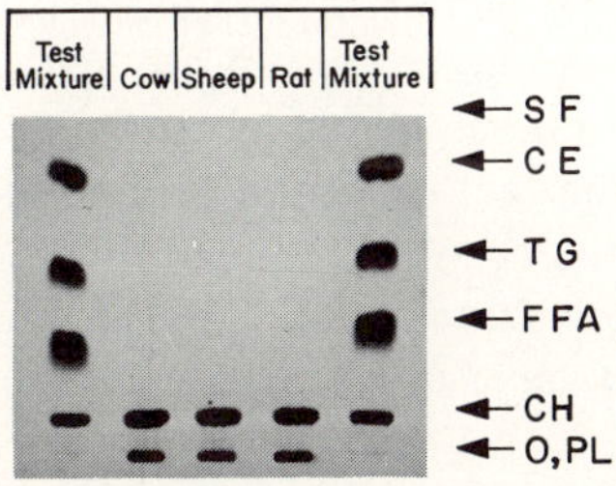

Fig. 1 Thin-layer-chromatography separation of the neutral lipids from cow, sheep, and rat erythrocytes. About 1.5 mg of each total-lipid extract was applied to the center lanes; the test mixture (400 μg) applied to the two outside lanes contained 100 μg each of cholesterol (CH), cholesteryl oleate (CE), triolein (TG), and oleic acid (FFA). The spots were visualized by charring with 50% sulfuric acid containing 0.6% potassium dichromate. No spots for neutral lipids other than cholesterol could be detected after charring, but faint spots for CE, TG, and FFA could be detected under ultraviolet light. SF, solvent front; O, origin; PL, phospholipids. [Reproduced from *J. Lipid Res.* **8**, 374–379 (1967).]

molecules (82). The washing procedure, the plasma free-fatty-acid level, and the pH of the wash medium can greatly influence the amount of free fatty acids remaining bound to the cell. In all probability the free fatty acids are not an integral part of the membrane structure. In well-washed cell preparations they amount to less than 0.1% of the total neutral lipids (58).

Triglycerides and cholesteryl esters may be in equilibrium between the plasma lipoproteins and the cells. Possibly the cholesteryl esters are formed in the membrane by a transferase reaction similar to that observed in plasma by Glomset (83). If so, they are transferred quickly to plasma lipoproteins, leaving only a low steady-state level in the membrane (see Chapter 14 for further speculation on this phenomenon).

Other factors affecting the values for neutral lipids in erythrocytes are the purity of the sample and the analytical methodology. Reticulocytes may be present in sufficient amount to contribute measurable quantities of neutral lipids to the extract. Leukocytes and platelets not adequately removed from the packed-cell preparation are other possible contaminants. The lipid compositions of these cells are described in Chapters 8 and 9, respectively.

Nelson (58) calculated that if only 0.1% of the original lipoproteins of plasma remained bound to erythrocytes, most of the neutral lipids other than cholesterol could be attributed to lipoprotein contamination. When sheep erythrocytes were washed 10 times with isotonic phosphate buffer (pH 7.4), the quantities of cholesteryl esters, triglycerides, and free fatty acids were below the levels of detection, about 0.2% of the total lipids extracted.

Although the reports by earlier investigators (76–79) that erythrocytes contain relatively large amounts of neutral lipids other than cholesterol may be in error, the presence of small amounts of these substances is still an open question. The fact that these compounds are not integral parts of the molecular architecture of the membrane does not preclude the possibility that plasma lipoproteins and plasma lipids are bound to the cell *in vivo*, or that they may have undiscovered physiological and biochemical significance.

D. Glycosphingolipids

Glycosphingolipids constitute a major fraction of red-cell lipids, estimated as between 10 and 20% of the total stromal lipids, depending on the species (73). However, their role and arrangement in the cell are not well defined (84). In addition, the quantitative data for this fraction are less definitive than those for neutral lipids and phospholipids, because of

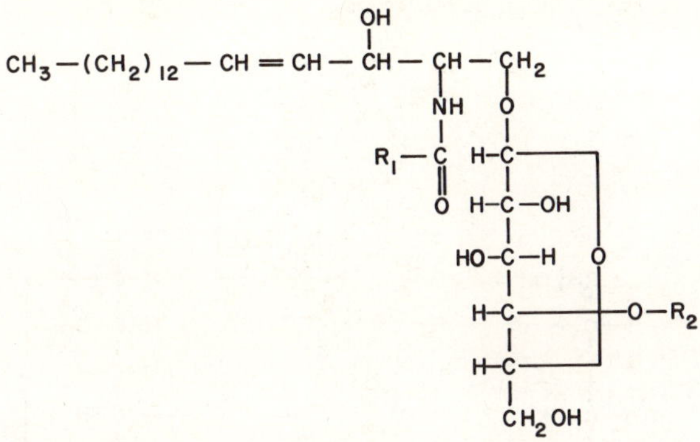

I

Oligoglycosyl ceramide; R_1 = acyl group; R_2 = H or carbohydrate residues

the lack of simple and rapid methods of analysis. Even the structures of many of the glycosphingolipids are as yet unknown (85).[2]

1. Glycosphingolipid Structure. All glycosphingolipids contain one ceramide group (sphingosine with a fatty acid in an amide linkage) and one or more carbohydrate residues. The simplest glycosphingolipids, cerebrosides, contain one sphingosine, one fatty acid, and one hexose residue; they are present in red cells (87) but usually as minor constituents.

The glycosphingolipids are usually divided into three groups: neutral glycosphingolipids, hexosamine-containing glycosphingolipids without sialic acid, and gangliosides, which contain one or more sialic acid residues.

The neutral glycosphingolipids (**I**) contain only sphingosine, fatty acids, and unsubstituted hexoses, usually glucose or galactose; this group is also termed ceramide monohexosides or polyhexosides.

The hexosamine glycosphingolipids (**II**) are a diverse group of substances that always contain at least two or more carbohydrate residues, one of which is a hexosamine, such as galactosamine or glucosamine (85, 88–90); Yamakawa suggested the name "globosides" for this class (91).

The third group of glycosphingolipids, usually termed gangliosides (**III**), are polyhexosides that usually contain several hexose residues and neuraminic acid (92). Some erythrocyte gangliosides contain two sialic acid residues (**IV**).

[2] After this chapter was completed, a very interesting study concerned primarily with erythrocyte glycosphingolipids was published by Sweeley and Dawson (86). The reader who wants much additional information on these compounds and their role in antigenicity and immunochemistry is urged to consult it.

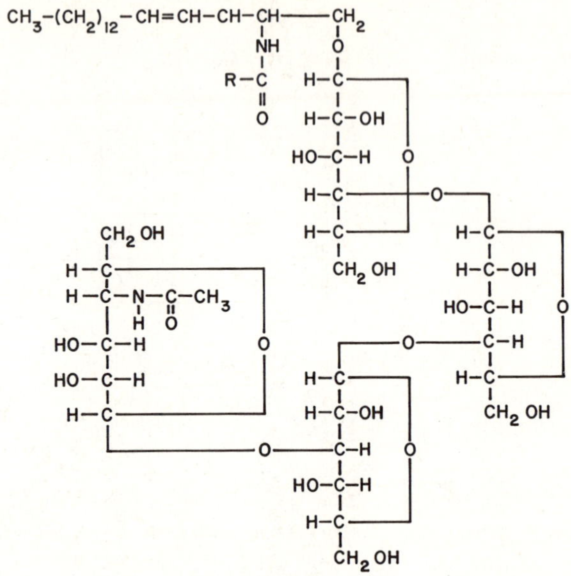

II

Globoside (hog and man); R = acyl group

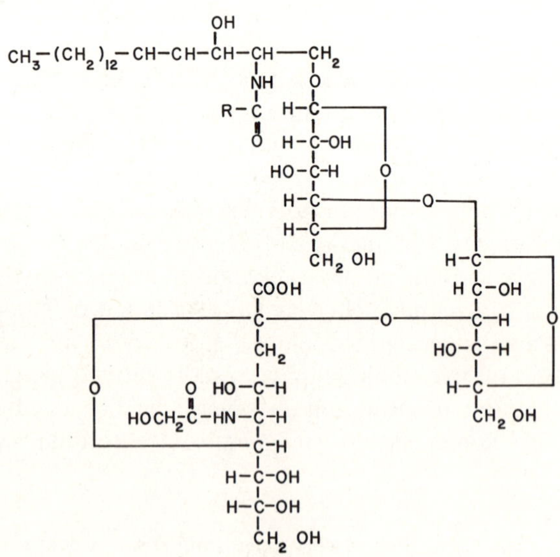

III

Ganglioside (horse); R = acyl group

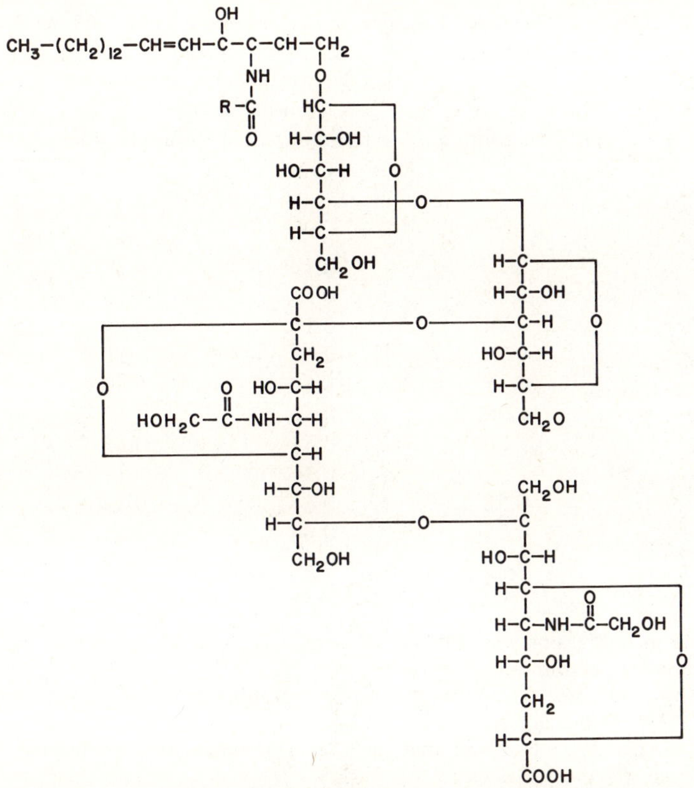

IV

Ganglioside (cat); R = acyl group

Table III lists some of the available data on the glycosphingolipid content of mammalian erythrocytes, and Table IV shows the proportions of glycosphingolipids in several species. The variations in the amounts and the types of glycosphingolipids in erythrocytes are rather perplexing. The glycosphingolipids exhibit the most remarkable species variation of any class of lipids, due perhaps to involvement with the immunological reactions of the cell (86).

2. Human Glycosphingolipids. The glycosphingolipids of human erythrocytes have been examined in somewhat greater detail than those of other species (89, 93, 96, 97, 99, 101). Klenk and Lauenstein (89) were unable to find gangliosides in human erythrocytes. This finding was confirmed by Yamakawa and co-workers (90, 99). The main glycosphingolipids of human erythrocytes are ceramide polyhexosides and globosides

Table III. Glycosphingolipid Content of Erythrocytes from Various Species[a]

Species	Total Glyco-sphingolipids	Neutral Glyco-sphingolipids	Gangliosides	Ref.
Man		1.09[b]		93
			0.17	94
			1.00	95
	2.52[b,c]	2.19[b]	0.34[b]	96
Cat	0.72[d]	0.19	0.53	73
Cow	0.34[e]	0.10	0.24	73
Dog	1.31	0.63	0.68	73
Goat	1.45	1.10	0.35	73
Guinea pig	1.00	0.87	0.13	73
Horse	1.26	0.43	0.83	73
		0.34		100
Pig	0.58	0.44	0.14	73
Rabbit	0.25	0.04	0.21	73
Rat	0.42	0.10	0.32	73
Sheep	0.50	0.12	0.38	73

[a] Measured in milligrams per milliliter of packed cells, unless otherwise indicated.
[b] In micromoles per milliliter.
[c] Yamakawa et al. (97) found that the total glycosphingolipids of human erythrocytes comprise 1.1% of the dry stroma.
[d] Handa and Handa (98) found that the total glycosphingolipids comprise 0.3% of the total lipids in cat erythrocytes.
[e] According to Yamakawa et al. (99) glycosphingolipids comprise 0.7% of the dry stroma of cow erythrocytes.

(87, 90, 97, 99). Recently Vance and Sweeley (87, 93) reported detailed analyses of human-erythrocyte neutral glycosphingolipids. The simplest type of glycosphingolipid detected was a cerebroside containing only glucose.[3] Ceramide dihexoside and trihexoside were present, but the main component was a globoside whose structure was determined by Yamakawa and co-workers (99).[4] Vance and Sweeley estimated that the four types of glycosphingolipids were present in mole ratios of 3.7 : 15.1 : 11.7 : 69.5 for the monohexoside, dihexoside, trihexoside, and globoside, respectively (87).

Although the early work of Klenk and Lauenstein (89) and Yamakawa et al. (90) yielded no evidence of sialic acid in human red cells, more

[3] See structure **I** in the preceding subsection.
[4] See structure **II** in the preceding subsection.

Table IV. Characteristics of Erythrocyte Glycosphingolipids in Various Species

Species	Amino Sugar in Major Glyco-sphingolipid[a]	Other Glyco-sphingolipids Detected	Carbohydrates Other than Galactose	References
Man	Galactosamine	Mono-, di-, tri-, oligo-hexose ceramides; gangliosides	Lactose, mannose, glucose, fucose, arabinose	23, 85, 93, 96, 97, 99–103
Cow	Neuraminic acid	Ceramide oligo-hexosides	Lactose, mannose, glucose, arabinose	23, 85, 88, 100, 103, 104
Horse	Neuraminic acid	Ceramide oligo-hexosides	Glucose, mannose, fucose	23, 85, 88, 100, 103, 105
Rabbit	Glucosamine	Mono-, di-, tri-hexose ceramides	Glucose	85, 88, 94
Hog	Galactosamine	Di-, tri-hexose ceramides; globosides	Glucose, fucose, mannose	23, 85, 88, 103, 106
Cat	Neuraminic acid	Mono-, di-hexose ceramides	Glucose	85, 98
Dog	*N*-glycolyl and *N*-acetyl neuraminic acids		Glucose	85, 105
Sheep	Hexosamine		Glucose	85, 88
Guinea pig	Galactosamine	Ceramide oligo-hexosides	None	85

[a] The structures of major glycosphingolipids are known for all species listed except sheep and guinea pig.

recent work from Yamakawa's laboratory (99) and others (96, 101) has established that sialolipids are indeed present in the red cell. Wherrett and Brown (96) estimated that glycosphingolipids containing sialic acid make up 15% of the total glycosphingolipid fraction. Yamakawa and co-workers (99) have reported evidence of two and perhaps more sialic-acid-containing lipids in human erythrocytes. The structures of these compounds have not been established, except that they contain hexosamine as well as sialic acid.

Sialic acid is also present in human red cells in the form of glycoproteins, or mucopolysaccharides (94). As the sialic acid fraction is small, cross contamination of the lipid extract by nonlipid sialic acid must be considered (94). Further work will be needed to clarify this point.

3. Glycosphingolipids of Other Species. The structures of the major glycosphingolipids in rabbit (107), dog (105), horse (100, 105), hog (106), cow (89), and cat (98) erythrocytes have been determined, primarily by members of Yamakawa's group in Japan. These workers have also partially characterized the main glycosphingolipids in sheep and guinea pigs (85). Rabbit erythrocytes contain a globoside that has five hexose residues along with smaller amounts of monohexosyl, dihexosyl, and trihexosyl ceramides. No sialic acid has been detected in the erythrocyte glycosphingolipids of rabbits, hogs, or sheep. The structure of the major glycosphingolipid of the hog erythrocyte is identical with that of man (99, 106).[5] Lesser amounts of monohexosyl and dihexosyl ceramides are also present in hog-erythrocyte lipids.

In the erythrocytes of cat, horse, cow, and dog the major glycosphingolipids are gangliosides that often contain both sialic acid and hexosamine. Cat erythrocytes have a disialoglycosphingolipid that does not contain hexosamine.[6] Horse erythrocytes have a monosialoglycosphingolipid without hexosamine; it was one of the first gangliosides isolated from erythrocytes for which the complete structure was determined (89).[7] The glycosphingolipid of dog erythrocytes is similar to that of the horse except that it contains both *N*-glycolylneuraminic and *N*-acetylneuraminic acids; the horse glycosphingolipid contains only *N*-glycolylneuraminic acid. The glycosphingolipid of bovine erythrocytes contains both neuraminic acid and hexosamine in a 1 : 1 molar ratio.

4. Fatty Acid Composition of the Glycosphingolipids. Table V lists some data on the fatty acid composition of the main glycosphingolipids from several species. As is typical of sphingolipids in general, the glycosphingolipids contain only saturated and singly unsaturated fatty acids. The straight-chain fatty acids are mainly 16, 18, 22, 23, and 24 carbon atoms in length. The dog has 45% palmitic acid (105); lignoceric and nervonic acids predominate in the glycosphingolipids of all other species for which data are currently available.

[5] See structure **II** in subsection 1.

[6] See structure **IV** in subsection 1.

[7] See structure **III** in subsection 1.

Table V. Fatty Acid Composition of Erythrocyte Glycosphingolipids

Fatty Acid[b]	Quantity (%)[a] Man (90)	Cat (98)	Horse (105)	Dog (105)	Hog (106)	Rabbit (107)
16:0	4.0	2.0	2.0	6.0	2.6	10.1
18:0	3.0	2.0	6.0	45.0	2.1	18.8
18:1	—	—	2.0	2.0	—	5.9
20:0	—	0.9	3.0	—	—	1.0
20:1	—	—	—	—	—	1.0
22:0	14.0	9.0	7.0 14.2[c]	6.0	32.7	7.5
22:1	—	0.9	4.0	—	—	—
23:0	—	3.0	— 3.0[c]	—	4.2	6.8
24:0	78.0	33.0	64.0 76.4[c]	15.0	41.7	9.6
24:1	—	49.0	2.0 6.0[c]	27.0	9.6	30.5
26:0	—	—	11.0	—	—	2.4

[a] The reference number of the source of data is shown below the name of the species. A dash stands for "not reported in the original reference."
[b] Fatty acids are described by two quantities: the number of carbon atoms and the number of double bonds (e.g., 16:0).
[c] Data from Ref. 104.

E. Phospholipids

In comparison with the glycosphingolipids the phospholipids of mammalian erythrocytes show less species variation in structure. However, the relative proportions of individual phospholipids, especially lecithin and sphingomyelin, do vary considerably from species to species (108, 109).

The major phospholipids so far detected in erythrocytes are lecithin, sphingomyelin, phosphatidylserine, phosphatidylethanolamine, and phosphatidylinositol, which together account for over 90% of the total phospholipids in all species for which data are now available. Phosphatidic acid, lysolecithin, and many unidentified phospholipids are present (110). Recently Nelson (111) reported the isolation and identification of a new phospholipid from sheep erythrocytes, an *N*-substituted phosphatidylserine (structure **V**).

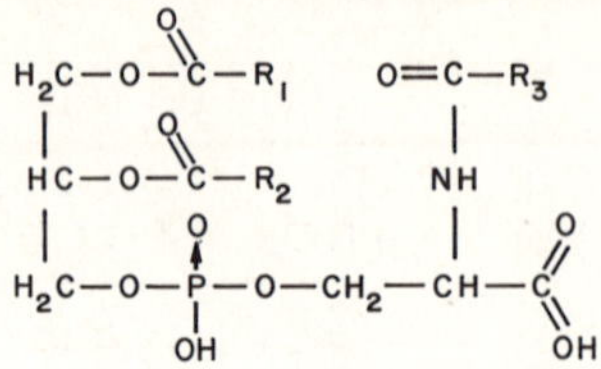

V

N-Acylphosphatidylserine; R_1, R_2, R_3 = acyl groups

The name proposed is *N*-acylphosphatidylserine. It comprises between 2 and 4% of the total phospholipids in sheep erythrocytes and is also present in smaller amounts in the erythrocytes of cows and goats (111). Figure 2 shows a two-dimensional thin-layer-chromatography (TLC) separation of the total phospholipids of sheep erythrocytes. The *N*-acylphosphatidylserine is clearly visible as a separate spot. Note the absence of a lecithin spot in this sample (see Fig. 3 for examples of TLC separations of phospholipids from the erythrocytes of other species).

Phosphatidylglycerol and cardiolipin have not been detected in red cells. This does not exclude the possibility that they are present in trace amounts, although cardiolipin is apparently exclusively associated with mitochondria (13); hence its absence in erythrocytes, which lack mitochondria, is expected.

One characteristic species variation in the erythrocyte phospholipids that is relatively unexplored is the nature of phosphatidylethanolamine. The ethanolamine lipids can exist in three forms: the diacyl; the monoacyl, alk-1-enyl ether; and the monoacyl, alkyl ether. Apparently the diacyl form and one, but not both, of the other forms can coexist in the cell; there is no evidence suggesting that the alk-1-enyl and alkyl ether forms are both present in the same species.

Hanahan and co-workers (112, 113) first reported the isolation and the structural characterization of the alkyl ether phospholipids in the erythrocytes of cows, the only species for which the structure of the ethanolamine ether phospholipid has been rigorously proved. Human erythrocytes contain the alk-1-enyl ethanolamine phospholipid along with the diacyl form (114, 115). In most studies in the literature the ethanolamine fraction is not separated into its subgroups but simply reported as phosphatidylethanolamine.

There is some indication that plasmalogen is a component of the lecithin fraction in human erythrocytes (114), but later reports indicate that it makes up only 1% or less of the lecithin (116, 117). The phosphatidyl-

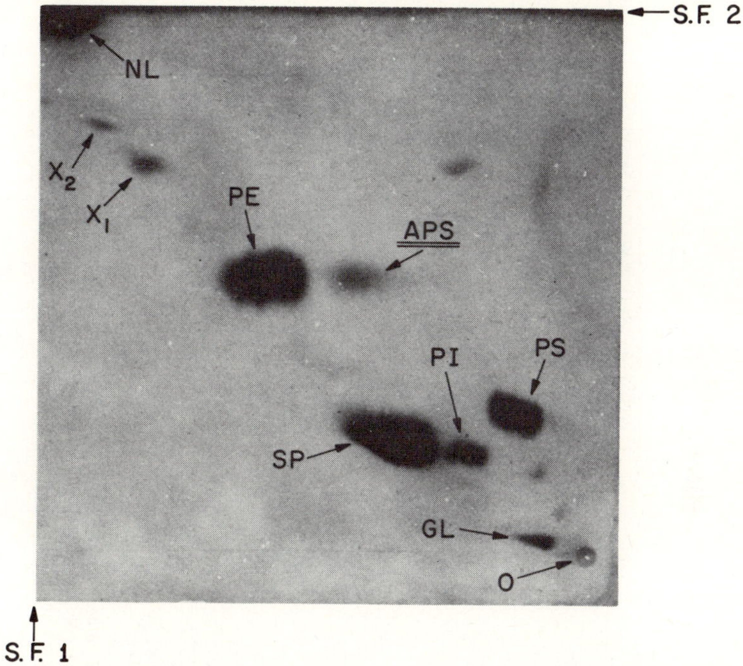

Fig. 2 A two-dimensional TLC separation of sheep-erythrocyte phospholipids. The spot for *N*-acylphosphatidylserine (APS) is clearly separated from the other major phospholipids. The spots were made visible by charring with 50% sulfuric acid containing 0.6% potassium dichromate. Solvents used to obtain separation were (a) chloroform–methanol–aqueous ammonia, 65 : 25 : 5 (by volume); and (b) chloroform–methanol–acetone–acetic acid–water, 5 : 2 : 1 : 1 : 0.5 (by volume). Abbreviations: S.F., solvent front, NL, neutral lipid components; PE, phosphatidylethanolamine; SP, sphingomyelin; PI, phosphatidylinositol; PS, phosphatidylserine; GL, glycosphingolipids; O, origin; X_1, X_2, unknown lipids. [Reproduced from *Biochem. Biophys. Res. Commun.* **38**, 261–265 (1970).]

serine fraction is entirely in the diacyl form in the erythrocytes of humans (117) as well as other species (73).

1. Phospholipid Composition of Human Erythrocytes. Table VI lists a number of recent analyses of the phospholipid composition of human erythrocytes. The various plasmalogen forms of the individual phospholipids are not distinguished in this table. The final column gives an average value for all the analyses. When the results in this table are compared with similar summaries in earlier reviews (14–16), it is immediately obvious that the agreement among values from different laboratories has improved dramatically in recent years. This is undoubtedly due to improvements in

Table VI. Phospholipid Composition of Human Erythrocytes

Year	Percentage of Total Phospholipids[a,b]								Ref.
	LPC	PI	PS	Sph	PC	PE	PA	Other	
1965	2.9	—	13.3	24.9	30.5	27.5	—	1.2	30
	—	—	14.8	25.3	29.9	24.3	(c)	(c)	31
	—	—	16.0	25.0	34.0	25.0	—	—	116
	1.6	3.2	9.2	31.3	35.4	19.4	—	—	35
1966	—	2.5	4.0	28.9	36.2	28.4	—	—	38
1967	1.1	1.3	13.0	26.9	28.9	27.2	2.2	—	13
	1.0	0.6	14.8	25.4	29.2	27.5	—	1.5	40
	—	—	15.0	22.3	32.7	34.0	—	—	42
1968	—	—	17.4	24.2	28.6	24.1		5.7	46
	1.2	(d)	(d)	24.1	29.5	31.2	1.0	—	48
	1.9	1.7	11.7	24.0	25.2	27.1	1.2	0.5	49
	2.1	1.6	14.0	25.9	27.4	29.0	—	—	43
	—	—	14.7	27.4	31.9	28.3	—	—	118
	—	—	11.6	29.0	33.1	26.1	—	—	51
	1.4	(e)	(e)	26.0	28.2	29.5	1.0	—	45
	9.9	—	10.6	23.7	28.3	25.6	—	—	119
1969	1.4	1.9	12.7	25.8	28.3	26.7	1.0	2.8	54
	—	—	14.5	23.4	32.8	28.3	—	—	117
Average ±S.D.	1.62 ± 0.57[f]	1.83 ± 0.77	12.96 ± 3.06	25.75 ± 2.20	30.56 ± 2.89	27.18 ± 3.01	1.78 ± 0.47	1.50 ± 0.83	

[a] Abbreviations: LPC, lysolecithin; PI, phosphatidylinositol; PS, phosphatidylserine; Sph, sphingomyelin; PC, lecithin; PE, phosphatidylethanolamine; PA, phosphatidic acid.

[b] A dash stands for "not reported in reference."

[c] Crowley et al. (31) report a combined value of 5.4% for phosphatidic acid and "other" phospholipids.

[d] Neerhout (48) reports a combined value of 13.1% for phosphatidylinositol and phosphatidylserine.

[e] Jaffe and Gottfried (45) report a combined value of 13.8% for phosphatidylinositol and phosphatidylserine.

[f] Average excludes value from reference 119.

techniques, in particular the almost universal replacement of paper, column, and hydrolytic techniques by thin-layer chromatography. The values that deviate most from the averages are those obtained by methods other than thin-layer chromatography. Another factor that has contributed to greater accuracy is the use of antioxidants and other precautions to prevent the degradation of samples during analysis (120, 121).

The average values given in Table VI are a good reference standard against which the reliability of other literature values can be checked. This is important, particularly in the burgeoning field of red-cell-lipid abnormalities, which is discussed in more detail in Section IV.C. Reports of "normal" values not in essential agreement with the averages in Table VI should be viewed with care, because these averages probably are very close to the true normal values for human erythrocytes. Future developments in the quantitation of human-red-cell lipids should not produce any significant changes in these values, only minor refinements.

2. Erythrocyte Phospholipid Composition in Animals. Table VII lists the phospholipid compositions of the erythrocytes of a number of species. Those of rabbits, cows, sheep, and rats have been studied most frequently. It is interesting that the data of Nelson (73) and Gercken and Brockman (67, 132) are in excellent agreement despite the wide differences in location and times of the analyses. This substantiates the idea that many of the variations in phospholipid composition in the same species are due to differences in procedure rather than individual variations among the animals.

As Turner (108) first reported, the phospholipid distribution in red cells shows wide variations among different species, but the differences are confined primarily to the amounts of lecithin and sphingomyelin in the stroma. For instance, the erythrocytes of ruminants contain little or no lecithin, which accounts for 50% of the total phospholipids in rat and dog erythrocytes. The amount of sphingomyelin is reduced in species with large amounts of lecithin but is never less than 10% of the total phospholipids. The major acidic phospholipids are less variable in composition than the choline-containing molecules.

Figure 3 presents some typical two-dimensional TLC separations of the phospholipids of various species. All of the plates were spotted with equal amounts of lipid phosphorus. Differences in the distribution of the phospholipids and glycosphingolipids are readily apparent. Also compare these patterns with Fig. 2, an example of the pattern obtained from ruminant erythrocytes.

Several attempts have been made to correlate phospholipid distribution in the erythrocyte with other physiological parameters of the cell (122,

Table VII. Phosphopipid Composition of Erythrocytes from Various Species

Species	Percentage of Total Phospholipids[a,b]								Ref.
	LPC	PI	PS	Sph	PC	PE	PA	Other	
Cat	0.3	7.4	13.2	26.1	30.5	22.2	0.8	—	73
Chicken	2.6	2.0	4.8	21.4	42.0	23.5	1.0	2.3	69
Cow	—	3.2	6.7	48.2	11.7	8.8	0.5	2.4	25
	—	—	17.0	50.0	6.0	21.0	—	6.0	57
	—	3.7	19.3	46.2	0.0	29.1	0.3	1.7	73
	—	—	3.0	61.0	7.0	29.0	—	—	122
	—	(c)	(c)	60.0	0.0	26.0	—	—	60
	—	—	(d)	49.5	13.6	36.9	—	—	123
Dog	1.8	2.2	15.4	10.8	46.9	22.4	0.5	—	73
Dolphin	0.5	7.5	16.7	27.8	18.1	24.6	0.1	4.5	(e)
Goat	—	6.4	17.1	33.1	14.2	9.5	—	2.7	25
	—	4.6	20.8	45.9	0.0	27.9	0.3	0.8	73
Guinea pig	0.3	2.4	16.8	11.1	41.1	24.6	4.2	—	73
Horse	—	4.8	9.4	23.8	45.0	13.6	1.6	3.4	25
	1.7	0.3	18.0	13.5	42.4	24.3	0.3	—	73
Monkey	2.1	5.1	11.0	16.1	34.0	28.1	1.8	1.8	75
Pig	—	2.9	16.2	12.7	30.0	27.9	0.8	1.1	25
	0.9	1.8	17.8	26.5	23.3	29.7	0.3	—	73
	—	—	1	36	29	31	—	—	122
Rabbit	0.3	1.6	12.2	19.0	33.9	31.9	1.6	—	73
	0.1	1.3	12.4	15.7	36.3	32.6	1.6	—	67
	—	—	1	29	44	26	—	—	122
	—	—	13.8	19.8	33.7	32.6	—	—	124
Rat	3.8	3.5	10.8	12.8	47.5	21.5	0.3	—	73
	—	—	1	26	56	17	—	—	122
	—	—	15.6	12.8	44.7	26.8	0.1	—	125
	4.8	—	—	13	52	17	—	—	61
	5.9	—	—	16.4	38.9	38.8	—	—	126
Seal:									
Elephant	1.2	1.6	18.9	19.4	33.3	25.2	0.2	1.4	74
Harp	1.7	2.4	15.2	21.3	32.9	24.2	0.4	2.1	74
Sheep	0.0	3.8	13.4	48.0	12.1	5.6	0.3	1.6	25
	0.0	2.9	14.1	51.0	0.0	26.2	0.3	4.8	73
	—	—	1	63	1	35	—	—	122
	0.0	3.5	12.9	48.5	0.0	28.2	0.3	2.9	127
	(f)	(f)	15.0	50.0	0.0	34.7	—	3.5	128
	—	—	2.1	53.2	0.9	39.3	—	—	129
	—	—	—	50	5	38	—	—	130
	1.5	0.0	10.5	54.5	7.3	23.9	2.3	—	131

[a] Abbreviations: LPC, lysolecithin; PI, phosphatidylinositol; PS, phosphatidylserine; Sph, sphingomyelin; PC, lecithin; PE, phosphatidylethanolamine; PA, phosphatidic acid.

[b] A dash stands for "not reported in reference."

[c] A combined value of 12.0% is given for PI + PS (60).

[d] Included in PE value.

[e] G. J. Nelson, unpublished information, 1970.

[f] A combined value of 4.50% is given for LPC + PI (128).

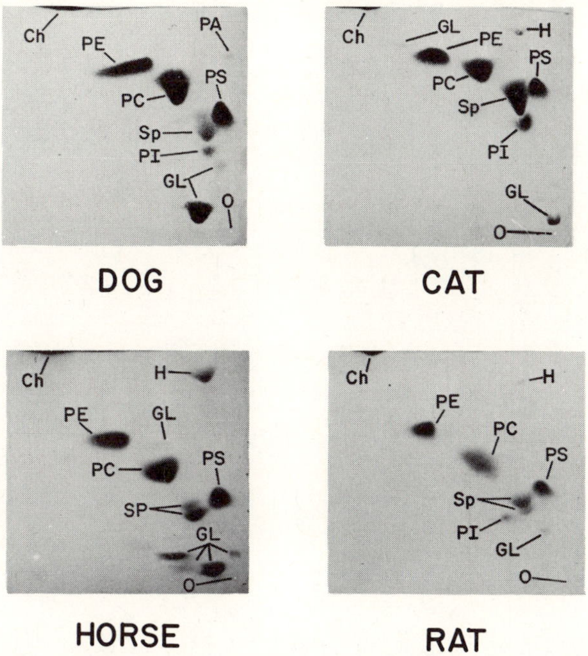

Fig. 3 Thin-layer-chromatography separations of dog, cat, horse, and rat erythrocyte lipids. Species variations in the distribution of the various lipids are readily apparent. Spots were made visible by charring with 50% sulfuric acid containing 0.6% potassium dichromate. Solvents: chloroform–methanol–aqueous ammonia, 65 : 25 : 5 (by volume), and chloroform–methanol–acetone–acetic acid–water, 5 : 2 : 1 : 1 : 0.5 (by volume). Compare with Figs. 2 and 4, which show the patterns obtained from sheep-erythrocyte lipids, which do not contain lecithin. Abbreviations: Ch, cholesterol; PE, phosphatidylethanolamine; PA, phosphatidic acid; PC, lecithin; PS, phosphatidylserine; Sp, sphingomyelin; PI, phosphatidylinositol; GL, glycosphingolipids; O, origin; H, heme pigments. [Reproduced from *Biochim. Biophys. Acta* **144**, 221–232 (1967).]

133–135), but these attempts have been unrewarding. The erythrocytes of different species are distinctly different in permeability (134); however, no exact correlation with lipid composition is possible, except that cells high in lecithin tend to be slightly more permeable to glycerol than those high in sphingomyelin (122, 135). The only firm conclusion to be drawn concerning the red-cell phospholipid distribution is that the sum of the choline-containing phospholipids is always between 40 and 60% of the total phospholipids, and the acidic phospholipids (primarily phosphatidylethanolamine and phosphatidylserine) contribute the rest of the total. The variation in the proportion of the glyceryl ether phospholipid to the diacyl type in the phosphatidylethanolamine fraction has not been studied in

Table VIII. Total Fatty Acid Composition of Normal Human Erythrocytes

Fatty Acid	Percentage of Total Fatty Acids[a]																	
	Year and Reference																	
	1962 (114)	1964 (32)	1964 (136)	1965 (31)	1965 (137)	1965 (138)	1967 (40)	1967 (139)	1967 (140)	1968 (43)	1968 (45)	1968 (51)	1968 (141)	1968 (142)	1968 (143)	1968 (144)	1968 (145)	1968 (146)
12:0	0.1	—	0.3	—	0.5	0.2	—	—	—	—	—	—	—	—	0.4	—	—	0.7
14:0	0.5	—	1.0	0.7	1.6	1.1	—	—	—	—	0.4	—	T	0.2	0.6	—	0.2	1.2
15:0	—	—	—	—	—	—	0.16	—	—	—	—	—	—	—	—	—	—	0.7
16:0	28.8	20	27.1	24.5	25.9	29.5	21.4	20.2	31.8	21.0	20.3	35.3	27.5	17.0	26.9	19.9	21.3	27.1
16:1	0.8	—	3.4	0.2	3.7	2.4	0.88	—	2.8	—	—	—	T	0.7	—	—	1.0	1.6
17:0	—	—	—	—	—	—	0.44	—	—	—	—	—	—	0.2	—	—	0.1	0.9
18:0	15.1	5	9.4	19.6	8.4	17.1	14.0	16.1	16.6	14.9	15.0	11.9	16.5	15.3	18.2	15.6	16.3	19.6
18:1	18.3	20	19.5	16.4	19.3	13.5	12.9	10.7	27.8	18.4	17.0	22.7	18.8	14.6	20.3	12.9	11.9	17.0
18:2	10.6	19	16.5	11.2	16.7	3.9	9.0	2.8	8.1	10.3	9.1	21.4	9	10.9	11.8	9.0	3.4	9.8
18:3	—	—	0.5	—	0.5	1.5	—	—	2.1	—	—	—	T	0.3	—	—	0.3	0.3
20:0	0.1	—	0.2	—	0.4	1.4	0.40	—	—	2.6	—	—	1.0	—	—	—	—	0.7
20:1	—	—	—	—	—	—	0.37	—	—	—	—	—	—	—	—	—	—	—
20:2	0.1	—	—	—	—	0.2	0.55	—	—	—	—	—	—	0.1	0.78	—	0.5	—
20:3	1.6	—	1.4	1.5	2.1	1.1	1.5	2.8	—	—	1.8	1.2	—	1.4	—	3.6	2.7	3.9
20:4	10.8	—	19.5	15.1	18.3	2.3	12.2	14.5	12.6	13.7	12.9	5.3	11.0	17.4	13.1	14.9	19.6	11.7
22:0	—	—	—	—	—	—	1.7	—	—	—	—	—	2.8	—	7.7	—	—	—
22:1	—	—	—	—	—	—	0.25	—	—	—	—	—	—	—	—	—	—	—
22:2	—	—	—	—	—	—	0.46	—	—	—	↑	—	—	—	—	—	—	—
22:4	—	—	—	—	—	—	2.6	13.2[b]	—	↑		—	↑	—	—	—	—	—
22:5	4.0	—	—	1.6	—	0.4	2.4	4.9	—		23.0	—	4.0	2.5	—	2.5	0.8	—
22:6	2.0	—	—	3.5	—	0.4	3.6	4.0	—	16.2		—	↓	4.8	—	5.0	6.6	3.1
24:0	—	—	—	2.4	—	2.1	3.7	3.6	—			—	4.2	4.9	—	4.2	5.5	—
24:1	—	—	—	3.3	—	2.1	3.8	—	—	↓	↓	—	5.2	2.6	—	7.6	3.4	—
Other	5.5	26	—	—	2.7	—	—	7.2	—	2.1	—	—	—	1.5	—	—	1.3	2.84

[a] A dash stands for "not reported in reference"; T stands for "trace, not reported as percentage in reference."

[b] Includes 24:1.

enough detail to permit any significant conclusion, but it is an interesting area for further exploration.

F. Fatty Acids

Fatty acid distribution in erythrocytes has been studied extensively, but work prior to 1963 is primarily of historical value, except that certain trends were established. The red-cell fatty acids are not unique. The fatty acid composition of the whole cell has only a small contribution from glycosphingolipids and reflects primarily the phospholipid fatty acid composition. Depending to some extent on the species studied, the major fatty acids in erythrocyte phospholipids are 16:0, 18:0, 18:1, 18:2, 20:3, 20:4, 22:5, 22:6, 24:0, and 24:1.

1. Human-Erythrocyte Fatty Acids. Table VIII lists some current values for the total fatty acid composition of human erythrocytes. The major fatty acids are typical of those found in the phospholipids of other human tissues. They differ significantly from the fatty acids found in plasma phospholipids (147, 148); plasma, of course, reflects the dietary intake of fatty acids more than other tissues.

Recent reports agree quite well (38, 40, 48, 117). Perhaps the most detailed report is that by Dodge and Phillips (40), which includes data on the positional isomers of the unsaturated fatty acids. A number of workers have studied the influence of dietary fats on the fatty acid composition of erythrocytes (59, 149, 150). Their reports are discussed in Section IV.

Tables IX, X, and XI present data on the fatty acid compositions of the individual phospholipids of the human erythrocyte. There is some variation among reports from different laboratories, but the overall pattern is similar in all cases, and each phospholipid has a distinct fatty acid composition.

Phosphatidylethanolamine and phosphatidylserine are less saturated than lecithin. Furthermore, phosphatidylserine contains 40% stearic acid and only 5% palmitic acid, whereas phosphatidylethanolamine contains 10 to 25% palmitic acid and only 10 to 15% stearic acid. Phosphatidylserine has only small amounts of 18-carbon unsaturated fatty acids like oleic and linoleic, which are relatively abundant in phosphatidylethanolamine. The biochemical significance of these differences is unknown, but they certainly represent an important aspect of lipid biochemistry.

Palmitic, stearic, and oleic acids contribute 50% of the total fatty acids of lecithin (Table X). Sphingomyelin contains very little polyunsaturated fatty acid (Table XI); early reports indicating otherwise (28, 31) may be attributed to experimental error. Palmitic, nervonic, and lignoceric acids

Table IX. Fatty Acid Composition of Phosphatidylethanolamine and Phosphatidylserine from Normal Human Erythrocytes

Fatty Acid	Percentage of Total Fatty Acids in Phosphatidylethanolamine[a]							Percentage of Total Fatty Acids in Phosphatidylserine[a]				
	Year and Reference							Year and Reference				
	1962 (114)	1965 (31)	1966 (38)	1967 (40)	1968 (141)	1968 (143)	1969 (117)	1962 (114)	1965 (31)	1966 (38)	1967 (40)	1968 (141)
12:0	—	—	0.4	—	—	1.4	—	—	—	0.9	—	—
14:0	0.2	0.3	0.2	—	—	2.3	—	—	0.3	2.4	—	—
15:0	0.2	—	0.3	—	—	—	—	—	—	2.6	—	—
16:0	18.9	24.4	12.6	12.9	18.3	27.5	16.6	7.1	4.9	12.5	2.7	13.7
16:1	0.6	2.1	0.9	—	0.7	4.2	—	0.4	1.0	0.2	—	0.8
17:0	—	—	0.2	0.33	1.5	—	—	0.3	—	1.0	0.4	3.5
18:0	8.0	12.0	8.0	11.5	13.0	17.1	11.2	41.6	46.4	11.3	37.5	26.5
18:1	25.2	18.3	20.2	18.1	23.5	21.7	15.6	13.0	5.4	19.1	7.8	20.0
18:2	7.0	2.5	7.6	7.1	6.5	7.5	4.7	2.8	1.4	6.2	1.8	4.2
18:3	—	—	0.1	—	—	—	—	—	—	—	—	—
20:0	—	—	1.4	0.3	2.0	0.9	—	—	—	0.7	0.3	3.0
20:1	0.3	—	—	0.7	—	—	1.5	—	—	—	0.4	—
20:2	0.1	1.2	—	1.3	—	—	—	—	0.8	—	0.8	—
20:3	1.0	2.4	0.5	1.5	2.8	—	1.3	2.1	—	0.8	2.6	3.5
20:4	21.9	20.0	26.4	23.7	18.4	16.4	24.8	19.7	21.7	22.0	24.2	16.8
22:0	—	—	—	—	2.0	0.9	—	—	2.6	0.3	—	—
22:1	—	—	0.4	—	—	—	—	—	—	0.4	—	—
22:2	—	—	—	1.2	—	—	—	—	—	—	0.3	—
22:4	—	1.9	7.3	7.5	↑	—	7.6	—	3.5	8.1	4.0	
22:5	3.1	8.6	4.3	5.3	11.3	—	7.0	2.9	—	5.2	4.9	8.0
22:6	3.9	—	7.5	8.2	↓	—	5.1	4.2	7.6	5.0	10.1	
24:0	—	6.3	0.3	0.3		—	—	—	4.3	0.6	—	—
24:1	—	—	—	—	—	—	—	—	—	—	—	—
Other	6.1	—	0.5	0.2	—	—	1.8	2.5	—	—	0.5	—

	Percentage of Total Fatty Acids in[a]											
	Lecithin									Lysolecithin		Phosphatidylinositol
Fatty Acid	1962 (114)	1965 (31)	1966 (38)	1967 (40)	1967 (151)	1968 (152)	1968 (143)	1969 (117)	1969 (153)	1966 (38)	1968 (141)	1966 (38)
12:0	0.1	—	0.4	—	—	—	0.7	—	—	2.7	—	0.7
14:0	0.5	0.6	0.5	—	0.2	0.7	1.8	—	0.5	3.8	—	0.8
15:0	0.3	—	0.2	—	—	0.2	—	—	0.4	3.1	—	2.7
16:0	33.0	39.0	33.0	31.2	33.7	30.5	28.1	33.6	32.9	48.9	47.0	10.5
16:1	1.0	1.8	1.4	—	2.4	5.4	2.7	—	1.0	2.5	4.0	0.8
17:0	0.5	—	0.5	0.7	—	—	—	—	—	1.3	2.0	1.0
18:0	11.7	10.4	9.8	11.8	13.5	11.6	20.9	12.7	13.6	7.7	26.0	24.3
18:1	20.3	17.5	18.9	18.9	18.4	21.8	25.3	19.7	17.8	15.4	12.0	13.5
18:2	18.2	7.0	23.5	22.8	23.1	22.6	11.3	22.8	16.1	14.0	1.0	4.6
18:3	—	—	—	—	0.3	—	—	—	—	—	—	—
20:0	0.2	—	0.2	0.2	—	—	2.1	—	—	3.9	5.0	8.0
20:1	0.2	—	—	0.5	—	0.4	1.3	0.3	0.3	—	—	—
20:2	0.2	—	0.1	1.1	—	—	—	—	0.8	—	—	0.9
20:3	1.6	3.7	1.4	1.9	2.1	1.3	—	1.9	2.0	1.3	1.0	2.1
20:4	5.0	13.8	6.3	6.7	6.3	5.5	5.4	6.2	9.3	0.6	—	21.1
22:0	—	—	—	—	—	—	0.9	—	0.6	0.5	—	0.4
22:1	—	—	—	—	—	—	—	—	—	—	—	0.1
22:2	—	—	—	0.3	—	—	—	—	—	—	—	—
22:4	—	1.1	0.6	0.4	—	—	—	0.3	0.4	—	—	3.4
22:5	5.4	4.0	0.9	0.8	—	—	—	0.8	0.6	—	(b)	1.7
22:6	1.1	1.4	2.1	2.1	—	—	—	1.2	2.0	—	(b)	2.3
24:0	—	—	—	—	—	—	—	—	—	0.9	—	1.1
24:1	—	—	0.2	—	—	—	—	—	0.2	1.3	—	—
Other	0.8	—	—	0.2	—	—	—	0.5	0.9	2.1	—	—

[a] A dash stands for "not reported in reference."
[b] Combined value for 22:5 and 22:6 listed as 2.0% (141).

Table XI. Fatty Acid Composition of Sphingomyelin from Normal Human Erythrocytes

	Percentage of Total Fatty Acids in Sphingomyelin[a]					
	Year and Reference					
Fatty Acid	1965 (31)	1966 (38)	1967 (40)	1968 (143)	1968 (152)	1968 (154)
12:0	—	—	—	1.1	—	—
14:0	1.2	—	—	1.5	1.4	—
15:0	—	0.5	—	—	0.2	—
16:0	44.9	45.7	23.6	29.8	15.0	36.3
16:1	0.7	1.1	—	1.5	3.7	—
17:0	0.5	0.6	0.6	—	—	—
18:0	12.9	7.3	5.7	18.9	8.7	11.0
18:1	7.4	1.1	0.8	18.6	8.6	6.0
18:2	—	0.3	0.2	6.4	—	3.8
20:0	2.8	1.3	1.9	—	1.3	1.1
20:1	—	—	0.2	—	0.7	1.8
21:0	—	—	—	1.7	—	—
22:0	5.5	8.7	9.5	—	10.1	7.2
22:1	—	—	—	—	4.1	—
23:0	—	0.9	2.0	—	2.0	—
23:1	—	—	—	—	0.4	—
24:0	14.4	17.1	22.8	10.5	15.5	14.4
24:1	11.9	15.4	24.0	10.2	24.2	16.8
26:0	—	—	1.0	—	—	—
26:1	—	—	14.0	—	—	—
Other	2.4	—	5.6	—	3.6	1.1

[a] A dash stands for "not reported in reference."

account for 70% of the total fatty acids of sphingomyelin from human erythrocytes (40, 154). Dodge and Phillips (40) report that the 24:0 and 24:1 fatty acids of human-erythrocyte phospholipids occur exclusively in the sphingomyelin fraction.

The fatty acid compositions of the minor phospholipids, such as phosphatidylinositol, lysolecithin, phosphatidic acid, and lysophosphatidylethanolamine, have not been studied as frequently as the major phospholipids of human erythrocytes. Soula et al. (141) report data indicating that the fatty acid compositions of lysolecithin and lysophosphatidylethanolamine are similar to those of the diacyl lipids but are more saturated.

Current advances in methodology, such as those discussed in earlier chapters of this volume and elsewhere (155), allow the analysis of the individual molecular species of each class of phospholipid. Van Golde et al. (151) and Marai and Kuksis (153) recently reported data on the composition of the molecular species in lecithin from human erythrocytes. Both reports indicate that lecithin molecules with a saturated fatty acid in position 1 usually contain an unsaturated fatty acid in position 2. Saturated fatty acids are uncommon in position 2. The major species with

Table XII. Major Molecular Species of Lecithin in Human, Rat, and Rabbit Erythrocytes

Fatty Acids		Quantity (mole %)[a]			
		Species and Reference			
		Man		Rat	Rabbit
1[b]	2[c]	(151)	(153)	(156)	(153)
16:0	16:0	9.5	4.2	20.2	10.3
18:0	16:0	3.7	1.3	4.3	3.0
16:0	16:1	1.8	—	—	1.0
16:0	18:1	14.0	27.2	14.5	19.5
18:0	16:1	1.8	—	—	1
18:0	18:1	4.4	5.5	4.4	3.4
18:1	18:1	4.8	2.3	0.8	—
16:0	18:2	20.4	19.5	12.4	24.0
18:0	18:2	11.3	8.5	5.6	17.8
18:1	18:2	9.3	1.4	0.7	8.2
16:0	18:3	1.0	—	—	2.8
18:0	18:3	1.0	—	—	
16:0	20:3	3.5	2.1	0.4	4.1
18:0	20:3	1.3	0.5	0.3	
16:0	20:4	6.6	8.5	5.4	2.0
18:0	20:4	3.4	3.6	7.5	1.4
18:1	20:3	—	0.4	0.8	—
18:2	18:2	—	0.6	2.7	—
16:0	20:5	—	0.8	0.5	—
18:1	20:4	—	1.1	0.8	—
16:0	22:6	—	2.7	4.0	—
18:0	22:6	—	0.6	2.3	—
18:2	20:4	—	0.7	3.0	—

[a] Values are estimated best fit only, not absolute identities or proportions.
[b] Fatty acids in position 1 of the lecithin molecule.
[c] Fatty acids in position 2 of the lecithin molecule.

Table XIII. Fatty Acid Composition of Total Erythrocyte Lipids from Rats, Sheep, and Chickens

	Percentage of Total Fatty Acids[a]											
	Species and Reference[b]											
	Rat							Sheep				Chicken
Fatty Acid	(158)	(159)	(135)	(160)	(139)	(44)	(161)	(162)	(163)	(135)	(164)	(69)
12:0	0.7	—	—	—	—	—	—	0.6	—	—	—	0.2
14:0	1.4	0.5	—	—	—	—	—	1.6	0.6	—	—	—
16:0	20.6	40.7	28.7	24.4	25.0	29.2	27.0	16.0	13.0	15.7	8.7	28.7
16:1	2.3	2.7	1.8	0.3	—	4.1	—	2.3	1.3	1.6	0.6	0.8
17:0	—	0.6	—	—	—	—	—	—	—	—	0.9	0.1
18:0	9.8	16.1	12.1	16.9	15.7	17.9	11.2	9.7	18.7	9.6	8.3	8.8
18:1	16.9	18.6	14.5	8.3	11.7	11.7	12.3	49.6	45.8	52.3	40.3	21.7
18:2	4.3	3.6	6.4	10.6	5.7	10.8	10.0	11.5	10.3	14.6	8.5	31.8
18:3	—	0.1	—	—	—	—	2.9	0.7	1.0	—	—	1.0
20:0	0.3	—	—	—	—	—	1.1	0.9	1.7	—	1.2	—
20:2	0.1	—	—	—	—	—	—	—	0.9	—	—	—
20:3	5.1	—	—	—	—	—	—	1.9	—	—	—	0.6
20:4	24.5	15.3	33.8	30.9	24.5	26.4	12.5	1.4	1.3	2.9	—	4.6
22:0	—	—	—	—	—	—	1.9	—	—	—	1.8	—
22:4	—	—	—	3.8	5.9	—	8.9	—	—	—	—	—
22:5	0.3	—	—	1.8	1.9	—	1.4	—	—	—	—	1.2
24:0	5.0	—	—	—	1.7	—	2.0	—	—	—	2.0	3.2
24:1	0.8	—	—	—	1.6	—	0.9	—	—	—	16.3	—
25:0	—	—	—	—	—	—	—	—	—	—	1.8	—
Other	22.5	—	—	—	6.3	—	7.9	3.7	5.6	—	9.6	—

[a] A dash stands for "not reported in reference."

[b] Data are arranged in chronological sequence from left to right.

two saturated fatty acids is dipalmitoyl lecithin; however, palmitic acid is usually associated with oleic or linoleic acid. No distearoyl lecithin was detected.

Marai and Kuksis (153) indicated that 90% or more of the total saturated fatty acids of lecithin is located in position 1. Except for a small amount of linoleic acid in position 1, all the polyunsaturated fatty acids are located in position 2.

Table XII summarizes the data on position distribution of molecular species found in human-erythrocyte lecithin. This table (modified, with permission, from Ref. 153) also presents data on the molecular species of lecithin in rat and rabbit erythrocytes for further comparison. Note that the major molecular species are similar in human, rat, and rabbit erythrocytes.

The biological significance of the fatty acid distribution in lecithin is unknown. However, according to Trewhella and Collins (157), the molecular species of lecithin have distinctly different turnover rates in the liver; hence it is possible that each specific molecular species has a separate function.

2. Fatty Acid Compositions of Animal Erythrocytes. The fatty-acid compositions of erythrocytes from various species differ quantitatively, but not qualitatively, from those of human erythrocytes. Tables XIII and XIV list some current data on the fatty acid composition of erythrocytes in a number of species.

In general carnivores and omnivores have more unsaturated fatty acids in their erythrocyte lipids than do herbivores. The rat erythrocyte is exceptionally high in arachidonic acid (158, 170). In ruminants the polyunsaturated fatty-acid content of the erythrocytes is reduced, the content of monounsaturated acids being proportionally increased (164). The hydrogenating bacteria in the rumens of ruminants may limit the availability of dietary polyunsaturated fatty acids.

Data on the fatty acid composition of individual erythrocyte phospholipids in various species are limited. Van Deenen and co-workers (162, 171) reported data for individual phospholipids in several species, but they only listed values for a few fatty acids and grouped all the acidic lipids under a "cephalin" heading. Most reports have been restricted to a single species (125, 132, 161, 163, 168) or a few species (44, 172). Nelson (164) recently reported a detailed study of sheep erythrocytes. It is apparent that each phospholipid has a characteristic fatty acid composition. Tables XV, XVI, and XVII summarize some of the recent data on the fatty acid composition of the major phospholipids in several common species.

The acidic lipids, such as phosphatidylserine, phosphatidylethanolamine,

Table XIV. Fatty Acid Composition of Total Erythrocyte Lipids from Various Species

Fatty Acid	Percentage of Total Fatty Acids[a] — Species and Reference: Guinea Pig			Rabbit		Monkey		Dog		Pig	Ox	Hamster	Cat	Mink
	(72)	(165)	(135)	(135)	(132)	(166)	(167)	(135)	(65)	(135)	(135)	(168)	(135)	(169)
12:0	—	—	—	—	0.4	0.3	—	—	—	—	—	—	—	0.1
14:0	—	—	—	—	—	—	—	—	0.8	—	—	—	—	0.4
15:0	—	—	—	—	—	—	—	—	—	—	—	—	—	0.2
16:0	11.1	9.9	16.1	22.3	23.5	15.6	23.8	16.9	19.1	21.4	12.1	19.0	20.1	20.5
16:1	—	0.7	2.6	3.3	1.8	0.5	2.2	1.7	1.6	2.4	2.7	4.9	2.6	0.8
17:0	—	—	—	—	—	—	—	—	—	—	—	—	—	0.5
18:0	27.4	37.3	26.6	10.5	11.7	15.2	15.3	19.0	27.4	10.4	14.1	14.7	17.8	20.0
18:1	7.0	9.8	12.3	11.8	17.9	15.7	13.4	14.2	14.5	32.1	34.5	22.6	11.0	15.8
18:2	19.5	9.1	15.7	32.0	25.5	11.0	14.5	12.9	10.7	23.2	21.1	18.1	21.5	11.3
18:3	—	—	—	—	1.7	—	—	—	—	—	—	1.1	—	0.8
20:0	—	—	—	—	—	—	—	—	—	—	—	—	—	0.2
20:2	—	—	—	—	0.7	—	—	—	—	—	—	—	—	0.1
20:3	2.8	1.5	—	—	1.7	1.0	1.8	—	—	—	—	—	—	0.8
20:4	23.2	19.3	16.1	6.6	7.6	12.3	25.0	30.8	22.8	6.4	4.8	19.0	18.5	22.2
22:4	10.2	—	—	—	1.0	4.2	—	—	—	—	—	—	—	1.5
22:5	—	2.5	—	—	0.5	10.8	—	—	—	—	—	—	—	0.8
24:0	—	1.6	—	—	2.4	—	—	—	—	—	—	—	—	1.7
24:1	—	—	—	—	0.5	—	—	—	—	—	—	—	—	0.4
Other	—	—	—	—	1.4	—	3.4	—	—	—	—	—	—	2.6

[a] A dash stands for "not reported in reference."

Table XV. Fatty Acid Composition of Lecithin in the Erythrocytes of Various Species

Fatty Acid	Percentage of Total Fatty Acids in Lecithin[a]							
	Species and Reference							
	Rat				Rabbit		Cow	Pig
	(62)	(126)	(125)	(156)	(151)	(132)	(16)	(16)
14:0	0.4	—	—	0.4	—	2.3	—	—
15:0	0.5	—	—	—	—	0.5	—	—
16:0	38.8	45.7	53.3	42.3	33.6	34.9	34.9	22.7
16:1	1.1	0.8	—	1.0	—	—	—	3.5
17:0	0.9	—	—	—	—	—	—	—
18:0	18.0	30.3	14.7	13.0	16.9	10.1	31.9	23.9
18:1	10.3	5.1	8.0	12.7	15.3	18.2	20.2	21.6
18:2	13.8	6.7	14.5	13.7	27.4	23.8	10.5	22.0
18:3	—	—	—	—	2.5	1.0	—	—
20:2	—	—	—	0.6	—	0.8	—	—
20:3	—	—	—	1.0	1.5	1.2	—	—
20:4	7.7	5.7	6.3	8.9	2.8	4.8	—	6.2
20:5	—	—	—	1.3	—	1.5	—	—
22:0	—	—	—	0.4	—	—	—	—
22:5	—	—	—	1.3	—	—	—	—
22:6	—	—	—	3.3	—	—	—	—
24:0	4.6	—	—	—	—	0.8	—	—
24:1	3.8	—	—	—	—	—	—	—
Other	—	4.0	—	0.3	2.5	—	—	—

[a] A dash stands for "not reported in reference."

and phosphatidylinositol, tend to be more unsaturated than the neutral phospholipids. This is true regardless of the overall degree of unsaturation present in the erythrocyte. In sheep erythrocytes, for instance, phosphatidylserine and phosphatidylethanolamine carry essentially all of the polyunsaturated fatty acids. Phosphatidylserine, regardless of the species, is always characterized by a low palmitate, and a high stearate, content. Apparently the palmitic acid is replaced by longer chain polyunsaturated fatty acids like 20:4 and 22:6. In sheep erythrocytes, in which the majority of the phosphatidylethanolamine molecules are of the alkyl ether variety (164), oleic acid accounts for more than 75% of the total phosphatidylethanolamine fatty acids and is located in the 2-position. The glycerol ether has not yet been determined, but presumably it has a saturated hydrocarbon residue.

Kuksis et al. (156) and Van Golde et al. (151) analyzed the molecular

Table XVI. Fatty Acid Composition of Various Phospholipids in the Erythrocytes of Various Species[a]

	Percentage of Total Fatty Acids in [b,c]								
	Phosphatidylethanolamine			Phosphatidylserine			Lysolecithin, Rat		Phosphatidylinositol, Sheep
Fatty Acid	Rat (125)	Rabbit (132)	Sheep (164)	Rabbit (132)	Sheep (164)	Pig (173)	(62)	(126)	(164)
12:0	—	—	—	—	—	—	0.3	—	—
14:0	—	0.3	—	1.2	—	—	1.5	—	—
15:0	—	0.2	—	0.1	—	—	1.0	—	—
16:0	14.9	24.2	2.1	5.5	6.4	5.3	22.0	16.1	9.6
16:1	—	0.1	1.1	—	—	—	4.0	5.9	—
17:0	—	0.3	—	0.7	—	—	1.1	—	—
18:0	11.7	10.0	79.5	23.2	19.3	31.4	33.7	15.8	28.7
18:1	16.0	21.4	8.8	12.2	49.6	54.5	9.4	9.3	33.0
18:2	7.4	27.2	—	31.1	17.1	5.2	6.3	0.6	12.5
18:3	—	—	—	3.7	—	0.6	1.2	—	—
20:0	—	—	1.6	—	1.5	1.5	1.1	—	2.7
20:2	—	0.5	—	2.2	—	—	—	—	—
20:3	—	0.6	—	2.1	—	—	1.1	—	—
20:4	50.0	7.4	—	11.1	—	0.9	3.1	—	—
20:5	—	0.8	—	0.4	—	—	—	—	—
22:0	—	—	1.1	—	1.2	—	1.5	—	2.5
22:4	—	1.2	—	0.6	—	—	—	—	—
22:5	—	0.5	—	0.3	—	—	—	—	—
22:6	—	2.1	—	2.7	—	—	—	—	—
Other	—	1.1	5.9	—	4.9	—	10.5	—	11.0

[a] See Tables XV and XVII for the fatty acid composition of erythrocyte lecithin and sphingomyelin, respectively.
[b] The reference number is shown below the name of the species.
[c] A dash stands for "not reported in reference."

species of rat and rabbit erythrocyte lecithin, respectively (see Table XII). Their reports are essentially in agreement, except for relatively minor quantitative differences, and indicate that the same molecular species exist in both animals and are similar to those found in man. These data, along with the total fatty acid composition of the individual phospholipids, suggest that each phospholipid is associated with specific fatty acids regardless of species (and tissue). This in turn supports the idea that each phospholipid has a specific function or a specific synthetic pathway that may or may not be related to its function in the membrane.

G. Fatty Aldehydes

The fatty aldehyde composition of human erythrocytes has been studied by several investigators (40, 114, 117). Farquhar (114) reported that the major fatty aldehydes were palmitaldehyde and stearaldehyde and their monounsaturated homologs. More recent reports (40, 117) suggest

Table XVII. Fatty Acid Composition of Sphingomyelin from the Erythrocytes of Various Species

Fatty Acid	Percentage of Total Fatty Acids in Sphingomyelin[a] — Species and Reference: Rat (62)	Rat (126)	Rabbit (132)	Cow (79)	Sheep (164)
12:0	0.4	—	—	—	—
14:0	1.5	—	1.1	—	—
15:0	1.1	—	1.2	—	—
16:0	32.9	17.2	23.9	40.0	20.6
16:1	3.0	4.5	0.3	1.0	—
17:0	1.4	—	0.4	—	—
18:0	21.1	21.6	11.7	4.0	2.9
18:1	7.5	6.9	9.6	1.0	1.5
18:2	4.0	4.8	4.2	4.0	—
20:0	1.1	—	1.3	—	1.0
20:1	—	—	1.6	—	—
22:0	4.3	—	3.5	—	2.7
22:1	—	—	1.2	—	1.1
23:0	—	—	1.7	—	1.3
23:1	—	—	—	—	1.9
24:0	11.2	—	4.3	31.0	5.6
24:1	4.9	—	21.8	10.0	52.3
25:0	—	—	—	—	1.8
Other	5.1	36.8	6.1	13.0	7.2

[a] A dash stands for "not reported in reference."

that the amount of plasmalogens in human erythrocytes is somewhat lower than that originally reported (114). Table XVIII lists some current values for the fatty aldehyde composition of human erythrocytes.

Kates and James (69) reported the fatty aldehyde composition of fowl erythrocytes. Hanahan et al. (113) and Thompson and Hanahan (175) gave values for the hydrocarbon moiety of the glyceryl ether in bovine erythrocytes and bone marrow, respectively. More recent reports are lacking. Since the ether phospholipids are located primarily in the ethanolamine fraction, analysis of the total erythrocyte lipids is adequate for characterizing this group. The data suggest that the hydrocarbon residues in the glyceryl ethers are saturated 16- and 18-carbon compounds. If a double bond is present in the molecule, it is usually in the 18-carbon chain in the Δ^{9-10}-position. Much further work is necessary to elucidate the functional significance of the alkyl and alk-1-enyl phospholipids. Only

Table XVIII. Fatty Aldehyde Composition of Normal Human Erythrocytes

	Percentage of Total Fatty Aldehydes[a]				
	Year and Reference				
Fatty Aldehyde	1961 (69)	1962 (114)	1967 (40)	1968 (48)	1969 (174)[b]
15:0	1.4	2.2	—	—	—
16:0	24.2	19.3	30.9	30.9	24.4
16:1	0.4	0.2	—	—	—
18:0	42.5	44.1	49.2	69.1	53.1
18:1	8.8	20.7	18.3	—	18.1
20:0	5.6	—	0.8	—	—
20:1	5.1	—	0.8	—	—
Other	13.4	13.5	—	—	4.4

[a] A dash stands for "not reported in reference."
[b] Data for phosphatidylethanolamine only.

recently Snyder and co-workers (176–178) demonstrated the primary metabolic pathways for the synthesis of these compounds.

III. METABOLISM OF LIPIDS IN ERYTHROCYTES

A. Lipid Synthesis in Erythrocytes

There is no net synthesis of the major lipids in mature cells (57, 179–182), and no catabolism of the membrane lipids (183, 184). This does not imply that the red-cell lipids are entirely static during the lifespan of the cell. Exchange of red-cell lipids is well documented (185–188) and is discussed further below. In addition, a limited amount of metabolic activity has been demonstrated in the cellular lipids (80, 189–191), but it generally involves modification of intact lipids rather than de novo synthesis.

Carbon from glucose or acetate is not incorporated into the lipids (including the fatty acid chains, the glycerol moiety, and cholesterol) of the mature erythrocyte under any conditions (181, 192, 193). Pittman and Martin (194) detected the remnants of a *de novo* fatty-acid-synthesizing system in human red cells. It could convert acetate to palmitic acid when acetyl-coenzyme A carboxylase was added to mature cells *in vitro*. Palmitate synthetase and acetyl-coenzyme A synthetase were found in the red cell.

Some early reports of fatty acid oxidation in mature erythrocytes (195, 196) were found to be in error by Rosenzweig and Ways (183), who attribute the error to the contamination of cell preparations with leukocytes. No metabolic breakdown of the carbon skeleton of the lipids has been demonstrated in mature erythrocytes.

B. Incorporation of Inorganic Phosphorus into Erythrocyte Phospholipids

Incorporation of inorganic phosphorus-32 into the phospholipids of mature erythrocytes is still a subject of controversy. The earliest investigations found no evidence that red cells could incorporate inorganic phosphate into their phospholipids (197–199). Agren and Ronquist (200), however, reported some incorporation into glycerylphosphorylcholine (GPC) and glycerylphosphorylethanolamine (GPE) when whole cells were incubated with inorganic phosphate. It was not clear from their data whether the labeled GPC and GPE were actually derived from the phospholipids of the cell; the existence of free GPC and GPE in the cell has not been established.

Hokin and Hokin (189) found that human-red-cell ghosts incorporated phosphorus-32 into phosphatidic acid as well as diphosphoinositol and triphosphoinositol when incubated in the presence of adenosine triphosphate (ATP) labeled in the terminal phosphate. They found no labeling of the major phospholipids of the ghosts, including monophosphoinositol. They suggested that the labeling of phosphatidic acid reflected a diglyceride kinase reaction, but the mechanism of the diphosphoinositol and triphosphoinositol labeling was not apparent. This work suggests that the red cell can synthesize these compounds *in vivo,* since ATP is readily available.

Westerman and Jensen (201) also confirmed the labeling of phosphatidic acid in mature erythrocytes. Paysant and co-workers (202, 203) found similar patterns of phosphate incorporation; their phosphatidic acid accumulated label 50 to 100 times more rapidly than did the inositol phosphatides. Thus from the 1950s to 1964 it was generally held that phosphate was incorporated only into the phosphatidic acid and polyphosphoinositols of the mature cell. These are very minor cellular components, whose physiological roles are probably very different from those of the major lipids of the cell membrane.

In 1965 Grossman et al. (204) published data indicating that red-cell phosphatidylethanolamine did indeed incorporate inorganic phosphorus-32 *in vitro* when incubated in a plasma-free medium. They suggested that plasma the incubation medium used by most previous investigators, inhibited the reaction. In a later publication Grossman et al. (205) elaborated some of the conditions necessary for incorporation *in vitro* into mature erythrocytes. It should be noted that the overall level of incorporation reported (204,

205) was very low in comparison with those observed in other tissues, such as liver or leukocytes.

Jacobs and Karnovsky (41) observed the *in vitro* incorporation of inorganic phosphate into the phospholipids of red cells obtained from normal human subjects and patients with hereditary spherocytosis. The diseased cells had a significantly higher rate of incorporation than did the normal ones. Phosphatidylserine and phosphatidic acid were the most highly labeled fractions, but again the total amount incorporated was small. Hence the picture was confusing, since earlier work showed no significant incorporation into any major phospholipid, and later Grossman (204, 205) and Jacobs and Karnovsky (41) published conflicting reports on whether phosphatidylserine or phosphatidylethanolamine was labeled.

Nelson (206) concluded that sheep erythrocytes incorporate inorganic phosphate only into phosphatidic acid and some other unidentified substances present in trace amounts. Figure 4 shows the TLC pattern of sheep-erythrocyte phospholipids, along with a radioautograph made from the TLC plate, from cells that had been incubated with inorganic phosphorus-32. It is obvious that the phosphorus-32 activity is not associated with any of the major phospholipids of the cell. Only phosphatidic acid had enough radioactivity to darken the film. Absolutely no label could be detected in either the phosphatidylethanolamine or the phosphatidylserine fraction. The pattern of incorporation was very similar to that found by Hokin and Hokin (189) for human erythrocytes.

In a study resembling that of Jacobs and Karnovsky (41) Reed (71) also used red cells from normal individuals and patients with hereditary spherocytocis. He could not confirm their results but in fact substantially duplicated the findings of Hokin and Hokin (189). He could suggest no obvious reason for the discrepancy between his results and those reported by Jacobs and Karnovsky. Furthermore, he found no labeling of phosphatidylserine, phosphatidylethanolamine, or lecithin, thus failing to confirm the report of Grossman et al. (205).

After reviewing these papers, I conclude that the preponderance of evidence supports the contention that mature mammalian erythrocytes do not incorporate inorganic phosphate into their major phospholipids in detectable amounts.

In vivo, de novo synthesis of red cells occurs in the marrow. Soula and associates (207) and Misra (208) followed the incorporation of phosphate into the newly formed red cells of rabbits and chickens, respectively. Red cells can also be labeled *in vivo* by exchange reactions with plasma and tissue phospholipids. Soula et al. (207) found that the inositol phospholipids are labeled most rapidly, then lecithin, then the acidic lipids.

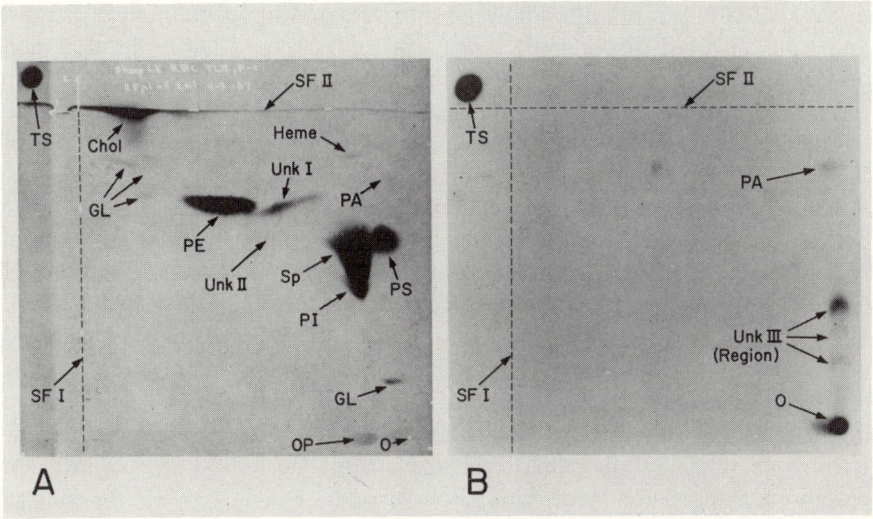

Fig. 4 (*A*) Thin-layer chromatography separation of the total-lipid extract from sheep erythrocytes after a 4-hr incubation with inorganic phosphate ^{32}P; (*B*) the radioautograph of the same sample prepared concurrently and exposed for 4 weeks. Spots were visualized by charring in (*A*). It is obvious that the major phospholipids of the sheep erythrocyte do not incorporate inorganic phosphate to any appreciable extent *in vitro*. Unk I in (*A*) has been identified as *N*-acylphosphatidylserine (see text). Solvents: chloroform–methanol–aqueous ammonia, 65 : 25 : 5 (by volume), and chloroform–methanol–acetone–acetic acid–water, 5 : 2 : 1 : 1 : 0.5 (by volume). Abbreviations: SF, solvent front; TS, total sample spot; Chol, cholesterol; Unk, unknown or identified; GL, glycosphingolipids; PA, phosphatidic acid; PE, phosphatidylethanolamine; Sp, sphingomyelin; PS, phosphatidylserine; PI, phosphatidylinositol; O, origin; OP, oxidation products. [Reproduced from *Lipids* **4**, 350–355 (1969).]

Sphingomyelin is labeled least rapidly. This sequence is common for other tissues besides erythrocytes.

C. Exchange of Cholesterol

The exchange of lipids between red cells and plasma was first reported by Hagerman and Gould (209) in 1951. They incubated red cells and plasma containing ^{14}C-labeled cholesterol with unlabeled plasma or red cells and found rapid equilibration of the labeled cholesterol in both systems. London and Schwarz (210) later demonstrated the same mechanism *in vivo*. Other authors have confirmed these results (211–213).

More recently Green and co-workers (214–217) found rapid exchange of red-cell cholesterol with whole plasma, isolated lipoprotein subfractions, and artificial lipid dispersions. Ashworth and Green (214) reported that only a portion of the cholesterol in human α-lipoproteins exchanges with red-cell cholesterol, and Basford, Glover, and Green (186) found that all of the β-lipoprotein cholesterol was exchangeable, but in both cases all of the erythrocyte cholesterol was exchanged.

In a later work Bruckdorfer and Green (216) found the exchange mechanism to be dependent on pH, but not on temperature. This would indicate that the phenomenon is not simply a collision displacement process. Organic solvents greatly increased the exchange rate. Bruckdorfer et al. (217) noted that if the plasma or source of cholesterol to be exchanged with the cell is deficient in cholesterol, the cells lose cholesterol to the medium. In another paper Bruckdorfer, Graham, and Green (218) found that cholesta-4,6-dien-3-one could be exchanged with erythrocyte cholesterol more rapidly than cholesterol itself. Most steroids, however, are not readily exchanged for membrane cholesterol.

Bruckdorfer and co-workers also noted that cholesterol-deficient cells removed cholesterol from β-lipoproteins only when dimethyl sulfoxide was added to the medium. This suggests different bonding arrangements for cholesterol in α- and β-lipoproteins. Bruckdorfer and co-workers (219) also replaced red-cell cholesterol with several other steroids. The rate of replacement as well as the amount accepted by the cell varied with the compound. The replacement of the cellular cholesterol had only a small effect on the osmotic fragility of the cell.

The conclusions to be derived from these studies are (a) the cholesterol in the cell readily exchanges with plasma or tissue in a 1 : 1 ratio, provided that neither the cell nor the plasma is deficient in cholesterol, and (b) the process is not energy dependent but is related to the architecture of the membrane. In the cellular exchange of cholesterol equilibrium is reached in 8 hr *in vitro* and may be more rapid *in vivo*. The function of the exchange is unknown, but the rapidity of the process suggests that the cholesterol molecule is readily exposed on the cell surface.

D. Exchange of Phospholipids

The phospholipids as well as the cholesterol in the erythrocyte can exchange with plasma lipoproteins. Sakagami, Minari, and Orii (185) demonstrated that most of the phospholipids in the rat erythrocyte exchange *in vitro* at a rate that varies with the individual phospholipid. Klibansky and De Vries (220) observed that lysolecithin exchanges very rapidly between cells and plasma; lecithin and sphingomyelin exchange more slowly, and the acidic phospholipids show little or no exchange capability.

The exchange of lecithin is a complicated and perhaps step-wise reaction, which may have two independent pathways. The lecithin:cholesterol acyltransferase reaction described by Glomset (83) may be operative (see Chapter 14) and may be the source of cellular lysolecithin. A number of investigators have reported that no phospholipase A activity can be detected in mature erythrocytes (190, 221, 222). Sakagami and associates (185) could not detect, in the rat, any conversion of labeled serum lysolecithin into erythrocyte lecithin. Similar results were obtained by Soula et al. (223), who studied the exchange of phospholipids between rabbit plasma and erythrocytes; they also noted that lecithin exchanged primarily with the β-lipoproteins. The general order was lysolecithin $>$ lecithin $\gg$ acidic phospholipids $\gg$ sphingomyelin.

Reed (188) recently investigated the *in vitro* exchange of phospholipids between erythrocytes and plasma in samples from humans and dogs. Besides confirming most of the previous findings (185, 223) he reported that phosphatidylserine is not exchanged, undoubtedly due to its absence from plasma. Phosphatidylethanolamine is exchanged only very slowly; it is present in small amounts in plasma (127, 224, 225). Lecithin and sphingomyelin are exchanged at significantly different rates (lecithin much more rapidly), but both reached equilibrium in 5 days, because of the smaller sphingomyelin pool. A certain fraction of the erythrocyte lecithin and sphingomyelin did not participate in the exchange reactions; Reed (188) assumed that only intact molecules are involved in the reactions. The significance of the exchange is unknown, but this phenomenon may be important in the diseased states discussed in Section IV.

E. Fatty Acid Exchange

Fatty acids cannot be synthesized in the mature red cell, but animals fed diets high in a particular fatty acid show rapid incorporation of the dietary fatty acids into the circulating cell *in vivo* (32, 116, 149, 226–228). This incorporation cannot be explained by the release of newly matured cells into the circulation.

Horwitt, Harvey, and Century (226) had observed that the linoleic acid of human red cells could be doubled over a 2-year period in subjects eating a corn-oil supplemental diet; they assumed that the changes were due solely to the incorporation of linoleic acid into newly formed cells. Leibetseder and Ahrens (227) confirmed this result but noted that erythrocytes showed changes in their total fatty acid composition within 10 days after patients had been placed on the diet. Hill et al. (32) reported changes within 8 days. These results proved that *de novo* synthesis of new erythrocytes could not be the only cause of the altered fatty acid composition, since the average lifespan of human erythrocytes is 120 days. Farquhar and Ahrens (149) reported that total equilibrium between the diet and circulating erythrocytes was established within 6 weeks; the red cells equilibrated somewhat more slowly than plasma but more rapidly than adipose tissue. Like the other workers (32, 116), Farquhar and Ahrens could detect no changes in the amount of lipid in the cell.

Whereas Farquhar and Ahrens assumed that all the phospholipids participated in the fatty acid turnover, Hill and co-workers (32) found that only lecithin was involved in short-term fatty acid exchange. They suggested that a specific reaction involving red-cell lecithin and plasma fatty acids was responsible for the changes observed in short-term feeding studies. The general shift in fatty acid composition observed by Farquhar and Ahrens (149) probably involved both exchange with plasma and synthesis of new blood cells, because their subject was followed for longer periods. Farquhar (228) also reported that human-erythrocyte lecithin was strongly affected by diet on short-term feeding, and furthermore, only the unsaturated fatty acids were affected. He suggested that the exchange mechanism could be either the substitution of a diacyl precursor of specific fatty acid composition or a deacylation and reacylation within the cell by the mechanism proposed by Robertson and Lands (222).

Oliveira and Vaughan (190) demonstrated *in vitro* that only lecithin participated in fatty acid exchange when washed erythrocytes were incubated with free fatty acids, ATP, and coenzyme A. Washed sheep cells, which contain no lecithin, did not incorporate fatty acids under identical conditions. They also found that linoleic acid was preferentially incorporated into the red-cell lecithin; this they assumed was related to the specificity of the enzyme system of the exchange reaction.

In a series of experiments Mulder and co-workers (171, 221, 229, 230) were able to define the biochemical mechanisms of the fatty acid–lecithin exchange reaction in the erythrocyte. Lysolecithin was an obligatory intermediate, its acylation being an energy-dependent step. They also discovered an energy-independent process by which two lysolecithin molecules could be converted to lecithin and glycerolphosphorylcholine. It was established that no phospholipase A activity exists in the cell; hence lysolecithin cannot be formed in the membrane directly.

Mulder and Van Deenen (229, 230) formulated the following general sequence for the overall reaction:

1. Plasma lysolecithin is adsorbed on the red cell.

2. Lysolecithin is acylated to lecithin.
3. A lecithin molecule is released from the cell.
4. Plasma lecithin is deacylated to lysolecithin.

Only step 2 is energy dependent. Step 4 probably involves the lecithin: cholesterol acyltransferase reaction (83).

Obviously this system cannot operate in the blood of cows or sheep, whose red cells contain no lecithin. Indeed, Winterbourn and Batt (57) found little incorporation of ^{14}C-palmitate into bovine red cells. Shastri and Rubenstein (193), in a detailed study of the incorporation of linoleate into human red cells *in vitro,* determined that the rate-limiting step may be an energy-dependent transport of free acids into a metabolic pool in the cell, as suggested by Shohet et al. (231), rather than step 2. This assumption needs further experimental proof.

Ferber and associates (232) reported a marked reduction in the ability of old cells to incorporate free fatty acids into lecithin by the above scheme. The ATP content of older cells was also reduced. Cells aged *in vitro* had very little ATP but could incorporate free fatty acids at a rate comparable to that of young cells, suggesting that lack of ATP is not the limiting function in the reaction. Both Shohet et al. (231) and Payne and Masters (81) concluded that the binding of free fatty acids to the erythrocyte involves an energy-dependent step, at least after the initial absorption. Only the fatty acids that are transferred to the energy-dependent pool can participate in the fatty acid–phospholipid exchange process. Oliveira and Nason (233) noted that in vitamin E deficiency red cells incorporate free fatty acids at the same rate as normal cells. This may indicate that the incorporation of new fatty acids into the cell is not related to autoxidation of red-cell lipids.

F. Lipid Loss and Aging of Erythrocytes

Normal erythrocytes lose lipid as they age. Reports (27, 137) indicate that young cells have more total lipid per cell than do older cells. Westerman et al. (27) found that for comparable packed-cell volumes the differences in lipid content disappeared. They concluded that the changes in lipid content were related to changes in cellular dimensions. Reticulocytes are richer in lipids than mature cells (234, 235). Raderecht and Scholzel (235) estimated that rabbit reticulocytes have four to five times as much lipid as mature cells. Although the total amount of lipid in the young cells is higher, the lipid-class distributions are unchanged (27, 137), suggesting that the loss with aging is uniform.

Phillips, Dodge, and Howe (236) recently reported a detailed analysis of the fatty acid composition of young and old human erythrocytes. They also analyzed the phospholipid-class distribution and found no significant differences between old and young cells, in agreement with the reports of Westerman et al. (27) and Van Gastel et al. (137). The main differences observed by Phillips et al. (236) were that the 20- and 22-carbon polyunsaturated fatty acids were lower, and the 18-carbon unsaturated fatty acids higher, in old cells than in young ones. A similar trend was noted by Van Gastel et al. (137).

Phillips et al. (236) could not account for the observed alteration in fatty acid distribution by changes in the phospholipid-class distribution, although they did see a slight diminution in phosphatidylserine, which would change the overall fatty acid composition in the observed direction. They also felt that several factors could be involved in the changes that occur with age in the fatty acid composition of erythrocytes: the lecithin: cholesterol acyltransferase reaction, phospholipid exchange, selective loss of phospholipid, and alterations in the affinity of erythrocytes for binding phospholipids.

Red cells survive much longer *in vivo* than they do *in vitro* (237). The reason for this is not clear, although a number of hypotheses have been suggested. Autoxidation of membrane lipids has been implicated by several authors (61, 237–241), but the addition of antioxidants to stored blood does not appreciably prolong storage life (237). Failure to remove metabolic waste *in vitro* is a more likely cause of rapid cell deterioration.

Whatever the cause, stored red cells lose lipid quite rapidly in most preservative solutions. Rimon, Brok, and Rimon (242) found rapid loss of lipid up to 11 days at 4°C, and then no change up to 42 days. Langley and Axell (46) showed that loss of lipid began immediately from defibrinated blood, cholesterol being the initial component lost. Lipid loss occurred even though sufficient glucose to sustain metabolic activity was present in the medium. If glucose was not provided, however, the lipid loss was appreciably greater, particularly from the phospholipid fraction of the erythrocyte. All cellular phospholipids were lost in direct proportion to their initial concentration in the membrane. Langley and Axell (46) observed no loss of protein during the same period.

Almond and Valeri (39) could see no loss of lipid from cells that had been frozen in glycerol solutions for 6 to 7.5 months. However, their individual values for glycerol-preserved cells varied widely, even though the mean values were close to the values for fresh cells. In agreement with previous work (46, 242) they found considerable loss of lipid in cells preserved with acid citrate dextrose after 7 days of storage, and most of the lipid lost was cholesterol.

Plasma-free erythrocytes that had been frozen in isotonic saline solution and stored at −20°C for 2 to 6 months were reported by Ways (243) to lose glycerophosphatides when thawed. Ghosts preserved in the same manner for an equal time did not lose lipid on thawing. Ways attributed the loss to a slow, hemoglobin-catalyzed autoxidation of the unsaturated fatty acids. The data of Almond and Valeri (39) suggest that glycerol acts to inhibit the reaction observed by Ways (243).

In a study similar to that of Langley and Axell (46) Cooper and Jandl (244) found that only cholesterol is lost from erythrocytes under conditions that are homeostatic for glucose. They suggested that the initial step in the loss of cholesterol during storage is the lecithin:cholesterol acyltransferase reaction. This reaction operates somewhat abnormally *in vitro* because of the altered ratio of free cholesterol to esterified cholesterol in plasma lipoproteins, which disturbs cholesterol exchange between the cell and plasma. Cooper and Jandl (244) also observed the erythrocyte's loss of both cholesterol and phospholipids in the absence of glucose.

We can construct the following hypothetical sequence of events that occur in stored erythrocytes:

1. Membrane cholesterol is lost because of the cholesterol:lecithin acyltransferase reaction.
2. The cell then loses its ability to oxidize glucose.
3. Depletion of cellular energy sources prevents the cell from maintaining the integrity of the membrane.
4. Phospholipids are lost from the membrane, followed by rapid hemolysis and cell destruction.

The cause of failure of the glycolytic apparatus is unknown; it could be autoxidation of cell lipids or accumulation of metabolic wastes in the medium. The latter is the more probable, but the two mechanisms could operate simultaneously.

IV. INFLUENCE OF DIET AND DISEASE ON ERYTHROCYTE LIPIDS

A. Dietary Influences on Lipid Class Composition

The lipid compositions of most tissues, except perhaps the central nervous system, vary with diet. These changes are reflected mainly in the fatty acid composition since the phospholipid-class distribution is more resistant to dietary influence (32, 116). The discussion of fatty acid exchange in Section III.C covered one aspect of dietary effects on the lipids of the erythrocyte. Human-erythrocyte lipids have been investigated in subjects on controlled diets (32, 116, 226, 227); the levels of phospholipid and cholesterol were unaffected. In a related study of hyperlipemic subjects Neerhout (142) could find no abnormalities in the erythrocyte lipids. Thus elevated plasma-lipid levels are not reflected in the erythrocyte lipids in humans, but this observation does not hold for all species (65).

The effects of fat-free and fat-supplemented diets on red-cell lipids have been investigated in several animal species (126, 166, 167, 245–249). The lipid composition was relatively unaffected by fat intake except in rodents. Silver, McMillan, and Silver (250) found that rabbits on high-cholesterol diets developed hemolysis and morphologically abnormal erythrocytes, but they did not study the erythrocyte lipid composition. Hestorff et al. (68) fractionated the lipids of erythrocytes from rabbits fed high-fat diets and confirmed a speculation of Silver et al. (250) that the lipid composition of the cells was altered. Hestorff et al. (68) reported that the red cells of anemic rabbits contained twice as much cholesterol as the cells of normal animals. Ostwald and Shannon (72) obtained similar results from guinea pigs fed 1% cholesterol diets: the red-cell cholesterol went from 1.36 to 3.76 mg/ml of packed cells, and the phospholipid-to-cholesterol ratio dropped from 1.9 to 1.5.

Thus in rodents cholesterol feeding appears to alter the lipid composition of the erythrocyte. The changes cannot be induced by feeding triglycerides or fatty acids only. Van Deenen (251) fed diets supplemented with corn oil and coconut oil, but no cholesterol, to several species without detecting any changes either in the phospholipid or in the cholesterol content of the erythrocytes.

Several authors (44, 62, 125, 245, 252) have studied the influence of diet on the erythrocyte lipids of rats. Studies by Menchaca and Arai (125) and Hollan and Breuer (44) indicate that the rat-erythrocyte lipids are quite resistant to dietary effects. The slight increase in cellular cholesterol observed by Menchaca and Arai is consistent with data on other rodents (68, 72, 250), but the rat is a very atypical rodent. For instance, though hypercholesterolemia is easily induced in most rodents, it is almost impossible to induce it in rats without adding thiouracil or other agents to the diet (253–255). Most studies with rats indicate that dietary fat does not alter red-cell cholesterol levels (245, 256).

B. Dietary Influences on Fatty Acid Composition and Cell Permeability

Dietary fatty acid acids are incorporated into the circulating red cells by exchange (see Section III.C) and by synthesis of new cells in the marrow. Exchange phenomena influence only the fatty acid composition of lecithin, but *de novo* synthesis influences all of the phospholipids in the cell. Walker,

Yurkowski, and Kummerow (158, 160, 257–260) have made extensive studies on rats, covering a variety of special diets and supplements. The level of arachidonic acid, which is high in normal rat erythrocytes, is relatively unaffected in essential fatty acid deficiency, yet the levels of oleic and linoleic acids are decreased. Essential fatty acid deficiency in other species produces similar effects (65, 246).

The erythrocyte stroma behaves like a semipermeable membrane. A number of investigators have studied the effect of diet on the permeability of the red cell *in vitro* in relation to changes in its fatty acid composition. De Gier et al. (135) separated a number of mammalian species into two groups based on the permeability characteristics of their erythrocytes. In the presence of glycerol the erythrocytes of man, rat, rabbit, and guinea pig were hemolyzed rapidly; those of pig, dog, cat, sheep, and cow, much more slowly. The fatty acid composition of the whole cell gave no basis for separating the two groups. The rapidly hemolyzing cells had more lecithin than the resistant groups except in the dog and the pig, and the rate of hemolysis was strongly dependent on the pH of the medium.

Walker and Kummerow (256) showed that in rats diet-induced changes in the fatty acid composition of erythrocytes were accompanied by changes in the apparent permeability of the cells, as measured by the rate of hemolysis in isotonic solutions of nonelectrolytes. Higher levels of essential fatty acids in the erythrocytes were associated with osmotic stability. There was an approximately linear relationship between the relative rate of hemolysis and the amount of essential fatty acids. In a study of vitamin E deprivation the same authors (257) found the erythrocytes of rats deficient in vitamin E to be more susceptible to copper- or iron-induced hemolysis than the cells of rats on normal diets. Corn oil in the diet increased the rate of hemolysis in the deficient animals. Others have noted that the erythrocyte lipids of animals on diets deficient in vitamin E have an increased susceptibility to autoxidation (161, 261).

The physiological significance of these observations is not clear. Most alterations in its normal fatty acid composition—induced by diet or other means—appear to be deleterious to the erythrocyte, at least as measured by the *in vitro* hemolysis rate. The effects *in vivo* have not been studied sufficiently to warrant any firm conclusion.

C. Erythrocyte Lipids in Disease

The study of erythrocyte lipids in various diseases has produced an enormous literature. Early reports suggested that specific diseases like anemia (262) and paroxysmal nocturnal hemoglobinuria (263) produced alterations in erythrocyte lipids. When some of the early work was shown to be in error, a counterreaction developed, holding that red-cell lipids were not affected by systemic disorders (16). Now, however, it is apparent that erythrocyte lipids are indeed affected in certain specific diseases like liver disorders and acanthocytosis.

One of the reasons for this confusion, particularly in anemias, was the increased number of reticulocytes in the circulation of such patients. Since reticulocytes may differ from mature cells in lipid composition, one must be cautious in interpreting data from patients in the absence of adequate information on the cell populations.

Raderecht et al. (234, 235), induced reticulocytosis in rabbits by repeated hemorrhage; they found a marked increase in the lipid phosphorus of the total red-cell population and concluded that young cells contain four to five times as much phospholipid as mature cells. Other investigators (27, 137) reported similar results for human red cells separated by centrifugal techniques. The mechanism by which cells lose lipid is not understood (see Section III.F).

D. Specific Diseases

1. Anemias. Anemias lead to rapid cell destruction and increased reticulocyte levels in the blood; hence reports suggesting associated abnormal lipid compositions must be viewed with caution. In most nonspecific anemias there is little or no difference in lipid composition between the anemic and normal cell populations (50, 52, 53, 55, 56, 136, 264–266). Most anemias can be related to the inability of the cells to obtain metabolic energy, that is, to metabolize glucose. Reports on the fatty acid composition of red cells from anemic subjects have been unremarkable (50, 266).

However, although several of the typical anemias, such as sickle cell anemia (267), hereditary elliptocytosis (268), primary refractory anemia (50), and pernicious anemia (50), are not associated with abnormalities in red-cell lipids, some recently characterized anemias of nonspecific origin do involve alterations of the red-cell lipids (53, 55, 269).

Brabec et al. (53) found lower than normal total-lipid levels in autoimmune hemolytic anemia; the phospholipid distribution was normal. Jaffe and Gottfried (45) reported a newly discovered nonspherocytic anemia in which the erythrocyte's lecithin level is significantly elevated whereas the remaining lipids are normal. Cooper (55) has discovered a spur cell anemia in which the cholesterol of the cell is elevated without a concomitant increase in phospholipids. (This disorder, however, may be related to the lecithin:cholesterol acyltransferase system in plasma and to a chronic liver malfunction of unknown origin; the red cell may be a secondary, rather than primary, source of the disease.) Similarly in patients with Zieve's syndrome (269), which is characterized by alcoholic cirrhosis, hyperlipemia, and hemolytic anemia, there is an elevation of erythrocyte cholesterol and phospholipids.

Hereditary spherocytosis has been the subject of many studies (37, 115, 262, 268, 270–272). Early reports indicating alteration in the phospholipids of the red cell (115, 262) were not confirmed by later work (37, 268). However, more recent studies have shown that in this condition lipids are easily lost from erythrocytes (270, 271). The observation of Jacobs and Karnovsky (41) that phospholipid synthesis in these cells is elevated has been refuted by Reed (71). The biochemical studies support the ideas of Cooper and Jandl (55, 270) that the lipid distribution in the cell is normal, and the loss of membrane lipid is due to some primary defect in the membrane, probably in the glycolytic energy system; the loss of lipid reduces the stability of the membrane, and the cells change shape and hemolyze rapidly. The work of Cooper and Jandl (270) showed that normal cells lose lipid when incubated *in vitro* in the absence of glucose in much the same manner as the cells from patients with hereditary spherocytosis.

2. Acanthocytosis. This is a rare disease that, unlike many of the anemias discussed above, does involve a true *in vivo* alteration in the lipid composition of the red cell. The etiology of the disorder is fairly well understood. It involves a genetic defect in the ability of the patient to synthesize the polypeptides necessary for the formation of low-density lipoproteins. Phillips and Roome reported (265), and Ways, Reed, and Hanahan confirmed (273), that the erythrocytes of patients with acanthocytosis have reduced lecithin, and elevated sphingomyelin, levels. Since the erythrocytes have normal total-lipid levels, lecithin must be selectively replaced by sphingomyelin.

Ways, Reed, and Hanahan (273), investigating the fatty acid composition of acanthocytotic cells, found greatly reduced linoleic acid levels. Phillips and Dodge (274) confirmed this result in a more extensive study of the fatty acid composition of acanthocytotic erythrocytes. They suggested that the patients suffer from an essential fatty acid deficiency that is a secondary effect of their fat-malabsorption syndrome. The intestinal cells cannot form chylomicrons or very low-density lipoproteins, nor can the liver synthesize low-density lipoproteins in the S_f 0–400 class. Kayden and Silber (275) observed that patients with this disease also suffer a vitamin E deficiency that may be an additional consequence of the fat-malabsorption syndrome. In a follow-up study Dodge et al. (139) found that in acanthocytosis the erythrocytes are more susceptible to autoxidation and peroxidation with hydrogen peroxide. It would appear that the red-cell-lipid alterations are again a secondary feature of this disorder rather than the primary source of the defect (29, 276, 277).

3. Hepatic Disease. Disorders of the liver profoundly affect the erythrocyte lipids (36, 42, 48, 266, 278–281). Nye and Marinetti (42) observed in subjects with liver disease and jaundice (unspecified) a markedly abnormal erythrocyte phospholipid distribution that usually involved elevated red-cell lecithin, and decreased phosphatidylethanolamine, levels. The total-lipid level was either slightly elevated or normal. Neerhout (48) also reported similar findings, adding that the red-cell cholesterol was elevated and the fatty acid composition altered. Mihaesco et al. (36) detected similar changes in patients with anemia induced by cirrhosis.

An interesting aspect of these results is that the erythrocytes in these subjects are completely normal until the liver malfunction appears. Indeed Neerhout (280) has shown that the red-cell lipids return to normal levels after the patients have recovered. Hence the changes in the red-cell lipids are undoubtedly acquired in the circulation either through interaction with altered plasma lipids (42) or in the passage of the cells through the hepatic circulation. It is interesting that cholesterol and lecithin are primarily involved in these alterations. These two lipids are much more susceptible to change in all of the defects of the erythrocyte. The reason for this is unknown, but the lecithin:cholesterol acyltransferase system is strongly implicated.

4. Paroxysmal Nocturnal Hemoglobinuria (PNH). This rather rare disease has attracted several studies, perhaps more because of its rarity than for any other reason (30, 50, 227, 266, 282). Some of the earlier work (227, 263) suggested that this disease is manifested by alterations in the lipid composition of erythrocytes, but later investigations (50, 266) failed to confirm this. Moreover, Weinstein and Williams (283) have reported that PNH red cells are morphologically normal, contradicting some previous reports of visible membrane lesions (284–286). Thus in this red-cell disorder the lipids are normal and clearly do not play a significant role in the hemolytic sequence.

5. Miscellaneous Sphingolipidoses. The sphingolipidoses most often manifest themselves in the nervous tissue, spleen, or liver, yet it has often been suspected that red cells are affected also. Hooghwinkel et al. (287) investigated a large series of lipidoses including Nieman–Pick disease, Gaucher's disease, metachromatic leukodystrophy, and others. They concluded that the sphingomyelin of the erythrocyte was depressed in most disorders but normal in juvenile amaurotic idiocy. In Fabry's disease Vance and Sweeley (93) found higher than normal values for the neutral glycosphingolipids of erythrocytes. On the other hand, gangliosides are normal in amaurotic familial idiocy (94) despite a previous report to the contrary (95).

6. Lecithin:Cholesterol Acyltransferase (LCAT) Deficiency. This rare but extremely interesting disorder was discovered recently in Norway by Norum and Gjone (288, 289). The complete elucidation of its pathology may have great importance to the understanding of other disorders of the erythrocyte membrane. In certain aspects the symptoms mimic those of liver malfunctions. The erythrocytes have elevated cholesterol and lecithin levels (290); the other phospholipids are present in either normal or slightly reduced amounts. The cells exhibit increased osmotic fragility.

In a very interesting study Gjone et al. (43) showed that on incubation with plasma from normal subjects cells from LCAT-deficient subjects assume a normal lipid distribution and their osmotic and permeability characteristics return to normal. Conversely, when cells from normal subjects are incubated with plasma from LCAT-deficient patients, they take on the characteristics of the diseased cells.

These observations support the idea that red-cell-lipid distributions can be influenced greatly by the external environment. The anemias observed in many of these diseases are caused by disturbances in plasma or liver enzymes and are not directly related to the production of erythrocytes in the patient.

7. Other Diseases. The literature includes reports on the erythrocyte lipids in a variety of other diseases, including polycythemia vera (143, 236), Huntington's chorea (152), hyperthyroidism and hypothyroidism (119), glucose-6-phosphate dehydrogenase deficiency (35), acrodermatitis enteropathica (140), leprosy (291), leukemia (292), atherosclerosis (293), cancer (118), Wolman's disease (294), paroxysmal cold hemoglobinuria (295), hyperlipemia (142, 266, 278), and diabetes (53, 278).

It is unnecessary to detail the results of all of these investigations, but in general they indicate that the red-cell-lipid composition is normal in these disorders. Thus the red-cell lipids are influenced only in diseases in which specific enzymes are disturbed (e.g., LCAT deficiency). Hyperlipemia alone does not appreciably affect red-cell lipids in humans (42, 142, 266). It appears that as long as the enzyme system that controls the lipid exchange between the cell and its environment is functioning normally, the erythrocyte can maintain its lipid balance even when the environmental lipid levels are drastically altered.

Apparently alterations in the erythrocyte cholesterol and lecithin levels result in increased osmotic fragility and premature destruction, even when the cells are essentially normal in other respects (e.g., in ATPase level and glucose metabolism). In acanthocytosis decreased lecithin, and increased sphingomyelin, levels also reduce the lifespan of the cell, although in this particular disease the complete syndrome is very complex and there may be other defects in the cell membrane. Nevertheless, it is apparent that changes in red-cell-lipid composition are deleterious to the stability of the cell membrane and hence to the longevity of the cell.

The role of the acidic phospholipids, which seem to be unaffected in the disorders discussed here, is unclear at present. To a certain extent they are more labile and difficult to analyze than the neutral phospholipids and hence have not been studied as thoroughly. However, it is possible that the role of the acidic phospholipids in the structure of the membrane is fundamentally different from that of the neutral phospholipids and its disturbance would lead to immediate cell destruction. It would be difficult to detect such disturbances if, indeed, they do occur.

V. THE ROLE OF LIPIDS IN MEMBRANE FUNCTION AND STRUCTURE

First with Gorter and Grendal (1), Danielli and Davson (2), and continuing up to the present with such investigators as Zahler (296), Chapman (297), Van Deenen (298), and others (299, 300), the red cell has been a prime source of biological membranes for chemical and physical studies of membrane structure and function. It is not appropriate in a chapter devoted primarily to quantification to give much space to biophysical and biochemical studies of membrane structure. These subjects are well covered elsewhere (297, 298, 301). This section simply mentions a few examples of work specifically related to erythrocytes in order to demonstrate recent advances in this area.

A. Physical Studies on Erythrocyte Membranes

1. X-Ray Diffraction. This technique has been very useful in the study of myelin, which is a very highly ordered system. The erythrocyte has proved to be not quite so amenable, but it has yielded some data to X-ray studies. Finean and co-workers (302) described the X-ray scattering of erythrocyte ghosts. The pattern is characterized by a 10-Å peak, which was assigned to protein, and a 4- to 5-Å peak, assigned to lipids; both peaks are very broad. Similar results were reported by Segerman (303), who also observed a side peak of 2.1 Å in ghost–water preparations. Segerman concluded that the side peaks at 2.1 and 5 Å are both from scattering that involves both lipids and proteins, whereas the 10-Å peak is produced solely by the proteins of the membrane. His most significant finding may be his conclusion that the cholesterol present is not in a condensed phase. He suggested that the cholesterol is arranged in rows that divide paracrystalline lipid regions into cells or ribbons. This intriguing idea should be explored further.

In an X-ray diffraction study of lipids extracted from erythrocytes Rand and Luzzati (304) obtained evidence suggesting that the liquid crystals formed by the extracted lipids in water are arranged in a lamellar structure. The liquid-crystal layers are separated by water layers of varying thickness, and the hydrophobic chains of the lipids are associated, with the polar ends facing the water phase. The cholesterol is oriented like the phospholipid molecules. The important question, of course, is whether this arrangement has any significance to the native membrane, but it cannot be answered yet.

2. Electron Microscopy. Electron microscopy of fixed, stained, whole erythrocytes or ghost preparations has shed little or no light on the structure of the membrane (301, 305). The newer "freeze etching or cleaving" technique has yielded more informative micrographs (283, 301, 306). Weinstein and Bullivant (307) observed small bumps or spheres on the surface of human erythrocytes and thought that they might be the sites of specific antigens or enzymes. These authors could not split the hypothetical lipid bilayer of the cell membrane as Branton (308) has claimed to do in plant cells. Their failure to do so may be due to differences between plant and animal membranes or may indicate that the lipids in the erythrocyte do not form a classic bilayer.

Weinstein and Koo (309) showed that the particulate components previously thought to be located only on the inner and outer surfaces of the cell actually penetrate from the inner to the outer surface of the membrane. If these structures are not artifacts, they suggest morphological discontinuity of the membrane and could be related to such membrane functions as transport and antigenicity. Whether the particles are related specifically to the lipids of the membrane is unknown. However, it is significant that myelin is one substance that shows little if any of these particles (310) and myelin is a protein-poor tissue (311). Membrane-associated particles have been demonstrated in nonmammalian erythrocytes by Koehler (312) as well as in those of mammals.

Other authors have described the effects of various agents, such as phospholipase C (313) or polyene antibiotics (314), on the red cell. Interpretations of the unusual structures that result from such treatments are limited only by the imagination of the investigators and are hence of somewhat limited value. Until more is known of the molecular architecture of the membrane such studies tend more to confuse than to illuminate.

Weinstein (301) has published an excellent monograph reviewing most of the recent advances in the study of the red-cell membrane by electron microscopy. The reader is referred to this work for further details.

3. Optical Rotary Dispersion and Circular Dichroism. Measurements of optical rotatory dispersion (ORD) and circular dichroism (CD) yield information primarily on the protein moiety of the membrane. Lipids, however, can cause shifts in absorption maxima or intensity differences that contribute to the information on membrane structure.

Lenard and Singer (315) interpreted their ORD data to mean that protein–lipid interactions occur through the hydrocarbon chains of the lipids. However, the interpretation of optical data on intact membranes is complicated by light-scattering effects attributed to the clumping of ghosts and the absence of a true solution (316). Gordon, Wallach, and Straus (317) claimed that such effects are negligible, however, and stated that shifts in the ORD and CD spectra of erythrocytes are in fact due to the presence of lipids in the membrane. These authors could not determine the specific interaction but suggested the following possibilities:

1. The hydrocarbon portion of the lipid might create an environment conducive to high polarizability and low polarity for portions of the protein molecule.
2. The quaternary structure of the protein depends on the lipids.
3. The secondary structure of the protein depends on the lipids.

All three possibilities could contribute to the observed phenomena.

4. Nuclear-Magnetic-Resonance Spectroscopy. Chapman et al. (318, 319) were unable to obtain nuclear-magnetic-resonance (NMR) spectra on whole ghosts with a 60-MHz instrument. They obtained good spectra on sonicated ghost preparations, but these were presumably disrupted membranes. Better results were obtained by Kamat and Chapman (320) with a 220-MHz instrument, which yielded good spectra from fresh, unsonicated ghosts. The results, though inconclusive, do suggest that the hydrocarbon portion of the lipid molecule is associated with the proteins in the membrane. From NMR spectra Clifford, Pethica, and Smith (321) deduced that most of the "bound" water in the membrane is associated with the protein. This suggests that the protein may have both hydrophilic and hydrophobic regions in the membrane—a reasonable idea, until now without any experimental basis.

5. Infrared Spectroscopy. Chapman, Kamat, and Levene (322) and Maddy and Malcolm (323) have recorded the infrared spectra of intact ghosts. Chapman et al. (322) interpreted their spectra to mean that the hydrocarbon chains of the lipids are much more disordered in the ghosts than in thin films prepared from the phospholipids extracted from the erythrocyte. The data argue against the idea that the lipids in the membrane exist in a highly ordered structure, such as a tightly packed bilayer. There is a suggestion in the infrared data that the hydrocarbon parts of the lipids are strongly associated with the polypeptide chains of the proteins; this assumption agrees with the NMR data.

6. Spin-Labeling Electron Spin Resonance. This is a new physical technique that has only recently been applied to biological membranes (324, 325). Two recent reports are available on spin-labeled erythrocyte membranes (326, 327). Chapman, Barratt, and Kamat (326) used a maleimide derivative rather unrelated to the membrane lipids, but Hubbell and McConnell (327) used a ketostearic acid derivative that is structurally similar to the fatty acids of natural membranes.

The study of red cells by this technique is difficult because the cells must be oriented with respect to the instrument and the applied magnetic fields. Hubbell and McConnell used a shear-orientation method that, while not giving absolute orientation, aligns a reasonably good percentage of the cells in the same direction. They concluded that the lipids in the erythrocyte are packed in an arrangement somewhat like a classical bilayer but that the hydrocarbon chains show less mobility than would be expected in a pure lipoid phase.

B. Biochemical Studies on Erythrocyte Membranes

Besides the physical techniques for the study of membrane structure, a number of biochemical approaches to the problem have been made. They are discussed only briefly here.

1. Solubilization of the Erythrocyte Stroma. A major impediment to the study of membrane proteins has been their insolubility. Maddy (328, 329) was able to dissolve the stroma of ox erythrocytes in *n*-butanol. Morgan and Hanahan (330) found that a soluble lipoprotein could be obtained by sonication of human-erythrocyte ghosts. However, only 6% of the total protein was recovered in this fraction, which contained 94% of the total lipids. The structure of the membrane may have been destroyed, yielding a micellar lipid form that contained entrapped protein.

In more recent work Zwaal and Van Deenen (331) completely solubilized human-erythrocyte ghosts in *n*-pentanol. Lauf and Poulik (332) described procedures for the solubilization of human-erythrocyte ghosts in 8 *M* urea. They found that the urea treatment did not remove lipid from the protein, which suggests that the lipid–protein interactions are nonionic.

2. Partial Extraction of Erythrocyte Lipids. Lipids can be partially extracted from red cells under rather mild conditions. Some investigators have used such procedures in the hope of elucidating the lipid-to-protein binding (333, 334). Roelofsen, De Gier, and Van Deenen (333) found that only a portion of the total lipids was extracted from lyophilized ghosts with dry ether. Repeated extraction with ether did not remove additional lipids. The remaining lipids could only be extracted from the ghost by more polar solvents, such as chloroform or alcohols. The ether-extracted lipids consisted of cholesterol and part of the acidic lipids; lecithin and sphingomyelin were not extracted. The nonphysiological conditions of this experiment make it difficult to relate the results to the structure of the native membrane.

In a related experiment Haahti, Nanto, and Viikari (334) extracted fresh ghosts with a continuous gradient of solvents going from nonpolar to polar. The results were similar to those reported by Roelofsen et al. (333). All of the cholesterol and a portion of the acidic phospholipids were removed by the nonpolar solvents. The remaining phospholipids could be removed only by polar solvents.

The results of these experiments cannot be interpreted as simply showing that some lipids are bound to the protein by polar bonds while other lipids are bound by nonpolar forces. If the removal of lipid from the membrane requires unfolding of the protein, then a polar solvent may be necessary regardless of lipid-to-protein binding. Also, bound water in the membrane could be a barrier to nonpolar solvents. Zamudio, Cellino, and Canessa-Fischer (335) reported that only polar solvents inactivated the enzymes of the membrane.

3. Surface Area of Lipids Extracted from Erythrocytes. The classic experiment of Gorter and Grendal (1) on the surface area of a monolayer formed by the lipids extracted from erythrocytes has been repeated with modern methods (6, 32). Despite the now obvious errors, in the original experiment, both Hill et al. (32) and Bar et al. (6) found that the conclusion of Gorter and Grendal was essentially correct.

Bar et al. (6) extended the scope of the experiment by measuring force-area curves for the lipid films. They found the surface pressure necessary to create a monolayer to be unrealistically high (above the collapse pressure of the film), but pressure in the range of 5 to 10 dynes/cm^2 was adequate to reduce the surface of the film well below that needed for a bilayer. Such pressures are perfectly realistic for a biological membrane, as determined by osmotic pressure calculation on erythrocytes. Hence the data are not conclusive for a bilayer, although a monolayer appears to be unlikely.

4. Permeability Studies. Experiments on the water permeability of the erythrocyte led to the concept of physical pores in the membrane. Rich and associates (336) estimated that the dog red cell behaved as though it had pores of 6-Å radius. Since this is below the resolving power of existing electron microscopes, the physical reality of such pores cannot be ruled out at present.

Finkelstein and Cass (337) showed that in thin lipid films permeability to water changes in direct proportion to the cholesterol content of the film. Sha'afi et al. (338), extended these experiments to erythrocytes and found no dependence of hydraulic conductivity of the cell on the cholesterol content of the membrane. With the technique described by Murphy (339), they varied the cholesterol content from 1.24 to 0.54 times the normal. This observation supports the contention that membrane lipids do not act as a simple barrier to diffusion, just as they do not contribute to the charge on the membrane. Eylar et al. (340) established that the charge on human erythrocytes is produced by sialic acid residues bound to protein, not lipid.

5. Immunochemical Studies on Erythrocyte Membranes and Lipids. It is usually assumed that antibody–antigen reactions occur on the cell surface, at distances no deeper than one molecular radius (341). Casu, Nanni, and co-workers (9, 342, 343) have made antigens reactive to sheep-erythrocyte lipids and then attempted to cross-react these antigens with fresh sheep erythrocytes. They concluded from this work that sphingomyelin is located on the outer surface of the membrane and the acidic lipids on the interior side. Immunological studies like these, particularly when antibodies to lipids are prepared, are fraught with difficulties in procedure and interpretation. Nevertheless, radial asymmetry in the distribution of lipids in the membrane could explain why the lipid composition is diverse and, perhaps, why approximately 50% of the membrane phospholipids are acidic and 50% are zwitterions.

Kinsky and co-workers (11, 12, 344) showed that liposomes prepared from sheep-erythrocyte lipid extracts can be used as a model membrane system in some immunological systems. They showed that immunological responses can be generated by liposomes into which are incorporated compounds of known antigenicity, such as Forssman hapten (11). Such artificial systems may greatly facilitate studies in immunological specificity, but their relevance to native membranes remains questionable because of the absence of protein in such preparations. However, the future of this approach to the study of the erythrocyte membrane appears to be promising.

6. Enzymatic Studies on Erythrocyte Lipids. Most studies on the enzymes of the erythrocyte are concerned solely with enzymic properties (345), but enzymes have also been used to study the lipids and structure of the cell (9, 317, 335, 346). Casu et al. (9) found that phospholipase A had no effect on intact sheep erythrocytes, but it did hydrolyze phospholipids of ghosts prepared from sheep cells. Phospholipase C hydrolyzed only sphingomyelin in whole cells. The authors concluded that the fatty acids of glycerol phospholipid are buried in the membrane, which agrees with some of the physical evidence described earlier.

C. Summary: Bilayer or ?

In an excellent review of the structure of the erythrocyte membrane Zahler (347) recently pointed out several features that must be satisfied by any satisfactory model. These are as follows:

1. The proteins of the membrane are 50% or more α-helical.
2. Lipoprotein subunits exist in the membrane.
3. Hydrophobic regions must exist in the membrane.
4. Hydrophobic interactions occur between the lipids and the proteins, probably through the fatty acid portions of the lipid molecules.

Zahler then goes on to state, after various experimental data for the above features, that ". . . recent data on membrane chemistry and physics have given rise to serious doubts against the unit membrane theory. . . ." Of course, no one seriously believed that the simple unit membrane–lipid bilayer concept was the ultimate answer to the problem of membrane structure. It has served a very useful purpose, but now the evidence suggests that it should either be discarded or drastically modified. Such an arrangement may exist in myelin, a protein-poor tissue, but in the erythrocyte one must search for more attractive hypotheses. Zahler suggests several, his own and those of other theorists, in his review (347). One feature that should be considered in future models is lipid asymmetry (8, 342, 343) and surface heterogeneity (306). No doubt the final answer to this problem will show a very complex structure for the native membrane.

VI. SUMMARY AND CONCLUSIONS

The systematic and careful analysis of red-cell lipids has made great progress in the last decade. This is particularly true of the erythrocyte phospholipids in several species (73, 110). The remaining problems in the quantitation of erythrocyte phospholipids center on the identification of the minor components (110) and the fatty acids associated with the phospholipids, particularly in nonhuman species.

From the average phospholipid distributions in human erythrocytes presented in Table VI it is possible to judge the relative accuracy of most of the current literature values. Wide deviations from the averages in Table VI for normal values suggest methodological difficulties in the analytical procedures. Figure 5 graphically presents the lipid distribution in human erythrocytes. Comparison with a similar presentation in the review of Van Deenen and De Gier (16) prepared in 1964 demonstrates significant advances in the analysis of red-cell lipids during the intervening period, particularly with respect to the acidic phospholipids, neutral lipids, and glycosphingolipids. It is doubtful that a similar figure prepared 8 years from now would show as many changes. Further advances are more likely to be in the areas of metabolism and membrane structure.

The vinyl and alkyl ethers, which exist mainly in the phosphatidylethanolamine fraction of erythrocyte lipids, represent another area that has not been fully explored. Quantitative data are either lacking or out of date. Although their biochemical and physiological significance is unknown, these compounds must play an important role in the cell membrane, and further analytical as well as biochemical data are urgently needed.

The quantitation of the erythrocyte glycosphingolipids has progressed less rapidly than that of the phospholipids. These compounds must have important implications in biochemical genetics and immunology. The studies of Kinsky and co-workers (11, 12, 344) show that antigenicity reaction can be obtained with lipid haptens and protein-free liposomes. This may have important consequences for models of the red-cell membrane.

The advances in the quantitation of red-cell lipids have obviously had major significance in the study of certain disorders of the red cell. The lipids can no longer be considered to be passive components of the erythrocyte during its lifespan. The work of Neerhout (48, 280) and others (42) has shown that disorders of the liver cause dramatic alterations in cellular lipids. These alterations may result subsequently in hemolysis of the cells, even though the erythropoietic system in these patients is presumably normal. It is now apparent that several other red-cell abnormalities are associated with disturbances of membrane lipid (270, 274, 275, 278). In many of these conditions the alterations in the red-cell lipids are secondary manifestations of diseases involving the plasma lipids or liver function.

What remains to be explained in the pathology of these disorders is the mechanism by which red-cell lipids are altered. Hyperlipemia alone has little or no effect on the erythrocyte lipids (142), unless it is a symptom of some other disturbance, such as that in Zieve's syndrome (269).

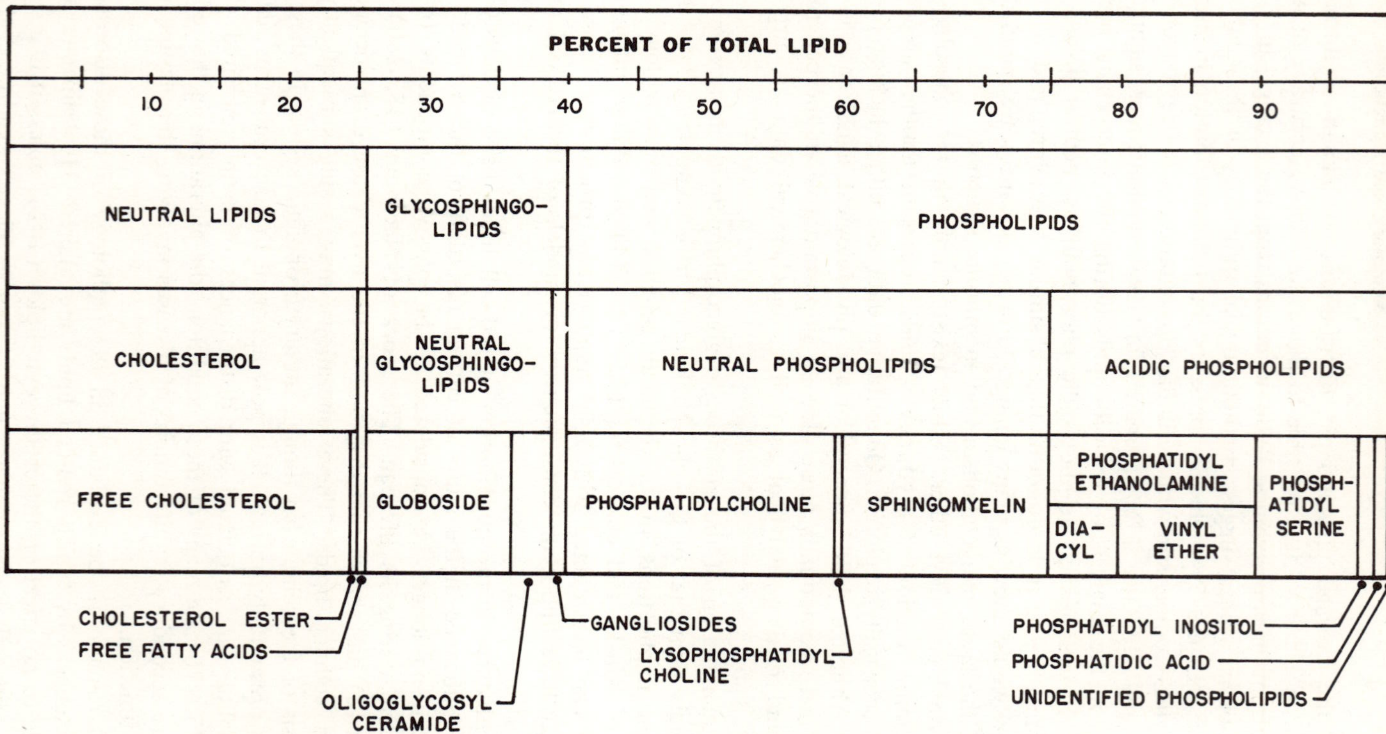

Fig. 5 Graphic illustration of the distribution of lipids in normal human erythrocytes

The lecithin:cholesterol acyltransferase system appears to be intimately involved in some red-cell-lipid alterations (43, 290); in others the glycolytic energy metabolism is implicated (55).

The cell needs energy to maintain the homeostasis of the membrane, including its lipid composition. Cholesterol and, to a lesser degree, phospholipids are rapidly lost from the membrane *in vitro* when the medium lacks a source of metabolic energy (46). Just how the cells translate metabolic energy into maintenance of membrane integrity is a mystery and a major problem in membrane biochemistry. Also, the exchange of some red-cell lipids is an energy-dependent process (231).

The metabolism of erythrocyte lipids has been studied extensively (183, 189, 190–192) and is basically well understood at present. Major lipids are neither synthesized nor catabolized by mature red cells. The cell does synthesize a very small amount of some of the trace phospholipids, such as phosphatidic acid. Cholesterol, lecithin, and sphingomyelin in the cell are continuously exchanged, as are some of the cellular fatty acids, particularly the unsaturated fatty acids of lecithin. The significance of these exchange reactions is unknown.

The structure of the red-cell membrane is still a mystery. The simple unit-membrane theory of a lipid bilayer sandwiched between protein is difficult to support with current physicochemical data. The lipid–protein interaction would appear to be through the hydrocarbon chains of the lipids and the hydrophobic regions of the polypeptide chains. It has been suggested that the lipids are asymmetrically distributed in the membrane (8, 9, 342). Although it is an interesting speculation, this idea remains unproved.

A lipoprotein subunit structure is a model with considerable appeal. It is supported by experiments that have succeeded in solubilizing the membrane in various solvents (328–332), but it is certainly not proved. Obviously our knowledge of the proteins of the red cell (see Chapter 10) must be enlarged for the ultimate answer to this problem; it is unlikely that further studies of the lipids alone can contribute significantly to the solution.

VII. ACKNOWLEDGMENTS

Some of the work cited in this chapter was supported by the U.S. Atomic Energy Commission. I am grateful to the various authors and publishers for permission to quote various publications and to reproduce Figs. 1 through 4 in the text. I would also like to thank Mr. R. A. Booth for his excellent technical assistance in the experimental work.

REFERENCES

1. Gorter, E., and F. Grendal, *J. Exp. Med.* **41**, 439–443 (1925).
2. Danielli, J. F., and H. Davson, *J. Cell. Comp. Physiol.* **5**, 495–508 (1935).
3. Robertson, J. D., *Biochem. Soc. Symp.* **16**, 3–43 (1959).
4. Green, D., and S. Fleischer, *Biochim. Biophys. Acta* **70**, 554–582 (1963).
5. Korn, E. D., *Science* **153**, 1491–1498 (1966).
6. Bar, R. S., D. W. Deamer, and D. G. Cornwell, *Science* **153**, 1010–1012 (1966).
7. Erickson, B. N., H. H. Williams, S. S. Bernstein, I. Avrin, R. I. Jones, and I. G. Macy, *J. Biol. Chem.* **122**, 515–528 (1938).
8. Murphy, J. R., *J. Lab. Clin. Med.* **65**, 756–774 (1965).
9. Casu, A., G. Nanni, and V. Pala, *Ital. J. Biochem.* **17**, 301–311 (1968).
10. Casu, A., G. Nanni, V. M. Marinari, V. Pala, and R. Menacelli, *Ital. J. Biochem.* **18**, 153–165 (1969).
11. Kinsky, S. C., J. A. Haxby, D. A. Zopf, C. R. Alving, and C. B. Kinsky, *Biochemistry* **8**, 4149–4158 (1969).
12. Alving, C. R., S. C. Kinsky, J. A. Haxby, and C. B. Kinsky, *Biochemistry* **8**, 1582–1587 (1969).
13. Rouser, G., G. J. Nelson, S. Fleischer, and G. Simon, in *Biological Membranes*, D. Chapman, Ed., Academic Press, New York, 1968, pp. 5–69.
14. Parpart, A. K., and R. Ballentine, in *Modern Trends in Physiology and Biochemistry*, E. S. G. Barron, Ed., Academic Press, New York, 1952, pp. 135–148.
15. Douste-Blazy, L., in *Exposés annuel de biochimie medicale*, P. Boulanger, M. F. Jayle, and J. Roche, Eds., Masson, Paris, 1959, pp. 187–213.
16. Van Deenen, L. L. M., and J. de Gier, in *The Red Blood Cell*, C. Bishop and D. M. Surgenor, Eds., Academic Press, New York, 1964, pp. 243–307.
17. Firkin, B. G., and J. S. Wiley, in *Progress in Hematology*, E. B. Brown and C. V. Moore, Eds., Grune and Stratton, New York, 1966, pp. 26–59.
18. De Gier, J., *Bibl. Haematol,* **29**, 158–167 (1968).
19. Pennell, R. B., in *The Red Blood Cell*, C. Bishop and D. M. Surgenor, Eds., Academic Press, New York, 1964, pp. 29–69.
20. Beilin, L. J., G. J. Knight, A. D. Munro-Favre, and J. Anderson, *J. Clin. Invest.* **45**, 1817–1825 (1966).
21. Dodge, J. T., C. Mitchell, and D. J. Hanahan, *Arch. Biochem. Biophys.* **100**, 119–130 (1963).
22. Mitchell, C. D., W. B. Mitchell, and D. J. Hanahan, *Biochim. Biophys. Acta* **104**, 348–358 (1965).
23. Relander, A., *Scand. J. Haematol.* **5**, 321–324 (1968).
24. Anderson, H. M., and J. C. Turner, *J. Clin. Invest.* **39**, 1–7 (1960).
25. Dawson, R. M. C., N. Hemington, and D. B. Lindsay, *Biochem. J.* **77**, 226–230 (1960).
26. Ponder, E., *Hemolysis and Related Phenomena*, Grune and Stratton, New York, 1948.
27. Westerman, M. P., L. E. Pierce, and W. N. Jensen, *J. Lab. Clin. Med.* **62**, 394–400 (1963).
28. Ways, P., and D. J. Hanahan, *J. Lipid Res.* **5**, 318–328 (1964).
29. Simon, E. R., and P. Ways, *J. Clin. Invest.* **43**, 1311–1321 (1964).

30. Bradlow, B. A., J. Lee, and R. Rubenstein, *Brit. J. Haematol.* **11**, 315–322 (1965).
31. Crowley, J., P. Ways, and J. W. Jones, *J. Clin. Invest.* **44**, 989–998 (1965).
32. Hill, J. G., A. Kuksis, and J. M. R. Beveridge, *J. Amer. Oil. Chem. Soc.* **41**, 393–397 (1964).
33. Iacona, J. M., J. F. Mueller, and D. C. Zellner, *Amer. J. Clin. Nutr.* **16**, 165–172 (1965).
34. Rose, H. G., and M. Oklander, *J. Lipid Res.* **6**, 428–431 (1965).
35. Szeinberg, A., J. Zaidman, and L. Clejan, *Biochim. Biophys. Acta* **98**, 598–606 (1965).
36. Mihaesco, E., P. Boivin, and R. Fauvert, *Nouv. Rev. Fr. Hematol.* **6**, 556–559 (1966).
37. Reed, C. F., and S. N. Swisher, *J. Clin. Invest.* **45**, 777–781 (1966).
38. Williams, J. H., M. Kuchmak, and R. F. Witter, *Lipids* **1**, 391–398 (1966).
39. Almond, D. V., and R. C. Valeri, *Transfusion* **7**, 10–16 (1967).
40. Dodge, J. T., and G. B. Phillips, *J. Lipid Res.* **8**, 667–675 (1967).
41. Jacobs, H. S., and M. L. Karnovsky, *J. Clin. Invest.* **46**, 173–185 (1967).
42. Nye, W. H. R., and G. V. Marinetti, *Proc. Soc. Exp. Biol. Med.* **125**, 1220–1224 (1967).
43. Gjone, E., H. Torsvik, and K. R. Norum, *Scand. J. Clin. Lab. Invest.* **21**, 327–332 (1968).
44. Hollan, S. R., and J. H. Breuer, *Acta Med. Acad. Sci. Hung.* **25**, 421–432 (1968).
45. Jaffe, E. R., and E. L. Gottfried, *J. Clin. Invest.* **47**, 1375–1388 (1968).
46. Langley, G. R., and M. Axell, *Brit. J. Haematol.* **14**, 593–603 (1968).
47. Moore, T. J., *J. Lipid Res.* **9**, 642–646 (1968).
48. Neerhout, R. C., *J. Lab. Clin. Med.* **71**, 438–447 (1968).
49. Pohl, A., and K. Moser, in *Metabolism and Membrane Permeability of Erythrocytes and Thrombocytes,* E. Deutsch, E. Gerlach, and K. Moser, Eds., Thieme, Stuttgart, 1968, pp. 357–360.
50. Sen, S. K., M. L. Mehrotra, A. Kumar, D. Chandra, and M. P. Singh, *Indian J. Med. Res.* **56**, 1232–1240 (1968).
51. Shacklady, M. M., E. M. Djardjouras, and J. K. Lloyd, *Lancet* **ii**, 151–153 (1968).
52. Zarkowsky, H. S., F. A. Oski, R. Sha'afi, S. B. Shohet, and D. G. Nathan, *New Engl. J. Med.* **278**, 593–600 and 652–657 (1968).
53. Brabec, V., C. Michalec, J. Palek, and M. Kout, *Blood* **34**, 414–420 (1969).
54. Broekhuyse, R. M., *Clin. Chim. Acta* **23**, 457–461 (1969).
55. Cooper, R. A., *J. Clin. Invest.* **48**, 1820–1831 (1969).
56. Palek, J., V. Brabec, M. Vopatova, C. Michalec, and L. Mircevova, *Clin. Chim. Acta* **23**, 133–138 (1969).
57. Winterbourn, C. C., and R. D. Batt, *Biochim. Biophys. Acta* **152**, 255–265 (1968).
58. Nelson, G. J., *J. Lipid Res.* **8**, 374–379 (1967).
59. Cornwell, D. G., R. E. Heikkila, R. S. Bar, and G. L. Biagi, *J. Amer. Oil Chem. Soc.* **45**, 297–304 (1968).
60. Burger, S. P., T. Fujii, and D. J. Hanahan, *Biochemistry* **7**, 3682–3700 (1968).
61. Haude, W., H. Oginscius, and E. Goetze, *Acta Biol. Med. Ger.* **18**, 589–595 (1967).
62. Watson, W. C., *Brit. J. Haematol.* **9**, 32–38 (1963).

63. Hallinan, T., and E. Eden, *Blood* **20**, 557–565 (1962).
64. D'Hollander, F., and F. Chevallier, *Biochim. Biophys. Acta* **176**, 146–162 (1969).
65. Ehrhart, L. A., A. Butkus, A. L. Robertson, and I. H. Page, *Lipids* **3**, 84–87 (1968).
66. Osmond, D. H., R. R. Smeby, and F. M. Bumpus, *J. Lab. Clin. Med.* **73**, 795–808 (1969).
67. Gercken, G., and U. Brockman, in *Metabolism and Membrane Permeability of Erythrocytes and Thrombocytes*, E. Deutsch, E. Gerlach, and K. Moser, Eds., Thieme, Stuttgart, 1968, pp. 352–356.
68. Hestorff, R., P. O. Ways, and S. Palmer, *J. Clin. Invest.* **44**, 1059 (1965).
69. Kates, M., and A. T. James, *Biochim. Biophys. Acta* **50**, 478–485 (1961).
70. Leveille, G. A., J. W. Shockley, and H. E. Sauberlich, *Proc. Soc. Exp. Biol. Med.* **109**, 345–347 (1962).
71. Reed, C. F., *J. Clin. Invest.* **47**, 2630–2638 (1968).
72. Ostwald, R., and A. Shannon, *Biochem. J.* **91**, 146–154 (1964).
73. Nelson, G. J., *Biochim. Biophys. Acta* **144**, 221–232 (1967).
74. Nelson, G. J., *Comp. Biochem. Physiol.* **34**, 109–116 (1970).
75. Portman, O. W., and M. Alexander, *Arch. Biochem. Biophys.* **117**, 357–365 (1966).
76. Hawthorne, B. E., E. Smith, and J. O. Pescador, *J. Nutr.* **81**, 241–248 (1963).
77. Reed, C. F., S. N. Swisher, G. V. Marinetti, and E. G. Eden, *J. Lab. Clin. Med.* **56**, 281–289 (1960).
78. Irie, R., M. Iwanaga, and T. Yamakawa, *J. Biochem.* (*Tokyo*) **50**, 122–127 (1961).
79. Hanahan, D. J., R. M. Watts, and D. Pappajohn, *J. Lipid Res.* **1**, 421–432 (1960).
80. Donabedian, R. K., and A. Karmen, *J. Clin. Invest.* **46**, 1017–1027 (1967).
81. Payne, E., and C. J. Masters, *Comp. Biochem. Physiol.* **29**, 717–729 (1969).
82. Smith, J. K., *J. Immunol.* **100**, 863–872 (1968).
83. Glomset, J. A., *Biochim. Biophys. Acta* **65**, 128–135 (1962).
84. Wintzer, G., and G. Uhlenbruck, *Z. Immunitatetforsch. Allergie Klin. Immunol.* **133**, 60–67 (1967).
85. Yamakawa, T., R. Irie, and M. Iwanaga, *J. Biochem.* (*Tokyo*) **48**, 490–507 (1960).
86. Sweeley, C. C., and G. Dawson, in *Red Cell Membrane, Structure and Function*, G. A. Jamieson and T. J. Greenwalt, Ed., Lippincott, Philadelphia, 1969, pp. 172–227.
87. Vance, D. E., and C. C. Sweeley, *J. Lipid Res.* **8**, 621–630 (1967).
88. Yamakawa, T., M. Matsumoto, and S. Suzuki, *J. Biochem.* (*Tokyo*) **43**, 63–72 (1956).
89. Klenk, E., and K. Lauenstein, *Z. Physiol. Chem.* (*Hoppe-Seyler's*) **291**, 249–258 (1952).
90. Yamakawa, T., T. Yokoyawa, and N. Handa, *J. Biochem.* (*Tokyo*) **53**, 28–36 (1963).
91. Yamakawa, T., and S. Suzuki, *J. Biochem.* (*Tokyo*) **39**, 393–402 (1952).
92. Yamakawa, T., and S. Suzuki, *J. Biochem.* (*Tokyo*) **38**, 199–212 (1951).
93. Vance, D. E., W. Krivit, and C. C. Sweeley, *J. Lipid Res.* **10**, 188–192 (1969).
94. Booth, D. A., *Lancet* **i**, 626 (1967).
95. Edgar, G. W. F., G. J. M. Hooghwinkel, and P. Borri, *Lancet* **ii**, 693 (1965).

96. Wherrett, J. R., and B. L. Brown, *Neurology* **19**, 489–493 (1969).
97. Yamakawa, T., N. Kiso, S. Handa, A. Makita, and S. Yokoyama, *J. Biochem. (Tokyo)* **52**, 226–227 (1962).
98. Handa, N., and S. Handa, *Jap. J. Exp. Med.* **35**, 331–341 (1965).
99. Yamakawa, T., S. Nishimura, and M. Kamimura, *Jap. J. Exp. Med.* **35**, 201–207 (1965).
100. Klenk, E., and G. Padberg, *Z. Physiol. Chem.* (*Hoppe-Seyler's*) **327**, 249–255 (1962).
101. Booth, D. A., *Biochim. Biophys. Acta* **70**, 486–487 (1963).
102. Yamakawa, T., S. Yokoyawa, and N. Kiso, *J. Biochem.* (*Tokyo*) **52**, 228–229 (1962).
103. Relander, A., *Scand. J. Haematol.* **5**, 313–320 (1968).
104. Kuhn, R., and H. Wiegandt, *Z. Naturforsch.* **B19**, 80–81 (1964).
105. Handa, S., and T. Yamakawa, *Jap. J. Exp. Med.* **34**, 293–304 (1964).
106. Miyatake, T., S. Handa, and T. Yamakawa, *Jap. J. Exp. Med.* **38**, 135–138 (1968).
107. Eto, T., Y. Ichikawa, K. Nishimura, S. Ando, and T. Yamakawa, *J. Biochem. (Tokyo)* **64**, 205–213 (1968).
108. Turner, J. C., *J. Exp. Med.* **105**, 189–193 (1957).
109. Turner, J. C., H. M. Anderson, and G. P. Gandel, *Biochim. Biophys. Acta* **30**, 130–134 (1958).
110. Turner, J. D., and G. Rouser, *Anal. Biochem.* **38**, 423–436 (1970).
111. Nelson, G. J., *Biochem. Biophys. Res. Commun.* **38**, 261–265 (1970).
112. Hanahan, D. J., and R. M. Watts, *J. Biol. Chem.* **236**, P.C. 60 (1961).
113. Hanahan, D. J., J. Ekholm, and C. M. Jackson, *Biochemistry* **2**, 630–641 (1963).
114. Farquhar, J. W., *Biochim. Biophys. Acta* **60**, 89–89 (1962).
115. Kates, M., A. C. Allison, and A. T. James, *Biochim. Biophys. Acta* **48**, 571–582 (1961).
116. Hill, J. G., A. Kuksis, and J. M. R. Beveridge, *J. Amer. Oil Chem. Soc.* **42**, 137–141 (1965).
117. Cohen, P., and A. Derksen, *Brit. J. Haematol.* **17**, 359–371 (1969).
118. Christian, J. C., K. W. Kang, and Y. C. Poon, *Clin. Chim. Acta* **21**, 289–290 (1968).
119. Ishii, J., and K. Nakao, *Tohoku J. Exp. Med.* **94**, 169–175 (1968).
120. Rouser, G., G. Kritchevsky, and A. Yamamoto, in *Lipid Chromatographic Analysis, Vol. I*, G. V. Marinetti, Ed., Dekker, New York, 1967, pp. 99–162.
121. Dodge, J. T., and G. B. Phillips, *J. Lipid Res.* **7**, 387–395 (1966).
122. De Gier, J., and L. L. M. van Deenen, *Biochim. Biophys. Acta* **49**, 286–296 (1961).
123. Schrader, G. J., and G. T. Dimopoullos, *Amer. J. Vet. Res.* **24**, 283–286 (1963).
124. Brockman, U., and G. Gercken, *Clin. Chim. Acta* **23**, 489–494 (1969).
125. Menchaca, J. A., and K. Arai, *Tex. Rep. Biol. Med.* **25**, 74–82 (1967).
126. Farnsworth, P., D. Danon, and A. Gellhorn, *Brit. J. Haematol.* **11**, 200–205 (1965).
127. Nelson, G. J., in *Drugs Affecting Lipid Metabolism,* W. L. Holmes, L. Carlson, and R. Paoletti, Eds., Plenum Press, New York, 1969, pp. 583–596.
128. Casu, A., V. Pala, R. Menacelli, M. Ferro, and G. Nanni, *Ital. J. Biochem.* **17**, 77–89 (1968).
129. Maheswaran, S. K., and R. K. Lindorfer, *J. Bacteriol.* **94**, 1313–1319 (1967).
130. Smith, J. K., and E. L. Becker, *J. Immunol.* **100**, 459–474 (1968).

131. Sloviter, H. A., and S. Tanaka, *J. Cell. Comp. Physiol.* **63**, 261–266 (1964).
132. Gercken, G., and U. Brockman, *Eur. J. Biochem.* **8**, 489–494 (1969).
133. Jacobs, M. H., H. N. Glassman, and A. K. Parpart, *J. Cell Comp. Physiol.* **7**, 197–225 (1935).
134. Jacobs, M. H., H. N. Glassman, and A. K. Parpart, *J. Exp. Zool.* **113**, 277–300 (1950).
135. De Gier, J., L. L. M. van Deenen, and K. G. van Senden, *Experientia* **22**, 20–21 (1966).
136. De Gier, J., L. L. M. van Deenen, M. C. Verloop, and C. van Gastel, *Brit. J. Haematol.* **10**, 246–256 (1964).
137. Van Gastel, C., D. van den Berg, J. de Gier, and L. L. M. van Deenen, *Brit. J. Haematol.* **11**, 193–199 (1965).
138. Introzzi, P., A. Notario, N. di Marco, G. Doneda, and D. Meduri, *Haematology (Pavia)* **50**, 323–358 (1965).
139. Dodge, J. T., G. Cohen, H. J. Kayden, and G. B. Phillips, *J. Clin. Invest.* **46**, 357–368 (1967).
140. Robertson, A. F., and J. Putz, *J. Pediat.* **70**, 279–281 (1967).
141. Soula, G., P. Valdiguie, and L. Douste-Blazy, *Bull. Soc. Chim. Biol.* **50**, 1331–1339 (1968).
142. Neerhout, R. C., *J. Lab. Clin. Med.* **71**, 448–454 (1968).
143. Dhopeshwarkar, G. A., and U. N. Sukhatankar, *Brit. J. Haematol.* **14**, 51–56 (1968).
144. Phillips, G. B., J. T. Dodge, and C. S. Rockmore, *J. Lipid Res.* **9**, 285–286 (1968).
145. Neerhout, R. C., *Pediat. Res.* **2**, 172–178 (1968).
(1968).
146. Olivi, O., R. Genova, C. Mussini, and E. Manzini, *Haematology* **53**, 334–343
147. Dodge, J. T., and G. B. Phillips, *J. Lipid Res.* **8**, 676–681 (1967).
148. Samuelsson, B., and K. Samuelsson, *J. Lipid Res.* **10**, 47–55 (1969).
149. Farquhar, J. W., and E. H. Ahrens, Jr., *J. Clin. Invest.* **42**, 675–685 (1963).
150. Salvioli, G. P., G. Ambrosioni, and G. Allocca, *Clin. Pediat.* (*Bologna*) **48**, 429–444 (1966).
151. Van Golde, L. M. G., V. Tomasi, and L. L. M. van Deenen, *Chem. Phys. Lipids* **1**, 282–293 (1967).
152. Borri, P. F., G. J. M. Hooghwinkel, and G. W. Bruyn, *Psychiat. Neurol. Neurochir.* **69**, 143–148 (1966).
153. Marai, L., and A. Kuksis, *J. Lipid Res.* **10**, 141–152 (1969).
154. Soula, G., P. Valdiguie, and L. Douste-Blazy, *Bull. Soc. Chim. Biol.* **50**, 887–896 (1968).
155. Renkonen, O., and P. Varo, in *Lipid Chromatographic Analysis, Vol. I,* G. V. Marinetti, Ed., Dekker, New York, 1967, pp. 41–98.
156. Kuksis, A., L. Marai, W. C. Breckenridge, D. A. Gornall, and O. Stachnyk, *Can. J. Physiol. Pharm.* **46**, 511–524 (1968).
157. Trewhella, M. A., and F. D. Collins, *Lipids* **4**, 304–307 (1969).
158. Walker, B. L., and F. A. Kummerow, *J. Nutr.* **82**, 329–332 (1964).
159. Voight, K. D., M. Apostolakis, and G. Grimmer, *Klin. Wochenschr.* **43**, 732–737 (1965).
160. Walker, B. L., and M. L. Yurkowski, *Biochem. J.* **103**, 218–224 (1967).
161. Carroll, R. L., *Aerosp. Med.* **39**, 1290–1293 (1968).
162. De Gier, J., and L. L. M. van Deenen, *Biochim. Biophys. Acta* **84**, 294–304 (1964).

163. Connellan, J. M., and C. J. Masters, *Aust. J. Biol. Sci.* **18**, 445–447 (1965).
164. Nelson, G. J., *Lipids* **4**, 350–355 (1969).
165. Reid, M. E., J. G. Bieri, P. A. Plack, and E. L. Andrews, *J. Nutr.* **82**, 401–408 (1964).
166. Fitch, C. D., J. S. Dinning, L. A. Witting, and M. K. Horwitt, *J. Nutr.* **75**, 409–413 (1961).
167. Greenberg, L. D., and H. D. Moon, *Arch. Biochem. Biophys.* **94**, 405–416 (1961).
168. Chaffee, R. R. J., W. S. Platner, J. Potter, and C. Jenny, *Proc. Soc. Exp. Biol. Med.* **127**, 102–106 (1968).
169. Walker, B. L., and V. F. Lishchenko, *Can. J. Biochem.* **44**, 179–185 (1966).
170. Bieri, J. G., and R. K. H. Poukka, *J. Nutr.* **100**, 557–564 (1970).
171. Mulder, E., J. de Gier, and L. L. M. van Deenen, *Biochim. Biophys. Acta* **70**, 94–96 (1963).
172. Kogl, F., J. de Gier, I. Mulder, and L. L. M. van Deenen, *Biochim. Biophys. Acta* **43**, 95–103 (1960).
173. Shimojo, T., and K. Ohno, *J. Biochem.* (*Tokyo*) **60**, 228–230 (1966).
174. Panganamala, R. V., D. W. Buntine, J. C. Geer, and D. G. Cornwell, *Chem.*
175. Thompson, G. A., and D. J. Hanahan, *Biochemistry* **2**, 641–646 (1963).
Phys. Lipids **3**, 401–404 (1969).
176. Snyder, F., B. Malone, and R. L. Wykle, *Biochem. Biophys. Res. Commun.*
177. Snyder, F., B. Malone, and M. L. Blank, *J. Biol. Chem.* **245**, 1790–1799 (1970).
34, 40–47 (1969).
178. Snyder, F., M. L. Blank, B. Malone, and R. L. Wykle, *J. Biol. Chem.* **245**,
179. Van Deenen, L. L. M., J. de Gier, and J. H. Veerkamp, in *Biochemical Prob-*
1800–1805 (1970).
180. Paysant-Diament, M., and J. Polonovski, *Bull. Soc. Chim. Biol.* **42**, 337–350
lems of Lipids, P. Desnuelle, Ed., Pergamon Press, New York, 1961, pp. 32–38.
181. Dimopoullos, G. T., and A. T. James, *Proc. Soc. Exp. Biol. Med.* **125**, 569–
(1960).
182. McLeod, M. E., and R. Bressler, *Biochim. Biophys. Acta* **144**, 391–396 (1967).
574 (1967).
183. Rosenzweig, A., and P. Ways, *Blood* **27**, 57–64 (1966).
184. Hrachovec, J. P., *Proc. Soc. Exp. Biol. Med.* **118**, 328–333 (1965).
185. Sakagami, T., O. Minari, and T. Orii, *Biochim. Biophys. Acta* **98**, 356–364
186. Basford, J. M., J. Glover, and C. Green, *Biochim. Biophys. Acta* **84**, 764–766 (1965).
187. Reed, C. F., *J. Clin. Invest.* **38**, 1032–1033 (1959).
(1964).
188. Reed, C. F., *J. Clin. Invest.* **47**, 749–760 (1968).
189. Hokin, L. E., and M. R. Hokin, *Biochim, Biophys. Acta* **84**, 563–575 (1964).
190. Oliveira, M. M., and M. Vaughan, *J. Lipid Res.* **5**, 156–162 (1964).
191. Ferber, E., P. G. Munder, A. Kohlschutter, and H. Fischer, *Folia Haematol.* (*Leipzig*) **90**, 224–232 (1968).
192. Marks, P. A., A. Gellhorn, and C. Kidson, *J. Biol. Chem.* **235**, 2579–2583 (1960).
193. Shastri, K., and D. Rubinstein, *Can. J. Biochem.* **47**, 967–975 (1969).
194. Pittman, J. G., and D. B. Martin, *J. Clin. Invest.* **45**, 165–172 (1966).
195. Hrachovec, J. P., M. Leblanc, and M. Rockstein, *Proc. Soc. Exp. Biol. Med.* **107**, 205–207 (1961).
196. Binet, L., and M. Leblanc, *Compt. Rend.* **253**, 1022–1025 (1961).

197. Jossen, L., F. Steven, and R. Ruyssen, *Boll. Chim.-Farm.* **101**, 259–269 (1962).
198. Raderecht, H. J., S. Binnewies, and E. Scholzel, *Acta Biol. Med. Ger.* **8**, 199–208 (1962).
199. Sloviter, H. A., and R. K. Bose, *Biochim. Biophys. Acta* **116**, 156–158 (1966).
200. Agren, G., and G. Ronquist, *Acta Chem. Scand.* **18**, 2029–2043 (1964).
201. Westerman, M. P., and W. N. Jensen, *Proc. Soc. Exp. Biol. Med.* **118**, 315–319 (1965).
202. Paysant, M., B. Maupin, and J. Polonovski, *Bull. Soc. Chim. Biol.* **45**, 247–252 (1963).
203. Polonovski, J., and M. Paysant, *Bull. Soc. Chim. Biol.* **45**, 339–347 (1963).
204. Grossman, C. M., J. Horky, and R. Kohn, *Arch. Biochem. Biophys.* **117**, 18–27 (1966).
205. Grossman, C. M., F. Bartos, and J. Horky, *Folia Haematol.* **90**, 303–308 (1968).
206. Nelson, G. J., *Lipids* **3**, 267–274 (1968).
207. Soula, G., P. Valdiguie, and L. Douste-Blazy, *Bull. Soc. Chim. Biol.* **49**, 43–58 (1967).
208. Misra, U. K., *Can. J. Biochem.* **43**, 711–722 (1965).
209. Hagerman, J. S., and R. G. Gould, *Proc. Soc. Exp. Biol. Med.* **78**, 329–332 (1951).
210. London, I. M., and H. Schwarz, *J. Clin. Invest.* **32**, 1248–1252 (1953).
211. Gould, R. G., G. V. LeRoy, G. T. Okita, J. J. Kabara, P. Keegan, and D. M. Bergenstal, *J. Lab. Clin. Med.* **46**, 372–384 (1955).
212. Porte, D., and R. J. Havel, *J. Lipid Res.* **2**, 357–362 (1961).
213. Murphy, J. R., *J. Lab. Clin. Med.* **60**, 571–578 (1962).
214. Ashworth, L. A. E., and C. Green, *Biochim. Biophys. Acta* **70**, 68–74 (1963).
215. Ashworth, L. A. E., and C. Green, *Biochim. Biophys. Acta* **84**, 182–187 (1964).
216. Bruckdorfer, K. R., and C. Green, *Biochem. J.* **104**, 270–277 (1967).
217. Bruckdorfer, K. R., P. A. Edwards, and C. Green, *Eur. J. Biochem.* **4**, 506–511 (1968).
218. Bruckdorfer, K. R., J. M. Graham, and C. Green, *Eur. J. Biochem.* **4**, 512–518 (1968).
219. Bruckdorfer, K. R., R. A. Demel, J. de Gier, and L. L. M. van Deenen, *Biochim. Biophys. Acta* **183**, 334–345 (1969).
220. Klibansky, C., and A. de Vries, *Biochim. Biophys. Acta* **70**, 176–187 (1963).
221. Mulder, E., J. W. O. van den Berg, and L. L. M. van Deenen, *Biochim. Biophys. Acta* **106**, 118–127 (1965).
222. Robertson, A. F., and W. E. M. Lands, *J. Lipid Res.* **5**, 88–93 (1964).
223. Soula, G., P. Valdiguie, and L. Douste-Blazy, *Bull. Soc. Chim. Biol.* **49**, 1317–1330 (1967).
224. Nelson, G. J., *Lipids* **2**, 323–328 (1967).
225. Turner, J., and G. Rouser, *Anal. Biochem.* **38**, 437–445 (1970).
226. Horwitt, M. K., C. C. Harvey, and B. Century, *Science* **130**, 917–918 (1959).
227. Leibetseder, F., and E. H. Ahrens, Jr., *Brit. J. Haematol.* **5**, 356–364 (1959).
228. Farquhar, J. W., *J. Amer. Oil Chem. Soc.* **42**, 615–616 (1965).
229. Mulder, E., and L. L. M. van Deenen, *Biochim. Biophys. Acta* **106**, 106–117 (1965).
230. Mulder, E., and L. L. M. van Deenen, *Biochim. Biophys. Acta* **106**, 348–356 (1965).
231. Shohet, S. B., D. G. Nathan, and M. L. Karnovsky, *J. Clin. Invest.* **47**, 1096–1108 (1968).

232. Ferber, E., P. G. Munder, A. Kahlschutter, and H. Fischer, *Eur. J. Biochem.* **5**, 395–401 (1968).
233. Oliveira, M. M., and A. Nason, *Biochim. Biophys. Acta* **150**, 319–322 (1968).
234. Raderecht, H. J., E. Scholzel, and S. M. Rapport, *Klin. Wochenschr.* **38**, 824–825 (1960).
235. Raderecht, H. J., and E. Scholzel, *Folia Haematol.* **78**, 613–619 (1962).
236. Phillips, G. B., J. T. Dodge, and C. Howe, *Lipids* **4**, 544–549 (1969).
237. Gibson, J. G., in *The Red Blood Cell,* C. Bishop and D. M. Surgenor, Eds., Academic Press, New York, 1964, pp. 477–489.
238. Horwitt, M. K., C. C. Harvey, G. D. Duncan, and W. C. Wilson, *Amer. J. Clin. Nutr.* **4**, 408–419 (1956).
239. Zalkin, H., and A. L. Tappel, *Arch. Biochem. Biophys.* **88**, 113–117 (1960).
240. Weed, R. I., and C. F. Reed, *Amer. J. Med.* **41**, 681–698 (1966).
241. Smith, K. A., and C. E. Mengel, *J. Lab. Clin. Med.* **72**, 505–510 (1968).
242. Rimon, S., F. Brok, and A. Rimon, *Clin. Chim. Acta* **12**, 22–26 (1965).
243. Ways, P. O., *J. Lipid Res.* **8**, 518–521 (1967).
244. Cooper, R. A., and J. H. Jandl, in *Metabolism and Membrane Permeability of Erythrocytes and Thrombocytes,* E. Deutsch, E. Gerlach, and K. Moser, Eds., Thieme, Stuttgart, 1968, pp. 376–384.
245. Witting, L. A., C. C. Harvey, B. Century, and M. K. Horwitt, *J. Lipid Res.* **2**, 412–418 (1961).
246. Monsen, E. R., R. Okey, and R. L. Lyman, *Metabolism* **11**, 1113–1124 (1962).
247. Bournique, C., R. Portet, and L. Chevillard, *C.R. Seances Soc. Biol. Filiales* **158**, 954–958 (1964).
248. Notario, A., H. Zenetti, V. Ricotti, and G. Bosco, *Haematology* **50**, 1–32 (1965).
249. March, B. E., V. Coates, and J. Biely, *Can. J. Physiol. Pharmacol.* **44**, 379–387 (1966).
250. Silver, M. M., G. C. McMillan, and M. D. Silver, *Brit. J. Haematol.* **10**, 271–280 (1964).
251. Van Deenen, L. L. M., in *Regulatory Function of Biological Membranes,* J. Jarnefelts, Ed., Elsevier, Amsterdam, 1968, pp. 72–86.
252. Mohrhauer, H., and R. T. Holman, *J. Lipid Res.* **4**, 346–350 (1963).
253. Fillios, L. C., S. B. Andrus, G. V. Mann, and F. J. Stare, *J. Exp. Med.* **104**, 539–554 (1956).
254. O'Neal, R. M., W. A. Thomas, and W. S. Hartroft, *Amer. J. Cardiol.* **3**, 94–100 (1959).
255. Thomas, W. A., R. F. Scott, K. T. Lee, H. S. Doud, and R. M. Jones, in *Comparative Atherosclerosis,* J. C. Roberts and R. Straus, Eds., Harper and Row, New York, 1965, pp. 92–108.
256. Walker, B. L., and F. A. Kummerow, *J. Nutr.* **81**, 75–80 (1963).
257. Walker, B. L., and F. A. Kummerow, *J. Nutr.* **82**, 323–328 (1964).
258. Walker, B. L., and F. A. Kummerow, *Proc. Soc. Exp. Biol. Med.* **115**, 1099–1103 (1964).
259. Walker, B. L., *Arch. Biochem. Biophys.* **114**, 465–471 (1966).
260. Walker, B. L., *J. Nutr.* **92**, 23–29 (1967).
261. Mengel, C. E., and H. E. Kahn, *J. Clin. Invest.* **45**, 1150–1158 (1966).
262. Allison, A. C., M. Kates, and A. T. James, *Brit. Med. J.* **i**, 1766–1768 (1960).
263. Harris, I. M., T. A. J. Prankerd, and M. P. Westerman, *Brit. Med. J.* **ii**, 1276–1277 (1957).

264. Salvioli, G. P., G. Ambrosioni, and G. Allocca, *Haematology* **53**, 534–550 (1968).
265. Phillips, G. B., and N. S. Roome, *Proc. Soc. Exp. Biol. Med.* **109**, 360–364 (1962).
266. Neerhout, R. C., *Clin. Pediat.* **7**, 451–464 (1968).
267. Westerman, M. P., L. E. Pierce, and W. N. Jensen, *Blood* **23**, 200–205 (1964).
268. De Gier, J., L. L. M. van Deenen, R. A. Geerdink, K. Punt, and M. C. Ver-
269. Westerman, M. P., S. P. Balcerzak, and E. W. Heinle, *J. Lab. Clin. Med.* **72**,
270. Cooper, R. A., and J. H. Jandl, *J. Clin. Invest.* **48**, 736–744 (1969).
271. Cooper, R. A., and J. H. Jandl, *J. Clin. Invest.* **48**, 906–914 (1969).
272. Jacobs, H. S., *J. Clin. Invest.* **46**, 2083–2094 (1967).
273. Ways, P., C. F. Reed, and D. J. Hanahan, *J. Clin. Invest.* **42**, 1248–1260 (1963).
274. Phillips, G. B., and J. T. Dodge, *J. Lab. Clin. Med.* **71**, 629–637 (1968).
275. Kayden, H. J., and R. Silber, *Trans. Assoc. Amer. Physicians* **78**, 334–342 (1956).
276. Phillips, G. B., *J. Lab. Clin. Med.* **59**, 357–363 (1962).
277. Phillips, G. B., *Lipids* **3**, 385–386 (1968).
278. Nye, W. H. R., and G. V. Marinetti, *J. Clin. Invest.* **44**, 1081 (1965).
279. Boon, J., R. M. Broekhuyse, P. van Munster, and E. Schretlen, *Clin. Chim. Acta* **23**, 453–456 (1969).
280. Neerhout, R. C., *J. Pediat.* **73**, 364–373 (1968).
281. Salvioli, G. P., *Folia Haematol.* **83**, 295–297 (1965).
282. Meriwether, W. D., and C. E. Mengel, *Nature* **210**, 91–92 (1966).
283. Weinstein, R. S., and R. A. Williams, *Blood* **30**, 785–791 (1967).
284. Braunsteiner, H., E. Gisinger, and F. Pakesch, *Blood* **11**, 753–756 (1956).
285. Cecchi, E., and E. Conestabile, *Lancet* **ii**, 466–468 (1957).
286. Lewis, S. M., D. Danon, and Y. Marikovsky, *Brit. J. Haematol.* **11**, 689–695 (1965).
287. Hooghwinkel, G. J. M., H. H. van Gelderen, and A. Staal, *Arch. Dis. Child.* **44**, 197–202 (1969).
288. Norum, K. R., and E. Gjone, *Scand. J. Clin. Lab. Invest.* **20**, 231–243 (1967).
289. Norum, K. R., and E. Gjone, *Biochim. Biophys. Acta* **144**, 698–700 (1967).
290. Norum, K. R., and E. Gjone, *Scand. J. Clin. Lab. Invest.* **22**, 94–98 (1968).
291. Nath, R. L., and A. Chatterjee, *Bull. Calcutta Sch. Trop. Med.* **10**, 82 (1962).
Sper. **38**, 204–206 (1962).
292. Ioppolo, C., G. Antognoni, O. Coppola, and E. Bottini, *Boll. Soc. Ital. Biol.*
293. Nothman, M. M., and S. Proger, *Med. Welt* **4**, 190–194 (1965).
(1968).
294. Sloviter, H. A., V. Janic, and J. L. Naiman, *Clin. Chim. Acta* **20**, 423–426
295. Scott, J. G., R. I. Weed, and S. N. Swisher, *Vox Sang.* **13**, 308–313 (1967).
296. Zahler, P., *Vox Sang.* **15**, 81–101 (1968).
297. Chapman, D., in *Biological Membranes*, D. Chapman, Ed., Academic Press, New York, 1968, pp. 125–202.
298. Van Deenen, L. L. M., in *Progress in the Chemistry of Fats and Other Lipids*, Vol. VIII, Part I, R. T. Holman, Ed., Pergamon Press, Oxford, 1965, pp. 1–126.
299. Vandenheuvel, F. A., *J. Amer. Oil Chem. Soc.* **40**, 455–471 (1963).
300. Jung, F., *Folia Haematol.* **90**, 182–195 (1968).
301. Weinstein, R. S., in *Red Cell Membrane, Structure and Function,* G. A. Jamieson and T. J. Greenwalt, Eds., Lippincott, Philadelphia, 1969, pp. 36–76.

302. Finean, J. B., R. Coleman, W. G. Green, and A. R. Limbrick, *J. Cell. Sci.* **1**, 287–296 (1966).
303. Segerman, E., in *Membrane Models and the Formation of Biological Membranes,* L. Bolis and B. A. Pethica, Eds., North-Holland, Amsterdam, 1968, pp. 52–75.
304. Rand, R. P., and V. Luzzati, *Biophys. J.* **8**, 125–137 (1968).
305. Finean, J. B., in *Progress in Biophysics and Molecular Biology,* Vol. 16, J. A. V. Butler and H. E. Huxley, Eds., Pergamon Press, London, 1966, pp. 145–170.
306. Weinstein, R. S., and F. B. Merk, *Proc. Soc. Exp. Biol. Med.* **125**, 38–40 (1967).
307. Weinstein, R. S., and S. Bullivant, *Blood,* **29**, 780–789 (1967).
308. Branton, D., *Proc. Natl. Acad. Sci. U.S.* **55**, 1048–1056 (1966).
309. Weinstein, R. S., and V. M. Koo, *Proc. Soc. Exp. Biol. Med.* **128**, 353–357 (1968).
310. Branton, D., *Exp. Cell Res.* **45**, 703–707 (1967).
311. Smith, M. E., in *Advances in Lipid Research*, Vol. 5, R. Paoletti and D. Kritchevsky, Eds., Academic Press, New York, 1967, pp. 241–278.
312. Koehler, J. K., *Z. Zellforsch. Mikroskop. Anat.* **85**, 1–17 (1968).
313. Kemp, C. L., and A. F. Howatson, *Virology* **30**, 147–151 (1966).
314. Kinsky, S. C., S. A. Luse, D. Zopf, L. L. M. van Deenen, and J. Haxby, *Biochim. Biophys. Acta* **135**, 844–861 (1967).
315. Lenard, J., and S. J. Singer, *Proc. Natl. Acad. Sci. U.S.* **56**, 1828–1835 (1966).
316. Urry, D. W., M. Mednieks, and E. Bejnarowicz, *Proc. Natl. Acad. Sci. U.S.* **57**, 1043–1049 (1967).
317. Gordon, A. S., D. F. H. Wallach, and J. H. Straus, *Biochim. Biophys. Acta* **183**, 405–416 (1969).
318. Chapman, D., V. B. Kamat, J. de Gier, and S. A. Penkett, *Nature* **213**, 74–75 (1967).
319. Chapman, D., V. B. Kamat, J. de Gier, and S. A. Penkett, *J. Mol. Biol.* **31**, 101–114 (1968).
320. Kamat, V. B., and D. Chapman, *Biochim. Biophys. Acta* **163**, 411–414 (1968).
321. Clifford, J., B. A. Pethica, and E. G. Smith, in *Membrane Models and the Formation of Biological Membranes,* L. Bolis and B. A. Pethica, Eds., North-Holland, Amsterdam, 1968, pp. 19–42.
322. Chapman, D., V. B. Kamat, and R. J. Levene, *Science* **160**, 314–316 (1968).
323. Maddy, A. H., and B. R. Malcolm, *Science* **150**, 1616–1617 (1965).
324. Libertini, L. J., A. S. Waggoner, P. C. Jost, and O. H. Griffith, *Proc. Natl. Acad. Sci. U.S.* **64**, 13–19 (1969).
325. Hubbell, W. L., and H. M. McConnell, *Proc. Natl. Acad. Sci. U.S.* **63**, 16–22 (1969).
326. Chapman, D., M. D. Barratt, and V. B. Kamat, *Biochim. Biophys. Acta* **173**, 154–157 (1969).
327. Hubbell, W. L., and H. M. McConnell, *Proc. Natl. Acad. Sci. U.S.* **64**, 20–27 (1969).
328. Maddy, A. H., *Biochim. Biophys. Acta* **88**, 448–449 (1964).
329. Maddy, A. H., *Biochim. Biophys. Acta* **117**, 193–200 (1966).
330. Morgan, T. E., and D. J. Hanahan, *Biochemistry* **5**, 1050–1059 (1966).
331. Zwaal, R. F. A., and L. L. M. van Deenen, *Biochim. Biophys. Acta* **150**, 323–325 (1968).
332. Lauf, P. K., and M. D. Poulik, *Brit. J. Haematol.* **15**, 191–202 (1968).

333. Roelofsen, B., J. de Gier, and L. L. M. van Deneen, *J. Cell Comp. Physiol.* **63**, 233–243 (1964).
334. Haahti, E. O., V. Nanto, and J. Viikari, *Acta Chem. Scand.* **21**, 2773–2780 (1967).
335. Zamudio, I., M. Cellino, and M. Canessa-Fischer, *Arch. Biochem. Biophys.* **129**, 336–345 (1969).
336. Rich, G. T., R. I. Sha'afi, T. C. Barton, and A. K. Solomon, *J. Gen. Physiol.* **50**, 2391–2405 (1967).
337. Finkelstein, A., and A. Cass, *Nature* **216**, 717–718 (1967).
338. Sha'afi, R. I., C. Gary-Bobo, and A. K. Soloman, *Biochim. Biophys. Acta* **173**, 141–142 (1969).
339. Murphy, J. R., *J. Lab. Clin. Med.* **60**, 86–109 (1962).
340. Eylar, E. H., M. A. Madoff, O. V. Brody, and J. L. Oncley, *J. Biol. Chem.* **237**, 1992–2000 (1962).
341. Zmijewski, C. M., *Immunohematology*, Appleton-Century-Crofts, New York, 1968.
342. Nanni, G., A. Casu, V. M. Marinari, and I. Baldini, *Ital. J. Biochem.* **18**, 25–34 (1969).
343. Nanni, G., V. M. Marinari, I. Baldini, M. Ferro, and A. Casu, *Ital. J. Biochem.* **18**, 123–132 (1969).
344. Haxby, J. A., C. B. Kinsky, and S. C. Kinsky, *Proc. Natl. Acad. Sci. U.S.* **61**, 300–307 (1968).
345. Marks, P. A., in *The Red Blood Cell,* C. Bishop, and D. M. Surgenor, Eds., Academic Press, New York, 1964, pp. 211–241.
346. Marchesi, V. T., and G. E. Palade, *J. Cell. Biol.* **35**, 385–404 (1967).
347. Zahler, P., *Experientia* **25**, 449–456 (1969).

8. Lipid Composition and Metabolism of Leukocytes

EUGENE L. GOTTFRIED

Department of Medicine, Cornell University Medical College, New York, New York

I. INTRODUCTION

A growing awareness of the complexity of the leukocytes and their importance in mammalian physiology has stimulated interest in the structure and metabolism of these cells. The phagocytic role has long been recognized as a key factor in defense against bacterial infection, but the far-reaching effects of cellular immunity under the control of the lymphoid cells have only recently been fully appreciated. Improvements in the methods of handling and isolating leukocytes have helped to overcome some of the difficulties and unreliability of the earlier studies. Nevertheless, in comparison with work on the lipid composition and lipid metabolism of erythrocytes, reports describing these properties in leukocytes, particularly human leukocytes, have been very few indeed.

An important factor that has delayed the accumulation of information about leukocytes is the difficulty in obtaining adequate amounts of suitably pure cell samples for study. Though they contain as much as 5% of all the blood cellular lipids (1) and are responsible for most of the lipid-metabolism activity in whole blood (2–4), leukocytes are about 800 times less numerous than erythrocytes in circulating blood—normally 5×10^6 to 10×10^6 cells/ml. They are sensitive to handling methods and tend to adhere to the surfaces of glassware used in isolation procedures.

Many studies of leukocyte lipids, particularly the earlier ones, have utilized mixed cell suspensions of varying degrees of purity (2–11) or samples from patients with abnormally high leukocyte counts (leukocytosis, leukemia) (12–17). The specificity of such observations is limited by the heterogeneity of the cell populations under investigation.

The term "leukocytes" represents, in fact, a mixed group of cells, alike only in that they are all nucleated, non-hemoglobin-bearing cells that spend at least a fraction of their lifespan circulating in the peripheral blood. There are major differences—especially between the myeloid and lymphoid groups of leukocytes—in many characteristics, including origin, functions, morphology, and lifespan (18). It is not at all surprising that there are differences in chemical composition and metabolic activity as well. Significant differences in lipid composition have been found not only between normal human leukocytes of different morphological type but also between normal and leukemic leukocytes of the same apparent morphological series (1).

Analytical methods useful in studying the lipid composition and metabolism of blood cells have been discussed in Part I. Microanalytical techniques are especially valuable in the case of leukocytes, where the sample size may be very small.

A word should be said about histochemical methods, which have been employed from time to time in an effort to uncover information about the lipids of leukocytes, normal and abnormal. Though such an approach has been greeted occasionally with enthusiasm—or at least with cautious optimism (19)—many pitfalls are associated with the preparation and fixation of tissues, and the staining techniques are all too often nonspecific. We agree with Pearse (20), who concludes that "no satisfactory histochemical technique for fatty acids exists, and that by staining methods alone absolute distinction between the various groups of lipids is sometimes a matter of great difficulty."

II. PREPARATION OF LEUKOCYTE SAMPLES

A. Isolation of Leukocytes from Normal Blood

Because of the known heterogeneity of the leukocyte population in circulating blood, metabolic or chemical investigations of specific leukocytes generally require not only separation of these cells from plasma, erythrocytes, and blood platelets but also isolation of the specific morphologic type under investigation. Many methods have been proposed, based on such diverse characteristics as differences in resistance to lytic agents, cell density, phagocytic ability, adhesiveness to glass or other surfaces, and surface charge. Some of these are listed in Table I.

Table I. Isolation of Leukocytes from Blood and Other Sources

Characteristic	Techniques	Cells Obtained	Refs.
Resistance to lysis	Hypotonic solutions, gramicidin, lysolecithin, acetic and tartaric acids, saponins, etc.	Leukocytes (mixed population)	21–26
Cell density	Sedimentation, centrifugation (with or without density gradients)	Erythrocytes ($\rho = 1.079$) > granulocytes ($\rho = 1.075$) > lymphocytes ($\rho = 1.063$) > platelets ($\rho = 1.030$)	27–46
Adhesiveness to surfaces	Glass vessels, glass beads; glass, cotton, or nylon-mesh columns	Lymphocytes (pass through); granulocytes, monocytes (adhere)	47–51
Phagocytosis	Ingestion of iron particles followed by centrifugation, sedimentation, or magnetic fields	Granulocytes (bottom); lymphocytes (in supernatant)	52–54
Surface charge	Electrophoresis, countercurrent distribution	Leukocytes (incomplete separation of types)	55, 56
Extravascular sources:			
Inflammatory exudates		Granulocytes, monocytes	57–66
Thoracic-duct lymph, lymph nodes, thymus		Lymphocytes	67–70
Tissue culture		Immature lymphoid or myeloid cells	71
Disease states		Abnormal leukocytes	12–17

The great variety of methods offered by different authors is a good indication of the technical difficulty involved in isolating a pure population of cells with high yields and minimal cell damage.

1. Removal of Erythrocytes by Lysis. One method commonly recommended for obtaining mixed populations of leukocytes from whole blood is to hemolyze the erythrocytes by brief exposure to distilled water or hypotonic saline solutions (21–23). Hemolytic agents—such as gramicidin, lysolecithin, saponin, acetic acid, and tartaric acid—have been recommended in the past (24–26). The lipid-containing erythrocyte ghosts are of low density and can easily be separated from the intact leukocytes, along with blood platelets, by low-speed centrifugation (150–250 *g*). It is essential, of course, that the leukocytes remain unharmed by the procedure employed to lyse the erythrocytes. We have had very satisfactory results with the method of Fallon et al. (21), in which the cell mixture is suspended for 30 to 45 sec in hypotonic saline solution, after which isotonicity is restored by adding hypertonic saline. This approach is particularly useful for cleaning up a mixed leukocyte suspension after the bulk of the erythrocytes have been removed by sedimentation.

2. Differential Centrifugation or Sedimentation. A gentle centrifugation or differential sedimentation method would appear to offer the best possibility of separating blood cells with the least amount of cell damage, on the basis of their known differences in density (Table I). A large number of procedures have been proposed (72), utilizing a variety of operating conditions, including special mechanical devices, various suspending media, and density gradients of sucrose, albumin, Ficoll, silicone fluids, and similar materials (32–44). Elaborate continuous-flow centrifuge cell separators have been designed for blood (27, 45, 46), permitting the selective removal of leukocytes from human or animal blood by continuous centrifugation. Large yields of cells have been obtained with such apparatus, but individual leukocyte types are not well separated (45).

To increase the rate of erythrocyte sedimentation by rouleau formation, a variety of additives have been used, including dextran of high molecular weight, fibrinogen, γ-globulin, polyvinylpyrrolidone, phytohemagglutinin, gum acacia, and others. The relative effectiveness of these agents has been compared by several workers (25, 27, 72, 73). Tullis (27) suggested that, regardless of the sedimenting agent selected, a certain minimum concentration of erythrocytes is reached (usually at an erythrocyte-to-leukocyte ratio of about 1 : 1) below which these cells are too widely dispersed for effective aggregation.

3. Adhesiveness to Foreign Surfaces. In 1926 Fleming (47) described a simple method for removing the bulk of leukocytes (chiefly granulocytes and monocytes) from whole blood by passing the sample through a U-tube filled with cotton or glass wool. Numerous variations of this technique have since been employed to remove granulocytes from mixed-cell suspensions, using columns of finely divided cotton, nylon, or glass wool or glass beads. Other workers have collected the leukocytes adhering to glass vessels of large surface area after first washing off contaminating erythrocytes (48). Detailed studies of factors that affect the adhesiveness of leukocytes to glass beads have been made by Garvin (49) and Kvarstein (50), who have demonstrated the significant effects of temperature, flow rate, plasma proteins, and anticoagulants on the adhesiveness of granulocytes. The ability of ethylenediaminetetraacetic acid (EDTA) to diminish leukocyte adhesiveness to glass beads has been exploited by Rabinowitz (51) to obtain pure leukocyte types with fairly good yields. In this method leukocyte-rich plasma is passed through a glass-bead column, and lymphocytes (which pass through freely) are collected in the initial fraction. Granulocytes and monocytes are then eluted sequentially with saline solutions containing EDTA.

4. Other Methods. Their capacity to ingest foreign particles distinguishes granulocytes from lymphocytes. This characteristic has encouraged attempts to remove these phagocytic cells from mixed populations of leukocytes by first loading them with fine particles of metallic iron and then collecting them by sedimentation (52), centrifugation (53), or exposure to magnetic fields (54). Blood cells are known to differ in surface-charge density (55). It is thus possible to achieve some degree of separation of specific cell types by electrophoresis.[1] Countercurrent distribution has also been suggested as a potentially useful way of separating lymphocytes from polymorphonuclear leukocytes (56).

B. Abnormal Circulating Leukocytes

The use of blood samples containing abnormally high numbers of leukocytes (as in certain infectious diseases, allergic states, or leukemia) offers apparent advantages over the routine study of normal blood leukocytes. In some conditions the white-blood-cell count may be extremely high; for example, in chronic lymphocytic or myelocytic leukemia it is not unusual to find 50 times the normal number of circulating leukocytes in the blood. Moreover, a single cell type may predominate, thus reducing the need for rigorous separation procedures in the isolation of leukocytes. Leukocyte types not readily available under normal conditions are more easily har-

[1] A free-flowing preparative electrophoretic separator currently available is said to be capable of satisfactorily separating some leukocyte types. (Brinkmann Instruments, Westbury, N.Y.)

vested from blood in certain conditions (e.g., eosinophilia). So it is that the earliest reports of lipid composition and metabolism of leukocytes contained a high proportion of studies based on abnormal blood specimens (12–17).

The main problem encountered in the use of abnormal blood as a source of cells is in the interpretation of the results in relation to normal leukocytes. In leukocytosis secondary to bacterial infection, for example, there is generally an increase in the relative proportion of polymorphonuclear leukocytes and at the same time a greater proportion of immature cells. The difficulties of interpretation are compounded in the case of leukemic leukocytes. Any deviation from expected normal values may be the result of either a shift in the differential cell count (when mixed leukocyte populations are compared), a nonspecific reflection of cell immaturity, or an alteration of structure or function specifically related to the disease process in question.

C. Extravascular Sources

Cells resembling the leukocytes of circulating blood can be obtained from sources other than blood, often in a relatively pure state. Lymphocytes have been successfully obtained from thoracic-duct lymph (67, 68) as well as from lymph nodes and the thymus (69, 70). Peritoneal exudates have provided a ready source of polymorphonuclear leukocytes or macrophages (depending on the procedure used for inducing the peritoneal inflammatory response and the time at which cells are harvested), and alveolar macrophages have been obtained from lung tissue (57–60). These macrophages are generally considered to be similar to the monocytes, which they resemble morphologically, but there is some disagreement about their actual origin (74). As in the case of abnormal blood leukocytes, cells derived from extravascular sources are not necessarily identical with morphologically similar leukocytes circulating in blood. Indeed it has been suggested that significant metabolic differences may exist (75). Recently tissue-culture techniques have made possible the large-scale production of immature cells of lymphoid or myeloid origin (71).

It is especially important to distinguish between leukocytes from man and other mammals. The granulocytic cells (heterophils) of some animals, such as the rabbit, have clearly demonstrable morphological differences from their human counterparts. But even morphologically similar cells derived from different species may have chemical and metabolic differences of considerable magnitude. In the analogous case of erythrocyte-membrane composition striking species differences in lipid composition have been demonstrated (76, 77) (see Chapter 7).

D. Processing Leukocyte Samples

The general problem of processing blood for investigation of the formed elements has been discussed in Chapter 1. The handling of leukocytes presents some special problems.

1. Choice of Anticoagulant. Leukocytes are particularly sensitive to the method chosen to prevent the blood from clotting during the separation process. The choice of anticoagulant depends in large measure on the procedure to be employed for cell separation.

Ethylenediaminetetraacetic acid, usually employed as the disodium or tripotassium salt, is a chelating agent that appears to be especially suitable for processing leukocytes. Clumping of cells, a troublesome factor particularly when the leukocytes must be centrifuged, is minimized with EDTA. In the recommended concentration of 1 mg/ml the effect on cellular lipids is probably small. However, like any anticoagulant that acts by binding calcium, EDTA has a profound effect on the functional state of the cell surface and interferes with the capacity of granulocytes to adhere to glass (49–51). When separation procedures like glass-bead columns are to be used for the isolation of specific leukocyte types, virtually the only agent suitable for initial anticoagulation is heparin. When used in high concentration, however, heparin may have deleterious effects on cell lipids (78, 79).

Defibrination has the advantage of avoiding the introduction of potentially toxic foreign substances, but this procedure itself leads to reduced yields of leukocytes, particularly granulocytes, which tend to become entangled in the fibrin clot.

2. Siliconized Glassware. Although opinion differs on the importance of siliconized glassware in processing leukocytes, we concur with the general impression that yields are considerably improved when all glass surfaces in contact with intact cells are siliconized (80). Nonwettable vessels of cellulose nitrate, Teflon, and polyethylene are also convenient and efficient.

The decision to use siliconized glassware in a lipid laboratory poses a problem, because there is a real hazard of generalized contamination with silicones and interference with analytical procedures. For this reason we siliconize only glassware that will actually be in contact with cells during separation procedures prior to extraction. This siliconized glassware is carefully segregated from all other laboratory ware at every stage of handling and washing.

3. Evaluation of Viability. Determination of viability in leukocyte preparations is commonly made by exclusion of such dyes as trypan blue or eosin (21, 81, 82), to which the cells are normally impermeable, because of the convenience and simplicity of this method. As emphasized by Tullis (83), however, some damaged cells may escape detection by dye-exclusion methods. Tullis noted that degenerating leukocytes undergo loss of their characteristic properties in stages, in the following order: oxidative metabolism, phagocytic ability, ameboid motility, Brownian motion, impermeability to certain dyes, and morphologic integrity.

III. LIPID COMPOSITION OF LEUKOCYTES

A. Major Lipid Classes of Normal Leukocytes

Of the lipid content of normal circulating leukocytes, most is known about lymphocytes and polymorphonuclear leukocytes, which have been isolated in sufficiently large numbers for the required analytical procedures. There is little consistent information regarding the less numerous leukocyte types.

Lipids constitute about 5% of the wet weight of normal human lymphocytes and polymorphonuclear leukocytes; erythrocytes have a total lipid content of only about 0.5% of the whole cell weight (Table II). Polymorphonuclear leukocytes have about twice as much lipid per cell as lymphocytes, in approximate proportion to the cell mass. Since the granulocytes

Table II. Lipid Composition of Normal Circulating Human Blood Cells (1, 84)

Characteristic	Polymorphonuclear Leukocytes ($n = 6$)[a]	Lymphocytes ($n = 5$)[a]	Erythrocytes ($n = 10$)[a]
Wet weight[b] ($\times 10^{-12}$ g)	430	212	97
Total lipids ($\times 10^{-12}$ g)	21.5	10.0	0.50
Percentage of wet weight	5.0	4.7	0.52
Cholesterol ($\times 10^{-15}$ mole)	5.33	3.24	0.34
Percentage of total lipids	10	12.5	27
Phospholipids ($\times 10^{-15}$ mole)	9.67	4.73	0.36
Percentage of total lipids[c]	34	35	55
Cholesterol/phospholipid molar ratio	0.55	0.68	0.94
α,β-Unsaturated ether/phospholipid molar ratio	0.24	0.14	0.17

[a] Mean values per cell.
[b] Calculated from Ref. 44.
[c] Calculated on the basis of an estimated average molecular weight of 750.

contain over 40 times as much lipid per cell as erythrocytes, the leukocytes, despite their comparatively small numbers, contribute a substantial proportion of the total circulating cellular lipids.

About one-third of the total lipid content (by weight) of polymorphonuclear leukocytes and lymphocytes is phospholipid, presumed to be associated with the structural lipoproteins. Another one-third consists of neutral lipids, primarily triglycerides and free cholesterol. An unusual feature of both granulocytes and lymphocytes is the presence of substantial amounts of glycolipids, predominantly ceramide dihexoside, which may amount to one-sixth of the total lipid weight in mixed leukocyte preparations (85).

B. Neutral Lipids

About 10 to 12% of the total lipids in human leukocytes is free cholesterol (1). Like the phospholipids with which it is closely linked, cholesterol appears to be concerned primarily with the organization of the cell's membranous structures. The cholesterol-to-phospholipid molar ratio is 0.68 for human lymphocytes and 0.55 for polymorphonuclear leukocytes, in contrast to the much higher ratio (0.94) found in erythrocytes (84). The cholesterol-to-phospholipid ratio of polymorphonuclear leukocytes is similar to that of platelet membranes (0.53) (86). Granulocytes and platelets, which have a common origin in the bone marrow, appear to have other similarities in their lipid patterns, including phospholipid distribution (see Fig. 1 and also Chapter 9).

Substantial amounts of triglycerides (about 20% of the total lipid weight) may be present in both lymphocytes and polymorphonuclear leukocytes (1, 57, 68). Diglycerides in small amounts and traces of monoglycerides have been reported (8, 60, 69), as well as small amounts of free fatty acids and hydrocarbons (8, 57, 69).

There is considerable disagreement in published reports regarding the presence of esterified cholesterol (8, 10, 11, 57, 68, 69). We have found only very small amounts of cholesteryl esters in human lymphocytes and granulocytes (1).

The distribution of fatty acids has not been studied extensively in purified leukocyte cell types. Elsbach (57) found granulocytes from rabbit peritoneal exudate to have a total fatty acid pattern similar to the erythrocytes, with a predominance of linoleic (18:2), palmitic (16:0), oleic (18:1), and stearic (18:0) acids. The phospholipid fraction contained mostly linoleic (40%) and palmitic (20%) acids, whereas the neutral-lipid fraction contained predominantly oleic and palmitic acids (about 26% each). Blomstrand (68) studied the fatty acid distribution of isolated human lymphocytes and found that both the phospholipid and triglyceride fractions contained large

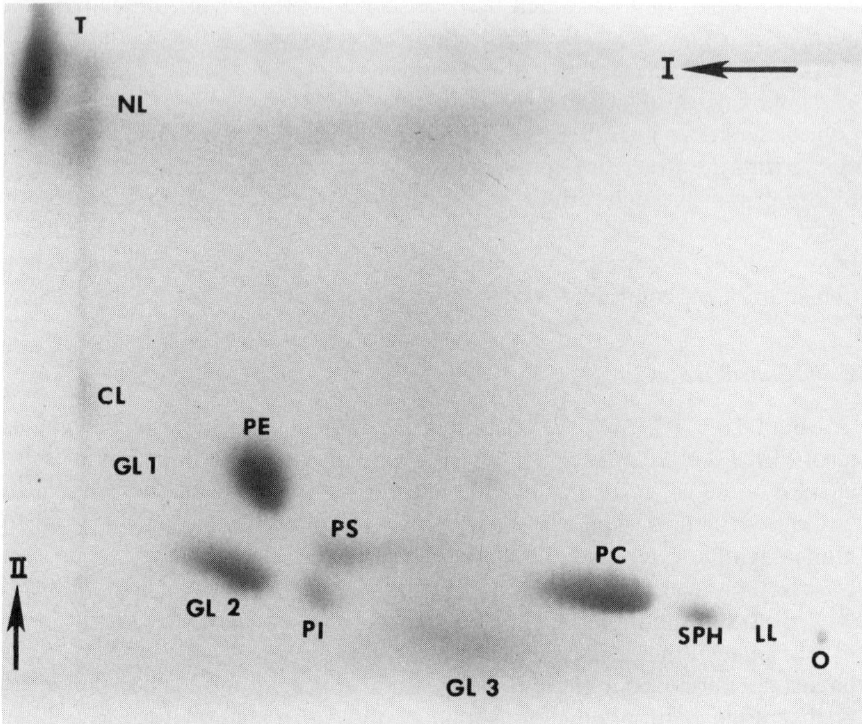

Fig. 1 Two-dimensional thin-layer chromatogram of the lipids in human polymorphonuclear leukocytes (570-μg sample). Silica gel H chromatoplate of 0.25 mm thickness, prepared with 0.001 *M* sodium carbonate (92, 93). Solvent I : chloroform–methanol–acetic acid–water, 50 : 30 : 4 : 4 (by volume), with 0.01% α-tocopherol added. Solvent II : diisobutyl ketone–acetic acid–water, 40 : 25 : 5 (by volume). Abbreviations: O, origin; LL, lysolecithin; SPH, sphingomyelin; PC, lecithin (phosphatidylcholine); PS, phosphatidylserine; PI, phosphatidylinositol; PE, phosphatidylethanolamine; CL, cardiolipin; GL 1, cerebrosides; GL 2, ceramide dihexoside; GL 3, unidentified glycolipid; NL, neutral lipids (phosphatidic acid also runs in this region); T, α-tocopherol (added to solvent I).

amounts of palmitic (20–25%), oleic (17–19%), and stearic (14–16%) acids, but only 9% linoleic acid. The lymphocyte phospholipid fraction had in addition an arachidonic acid (20:4) content of 18%.

C. Phospholipids

The phospholipids of leukocytes have been studied in considerable detail, particularly in regard to the differences between cell types and to the possible effects of phagocytosis and disease states. A number of attempts have been made to seek specific alterations of phospholipid content or metabolism in relation to disease states (1, 17, 87, 88) or physiological conditions like phagocytosis (57–59, 61–66) or blast transformation (70, 89–91).

Phospholipids constitute about 35% of the total lipid weight of normal human lymphocytes and polymorphonuclear leukocytes (1). The major phospholipids (Figs. 1 and 2) are lecithin, phosphatidylethanolamine, sphingomyelin, phosphatidylserine and phosphatidylinositol. Small amounts of cardiolipin and lysolecithin are detectable, as well as traces of phosphatidic acid. In normal cells the proportions of the major phospholipids appear to be quite constant.

Figure 2 shows the phospholipid distribution in human lymphocytes, polymorphonuclear leukocytes, erythrocytes, and platelets. These cellular

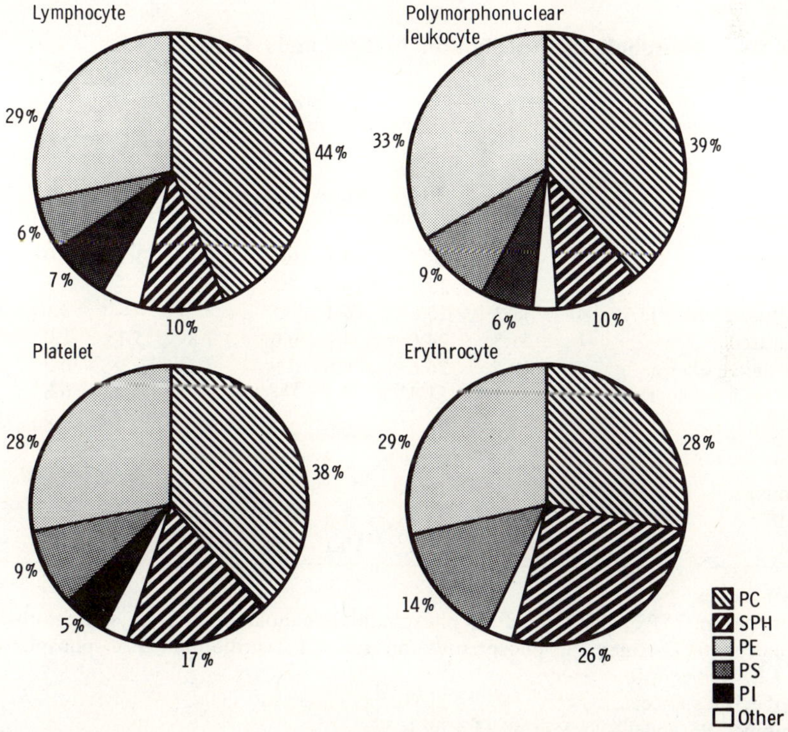

Fig. 2 Phospholipid patterns of human blood cells. Abbreviations: PC, lecithin (phosphatidylcholine); SPH, sphingomyelin; PE, phosphatidylethanolamine; PS, phosphatidylserine; PI, phosphatidylinositol; "other" includes cardiolipin, phosphatidic acid, lysolecithin, and unidentified phospholipids. (From Refs. 1, 84, 86, and unpublished observations.)

elements of circulating blood all have close to 30% phosphatidylethanolamine, most of which is in the plasmalogen form (α-alkenyl, β-acyl glycerophosphorylethanolamine). The lecithin content differs considerably among the four cell types (from 28% in erythrocytes to 44% in lymphocytes). There appears to be a reciprocal relationship between lecithin and sphingomyelin, and the total content of these two choline phospholipids is close to 55% in all cells except polymorphonuclear leukocytes, in which it is 49%. A similar relationship between lecithin and sphingomyelin has been demonstrated in the erythrocytes of various mammals (76). An inverse correlation between phosphatidylserine and phosphatidylinositol content also seems to be present, the total content of these two phosphatides being 13 to 15% in each cell type.

Table III compares the phospholipid distribution in lymphoid cells of various types. Because of differences in methodology, reports from different

Table III. Phospholipid Distribution in Lymphoid Cells

		Quantity (mole %)[a,b]							
Cell	n[c]	PC	PE	Sph	PS	PI	CL + PA	LL	Ref.
Human lymphocytes:									
Normal	8	43.6	28.7	10.1	(d)	(d)	3.2	1.0	1
	4	39.9	28.8	16.5	(e)	(e)	—	2.5	89
Cultured with PHA[f]	4	41.3	25.6	16.1	(g)	(g)	—	3.0	89
Cultured	1	51.3	24.0	4.8	6.0	7.8	5.1	1.0	93
Chronic leukemia	6	49.5	26.6	6.6	5.9	7.3	3.9	0.3	1
	3	38.3	21.4	9.1	(h)	(h)	4.2	6.3	17
Lymphoblasts, acute leukemia	4	48.7	26.2	6.6	3.2	9.4	5.3	0.5	1
Thymus:									
Calf	3	57.2	34.2	5.8	0.2	0.3	2.1	—	70
Rat	2	49.5	19.1	10.1	5.9	11.9	2.3	1.2	69

[a] Mean values.
[b] Abbreviations: PC, lecithin; PE, phosphatidylethanolamine; Sph, sphingomyelin; PS, phosphatidylserine; PI, phosphatidylinositol; CL, cardiolipin; PA, phosphatidic acid; LL, lysolecithin.
[c] Number of subjects.
[d] Combined PS and PI content of 13.4 mole %.
[e] Combined PS and PI content of 12.2 mole %.
[f] Phytohemagglutinin.
[g] Combined PS and PI content of 12.9 mole %.
[h] Combined PS and PI content of 18.1 mole %.

laboratories may not be directly comparable, but there appears to be fairly good general agreement.

In comparison with normal, mature, human lymphocytes, cells derived from patients with acute or chronic leukemia show considerable reduction in sphingomyelin content, with a corresponding increase in lecithin levels. A slight reduction in phosphatidylethanolamine content may also be observed. Although no such change was observed by Huber et al. in lymphocytes cultured with phytohemagglutinin (89), lymphoblasts from a cultured normal human lymphocyte line (93) showed a phospholipid pattern similar to that of leukemic lymphoblasts.

Table IV compares the corresponding phospholipid distribution in myeloid cells from various sources. Here too the leukemic myeloblasts have a higher proportion of lecithin than do normal polymorphonuclear leukocytes.

Table V shows the absolute content of phospholipids and cholesterol in normal and leukemic leukocytes. In both the lymphoid and myeloid series leukemic cells show little change in total phospholipid content but a striking

Table IV. Phospholipid Distribution in Myeloid Cells

		Quantity (mole %)[a,b]						
Cell	*n*[c]	PC	PE	Sph	PS + PI	CL + PA	LL	Ref.
Polymorphonuclear leukocytes:								
Circulating human	5	38.6	33.4	10.5	15.0	1.3	1.1	1
Human peritoneal exudate	1	46.4	29.6	7.7	15.6[d]	0.6	0.1	1
Guinea-pig peritoneal exudate	14	35	35	18	8[e]	4	—	59
Chronic myelocytic leukemia	2	39.9	31.3	10.2	14.4	2.2	2.0	1
	11	37.7	24.0	13.2	14.7	4.3	3.5	17
	5	42	29	10	15[f]	4	—	87
Myeloblasts, acute leukemia	2	48.8	28.6	8.8	10.8	2.3	0.8	1
Mitochondrial fraction, chronic leukemia	1	38.8	31.2	20.2	9.9	—	—	94
Lysosomal membranes, rabbit granulocytes	1	21.4	25.3	35.7	12.4	2.0	—	95

[a] Mean values.
[b] Abbreviations: PC, lecithin; PE, phosphatidylethanolamine; Sph, sphingomyelin; PS, phosphatidylserine; PI, phosphatidylinositol; CL, cardiolipin; PA, phosphatidic acid; LL, lysolecithin.
[c] Number of subjects.
[d] Reported as 9.5 mole % PS and 6.1 mole % PI.
[e] Reported as 4 mole % PS and 4 mole % PI.
[f] Reported as 9 mole % PS and 6 mole % PI.

Table V. Total-Lipid, Phospholipid, and Cholesterol Content of Leukocytes in Leukemia[a]

Cell	n[b]	Total Lipids ($g \times 10^{-12}$)	Phospholipids (moles $\times 10^{-15}$)	Cholesterol (moles $\times 10^{-15}$)	C/PL[c]
Lymphocytes:					
Normal	5	10.0	4.73	3.24	0.68
Chronic lymphocytic leukemia	6	5.44	4.00	1.54	0.38
Lymphoblasts:					
Acute lymphoblastic leukemia	2	5.96	4.28	1.08	0.25
Cultured lymphocytes[d]	1	19.6	17.2	7.00	0.41
Monoblasts, acute monoblastic leukemia	1	19.6	19.0	5.92	0.31
Polymorphonuclear leukocytes:					
Normal	6	21.5	9.67	5.33	0.55
Chronic myelocytic leukemia	2	13.4	10.2	4.98	0.49
Myeloblasts, acute myeloblastic leukemia	2	15.0	9.97	4.15	0.42

[a] Mean values per cell; data from Refs. 1 and 93.
[b] Number of subjects.
[c] Cholesterol-to-phospholipid molar ratio.
[d] Obtained from Associated Biomedic Systems, Inc., Buffalo, N.Y. (RPMI #1788).

decrease in total lipid weight and cholesterol content. The cultured lymphoid cells (RPMI #1788) are not directly comparable with the much smaller lymphoblasts isolated from leukemic blood, but the gross lipid pattern bears some resemblance to that of a case of monoblastic leukemia.

The significance of this lipid-pattern variance between normal and leukemic leukocytes is not clear. The observed differences may reflect changes in the relative content of various intracellular organelles, each with its own characteristic composition, or actual alterations of membrane-lipid patterns. Available evidence does not yet permit a conclusion on this point. Huber and co-workers (89) were unable to find a difference in the phospholipid patterns of separated mitochondrial and microsomal fractions of human lymphocytes. Granda and Posner (95) isolated from rabbit granulocytes lysosomal membranes that showed a very high proportion of sphingomyelin and a low lecithin content (Table IV), but their report shows no control values for whole-cell phospholipids. In an analogous study with blood platelets of human origin, Marcus, Ullman, and Safier (86) found very little difference between whole-platelet and isolated-membrane phospholipids, whereas isolated-platelet granules showed a distinct decrease in lecithin, and an increase in sphingomyelin, levels. The definitive answer to this question must await further studies with purified fractions of leukocyte subcellular components. The lipid pattern of cultured human lymphocytes of nonleukemic origin suggests that immaturity, rather than a specific defect in leukemia, is responsible for the altered lipid composition observed in these cells.

D. Glycolipids

Both lymphocytes and granulocytes contain substantial quantities of glycolipids—as much as 18% of the total lipid weight of mixed leukocyte preparations (85). Miras, Mantzos, and Levis (85), studying mixed human-leukocyte lipids by Florisil and silicic acid column separation methods, found most of the glycolipids to be in the form of ceramide dihexosides, with only small amounts of monohexosides and trihexosides (3.6 and 1.6% of total hexose, respectively). The main fatty acids of the major glycolipid were reported to palmitic (16:0) and nervonic (24:1). The ratio of galactose to glucose was 2:1, indicating a mixture of dihexosides—probably galactose–galactose plus galactose–glucose. Kampine and co-workers (96), on the other hand, working with borate-impregnated thin-layer plates and ^{14}C-labeled sugars, concluded that virtually all the dihexoside was in the form of lactose ceramide, with only traces of galactose–galactose ceramide. They also found that the small amount of ceramide monohexosides present in their leukocyte extracts was in the form of glucose ceramide, not galactose [as suggested, but not actually demonstrated, by Miras et al. (85)].

Although such studies with mixed cell populations reflect primarily the lipid content of the larger, more numerous granulocytes, we have confirmed (E. L. Gottfried and N. A. Robertson, unpublished observations) the presence of large amounts of glycolipids, mostly ceramide dihexosides, in isolated polymorphonuclear leukocytes and lymphocytes, as well as in a variety of leukemic cells[2].

As emphasized by Miras et al. (85), the unusual feature of the glycolipid content of leukocytes is that ceramide dihexosides comprise such a high proportion of the total lipid content. This finding suggests that these glycolipids may play a special role in the function of leukocytes, perhaps

[2] Hildebrand, Stryckmans, and Stoffyn (96a) recently reported that leukemic cells consisting mainly of myeloid or blastic forms contained lactose ceramide as the major glycolipid, whereas normal or leukemic lymphocytes contained only glucose ceramide.

related to immunological properties. Indeed the glycolipid content of a single polymorphonuclear leukocyte is nearly 400 times as great as that of an erythrocyte, a fact that may be of particular significance in the mechanism of Gaucher's disease (see Section IV.E.1).

IV. LIPID METABOLISM OF LEUKOCYTES

In comparison with the small number of available reports on the lipid composition of leukocytes, there is an impressive number of reports on the synthesis of lipids in leukocytes from isotopically labeled precursors and on the metabolic fate of labeled lipids. The majority of these investigations are based on cell preparations derived from the peritoneal exudates of animals (57–59, 61–66) as a model of the polymorphonuclear leukocyte or on mixed cell populations derived from blood (2–4, 7, 8, 97–101). It is now generally agreed (2, 3) that observations of lipid metabolism made on whole-blood specimens reflect primarily the metabolic activity of the leukocytes and, to a lesser extent, the platelets. Most likely, studies of mixed leukocyte populations in turn reflect primarily the lipid metabolism of the polymorphonuclear leukocytes, since these cells predominate in number, size, and total lipid content. Nevertheless, it must be emphasized that studies of lipid metabolism in mixed cell populations are even more susceptible than static structural analyses to distortion by an inconspicuous, but disproportionately active, cell type. Conclusions based on work with leukemic or other abnormal cells (8, 13, 14, 87, 102–105) must be limited to these specific cell types, since it may be presumed that such cells behave at least a little differently from their normal counterparts.

A. Polymorphonuclear Leukocytes

Subject to the limitations discussed above, work based on animal peritoneal exudates and mixed cell populations suggests certain general metabolic characteristics of polymorphonuclear leukocytes.

It has been found that 1-^{14}C-acetate, ^{14}C-glucose, and inorganic $^{32}PO_4$ are readily incorporated into the lipids of resting and phagocytizing cells (2–4, 13, 57, 59, 64–66, 98, 101). Phagocytosis markedly enhances the turnover of cell lipids, as shown by the increased uptake of label, but there is no actual net synthesis of lipids during this process (57, 59, 64–66). A plausible explanation is that breakdown and reformation of the cell membranes are closely related to the process of phagocytosis. Sbarra and Karnovsky (64) found no similar increase in the incorporation of L-leucine-^{14}C into protein or of ^{14}C-glucose into glycogen during phagocytosis; this suggests that the observed lipid stimulation is not simply a general manifestation of increased cell activity.

It has been found that 1-^{14}C-acetate is incorporated into fatty acids, especially the long-chain fatty acids with 20 to 24 carbon atoms (57, 98, 101), and the label is found about equally in the triglyceride and phospholipid fractions. The mechanism involved in the incorporation of acetate into the lipids of mature polymorphonuclear leukocytes is exclusively that of chain elongation (106), and the label is found only in the carbonyl groups. Majerus and Lastra (101) found that human-leukocyte extracts lack the first enzyme unique to the pathway of fatty acid synthesis, acetyl-coenzyme A carboxylase, thus eliminating the possibility of de novo synthesis via malonyl-coenzyme A. On the other hand, these authors were able to find evidence of other enzymes necessary for fatty acid synthesis, such as fatty acid synthetase. They also noted that leukemic blast cells showed acetyl-coenzyme A carboxylase activity, which suggests that precursor hematopoietic cells are capable of de novo fatty acid synthesis.

Miras, Legakis, and Levis (104) showed that glucose is utilized for lipid synthesis mainly via the triose phosphate intermediate. Uniformly labeled ^{14}C-glucose is incorporated primarily into the glycerol portion of phospholipids and triglycerides (about 85% of the total incorporated), with smaller amounts of label appearing in the hexose of glycolipids and in fatty acids.

Incorporation of inorganic $^{32}PO_4$ into phospholipids is readily demonstrated *in vitro,* most prominently into the fractions identified as phosphatidylinositol and phosphatidic acid (59, 66, 99). These phospholipids in particular have been found to exhibit the greatest increase (threefold to sixfold) in specific activity during phagocytosis (59). Sastry and Hokin (66) attributed the rapid incorporation of $^{32}PO_4$ into phosphatidic acid to the direct activity of diglyceride kinase (or possibly monoglyceride kinase plus lysophosphatidic acid acylase). These authors also found evidence of the formation of phosphatidic acid in polymorphonuclear leukocytes by acylation of α-glycerophosphate, but this route is not stimulated by phagocytosis.

Lysolecithin is acylated to form lecithin by several mechanisms described in detail in a series of reports by Elsbach (57, 58, 61, 62), who used rabbit peritoneal exudates in his studies.

At low pH and relatively high concentrations of lysolecithin the transacylation mechanism of Erbland and Marinetti (107) is most prominent in cell homogenates:

$$\text{2 lysolecithin} \longrightarrow \text{lecithin} + \text{glycerophosphorylcholine} \qquad (1)$$

This pathway produces large amounts of lecithin, does not require adenosine triphosphate (ATP) or coenzyme A (CoA), and appears to be associated with the 100,000-*g* supernatant fraction of cell homogenates. This route is evidently inoperative in the intact cell (62).

At physiological pH (~7.4) and low concentrations of lysolecithin direct acylation by the mechanism of Lands (108) prevails:

$$\text{lysolecithin} + \text{free fatty acid} \xrightarrow{\text{ATP, CoA}} \text{lecithin} \qquad (2)$$

In contrast to the transacylation pathway, this route requires ATP and coenzyme A. In cell homogenates the acylating activity is found in the particulate cell fractions.

During phagocytosis conversion of medium lecithin to cellular lecithin is stimulated. Surprisingly, there is no concomitant increase in the incorporation of free fatty acids in the medium (66, 109). In explanation of this observation Elsbach and Farrow (63) confirmed that direct acylation is the major route for stimulated conversion of lysolecithin, but endogenous triglycerides, rather than free fatty acids in the medium, are the fatty acid reservoir in this reaction. Triglycerides are hydrolyzed during phagocytosis by lipases, which appear to be lysosomal enzymes. A similar finding was reported by Shohet in a study made with human myelocytic leukemia cells (105). Elsbach and Farrow (63) concluded that endogenous triglycerides serve primarily as a reservoir for increased phospholipid synthesis during phagocytosis, rather than as an additional source of energy. This acylation pathway was intact in a case of chronic granulomatous disease of childhood, a fatal inherited disorder in which the polymorphonuclear leukocytes exhibit apparently normal phagocytosis but decreased bactericidal activity (88).

Thus in phagocytosis the following reaction sequence appears to be favored:

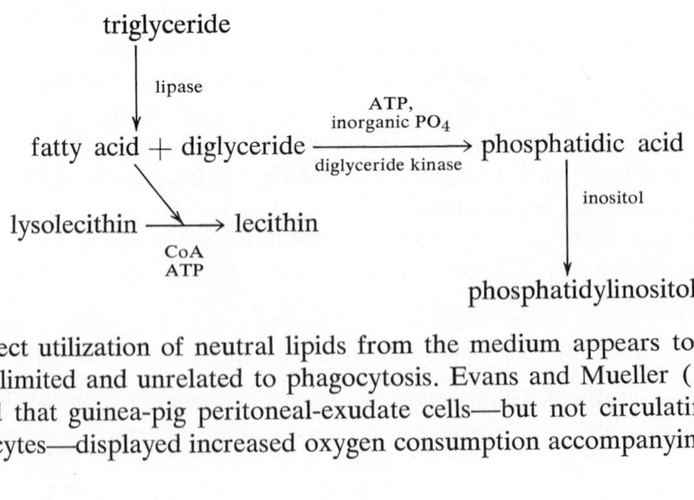

(3)

Direct utilization of neutral lipids from the medium appears to be relatively limited and unrelated to phagocytosis. Evans and Mueller (110) reported that guinea-pig peritoneal-exudate cells—but not circulating blood leukocytes—displayed increased oxygen consumption accompanying uptake of palmitate. This process appeared to be independent of phagocytosis but sensitive to inhibitors of glycolysis (sodium fluoride, iodoacetic acid).[3] Rosenzweig and Ways (100) showed that mixed-leukocyte preparations derived from blood are capable of oxidizing free fatty acids from the surrounding medium. Elsbach (111) compared the rates of uptake and incorporation of palmitic, stearic, oleic, and linoleic acids and found that uptake is nonspecific and depends primarily on concentration. In these experiments fatty acids were incorporated as esters into both phospholipid and neutral-lipid (primarily triglyceride) fractions. The relative distribution between these fractions was highly specific for each fatty acid, however.

In contrast to the utilization of free fatty acids, uptake of triglycerides and mixed phospholipids from the medium is apparently due to nonspecific adherence of these lipids to the cell's surface (112). Elsbach (112) concluded that phagocytosis as a mechanism for the uptake of complex lipid molecules is not quantitatively important. Under appropriate conditions, however, lysosomal enzymes in rabbit granulocytes may be capable of splitting off free fatty acids from exogenous triglycerides (113). The liberated fatty acids presumably are then available for utilization by the leukocytes.

Incorporation of L-(3-^{14}C)-serine into microsomal phosphatidylserine and phosphatidylethanolamine was found by Miras, Mantzos, and Levis (114) to occur by the following two mechanisms:

1. A system requiring added ATP, CoASH, and Mg^{2+}, but not exogenous cytidine nucleotides.
2. A system activated by Ca^{2+}.

This study was based on mixed leukocyte populations.

B. Macrophages

Metabolic studies of macrophages are based largely on cell specimens derived from chronic peritoneal (60, 65, 110, 115–119) or alveolar (58) exudates—most commonly from rabbits or guinea pigs. Relatively little is known about these cells in comparison with granulocytes, and in any event their suitability as models for the monocytes of circulating blood must be considered to be tentative.

Macrophages are much more active metabolically than granulocytes, demonstrating nine to ten times as much uptake of oxygen and glucose and

[3] These experiments have been cited as an example of differences in metabolic activity between circulating blood leukocytes and exudate cells, but it should be noted that the experimental conditions were not directly comparable.

four times the uptake of palmitic acid for the oxidation of free fatty acids (110).

It has been found that 1-^{14}C-acetate, ^{14}C-glucose, and inorganic $^{32}PO_4$ are readily incorporated into the lipids of these cells (65, 115–118). Glucose is incorporated almost entirely (95%) into the glycerol portion of triglycerides and phospholipids (117), as in granulocytes.

In contrast to the pattern of acetate incorporation into the fatty acids of granulocytes, 1-^{14}C-acetate was found by Day and Fidge (115) to be incorporated predominantly (70–80%) into cholesterol, with lesser amounts (20–30%) appearing in the fatty acid fraction.

Inorganic $^{32}PO_4$ is incorporated readily into the phospholipids of macrophages. Day, Fidge, and Wilkinson (118) found most of the label in lecithin and sphingomyelin, with lesser amounts in the phosphatidylinositol and phosphatidylethanolamine fractions of rabbit peritoneal macrophages. Karnovsky et al. (65), on the other hand, reported that in guinea-pig monocytes the highest specific activity appeared in the fraction containing phosphatidylinositol plus phosphatidylserine.

The formation of lecithin from lysolecithin in alveolar macrophages occurs mainly by direct acylation (58). Elsbach found that in these cells, as in granulocytes, transacylation is not a prominent mechanism (58).

As in the case of polymorphonuclear leukocytes, ^{14}C-labeled fatty acids are readily incorporated into the triglyceride and phospholipid fractions of macrophages (60). Cholesterol appears to be esterified directly in the presence of free fatty acids, but not with lecithin alone, indicating the absence of lecithin:cholesterol acyltransferase (119).

C. Lymphocytes

There have been few studies on lipid metabolism in purified lymphocyte preparations. There is accumulating evidence that the group of morphologically similar cells classified as lymphocytes may actually include members with rather diverse functions (120). It is quite possible that future studies will reveal differences in metabolic patterns as well.

Blomstrand (68) studied the incorporation of 1-^{14}C-acetate into the lipids of lymphocytes isolated from human thoracic-duct lymph. As in the case of polymorphonuclear leukocytes (98, 101), acetate was incorporated mainly into the fatty acids of phospholipids and triglycerides by chain elongation of preexisting fatty acids. Longer chain fatty acids (C_{20}–C_{22}) contained most of the radioactivity, and 80% of the label was found in the phospholipid fraction.

Generally similar results were reported by Miras, Mantzos, and Levis (121) for cell-free fractions of rabbit thymus. The mitochondrial fraction incorporated 1-^{14}C-acetate into longer chain fatty acids, whereas the 93,000-*g* supernatant utilized both 1-^{14}C-acetate and 2-^{14}C-malonate for the production of shorter chain fatty acids, particularly myristic (14:0) and palmitic (16:0) acids.

Phytohemagglutinin, a glycoprotein derived from the kidney bean *Phaseolus vulgaris,* induces in cultures of small lymphocytes a sharp increase in metabolic activity, accompanied by a morphologic transformation to a "blastoid" appearance. Huber et al. (89) found that phytohemagglutinin-stimulated human lymphocytes incorporated ^{14}C-acetate into lipids more than seven times faster than did unstimulated cells. The label was evenly distributed among all the phospholipids. Fisher and Mueller (90, 91) found a stepwise pattern of incorporation of labeled inorganic phosphate, choline, and methionine into the phospholipids of lymphocytes stimulated by phytohemagglutinin, as follows:

1. In the first 10 min phosphatidylinositol synthesis was stimulated, with no associated increase in protein synthesis.
2. From 1 to 24 hr, all phospholipids accumulated, particularly phosphatidylserine and phosphatidylethanolamine, concomitant with the activation of RNA synthesis.
3. From 24 to 48 hr, a dramatic rise in lecithin synthesis occurred. This last peak of phospholipid synthesis was dependent on protein synthesis.

Fisher and Mueller concluded (91) that phospholipid synthesis in the intermediate period from 1 to 24 hr was related primarily to new membrane production associated with RNA formation, whereas that in the late period was associated with general cellular hypertrophy and protein production.

D. Leukemic Cells

As already mentioned, metabolic studies of leukocytes derived from patients with leukemia pose a special problem in the interpretation of results. In the majority of published reports it is not possible to separate the effects related to (a) shifts in the distribution of various cell types (differential cell count), (b) cell immaturity, or (c) alterations specifically attributable to the disease process itself.

The incorporation of 1-^{14}C-acetate into cell lipids has been observed by O'Donnell et al. (102) in the leukemic cells of chronic myelocytic leukemia and monocytic leukemia, but not chronic lymphocytic leukemia. Kidson (14) reported that acetate incorporation occurred at an increased rate in acute myeloblastic leukemia and at a reduced rate in acute lymphoblastic leukemia and myeloproliferative states. Distribution of the ^{14}C label in leukemic cells was found by Malamos et al. (8) to favor phospholipids over neutral lipids, in contrast to the incorporation pattern in normal mixed cell populations. This observation may help to explain the fact that leukemic cells of a given morphological type frequently have a considerably lower neutral-lipid content than their normal counterparts (1).

Majerus and Lastra (101) have reported the presence of fatty acid synthetase in a variety of leukocyte preparations, but acetyl-coenzyme A carboxylase only in leukemic blast cells (one case of monomyelocytic leukemia, two cases unspecified):

$$\text{acetyl-CoA} \xrightarrow[\substack{\text{acetyl-CoA carboxylase} \\ \text{A}}]{} \text{malonyl-CoA} \xrightarrow[\substack{\text{fatty acid synthetase} + \\ \text{NADPH} + \text{acetyl-CoA} \\ \text{B}}]{} \text{palmitic acid} \qquad (4)$$

Only the most immature cells were capable of *de novo* synthesis by reactions A and B, although normal-mixed-leukocyte preparations readily incorporated malonyl-coenzyme A into palmitic acid by reaction B. Majerus and Lastra (101) thus confirmed previous observations (98) that 1-^{14}C-acetate is incorporated into longer chain fatty acids in mature leukocytes only by the chain-elongation mechanism.

Incorporation of inorganic ^{32}P into the phospholipids of leukemic cells (principally chronic myelocytic leukemia) was studied by Firkin and Williams (87), who found rapid *in vitro* labeling of the phosphatidylinositol and phosphatidic acid fractions, and much smaller degrees of labeling of the other leukocyte phospholipids, in agreement with the results of similar studies on normal polymorphonuclear leukocytes (59, 66, 99). In contrast, when a patient with chronic myelocytic leukemia was given a therapeutic dose of ^{32}P, *in vivo* labeling was detectable only after 18 hr, and the label was evenly distributed among phosphatidylinositol, lecithin, and phosphatidylethanolamine. There was relatively little radioactivity in sphingomyelin and phosphatidylserine, and none at all in phosphatidic acid. The differences between *in vivo* and *in vitro* labeling patterns are not surprising, in view of the considerable differences in environmental conditions and length of cell exposure to the ^{32}P label. Presumably prolonged exposure of younger cells to ^{32}P *in vivo* is reflected in greater labeling of structural lipids, whereas *in vitro* experimental conditions (high specific activity, short time periods) favor selective incorporation into components with a small total content but rapid turnover (87).

Miras et al. (104) studied the incorporation of uniformly labeled ^{14}C-glucose into the lipids of a variety of leukemic leukocytes and found most of the label in the glycerol of phospholipids and triglycerides. In comparison with normal mixed populations, however, leukemic cells of the myelocytic and monocytic series incorporated much more label into glycolipids. This finding was attributed to the increased content in leukemic leukocytes of uridine diphosphate glucose (122), which is involved in glycolipid biosynthesis (123).

E. Hereditary Disorders

1. Sphingolipidoses. A number of hereditary metabolic disorders are characterized by the accumulation in tissues of abnormal amounts of sphingolipids. There is evidence that each of these disorders is the result of a deficiency of a single catabolic enzyme, with consequent inability to provide for the disposal of normally produced lipid by-products (124). Included in this group are disorders involving glucocerebrosides (Gaucher's disease), sphingomyelin (Niemann–Pick disease), gangliosides (Tay–Sachs disease), sulfatides (metachromatic leukodystrophy), and ceramide trihexosides (Fabry's disease).

In certain of these disorders engorgement of reticuloendothelial cells results in a characteristic histologic picture of lipid-laden cells in the bone marrow, spleen, and other organs. In Niemann–Pick disease accumulation of sphingomyelin and cholesterol in reticuloendothelial cells produces "foam cells" with a nonspecific pattern. In Gaucher's disease, on the other hand, the glucocerebroside-filled Gaucher cell has a typical appearance that until recently was considered to be diagnostic of this familial disorder (125).

Kampine et al. (126) demonstrated that leukocytes of peripheral blood have measurable amounts of sphingomyelinase and glucocerebrosidase, and that these enzymes are deficient or absent in Niemann–Pick and Gaucher's diseases, respectively. This finding has provided a practical biochemical means for confirming the diagnosis of these two disorders and has pointed the way for the investigation of analogous conditions (127). The same group (103) found increased activity of sphingomyelinase and glucocerebrosidase (but not of galactocerebrosidase) in acute and chronic myelocytic leukemia, as compared with normal mixed leukocyte populations. The relative effects of cell immaturity and altered differential count were not adequately evaluated, however.

Speculation regarding the source of the glycolipids that accumulate in Gaucher's disease has centered around the erythrocytes, with the presumption (128) that erythrocyte glycolipids are normally broken down in the spleen in large quantities. Fredrickson calculated this amount to be 500 mg/kg body mass per year (125), but recent studies (129) suggest that this estimate may be as much as 50 times too high.

Several reports of typical Gaucher cells in the bone marrow of patients with chronic myelocytic leukemia (130–134) have stimulated a fresh look at this problem. The conclusion is now inescapable that the granulocytes not only contain glycolipids in quantities sufficient to produce Gaucher-like cells in myelocytic leukemia but also are far more likely than erythrocytes to be the source of accumulated glucocerebrosides even in the classic familial form of Gaucher's disease.

Kattlove and co-workers (132) studied in detail a patient with chronic myelocytic leukemia and typical Gaucher-like cells in the bone marrow. The blood glucocerebrosidase activity was elevated to three times the normal level. This finding is common in myelocytic leukemia (103) but contrasts sharply with the expected decrease in classical Gaucher's disease. Kattlove et al. calculated that for a normal 70-kg man, with a leukocyte turnover of about 10^{11} cells per day (135) and an erythrocyte turnover of about 2×10^{11} cells per day (136), the daily contribution to glycolipid turnover would be 387 mg from granulocytes and only 5 to 10 mg from erythrocytes. If the figures of Vance and Sweeley (129) are used as an estimate of erythrocyte-glycolipid content, daily erythrocyte-glycolipid turnover amounts to only 2 mg. Thus, even in the normal state, granulocytes contribute about 200 times as much to the glycolipid pool as erythrocytes. In myelocytic leukemia, with a sharply elevated leukocyte count, a vastly increased load of glycolipids may easily overwhelm the normal catabolic mechanisms of the reticuloendothelial system.

2. Chediak–Higashi Syndrome. The Chediak–Higashi syndrome is an inherited disorder marked by distinctive morphological changes in leukocytes, including giant granulations in granulocytes and inclusions in lymphocytes and monocytes. Kritzler and co-workers (137) reported, on the basis of staining characteristics, an increased glycolipid content in leukocytes. Kanfer et al. (138), on direct analysis of the leukocytes in this disorder, reported not an increase, but rather a 50% decrease, in glycolipid and sphingomyelin content. In another study this group (139) demonstrated an accelerated turnover of leukocyte sphingolipids. It is likely that the observed increase in lipid turnover is a nonspecific reflection of accelerated leukocyte destruction, rather than a specific biochemical defect.

V. SUMMARY AND CONCLUSIONS

The leukocytes are a diverse group of cells with a wide range of metabolic activity. Compared with erythrocytes, these cells have a broader range of functions, but much less is known about them.

For proper evaluation of the lipid composition and metabolism of leukocytes and the effects of disease it is essential to study the cells of a specific morphological type. Of the many methods that have been proposed for the isolation of pure leukocyte types from blood, none is ideal, but a few offer a practical means of obtaining useful quantities of individual cell types. Lymphoid and myeloid cells have different lipid patterns, and leukemic cells show important lipid-content differences from their normal counterparts of the same morphological series. Whether these changes are specifically related to the disease process or (as is more likely) are a nonspecific reflection of cell immaturity is not yet certain.

An unusual feature of leukocyte lipid composition is the very high content of glycolipids, particularly the ceramide dihexoside fraction.

It is probable that granulocytes, rather than erythrocytes as previously believed, are the source of the glucocerebrosides that accumulate in abnormally large quantities in Gaucher's disease.

Techniques have been developed for measuring the levels of lipid-metabolism enzymes in the leukocytes of peripheral blood. These methods are being applied to the investigation of sphingolipidoses. As better methods become available for the separation and handling of leukocytes, we can expect to find increased usefulness of these cells as a diagnostic tool.

VI. ACKNOWLEDGMENTS

Investigations of the author cited in this review have been supported in part by a grant from the U.S. Public Health Service (HE 12762). The author is a Career Scientist of the Health Research Council of the City of New York under contract I-638. The expert assistance of Mrs. Norma Robertson is gratefully acknowledged.

REFERENCES

1. Gottfried, E. L., *J. Lipid Res.* **8**, 321–327 (1967).
2. Buchanan, A. A., *Biochem. J.* **75**, 315–320 (1960).
3. Marks, P. A., A. Gellhorn, and C. Kidson, *J. Biol. Chem.* **235**, 2579–2583 (1960).
4. Rowe, C. E., A. C. Allison, and J. E. Lovelock, *Biochim. Biophys. Acta* **41**, 310–314 (1960).
5. Boyd, E. M., *J. Biol. Chem.* **101**, 623–633 (1933).
6. Boyd, E. M., and D. J. Stephens, *Proc. Soc. Exp. Biol. Med.* **33**, 558–560 (1936).
7. Rowe, C. E., *Biochem. J.* **73**, 438–442 (1960).
8. Malamos, B., C. Miras, G. Levis, and J. Mantzos, *J. Lipid Res.* **3**, 222–228 (1962).

9. Finke, S. R., G. B. Phillips, and E. Middleton, Jr., *J. Lab. Clin. Med.* **67**, 601–609 (1966).
10. Schwandt, P., J. Birk, and H. Ehrhart, *Klin. Wochenschr.* **45**, 1008–1009 (1967).
11. Kim, H.-S., M. Suzuki, and R. O'Neal, *Amer. J. Clin. Pathol.* **48**, 314–319 (1967).
12. Boyd, E. M., *Arch. Pathol.* **21**, 739–748 (1936).
13. Kidson, C., *Brit. J. Exp. Pathol.* **42**, 597–602 (1961).
14. Kidson, C., *Australas, Ann. Med.* **10**, 282–287 (1961); *ibid.,* **11**, 50–54 (1962).
15. Chiarioni, T., E. Nardi, F. Ronchi, and L. Guacci, *Progr. Med.* **19**, 754–759 (1963).
16. Schwandt, P., J. Birk, and H. Ehrhart, *Klin. Wochenschr.* **46**, 687–689 (1968).
17. Schwandt, P., J. Birk, and H. Ehrhart, *Klin. Wochenschr.* **47**, 111–112 (1969).
18. Wolstenholme, G. E. W., and M. O'Connor, Eds., *Biological Activity of the Leucocyte,* Ciba Foundation Study Group No. 10, Little, Brown & Co., Boston, 1961.
19. Tanaka, Y., and T. J. Liddy, *Lab. Invest.* **15**, 455–463 (1966).
20. Pearse, A. G. E., *Histochemistry, Theoretical and Applied,* Little, Brown & Co., Boston, 1960, p. 329.
21. Fallon, H. J., E. Frei III, J. D. Davidson, J. S. Trier, and D. Burk, *J. Lab. Clin. Med.* **59**, 779–791 (1962).
22. Bertino, J. R., R. Silber, M. Freeman, A. Alenty, M. Albrecht, B. W. Gabrio, and F. M. Huennekens, *J. Clin. Invest.* **42**, 1899–1907 (1963).
23. Behrens, M., and F. Esch, *Experientia* **19**, 406–407 (1963).
24. Singer, T. P., I. Silberbach, and S. Schwartz., *Blood*, special issue No. 1, 88–97 (1947).
25. Seabright, M., *J. Med. Lab. Technol.* **14**, 85–100 (1957).
26. Schwartz, S., L. Graxie, K. Cheney, M. B. Hasenfus, and S. Cohen, U.S. Atomic Energy Commission Tech. Info. Dir. Series MDDC, #267 (1946).
27. Tullis, J. L., *Blood* **7**, 891–896 (1952).
28. Ottesen, J., *Acta Physiol. Scand.* **32**, 75–93 (1954).
29. Maupin, B., and R. Chary, *Le Sang* **23**, 336–340 (1952).
30. Juhlin, L., and W. B. Shelley, *Blood* **18**, 477–480 (1961).
31. Green, I., and W. Solomon, *J. Clin. Pathol.* (*London*) **16**, 180–182 (1963).
32. Vallee, B. L., W. L. Hughes, Jr., and J. G. Gibson 2nd, *Blood,* special issue No. 1, 82–87 (1947).
33. Agranoff, B. W., B. L. Vallee, and D. F. Waugh, *Blood* **9**, 804–809 (1954).
34. Jago, M., *Brit. J. Haematol.* **2**, 439–444 (1956).
35. Lapin, J. H., A. Horonick, and R. H. Lapin, *Blood* **13**, 1001–1005 (1958).
36. Ventzke, L. E., S. Perry, and G. Crepaldi, *J. Lab. Clin. Med.* **53**, 318–321 (1959).
37. Lalezari, P., *Blood* **19**, 109–114 (1962).
38. Coulson, A. S., and D. G. Chalmers, *Lancet* **i**, 468–469 (1964).
39. Böyum, A., *Scand. J. Clin. Lab. Invest.* **21** (suppl. 97), 1–109 (1968).
40. Noble, P. B., J. H. Cutts, and K. K. Carroll, *Blood* **31**, 66–73 (1968).
41. Perper, R. J., J. W. Zee, and M. M. Mickelson, *J. Lab. Clin. Med.* **72**, 842–848 (1968).
42. Boyle, W., and A. Chow, *Transfusion* (*Philadelphia*) **9**, 151–155 (1969).
43. Brubaker, L. H., and W. H. Evans, *J. Lab. Clin. Med.* **73**, 1036–1041 (1969).
44. Zucker, R. M., and B. Cassen, *Blood* **34**, 591–600 (1969).
45. Freireich, E. J., G. Judson, and R. H. Levin, *Cancer Res.* **25**, 1516–1520 (1965).

46. Buckner, D., R. Eisel, and S. Perry, *Blood* **31**, 653–672 (1968).
47. Fleming, A., *Brit. J. Exp. Pathol.* **7**, 281–286 (1926).
48. Wildy, P., and M. Ridley, *Nature* **182**, 1801–1803 (1958).
49. Garvin, J. E., *J. Exp. Med.* **114**, 51–73 (1961).
50. Kvarstein, B., *Scand. J. Clin. Lab. Invest.* **23**, 259–270 (1969).
51. Rabinowitz, Y., *Blood* **23**, 811–828 (1964).
52. Thierfelder, S., *Vox Sang.* **9**, 447–454 (1964).
53. Cassen, B., J. Hitt, and E. F. Hays, *J. Lab. Clin. Med.* **52**, 778–783 (1958).
54. Levine, S., *Science* **123**, 185–186 (1956).
55. Bazin, S., and R. Robineaux, *C. R. Seances Soc. Biol. Filiales* **144**, 957–959 (1950).
56. Walter, H., E. J. Krob, and G. S. Ascher, *Exp. Cell Res.* **55**, 279–283 (1969).
57. Elsbach, P., *J. Exp. Med.* **110**, 969–980 (1959).
58. Elsbach, P., *Biochim. Biophys. Acta* **125**, 510–524 (1966).
59. Karnovsky, M. L., and D. F. H. Wallach, *J. Biol. Chem.* **236**, 1895–1901 (1961).
60. Day, A. J., and N. H. Fidge, *J. Lipid Res.* **3**, 333–338 (1962).
61. Elsbach, P., J. W. O. van den Berg, H. van den Bosch, and L. L. M. van Deenen, *Biochim. Biophys. Acta* **106**, 338–347 (1965).
62. Elsbach, P., *J. Clin. Invest.* **47**, 2217–2229 (1968).
63. Elsbach, P., and S. Farrow, *Biochim. Biophys. Acta* **176**, 438–441 (1969).
64. Sbarra, A. J., and M. L. Karnovsky, *J. Biol. Chem.* **235**, 2224–2229 (1960).
65. Karnovsky, M. L., A. W. Shafer, R. H. Cagan, R. C. Graham, M. J. Karnovsky, E. A. Glass, and K. Saito, *Trans. N.Y. Acad. Sci.* (Ser. 2) **28**, 778–787 (1966).
66. Sastry, P. S., and L. E. Hokin, *J. Biol. Chem.* **241**, 3354–3361 (1966).
67. Bollman, J. L., J. C. Cain, and J. H. Grindley, *J. Lab. Clin. Med.* **33**, 1349–1352 (1948).
68. Blomstrand, R., *Acta Chem. Scand.* **20**, 1122–1128 (1966).
69. Abramson, D., and M. Blecher, *Biochim. Biophys. Acta* **98**, 117–127 (1965).
70. Rose, H. G., and J. H. Frenster, *Biochim. Biophys. Acta* **106**, 577–591 (1965).
71. Moore, G. E., R. E. Gerner, H. Kitamura, J. Minowada, and A. Fjelde, in *Proceedings of the 3rd Annual Leucocyte Culture Conference*, W. O. Rieke, Ed., Appleton-Century Crofts, New York, 1969, pp. 177–198.
72. Walford, R. L., *Leukocyte Antigens and Antibodies*, Grune & Stratton, New York, 1960.
73. Skoog, W. A., and W. S. Beck, *Blood* **11**, 436–454 (1956).
74. Leder, L.-D., *Der Blutmonocyt*, Springer-Verlag, Berlin, 1967.
75. Antonioli, J. A., in *Biological Activity of the Leucocyte*, G. E. W. Wolstenholme and M. O'Connor, Eds., Ciba Foundation Study Group No. 10, Little, Brown & Co., Boston, 1961, pp. 92–99.
76. De Gier, J., and L. L. M. van Deenen, *Biochim. Biophys. Acta* **49**, 286–296 (1961).
77. Nelson, G. J., *Biochim. Biophys. Acta* **144**, 221–232 (1967).
78. Currie, G. A., *Nature* **215**, 164–165 (1967).
79. Chodirker, W. B., G. N. Bock, and J. H. Vaughan, *J. Lab. Clin. Med.* **71**, 9–19 (1968).
80. Athens, J. W., *Ann. Rev. Physiol.* **25**, 195–212 (1963).
81. Hanks, J. H., and J. H. Wallace, *Proc. Soc. Exp. Biol. Med.* **98**, 188–192 (1958).
82. Turk, A., P. R. Glade, and L. N. Chessin, *Blood* **33**, 329–340 (1969).
83. Tullis, J. L., *Blood* **8**, 563–575 (1953).

84. Jaffé, E. R., and E. L. Gottfried, *J. Clin. Invest.* **47**, 1375–1388 (1968).
85. Miras, C. J., J. D. Mantzos, and G. M. Levis, *Biochem. J.* **98**, 782–786 (1966).
86. Marcus, A. J., H. L. Ullman, and L. B. Safier, *J. Lipid Res.* **10**, 108–114 (1969).
87. Firkin, B. G., and W. J. Williams, *J. Clin. Invest.* **40**, 423–432 (1961).
88. Elsbach, P., D. Zucker-Franklin, and C. Sansaricq, *New Engl. J. Med.* **280**, 1319–1322 (1969).
89. Huber, H., N. Strieder, H. Winnler, G. Reiser, and K. Koppelstaetter, *Brit. J. Haematol.* **15**, 203–209 (1968).
90. Fisher, D. B., and G. C. Mueller, *Proc. Natl. Acad. Sci. U.S.* **60**, 1396–1402 (1968).
91. Fisher, D. B., and G. C. Mueller, *Biochim. Biophys. Acta* **176**, 316–323 (1969).
92. Skipski, V. P., R. F. Peterson, and M. Barclay, *Biochem. J.* **90**, 374–378 (1964).
93. Gottfried, E. L., *J. Lipid Res.* **12**, 531–537 (1971).
94. Massaro, E. J., Ph.D. thesis, University of Texas, University Microfilms, Ann Arbor, Mich., 1963 (*Diss. Abstr.* **24**, 495 (1963)).
95. Granda, J. L., and A. Posner, *Trans. N.Y. Acad. Sci.* (Ser. 2) **31**, 879–891 (1969).
96. Kampine, J. P., E. Martensson, R. A. Yankee, and J. N. Kanfer, *Lipids* **3**, 151–156 (1968).
96a. Hildebrand, J., P. Stryckmans, and P. Stoffyn, *J. Lipid Res.* **12**, 361–366 (1971).
97. Miras, C., J. Mantzos, and V. Samara, *Nature* **202**, 801–806 (1964).
98. Miras, C. J., J. D. Mantzos, and G. M. Levis, *Biochem. Biophys. Res. Commun.* **19**, 79–83 (1965).
99. Westerman, M. P., and W. N. Jensen, *Proc. Soc. Exp. Biol. Med.* **118**, 315–319 (1965).
100. Rosenzweig, A., and P. Ways, *Blood* **27**, 57–64 (1966).
101. Majerus, P. W., and R. Lastra R., *J. Clin. Invest.* **46**, 1596–1602 (1967).
102. O'Donnell, V. J., P. Ottolenghi, A. Malkin, O. F. Denstedt, and R. D. H. Heard, *Can. J. Biochem. Physiol.* **36**, 1125–1136 (1958).
103. Kampine, J. P., R. O. Brady, R. A. Yankee, J. N. Kanfer, D. Shapiro, and A. E. Gal, *Cancer Res.* **27**, 1312–1315 (1967).
104. Miras, C. J., N. J. Legakis, and G. M. Levis, *Cancer Res.* **27**, 2153–2158 (1967).
105. Shohet, S., *Abstr. XII Congr. Int. Soc. Hematol.*, New York, 1968, p. 35.
106. Wakil, S., *J. Lipid Res.* **2**, 1–24 (1961).
107. Erbland, J. F., and G. V. Marinetti, *Fed. Proc.* **21**, 295 (1962).
108. Lands, W. E. M., *J. Biol. Chem.* **235**, 2233–2237 (1960).
109. Elsbach, P., *Biochim. Biophys. Acta* **70**, 157–167 (1963).
110. Evans, W. H., and P. S. Mueller, *J. Lipid Res.* **4**, 39–45 (1963).
111. Elsbach, P., *Biochim. Biophys. Acta* **84**, 8–17 (1964).
112. Elsbach, P., *Biochim. Biophys. Acta* **98**, 402–419 (1965).
113. Elsbach, P., and H. J. Kayden, *Amer. J. Physiol.* **209**, 765–769 (1965).
114. Miras, C. J., J. Mantzos, and G. Levis, *Biochim. Biophys. Acta* **84**, 101–103 (1964).
115. Day, A. J., and N. H. Fidge, *J. Lipid Res.* **5**, 163–168 (1964).
116. Day, A. J., N. H. Fidge, and G. K. Wilkinson, *Biochim. Biophys. Acta* **84**, 149–153 (1964).
117. Day, A. J., and N. H. Fidge, *Biochim. Biophys. Acta* **106**, 19–24 (1965).
118. Day, A. J., N. H. Fidge, and G. N. Wilkinson, *J. Lipid Res.* **7**, 132–140 (1966).
119. Day, A. J., and R. K. Tume, *Biochim. Biophys. Acta* **176**, 367–376 (1969).
120. Elves, M. W., *The Lymphocytes*, Year Book Medical Publishers, Chicago, 1967.

121. Miras, C. J., J. D. Mantzos, and G. M. Levis, *Nature* **207**, 1090–1092 (1965).
122. Nakai, G. S., and C. G. Craddock, *Cancer Res.* **25**, 575–578 (1965).
123. Burton, R. M., M. A. Sodd, and R. O. Brady, *J. Biol. Chem.* **233**, 1053–1060 (1958).
124. Brady, R. O., *Clin. Chem.* **13**, 565–577 (1967).
125. Fredrickson, D. S., in *The Metabolic Basis of Inherited Disease*, 2nd ed., J. B. Stanbury, J. B. Wyngaarden, and D. S. Fredrickson, Eds., McGraw-Hill, New York, 1966, pp. 565–585.
126. Kampine, J. P., R. O. Brady, and J. N. Kanfer, *Science* **155**, 86–88 (1967).
127. Snyder, R. A., and R. O. Brady, *Clin. Chim. Acta* **25**, 331–338 (1969).
128. Philippart, M., and J. Menkes, *Biochem. Biophys. Res. Commun.* **15**, 551–555 (1964).
129. Vance, D. E., and C. C. Sweeley, *J. Lipid Res.* **8**, 621–630 (1967).
130. Albrecht, M., *Blut* **13**, 169–179 (1966).
131. Albrecht, M., *Klin. Wochenschr.* **47**, 778–784 (1969).
132. Kattlove, H. E., J. C. Williams, E. Gaynor, M. Spivack, R. M. Bradley, and R. O. Brady, *Blood* **33**, 379–390 (1969).
133. Rosner, F., H. Dosik, S. S. Kaiser, S. L. Lee, and A. N. Morrison, *J. Amer. Med. Ass.* **209**, 935–937 (1969).
134. Smith, W. C., M. M. Kaneshiro, B. D. Goldstein, J. W. Parker, and R. J. Lukes, *Lancet* **2**, 780–781 (1968).
135. Boggs, D. R., *Seminars Hematol.* **4**, 359–386 (1967).
136. Wintrobe, M. M., *Clinical Hematology*, 6th ed., Lea and Febiger, Philadelphia, 1967, p. 180.
137. Kritzler, R. A., J. Terner, J. Lindenbaum, J. Magidson, R. Williams, R. Preisig, and G. B. Phillips, *Amer. J. Med.* **36**, 583–594 (1964).
138. Kanfer, J. N., R. Richards, J. P. Kampine, S. Handmaker, and R. A. Yankee, *Life Sci.* **6**, 2661–2664 (1967).
139. Kanfer, J. N., R. S. Blume, R. A. Yankee, and S. M. Wolff, *New Engl. J. Med.* **279**, 410–413 (1968).

9. The Lipids of Human Platelets

AARON J. MARCUS, LENORE B. SAFIER and HARRIS L. ULLMAN

Hematology Section, Veterans Administration Hospital, and the Department of Medicine, New York Hospital-Cornell Medical Center, New York, New York

I. INTRODUCTION

It is now generally accepted that platelets play a number of important roles in physiological homeostasis. They perform several unique functions, such as aggregation, participation in blood coagulation, and maintenance of vascular integrity. They may also be involved pathologically in the formation of occlusive arterial thrombi. Other interesting properties include the ability to take up and transport serotonin and produce clot retraction; furthermore, if administered in the "living" state, they can arrest hemorrhage that has occurred in their absence. Recent developments in our knowledge of platelet function have been summarized by Marcus (1) and Marcus and Zucker (2).

Some years ago a number of investigators observed that certain lipids

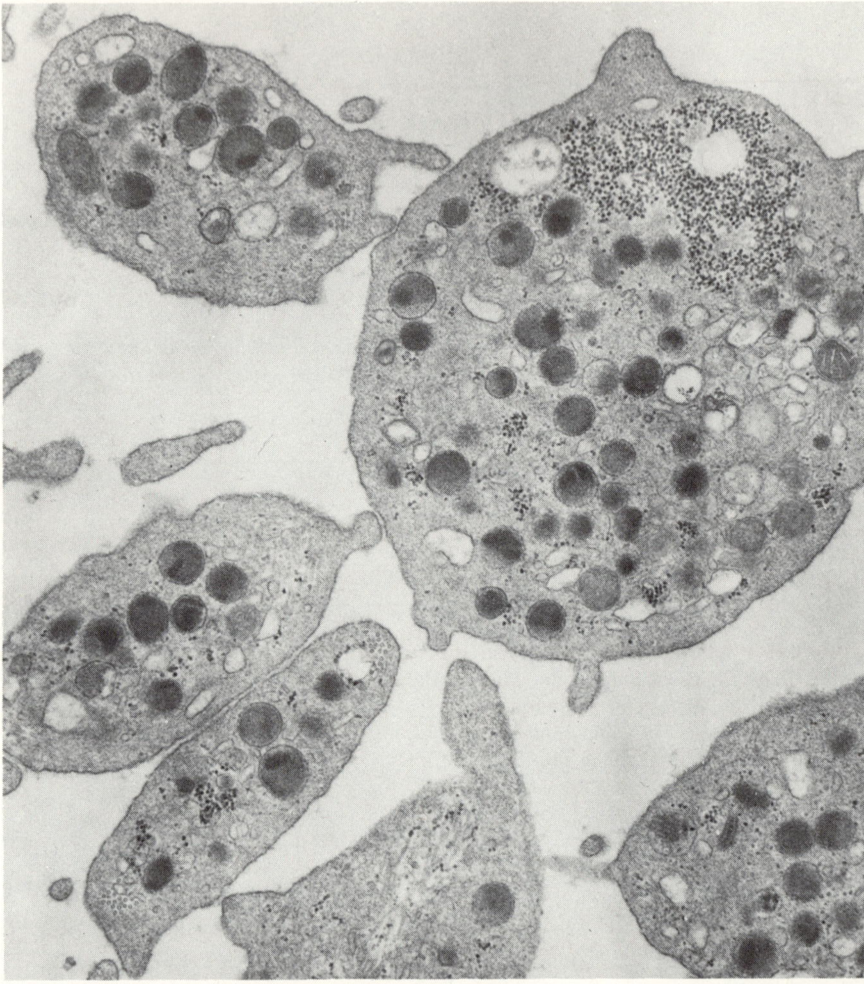

Fig. 1 Electron micrograph of a human platelet (courtesy of Dr. Dorothea Zucker-Franklin). Platelets are devoid of nuclei. They have no DNA and very little RNA. The endoplasmic reticulum is mainly of the smooth type. The major intracellular components are granules, some of which have an eccentric circular dark-staining area and have been termed bull's-eye granules. Other granules appear to have a homogeneous interior and have been called α-granules. Among the granules mitochondria can also be seen. Platelet mitochondria have few cristae in comparison with the mitochondria of other tissues. The dark-staining material between the granules is glycogen. Lysosomal enzyme activity has been found in isolated-platelet-granule preparations.

could substitute for platelets in *in vitro* coagulation test systems. It was then postulated that these lipids might be capable of arresting hemorrhage or producing a "hypercoagulable" state *in vivo*. As will be mentioned later, both of these assumptions proved to be incorrect (1, 2). Only a living and "intact" platelet can aggregate and arrest bleeding.

Advances in lipid methodology in the last 10 years have made it possible to study platelets in great detail. Contributions from many laboratories have already been surveyed (3, 4). In this chapter we summarize some of the techniques employed in our laboratory specifically for the preparation and study of whole-platelet lipids and the lipids of subcellular platelet particles. Figure 1 is an electron micrograph of a platelet fixed in osmic acid.

II. ANALYTICAL PROCEDURES

A. Collection, Processing, and Storage of Human Platelets

In general it is preferable to use large amounts of platelets for initial experiments because otherwise minor platelet constituents may be overlooked. Subsequently, when the exact amount of starting material is determined for a given study, smaller quantities of platelets may be employed. This is also important if metabolic studies on platelets are contemplated. For these reasons we collect approximately 425 ml of whole blood for each experiment. A plastic bag containing 75 ml of acid-citrate-dextrose (code JA-2C, Fenwal Laboratories, Morton Grove, Ill.) is used. If possible, the donor should be in good health, and a platelet count should be performed prior to collection. Blood with platelet counts below 200,000 per cubic millimeter should not be used because the final platelet yield will be relatively poor. The blood collection is made after an overnight fast since platelets are more difficult to isolate from lipemic plasma than are other cells. The subject should be in the supine position and requested to remain so for 45 min after the blood is obtained. During this time fluids, such as water, fruit juice, or whiskey, may be administered. If the donor is anemic, the red cells are returned after separating the platelet-rich plasma.

It is imperative that a clean venipuncture be made and that the flow of blood into the bag be rapid and continuous. The bag should be full, as evidenced by slight bulging before the collection is terminated. Deviations from this procedure will result in platelet clumping and contamination with red cells during the isolation process. Prior to centrifugation the tubing leading to the bag should be sealed or knotted as close to the bag as possible.

If metabolic studies are planned, especially those involving radioisotopes, the pH of the anticoagulant, which is ordinarily 7.1, should be reduced to 6.5 (5, 6). This can be done by injection approximately 22 ml of 0.15 *M* citric acid into the standard bag immediately before collection. If the platelets are to be washed, the washing fluid should also be held at a pH of 6.5. At this pH aggregation due to traces of adenosine diphosphate (ADP) that has escaped from red cells and the platelets themselves is inhibited. Platelets clumped even on the microscopic level can result in reduced uptake of radioisotopes (6; also P. Elsbach and A. J. Marcus, unpublished observations). In some cases it may be necessary to devise special washing media that are more suitable for the experiment—for example, a medium containing ethylenediaminetetraacetic acid (EDTA). In such instances the platelets must be monitored for clumping by phase microscopy.

The bag is centrifuged at 800 *g* for 20 min at 5°C. The temperature of centrifugation is varied according to the purpose of the experiment. Platelets spun in the cold undergo a change in shape, which, though reversible (1), may have a deleterious effect on platelet metabolism. For incubation studies and experiments in which platelets are readministered *in vivo* it is probably better to centrifuge the platelets at room temperature or perhaps at 15°C. The disadvantage of this procedure is that platelet preparations obtained at temperatures higher than 5°C are contaminated with erythrocytes, which are difficult to sediment from plasma that is not refrigerated.

After centrifugation the platelet-rich plasma is expressed from the bag with a spring-loaded instrument (plasma extractor BM-1, Fenwal) into 50-ml conical polypropylene tubes. A leukocyte layer is visible above the sedimented red cells. Care should be taken to avoid expressing this fraction along with the platelet-rich plasma. This is achieved by terminating the plasma collection when its level is within 1.5 in. of the packed white cells. The plasma may be used directly for incubation experiments or other procedures for which a plasma milieu is desirable. For lipid work the plasma must be removed by washing. A platelet button is prepared by centrifuging the platelet-rich plasma at 5000 *g* for 20 min at 5°C. Lower speeds (1500 *g*) can be used without significant loss of platelet material. About 10 ml of wash fluid is added, and the platelet button is gently resuspended by a combination of mixing and aspiration with a polypropylene medicine dropper. Additional washing fluid is added, and the resuspending maneuver is continued until the tube is filled with an even suspension of platelets. The tube is then spun for 15 min at the same speed as that used for preparing the initial button. The entire procedure is then repeated once or twice, depending on the desired degree of washing. Occasionally a small red-cell button may be seen to be trapped in the cone of the centrifuge tube, in which case the suspended platelets should be transferred to another tube and the procedure continued. As the washing proceeds it is advisable to combine the suspensions into one or two tubes. The final platelet button derived from a single unit of blood will vary from 1 to 2 ml ($\sim$ 2 g wet weight) of packed platelets. The average yield of crude platelet lipid from a single unit is about 31 mg (2).

The washing medium that is used depends on the ultimate goal of the investigation. We use a glucose-containing buffered saline solution (7), pH 7.6, with or without added EDTA. In metabolic experiments the pH is brought to 6.5.

When lipid analyses are to be carried out on a large scale, platelet buttons are frozen, preferably at −85°C. This minimizes the oxidative changes that take place in platelets stored at conventional freezer temperatures after short periods of time. A useful procedure for obtaining the frozen pellet before thawing takes place is to remove the tube from the freezer, place it on its side on a table, and strike it with a hammer. The frozen pellet that is dislodged can then be immediately extracted with appropriate solvents. Furthermore, any traces of contaminating erythrocytes still remaining on the pellet can be quickly sliced off with a razor blade.

B. Preparation of Platelet-Lipid Extracts

The basic technique for the preparation of platelet-lipid extracts is a variation of the procedure originally described by Folch, Lees, and Sloane-Stanley (8). The major change involves its application to small amounts of tissue.

The platelet material is placed in a glass-stoppered graduated centrifuge tube, and aliquots are taken for protein analyses (9). It is then transferred to a glass-stoppered Erlenmeyer flask with a Pasteur pipette. Nineteen volumes of chloroform–methanol, 2 : 1 (v/v), are added to the tissue, part of the solvent being used to rinse the original centrifuge tube and pipette. The extraction is allowed to proceed at room temperature for 30–60 min, depending on the amount of material to be extracted. All operations are carried out under cover of prepurified nitrogen. The extract is filtered through solvent-washed Whatman No. 1 filter paper into a glass-stoppered graduated cylinder. The flask and filter paper are washed with fresh solvent consisting of 19 parts chloroform–methanol, 2 : 1, to 0.8 part water. A solution of 0.05% calcium chloride equivalent to one-fifth of the filtrate is added, and the mixture is shaken, thus producing the classical two-phase system. The two phases can be sharply demarcated if the mixture is centrifuged (5°C for 15 min at 350 *g*). The aqueous top layer is carefully removed, and the remaining top layer near the interphase is rinsed off with 3 ml of a mixture containing 0.02% calcium chloride in chloroform–methanol–water, 3 : 48 : 47 (pure-solvents upper phase) (8). The lower phase is then washed three times with the calcium-containing pure-solvents upper phase, using 40 parts of pure solvents per 60 parts of lower phase. After shaking and centrifugation, the aqueous layer is discarded. The interphase is rinsed once after each wash and three times after the final wash. The aqueous layer is removed as completely as possible. Under certain circumstances it may be advisable to avoid the formation of calcium–lipid complexes. For this reason sodium chloride may be substituted for calcium chloride. However, the quantities required are different (8). The lipid is then taken to dryness under nitrogen at 37°C and redissolved to any desired volume in chloroform–methanol, 2 : 1.

C. Silicic-Acid-Column Chromatography

Crude platelet-lipid extracts are first separated into a phospholipid fraction and a "neutral" lipid component. For example, in a typical experiment about 200 mg of whole-platelet lipid in 5 ml of chloroform is applied to a 60-g silicic acid column (Mallinckrodt SilicAR CC-7, 100–200 mesh). The neutral lipids are eluted first with 700 ml of chloroform. Fractions are monitored by the glass-paper char test (10). The emergence of the neutral-lipid fraction from the column is conveniently indicated by a sharp band of platelet pigment, at which time the charring test becomes positive.

When the char test becomes negative, the phospholipid fractions are ready for separation. About 500 ml of chloroform–methanol, 4 : 1, is added to the column. This will elute phosphatidylethanolamine, phosphatidylserine, and some phosphatidylinositol. The fractions can be monitored by a ninhydrin reaction (11, 12). The next solvent pair is chloroform–methanol, 5 : 4. The mixture first elutes the remainder of the phosphatidylinositol (containing small amounts of phosphatidylserine) and then the bulk of the lecithin. The separation is completed with 500 ml of chloroform–methanol, 1 : 9—which elutes most of the sphingomyelin—and finally 100 ml of methanol. There is invariably some overlapping between lecithin and sphingomyelin, but these compounds are easily separated by thin-layer chromatography.

The precise distribution of all phosphatides in the column eluates always varies slightly. For this reason a combination of all identification procedures is necessary, especially the first few times these separations are carried out. All fractions containing phosphatidylethanolamine, phosphatidylserine, and phosphatidylinositol are pooled and separated 24 hr later by the ammoniated-silicic-acid-column technique devised by Rouser, O'Brien, and Heller (11, 13).

It is advisable to study the phospholipid components first because of their known lability in storage and handling.

For the neutral-lipid separation the basic scheme of Hirsch and Ahrens (14) can be simplified. The principal neutral lipid in platelets is free cholesterol (about 90%), whereas triglycerides, free fatty acids, and chloestryl esters are very minor components (12). Thus approximately 65 mg of neutral lipid is added to a 21-g silicic acid column (Bio-Sil HA, — 325 mesh, Bio-Rad Laboratories, Richmond, Calif.), and hydrocarbons, cholesteryl esters, triglycerides, and some free fatty acids are collected as a pool with 4% ethyl ether in petroleum ether (approximately 300 ml). The components of this pool are subsequently separated by thin-layer chromatography. A mixture of 8% ethyl ether in petroleum ether (about 650 ml) is then added, and individual fractions are collected. These fractions contain additional amounts of free fatty acids, traces of triglycerides, and possibly diglycerides. Cholesterol begins to emerge in this solvent mixture and is obtained in relatively pure form. Elution of this lipid is completed with about 450 ml of 25% ethyl ether in petroleum ether.

The char test is particularly useful for monitoring cholesterol since the charring reaction is preceded by a pink color. At this point the bulk of the cholesterol can be collected as a pool. As the char test becomes negative, collection in tubes is resumed. This is done to avoid mixing the cholesterol with the series of pigments that emerge with succeeding solvents. One pigment is eluted with 100% ether (150 ml) and the other with methanol. These pigments have not as yet been identified. Final verification of column eluates is made by thin-layer chromatography.

D. Thin-Layer Chromatography

Accurate qualitative and quantitative analyses of platelet phospholipids can be achieved by thin-layer chromatography (TLC). Complete separation of the five main platelet phospholipids requires careful attention to detail. The separation of phosphatidylserine from phosphatidylinositol can be extremely difficult if certain precautions are not taken. Quantitative analysis is of little value unless all components are completely and reproducibly separated. In general, tanks measuring 8.5 × 4.5 × 8.5 in. are used. We have found it unnecessary to line the tanks with filter paper. Only the four corners of the cover are lightly coated with silicone grease. In our procedure it is important to make the chromatography run with the tank sealed in a plastic bag by means of a screw clamp. Evaporation of solvent during the run may result in incomplete separation. The techniques devised by Skipski and associates have been used (15, 16).

The best phospholipid separations are achieved with Kieselgel D-O (Camag, distributed by Arthur H. Thomas Co., Philadelphia, Pa.), which contains *no binder*. Plates of 0.5-mm thickness are prepared as follows: Silica gel (40 g) is mechanically stirred with 90 to 100 ml of 0.001 *M* sodium carbonate for 3 to 5 min, at which time a smooth slurry is obtained. The slurry is then poured into an adjustable applicator (Desaga/Brinkmann), and the plates are coated in the usual manner. The plates are air dried and stored in a desiccating cabinet. Prior to use, the plates are activated at 110°C for 1 hr. They are then allowed to cool in a desiccator for about 20 min before the sample is applied. Lipids are applied to the plate while it is enclosed in a box with nitrogen flowing (Model DB, Brinkmann Instruments). This serves to retard spreading of the solvent and possible oxidative changes during the application period. The lipid is applied in 5-μl amounts with a Hamilton 5-μl syringe in a concentration not exceeding 10 μg of lipid phosphorus. For this purpose the most useful solvent has been chloroform–methanol, 2 : 1.

A good solvent system for phospholipid separations is chloroform–methanol–acetic acid–water, 50 : 28 : 10 : 5 (16). The tanks are equilibrated with the solvent for at least 1 hr before development. It is also helpful to produce individual lanes on the TLC plates by drawing several vertical lines about 2 cm apart and one horizontal line about 15 cm from the origin with a sharply pointed instrument. A typical run takes an average of 2.5 hr. On completion of the run the plates are carefully dried under nitrogen for 10 min, and the separated components are identified by charring with 50% sulfuric acid or by exposure to iodine vapor.

For accurate quantitative analysis of phospholipids, further precautions are necessary. The silica gel must be washed prior to use because it contains substances that give rise to high blank readings in phosphorus analysis. The procedure is carried out as follows: Silica gel (60 g) is washed with 600 ml of distilled water through a coarse-porosity fritted-glass funnel. The water is removed by gentle suction. This is followed by 600 ml of acetone, then 500 ml of chloroform–methanol, 4 : 1, and finally 100 ml of methanol. The dry powder is transferred to a glass tray lined with aluminum foil and finally heated for 1 hr at 110°C. Phosphorus analyses are carried out by the method of Parker and Peterson (17), with slight modifications (12), on material that has been scraped from the plates along with blanks of comparable size.

Thin-layer chromatography can be supplemented by analyzing phospholipids on filter paper coated with silica gel (12, 18, 19). Phosphorus analyses are carried out by directly digesting the paper. The method is particularly useful if one is interested in studying cardiolipin, a lipid prominent in mitochondria.

Neutral lipids in whole platelets can be qualitatively identified on Camag silica-gel plates prepared as described above except that distilled water is substituted for sodium carbonate. The two-step development system of Skipski and associates (20) is excellent. The precautions cited by these authors should be scrupulously observed.

A useful solvent system for the separation of the pool containing platelet hydrocarbons, cholesteryl esters, triglycerides, and free fatty acids is petroleum ether–diethyl ether–glacial acetic acid, 82 : 18 : 1 (21).

The results of quantitative analyses of platelet lipids separated by these techniques are shown in Table I.

Table I. Lipids of Human Platelets

Component	Percentage of Total Lipids in		
	Whole Platelets	Membranes	Granules
Neutral lipids	21.0	22.0	25.0
Ethanolamine phosphoglycerides	20.0	20.7	20.3
Serine phosphoglycerides	8.0	6.4	8.6
Inositol phosphoglycerides	3.4	3.3	2.9
Choline phosphoglycerides (lecithin)	31.4	32.5	25.1
Sphingomyelin	14.5	13.4	15.0
Lysolecithin	0.6	0.2	1.4
Cardiolipin	0.4	0.2	1.0
Gangliosides	0.5		

E. Gas–Liquid Chromatography

The fatty acids (and aldehydes) of all platelet-lipid classes can be studied by means of gas–liquid chromatography (11, 12). We use a Barber-Colman Model 10 chromatographic apparatus, which accommodates two columns and two strontium ionization-detection cells.[1] Our glass columns are U-shaped and 6 ft in overall length, with an internal diameter of 4 mm. For accurate quantitative analysis the linearity of detector response must be checked. This can be done with the use of known model mixtures available from various commercial sources (for example, mixtures KA-D, Applied Science Laboratories, State College, Pa.).

The reliability of quantitative fatty acid analysis is enhanced if the gas–liquid chromatography is carried out on polar and nonpolar columns. Thus the platelet fatty acids are analyzed on columns coated with Apiezon L (nonpolar) as well as columns coated with ethylene glycol adipate (polar)

[1] More recently a Hewlett-Packard Model 7620A Gas-Chromatograph has been used.

(11). Fatty acid methyl esters and fatty aldehyde dimethyl acetals (DMA) are prepared from lipids separated on either columns or TLC plates. Lipids from TLC separations are scraped directly from the plate and esterified. Appropriate blanks are always included. Methyl esters are formed with the boron trifluoride–methanol reagent (22, 23) (Applied Science Laboratories).

Since phospholipids are known to contain highly unsaturated fatty acids, it is necessary to use an antioxidant like 2,6-di-*tert*-butyl-*p*-cresol (BHT), especially during TLC separations of phosphatidylinositol and phosphatidylserine. It is also used whenever the TLC procedure takes more than 30 min. The antioxidant is added to the developing solvents in a concentration of 50 mg per 100 ml (23).

The presence of BHT creates a problem during GLC analysis. Artifactual peaks appear on the polar columns and to some extent on the nonpolar columns. These can be avoided by a rapid TLC procedure using silica gel HR (Brinkmann) and a solvent system consisting of hexane–diethyl ether–acetic acid, 90 : 10 : 1 (24). This separates the BHT from the methyl esters, which are then eluted with chloroform (22) (BHT migrates at or near the solvent front). This solvent system is also useful for purifying methyl esters formed from free fatty acids and triglycerides. It also separates free cholesterol from the methyl esters of fatty acids produced during the methanolysis of cholesteryl esters.

F. Subcellular Platelet Particles

The methods described in the preceding sections have recently been adapted for the study of platelet membranes and granules. For reasons that are not clear, washed platelets cannot be physically disrupted by classical techniques. For example, freeze-thawing, glass homogenization, blendorizing, osmotic lysis, and nitrogen-bomb cavitation all result in unsatisfactory platelet homogenates (25).

Hence it was necessary for us to devise a special type of homogenizing apparatus. It consists of a no-clearance Teflon plunger that fits into a clear-walled glass tube only after 15 min at 4°C (No. K88600, size D, Kontes Glass Co., Vineland, N.J.). The shaft of the plunger is inserted into a motor that can revolve at a speed of approximately 1700 rpm. A platelet button from 1 unit of freshly collected blood, prepared as described in Section II.A, is transferred to the clear-walled glass receptacle of the homogenizing apparatus. This is done by adding about 1 ml of the homogenizing medium (usually 0.44 *M* sucrose containing 0.001 *M* EDTA) to the packed platelets and gently aspirating back and forth until all of the platelets are removed. This procedure also allows any residual contaminating red cells to be left behind.

Homogenization is carried out by a vigorous up-and-down motion for 5 min. After 3 min have elapsed, the glass tube may become warm, in which case it is placed in a large paper cup filled with ice. Cell disruption is accomplished by virtue of the shearing force of the no-clearance action of the Teflon plunger. After the homogenization period, the contents of the tube are transferred, and the tube is carefully washed with about 10 ml of the homogenizing medium. At this point "intact" platelets that have escaped homogenization are removed by centrifugation for 30 min at 2000 *g*. A pellet of relatively intact platelets results, but the supernatant contains granules, membranes, and the soluble components. The homogenate is now ready for further fractionation.

For this purpose isopycnic ultracentrifugation in a continuous sucrose gradient is the procedure of choice. The sucrose solutions required for adequate separation are unfortunately hypertonic and quite viscous (a better alternative has not been found so far). The platelet homogenate is layered on a continuous sucrose gradient ranging from 30 to 60%. A centrifuge rotor with either a 5-ml (SW39) or a 14-ml (SW41) tube capacity can be used for these separations. One to two hours of ultracentrifugation at the highest speed obtainable with the rotor is necessary.

On completion of the ultracentrifugation step, it is best to collect the fractions by aspiration from above with a Pasteur pipette. In most instances it is then advisable to remove the sucrose by washing or dialysis.

Three main subcellular "compartments" have been arbitrarily defined. The material at the top of the gradient is known as the soluble fraction. It contains many platelet proteins and enzymes. It is difficult to characterize the soluble compartment adequately, since many of its components may have originally been bound to a particle and released during homogenization or ultracentrifugation (or both).

The next compartment has a density range of 1.12 to 1.13. It consists of platelet membranes in a characteristic vesicular form of varying size (Fig. 2). There are probably two separate bands in this fraction, which await further characterization. The membrane compartment is thought to consist mainly of plasma membranes, as well as membranes derived from damaged granules and the smooth endoplasmic reticulum.

The third compartment has a density range of 1.17 to 1.21. The platelet granules and mitochondria are found in this band (Fig. 3). The granule fraction has high lysosomal enzyme activity. It is clear, however, that not all of the platelet granules are classical lysosomes. The function of platelet granules is currently under intensive research in several laboratories.

Some investigators have suggested that platelet granules are responsible for the platelet contribution to blood coagulation. It is proposed that these granules are discharged into the surrounding medium during the early phases of coagulation. Although it is true that procoagulant activity can

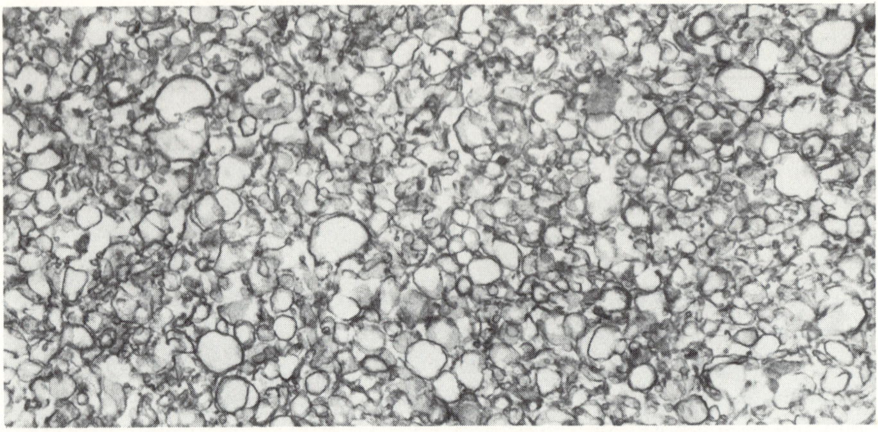

Fig. 2 Representative electron micrograph (×24,000) of platelet membrane fraction obtained by continuous-density-gradient ultracentrifugation in sucrose. The density range of this fraction is 1.12 to 1.13. It consists mainly of platelet plasma membranes and membranes from disrupted granules. No formed intracellular organelles were present in this fraction. (Electron micrograph supplied by Dr. Dorothea Zucker-Franklin. Reprinted from Ref. 25 by permission from the *Journal of Clinical Investigation.*)

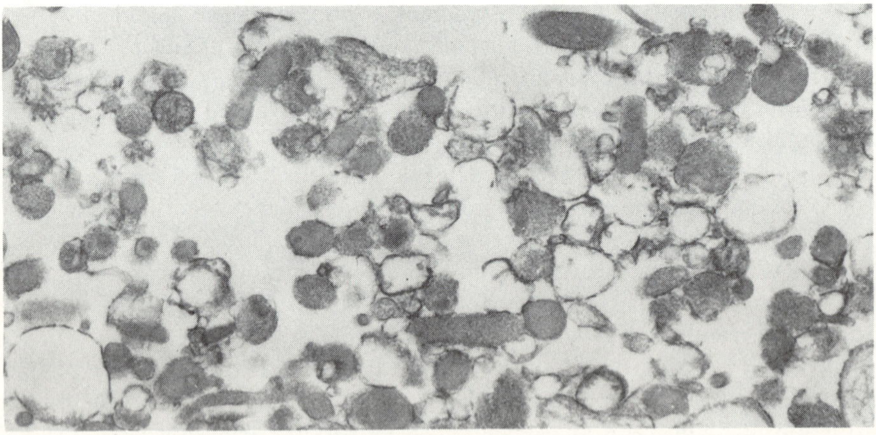

Fig. 3 Electron micrograph (×24,000) of platelet granule fraction obtained by continuous density-gradient ultracentrifugation in sucrose. The density range is 1.17 to 1.21. The scattered membrane fragments that can be seen probably originated from ruptured granules. Mitochondria and bull's-eye granules are present. (Electron micrograph supplied by Dr. Dorothea Zucker-Franklin. Reprinted from Ref. 25 by permission from the *Journal of Clinical Investigation.*)

be found in isolated platelet granules, most electron microscopists have not observed platelet granules in the surrounding medium prior to the formation of thrombin. We believe that platelet granules function principally as lysosomes and "metabolic storehouses." In our view it is the plasma membrane of the platelet that furnishes the proper catalytic lipoprotein surface for interaction with blood coagulation factors.

Two outstanding monographs that have recently appeared provide extensive information on subcellular platelet particles and their constituent enzymes (26, 27).

Table II. Phospholipid Fatty Acids and Aldehydes of Whole Platelets[a,b]

	Quantity (wt %) in				
Fatty Acid[c]	PE	PS	PI	PC	Sph
16:0[d]	9.2	0.60	0.92	0.80	
16:0	3.4	0.97	1.6	34.1	24.6
16:1	0.26	0.67	0.46	1.6	1.2
18:0[d]	17.9	0.19	0.12	(e)	
18:0	13.7	44.7	44.7	14.1	5.8
18:1[d]	2.7				
18:1	5.9	26.7	8.7	27.0	1.3
18:2	2.3		0.05	6.9	
18:3	1.6				
20:0	0.64	1.6	0.84	0.38	9.4
20:4	31.8	22.6	41.8	12.0	(e)
22:0					29.3
22:1					2.0
22:4[f]	4.4				
22:5	1.8	(e)		(e)	
22:6	1.2	(e)			
23:0					1.2
24:0					10.9
24:1					12.8

[a] For further details see Ref. 12.
[b] Abbreviations: PE, phosphatidylethanolamine; PS, phosphatidylserine; PI, phosphatidylinositol; PC, phosphatidylcholine (lecithin); Sph, sphingomyelin.
[c] Fatty acids are designated by two quantities: the number of carbon atoms and the number of double bonds (e.g., 16:0). Besides those shown, the following acids were detected in small ($< 1.5\%$) amounts: 12:0, 14:0, 15:0, 17:0 (dimethyl acetal), 17:0, 20:1, 20:2, 20:3, and one with a probable carbon number of 22 on Apiezon.
[d] Dimethyl acetal.
[e] Trace.
[f] In this fatty acid there are six carbon atoms from the methyl end of the chain to the center of the nearest double bond.

III. THE LIPIDS OF SUBCELLULAR PLATELET PARTICLES

As already mentioned, human platelets can be fractionated into three main subcellular compartments (25). The lipids in the granule and membrane compartments have been studied in great detail, although the lipids of the soluble layer remain to be explored. In addition, quantitative relationships between lipids and proteins in these particles have been examined and compared with the lipids and proteins of other tissues.

Table III. Phospholipid Fatty Acids and Aldehydes of Platelet Membranes[a,b]

	Quantity (wt %) in				
Fatty Acid[c]	PE	PS	PI	PC	Sph
16:0[d]	8.7		2.0	0.36	
16:0	3.5	0.36	1.4	31.0	21.9
16:1	0.51	0.51	0.55	1.4	0.15
18:0[d]	18.2	0.15			
18:0	14.1	46.5	44.4	15.7	5.6
18:1[d]	3.1				
18:1	5.5	25.0	9.2	27.4	0.72
18:2	2.2	(e)	0.33	7.5	0.12
18:3	1.5				
20:0	0.52	1.7	0.47	0.51	9.8
20:4	31.6	24.7	41.2	12.5	
22:0					31.5
22:1					5.8
22:4[f]	3.8				
22:5	1.1	(e)		0.81	
22:6	1.2	(e)		(e)	
23:0					2.1
24:0					7.7
24:1					12.0

[a] For further details see Ref. 12.
[b] Abbreviations: PE, phosphatidylethanolamine; PS, phosphatidylserine; PI, phosphatidylinositol; PC, lecithin; Sph, sphingomyelin.
[c] Fatty acids are designated by two quantities: the number of carbon atoms and the number of double bonds (e.g., 16:0). Besides those shown, the following acids were detected in small ($< 1.5\%$) amounts: 12:0, 14:0, 15:0, 17:0 (dimethyl acetal), 17:0, 20:1, 20:2, 20:3, and one with a probable carbon number of 22 on Apiezon.
[d] Dimethyl acetal.
[e] Trace.
[f] In this fatty acid there are six carbon atoms from the methyl end of the chain to the center of the nearest double bond.

In contrast to whole cells or tissues, special precautions are required for the study of subcellular lipids. More preparative work is frequently necessary in order to obtain sufficient material for analysis, thereby creating a storage problem. At ordinary freezer temperatures (−20°C) subcellular particles gradually discolor, presumably due to lipid peroxidation. It is therefore necessary to store the particles at temperatures in the vicinity of −85°C, at which these changes do not occur.

A second problem is the presence of sucrose in the fractions. Sucrose is

Table IV. Phospholipid Fatty Acids and Aldehydes of Platelet Granules[a,b]

	Quantity (wt %) in				
Fatty Acid[c]	PE	PS	PI	PC	Sph
16:0[d]	8.7			0.47	
16:0	3.0		0.94	31.0	22.5
16:1	0.24	0.2	0.24	1.8	0.26
18:0[d]	17.8	(e)	(e)		
18:0	13.8	44.2	44.3	15.6	5.7
18:1[d]	4.7				
18:1	5.8	26.0	9.0	27.5	0.83
18:2	2.1	(e)	0.44	7.2	0.16
18:3	1.4				
20:0	0.41	1.5	0.48	0.94	9.6
20:4	28.9	25.2	44.1	11.8	(e)
22:0					29.2
22:1					4.0
22.4[f]	5.6				
22:5	2.0	(e)			
22:6	1.6	(e)			
23:0					2.9
24:0					7.3
24:1					15.4

[a] For further details see Ref. 12.

[b] Abbreviations: PE, phosphatidylethanolamine; PS, phosphatidylserine; PI, phosphatidylinositol; PC, lecithin; Sph, sphingomyelin.

[c] Fatty acids are designated by two quantities: the number of carbon atoms and the number of double bonds (e.g., 16:0). Besides those shown, the following acids were detected in small (< 1.5%) amounts: 12:0, 14:0, 15:0, 17:0 (dimethyl acetal), 17:0, 20:1, 20:2, 20:3, and one with a probable carbon number of 22 on Apiezon.

[d] Dimethyl acetal.

[e] Trace.

[f] In this fatty acid there are six carbon atoms from the methyl end of the chain to the center of the nearest double bond.

partially soluble in lipid solvents and thus interferes with weight determinations as well as many analytical procedures. There are two main approaches to this difficulty, both of which necessitate further handling of the fractions. The first entails washing in water or appropriate buffers, followed by repeated ultracentrifugation. Two washes are frequently necessary, and this, in our experience, produces an ill-defined change in the consistency of the particles. For example, the original membrane pellet is glossy and translucent, but after a second wash it takes on an opaque, whitish appearance. An alternative procedure is that of dialysis, which has proved to be successful in certain instances (28). During the dialysis procedure it is important to allow for large increases in the volume of the dialysis bag.

Despite these measures the washed particles may still contain traces of sucrose. Thus it is always necessary to wash the extracted lipids by the

Table V. Neutral-Lipid Fatty Acids of Whole Platelets[a]

	Quantity (wt %) in		
Fatty Acid[b]	Cholesteryl Esters	Triglycerides	Free Fatty Acids
12:0	2.7	0.82	1.2
14:0	6.4	7.0	4.8
14:0[c]	1.4	1.5	0.54
15:0	0.78	2.7	1.6
15:0[c]	4.8	0.71	0.16
16:0	16.6	29.8	38.6
16:1	34.5	11.6	4.1
17:0	2.9	0.91	0.97
17:0[d]	(e)	1.8	0.36
?	(e)	1.3	0.45
18:0	2.3	10.1	20.2
18:1	27.6	23.1	23.2
18:2	(e)	8.5	1.8
18:3			(e)
20:0			0.86
20:1		0.21	0.50
20:3			0.59

[a] For further details see Ref. 12.

[b] Fatty acids are designated by two quantities: the number of carbon atoms and the number of double bonds (e.g., 12:0).

[c] Branched chain.

[d] *Anteiso* (terminal isobutyl group).

[e] Trace.

Folch technique (8), which also serves to remove other nonlipid contaminants.

One of the principal reasons for studying subcellular platelet lipids is to learn whether intracellular organelles that have specialized functions are endowed with a specific lipid or fatty acid. In the case of platelets the particles studied so far have been very similar with regard to qualitative and quantitative lipid composition. However, to date platelet mitochondria have not been isolated in pure form, nor have the various types of granules been satisfactorily separated from each other. Finally, the platelet membrane fraction does not consist of pure plasma membranes. It is possible that when such separations become feasible, particle-specific lipids may be found.

Table VI. Neutral-Lipid Fatty Acids of Platelet Membranes[a]

	Quantity (wt %) in		
Fatty Acid[b]	Cholesteryl Esters	Triglycerides	Free Fatty Acids
12:0	0.21	0.6	0.71
14:0	1.6	4.0	3.7
14:0[c]	4.7	1.6	0.51
15:0	2.9	1.6	1.4
15:0[c]	1.2	0.57	0.29
16:0	17.4	22.7	26.4
16:1	37.3	7.5	4.4
17:0	4.4	0.81	1.2
17:0[d]	(e)	1.5	1.2
?	(e)	0.96	1.4
18:0	4.4	13.6	22.6
18:1	26.0	30.1	27.8
18:2		7.8	3.5
18:3		0.45	0.3
20:0		2.2	1.6
20:1		1.4	1.1
20:3		0.58	1.7
20:4		2.2	0.2

[a] For further details see Ref. 12.

[b] Fatty acids are described by two quantities: the number of carbon atoms and the number of double bonds (e.g., 12:0).

[c] Branched chain.

[d] *Anteiso* (terminal isobutyl group).

[e] Trace.

The results of GLC studies on the fatty acid and aldehyde composition of platelet lipids are given in Tables II through VII.

Some recent analytical findings are as follows: phospholipids comprise 79, 78, and 75% of the total lipids in whole platelets, membranes, and granules, respectively. Platelet granules contain less lecithin than do the membranes or whole platelets. This decrease in lecithin is accompanied by a reciprocal increase in granule sphingomyelin and agrees with findings in other tissues in which the sum of the lecithin and sphingomyelin fractions is usually constant. As in most other mammalian tissues, lecithin is the predominant phospholipid. Although each platelet phospholipid class has a distinctive fatty acid composition, the fatty acid composition of the granules and membranes was virtually identical with that of whole platelets (11, 12).

The molar ratios of cholesterol to phospholipid and lipid to protein are of interest. The original idea that the molar ratio of cholesterol to phospho-

Table VII. Neutral-Lipid Fatty Acids of Platelet Granules[a]

	Quantity (wt %) in		
Fatty Acid[b]	Cholesteryl Esters	Triglycerides	Free Fatty Acids
12:0		0.8	0.3
14:0	1.3	4.7	1.8
14:0[c]	1.3	1.6	0.25
15:0	1.3	2.2	0.68
15:0[c]	2.5	0.85	0.08
16:0	15.5	24.1	19.4
16:1	44.0	8.2	3.0
17:0	7.9	1.5	0.89
17:0[d]	(e)	1.7	0.96
?		1.7	0.36
18:0	7.5	11.9	34.1
18:1	18.7	28.1	21.1
18:2	(e)	8.7	6.2
18:3		0.79	0.13
20:0		1.0	1.2
20:1		0.37	0.46
20:3		(e)	0.34
20:4		1.8	8.8

[a] For further details see Ref. 12.

[b] Fatty acids are designated by two quantities: chain length and the number of double bonds (e.g., 12:0).

[c] Branched chain.

[d] *Anteiso* (terminal isobutyl group).

[e] Trace.

lipid in a cell membrane should be unity is probably no longer tenable. In platelet membranes the ratio is 0.53. Other cell membranes have also been reported to vary from the "classical" ratio of unity (12).

IV. OTHER ANALYTICAL TECHNIQUES

We have measured proteolipids in human platelets by the method of Hess and Lewin (29) as modified by Lees (30). Whole-platelet lipids contain 1.8% proteolipid protein. A functional role for proteolipid in platelets remains to be defined.

For cholesterol determinations the method of Zak and associates (31) has been employed. The color is allowed to develop at 4°C for 1 hr in the dark. When saponification is required, the procedure of Abell and co-workers (32) is used. It is slightly modified in that it is carried out in a 60°C water bath for 60 min.

Attempts have been made to identify cerebroside and cerebroside sulfate in human platelets. Thus far these compounds have not been detected by TLC techniques (12). On the other hand, gangliosides are present in platelets. They appear to comprise less than 1% of the total lipid fraction. Preliminary TLC studies indicate that the principal platelet ganglioside is probably "hematoside." Studies on this interesting group of compounds are now in progress.

V. THE ROLE OF PLATELETS AND PLATELET LIPIDS IN BLOOD COAGULATION

That platelets play an important role in blood coagulation is a well-established fact (1, 2). If platelets are carefully removed from "native" plasma (no anticoagulant), the clotting time is markedly prolonged. This "defect" can be corrected if the platelets are added back to the plasma. It is of interest that one need not add back the platelets but merely certain phosphatides or a crude mixture of phospholipids. Phosphatidylserine is the best platelet substitute in *in vitro* clotting systems. Also active but less effective are phosphatidylethanolamine and inositol phosphatides. Lecithin and sphingomyelin are inactive. If the active lipids are present in excess, they act as anticoagulants.

When the clot-promoting properties of lipids derived from platelets and other tissues were discovered, it was anticipated that these lipids might function *in vivo* as hemostatic agents. Unfortunately this was not the case, and on the basis of our current concepts of the role of platelets in hemostasis this would have been predictable. The immediate arrest of bleeding (primary hemostasis) can only be accomplished by intact "living" platelets. The coagulation mechanism is involved in a secondary manner. For example, a patient with hemophilia in whom the blood-coagulation mechanism is impaired still has normal primary hemostasis (normal bleeding time). Thus platelet lipids or platelet subcellular particles do not function in primary hemostasis. They do, however, participate in an important manner in the formation of thrombin, which in turn results in the production of fibrin. Fibrin serves to "consolidate" the initial platelet plug and to permanently seal the opening in the blood vessel.

The clot-promoting properties of platelet lipids are even more striking if they are used in the form of lipoprotein particles in *in vitro* coagulation systems. If one quantifies the amount of lipid phosphorus required to achieve a given clotting time in a standard *in vitro* test system, it will be observed that 20 times less lipid phosphorus is required when the lipid is in the form of a lipoprotein (25).

Clot-promoting lipids and lipoproteins can be found in a wide variety of tissues and blood cells, but they do not appear to be involved in the intrinsic coagulation system (1). Furthermore, platelets also contain a soluble lipoprotein that is nonsedimentable and is capable of participating in the coagulation process (33). However, this activity can be demonstrated only after platelets have been treated with thrombin. On the other hand, tissues contain a lipoprotein, known as "tissue factor," that functions in the extrinsic coagulation system. This contributes to thrombin formation and has great importance for *in vivo* coagulation. It differs from the lipoprotein found in platelets. For further details see Refs. 1 and 34.

The platelet contribution to blood coagulation has been called platelet factor 3 (PF-3)—a term that we feel is inappropriate. There is no such biochemical factor. The term "PF-3" actually designates the platelet-lipoprotein contribution to the intrinsic prothrombin-activation system. It is in the form of a catalytic lipoprotein surface on which the plasma coagulation factors interact with the platelet membrane. In our view this activity is manifest before thrombin has formed. Clotting activity measured after the appearance of thrombin may not be platelet factor 3. It is conceivable that biochemical substances such as ADP affect the platelet membrane in such a way that aggregation is produced and membrane lipoprotein is made "available" for interaction with plasma coagulation factors.

VI. LIPID METABOLISM IN HUMAN PLATELETS

When platelets are incubated with acetate-1-^{14}C, 75% of the label is recovered in three platelet-lipid classes: lecithin, free fatty acids, and ceramide. If the incubation is carried out in plasma, 40% of the newly formed lipid appears in the medium (6). It is also interesting that platelets can form fatty acids by both *de novo* synthesis and chain elongation (6, 35, 36). Unlike platelets, mature leukocytes and erythrocytes do not contain acetyl-coenzyme A carboxylase and therefore form fatty acids only by chain elongation (36).

Several observations on the pathways of fatty acid metabolism in platelets have recently been reported (37). Incubation of platelets with tracer amounts of 16:0, 18:0, 18:1, and 18:2 fatty acids showed interesting patterns of uptake among the neutral lipids and phospholipids. The phospholipid distribution, for example, resembled that of the natural platelet phospholipids. It was also shown that a de novo pathway for lecithin renewal is present in platelets. Furthermore, the capacity of platelets to oxidize glucose as well as long-chain fatty acids has been demonstrated (38). As in other mammalian tissues, the rate at which platelets oxidize these fatty acids is regulated by carnitine. After 24 hr of storage at 4°C, the platelet capacity for glucose oxidation is reduced by 25% and long-chain fatty acid oxidation by 50%. Thus the respiratory capacity of platelets after storage at 4°C gradually becomes impaired. This information is of importance for the ever expanding clinical use of platelets for transfusion purposes.

VII. SUMMARY

Sophisticated techniques in lipid methodology have afforded us considerable information concerning the lipid composition of platelets and subcellular platelet particles. Until relatively recently, however, most of the work has been of a "descriptive" nature. This era is gradually coming to a close and will soon be superseded by studies of the dynamic aspects of platelet lipid and lipoprotein metabolism. We still do not know the precise mechanism by which platelet-membrane lipoprotein interacts with plasma coagulation factors. The dynamics of platelet adhesion to blood vessels and cohesion to each other—reactions that appear to involve cell surfaces and offer intriguing challenges to investigators—are as yet ill defined. It is hoped that information gleaned in the near future will illuminate the nature of occlusive vascular disease—a problem of the greatest urgency in clinical medicine.

VIII. ACKNOWLEDGMENTS

Our work has been supported by grants from the National Institutes of Health (HE 09070-06), the Veterans Administration, and the New York Heart Association.

We are grateful to Dr. Dorothea Zucker-Franklin for supplying the three electron micrographs shown in Figs. 1, 2, and 3.

REFERENCES

1. Marcus, A. J., *New Engl. J. Med.* **280**, 1213–1220, 1278–1284, and 1330–1335 (1969).
2. Marcus, A. J., and M. B. Zucker, *The Physiology of Blood Platelets,* Grune and Stratton, New York, 1965.
3. Marcus, A. J., *Advances in Lipid Research,* Vol. 4, R. Paoletti and D. Kritchevsky, Eds., Academic Press, New York, 1966, pp. 1–37.
4. Merskey, C., and A. J. Marcus, *Ann. Rev. Med.* **14**, 323–328 (1963).
5. Aster, R. H., and J. H. Jandl, *J. Clin. Invest.* **43**, 843–855 (1964).
6. Deykin, D., and R. K. Desser, *J. Clin. Invest.* **47**, 1590–1602 (1968).
7. Gaintner, J. R., D. P. Jackson, and E. W. Maynert, *Bull. Johns Hopkins Hosp.*
8. Folch, J., M. Lees, and G. H. Sloane-Stanley, *J. Biol. Chem.* **226**, 497–509 **111**, 185–197 (1962).
9. Miller, G. L., *Anal. Chem.* **31**, 964 (1959). (1957).
10. Ways, P., *J. Lipid Res.* **4**, 101–106 (1963).
11. Marcus, A. J., H. L. Ullman, L. B. Safier, and H. S. Ballard, *J. Clin. Invest.* **41**,
12. Marcus, A. J., H. L. Ullman, and L. B. Safier, *J. Lipid Res.* **10**, 108–114 (1969). 2198–2212 (1962).
13. Rouser, G., J. O'Brien, and D. Heller, *J. Amer. Oil Chem. Soc.* **38**, 14–19 (1961).
14. Hirsch, J., and E. H. Ahrens, Jr., *J. Biol. Chem.* **233**, 311–320 (1958).
15. Skipski, V. P., R. F. Peterson, and M. Barclay, *Biochem. J.* **90**, 374–378 (1964).
16. Skipski, V. P., M. Barclay, R. K. Barclay, V. A. Fetzer, J. J. Good, and F. M. Archibald, *Biochem. J.* **104**, 340–352 (1967).
17. Parker, F., and N. F. Peterson, *J. Lipid Res.* **6**, 455–460 (1965).
18. Marinetti, G. V., *J. Lipid Res.* **6**, 315–317 (1965).
19. Letters, R., *Biochem. J.* **93**, 313–316 (1964).
20. Skipski, V. P., A. F. Smolowe, R. C. Sullivan, and M. Barclay, *Biochim. Biophys.*
21. Schlierf, G., and P. Wood, *J. Lipid Res.* **6**, 317–322 (1965). *Acta* **106**, 386–396 (1965).
22. Morrison, W. R., and L. M. Smith, *J. Lipid Res.* **5**, 600–608 (1964).
23. Dodge, J. T., and G. B. Phillips, *J. Lipid Res.* **8**, 667–675 (1967).
24. Mangold, H. K., *Thin-Layer Chromatography: A Laboratory Handbook,* E. Stahl, Ed., Academic Press, New York, 1965, pp. 137–186.
25. Marcus, A. J., D. Zucker-Franklin, L. B. Safier, and H. L. Ullman, *J. Clin. Invest.* **45**, 14–28 (1966).
26. Day, H. J., H. Holmsen, and T. Hovig, *Scand. J. Haematol.* Suppl. 7, 3–35 (1969).
27. Holmsen, H., H. J. Day, and H. Stormorken, *Scand. J. Haematol.* Suppl. 8, 3–26 (1969).
28. Bradlow, B. A., and A. J. Marcus, *Proc. Soc. Exp. Biol. Med.* **123**, 889–893 (1966).
29. Hess, H. H., and E. Lewin, *J. Neurochem.* **12**, 205–211 (1965).
30. Lees, M. B., *J. Neurochem.* **13**, 1407–1420 (1966).

31. Zak, B., R. C. Dickenman, E. G. White, H. Burnett, and P. J. Cherney, *Amer. J. Clin. Pathol.* **24**, 1307–1315 (1954).
32. Abell, L. L., B. B. Levy, B. B. Brodie, and F. E. Kendall, *J. Biol. Chem.* **195**, 357–366 (1952).
33. Horowitz, H. I., and M. F. Papayoanou, *J. Lab. Clin. Med.* **69**, 1003–1012 (1967).
34. Nemerson, Y., *J. Clin. Invest.* **47**, 72–80 (1968).
35. Hennes, A. R., K. Awai, K. Hammarstrand, and G. Duboff, *Nature* **210**, 839–841 (1966).
36. Majerus, P. W., M. B. Smith, and G. H. Clamon, *J. Clin. Invest.* **48**, 156–164 (1969).
37. Cohen, P., A. Derksen, and H. van den Bosch, *J. Clin. Invest.* **49**, 128–139 (1970).
38. Cohen, P., and B. Wittels, *J. Clin. Invest.* **49**, 119–127 (1970).

10. Protein Components and Their Role in the Structure of Red-Cell Membranes

VIRGIE G. SHORE and BERNARD SHORE

Bio-Medical Division, Ernest O. Lawrence Livermore Laboratory, Livermore, California

I. INTRODUCTION

Erythrocyte-membrane structure is the object of numerous investigations by a wide variety of physical and chemical methods. It appears that information gained from many disciplines will be necessary to understand the organization and molecular interactions in a biological structure as complex as the cell membrane. Such studies have been applied to whole membranes, either intact or modified (e.g., treated with heat, chemicals, or enzymes), to macromolecular fragments of membranes or lipoprotein complexes, and to the individual lipids, proteins, and glycoproteins isolated from the membranes.

Electron microscopy is still a major physical method for the study of membrane ultrastructure, but it alone, at least at the present state of development, cannot reveal membrane structure on the molecular level. The physical techniques of optical rotatory dispersion, circular dichroism, infrared spectroscopy, nuclear magnetic resonance, X-ray diffraction, and differential-scanning calorimetry are being applied to the problem of protein and lipid conformation in membranes. Information from these physical studies must be supplemented by studies on the isolated lipids, proteins, and glycoproteins. Knowledge of the lipid moiety of membranes has increased tremendously in recent years, as demonstrated by Nelson's review in Chapter 7. The structures of the individual proteins and of their protein–protein and protein–lipid interactions are necessary information for the elucidation of membrane structure. Not all of the proteins have yet been isolated, and no sequence work has yet been undertaken. Ultimately we would like to know the primary, secondary, and tertiary structures of the membrane polypeptides and their roles in membrane structure and function.

II. ERYTHROCYTE-MEMBRANE PROTEINS

The erythrocyte membrane contains a number of different proteins and glycoproteins, which account for about 55% of its mass. The number is not yet known, but it includes many enzymes that are minor components of the membrane protein as well as the major polypeptides, which are determinants of the architecture of the membrane as well as its physical and chemical properties, permeability, and functions. Several different experimental procedures have yielded soluble membrane protein and lipoprotein preparations. Fractions differing in amino acid and carbohydrate composition have been obtained from membranes, but it has not been conclusively demonstrated that any of the isolated fractions contain only one kind of polypeptide; many of them are clearly heterogeneous. It is difficult to dissociate the proteins into monomolecular species and to prevent intermolecular associations even in soluble membrane preparations. There is considerable evidence that much of the protein is relatively small in molecular weight, however.

The membrane proteins can be regarded, in part at least, as the apoproteins of an insoluble lipoprotein complex. Their amino acid compositions provide few clues to the properties that account for their characteristic aggregation and for the formation of an insoluble membrane. Unfractionated erythrocyte-membrane protein, though different, is not strikingly different in composition from the apoproteins of the soluble lipoproteins of human plasma (1–3). It contains a slightly higher proportion (39%) of hydrophobic residues than the plasma-lipoprotein proteins (34–37%). Membrane protein contains very little cystine; it has more cysteine and less lysine than the plasma lipoproteins; plasma high-density lipoproteins contain much less isoleucine than the membrane and low-density lipoproteins. Although plasma-lipoprotein proteins are not unusual in amino acid composition (1), they are made up of polypeptides that differ strikingly in composition and in secondary structure (4) (see also Chapter 15). Undoubtedly the membrane protein, like those of the various soluble lipoproteins, is a complement of unique polypeptides differing in amino acid composition and sequence, conformation, and capacity for interaction with lipids and other membrane components.

A. Heterogeneity of Membrane Proteins in Polyacrylamide Gel Electrophoresis

The erythrocyte-membrane protein may contain 15 to 20 different proteins, or even more, according to polyacrylamide gel electrophoresis patterns of membranes or the membrane proteins (5–11). Zahler and co-workers (5) observed that the soluble erythrocyte-membrane protein prepared with 2-chloroethanol gave 20 bands, of which five were major components in disc electrophoresis in polyacrylamide gels in acid urea. The molecular weights of most of the proteins in 90% 2-chloroethanol were estimated from sedimentation velocity experiments to be less than 20,000 (6). Demus and Mehl (7) resolved the membrane protein solubilized by phenol/formic-acid/water into 14 to 16 protein bands by electrophoresis in a 3.5 to 14% polyacrylamide gel gradient with phenol/formic-acid/water (14 : 3 : 3, w : v : v) as solvent. From the electrophoretograms, they estimated that over 90% of the protein had molecular weights in the range 26,000 to 65,000.

Polyacrylamide gel electrophoresis in the presence of sodium dodecyl sulfate also gives many bands (8, 9, 10, 11). Fairbanks and co-workers (8) found six major proteins that were estimated to range in molecular weight from 36,200 to 250,000, with much of the protein having molecular weights of 89,000 and 250,000. Similarly, Lenard (9) estimated that about two-thirds of the protein was contained in four bands, two of about 240,000 and 255,000 molecular weight and two of about 86,000 and 108,000 molecular weight. By similar means, under somewhat different conditions, Laico and co-workers (10) observed that more than half of the erythrocyte-membrane protein is made up of polypeptides and/or glycopeptides of molecular weight ~5000. Membranes were dissolved with 2.5% (w/v) sodium dodecyl sulfate—2.5% (v/v) β-mercaptoethanol and dialyzed against buffer of lower detergent and mercaptoethanol concentration. Polyacrylamide gel electrophoresis and gel filtration were carried out in the presence of sodium dodecyl sulfate.

B. Proteins Solubilized at Low Ionic Strength

Much of the protein in erythrocyte membranes can be dissociated in lipid-free, water-soluble form by gentle means. Low-ionic-strength and hypertonic saline solutions wash large amounts of protein off the membrane. Marchesi and co-workers (12) removed about 25% of the protein free of carbohydrate and lipid by dialysis of guinea pig erythrocyte membranes against 0.001 *M* ethylenediaminetetraacetic acid (EDTA), 0.005 *M* mercaptoethanol at pH 7.5 for 48 hr in the cold. The protein appeared to contain one major protein called spectrin, which was found in human, horse, sheep, rabbit, and rat red cells (12–15). After gel filtration on a Sephadex G200 column, the protein gave one major band, near the top of the separating gel, in disc electrophoresis at pH 8.4 in 5% polyacrylamide gels containing 8 *M* urea (12). By a similar dialysis procedure, Rosenberg and Guidotti (16) removed about 11% of the total membrane protein of human red cells. Without further purification, the amino acid composition was very similar to that of spectrin.

Using the EDTA procedure of Marchesi et al., Maddy and Kelly (17) extracted 30% of the total membrane protein from human, ox, and sheep cells. Their protein preparations gave numerous bands, including three or four major ones, on polyacrylamide gel electrophoresis in 0.26 *M* acetic acid. Under the electrophoresis conditions of Marchesi et al. (12), Maddy and Kelly found four major bands in the EDTA extract before and after gel filtration on a Sephadex G200 column. Dilute acetic acid also released 30 to 40% of the membrane protein, free of phospholipid and sialic acid, that resembled the EDTA-extracted protein in polyacrylamide gel electrophoresis, except that the former contained relatively more of the faster-moving components (17). Sedimentation velocity experiments on the acetic acid–extracted proteins showed heterogeneity and low sedimentation coefficients (~2S) in 0.26 *M* acetic acid and aggregation on addition of KC1 (0.01 or 0.1 *M*). Marchesi et al. (12) observed S_{20} values of 13 and 7 at pHs 7.5 and 9.5, respectively, for spectrin, which gave a single boundary. Trayer and co-workers (18) found that prolonged exposure to the EDTA-mercaptoethanol solvent of Marchesi et al. (12) dissolves over 90% of the protein of human membranes. The protein solubilized by EDTA during dialysis for 1 to 2 days at 4° was heterogeneous in molecular size according to their data from gel filtration on 4% agarose in 6 *M* guanidine hydrochloride. Trayer et al. believed that each agarose fraction represented a discrete polypeptide, but confirmatory chemical evidence was not presented. Guanidine hydrochloride (6 *M*) in the presence of 20 m*M* dithiothreitol did not completely dissociate erythrocyte-membrane proteins in the experiments of Maddy and Kelly (19).

In our previously unpublished experiments, about 20 to 25% of the protein of sheep-erythrocyte membranes was removed by washing with distilled water over a short period of time (<2 hr). The water wash was free of lipid and contained a number of minor proteins and two major ones that differed in amino acid composition, in circular dichroic spectrum, and in electrophoretic mobility at pH 8.5 in 7.5% polyacrylamide gels containing 8 *M* urea. One of the major proteins resembled spectrin in composition and mobility, and the other had a much faster mobility in gel electrophoresis.

The amino acid compositions of whole membranes, the water-soluble proteins dissociated from membranes, and carbohydrate-rich proteins are presented in Table I. Tillack and co-workers (14) noted that spectrins from human, sheep, horse, and guinea-pig erythrocytes are quite similar. The sheep-erythrocyte fraction (Table I, water-extracted protein 1) that was obtained by us and appears to correspond to spectrun is more similar to guinea-pig spectrin (Table I) than to the sheep spectrin of Tillack et al.

The second major component in the water wash of sheep erythrocytes (Table I, protein 2) differs considerably from spectrin in the content of glutamic acid, proline, glycine, and valine but is very similar to spectrin in the content of the other amino acids. The two major water-soluble proteins (1 and 2 of Table I) differ considerably in conformation and electrophoretic mobility. There were no differences between sheep–high-potassium and low-potassium erythrocytes in compositions of the two major water-soluble proteins.

One of the major water-soluble proteins (Table I, protein 1) is largely α-helical in structure (V. G. Shore and B. Shore, unpublished observation). In water solution it has a circular-dichroism spectrum, with minima at 208 and 222 nm, that is typically seen with α-helical structures. The molar ellipticity values at these wavelengths, when compared with those for polyglutamic acid (23), indicate about 70% α-helical structure in spectrin. The optical-rotatory-dispersion spectrum of the protein is consistent with this estimate. The conformation is helical to a much greater extent than the average for the protein in intact membranes (about 40% helical) or in

Table I. Amino Acid Composition of Erythrocyte-Membrane Proteins

	Quantity (moles per 1000 moles amino acids)							
	Glycoproteins			Water-Soluble Proteins				
Amino Acid	A[a]	B[b]	C[c]	Sp[d]	1[e]	2[e]	3[f]	UP[g]
Lysine	56	35	62	68	62	61	60	52
Histidine	32	38	40	25	24	24	27	27
Arginine	44	41	49	58	59	45	42	48
Aspartic acid	144	60	70	104	108	97	95	84
Threonine	63	138	101	41	37	55	64	58
Serine		136	122	56	59	66	77	65
Glutamic acid	141	100	123	185	188	126	118	130
Proline		65	66	29	23	49	61	55
Glycine	65	68	50	45	43	73	81	61
Alanine	96	68	52	82	82	83	81	76
Cystine (½ residue)			2	12	12	19	11	12
Valine	63	77	80	50	50	76	71	64
Methionine	41		13	22	24	19	13	22
Isoleucine	44	45	73	41	42	39	37	40
Leucine	97	45	63	112	108	97	93	121
Tyrosine	17	36	26	24	24	27	28	25
Phenylalanine	32	35	9	32	31	39	35	41
Tryptophan					31	10		18
Percentage of α-helix					72	35		40

[a] Extracted from human-erythrocyte membranes into ether–ethanol solvent (16).
[b] Isolated from human-erythrocyte membranes by Winzler (20).
[c] Isolated from human-erythrocyte membranes by Zvilichovsky et al. (21).
[d] Spectrin extracted by dialysis of guinea-pig-erythrocyte membranes against 0.001 *M* EDTA, pH 7.5, and 0.005 *M* mercaptoethanol; purified by gel fitration (12).
[e] Extracted from sheep-erythrocyte membranes by water and fractionated on diethylaminoethyl cellulose (V. G. Shore and B. Shore, unpublished data).
[f] The pH 4.5-soluble protein prepared from human-erythrocyte membranes by Hamaguchi and Cleve (22).
[g] Unfractionated sheep-erythrocyte membrane protein (V. G. Shore and B. Shore, unpublished data).

the membrane residue after extraction with water. The other major water-soluble membrane protein (Table I, protein 2) from sheep red cells is estimated from its optical-rotatory-dispersion and circular-dichroism spectra to be about 35% α-helical in structure.

Both water-soluble membrane proteins (Table I, proteins 1 and 2) readily aggregate to give high-molecular-weight polymers especially in the presence of salts. Marchesi and co-workers (12, 15) reported that the guinea-pig spectrin monomer has a molecular weight of 100,000 to 140,000.

They observed that molecular weight was a function of rotor speed in their sedimentation-equilibrium experiments. Urea, guanidine hydrochloride, and sodium dodecyl sulfate did not dissociate spectrin into smaller units. Spectrin in 6 *M* guanidine hydrochloride, 5 m*M* dithiothreitol had a molecular weight of 100,000 to 150,000 and a sedimentation coefficient of 1.9S. However, these solvents do not always dissociate soluble proteins to monomeric form. The molecular species of serum high-density-lipoprotein protein in sodium dodecyl sulfate is a dimer, and one of its purified polypeptides, which has no sulfhydryl or disulfide groups, is not dissociated completely in concentrated urea or guanidine hydrochloride solutions (24). In 0.1 *M* sodium chloride the molecular weight of spectrin was more than 10^6 (14). In our sedimentation experiment (V. G. and B. Shore, unpublished) the water-soluble proteins from sheep-erythrocyte membranes appeared to contain small subunits whose molecular weight is less than 20,000. During centrifugation the low-molecular-weight species and polymers of higher molecular weight underwent an association–dissociation reaction that depended on rotor speed. In some instances almost all of the protein that had been found to be small in molecular size appeared to have a molecular weight of 110,000 to 130,000.

A strong similarity between actin and spectrin in their intermolecular interactions to give fibrils in the presence of potassium and magnesium chlorides was noted by Steers and Marchesi (13). Their electron micrographs of spectrin resemble those of actin and show coiled filaments 50 to 60 Å in diameter.

Another soluble, lipid-free protein preparation, possibly different from the water-soluble proteins listed in Table I, was prepared by earlier investigators from human-erythrocyte membranes. It is insoluble in water at pH 6.5, unlike spectrin, and is soluble in salt solutions. It was called S-protein by its discoverers, Moskowitz and co-workers (25, 26), who obtained it from membranes during the preparation of the lipoprotein elinin. A flocculent precipitate of S-protein, obtained by lowering the pH to 6.5, dissolved at pH 7.3 or higher and was soluble in 0.15 *M* sodium chloride at pH 6.5. Unfortunately information on the composition and structure of the S-protein is not available, and hence comparison with membrane-protein fractions prepared by other methods is difficult.

C. Proteins Solubilized by Hypertonic Salt Solutions

Hypertonic sodium chloride solutions dissociate lipid-free protein and lipoprotein in soluble form from erythrocyte membranes (27). Insufficient information is available for comparison of this salt-soluble protein, prepared by Mitchell and Hanahan, with the S-protein, but they may be the same. Mitchell and Hanahan (27) found that increasing amounts of soluble protein, lipid, and acetylcholinesterase were removed from human-erythrocyte membranes as the concentration of sodium chloride in the wash solution was increased up to 1.2 *M*. The solubilization was about the same over a pH range of 6.2 to 8.2, but tris buffer (0.005 *M*, pH 8.2) decreased the solubilization of the membrane components, and the maximum release occurred at a lower salt concentration (0.6 *M*). The lipid-free-protein component accounted for most of the salt-dissociated protein (20–30% of the membrane protein) and did not contain the acetylcholinesterase activity. Mitchell and Hanahan did not investigate the amino acid composition and structure of their lipid-free protein. However, the composition of a protein fraction of human-erythrocyte membranes obtained by a similar procedure has been reported by Rosenberg and Guidotti (16). The protein was extracted with 0.8 *M* sodium chloride from the membrane residue after extraction of the water-soluble protein by 0.001 *M* EDTA and 0.05 *M* β-mercaptoethanol. The fraction, about 40% of the total membrane protein, contained a small amount (1.5% by weight) of neutral sugars and little or no sialic acid. Its amino acid composition resembles, but is not identical with, that of the water-soluble protein(s) obtained by washing the membranes with a solution of EDTA and mercaptoethanol. The extent of heterogeneity and the size and conformation of the proteins in the salt-soluble protein fraction have not yet been reported.

Moore et al. (28) found that a proteinase together with other proteins and lipoproteins could be extracted by 1*M* sodium chloride or 1 *M* potassium thiocyanate from human stroma suspended in a Dounce tissue grinder. The enzyme was activated by potassium thiocyanate and was associated with one or more lipoprotein species. The enzyme hydrolyzed casein, hemoglobin, stroma proteins, and stroma. It corresponds to one of three erythrocyte proteinases described earlier by Morrison and Neurath (29).

D. Glycoproteins Solubilized by Organic-Solvent Mixtures

The membrane glycoproteins can be isolated by phenol-water (1 : 1) extraction of membranes followed by alcohol precipitation, gel filtration, and use of the Sevag procedure (20). Alternatively, they can be extracted into cold aqueous pyridine and remain in solution on dialysis against water. Further purification is carried out in two stages, both involving alcohol precipitation of other membrane proteins (21). Erythrocyte membrane contain about 8% carbohydrate (dry weight), much of which is covalently bound to protein (20). Almost all of the membrane sialic acid (2.1% by weight) is associated with a relatively small fraction, perhaps ~5%, of the membrane protein. The first method, that of Winzler and co-workers, yields a glycoprotein (or glycoproteins) containing 35.7% protein and 64.4% carbohydrate [galactose (13.2%), mannose (2.6%) fucose (1.2%), acetyl glucosamine (6.5%), acetyl galactosamine (13.2%), and *N*-acetyl neuraminic acid (27.8%)] (20). The carbohydrate is attached to the protein by O-glycosidic linkages between the anomeric carbon of acetyl-galactosamine and the hydroxyl groups of serine and threonine and by *N*-glycosidic linkage between the reducing group of acetyl glucosamine and the amide group of asparagine (20). The glycoprotein has a molecular weight of about 30,000 daltons (30, 31). It contains the *M* and *N* antigens and the myxovirus receptor site (30). Its amino acid composition is given in Table I.

The second isolation procedure, that of Zvilichovsky and co-workers (21), yields a glycoprotein preparation that is similar but not identical in composition (Table I) to that of Winzler et al. It contains two glycoproteins and glycolipid. The ratio of carbohydrate to protein was about 3 : 1, and the average molecular weight, by sedimentation equilibrium, was 22,000 (21).

Rosenberg and Guidotti (16) isolated from human-erythrocyte membranes a carbohydrate-rich protein fraction (Table I) that contained 7% of the membrane protein and about 0.6 g of neutral sugars and 0.1 g of sialic acid per gram of protein. Sialic acid was present in smaller amounts in four other protein fractions of a total of eight separated by Rosenberg and Guidotti. Together with the lipids, the carbohydrate-rich protein (fraction III) was extracted from the membrane residue by ethanol–ether (3 : 1) and ether after removal of fraction I by the method of Marchesi and co-workers (12) and fraction II by the method of Mitchell and Hanahan (27). Fractions IV through VIII were obtained by gel filtration of the solvent-extracted residue in a 3% sodium dodecyl sulfate solution. Fraction II contained 41% of the total membrane protein, each of the other fractions containing 5 to 13%.

All eight fractions differed in amino acid composition; Rosenberg and Guidotti (16) estimate that at least 12 different proteins are present in significant amounts. Some of the fractions were shown to be heterogeneous, and none was rigorously established to be homogeneous. The compositional differences among the eight fractions are significant. Fractions IV, V, and VI had a higher content of hydrophobic residues (about 47–50%) than the other fractions.

E. Solubilization of Protein-Lipid Complexes

Other soluble membrane fractions containing protein in association with considerable amounts of lipids have been derived from erythrocyte membranes by a variety of procedures. Study of such fractions may lead to elucidation of possible lipoprotein substructures and lipid–protein or lipid–glycoprotein interactions in the membrane as well as to the characterization of their protein moieties. Studies of the lipoprotein structures of membranes are more complicated than those of the lipid-free proteins because dissociation of some components, either protein or lipid, can occur during isolation; rearrangement of membrane components to give artifactual lipid–protein complexes is also possible. The fact that some proteins are easily dissociated from membranes in lipid-free form does not necessarily mean that they were derived from lipid-poor regions of the membrane. For example, the major polypeptide apo-HDL-Thr of plasma high-density lipoproteins is readily dissociated in lipid-free form from the lipoprotein (Chapter 15).

About twenty years ago Moskowitz, Calvin, and co-workers (25, 26, 32) prepared the lipoprotein elinin from the membrane residue remaining after ether extraction of the dry stroma of human erythrocytes. Elinin was isolated from a solution of the residue in water at pH 9 by alternate precipitation with 0.15 *M* sodium chloride and solution in water at pH 9. The protein is undoubtedly heterogeneous. It is a complex of lipids, carbohydrates, and proteins, and about 25% of it is material that is extractable with alcohol–ether. Electron micrographs show rods that are about 125 Å wide and vary in length from about 2500 to 10,000 Å (32). Moskowitz and Calvin (26) suggested that these long fibrils are parallel to the surface of the cell and are joined side by side by the ether-extractable lipids.

Mitchell and Hanahan (27) found that as much as half the lipids with about 20 to 30% of the protein was washed off erythrocyte membranes by hypertonic saline solution. Only a small fraction of the protein appears to be associated with the extracted lipids, since most of it sedimented in sodium bromide solution of 1.21-g/ml density. Acetylcholinesterase, up to 70% of which was extracted by hypertonic sodium chloride, floated with the lipids or lipoproteins during centrifugation. There was no selection in the kinds of phospholipids extracted by hypertonic saline, but the phospholipid-to-cholesterol ratio was higher in membranes than it was in the extract. The nature of the protein associated with the lipids in the salt extract was not investigated, so it is not known how many proteins besides acetylcholinesterase are present or whether any of them are present also in the lipid-free protein.

Ultrasonic irradiation was used by Morgan and Hanahan (33) to prepare a soluble lipid–protein complex from human-erythrocyte membranes. Sonication of the stroma, which had been frozen and thawed, at 4°C for 30 min in a 10% 1-butanol solution gave a suspension of membrane lipid and protein in addition to a small amount of insoluble material. The soluble material was separated by preparative centrifugation at $d > 1.063$ g/ml into a protein-rich fraction and a lipoprotein consisting of 94% lipid and 6% protein. The lipid distribution of the lipoprotein was that of the erythrocyte membrane, but its protein moiety differed in amino acid composition from the other membrane proteins. This work indicates, as might be expected, that some of the membrane proteins have a greater affinity for lipids than others. Unfortunately there are no data for comparing the protein moiety of the lipoprotein of this investigation with that prepared by Mitchell and Hanahan (27) or with the membrane glycoprotein that was extracted together with the membrane lipids into ether and alcohol by Rosenberg and Guidotti (16). The latter protein may have been extracted as a lipid–protein complex, or the lipid-free glycoprotein may have been soluble in the organic solvent.

Soluble lipoprotein complexes have been obtained from membranes exposed to detergents and other solvents. Concentrated urea solutions and detergents like sodium dodecyl sulfate and Kyro EO (an alkylphenol–ethylene oxide polymer) almost completely dissolve the membranes (34). Urea or detergents (or both) may disrupt hydrophobic interactions and dissociate not only lipids from proteins but also protein aggregates. Partial to almost complete delipidation by detergents has been observed in lipoproteins by several investigators (35–37).

Bakerman and Wasemiller (34) used polyacrylamide-gel filtration to separate human-erythrocyte membranes that had been dissolved in 0.5% sodium dodecyl sulfate at pH 11 into two fractions, retarded or excluded on the basis of size by the gel. The components were lipoglycoproteins whose proportions of lipids, carbohydrates, and proteins were similar to those of the membranes. All six fractions (two from the original fractionation and four from rechromatography experiments) differed in amino acid composition. The fractions were heterogenous with respect to size. Weight-average molecular weights for the smaller components of 40,000 and 70,000 were obtained at the meniscus and bottom of the centrifuge cell, respectively, during the approach to sedimentation equilibrium. Since the material was 55% protein, the protein moiety had a molecular weight of about 22,000.

These experiments indicate that the membrane protein is heterogeneous and that a considerable portion of it is rather small in molecular weight. However, there is no indication that the protein in any of the fractions is homogeneous or that the extended exposure (2 days to 1 week) of the membrane to alkaline conditions did not cleave covalent bonds or cause a rearrangement of membrane components. Hence Bakerman and Wasemiller's conclusion that the different molecular-weight classes are different repeating units of erythrocyte structural membrane is perhaps premature.

F. Nonselective Solubilization of the Membrane

Other procedures convert a high percentage of membrane protein into water-soluble form. However, it seems that strong protein–protein interactions persisting after solubilization of the membrane protein may account for the apparent high molecular weights and for the difficulty in fractionating the protein by such means as gel filtration and ion-exchange chromatography on carboxymethyl or DEAE-cellulose columns.

Zahler and co-workers (6) have investigated the solubility of stroma and stroma proteins in a number of organic solvents and in dilute acids, base, tris, or salt and in urea and guanidine solutions. Erythrocyte stroma were very soluble in 2-chloroethanol at pH 2 to 3, in acetic acid, in methyl cellosolve at solvent concentrations between 90 and 100%, and in ethylene glycol monobutyl ether at 50 to 60% (v/v). Sedimentation velocity experiments indicated that 2-chloroethanol was very effective in dissociating the protein and that methyl cellosolve and acetic acid were somewhat less effective. The membrane proteins were completely soluble in acidified urea, in neutral 20% (v/v) methyl cellosolve, and in dilute acetic acid, suggesting to the authors that the lipid-free proteins are quite hydrophobic in nature. Chloroethanol dissociates lipids from the membrane proteins, but the protein, after dialysis, can recombine with lipids to give membranelike structures (38). The protein in 2-chlorethanol retains its secondary structure (39).

At least 90% of the protein of ox-erythrocyte membranes was solubilized by the extraction of lipids from an aqueous suspension of salt-free membranes with 1-butanol in the cold (40). The soluble protein of the aqueous phase contained 5% lipid and 8% carbohydrate. The protein is obtained as aggregates of high molecular weight. Electrophoresis of the protein in phosphate buffer (pH 7.0, $\mu = 0.1$) in a Tiselius apparatus showed one major component with a mobility of -9×10^{-5} cm^2/sec-V and three very minor components. Sedimentation-velocity experiments separated the protein into fractions of 5 and 10S, both of which were heterogeneous in size, and a small amount of larger particles. The molecular weight of the protein was estimated to be on the order of 300,000 daltons. The observations of Rega and co-workers (41) on the membrane protein of human erythrocytes were similar to those of Maddy (40).

A soluble protein preparation containing more than 80% of the membrane protein was prepared by Mazia and Ruby from ox erythrocytes with the aid of detergent and high pH (42). The cells, which had been washed with isotonic sucrose, were lysed by a water solution of the nonionic detergent Triton X 100 (0.1%) in the presence of a mixed-bed ion-exchange resin. As in the butanol-extraction procedure, salt must be excluded. A membrane pellet was obtained by centrifugating the lysate after removing the resin and adjusting the pH to 6.5. The soluble protein was obtained by dialyzing the suspended membranes (previously washed with ammonium acetate, 20 m*M*, pH 6.5) at pH 9.3 to 9.5. It was separated from insoluble membrane material by centrifugation at 100,000 *g* for 1 hr. Most of the membrane lipid was presumed to be in the insoluble sediment. The nitrogen-to-phosphorus ratio (mole/mole) was 55 for the soluble protein fraction and 15.5 for whole membranes. Salt at low concentrations caused aggregation of the water-soluble protein, and it is likely that the material was not completely dissociated in water. There is heterogeneity due to the presence of different proteins also. In addition to quickly-sedimenting material, major and minor components with sedimentation coefficients of about 3 and 5.5S, respectively, were observed in water. Mazia and Ruby (42) were of the opinion, based at the time on quite limited evidence, that a large proportion of all membrane proteins are of a type (which they called tektins) that resembles the proteins of microtubules and the actin of muscles. More recently Steers and Marchesi (13) have suggested that the membrane protein spectrin resembles actin.

Hamaguchi and Cleve (22) applied the Mazia and Ruby method with minor modifications to the dissolution of human erythrocyte membranes. The yield (~40%) of soluble protein was about half that from beef erythrocyte membranes (42), but the amino acid compositions and N/P ratios of the human and beef soluble protein preparations were similar. At least 15 protein bands were seen in sodium-dodecyl-sulfate polyacrylamide-gel electrophoresis patterns of the soluble protein. Small amounts of Ca^{2+}, Mg^{2+}, Na^{+} or K^{+} ions caused protein aggregation. Most of the protein precipitated between pH 3.9 and 5.4. The pH 4.5 soluble protein, about 8% of the proteins, gave one major and two minor bands in sodium-dodecyl-sulfate polyacrylamide-gel electrophoresis. Its composition is given in Table I.

III. PHYSICOCHEMICAL STUDIES OF ERYTHROCYTE MEMBRANES

Much valuable information on erythrocyte-membrane structure has come from studies by such physicochemical techniques as optical rotatory dispersion (ORD), circular dichroism (CD), infrared spectroscopy (IR), electron-paramagnetic-resonance (EPR) spectroscopy, proton-magnetic-resonance (PMR) spectroscopy, X-ray diffraction, and differential-scanning calorimetry. In considering the results obtained in such studies it is important to realize that these techniques essentially depend on overall averages in the membrane and may not be sensitive enough to demonstrate functionally important centers. These studies must be coupled with information on the chemical properties of the membrane if one is to understand its functional properties. Only part of the membrane may be important for a given function.

A. Conformation Studies by Optical Rotatory Dispersion and Circular Dichroism

Studies of the optical rotatory dispersion (ORD—the wavelength dependence of optical rotation) and the optical circular dichroism (CD—the differential absorption by a medium of right and left circularly polarized light) of membranes have afforded a sensitive measure of the secondary structure of their proteins and a nondestructive probe of the structure of intact and perturbed membranes. Both measurements have been useful in discriminating between helical and nonhelical structures and in estimating the helical content of partially helical structures.

In general the ORD and CD spectra of membranes resemble those of an α-helix, but they differ from it in several respects: decreased amplitude of molar ellipticity and molar rotation, distortions in the relative intensity of the 208-nm $\pi \rightarrow \pi^*$ electronic transition, and a "red-shift" of the Cotton effect toward longer wavelengths. With respect to the latter phenomenon, a trough at 233 nm and a peak at 198 to 199 nm are observed in the rotatory dispersion of polypeptides and proteins and are characteristic of the α-helix. In most membrane preparations, however, the trough appears at 235 to 237 nm, and the peak is at 200 to 204 nm rather than at 198 to 199 nm; in addition the crossover of the spectrum from negative to positive rotation is also "red-shifted" to a longer wavelength (39, 43–46).

Several explanations have been advanced for the red shift. First, it has been suggested that it reflects protein association and aggregation phenomena, with the possible alignment of adjacent interacting α-helices (39, 43, 45). This explanation finds support in the observations of Cassim and Yang (47), who found that the entire Cotton effect and the CD bands of the helical polymer poly-α-glutamic acid shift about 1 nm toward longer wavelengths when the pH is lowered from 4.5 to 3.8. Light-scattering and hydrodynamic measurements indicate that the polymer aggregates as the pH is lowered below 4.5.

Interaction between the membrane proteins and lipids also has been suggested as an explanation for the red shift (45, 46). If a significant portion of the helical parts of the membrane proteins and their associated side-chain chromophores is located in regions of high refractive index, such as those observed in lipid bilayer membranes (48), a red shift in the spectrum could follow, analogous to that observed when aromatic chromophores are transferred to media of high polarizability, the interior of detergent micelles (49). The red shift is absent in the presence of 2-chloroethanol or sodium lauryl sulfate, media that affect protein–protein and protein–lipid interactions and the particulate nature of the membrane system. For example, in a typical experiment, λ_{min} and λ_{max} of the ORD spectrum of human-erythrocyte membranes in pH 7.7, 0.008 *M* phosphate were 235 to 235.5 and 201 to 202 nm, respectively, and the crossover wavelength λ_{co} was 226 to 227 nm. In membranes in 100% 2-chloroethanol, the values of λ_{min} and λ_{co} were 233 to 234 and 224 to 225 nm; in membranes in 0.05 *M* sodium dodecyl sulfate λ_{min}, λ_{co}, and λ_{max} were reduced to 233, 220 to 221, and 197 to 198 nm, respectively. There was a similar reduction in λ_{min} of the CD spectra: the two λ_{min} of 224 and 210 nm of membranes in the phosphate buffer were reduced to 221 and 207 nm in 0.05 *M* sodium lauryl sulfate and to 222 and 209 nm in 2-chloroethanol (39). In these studies Lenard and Singer concluded that the spectra of the membranes showed features indicating that about one-quarter to one-third of the membrane protein is α-helical, with the remainder of the membrane protein very probably being in the random-coil form.

Finally, it was proposed recently by Urry and Ji (50, 51) and confirmed and extended by Schneider et al. (52) and by Cauldwell and Schumaker (53) that the red shift and distortions in the membrane CD spectrum have two sources. The first of these is the flattening of the absorption spectra of suspensions in comparison with the spectra of solutions. As Duysens has shown (54), the absorption spectrum of a suspension of strongly absorbing particles, such as red-cell ghosts, even if corrected for light scattering, will appear flattened in comparison with the spectrum of a solution containing a homogeneous dispersion of the same molecules. This flattening is independent of concentration and is derived from the shadow of an opaque object (membrane in this case). The second source of the distortion of the CD pattern of membrane systems is the high degree of light scattering that is concentration dependent and results from the large size of the membrane particles. Urry and Ji have shown that both of these distortions come from wavelength-dependent changes in effective absorbing units and are dependent on particle size.

Schneider and co-workers (52) carried out three kinds of comparison between scattering and nonscattering systems (in using the term "scattering" they are referring to effects due to both scattering and absorption flattening). The results of these experiments were consistent with the hypothesis that the characteristic red-shifted and distorted spectrum represents superposition of the spectrum of a normal α-helical protein on optical artifacts due to scattering and flattening. Schneider and co-workers also analyzed the CD spectra of sonicated ghosts by the method of Greenfield and Fasman (55), using their data on polylysine as a reference. Their estimate of the average secondary structure of the membrane protein was that it was about 50% α-helix, 45% random coil, and 0 to 10% β, or pleated sheet.

In another study rabbit-erythrocyte ghosts were dispersed by intense shearing forces into a collection of randomly sized, disk-shaped fragments, 100 to 700 Å in diameter and with an average molecular weight on the order of 3×10^6 (53). These membrane fragments were completely soluble in dilute or concentrated salt solutions and behaved like a polydisperse collection of macromolecules in sedimentation, diffusion, viscometry, light-scattering, and CD studies. There were no significant changes in the quantities of protein, phospholipid, and cholesterol contained in ghosts that had been sheared and clarified. The CD experiments were performed on ghost fragments in dilute phosphate buffer in turbidity-free solutions, so that light-scattering corrections were not required. Under these conditions the material appeared to be about one-third α-helical, with no apparent evidence of β (pleated-sheet) structure.

To sum up the ORD and CD studies, it seems reasonable to conclude that one should not deduce from them that the membrane proteins strongly interact and aggregate with themselves and with other membrane proteins or that they are in hydrophobic interaction with the lipids of the membrane. Each of these kinds of interaction may in fact be occurring in erythrocyte membranes, but optical-activity measurements do not provide unequivocal evidence of this. It does seem likely, however, that the average secondary structure of the membrane protein is about one-third to one-half α-helix, with from none to one-tenth of the protein being in the β-conformation and the remainder in the random-coil form.

B. Conformation Studies by Infrared Spectroscopy

The technique of infrared spectroscopy complements that of optical rotatory dispersion and circular dichroism since it distinguishes between the α-helix and the β-conformation. Its usefulness in elucidating protein configuration arises from the observation that in the infrared spectra of peptides the portions of certain bands, the amide I and amide II bands, differ, depending on the conformation of the peptide chains. Thus the amide I band, which arises primarily from carbonyl stretching, occurs at about 1652 cm^{-1} for the α-helix and random-coil forms and at about 1628 cm^{-1} for the β-form in water. The amide II band at about 1535 cm^{-1} does not allow one to distinguish between the α-helix and the β-conformation.

Maddy and Malcolm (56, 57) have studied the infrared spectra of dried films of ox-erythrocyte ghosts; they found that the amide I band was symmetrical at about 1648 cm^{-1}, with no evidence of a strong band or shoulder in the 1630-cm^{-1} region. Their observations were confirmed by Chapman, Kamat, and Levene (58), who reported the amide I band to be at about 1652 cm^{-1}. These studies suggest that there is no extensive β-conformation in the protein structure; if it is present, it occurs in amounts that the infrared method cannot detect. The absence of β-conformation indications in the infrared spectra confirms the conclusion drawn from the ORD and CD spectra. Thus it is likely that the Cotton effects observed in optical-activity studies of membranes reflect the α-helical content of their proteins and that the average secondary structure of the protein can best be described as a mixture of the α-helical and random-coil conformations.

Studies of polypeptides isolated from membranes indicate that membrane protein is a complement of polypeptides varying widely in the proportions of helical structure and of hydrophilic residues. It is reasonable to expect that the hydrophilic polypeptides will be localized at the membrane surfaces in contact with an aqueous medium and that the unfolded and hydrophobic regions of proteins will be turned inward or in association with lipids. As Kauzmann (59) pointed out, the stable conformations of a protein in aqueous solution will be those in which nonpolar groups can come into contact with each other and are thus partially or completely removed from water. Because of these considerations, particularly the data on the helical content of membrane proteins, it also would seem that some modification is necessary for the models of membrane structure that are based on a bimolecular layer of lipids sandwiched between two layers of unfolded polypeptides (60).

C. Interactions between Lipids and Proteins in Membranes

Valuable information concerning the nature of the interactions between the proteins and the lipids has come from a number of recent studies, particularly those of Glaser et al. (61), Steim et al. (62), Metcalfe et al. (63, 64), and Engelman (65). The Glaser group has used chemical analyses and a coordinated CD and PMR study to investigate the effects of temperature and of purified phospholipase C on human-erythrocyte membranes. Steim and co-workers studied membrane structure by differential-scanning calorimetry. X-ray diffraction patterns at temperatures above and below the thermal phase transition of *Mycoplasma laidlawii* membrane lipids were investigated by Engelman and by Metcalfe and co-workers. Metcalfe et al. also used a fluorescent probe and nuclear magnetic relaxation measurements in a study of structural comparisons of native and reaggregated membranes from *Mycoplasma laidlawii* and erythrocytes.

1. Circular Dichroism and Nuclear Magnetic Resonance of Phospholipase- and Heat-Treated Membranes. Phospholipase C from *B. cereus* hydrolyzed the membrane phospholipids to diglycerides and water-soluble phosphorylated amines (61). No protease or nucleotidase activities were found in the purified enzyme, which was immunologically homogeneous. The cholesterol and diglycerides remained in the membrane after it had been exposed to the enzyme, but about 60% of the total phosphorus of the membranes was released. The phospholipids of intact erythrocytes are hydrolyzed by phospholipase C to the same extent (about 65–70%) as those of membranes (66). Phospholipase C causes hemolysis, but Bowman and co-workers (66) observed that lysis occurred only after extensive loss of membrane phosphorus. Lysis was preceded by a loss of lipid phosphorus, decreased cell volume, sphering, and increased susceptibility to osmotic shock. Bowman and co-workers suggested that the lesion in the red cell produced by phospholipase C is not instantly destructive, but alters membrane function so that the cell is destined to lysis (66).

The extensive hydrolysis of the membrane phospholipids by phospholipase did not detectably change the CD spectrum of the membrane (61), which reflects the average conformation of the proteins in the membrane. The ease of hydrolysis of the phospholipids suggested to Glaser and co-workers that in some positions in the membrane the phospholipids are probably in contact with the surrounding aqueous medium and that at these positions the polar groups are not bound to the protein. These results also suggested that electrostatic interactions between phospholipids and proteins play a secondary role, presumably to hydrophobic interactions, in determining the conformation of membrane proteins. The secondary structures of the proteins are probably determined by their compositions and sequences with perturbing and/or stabilizing effects by the local environment.

On the other hand, the PMR spectra, which measure essentially molecular motion and the relative immobility of protons in the membrane, indicated that the physical state of the fatty acid chains of the phospholipids had been changed by phospholipase C digestion. In the spectra of untreated, intact membranes, at room temperature, the line broadening was so pronounced that very little spectral detail was observed. However, after the phosphorylated amines had been released by the enzyme, there was a comparatively sharp resonance that accounted for about 75% of the methylene protons present in the fatty acid chains of the membrane phospholipids. These data indicate that after the enzyme treatment about three-quarters of the fatty acid chains became much more mobile than they were in the unmodified membrane.

When the intact, untreated membranes were examined at 82°C by PMR spectroscopy, there was no indication of the methylene-proton peak from the fatty acid chains of the lipids. These results suggest that the protein portion of the membrane might be primarily responsible for the spectrum at 82°C. The CD data indicate that the random coil is the predominant conformation of the proteins at 82°C and that about one-fifth of the protein changed from the α-helical to the random-coil conformation in the temperature interval from room temperature to 82°C. Accordingly, using the chemical shifts of the protons from the different amino acid residues in the random-coil conformation, Glaser and associates (61) computed the spectrum to be expected for the membrane proteins in the region of the methylene and methyl protons. The computed spectrum was very similar to the observed one; the observed intensity of the methyl-proton peak corresponded to one- to two-fifths of the total methyl protons of the membrane proteins. From these experiments Glaser et al. (61) concluded that a substantial fraction of the membrane proteins can change their physical state with increasing temperature, but that under these circumstances the fatty acid chains of the phospholipids do not change their mobility.

The work of Glaser's group can be summarized in their own words as follows:

> In the experiments involving phospholipase C, the chemical structure and physical state of about three-fourths of the phospholipids were radically altered, with no detectable effect on the gross physical state of the protein; conversely, in the experiments with untreated membranes raised to high temperatures, the physical state of as much as two-fifths of the protein was altered, with no indication of a change in the state of the lipid fatty acid chains. It is therefore reasonable to conclude that a substantial fraction of the phospholipids and the proteins of the red cell membrane can change structure independently of one another [61].

2. Differential Scanning Calorimetry of Membranes. Another study that bears on the nature of interactions among the membrane constituents is an investigation by differential-scanning calorimetry of the membranes of *Mycoplasma laidlawii* (62). If the membrane lipids occur as bilayers, differential thermal analysis should detect a characteristic property of the smectic mesophase, the reversible thermotropic transition between gel and liquid-crystal phase, as observed in synthetic phospholipid bilayers in water (67). The transition temperature is lowered by unsaturated fatty acid residues in the phospholipids and by cholesterol (62, 67), which also decreases the heat absorbed at the transition (67). Thus *M. laidlawii* membranes, which contain no cholesterol and whose fatty acid composition is a function of the growth medium, were selected for study so that a phase change above the ice point could be detected. Both the membranes of *M. laidlawii* and its protein-free lipids dispersed in water underwent endothermic phase transitions at the same temperature. The transitions were reversible and persisted after membrane-protein denaturation and digestion by pronase. In the phase changes the hydrocarbon core of the bilayer "melts" from a crystalline to a liquidlike phase; that is, the association between hydrocarbon chains is disrupted. The melts are cooperative phenomena; hence any interaction in the membrane between phospholipid fatty acid residues and protein should perturb the transition. By assuming that the enthalpy change was the same for lipids in the membranes and lipids dispersed in water, it was estimated that approximately one-fourth of the membrane lipids do not participate in the phase transition. These lipids could be hydrophobically bonded to the protein; however, most of the lipid hydrocarbon chains appear to associate with each other, rather than with proteins, to give a lamellar bilayer.

3. X-Ray Diffraction Patterns of Membranes. Engelman's X-ray diffraction patterns, a sharp wide-angle diffraction at 4.15 Å and low-angle patterns at temperatures above and below the phase transition of the membrane lipids and their differences, are consistent with a bilayer as the predominant lipid structure in *M. laidlawii* membranes (65). Engelman also concluded that most of the protein is not located in uniform layers on either side of the bilayer regions, that protein-lipid interactions do not greatly constrain the spacing of the lipid head groups, and that protein cannot penetrate the head-group layers below the transition temperature without disruption of the packing. Membrane particles, such as those seen in electron micrographs or nonlipid structures, could penetrate the bilayer but not in the ordered hydrocarbon regions below the thermal phase transition. The diffracting regions were relatively large, ~400Å in extent, in comparison with the membrane thickness, indicating that the regions are in the plane of the membrane with the fatty acid hydrocarbon chains approximately perpendicular to the membrane. Membranes enriched in palmitic, oleic, or erucic acid were studied. All the low-angle diffraction patterns showed characteristics of the patterns predicted and observed for the lipid bilayers above and below the phase transition. Each of the membranes irrespective of predominant lipid, gave a sharp 4.15 Å diffraction line below the thermal transition. It was ascribed to a hexagonal array of parallel hydrocarbon chains with an axis-to-axis spacing of 4.80 Å. Above the transition temperatures the chains show less long-range order and are in a more fluid state like that of a liquid hydrocarbon. The phase transition regions [extending 20 to 25°C below the upper temperature limits of 44, 37, and —15°C, respectively, for palmitate- erucate- and oleate-enriched membranes (65)] are within or below physiological temperatures so that both the tightly packed and more fluid conformations of the lipids may occur in living cells.

4. Nuclear Magnetic Resonance and Electron Spin Resonance Studies. It remains to be seen whether the conclusions about the state of the lipids and proteins of *M. laidlawii* membranes, which contain no cholesterol, can be extrapolated to red-cell membranes, which contain cholesterol. Studies by PMR and paramagnetic organic free radical spectroscopic techniques indicate that the extrapolation can be made with at least some degree of assurance.

Thus Chapman and co-workers (68) have shown by PMR techniques that the spectral peaks normally associated with signals from the —CH_2— and —CH=CH— groups of lipid hydrocarbon chains are weakened in, or absent from, human-red-cell ghosts. However, the hydrocarbon protons show a narrow resonance line after dispersal of the total lipids from the ghosts in water by sonication. Thus the spectroscopic evidence suggests that the hydrocarbon chains of the lipids are relatively immobilized in the red-cell membrane. This immobilization could reflect the restriction of the motion of fatty acid chains within bilayers, or it could arise from hydrophobic association of the lipids with proteins.

Data obtained with paramagnetic organic free radicals (spin labels) support the concept that the hydrocarbon portions of membranes are relatively fluid and are not extensively restricted in motion by association with proteins. Electron-spin-resonance techniques are often valuable in providing information about the freedom of molecular motion, the local environment, and the anisotropic motion of the spin-labeled molecule. Hubbell and McConnell (69) have studied the anisotropy of the paramagnetic resonance of nitroxide spin labels in human-erythrocyte membranes oriented by hydrodynamic shear. Their resonance spectra indicated that the hydrophobic regions in erythrocyte membranes are very similar to a bilayer.

As Glaser et al. (61) have pointed out, several different kinds of experiment seem to have resulted in alterations in a similar fraction of lipids. Thus about 70% of the lipid phosphorus of red-cell membranes can be removed from the membrane by phospholipase C. About 75% of the methylene protons of the lipids are melted after phospholipase treatment of red-cell membranes. In addition, enthalpy of transition of the lipids in the membranes of *M. laidlawii* is approximately 75% of that observed for the isolated lipids. These data are consistent with the hypothesis that about one-quarter of the phospholipids in red-cell membranes differ in physical state from the remainder of the lipids, involved perhaps in a relatively strong interaction with the membrane proteins.

5. Physical Studies of Native and Reconstituted Membranes. Membranes that have been separated into lipid and protein components can reaggregate under favorable conditions to give structures resembling the native membranes (38, 63, 64, 70). The native and reconstituted membranes were indistinguishable in composition, density, and appearance in electron micrographs, but the data of Metcalfe and co-workers (63, 64) indicate that the membrane proteins are incorrectly reassembled. Membranes of erythrocytes and *Mycoplasma laidlawii* were studied. They used a fluorescent probe (1-anilinonaphthalene-8-sulfonate) and nuclear magnetic resonance techniques. Benzyl alcohol was used as a structure-perturbing agent, which allowed direct comparison of native and reaggregated membranes by the two methods of study. X-ray diffraction patterns indicated that in *M. laidlawii* the lipid bilayer was reformed but that the bilayer regions were less extensive than in the native membranes (63). The broad band at 10 Å attributed to protein was relatively less in intensity in the reaggregated structures. Erythrocyte membranes were not subjected to X-ray diffraction. It is very possible, of course, that the methods for dissolving the membranes produced some irreversible changes in the proteins that prevented correct reassembly. However, the probability of correct reassembly of a structure containing so many proteins may be quite low under the experimental conditions used.

With regard to the nature of the lipids and proteins in membranes, a recent hypothesis of Glaser et al. (61) is of interest. They propose that the ionic and random-coil parts of the proteins are outside the membrane and the helical portions are inside, that large portions of the lipids and proteins of membranes are segregated, that in the membrane possibly only 25 to 30% of the phospholipids interact with the membrane proteins, that the phospholipids and proteins of membranes can change structure independently of one another, and that there may be a mosaic pattern for the organization of the lipids and proteins in membranes. In this model "globular protein molecules, perhaps noncovalently bound to about one-quarter of the phospholipids, are interspersed in a matrix that consists of the remaining lipids in a form similar to that of a discontinuous bilayer" (61).

A mosaiclike membrane makes it possible for chemical and conformational changes to occur independently in the proteins and to the lipids. With regard to the latter possibility, it is of interest that physiological cations like Na^+, K^+, Mg^{2+}, and Ca^{2+} can increase the anisotropy of lipid-bilayer-model membranes to an extent depending on their charge (71). Possibly Ca^{2+} and Mg^{2+} ions function physiologically by diminishing the charge repulsion between the ionic heads of the membrane phospholipids so that the lipid bilayers contract to constrain the motion of the hydrocarbon chains.

D. Electron Microscopy of Membranes and Membrane Proteins

Erythrocytes and their membranes have been examined by transmission and scanning electron-microscopy techniques involving a variety of preparative methods. In spite of resolution limitations with biological specimens and artifacts due to fixation, electron micrographs have revealed considerable information on erythrocyte-membrane substructure. Micrographs of freeze-cleaved red cells and membranes and pictures from the scanning electron microscope reveal very interesting aspects of the red cells (72, 73). Freeze-cleaving (the sample is frozen and then fractured or cleaved to expose new surfaces toward the interior of the cell) avoids dehydration, chemical fixing, and embedding. The scanning electron microscope is limited in resolution to about 100 Å and requires a specimen that is fixed by physical or chemical means and coated with a conductive material, such as a film of metal. Despite these limitations it gives a remarkable three-dimensional impression and a large depth of field, and covers a large specimen area. Application of the scanning method to cells that have been etched by ion bombardment gives below-the-surface views of the cell.

The negatively stained erythrocyte membrane is a trilaminar structure about 80 Å thick. Electron micrographs of air-dried and chromium-shadowed red-cell membranes show a surface layer of randomly distributed plaques (30 Å thick and 100–500 Å in diameter) on a network of fibers (20 Å in diameter) oriented tangentially to the cell surface (74, 75). After incubation with trypsin in the presence of ATP and Mg^{2+}, followed by negative staining with 2% potassium phosphotungstate, the membranes appear to contain long bundles of helically coiled filaments, resembling actin, across their surfaces (76).

The scanning electron microscope work of Baker (73) shows the human red cell (fixed with glutaraldehyde and coated with 100 Å of gold) to be a biconcave disk with a smooth surface. The unwashed cell has a shaggy coat of material (possibly plasma protein) that can be removed by washing with isotonic saline solution. Removal of a superficial layer of membrane from whole cells by etching for a brief period reveals a layer of particles about 500 Å diameter on the outer cell surface. Membranes briefly etched also show the surface layer of particles. Longer etching removes most of the membrane and exposes a porous interior.

In the electron micrographs of Weinstein and co-workers (72), freeze-cleaved human erythrocytes or membranes from osmotic lysis show a rather flat, thin surface, 60 to 100 Å thick, partially covered on the outside with clusters of small spherical particles, 80 to 130 Å in diameter. In the freeze-cleaved membrane similar particles are seen also on the inner surface. The flat area of the membrane appears to be made up of tightly packed subunits of 60 to 90 Å in diameter. Micrographs of red cells frozen and cleaved immediately after collection show the inner flat surface between the particles to be partially covered by long fibrils, 40 to 60 Å in diameter, lying parallel to the surface (72). Freeze-cleavage is thought by Pinto da Silva and Branton (77) to split membranes, exposing faces from the inner hydrophobic region. As in the above work, the electron micrographs of Pinto da Silva et al. (77, 78) showed relatively smooth areas with embedded particles, possibly protein, of 85 Å diameter which seem to protrude through the membrane surface. The numbers of particles per square micron of inner membrane face were 2800 and 1400, respectively, for the densely and thinly populated faces (79).

Isolated membrane proteins have been shown to form cylinders (80) and fibrils (76), which are thought to occur as such in the intact membrane. Harris (80) found that a protein released by dialysis of human erythrocyte membranes against distilled water occurred as torus or hollow-cylinder structures. About 10 to 20% of protein was released by dialysis. Possibly the major component corresponds to water-soluble protein #2 of Table I, which is released more readily by water than spectrin. The hollow cylinder rather than the torus is thought to be associated with the intact membrane (80). The protein spectrin, which forms actinlike fibrils, is thought to be derived from the inner surface of the membrane, possibly from a fibrous network (12).

IV. CONCLUSIONS

Electron microscopy suggests that much of the membrane protein occurs as spherical and fibrillar particles of protein or lipoprotein. The protein particles are made up of relatively small polypeptides which aggregate to give much larger structures. A considerable variety of proteins is present in membranes, so that some particles may contain more than one kind of polypeptide, and several kinds of particles differing in protein are possible. Some of the spherical particles appear to penetrate through the hydrophobic interior of the membrane, while others are localized at the surfaces. The studies of Engelman (65) indicate that the surface protein is not a continuous coat. They also indicate that protein could penetrate the bilayer in regions above the thermal phase transition; the bilayer very probably is the predominant lipid arrangement. Other evidence on the membrane phospholipids suggests that much of their polar moiety is exposed at the outer surface. The exposed phospholipid regions appear to be in a rectilinear array within or upon the membrane (81). The results of several other studies are consistent with asymmetric distribution of proteins across the membrane and with some proteins spanning the thickness of the membrane. Bretscher (82) and Steck and co-workers (83) have suggested, on the basis of results of experiments involving proteolysis of the proteins in erythrocyte membranes, that one or more of the proteins do extend through the membrane. All the sialic acid and much of the carbohydrate moiety are localized on the outer surface of the membrane (20). Trypsin splits off several different glycopeptides that have been characterized with respect to size and composition (20, 84).

Thus the bilayer theory of membrane structure is perhaps compatible with the existence of protein and/or lipoprotein subunits in the membrane. These subunit particles would lie upon or below or be interspersed with regions of lipid bilayer. Since many biochemical and physiological processes are carried out upon or within the membrane, its structure probably is not fixed but undergoes reversible changes in the living cell. An example of such a change in membrane structure was reported by Sonenberg (85). He observed that a conformational change in membrane proteins appears to occur on interaction of erythrocyte membranes with growth hormone or a fragment produced by tryptic digestion of the hormone.

Most of the membrane proteins have not been isolated. However, studies toward this end indicate a number of proteins that differ in composition and conformation. The water-soluble protein spectrin is largely α-helical in structure, whereas others are probably largely in the random-coil form. Much of the protein appears to be made up of small polypeptide subunits that interact strongly to give larger structures. Each of the different substructural components seen in electron micrographs would be expected to contain one or more proteins unique to it, but the characterization of these substructures in terms of their polypeptides, lipids, and sugars, and their interactions is largely yet to be done.

V. ACKNOWLEDGMENTS

This work was performed under the auspices of the U.S. Atomic Energy Commission. We thank Dr. Valeska Evertsbusch for editorial assistance.

REFERENCES

1. Oncley, J. L., and N. R. Harvie, *Proc. Natl. Acad. Sci. U.S.* **64**, 1107–1118 (1969).
2. Nichols, A. V., *Adv. Biol. Med. Phys.* **11**, 109–158 (1967).
3. Hatch, F. T., and A. L. Bruce, *Nature* **218**, 1166–1168 (1968).
4. Shore, B., and V. Shore, in *Proceedings of the Second International Symposium on Atherosclerosis,* R. Jones, Ed., Springer-Verlag, Heidelberg, 1970, pp. 144–150.
5. Zahler, P., *Experientia (Basel)* **25**, 449–456 (1969).
6. Zahler, P. H., D. H. F. Wallach, and E. F. Lüscher, in *Protides of the Biological Fluids,* H. Peeters, Ed., Elsevier Publishing Co., Amsterdam, 1968, pp. 69–78.
7. Demus, H., and E. Mehl, *Biochim. Biophys. Acta* **203**, 291–297 (1970).

8. Fairbanks, G., T. L. Steck, and D. F. H. Wallach, *Biochemistry* **10**, 2606–2617 (1971).
9. Lenard, J., *Biochemistry* **9**, 1129–1132 (1970).
10. Laico, M. T., E. I. Ruoslahti, D. S. Papermaster, and W. J. Dreyer, *Proc. Natl. Acad. Sci. U.S.* **67**, 120–127 (1970).
11. Carraway, K. L., and D. Kobylka, *Biochim. Biophys. Acta* **219**, 238–241 (1970).
12. Marchesi, V. T., E. Steers, Jr., T. W. Tillack, and S. L. Marchesi, in *Red Cell Membrane Structure and Function*, G. A. Jamieson and T. J. Greenwalt, Eds., Lippincott, Philadelphia, 1969, pp. 117–130.
13. Steers, E., and V. T. Marchesi, *J. Gen. Physiol.* **54**, 65*s*–71*s* (1969).
14. Tillack, T. W., S. L. Marchesi, V. T. Marchesi, and E. Steers, Jr., *Biochim. Biophys. Acta* **200**, 125–131 (1970).
15. Marchesi, S. L., E. Steers, V. T. Marchesi, and T. W. Tillack, *Biochemistry* **9**, 50–57 (1970).
16. Rosenberg, S. A., and G. Guidotti, *J. Biol. Chem.* **244**, 5118–5124 (1969).
17. Maddy, A. H., and P. G. Kelly, *Biochim. Biophys. Acta* **241**, 290–301 (1971).
18. Trayer, H. R., Y. Nozaki, J. A. Reynolds, and C. Tanford, *J. Biol. Chem.* **246**, 4485–4488 (1971).
19. Maddy, A. H., and P. G. Kelly, *Biochim. Biophys. Acta* **241**, 114–116 (1971).
20. Winzler, R. J., in *Red Cell Membrane Structure and Function,* G. A. Jamieson and T. J. Greenwalt, Eds., Lippincott, Philadelphia, 1969, pp. 157–171.
21. Zvilichovsky, B., P. M. Gallop, and O. O. Blumenfeld, *Biochem. Biophys. Res. Commun.* **44**, 1234–1243 (1971).
22. Hamaguchi, H., and H. Cleve, *Biochim. Biophys. Acta* **233**, 320–333 (1971).
23. Timasheff, S. N., H. Susi, R. Townend, L. Stevens, M. J. Gorbunoff, and T. F. Kumoshinski, in *Conformation of Biopolymers*, G. N. Ramachandran, Ed., Vol. I, Academic Press, New York, 1967, pp. 173–196.
24. Shore, V., and B. Shore, *Biochemistry* **7**, 3396–3406 (1968).
25. Moskowitz, M., W. B. Dandliker, M. Calvin, and R. S. Evans, *J. Immunol.* **65**, 383–392 (1950).
26. Moskowitz, M., and M. Calvin, *Exp. Cell Res.* **3**, 33–46 (1952).
27. Mitchell, C. D., and D. J. Hanahan, *Biochemistry* **5**, 51–57 (1966).
28. Moore, G. L., W. F. Kocholaty, D. A. Cooper, J. L. Gray, and S. L. Robinson, *Biochim. Biophys. Acta* **212**, 126–133 (1970).
29. Morrison, W. L., and H. Neurath, *J. Biol. Chem.* **200**, 39–51 (1953).
30. Kathan, R. H., R. J. Winzler, and C. A. Johnson, *J. Exp. Med.* **113**, 37–45 (1961).
31. Morawiecki, A., *Biochim. Biophys. Acta* **83**, 339–347 (1964).
32. Dandliker, W. B., M. Moskowitz, B. H. Zimm, and M. Calvin, *J. Amer. Chem. Soc.* **72**, 5587–5592 (1950).
33. Morgan, T. E., and D. J. Hanahan, *Biochemistry* **5**, 1050–1059 (1966).
34. Bakerman, S., and G. Wasemiller, *Biochemistry* **6**, 1100–1113 (1967).
35. Macheboeuf, M. A., and F. Tayeau, *Compt. Rend.* **206**, 860–862 (1938).
36. Scanu, A., and P. Oriente, *J. Exp. Med.* **113**, 737–757 (1961).
37. Gotto, A. M., R. I. Levy, F. T. Lindgren, and D. S. Fredrickson, *Biochim. Biophys. Acta* **176**, 667–669 (1969).
38. Zahler, P., and E. R. Weibel, *Biochim. Biophys. Acta* **219**, 320–338 (1970).
39. Lenard, J., and S. J. Singer, *Proc. Natl. Acad. Sci. U.S.* **56**, 1828–1835 (1966).
40. Maddy, A. H., *Biochim. Biophys. Acta* **117**, 193–200 (1966).
41. Rega, A. F., R. I. Weed, C. F. Reed, G. G. Berg, and A. Rothstein, *Biochim. Biophys. Acta* **147**, 297–312 (1967).

42. Mazia, D., and A. Ruby, *Proc. Natl. Acad. Sci. U.S.* **61**, 1005–1012 (1968).
43. Steim, J. M., and S. Fleischer, *Proc. Natl. Acad. Sci. U.S.* **58**, 1292–1298 (1967).
44. Urry, D. W., M. Mednieks, and E. Bejnarowicz, *Proc. Natl. Acad. Sci. U.S.* **57**, 1043–1049 (1967).
45. Wallach, D. F. H., and P. H. Zahler, *Proc. Natl. Acad. Sci. U.S.* **56**, 1552–1559 (1966).
46. Wallach, D. F. H., *J. Gen. Physiol.* **54**, (1), Part 2, 3S–26S (1969).
47. Cassim, J. Y., and J. T. Yang, *Biochem. Biophys. Res. Commun.* **26**, 58–64 (1967).
48. Huang, C., and T. E. Thompson, *J. Mol. Biol.* **13**, 183–193 (1965).
49. Yanari, S., and F. A. Bovey, *J. Biol. Chem.* **235**, 2818–2826 (1960).
50. Urry, D. W., and T. H. Ji, *Arch. Biochem. Biophys.* **128**, 802–807 (1968).
51. Ji, T. H., and D. W. Urry, *Biochem. Biophys. Res. Commun.* **34**, 404–411 (1969).
52. Schneider, A. S., M. J. T. Schneider, and K. Rosenheck, *Proc. Natl. Acad. Sci. U.S.* **66**, 793–798 (1970).
53. Cauldwell, C. B., and V. N. Schumaker, *Physiol. Chem. Phys.* **2**, 201–216 (1970).
54. Duysens, L. N. M., *Biochim. Biophys. Acta* **19**, 1–12 (1956).
55. Greenfield, N., and G. D. Fasman, *Biochemistry* **8**, 4108–4116 (1969).
56. Maddy, A. H., and B. R. Malcolm, *Science* **150**, 1616–1618 (1965).
57. Maddy, A. H., and B. R. Malcolm, *Science* **153**, 213 (1966).
58. Chapman, D., V. B. Kamat, and R. J. Levene, *Science* **160**, 314–316 (1968).
59. Kauzmann, W., *Adv. Protein Chem.* **14**, 1–63 (1959).
60. Danielli, J. F., and H. Davson, *J. Cell. Comp. Physiol.* **5**, 495–508 (1935).
61. Glaser, M., H. Simpkins, S. J. Singer, M. Sheetz, and S. I. Chan, *Proc. Natl. Acad. Sci. U.S.* **65**, 721–728 (1970).
62. Steim, J. M., M. E. Tourtellotte, J. C. Reinert, R. N. McElhaney, and R. L. Rader, *Proc. Natl. Acad. Sci. U.S.* **63**, 104–109 (1969).
63. Metcalfe, J. C., S. M. Metcalfe, and D. M. Engelman, *Biochim. Biophys. Acta* **241**, 412–421 (1971).
64. Metcalfe, S. M., J. C. Metcalfe, and D. M. Engelman, *Biochim. Biophys. Acta* **241**, 422–430 (1971).
65. Engelman, D. M., *J. Mol. Biol.* **58**, 153–165 (1971).
66. Bowman, M. H., A. C. Ottolenghi, and C. E. Mengel, *J. Membrane Biol.* **4**, 156–164 (1971).
67. Ladbrooke, B. D., R. M. Williams, and D. Chapman, *Biochim. Biophys. Acta* **150**, 333–340 (1968).
68. Chapman, D., V. B. Kamat, J. de Gier, and S. A. Penkett, *J. Mol. Biol.* **31**, 101–114 (1968).
69. Hubbell, W. L., and H. M. McConnell, *Proc. Natl. Acad. Sci. U.S.* **64**, 20–27 (1970).
70. Terry, T. M., D. M. Engleman, and H. J. Morowitz, *Biochim. Biophys. Acta* **135**, 391–405 (1967).
71. Butler, K. W., H. Dugas, I. C. P. Smith, and H. Schneider, *Biochem. Biophys. Res. Commun.* **40**, 770–776 (1970).
72. Weinstein, R. S., in *Red Cell Membrane Structure and Function,* G. A. Jamieson and T. J. Greenwalt, Eds., Lippincott, Philadelphia, 1969, pp. 36–76.
73. Baker, R. F., in *Red Cell Membrane Structure and Function,* G. A. Jamieson and T. J. Greenwalt, Eds., Lippincott, Philadelphia, 1969, pp. 13–35.
74. Hillier, J., and J. F. Hoffman, *J. Cell. Comp. Physiol.* **42**, 203–247 (1953).
75. Ponder, E., in *The Cell,* J. Brachet and A. E. Mirsky, Eds., Vol. 2, Academic Press, New York, 1961, pp. 1–84.

76. Marchesi, V. T., and G. E. Palade, *Proc. Natl. Acad. Sci. U.S.* **58**, 991–995 (1967).
77. Pinto da Silva, P., and D. Branton, *J. Cell. Biol.* **45**, 598–605 (1970).
78. Pinto da Silva, P., S. D. Douglas, and D. Branton, *Nature* **232**, 194–195 (1971).
79. Branton, D., *Annu. Rev. Plant Physiol.* **20**, 209–238 (1969).
80. Harris, J. R., *Biochim. Biophys. Acta* **188**, 31–42 (1969).
81. Remsen, C. C., S. W. Watson, and A. W. Bernheimer, *Biochem. Biophys. Res. Commun.* **40**, 1297–1304 (1970).
82. Bretscher, M. S., *J. Mol. Biol.* **59**, 351–357 (1971).
83. Steck, T. L., G. Fairbanks, and D. F. H. Wallach, *Biochemistry* **10**, 2617–2627 (1971).
84. Seaman, G. V. F., and L. J. Jackson, *Biochem. Biophys. Res. Commun.* **44**, 1050–1055 (1971).
85. Sonenberg, M., *Proc. Natl. Acad. Sci. U.S.* **68**, 1051–1055 (1971).

Part III

SOLUBLE LIPOPROTEINS

11 Lipid Composition of Lipoproteins in Normal and Diseased States

VLADIMIR P. SKIPSKI

Division of Experimental Chemotherapy, Sloan-Kettering Institute for Cancer Research, Walker Laboratory, Rye, New York

I. GENERAL CHARACTERISTICS OF PLASMA LIPOPROTEINS

A. Introduction

Many proteins have a tendency to form complexes with other types of compounds, including lipids. There are two main types of protein–lipid complexes, or molecules, that have been isolated and characterized: lipoproteins and proteolipids. Lipoproteins, in general, have the solubility properties of proteins; they are soluble in water or weak salt solutions. On the other hand, proteolipids have the solubility characteristics of lipids; they are insoluble in water and weak salt solutions but soluble in certain organic solvents. Proteolipids are not present under normal conditions in blood plasma. However, practically all the plasma lipids are found in the lipoproteins (1). The lipid composition of human-plasma lipoproteins is the subject of this chapter.

The first lipoproteins as an entity were isolated by Macheboeuf (2, 3) in 1929 from horse serum. Previously, however, it had been realized that various protein fractions isolated from plasma contained some lipids (4). Macheboeuf, who isolated lipoprotein by ammonium sulfate and sulfuric acid (0.2 *N* H_2SO_4) precipitation, found that it contains up to 40% lipid and 60% protein. The preparations had a relatively constant composition and, in spite of the high lipid content, were soluble in water at neutral and alkaline pH. Subsequently the results of many investigators, most of whom will be cited later, indicated that plasma contains several different types of lipoprotein.[1]

[1] The term "plasma" is used throughout this chapter when the discussion is general. When concrete data on lipid composition are presented, plasma and serum are differentiated.

One of the principal differences among the lipoprotein classes is their relative lipid content, or, more precisely, their lipid-to-protein ratio. Roughly, the ratios may vary from 99 : 1 in chylomicrons to 1 : 99 in the albumin–free fatty acid complex. The lipid-to-protein ratio determines the densities of lipoproteins. This property is used for separating lipoproteins into different classes by ultracentrifugation. In spite of the fact that lipoprotein classification is at least partially operational, it is justified physiologically since most of the lipoprotein classes have distinctly different roles in lipid transport. However, in some instances the borderline between lipoprotein classes is arbitrary.

On the basis of density lipoproteins can be divided into low- and high-density lipoproteins. The technical description of these separations is presented in detail in Chapter 5. However, a simplified description of lipoprotein classifications is presented here for those not familiar with the subject. Lipoproteins that float in a solution of 1.063-g/ml density (*d*) in the ultracentrifugal field are considered to be low-density lipoproteins, (LDL), and those with a tendency to sediment are high-density lipoproteins (HDL).

Low-density lipoproteins are usually divided into two classes: proper low-density lipoproteins (LDL, *d* 1.006–1.063 g/ml) and very-low-density lipoproteins (VLDL, $d < 1.006$ g/ml). These classes can be further characterized by their flotation rates in the analytical ultracentrifuge. Each class represents a group of closely related complexes that have different lipid-to-protein ratios and hence densities. Therefore, if low-density lipoproteins are centrifuged in a solution of 1.063-g/ml density, their velocities of flotation, or flotation rates, will differ because of the difference in their densities. The flotation rate, or S_f, is expressed in Svedberg flotation units (negative sedimentation Svedberg units, 10^{-13} cm/sec-dyne-g).

If the flotation rate of the LDL (*d* 1.006 to 1.0635 g/ml) is measured in NaCl solution of 1.063-g/ml density (at 26°C), the S_f-rate will be 0 to 20. In general practice the LDL and VLDL flotation rates are measured in a solution of 1.063-g/ml density and are designated simply S_f. However, some authors (5, 6) measure the flotation rates at the densities at which the particulate lipoprotein classes were isolated in the preparative ultracentrifuge. Thus $S_{f(1.006)}$ means that the flotation rates were measured in a solution of 1.006-g/ml density. Sometimes the subscript also includes the nature of the salt used to determine the particular density. Ewing, Freeman, and Lindgren (7) suggested designating the flotation rate at densities other than 1.063 g/ml by the symbol "F" with a subscript indicating the density.

The flotation rate of the VLDL class (*d* 1.006–0.97 g/ml) is S_f 20–400.

The $S_f > 400$ lipoproteins are visible in the dark-field microscope and are called particulate fat (8). They vary in origin, particle size, and physicochemical properties (8–10) in healthy subjects and are represented by chylomicrons, or primary particles, and secondary particles. Chylomicrons and secondary particles are present only after ingestion of fatty or mixed meals and are of exogenous (alimentary) origin. Under some pathologic conditions (carbohydrate-induced lipemia) a third form of particulate fat, called endogenous particles (11, 12), has been isolated (see Section II.D). These apparently represent the continuation of the VLDL spectrum, and, as the name indicates, their presence is unrelated to fat ingestion. Thus they may be considered VLDL with S_f-rates of 400 to 10^5 or even higher (13–16).

The $S_f > 400$ lipoproteins are not fractionated by conventional preparative ultracentrifugation. Usually they are removed from unaltered serum or plasma samples by a brief ultracentrifugation and further separated by special techniques, for example, density-gradient centrifugation, electrophoresis, or polyvinylpyrrolidone (PVP) density-gradient fluocculation (see Section II and Chapters 5 and 13). Unfortunately data on $S_f > 400$ lipoproteins are often reported without precise identification of the fractions.

High-density lipoproteins are represented in plasma by two well-defined and extensively studied classes: high-density lipoproteins-2 (HDL_2, *d* 1.063–1.125 g/ml) and high-density lipoproteins-3 (HDL_3, *d* 1.125–1.210 g/ml) (17). In the density range between 1.063 and 1.125 g/ml additional lipoproteins may be present in small amounts (5). Their individual chemical compositions are not known, and they are included in analyses with HDL_2. Another minor "class," high-density lipoproteins-1 (HDL_1), appears as a shoulder on the spectrum of LDL (Fig. 1), which it resembles in some respects (17, 18).

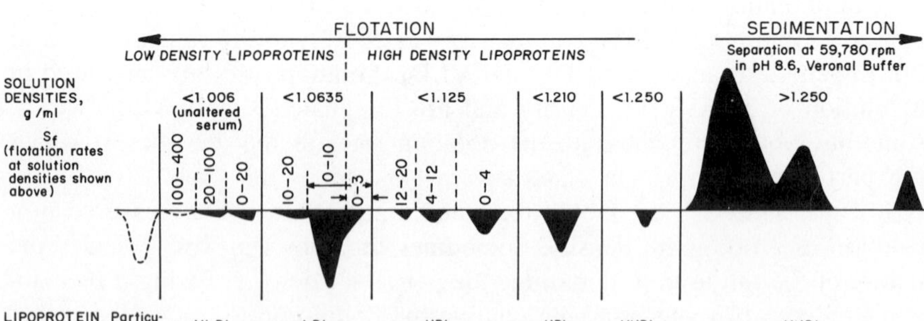

Fig. 1 Lipoprotein classes and subclasses separated by preparative and analytical ultracentrifugation. The solid vertical lines separate classes of lipoproteins isolated in the preparative ultracentrifuge. The broken lines separate the subclasses of lipoproteins observed in the analytical ultracentrifuge. (Adapted from Ref. 19.)

After all the above lipoproteins are separated, the remaining fraction is sedimented at *d* 1.21 g/ml. This $d > 1.21$ g/ml fraction is known as the ultracentrifugal residue (20). Alaupovic and co-workers (21) centrifuged this fraction again at *d* 1.250 g/ml and succeeded in separating a new HDL class, which they called very-high-density lipoproteins-1 ($VHDL_1$, *d*ensity 1.210–1.250 g/ml). The remaining ultracentrifugal residue with $d > 1.250$ g/ml still contains some lipoproteins. Apparently they are mostly a complex of albumin and free fatty acids or, probably more correctly, a complex of albumin, free fatty acids and lysolecithin. However, this fraction also contains high amounts of lipid-free proteins.

Figure 1 shows schematically the classification of lipoproteins separated by preparative and analytical ultracentrifugation.

B. General Physicochemical Characteristics of Lipoproteins

Table I shows the general physicochemical characteristics of the major human-plasma lipoprotein classes. Although for the chemical characterization of plasma lipoproteins conventional ultracentrifugal separation (based mainly on the hydrated densities of lipoproteins) is the most suitable method, other techniques, such as paper or starch-block electrophoresis, are important tools for separating some lipoproteins. The terminology used for the lipoprotein fractions separated by electrophoresis and ultracentrifugation differs and is presented in Table I. Pre-β-lipoproteins are the lipoproteins that have a somewhat higher mobility in paper electrophoresis than β-globulins and correspond to VLDL plus endogenous particles, if the latter are present. β-lipoproteins have the mobility of β-globulins and correspond to LDL. α-lipoproteins have the mobility of α-globulins in paper electrophoresis and correspond to HDL. "Albumins" correspond to lipoproteins with $d > 1.250$ g/ml.

The physicochemical data presented in Table I in most cases have been selected from published original values and from review articles (8–10, 18, 21–24).

As the hydrated density increases from that of particulate fat (*d* 0.93 g/ml) to that of $VHDL_1$ (*d* 1.155 g/ml), the protein content of the lipoproteins increases from 1 to 62%. The increase in the relative protein content and the respective decrease in the lipid content of lipoprotein molecules determine the alteration of density. Thus the density of particulate fat (primarily built up from triglycerides) is close to the density of triglycerides, which is near 0.92 g/ml. The density of proteins is on the order of 1.33 to 1.35 g/ml, and the density of the ultracentrifugal residue approaches this value. The alteration of density is accompanied by drastic changes in molecular weight. The molecular weights of particulate fat are expressed in

Table I. General Physicochemical Characteristics of Human-Plasma Lipoprotein Classes[a]

	Lipoprotein Class[b]				
	Particulate Fat[c]				
			VLDL		
Characteristic	Chylomicrons	Secondary Particles	Endogenous Particles	VLDL[e]	LDL[f]
Electrophoresis nomenclature	Chylomicrons		Pre-β-lipoproteins		β-Lipoproteins
Ultracentrifugal characteristics:					
Separation solution density, g/ml	1.006	1.006	1.006	1.006[j]	1.063
Density range, g/ml				0.94–1.006	1.006–1.063
Flotation rate:					
S_f[k]	400–15,000	400–15,000	>400	20–400	0–20
F[l]				43–770	20–43
Average hydrated density, g/ml	0.93	0.93		0.97	1.03
Electrophoretic mobility:					
Paper	Origin	Origin	Pre-β, with tailing	Pre-β	β
Starch block	α_2	β	α_2–β	α_2	β
Molecular weight	$(0.4–30) \times 10^9$	$(0.4–30) \times 10^9$		$(5–10) \times 10^6$	$(2.2–3.5) \times 10^6$
Diameter, Å[m]	750–6000	750–6000		250–750	170–260[o]
Shape	Spherical	Spherical	Spherical	Spherical	Spherical
Axes if not spherical, Å					
Lipid/protein ratio	99:1–98:2	99:1–98:2	97:3	92:8	79:21
Origin	Exogenous	Exogenous	Endogenous	Endogenous	Endogenous
Presence in blood	After fat ingestion	After fat ingestion	After meals; unrelated to fat ingestion	Usual	Usual

Characteristic	Lipoprotein Class[b]				
	HDL			Ultracentrifugal Residue[d]	
	HDL_1[g]	HDL_2	HDL_3	VHDL[h]	Albumin–FFA Complex[i]
Electrophoresis nomenclature		α-Lipoproteins			"Albumins"
Ultracentrifugal characteristics:					
Separation solution density, g/ml	1.063	1.125	1.210	1.250	1.250
Density range, g/ml		1.063–1.125	1.125–1.210	1.210–1.250	>1.250
Flotation rate:					
S_f[k]	0–3	Sediment	Sediment	Sediment	Sediment
F[l]		3.5–9	0–3.5		
Average hydrated density, g/ml	1.05	1.094	1.145	1.155	1.33
Electrophoretic mobility:					
Paper		α	α		Albumin
Starch block		α_1	α_1		Albumin
Molecular weight		3.86×10^5	1.86×10^5	1.51×10^5	69×10^3[n]
Diameter, Å[m]		60–140[p]	40–100[q]		
Shape		Built up from subunits; some are elongated			Ellipsoidal
Axes if not spherical, Å		64×95	64×65		38×150
Lipid/protein ratio		59:41	44:56	38:62	1:99[r]
Origin		Endogenous	Endogenous	Endogenous	Endogenous
Presence in blood		Usual	Usual	Usual	Usual

Notes to table on page 478.

NOTES TO TABLE 1

[a] Since values have been selected from many published results, they may not agree with data presented by any specific investigator.

[b] The lipoprotein classes are listed in the boxhead in accordance with the standard nomenclature used in ultracentrifugal studies. The corresponding electrophoresis terminology is shown in the body of the table. Abbreviations: VLDL, very-low-density lipoproteins; LDL, low-density lipoproteins; HDL, high-density lipoproteins; VHDL, very-high-density lipoproteins; FFA, free fatty acids.

[c] Chylomicrons (also known as primary particles), secondary particles, and endogenous particles are not separated by conventional ultracentrifugation. However, they can be separated by polyvinylpyrrolidone density-gradient flocculation or starch-block electrophoresis (11, 12). Endogenous particles are present in plasma in some forms of lipemia.

[d] The ultracentrifugal residue (lipoproteins with $d > 1.210$ g/ml) and the further purified albumin–free fatty acid complex ($VHDL_2$) also contain different plasma non-lipid-containing proteins.

[e] Also called LDL_2 by some investigators.

[f] Sometimes referred to as LDL_1.

[g] After preparative ultracentrifugation, HDL_1 is present in the fraction with *d* 1.006–1.063 g/ml as impurities of LDL.

[h] Also known as $VHDL_1$.

[i] Also known as $VHDL_2$.

[j] Some investigators draw the border line between VLDL and LDL at *d* 1.019 g/ml, rather than the more conventional *d* 1.006 g/ml. The lipoproteins with *d* 1.006–1.019 g/ml represent around 5% of total LDL (20).

[k] S_f denotes the negative sedimentation coefficient in Svedberg units at *d* 1.063 g/ml in NaCl solution at 26°C.

[l] Analogous to S_f measured at solution *d* 1.210 g/ml.

[m] Assuming spherical particles.

[n] Albumins.

[o] Average 216 Å.

[p] Average 95 Å; 77% of the molecules are 70 to 100 Å in diameter.

[q] Average 65 Å; 78% of the molecules have diameters of 60 to 80 Å.

[r] The albumin-free fatty acid complex represents a mixture of this lipoprotein and non-lipid-containing proteins. The given ratio is for the whole fraction.

billions, those of VLDL and LDL in millions, and those of HDL in the hundreds of thousands (16). There are concomitant changes in molecular size, the diameter diminishing from 6000 Å in particulate fat to an average of 86 Å in total HDL (25).

C. Structural Features

Hayes (26), Lossow (27), and their associates used electron microscopy to study the shape of lipoprotein molecules stained with osmium tetroxide. Chylomicrons and secondary particles from serum and chylomicrons from thoracic-duct lymph were found to be spherical, with some tendency to adhere to each other. These two fractions contain a similar wide range of particles of different sizes (Table I), indicating that lipoproteins in the same size range may differ significantly in their surface properties (electrophoresis). Forte, Nichols, and Glaeser (25), working in the same laboratories, negatively stained the lipoprotein molecules with sodium phosphotungstate. Electron-microscopic examinations of such preparations revealed that serum "chylomicrons" (apparently a mixture of primary and secondary particles) and VLDL are very diverse in size and shape. Smaller complexes were more or less spherical but easily deformed; larger ones often appeared to be amorphous. This may have resulted from a flattening of the structures during drying, since these lipoproteins contain very little protein and large amounts of triglycerides. No such phenomenon was observed in preparations stained with osmium tetroxide, which is also a fixative.

Low-density-lipoprotein molecules appeared to have a spherical shape with a mean diameter of 216 Å (range 170–260 Å). Since single LDL macromolecules never appeared elongated and were never seen on edge, there was no evidence that they may have an ellipsoid or disk shape. However, on contact with one another, the particles exhibited a polygonal shape (25). The LDL molecules appear granular, which is somewhat suggestive of substructure. Additional evidence that they have a spherical shape was provided by calculating their molecular weight. By assuming the molecule to be a sphere with a mean diameter of 216 Å and a density of 1.035 g/ml, a molecular-weight of 3.29×10^6 was obtained. This is in good agreement with the molecular weight of 3.5×10^6 determined by agarose-gel filtration (28). However, Scanu, Pollard, and Reader (29) reported that the average molecular weights of lipoproteins with *d* 1.019 to 1.063 g/ml (obtained by sedimentation equilibrium) are 2.1×10^6 to 2.3×10^6.

Concerning the LDL structural organization, on the basis of physical and chemical data Scanu et al. (29, 30) postulated that the apoproteins of this lipoprotein class are made from subunits and are held together, at least partly, by lipid bridges. Thus lipids play a stabilizing part in the protein conformation of the native lipoprotein complex. An LDL complex contains approximately 12 polypeptide subunits (29, 30).

High-density lipoproteins (*d* 1.063–1.210 g/ml) appear to be aggregations of subunits. A ringlike structure composed of four to five subunits was the configuration most frequently observed by Forte and associates (25). Occasionally two fused ringlike structures were seen where one of the subunits appeared to be shared by both rings. No single subunits were observed in electron micrographs. High-density lipoproteins had an average diameter of 86 Å.

Forte et al. (25) also investigated the HDL_2 and HDL_3 classes separately. The HDL_2 molecules had an average diameter of 95 Å (range 60–140 Å), 77% being between 70 and 100 Å in diameter. The HDL_3 molecules had an average diameter of 65 Å (range 40–100 Å), 78% being between 60 and 80 Å in diameter.

The molecular weights computed for these two classes of lipoproteins on the assumption that the molecules are spheres with the above mentioned mean diameters were significantly lower than those determined on the basis of ultracentrifugal data by Scanu and Granda (31). However, the molecular weights calculated on the assumption that the HDL_2 and HDL_3 molecules are cylinders with diameters of 95 and 65 Å, respectively, and heights (for both classes) of 65 Å (the estimated length of an individual subunit) were 407,000 and 202,000, respectively (25), in good agreement with the reported values of 360,000 ± 21,000 and 170,000 ± 21,000, respectively (31). The molecular weights calculated for cylindrical HDL_2 and HDL_3 molecules purposely ignored the fact that the molecules are most likely made up of several subunits.

Within the limit of negative-staining resolution Forte et al. (25) estimated that the HDL subunit is 36 × 64 Å, with molecular weights of 57,500 and 60,000 for the subunits of HDL_2 and HDL_3, respectively. On this basis the HDL_2 molecule may be composed of seven subunits, and the HDL_3 molecule may have three to four subunits. Scanu et al. (31, 32) demonstrated that acetylation, succinylation, or addition of 0.05 *M* sodium dodecyl sulfate to apoprotein (lipoprotein protein delipidated with ethanol–diethyl ether) caused its dissociation to subunits, with average molecular weights of 27,500. From the protein masses of HDL_2 and HDL_3 the authors concluded that HDL_2 has an average of six, and HDL_3 four, peptide subunits.

Most of the lipids present in plasma lipoproteins can be relatively easily extracted by solvent mixtures like chloroform–methanol (2:1 or 1:1, v/v) or diethyl ether–ethanol (1:2, v/v). This indicates that the mode of association between lipids and proteins is noncovalent (33, 34). Fisher and Gurin (35) demonstrated in 1964 that small amounts of lipids do associate with proteins by covalent bonds. This problem is discussed in some detail in Section VIII. Of course, these lipids cannot be extracted by solvents or removed by other physicochemical means without hydrolysis of lipoproteins. However, the main bulk of lipoprotein lipids do associate with proteins by forces weaker than those of covalent bonds. The amounts of lipids in some lipoprotein complexes are so high that not all lipids can associate directly with proteins, and there is also an association of lipids with lipids (36). Individual LDL complexes may contain 1000 to 2000 lipid molecules. The ratio of the number of lipid molecules per molecule of protein in VLDL and particulate fat is even higher. Only certain lipid molecules may have direct contact with the protein moieties of these lipoproteins. On the other hand, the protein molecules of such lipoproteins as the albumin–free fatty acid complex, or, probably more correctly, the albumin–free fatty acid–lysolecithin complex, apparently possess some individual sites with appropriate functional groups and steric orientation to bind individual fatty acids (see Section VII). This type of lipid binding probably is analogous to enzyme–substrate interactions. It appears that London–van der Waals, polarization, and electrostatic forces are responsible for the integrity of the lipoprotein molecules (36, 37). However, most of the evidence that supports this statement is indirect.

During the last 10 years several hypotheses have been proposed concerning the structural organization of lipoproteins. The essence of these hypotheses in regard to the VLDL, LDL, and HDL classes is discussed in this section. The probable structural organizations of particulate fat (chylomicrons) and the albumin–free fatty acid complex are considered in Sections II and VI, respectively.

Although the details of their hypotheses differ, Lindgren and Nichols (38), Cook and Martin (23, 39), and Vandenheuvel (40) proposed that VLDL and LDL molecules have a lipid core surrounded by a film of proteins and polar lipids like phospholipids and that HDL molecules have a protein matrix with which the lipid interacts without essentially altering the molecular integrity of the proteins. Generally the experimental evidence only partly supports the possibility of such organization.

In 1969 Day and Levy (41) evaluated new physicochemical and chemical data concerning lipoproteins and postulated a new hypothesis of their structure. The authors divided all lipoproteins into two groups: (1) molecules whose substructure is visible in the electron microscope and which have an invariable particle size and (2) molecules with no visible substructure and a wide variation in particle size. Thus the LDL, HDL_2, and HDL_3 classes are included in group 1, and VLDL and chylomicrons in group 2. Lipoproteins in group 1 are formed from repeating units that Day and Levy call lipotides. Each unit is built up of two helical peptide chains to which phospholipids are attached on one side predominantly by electrostatic forces. The phospholipid sides face each other. Between the two layers of phospholipids are the nonpolar lipids—such as triglycerides, cholesterol, and cholesteryl esters—which interact with the fatty acid chains of the phospholipids through hydrophobic forces and become bound to form a layer or several layers of these nonpolar lipids. Thus a lipotide unit represents a narrow sandwich (rather a stick) consisting of a helical peptide on the outside, then a layer of phospholipids, a layer (or several) of nonpolar lipids, a layer of phospholipids, and again a layer of helical peptide. In both sides of the nonpolar-lipid layers are embedded some polar lipids (phospholipids, free fatty acids), with their hydrophilic heads at the surface to stabilize the molecule. The two lipid-binding helical parts of the peptide chain of a lipotide are connected by the nonhelical, non-lipid-binding portion of the peptide chain. The chains of polypeptide with several lipotides are subsequently folded into a configuration allowing the whole molecule to be at its lowest energy state in a manner analogous to the tertiary structuring of globular proteins.

The simplest possible way for two polypeptides containing several lipotides in each chain to associate into a lipoprotein molecule would be the formation of an additional lipotide between two different peptide chains. One-half of the lipotide sandwich would be contributed by one peptide and the other half by a neighboring peptide chain. Thus a "lipid bridge" would be formed between two polypeptides containing lipotides. Some of the supporting evidence, without details, is presented here.

Optical-rotatory-dispersion analysis of HDL indicates that around 65% of their proteins are in the α-helix form. Delipidation decreases the content of helical structure in the protein moiety of these lipoproteins (42–44). Moreover, Scanu and Hirz (45) observed by circular-dichroism measurements that HDL_3 and apo-HDL_3 recombined with phospholipids are more resistant than delipidated lipoproteins to changes induced by alteration of pH, urea treatment, or chemical modification with succinic anhydride. On the basis of these observations it has been concluded that phospholipids play a structural role in stabilizing the predominantly α-helical configuration of the HDL polypeptide chains.

There is some controversy between Scanu's group (30, 44) and Fredrickson's group (46, 47) concerning the conformation of proteins in the LDL molecule. Scanu et al. (30, 44) consider, on the basis of physicochemical measurements, that the LDL protein exists as a combination of an α-helix and unordered chains. Delipidation decreases the helical content of the LDL molecule from 40 to 30%. On the other hand, Gotto and associates (46, 47) interpret the structure of LDL protein to be a combination of the β-structure (pleated sheet) of antiparallel chains and unordered chains. According to Day and Levy (41), both these structural organizations of proteins secure the regions for phospholipid binding.

Day and Levy (41) believe that the phospholipid–protein interaction is a mixed ionic–apolar binding: the charged portion of the phospholipid interacts with a charged amino acid group. One fatty acid of the same phospholipid molecule interacts with the hydrocarbon portion of the amino acid side chain, and another phospholipid fatty acid interacts with a nonpolar lipid. However, Scanu (43) considers that a nonpolar interaction between polypeptides and phospholipids is the predominant type of binding since changing the polypeptide charges by acetylation, succinylation, or other chemical means, as well as variations in the pH and ionic strength of the medium, does not prevent the binding of phospholipids by polypeptides.

The key role of phospholipids in the interaction between polypeptides and other lipids has been stressed by Sodhi and Gould (48), who observed that the HDL apoprotein combines with cholesterol alone in much smaller amounts than it does in the presence of phospholipids. This suggests rather strongly that the combination of phospholipids with apo-HDL is the primary step in HDL formation.

The results obtained by delipidating lipoproteins with organic solvents indicate that different lipid classes are differently bound in the lipoprotein molecules. Thus Avigan (49) extracted lipoproteins with diethyl ether and was able to remove all triglycerides, 25% of the cholesterol, and a small amount of phospholipids. However, more potent solvents (e.g., ethanol–diethyl ether) removed all triglycerides, cholesterol, and most of the phospholipids (42, 49).

The structural organization of chylomicrons is presented in Section II.C. Apparently VLDL molecules have a similar structure (41). Electron-microscopic studies of the latter (50) have shown the existence of an outer membranelike layer (surface coat) similar to that observed in chylomicrons. In spite of the fact that the VLDL protein content exceeds that of chylomicrons, the ratio of protein content to surface area is the same in chylomicrons and in S_f 90–400 lipoproteins, and only slightly higher in S_f 16–101 lipoproteins (27). It appears that both chylomicrons and VLDL molecules have globular lipid cores, 20 to 30% of which are covered with proteins.

The reader may find a detailed review on the structural organization of lipoproteins in *Structural and Functional Aspects of Lipoproteins in Living Systems,* edited by Tria and Scanu (51).

II. CHYLOMICRONS

A. General Remarks

Often present in human plasma and serum are the lipoproteins that are known as particulate fat and are larger than VLDL molecules. Their amount, chemical composition, and origin are determined by physiologic and pathologic conditions. A common characteristic is their size: these molecules can be observed in the dark-field microscope.

The most prominent particles in particulate fat are the chylomicrons. The term "chylomicron" was introduced by Gage (52, 53) about 50 years ago to describe the luminous lipid particles observed under the dark-field microscope in blood samples taken after the ingestion of fat. Subsequently it was found that chylomicrons are the principal form in which absorbed fat is transported from the intestinal cell through the lymph channels and eventually, via the thoracic lymph, into the bloodstream. From there they are removed by the liver as well as by adipose and other extrahepatic tissues (8, 54–57).

Chylomicrons that are built up primarily of exogenous fat are also called alimentary particles. They are present in lymph as well as in the bloodstream, but in the latter they are slightly different chemically because their surfaces acquire some components from blood. The amount of chylomicrons in the lymph and bloodstream is determined by the nature of digested food.

A detailed account of the formation and physiologic role of chylomicrons is presented in Chapter 13. In this chapter they are considered mainly as one form of serum or plasma lipoproteins, with emphasis on their chemical, and especially lipid, composition. Since chylomicrons, after entering the bloodstream, may undergo some chemical changes, the chemical composition of chyle (lymph) chylomicrons is also considered.

Particulate fat also contains particles known as lipomicrons (58). According to Frazer and Steward (58), lipomicrons are present even during complete starvation and are essentially unaffected by simple dietary changes or prolonged starvation. The only changes are in their relative and absolute numbers; for example, in certain forms of lipemia, they may be essentially increased.

Unlike chylomicrons, lipomicrons have an endogenous origin, and were therefore called nonalimentary particles by Dole and Hamlin (8). They are considered by some authors (59) to represent an extension of the VLDL spectrum with S_f-rates of 400 to 15,000. Until recently the average size of nonalimentary particles has been considered to be smaller than that of typical chylomicrons (12).

The borderline between particulate fat and the VLDL fraction is arbitrary and lacking in uniformity. Thus Lindgren and Nichols (38), on the basis of S_f-rates measured in 1.063-g/ml NaCl solution at 26°C, consider S_f 20–400 lipoproteins to belong to the VLDL class and S_f 400 lipoproteins to be the lowest limit for the particles (minimum diameter 75 mμ). On the other hand, Alaupovic et al. (59) consider all S_f 20–5000 lipoproteins to be in the VLDL class and S_f > 5000 lipoproteins (minimum diameter

200 mμ) to be chylomicrons. Hence this section covers such topics as the composition of particles, the specific conditions of isolation, and, when possible, size limits as well as centrifugation data (*g*-min values). Dole and Hamlin (8) consider that 10^6 *g*-min could be taken as a standard for the separation of particulate fat. This amount of centrifugation separates a mixture of particles with minimum diameters of about 75 mμ and S_f-rates of 400. These conditions coincide with those used by most lipoprotein specialists to separate the VLDL fraction from particles (10). For a detailed description of such separations see Chapters 5 and 13 or an extensive review, *Particulate Fat in Lymph and Blood,* by Dole and Hamlin (8).

B. Lipid Composition of Human Chylomicrons

Table II shows the lipid composition of human chylomicrons isolated, in most cases, from serum or plasma. In certain instances lymph was collected from the intestines of patients. Generally chylomicrons were collected during the absorption of fat meals.

Chylomicrons are composed mainly of lipids (97.5–99.2%) and small amounts of proteins. The data suggest that chylomicrons isolated from chyle have slightly less protein (0.8–1.7%) than those isolated from serum or plasma (2.0–2.5%). Possibly chylomicrons receive additional proteins later when circulating in the bloodstream. The bulk of the chylomicron lipids are triglycerides (81.3–89.4%). Apparently small amounts of diglycerides and monoglycerides are also present (65). On the average, phospholipids comprise 8.0% of total human plasma or serum chylomicrons.

The most variable lipid in chylomicrons is cholesterol, whose total amount varies from 0.5% in large chylomicrons isolated from chyle (59, 67) to 6.7% in chylomicrons isolated from pooled heterogeneous serum samples. In this combined sample, blood from fasting or semifasting subjects was not excluded (64). Other than these two extremes, most investigators reported that the total cholesterol content in chylomicrons is 2.5 to 5.6%. Whereas Jobst and Schettler (66) have reported that free cholesterol and esterified cholesterol are equally distributed (2.8%) in chylomicrons, all other authors have reported relatively higher values for esterified cholesterol.

Because of the relatively small amount of phospholipids in chylomicrons, their composition was until recently unknown. However, in 1964 Wood et al. (65) reported on the phospholipid composition of chylomicrons isolated from plasma, and in 1968 Alaupovic et al. (59), on those isolated from chyle (Table III). The total amounts of phospholipids reported by these authors are similar: 9.0 and 9.2%, respectively, of the total chylomicron weights.

Table II. Chemical Composition of Human Chylomicrons[a]

Variable	Reference 60	61	62, 63	64	65	66	59
Source	Chylous ascitic fluid	Serum	Serum	Serum[b]	Plasma	Serum	Chyle[c]
Physiologic conditions	Obstructed thoracic duct; accumulated chylomicrons	Absorptive phase (animal fat)	Absorptive phase (butter)		Absorptive phase (butter)	Absorptive phase (butter)	Absorptive phase (heavy cream)
Isolation procedure	Flocculation with protamine sulfate	Centrifugation (several washings)	Centrifugation	Spontaneous flotation, centrifugation	Centrifugation (several washings)	Centrifugation	Centrifugation (washed)
Centrifugation data:							
Amount of centrifugation, *g*-min		9×10^4[e]			8.6×10^5	1.3×10^6[e]	(9.5×10^4)
Particle size, mμ[d]		300				55	200–250
S_f-Rate[d]		10^4	400			300	5000
Chemical composition, wt %:							
Proteins	1.7	2.1	2.0	2.5	2.5		0.8
Lipids:[f]							
Total	98.3	97.9	98.0	97.5	97.5		99.2
Triglycerides	86.0	86.5	88.0	81.3	(84.0)[g]	86.5	89.4
Cholesterol:							
Total	5.2	4.4	(2.8)	(6.7)	(2.5)	(5.6)	0.5
Free	1.3		1.0	3.1	0.8	2.8	
Esterified	3.9		(1.8)	(3.6)	1.7	2.8	
Cholesteryl esters[h]	6.6		3.0	6.1	(2.9)	4.7	
Free fatty acids			1.0		Trace		
Phospholipids	7.3	9.3	8.0	7.1	9.0	5.8	9.2

[a] Values in parentheses were calculated by the author.
[b] Pooled heterogeneous samples. Blood from fasting or semifasting subjects not excluded.
[c] Patient with lung tumor.
[d] Lower limit.
[e] Estimated by Dole and Hamlin (8).
[f] Estimated by difference: 100% − protein %.
[g] Presence of diglycerides and traces of monoglycerides reported (65).
[h] In most cases presented as cholesteryl oleate.

Table III. Phospholipid Composition of Human Chylomicrons[a]

Variable	Reference 65	Reference 59
Source	Plasma	Chyle
Fat ingested	Butter	Heavy cream
Centrifugation data:		
Amount of centrifugation, *g*-min	8.6×10^5	(9.5×10^4)[b]
Particle size, mμ[c]		200–250
S_f-Rate[c]		5000
Total phospholipids, wt %	9.0	9.2
Phospholipid composition, % of total phospholipids:		
Phosphatidylethanolamine	5.6	6.9
Lecithin	78.5	56.9
Lysolecithin	4.2	10.2
Sphingomyelin	11.7	26.0

[a] Samples collected during absorptive phase. Chylomicrons isolated by centrifugation, with several washings.
[b] Calculated by the author.
[c] Lower limit.

The major phospholipid is lecithin. However, it constitutes 78.5% of the total phospholipids according to Wood et al. (65) and only 56.9% according to Alaupovic et al. (59). The quantity of sphingomyelin reported by Alaupovic et al. is more than twice the value reported by Wood et al. The total quantities of choline-containing phospholipids (lecithin, lysolecithin, and sphingomyelin) and phosphatidylethanolamine are similar in both reports.

Chylomicrons are the principal form of lipoproteins in which the absorbed triglycerides are transported from the intestines to various organs.

The earlier literature gave conflicting information on the extent to which the fatty acid composition of chylomicrons reflects the fatty acid composition of ingested fat (68). Since the development of chromatographic techniques for the separation of lipids during the last decade, it has become possible to answer this question more precisely. Dole et al. (68), using gas–liquid chromatography, compared the fatty acid composition of ingested fats (corn oil, coconut oil, and butter) with the fatty acid composition of plasma chylomicrons and some plasma-lipid fractions that remained after the isolation of chylomicrons. The chylomicrons were isolated under fasting conditions and at different stages of fat absorption (up to 9 hr after ingestion). They were isolated by centrifugation at 100,000 *g* for 30 min (3×10^6 *g*-min).

The fatty acid patterns of chylomicrons under fasting conditions and 3, 6, and 9 hr after corn-oil ingestion are shown in Table IV. The chief component of corn oil is linoleic acid (18:2, 55%). During absorption the proportion of this acid in chylomicrons rose moderately from 8.3% under fasting conditions to 24.1% 9 hr after corn-oil ingestion, remaining well below the linoleic acid concentration in corn oil. In the case of palmitic and stearic acids there was little, if any, effect of dietary fat on chylomicron composition. The results were approximately the same when other fats were administered.

Thus the pattern of chylomicron fatty acids tends to follow that of fasting samples, although there are some obvious effects of the dietary loads. Even lesser dietary effects were observed in lipid fractions extracted from plasma after the removal of chylomicrons. Dole et al. (68) consider that this is due to some extent to stabilization by equilibration with a large pool of tissue lipids. The smallness of the effect exerted by ingested fats on the fatty acid composition of chylomicrons can be partially explained by the fact that triglycerides were not separated from other chylomicron lipids, especially phospholipids. As will be noted later, the fatty acid composition of phospholipids is not affected by ingested fat. Moreover, the chylomicrons were isolated from blood plasma, but not from lymph. Contributions from other types of particulate fat to the fatty acid pattern of chylomicrons were not excluded; also the dietary load of fat was moderate in quantity (100 g).

On the other hand, a number of investigators have reported in the last decade that ingested fat affects the fatty acid composition of chylomicron triglycerides to a much higher degree than that observed by Dole et al. (68). Blomstrand and Dahlbäck (69) studied the effect of diet on the fatty acid composition of lymph lipids. The lymph was collected from the thoracic ducts of two patients with cancer. The same diet of known composition was used for several days before and during the experiment. The extracted samples contained all the lipids present in lymph, which of course included various lipoproteins of endogenous origin. Triglycerides and other lipids present in the extracts were separated by column chromatography, and their fatty acid patterns were investigated. Since the vast majority of triglycerides during the peak of absorption represent the chylomicron triglycerides, such observations are of some importance. The authors found that the fatty acid compositions of lymph and diet triglycerides were very similar. For example, oleic acid constituted 74.4% of the ingested triglycerides and 70.2% of the lymph triglycerides; palmitic and stearic acids were present in almost the same concentrations in both the lymph and the ingested triglycerides. However, lymph triglycerides contained 7.7% of linoleic acid

Table IV. Fatty Acid Composition of Human-Plasma Chylomicrons Before and After Ingesting 100 g of Corn Oil[a]

	Composition %				
		Chylomicrons			
Fatty Acid[b]	Corn Oil	Fasting	3 hr[c]	6 hr[c]	9 hr[c]
Saturated:					
12:0		1.8	0.7	0.1	1.5
14:0		3.6	2.6	1.5	1.5
15:0		0.8		0.3	
16:0	9.8	22.8	26.0	24.8	22.1
17:0		0.5	0.4	0.2	0.2
18:0	1.1	10.6	9.7	7.5	10.6
20:0			0.5		
Monounsaturated:					
12:1		0.6	0.4		0.6
14:1		1.4	1.0	0.4	0.4
16:1		2.6	2.2	3.2	3.9
18:1	33.9	18.4	21.3	26.5	25.6
Diunsaturated:					
18:2	55.1	8.3	11.6	21.7	24.1
Polyunsaturated:					
18:3					0.2
20:3		1.9	0.7	1.0	0.2
20:4		0.3	0.2	1.0	
Unidentified		12.8	19.3	3.3	5.2
Double-bond index[d]	51.3	34.1	43.9	33.3	35.6

[a] Data from Ref. 68.

[b] Fatty acids are described by two quantities: the number of carbon atoms and the number of double bonds.

[c] Time after corn-oil ingestion.

[d] Double-bond index =

$$\Sigma \frac{N_i W_i}{M_i}$$

where N_i is the number of double bonds in the fatty acid i, M_i is the molecular weight, and W_i is the percentage by weight of the fatty acid in a given mixture.

versus 0.5% in the diet, although the diet had been consumed several days before the collection of lymph.

Bragdon and Karmen (70, 71) investigated the effect of a single fat load on the total fatty acid pattern of chylomicrons rather than the patterns of individual lipid classes. Since on the average (Table II) triglycerides constitute 86% of the chylomicrons, the composition of the total lipid fatty acids practically reflects the composition of chylomicron triglycerides. When human subjects were fed corn oil, which contains exclusively long-chain acids, the fatty acid composition of chylomicrons was close to that of the corn oil itself. When the subjects ingested coconut oil, which contains 73% lauric acid (which is absorbed at least partially via the portal system), the fatty acid compositions of the chylomicron lipids and ingested fat were not similar.

Another series of experiments (71) covered the effect of feeding corn oil, which is characterized by a high content of linoleic acid, on the ratio of linoleic acid to oleic acid. The ratio in chylomicrons in the fasting state was 0.37; 6 hr after ingestion of corn-oil emulsion, though it increased to 1.81, it did not reach the ratio of these fatty acids in corn oil (2.28). When the ratios of these fatty acids in the various lipoprotein fractions are compared, it is obvious that the ratio closest to that of ingested oil is in the chylomicrons.

Kayden et al. (67, 72) investigated the acute effect of a single feeding (100 g) of various fats on the composition of human lymph and serum

Table V. Alteration of Total Fatty Acid Composition of Human-Lymph Chylomicrons After Corn-Oil Feeding[a]

	Composition (%)					
		Chylomicrons				
Fatty Acid[b]	Corn Oil	Fasting	2–4 hr[c]	8–10 hr[c]	11–23 hr[c]	35–47 hr[c]
10:0		2	0	0	0	0
12:0		3	0	0	0	2
14:0		10	1	0	0	4
16:0	11	37	16	10	14	29
18:0		8	3	1	3	8
18:1	27	32	31	26	34	38
18:2	61	8	49	63	49	19

[a] Data from Ref. 72.

[b] Fatty acids are described by two characteristics: the number of carbon atoms and the number of double bonds.

[c] Time after corn-oil feeding.

lipoproteins. Only the effect on chylomicrons is considered here. Lymph chylomicrons were collected from two patients, one with carcinoma of the lung, and the other with intermittent bouts of pancreatitis. Serum samples were obtained from a patient convalescing from pneumonia. Chylomicrons were isolated by centrifugation at 26,000 *g* for 30 min (7.8×10^5 *g*-min).

Table V shows the total-lipid fatty acid compositions of chylomicrons after 12 hr of fasting. Corn oil (100 g) was administered by stomach tube. The lymph was collected every 2 hr, as indicated. The patients were not given any food until after the 8- to 10-hr collection. The fatty acid composition of the chylomicrons collected 8 to 10 hr after administration of corn oil was practically identical with that of the ingested corn oil. After 47 hr the composition of the chylomicrons approximated the values obtained during the fasting state, although some aftereffect of ingested food was still observed.

The lipids of the chylomicrons that were collected between 8 and 10 hr after the administration of corn oil were separated into triglycerides and cholesteryl esters (Table VI). The fatty acid patterns of triglycerides and corn oil were similar as were those of cholesteryl esters and ingested fat. On the other hand, in fatty acid composition the serum-chylomicron total lipids and triglycerides resemble ingested fat to a much lesser degree than do the lymph chylomicrons (Table VI).

When patients were fed coconut oil (very saturated and rich in short-chain fatty acids), in general the pattern was the same as that observed

Table VI. Alteration of Fatty Acid Composition of Human Lymph and Serum Chylomicron Lipids After Corn-Oil Feeding[a]

		Composition (%)							
		Lymph chylomicrons[b]				Serum Chylomicrons			
		Triglycerides		Cholesteryl Esters		Total lipids		Triglycerides	
Fatty Acid[c]	Corn Oil	Fasting	8–10 hr[d]	Fasting	8–10 hr[d]	Fasting	8 hr[d]	Fasting	8 hr[d]
12:0		4	0	4	0	2	1	2	0
14:0		13	0	10	0	1	0	3	1
16:0	11	28	10	38	11	30	25	33	21
18:0		10	2	11	2	9	4	8	5
18:1	27	32	22	31	23	41	26	42	32
18:2	61	10	64	7	58	17	42	12	42

[a] Data from Ref. 72.
[b] Estimated by the author on the basis of data in Ref. 72.
[c] Fatty acids are described by two characteristics: the number of carbon atoms and the number of double bonds.
[d] Time after corn-oil feeding.

with corn oil. However, the similarity in composition between ingested fat and chylomicron lipids was less pronounced.

Wood et al. (65) studied in detail the effect of butter ingestion on the fatty acid composition of triglycerides, diglycerides, and individual phospholipids present in human-plasma chylomicrons (Table VII). In fatty acid composition chylomicron triglycerides and diglycerides showed a fairly close resemblance to butter, the content of palmitic, palmitoleic, and stearic acids being practically identical. The amounts of oleic and linoleic acids were higher in chylomicron glycerides than in butter. On the other hand, fatty acids with shorter chains than those of palmitic acid were either present in much smaller quantities in the triglycerides and diglycerides (myristic acid) or were practically absent (lauric acid). This observation supports the

Table VII. Fatty Acid Compositions of Butter and the Lipids in Human-Plasma Chylomicrons[a]

	Composition[b]						
				Phospholipids[c]			
Fatty Acid[d]	Ingested Butter	Triglycerides[e]	Diglycerides[f]	PC	PE	LL	Sph
12:0	3						
14:0	12	6	4				
16:0	33	30	28	34	13	23	28
16:1	3	3	4	1	3	4	2
18:0	13	13	12	16	24	37	10
18:1	24	31	31	13	19	14	4
18:2	3	7	7	25	15	7	2
20:0							4
20:3				2	1	1	
20:4				5	7	8	
22:0							13
22:6				1	2		
23:0							8
24:0							8
24:1							16

[a] Data from Ref. 65.
[b] In mass percent of the total methyl esters of each compound. Values quoted to nearest whole number.
[c] Pooled sample from 12 subjects. Abbreviations: PC, lecithin; PE, phosphatidylethanolamine; LL, lysolecithin; Sph, sphingomyelin.
[d] Fatty acids are described by two characteristics: the number of carbon atoms and the number of double bonds.
[e] Average of four experiments.
[f] Pooled sample from four subjects.

idea that lower fatty acids either are not transported in significant amounts in the chylomicrons or disappear from the chylomicrons in the bloodstream (70). Apparently the fatty acid compositions of phospholipids were only slightly affected by absorbed fatty acids.

Zilversmit (73) found that ingestion of corn oil and cream definitely affected the fatty acid composition of lymph chylomicrons isolated from a patient with diabetes mellitus. After ingestion of cream the composition of chylomicron triglycerides was similar to that of cream, which, however, had a much higher stearic acid content. Similarities in the fatty acid compositions of corn oil and chylomicron triglycerides were less pronounced. However, variations in the fatty acid composition of chylomicron triglycerides collected during the absorption of two different fats were much greater than the differences between chylomicron triglycerides and ingested fat. The fatty acid compositions of chylomicron phospholipids were only slightly affected by the nature of absorbed fat.

The reviewed literature indicates that ingested fat does affect the fatty acid composition of chylomicrons, mainly in the triglyceride fraction. However, the degree of such an effect in most cases is determined by the origin of the chylomicrons—that is, whether they were isolated from lymph or from plasma or serum. In plasma or serum alimentary chylomicrons may be diluted by other fat particles, as shown by Gordis (74) and Bierman et al. (12).

The heterogeneity of plasma or serum chylomicrons has long been recognized. Several attempts have been made to classify chylomicrons according to densities, electrophoretic mobilities, and so on (12, 74–77) in normal subjects and in patients.

Gordis (74) and Bierman et al. (12) succeeded in separating and characterizing two distinct groups of fat particles appearing in the plasma of subjects during alimentary lipemia. One type, which Bierman et al. (12) called primary particles, apparently originated in the intestines. It was constituted predominantly of triglycerides with a fatty acid pattern similar to that of ingested fat. Actually they were lymph chylomicrons that had been slightly modified in the bloodstream. The other type, secondary particles, was also predominantly composed of triglycerides. However, in composition these seemed to be a mixture of fatty acids originating in ingested and body fat.

The primary and secondary particles were separated on the basis of their surface properties (rather than size and density) by zone electrophoresis on starch granules (12) and differential flocculation in polyvinylpyrrolidone density-gradient columns (12, 74). The primary and secondary particles were eluted from starch blocks after separation by electrophoresis. The lipids were extracted and analyzed. In starch zone electrophoresis the primary particles migrated in the region of α_2-globulins (migration distance about 0.60, considering albumin migration to be 1.00). The secondary particles migrated in the region of β-globulins (migration distance about 0.23). On the other hand, fat particles from thoracic-duct lymph migrated as a single zone between α_2-globulins and albumin. Incubation of these particles with fasting plasma *in vitro* at 37°C affected their migration to some extent: they still migrated as a single zone, but to the region of α_2-globulins.

During fat absorption in normal subjects the concentrations of primary

Table VIII. Properties of Primary Particles and Secondary Particles[a]

Property	Primary Particles	Secondary Particles
Density, g/ml	<1.006	<1.006
S_f-Rate	>400	>400
Diameter, mμ	75–600	75–600
Electrophoretic mobility:		
Free	Between α_2-Globulin and albumin	β-Globulin
Paper	Origin	Origin
Starch	α_2-Globulin	β-Globulin
Migration distance[b]	0.60	0.23
Flocculation[c]	Top	Bottom
Lipid composition, wt %:		
Cholesterol	6	6
Phospholipids	10	7
Triglycerides	84	87
Fatty acid composition of phospholipids, %:[d]		
16:0 (12.4)[e]	40.0	37.7
18:0 (1.5)[e]	22.1	17.4
18:1 (31.5)[e]	18.1	29.3
18:2 (54.8)[e]	12.4	4.1
Other	7.4	11.5
Proteins, wt %	1	1

[a] Data from Refs. 11, 12, and 16.
[b] Assuming the migration distance of albumin to be 1.00.
[c] In 0 to 5% polyvinylpyrrolidone.
[d] Particulate fat was collected during alimentary lipemia caused by ingestion of corn oil.
[e] Concentration (%) in corn oil.

and secondary particles in plasma varied independently. The amounts of primary particles reached a maximum in 6 hr and then decreased. The secondary particles, however, gradually increased throughout alimentary lipemia. During the late stages of fat absorption only the secondary particles were observed in plasma.

The physicochemical and chemical characteristics of the primary and secondary particles are presented in Table VIII.

Originally Bierman et al. (12), on the basis of centrifugation data, estimated that the primary particles have a minimal diameter of 200 mμ and an S_f-rate of 1000, the corresponding values for secondary particles being 70 mμ and 400, respectively. However, recent, more detailed, studies undertaken by Bierman's group together with Lindgren's group (16) require some revision of this concept. The size of electrophoretically and ultracentrifugally fractionated primary and secondary particles from subjects fed corn oil were determined by the use of the electron microscope. Results indicated a considerably broader particle-size distribution than had been previously estimated. Clumping of particles during preparative centrifugation at low temperatures can yield operational estimates of size that differ from observations with the electron microscope. A comparison of the particle-size distribution of primary and secondary particles from the same plasma showed a range in diameter of 75 to 600 mμ for each type of particle. Apparently the secondary particles have a somewhat larger median particle diameter than the primary particles.

Both types of particles are rather similar in gross chemical composition (12). They are composed mainly of triglycerides and small amounts of cholesterol and phospholipids, the latter being somewhat more abundant in primary particles. However, their fatty acid compositions reflect the nature of ingested fat differently (12, 74), as shown in Fig. 2. During absorption the ratio of linoleic acid to oleic acid in the triglycerides of the primary particles in the peak of their formation practically reached the ratio of corn oil. However, in the triglycerides of the secondary particles this ratio was similar to that of body fat, and though it gradually shifted upward as absorption proceeded, it remained much lower than that of corn oil. The fatty acid composition of phospholipids in the primary and secondary particles from plasma practically did not reflect the fatty acid composition of ingested fat (Table VIII).

Whereas the origin of the primary particles in the bloodstream is, no doubt, the lymph chylomicrons, the origin of secondary particles is not clear. At first, Gordis (74) and Bierman et al. (12) considered the liver to be a possible origin, on the basis of experiments by Kay and Entenman (78). These authors observed the formation of "chylomicronlike" bodies in perfused rat livers. However, only livers from fed rats can synthesize

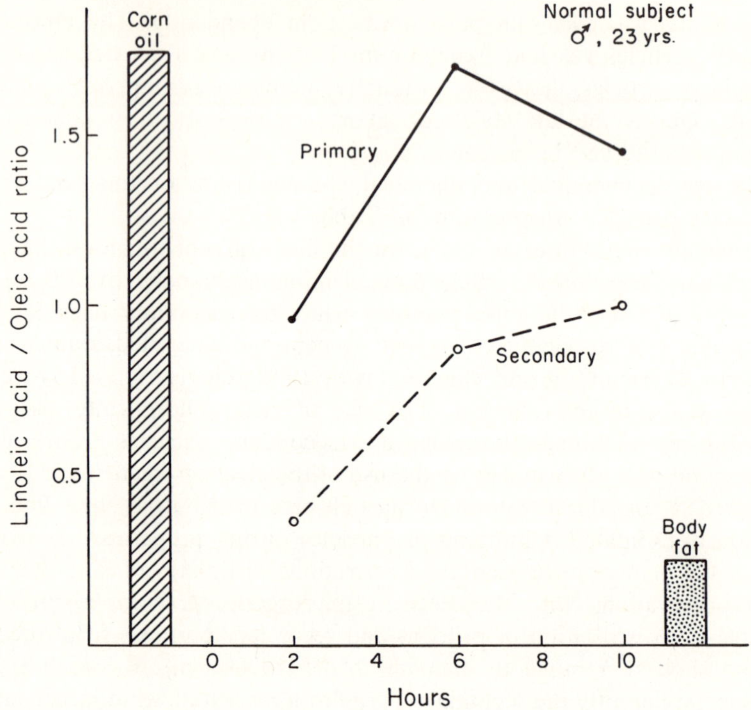

Fig. 2 Linoleic acid to oleic acid ratios in corn oil, in primary- and secondary-particle triglycerides after corn-oil feeding (normal 23-year-old male), and in body fat (adipose tissue). (Reproduced from Ref. 12 with permission.)

and release "chylomicronlike" bodies into perfusing blood. There was no net increase in glycerides in the perfusate when the livers of fasting rats were studied.

In 1966 Bierman and Strandness (79) concluded that secondary particles are derived from primary particles. This was based on experiments performed on dogs with ^{14}C-labeled chylomicrons (primary particles). A substantial number of radioactive secondary particles were isolated from hepatic vein plasma during constant intraperitoneal infusions of ^{14}C-labeled lymph containing primary particles almost exclusively. The specific activity of the secondary-particle triglycerides ranged from 50 to 80% of the infused lymph-chylomicron triglycerides, which indicated dilution with endogenous triglycerides. In each dog this specific activity remained constant throughout the infusion period of 1 to 1.5 hr. The extent of the conversion of primary particles to secondary particles varied during the perfusion period. At the beginning of the perfusion 70 to 100% of the primary particles were converted to secondary particles, but during the main course of the perfusion the conversion rate was only 40 to 50%. Again secondary particles predominated in the postinfusion samples. On the other hand, secondary particles were produced in a peripheral artery during infusion of the lymph into the femoral artery of a hepatectomized, partially eviscerated dog. A substantial number of secondary particles were demonstrated in the plasma sample obtained during the infusion of a distal arterial limb.

Secondary particles were also recovered from the thoracic-duct lymph of a dog during the earliest phases of fat absorption after a 72-hr fast. As absorption progressed, primary particles rapidly became predominant. Thus by the fifth hour virtually all the fat particles in the lymph were primary particles. Secondary particles also formed *in vitro* as lymph combined with particle-free plasma.

These observations indicate that the transformation of primary particles to secondary ones may occur without liver participation and strongly suggest that secondary particles are the result of the interaction of lymph primary particles (chylomicrons) with plasma triglyceride-containing lipoproteins. In general it appears that the fatty acid composition of lymph-chylomicron triglycerides tends to acquire the composition of the ingested fat, especially during the peak of absorption. However, if the compositions of the digested and body fats are extremely different (e.g., coconut oil with a high content of short-chain saturated fatty acids), the fatty acid compositions of lymph-chylomicron triglycerides and ingested fat are dissimilar. The triglycerides of chylomicrons isolated from the bloodstream have as a rule less resemblance to the fatty acid composition of ingested fat. This may result from the dilution of chylomicrons by nonalimentary particles or by other types of particulate fat, which in turn may be the altered chylomicrons (secondary particles). It seems that the experiments of Kay and Entenman (78) at least suggested the possibility that the liver in normal organisms forms some endogenous particulate fat (VLDL with $S_f > 400$).

C. Structure of Chylomicrons and Lipid Composition of Substructural Units

Electron-microscopic examination of chylomicrons has revealed their uniform structural organization. Each chylomicron appears to be a moderately dense globule with a core. It is bordered by a denser rim, or surface coat, which may be a continuous (80) or interrupted (81) structure. The appearance of this surface coat depends to some extent on the methods by which the chylomicrons are prepared and fixed and even on the type of fat digested during chylomicron collection (82, 83). The surface coat of rat chylomicrons collected from thoracic-duct lymph during corn-oil digestion measured 50 to 100 Å in width when sectioned transversely (83). The origin of the surface coat is subject to speculation. Is it a piece of plasma membrane pinched off during the extrusion of the lipid particles from the intestinal cell into the extracellular space or has it another origin? High-resolution electron micrographs do show the presence of a surface coat differing from the core material but not resembling plasma membrane (73, 82, 84). With rare exceptions, there are no structures that can be interpreted as the plasma "unit membranes" (83). Most likely, therefore, the chylomicron coat is not a modified plasma membrane.

Chylomicron coats, which apparently have a rather firm structure, have been successfully isolated by Zilversmit (73, 84, 85) and Huang and Kuksis (86). Chylomicrons, suspended in water, were frozen (—40°C) and thawed several times until a layer of oil floated on the top of the aqueous phase (73, 86). The oil was separated from the subnatant by low-speed centrifugation. This fraction represents the core material. When the aqueous subnatant was subjected to ultracentrifugation at 100,000 *g*, the surface-coat fraction formed a pellet in the bottom of the tube.

A second method of isolating the surface coat, referred to as rotary evaporation (85), consists of drying the washed chylomicron suspension in a flash evaporator rotated in a water bath. The residue is rehydrated by the addition of water, and the evaporation is repeated. This cycling is repeated several times until the chylomicrons have visibly broken up into an oil phase and a turbid aqueous layer. The oil, or core fraction, and the surface coat are separated by centrifugation, as in the first procedure.

The lipid compositions of lymph chylomicrons and of their cores and surface coats are presented in Table IX (from Zilversmit, 73, 84). On the average the surface coat represents 5% of the total chylomicron weight. The rest, which is core, consists of triglycerides, some cholesteryl esters, and a small amount of free cholesterol. Hardly any protein or phospholipid is present. On the other hand, the protein content of the surface coat is 5% (dog) to 12% (human). Among the lipids the most prominent are phospholipids which constitute from 53% (human) to 82% (rat) of the total lipids. Whereas the amounts of triglycerides and free cholesterol are substantial, cholesteryl esters are either present in rather small amounts or not at all (85).

Huang and Kuksis (86) obtained similar results when they studied the lipid composition of dog-chylomicron cores and surface coats: the core contained 90 to 96% triglycerides, 0.7 to 1.9% free cholesterol, 0.2 to 0.5% cholesteryl esters, 0.9 to 3.5% free fatty acids, and 1.4 to 6.1% diglycerides, but no phospholipids; the lipids of the surface coat contained 58 to 75% phospholipids, 20 to 35% triglycerides, 2 to 5% free cho-

Table IX. Lipid Composition of Lymph Chylomicrons and Their Cores and Surface Coats[a]

		Lipid Composition[b]					
Species	Fraction	TG	PL	TC	FC[b]	EC	Pr[c]
Man ($n^d = 1$)	Chylomicron	96.5	2.9	0.6			0.6
	Surface coat	43.0	52.8	4.8			11.5
Rat ($n^d = 2$)	Chylomicron	95.6	4.1	0.3			
	Surface coat	15.8	81.3	3.0			
Rat ($n^d = 2$)	Chylomicron	95.5	4.2	0.3	0.2	0.1	
	Surface coat	16.0	81.5	3.0	3.0	0.0	
Dog ($n^d = 4$)	Chylomicron	96.0	3.6	0.8			0.6
	Core	99.4	Traces	0.5			0.0
	Surface coat	17.0	74.6	8.5			5.4
Dog ($n^d = 2$)	Chylomicron	95.0	3.9	0.8	0.6	0.2	
	Core	99.0	0.0	0.5	0.2	0.3	
	Surface coat	20.0	72.0	7.9	7.9	0.0	

[a] Data from Refs. 73 and 84. Abbreviations: TG, triglycerides; PL, phospholipids; TC, total cholesterol; FC, free cholesterol; EC, esterified cholesterol; Pr, proteins.
[b] Percentage of total lipids.
[c] Percentage of total weight.
[d] Number of experiments; values for compositions are averages.

lesterol, 1 to 2% free fatty acids, and 2 to 3% diglycerides, but little or no cholesteryl esters.

The main difference between the data presented by Zilversmit (73, 84, 85) and Huang and Kuksis (86) is quantitative rather than qualitative; at least in some instances this may be due to small differences in the techniques of isolating the chylomicron core and surface coat. The amount of protein present in the surface coat according to Huang and Kuksis (86) is 20 to 30%, or two to three times the values reported by Zilversmit (73).

Experimental conditions (temperature) and the methods of isolation to some extent influence the lipid compositions of chylomicron cores and surface coats; for example, the triglycerides of surface coats prepared by freezing and thawing contain higher amounts of saturated fatty acids than does the same fraction isolated by rotary evaporation at room temperature (85). Moreover, surface coats prepared by freezing and thawing contain more triglycerides and total cholesterol, and less phospholipids, than do those prepared by rotary evaporation at room or higher temperatures. However, Zilversmit (85) observed such a shift between the core and the surface coat only for cholesteryl esters. Surface coats isolated by rotary evaporation at different temperatures also vary in their cholesteryl ester content, which is higher in coats isolated at 2°C than it is in those isolated at 25 or 40°C.

Nonetheless there are some intrinsic differences in the composition of chylomicron surface coats, and they are related to particle size (73, 84, 87). Chylomicrons isolated from the thoracic duct of dogs fed corn oil or cream were further fractionated to different particle sizes (140, 140–200, and 200 mμ) by centrifugation in a sucrose gradient (88). The small chylomicrons contained more proteins, phospholipids, free cholesterol, and cholesteryl esters than did the large ones. If proteins and polar lipids are concentrated on their surfaces, one would expect that with a decrease in particle size there would be an increase in surface area as well as an increase in the relative amounts of proteins and polar lipids.

Zilversmit (73) and Huang and Kuksis (86) studied the phospholipid composition of dog-chylomicron surface coats. Zilversmit found that the phospholipid fraction consisted of 75 mole % lecithin, 12 mole % phosphatidylethanolamine, 5 mole % sphingomyelin, and 3 mole % lysolecithin. This composition was the same regardless of change in diet (corn oil or cream). Huang and Kuksis reported almost identical results, lecithin accounting for an average of 85% of the phospholipids, the cephalins (mostly phosphatidylethanolamine) for an average of 10% and sphingomyelin and lysolecithin for an average of 3% each.

As indicated in Section II.B, the fatty acid composition of triglycerides in human-lymph chylomicrons actually mirrors the composition of ingested fat. The lipid cores of chylomicron triglycerides, diglycerides, and free fatty acids contain about the same proportions of fatty acids as the ingested fat (Table X). However, the triglycerides (also diglycerides and free fatty

Table X. Fatty Acid Composition of Triglycerides in Chylomicron Cores and Surface Coats after Corn Oil Feeding[a]

		Composition (%)					
		Dog Chylomicrons[b]		Human Chylomicrons		Rat Chylomicrons[b]	
Fatty Acid	Corn Oil	Core[c]	Surface[d]	Core	Surface	Core	Surface
14:0	<0.1	0.2 (12)	1.6 (13)	3.2	9.0	0.4	0.7
16:0	11	12 (31)	46.5 (39)	16	58	10.8	39.5
18:0	2.6	1.8 (14)	9.6 (19)	3.6	13	1.5	6.0
18:1	30	29 (30)	16 (22)	29	9.8	29.5	20
18:2	55	54.5 (1.9)	23.5	40	5.5	56.5	34
Saturated, total	14	14 (64)	57.7 (77)	27	84	12.7	46.2

[a] Data from Ref. 73.
[b] Average of two experiments.
[c] Values in parentheses represent concentrations reported for the whole chylomicron, rather than the core, after feeding cream with the following fatty acid composition: 14:0, 14%; 16:0, 31%; 18:0, 15%; 18:1, 28%; 18:2, 2.7%; saturated, 62%.
[d] Values in parentheses represent concentration after feeding cream (see footnote c).

acids) of the surface coat contain relatively more saturated fatty acids than does the core or ingested fat. The surface-coat triglycerides and diglycerides are characterized especially by an increased proportion of palmitic acid, regardless of whether the diet consists of corn oil or cream [or butterfat (86)]. However, the dietary influence on the fatty acid composition of surface-coat glycerides can be noted in the higher content of myristic or linoleic acid after cream or corn-oil feeding, respectively. The predominant accumulation of saturated glycerides in the surface coats of chylomicrons may be to some degree affected by the method of isolation, thus representing an artifact (85). However, it is not ruled out that this phenomenon is related in some way to the critical spatial requirements in the tightly packed surface coat (86).

In general the cholesteryl esters of the chylomicron core have the same fatty acid pattern as the surrounding glycerides (86). On the other hand, the fatty acid compositions of phospholipids in chylomicron surface coats and lymph-serum lipids after removal of the chylomicrons are relatively unaffected by the composition of ingested triglycerides. Zilversmit (85) used dogs to compare the fatty acid patterns of some phospholipids isolated from the chylomicron surface coat with those of lymph and plasma lipoproteins after the removal of chylomicrons (clear lymph and plasma). The lecithin of the chylomicron surface coat contains substantially more linoleic acid, and less arachidonic acid, than does the lecithin of lymph lipoproteins. Although the lecithin and phosphatidylethanolamine isolated from dog-chylomicron surface coats contain about equal proportions of saturated and unsaturated fatty acids, the sphingomyelin is composed primarily of saturated fatty acids (86). The sphingomyelin of the surface coat is unusual since it contains little long-chain fatty acids (fatty acids with 20 or more carbon atoms) compared with the sphingomyelin of plasma or clear lymph. It is also characterized by a high content of palmitic acid. The difference in the fatty acid composition of phospholipids from chylomicron surface coats and lymph subnatant indicates that at least a substantial portion of the surface lipids is not acquired by random absorption of extracellular phospholipids and that most likely the surface coat of chylomicrons originated intracellularly (85).

D. Alteration of the Chemical Composition of Chylomicrons under Pathologic Conditions

Most abnormalities in plasma-lipid concentrations can be accounted for by changes in lipoprotein concentrations and vice versa (89). It is believed that in most diseases the alteration of lipoprotein levels in plasma occurs without substantial alterations in chemical composition and structure. Therefore, in some instances, the plasma levels of the various lipoprotein classes are measured by determining either cholesterol or phosphorus in separated fractions. However, certain metabolic disorders are connected with alterations in the chemical compositions of lipoproteins, including particulate fats, and some of them are discussed in this section.

Swahn (76) observed that the serum chylomicrons of subjects with alimentary hyperlipemia migrate in free electrophoresis as α_2-globulins and that patients with essential hyperlipemia have two types of chylomicron: particles that migrate with α_2-globulins and particles that migrate with β-globulins. He also noted the presence of the α- and β-types of chylomicron in the lipemias of the nephrotic syndrome and diabetes. Patients with myxedema have the β-type of chylomicron only. Lipid analysis of total serum and serum after centrifugal removal of chylomicrons suggests that the lipid compositions of α- and β-chylomicrons are different.

Jobst and Schettler (66) also studied the electrophoretic pattern and chemical composition of serum particulate fat in different types of lipemia: alimentary lipemia in normal subjects and lipemias after fat load in patients with "essential hyperlipemia" and the nephrotic syndrome. In starch-block electrophoresis the mobility of particulate fats from pathologic sera is in the area between α_2- and β-globulins, whereas the mobilities of the particulate fats of normal subjects with alimentary lipemia are between those of α_1- and α_2-globulins.

The chemical compositions of particulate fats isolated from pathologic and normal serums are significantly different (Table XI). Particulate fats from normal subjects contain 87% triglycerides which comprise only 55 and 56% of the particulate fats of patients with essential hyperlipemia or the nephrotic syndrome, respectively. The latter disease is characterized by a high level of cholesteryl esters and somewhat higher levels of free cho-

Table XI. Lipid Composition of Particulate Fat in Essential Hyperlipemia and the Nephrotic Syndrome[a]

Condition	Particulate-Fat Composition (%) Triglycerides	Phospholipids	Free Cholesterol	Cholesteryl Esters
Essential hyperlipemia	55.6	11.7	6.0	26.7
Nephrotic syndrome	55.2	8.5	6.8	29.5
Normal subjects–chylomicrons	86.5	5.8	2.8	4.9

[a] Data from Ref. 66.

lesterol and phospholipids than those of particulate fats isolated from normal subjects. Cornwell et al. (90) observed that chylomicrons isolated from patients with idiopathic hyperlipemia or the hyperlipemia of diabetes mellitus had lower ratios of fatty acid esters to cholesterol than do chylomicrons isolated from normal subjects during alimentary lipemia. Also the ratios of cholesterol to phospholipids in the particulate fats of most patients were higher than those in normal subjects. The authors consider that particulate fats in patients are a mixture of alimentary chylomicrons and particulate fats of endogenous origin (VLDL).

Nye and Schultz (77) used polyvinylpyrrolidone gradient columns (74) to separate particulate fat from the plasma of patients with hyperlipemia of various etiologies into two types. Particulate fats that move to the top of the column were called α-particles due to their α-globulin mobility in starch-block electrophoresis (91). This type corresponds to the primary particles of Bierman et al. (12). The particulate fats that stay at the bottom of the column were called β-particles due to their electrophoretic mobilities. According to the method of isolation, the β-particles should be analogous to the secondary particles of Bierman et al. (12) isolated from normal subjects. However, in chemical compositions the α- and β-particles isolated by Nye and Schultz (77) differ significantly from the primary and secondary particles isolated by the same method from normal subjects, in spite of the fact that in starch-block electrophoresis they behave similarly to primary and secondary particles.

Plasma from subjects with hyperlipemia can be divided into two groups (77): in group 1 β-particles predominate or are present exclusively, whereas in group 2 α-particles predominate (Table XII). Patients with diabetes, carbohydrate induced hyperlipemia, and the nephrotic syndrome (not shown in the table) have predominantly or exclusively β-particles, which are characterized by a relatively high content of phospholipids (20% of total lipids) and cholesterol, both esterified and free. The amount of triglycerides varies from 47 to 58% of the total particle lipids. In patients with fat-induced hyperlipemia and severe hyperlipemia associated with alcoholism and probable pancreatitis α-particles predominate. They contain less phospholipids and cholesterol than do β-particles, and their triglyceride content varies from 60 to 73% of their total lipids. Thus α- and β-particles isolated from pathologic serum have different chemical compositions. Both of these types of particulate fat also differ from the primary and secondary particles isolated from the plasma of normal subjects by Bierman et al. (12) (Table VIII).

Ahrens et al. (92, 93) distinguish between two forms of primary hyperlipemia: fat-induced lipemia and carbohydrate-induced lipemia, identified by their response to a low-fat, high-carbohydrate diet. In fat-induced

Table XII. Particulate-Fat Composition in Hyperlipemic States[a]

Clinical Diagnosis	Particle Type	Total Lipid in 100 ml Plasma (mg)	Lipid Composition[b]			
			TG	PL	CE	FC
		Group I				
Diabetes	$\beta > \alpha$	1800	57	19	18	4
Diabetes	β	3540	47	21	18	
Carbohydrate-induced hyperlipemia	β	1530	58	20	13	5
		Group II				
Fat-induced hyperlipemia	$\alpha > \beta$	6000	62	16	13	4
Fat-induced hyperlipemia	$\alpha > \beta$	8620	73	11	9	3
Fat-induced hyperlipemia	$\alpha > \beta$	3420	71	11	11	4
Alcoholism, probable pancreatitis	$\alpha > \beta$	7100	60	16	11	7

[a] Data from Ref. 77.

[b] Percentage of total lipids; calculated by using a factor of 25 for converting phosphorus to phospholipids and 1.69 for converting esterified cholesterol to cholesteryl esters. Abbreviations: TG, triglycerides; PL, phospholipids; CE, cholesteryl esters; FC, free cholesterol.

lipemia plasma clears when fat intake is reduced. In carbohydrate-induced lipemia grossly visible lipemia is maintained despite a low-fat diet. Such diverse responses to diet suggest that the particulate fats accumulated in hyperlipemic patients may have different origins. Ahrens et al. concluded that "hyperlipemic chylomicrons" in fat-induced hyperlipemia [type I of the familial hyperlipoproteinemias of Fredrickson et al. (89, 94–96)] are indistinguishable by physicochemical behavior from the chylomicrons of normal subjects. In fatty acid compositions they mirror the ingested fat (corn oil).

On the other hand, Ahrens and Spritz (93) and Bierman et al. (11) demonstrated the presence of a specific form of particulate fat in the plasma of patients with carbohydrate-induced lipemia [type IV, probably also types III and V of the familial hyperlipoproteinemias of Fredrickson et al. (89, 94–96) and Kinsell et al. (97)]. When these patients consume an ordinary mixed diet (including fat and carbohydrates), two types of fat particle can be found. Their properties are similar to those of the primary and secondary particles present in normal subjects during alimentary lipemia (Section II.B). However, when the patients are placed on a fat-free, high-carbohydrate diet for a prolonged period, the plasma contains only one type of particulate fat—a type that is distinctly different from the primary and secondary particles recovered from plasma during fat ingestion (see Table XIII). This new type of particulate fat has been called hyperlipemic particles by Bierman et al. (11) and endogenous particles by Ahrens and Spritz (93). These particles were isolated on polyvinylpyrrolidone density-gradient columns.

Hyperlipemic particles have more than twice the cholesterol content of primary and secondary particles. Approximately two-thirds of the cholesterol is present in the esterified form, and the phospholipid content is elevated. Subsequently the content of triglycerides decreases to 70% of the total lipids of fat particles. The fatty acid composition of their triglycerides is characterized by a high content of saturated fatty acids, especially by the presence of a high amount of palmitic acid (11). Ahrens and Spritz (93) also observed a dramatic alteration in the fatty acid patterns in all

Table XIII. Physiochemical Properties of Hyperlipemic Particles, Other Fat Particles, and Very-Low-Density Lipoproteins[a]

Property	Primary Particles	Secondary Particles	Hyperlipemic Particles[b]	VLDL
S_f-Rate	>400	>400	>400	20–400
Electrophoretic behavior on starch:				
Migration distance[c]	0.60	0.23	0.51	0.57
Mobility	α_2	β	α_2–β	α_2
Migration in flocculation[d]	Top	Bottom	Diffuse spread from bottom	None–bottom
Lipid composition, wt %:				
Total cholesterol	8	7	20	32
Phospholipids	6	3	10	18
Triglycerides[e]	86	90	70	50
Proteins, wt %	1	1	3	9

[a] Data from Ref. 11.
[b] The endogenous particles of Ahrens and Spritz (93).
[c] Albumin = 1.00.
[d] In polyvinylpyrrolidone.
[e] See Table XIV for the fatty acid composition of triglycerides in hyperlipemic particles.

major serum-lipid classes in patients with carbohydrate-induced lipemia on a carbohydrate-rich diet. The content of linoleic acid decreases several times in triglycerides, cholesteryl esters, free fatty acids, and phospholipids, whereas the amounts of those fatty acids that may form by lipogenesis from carbohydrate in the mammalian organism (98, 99) increase several times.

According to Bierman et al. (11), there is a distinct difference between the fatty acid patterns of triglycerides isolated from hyperlipemic particles and those isolated from adipose tissue (Table XIV). An even greater

Table XIV. Fatty Acid Composition of the Triglycerides in Hyperlipemic Particles and Adipose Tissue[a]

	Concentration (%) in Triglycerides	
Fatty Acid	Hyperlipemic Particles	Adipose Tissue
14:0	3.8	2.7
16:0	38.6	25.4
16:1	7.5	7.4
18:0	6.2	3.4
18:1	37.4	48.2
18:2	7.3	12.3

[a] Data from Ref. 11.

difference has been observed in two patients by Ahrens and Spritz (93), who found adipose-tissue triglycerides to contain 30 and 36% of linoleic acid, whereas those of hyperlipemic (endogenous) particles contained only 5%. These observations indicate that the triglycerides of hyperlipemic particles do not originate in adipose-tissue lipids; most likely they are derived from hepatic lipogenesis, which is characterized by the biosynthesis of predominantly saturated fatty acids (99).

Fredrickson and associates (94, 100) reported that in type III hyperlipoproteinemia (carbohydrate-induced lipemia) the plasma contains an abnormal form of VLDL with β-globulin mobility in starch-block electrophoresis. The normal mobility of the VLDL class is α_2 (pre-β—see Section III.C). At present it is difficult to say whether there is any relationship between hyperlipemic particles and this unusual VLDL form.

The additional types of particulate fat in primary lipemias (essential hyperlipemias) or the lipemias of diabetes mellitus and the nephrotic syndrome require further study. At present the general picture is confusing due, in part, to poor documentation of the types of hyperlipemia studied as well as the exact conditions under which they have been investigated (diet). The appearance of hyperlipemic particles with an unusual chemical composition in patients with carbohydrate-induced lipemia is rather firmly established. However, the presence of such particulate fats in some other lipemias is yet to be established. Furthermore there are conflicting observations concerning the chemical alteration of particulate fats in fat-induced lipemias.

III. VERY-LOW-DENSITY LIPOPROTEINS

A. Definition

Very-low-density lipoproteins (VLDL) were also named (40) low-density lipoproteins-2, or LDL_2, in an attempt to unify the nomenclature of lipoproteins. Some authors (89, 101, 102) considered it necessary to emphasize the difference in VLDL and LDL mobilities in paper electrophoresis. The VLDL class was called pre-β-lipoproteins since they move slightly further from the origin than the LDL fraction, which in turn has the mobility of β-globulins. The α-globulins and α-lipoproteins move still further from the origin.

From the biophysical point of view the term "very-low-density lipoproteins" refers arbitrarily to lipoproteins with $d < 1.006$ g/ml. The border line between VLDL and LDL expressed as flotation rates is S_f 20. Thus lipoproteins with a flotation rate higher than 20, measured at a solution density of 1.063 g/ml, are considered VLDL; those with lower flotation rates are considered to be LDL. The border line between VLDL and lipoproteins whose density is even lower, mainly particulate fats, is rather confused. Gustafson, Alaupovic, and Furman (13) included in the VLDL class S_f 400–5000 and even $S_f > 5000$ particles. Hatch (103) excluded S_f 100–400 lipoproteins from VLDL because they trail in paper electrophoresis. Presently the tendency is to consider that all endogenous lipoproteins with $d < 1.006$ g/ml are VLDL with an S_f-rate of 20 to 10^5 (24) and that "proper" VLDL have an S_f-rate of 20 to 400. Most investigators (10) still consider the upper border line to be S_f 400 for VLDL and $S_f > 400$ lipoproteins to be particulate fats. These designations are followed in this chapter particularly because the electrophoretic mobilities of S_f 20–400 and $S_f > 400$ lipoproteins are different. Thus the term "very-low-density lipoproteins" is applied in this chapter to S_f 20–400 lipoproteins.

B. Lipid Composition of S_f 20–400 VLDL in Normal Subjects

Table XV shows the lipid compositions of VLDL reported by various authors. Lipoproteins in the VLDL class are composed of 8 to 10%

Table XV. Lipid Composition of Very-Low-Density Lipoproteins

	References										
Characteristic	64	104–106	62, 63, 107	108, 109	13, 14			7		20	19
Source	Serum[a]	Plasma[a]	Serum	Serum and plasma[a]	Serum			Serum		Serum	Serum
Physiologic conditions	Nonfasting[b]		Fasting		Normal subjects after high-fat meal and fasting hyperlipemic patients			Nonfasting		Fasting	Fasting females
Density, g/ml	<1.019	<1.005	<1.006	<1.019	<1.006[d]					<1.006	<1.006
S_f-Rates[c]	>10	10–100	20–400	12–400	100–400	50–100	20–50	20–400			0–400[e]
Chemical composition, %:											
Lipids	92.9	90.0	90	85	94.7	90.7	87.8			90.0	92.0
Proteins	7.1	10.0	10	15	5.3	9.3	12.2			10.0	8.0
Lipid composition, % of total lipids:											
Total glycerides	55.7	53.7	56	37.3[f]	68.3	59.3	56.8	58.0[g]	49.5[h]	56.7	49.3[i]
Cholesterol:											
Total	16.8	17.6	17	16.5	14.8	17.5	17.9			24.4	20.7
Free	6.5	7.5	8	7.5	3.9	4.2	4.4				9.0
Esterified	10.3	10.1	9	9.0	10.9	13.3	13.5				11.7
Cholesteryl esters	17.4	17.1	15	15.2	18.4	22.5	22.8	25.6[g]	17.9[h]		19.8
Free fatty acids			1–2								3.4
Hydrocarbons											2.7
Unidentified lipids				17.9							2.0
Total "neutral lipids"	79.6	78.3	80	77.9	90.6	86.0	84.1				86.2
Glycolipids											0.3
Phospholipids	19.3	20.9	20	19.4	11.6	13.9	13.1	19.6[g]	25.0[h]	18.9	12.4

[a] Pooled samples.
[b] May be slightly contaminated with fat particles.
[c] Measured at a solution density of 1.063 g/ml unless otherwise indicated.
[d] The anhydrous densities of S_f 100–400, S_f 50–100, and S_f 20–50 lipoproteins are reported to be 0.96, 0.98, and 0.99 g/ml, respectively.
[e] Measured at a solution density of 1.006 g/ml.
[f] Triglycerides only.
[g] Males.
[h] Females.
[i] The glyceride composition (in percentage of total lipids) is as follows: triglycerides, 45.6%; diglycerides, 2.3%; monoglycerides, 1.4%.

protein and 90 to 92% lipid. Reported values for the protein content vary from 7.1 to 15%. Where a protein content of 15% was observed, the analyzed fraction contained S_f 12–400 lipoproteins with $d < 1.019$ g/ml. Although on the border line between VLDL and LDL relatively small amounts of S_f 12–20 lipoproteins were reported, the high protein levels in these fractions can be partially explained by the contribution of these lipoproteins (*d* 1.006–1.019 g/ml). On the other hand, Bragdon et al. (64) indicated that their fraction, containing 7.1% protein, might have been slightly contaminated by fat particles.

The VLDL class is characterized by a high content of triglycerides. Since most investigators based triglyceride values on glycerol determinations in the neutral-lipid fraction, lower glycerides—diglycerides and monoglycerides—may also be included. According to Skipski et al. (19), lower glycerides represent 3.7% of the total VLDL lipids. Therefore the values reported for triglycerides should be considered as values for total non-phosphorus-containing glycerides. In Table XV they have been tabulated as "glycerides," rather than triglycerides, which in turn have a 3 to 4% lower value. The amount of VLDL triglycerides ranges from 41 to 54% of the total lipids. Ewing et al. (7) reported glyceride values of 49.5% in women and 58.0% in men. However, most determinations made on pooled samples from both sexes had values just between these two extremes. The average values for total glycerides, disregarding the sex difference, were 54 to 55% of the total lipids, and the values for triglycerides were 50 to 51%.

The lipid moiety of VLDL contains small amounts of free fatty acids (1–3.4% of the total lipids).

Total cholesterol was reported as 16.5 to 24.4% of the total VLDL lipids. With the exception of the values reported by Gustafson et al. (13, 14), the free-to-esterified cholesterol ratios were rather high, ranging from 1 : 1.1 to 1 : 1.7. They were much higher than those observed in total serum or plasma (1 : 2.4 to 1 : 2.5) (110).

The values reported for VLDL phospholipids vary. Gustafson et al. (13, 14) and Skipski et al. (19) reported low values, 12 to 14% of the total lipids, whereas Ewing et al. (7) reported 25% of the total lipids in VLDL isolated from females. Most authors reported 19 to 21%.

The data from three reports presented in Table XV require some additional comments. Ewing et al. (7) reported significant sex differences in the lipid composition of VLDL. The amounts of glycerides and cholesteryl esters in males were 58 and 25.6%, respectively; in females, 49.5 and 17.9%, respectively. On the other hand, females had significantly higher values for phospholipids.

Gustafson et al. (13, 14) studied the VLDL subclasses and observed that, as anhydrous density increased and S_f-values decreased, the amounts of protein increased and the total lipids decreased. The decreases in the total lipid content resulted mainly from a decrease in the glycerides.

Skipski et al. (19) demonstrated that the VLDL class contains some minor lipid components: diglycerides and monoglycerides, hydrocarbons, and glycolipids (cerebrosides).

Table XVI presents the phosholipid composition of VLDL. The most

Table XVI. Phospholipid Composition of Very-Low-Density Lipoproteins

	References			
Characteristic	111	112, 113	114	19
Source	Serum	Serum	Plasma	Serum
Physiologic conditions	Fasting	Postabsorptive		Fasting females
Density, g/ml	<1.019	<1.006	<1.007	<1.006
S_f-Rate[a]		20–400	20–400	0–400[b]
Phospholipids in total-lipid extract, %		18.9	21.0	12.4
Phospholipid composition, % of total phospholipids:				
Lecithin	66.2	74.0	65–70	59.7
Lysolecithin	5.1		2–15	5.0
Sphingomyelin	23.1	18.3	15–20	14.8
Phosphatidylethanolamine	5.7[c] (with phosphatidylserine)	7.7[c] (with phosphatidylserine)	2–10[c] (with phosphatidylserine)	4.6
Phosphatidylserine				1.5
Phosphatidylinositol				3.6
Polyglycerophosphatides and phosphatidic acid				7.6
Unidentified				3.2
Choline-containing phospholipids	94.4	92.3		79.5

[a] Measured at a solution density of 1.063 g/ml unless otherwise indicated.
[b] Measured at a solution density of 1.006 g/ml.
[c] "Cephalin" in original papers.

abundant phospholipids are lecithin and sphingomyelin (60–74% and 15–23% of the total phospholipids, respectively). All authors reported relatively low values for lysolecithin (about 5%) and moderate amounts of non-choline-containing phospholipids. Skipski et al. (19) demonstrated recently that approximately 20% of the total VLDL phospholipids consists of phosphatidylethanolamine, phosphatidylserine, phosphatidylinositol, and non-nitrogen-containing phospholipids (polyglycerophosphatide and phosphatidic acid), which were incompletely characterized.

In general the VLDL class has the highest triglyceride levels of all the lipoproteins, with the exception of particulate fats. In fasting conditions about 7.5% of the total plasma lipids are associated with VLDL (19).

C. Familial Hyperlipoproteinemia and VLDL

Familial hyperlipoproteinemia, or essential hyperlipemia, is a disease in which there is an abnormal increase in certain plasma lipids because of a hereditary defect in lipid or lipoprotein metabolism (94). Since all plasma lipids are present as lipid–protein complexes, or lipoproteins, an increase in lipid concentration actually represents an increase in one or more of the several classes of lipoproteins. Therefore the term "hyperlipoproteinemia" coined in 1966 by Fredrickson and Lees (94, 95) for this disease is more correct than the commonly used term "hyperlipemia." The word "familial" indicates that this disease is common in a family or is inheritable and distinguishes it from other lipemias (or, more correctly, hyperlipoproteinemias), which may be of physiologic (alimentary lipemia) or pathologic nature (as a secondary manifestation of other primary diseases: diabetes, the nephrotic syndrome). In familial hyperlipoproteinemia the levels of definite classes of lipoproteins (particulate fats, VLDL, LDL) are affected, as manifested by an increase in plasma triglycerides, cholesterol, or both. Other lipids may also be somewhat increased.

Although it is believed that in most cases only the levels of specific lipoprotein classes are affected, in some instances there is a substantial alteration in the lipid composition of lipoproteins; even new types of lipoproteins can be synthesized. In Section II.D I discussed the appearance of endogenous, or hyperlipemic, particles in serum from patients with carbohydrate-induced hyperlipemia (familial hyperlipoproteinemia, probably type IV of Fredrickson and Lees), and in Chapter 12, Section IX, a general and more detailed consideration of lipoproteins in familial hyperlipoproteinemia is presented. The present section covers an instance of lipoprotein abnormality, a hyperlipoproteinemia involving biochemical alterations in the lipid components. It can be caused by abnormalities in various parts of the lipid-transport system and lipid metabolism, and, on the basis of clinical and laboratory observations, can be separated into several familial types.

Ahrens et al. (92, 93) distinguished between two main clinical types of this disorder: fat-induced and carbohydrate-induced hyperlipoproteinemia (see Section II.D). More recently Fredrickson et al. (89, 94–96) proposed a classification based mainly on alterations in lipoprotein patterns which distinguished five types of hyperlipoproteinemia:

Type I: characterized by an increase in chylomicrons, but not pre-β-lipoproteins (VLDL). Because of the increase in chylomicrons, plasma levels of triglycerides are significantly elevated. This type of lipoproteinemia is fat induced.

Type II: characterized by an increase in β-lipoproteins (LDL). No lipoproteins are present in the fraction with $d < 1.006$ g/ml with β-globulin mobility in paper electrophoresis. Pre-β-lipoproteins (VLDL) may or may not be increased. Because of the increase in β-lipoproteins, there is a significant increase in serum cholesterol (familial hypercholesterolemia).

Type III: lipoproteins with β-globulin mobility are present in the ultracentrifugal supernatant fraction with $d < 1.006$ g/ml (see below); also the β- (LDL) and pre-β-lipoprotein (VLDL) levels are elevated. This type may be induced by a high-carbohydrate diet. The serum levels of cholesterol and, to a lesser extent, triglycerides are elevated (familial hypercholesterolemia with hyperglyceridemia).

Type IV: Pre-β-lipoproteins (VLDL) are increased, but typical chylomicrons are absent. The level of serum triglycerides (and cholesterol) is higher than normal. This is a carbohydrate-inducible form.

Type V: The levels of both chylomicrons and pre-β-lipoproteins (VLDL) are elevated. The amount of serum triglycerides, and to a lesser extent cholesterol, is increased. This is a fat- and carbohydrate-inducible form.

Whereas it is presently believed that most of the abnormalities in familial hyperlipoproteinemias are expressed as alterations in the levels of the various classes of lipoproteins, in type III hyperlipoproteinemia fraction an abnormal VLDL ($d < 1.006$ g/ml) has been found. Very-low-density lipoproteins from normal subjects and patients with other dyslipoproteinemias have α_2 (pre-β) mobility in preparative starch-block electrophoresis. In type III hyperlipoproteinemia there are two distinct VLDL components (94, 100): one with the usual α_2-mobility in electrophoresis (α-VLDL), and the other with a slower β-mobility (β-VLDL). The lipid and protein composition of α-VLDL is similar to that of conventional VLDL. The slower β-VLDL component has a different lipid and protein content. Partial delipidation of this lipoprotein revealed only β-lipoproteins (similar treatment of normal VLDL reveals both α- and β-lipoproteins). The β-VLDL resemble normal LDL with 4 to 10 times more triglycerides. The rate of triglyceride turnover in β-VLDL is very slow and comparable to that of LDL, whereas the turnover of α-VLDL in patients with hyperlipoproteinemia and in normal subjects is very rapid.

Hazzard, Lindgren, and Bierman (115) studied the lipid composition of VLDL isolated from patients with type III and type IV hyperlipoproteinemia. The authors analyzed the lipids of the whole S_f 20–400 VLDL fraction as well as the S_f 100–400, S_f 60–100, and S_f 20–60 subfractions. In the case of type IV hyperlipoproteinemia (endogenous hyperlipemia) the relative lipid composition of the whole VLDL fraction and the above mentioned subfractions was similar to that of normal subjects (see Table XV). On the other hand, in type III hyperlipoproteinemia ("broad-β disease") there was a definite alteration in lipid composition: in the whole VLDL fraction and in each subfraction the level of cholesteryl esters was approximately twice that of the corresponding fractions isolated from normal subjects, and there was a reciprocal decrease in triglyceride content. However, the total relative content of these two nonpolar lipids (cholesteryl esters + triglycerides) was similar in both type III and type IV hyperlipoproteinemia and in normal subjects. The relative content of polar lipids (phospholipids, cholesterol) and proteins was not affected in the patient with type III hyperlipoproteinemia.

Hazzard et al. (115) also observed an abnormal electrophoretic mobility (β instead of pre-β) in the S_f 20–60 subfraction isolated from the patient with type III hyperlipoproteinemia. The other two VLDL subfractions (S_f 60–100 and S_f 100–400) had the normal mobilities of pre-β-lipoproteins. It is obvious that the alteration in the electrophoretic mobility of the S_f 20–60 subfraction cannot be accounted for by changes in the level of cholesteryl esters since similar changes did not affect the electrophoretic mobilities of the S_f 60–100 and S_f 100–400 subfractions. It is more likely that the protein moiety of the S_f 20–60 subfraction is responsible.

The chemical alteration of particulate fats in familial hyperlipoproteinemia has been considered in Section II.D.

IV. LOW-DENSITY LIPOPROTEINS

A. General Characteristics

Low-density lipoproteins [LDL, or S_f 0–20 lipoproteins: $d = 1.006$–1.0635 g/ml, mean hydrated density 1.032 g/ml (105)] are also called β-lipoproteins because of their β-globulin mobility in paper, starchblock, and moving-boundary electrophoresis (38, 98). Vandenheuvel (40) classifies them as low-density lipoproteins-1, or LDL_1.

The LDL fraction isolated by ultracentrifugation at a solution density of 1.0635 g/ml contains small amounts of S_f 0–3 lipoproteins with a mean hydrated density of 1.05 g/ml (38) and α_2-mobility in starch-block (116) or free electrophoresis (104, 117). These are designated as high-density lipoproteins-1, or HDL_1. The amount of HDL_1 in the total LDL fraction does not exceed 5%. The lipid composition of HDL_1 as an entity, together with those of other HDL fractions, is discussed in Section V.

Table XVII. Lipid Composition of Low-Density Lipoproteins

Characteristic	References: 64	104, 105	62, 63, 107	108[a]	20	7	19
Source	Serum[b]	Plasma[c]	Serum	Serum and plasma[c]	Serum	Serum	Serum
Physiologic conditions	Mostly nonfasting		Fasting		Fasting	Nonfasting	Fasting females
Density, g/ml	1.019–1.063	1.038	1.006–1.063	1.019–1.063	1.006–1.063	1.006–1.063	1.006–1.063
S_f-Rate	0–10	3–9	0–20	0–12			0–20
Chemical composition, %:							
Lipids	79.4	78.1	75	80–83	78.0		79.2
Proteins	20.6	21.9	25	17–20	22.0		20.8
Lipid composition, % of total lipids:							
Total glycerides	9.1	11.4	16	(11.1)	9.0	7.8[d] 8.4[e]	7.3[f]
Cholesterol:							
Total	40.2	40.3	40	(35.6)[g]	58.8		39.9
Free	10.1	9.5	12	(10.2)			12.0
Esterified	30.1	29.8	28	(25.4)			27.9
Cholesteryl esters	50.8	50.4	47	(43.0)		55.6[d] 52.9[e]	47.1
Free fatty acids			1				1.1
Hydrocarbons							0.7
Unidentified lipids				(19.0)			2.2
Total "neutral lipids"	70.0	71.3	66				70.4
Glycolipids							0.2
Phospholipids	29.5	28.7	24	(21.0)	32.0	29.6[d] 30.4[e]	27.8

[a] Figures in parentheses are estimated by the author of this review.
[b] Pooled and individual samples.
[c] Pooled samples.
[d] Males.
[e] Females.
[f] The glyceride composition (in percentage of total lipids) is reported as follows: triglycerides, 6.2%; diglycerides, 0.4%; monoglycerides, 0.7%.
[g] Value not precise (estimated from a diagram of LDL lipid composition).

The LDL class represents a family of closely related lipoprotein complexes, rather than a well-defined chemical entity.

B. Lipid Composition of LDL in Normal Subjects

Low-density lipoproteins, the most abundant lipoproteins in human plasma or serum, are the major carriers of cholesterol, both esterified and free. The detailed composition of LDL is shown in Table XVII. The total amount of lipids in LDL ranges from 75 to 80% and that of proteins, from 20 to 25%.

The most abundant lipid in LDL is cholesterol, comprising 40 to 59% of the total lipids. From 24 to 31% of the total cholesterol is free cholesterol; the remaining is esterified.

The amount of phospholipids in the lipids of LDL is 28 to 30% according to the majority of the investigators. In earlier publications Lindgren and associates (62, 63, 107) reported that phospholipids comprised 24% of the total lipids. New values published from the same laboratory by Ewing, Freeman, and Lindgren (7) are 29.6% for males and 30.4% for females.

The amount of glycerides (mostly triglycerides) ranges from 7 to 11%. The higher values (16%), originally reported by Lindgren et al. (62, 63, 107), have also been revised to 7.8% for males and 8.4% for females (7).

The LDL lipids also contain some minor components: free fatty acids (1%), diglycerides and monoglycerides, hydrocarbons, and traces of glycolipids (ceramide monohexosides).

Levy and co-workers (118) separated LDL by polyanion (sulfated amylopectin) precipitation and studied their composition. Their values of 77.3 and 22.7% for the concentrations of lipids and proteins, respectively, are similar to those reported for LDL isolated by ultracentrifugation. However, the values reported by Levy et al. for the breakdown of the total-lipid fraction (phospholipids, 36.1%; cholesteryl esters, 37.3%; glycerides, 13.6%) substantially differ from those reported by the majority of the investigators who separated LDL by ultracentrifugation. The discrepancies may be due to the method of isolation or the relatively small number of experiments (duplicate determinations were made on a single pooled sample).

The phospholipids of LDL are characterized by high contents of lecithin and sphingomyelin (Table XVIII). The amounts of lecithin range from 64 to 69% of the total phospholipids according to the majority of reports, although Polonovski (114) observed a lower range (50–60%). Most authors agree that the amount of sphingomyelin ranges from 25 to 26%.

Table XVIII. Phospholipid Composition of Low-Density Lipoproteins

Characteristic	Reference 111	112	114		19
Source	Serum	Serum	Plasma		Serum
Physiologic conditions	Fasting	Postabsorptive			Fasting females
Density, g/ml	1.019–1.063		1.007–1.019	~1.040	1.006–1.063
S_f-Rate		0–20	12–20	2–12	0–20
Phospholipids in total-lipid extract, %		25.0	21.0		27.8
Phospholipid composition, % of total phospholipids:					
Lecithin	66.3	68.8	50–55	50–60	63.7
Lysolecithin	4.1		10–15	5–15	2.7
Sphingomyelin	25.3	25.6	25–35	25–35	25.9
Phosphatidylethanolamine	} 4.4[a]	} 5.6	} 2–10	} 5–10	2.2
Phosphatidylserine					0.8
Phosphatidylinositol					1.6
Polyglycerophosphatides and phosphatidic acid					2.0
Unidentified phospholipids					1.1
Choline-containing phospholipids	95.7	94.4			92.3

[a] "Cephalin" in the original paper.

These values correspond to the lowest range reported by Polonovski (114). Phillips (111) and Skipski et al. (19) reported that lysolecithin comprises 4 and 3%, respectively, of the total phospholipids, whereas Polonovski's (114) data show up to 15%.

The values of Polonovski may be unrealistic since Nelson (113) reported an average of 3% lysolecithin in whole serum, and Williams, Kuchmak, and Witter (119) reported 8.2%. Other authors found averages of 6.8% (120) and 6.2% (121) in the plasma of healthy subjects. Since lipoproteins with $d > 1.21$ g/ml are the major contributors of lysolecithin to whole serum (see Section VI), low values for LDL lysolecithin are more realistic. However, some loss of lysolecithin by washing lipid extracts is not excluded. On the other hand, some hydrolysis of lecithin with the production of lysolecithin during lipoprotein isolation, lipid extraction, and even storage of lipid extracts may be responsible for the high lysolecithin levels reported for LDL.

Choline-containing phospholipids comprise on the average 90 to 95% of the total LDL phospholipids. Small amounts (2–10%) of phosphatidylethanolamine and phosphatidylserine are also present. Skipski et al. (19) reported the presence of non-nitrogen-containing phospholipids: phosphatidylinositol (1.6%), a phospholipid of the cardiolipin type, and phosphatidic acid, averaging together 2%.

V. HIGH-DENSITY LIPOPROTEINS

A. General Characteristics

Lipoproteins that float between *d* 1.0635 and 1.210 g/ml are called high-density lipoproteins (HDL), or α-lipoproteins, since their mobilities are similar to those of α-globulins in paper, free, and starch-block electrophoresis (38, 122). Two main HDL classes are separated by ultracentrifugation: high-density lipoproteins-2 (HDL_2, $S_{f(1.125)}$ 0–4) and high-density lipoproteins-3 (HDL_3), with mean hydrated densities of 1.09 and 1.14 g/ml, respectively (123).

Ewing, Freeman, and Lindgren (7) suggested that the designation "S_f" be limited to flotation rates measured at a solution density of 1.063 g/ml and that flotation rates at other densities be designated by the symbol "F" with a subscript indicating the density. For HDL characterization these authors suggested using *d* 1.20 g/ml, at which the flotation rates of HDL_2 and HDL_3 are $F_{1.20}$ 3.5–9 and $F_{1.20}$ 0–3.5, respectively.

As stated in the preceding section, LDL separated at a solution density of 1.0635 g/ml contain a fraction classified by many workers as high-density lipoproteins-1 (HDL_1, S_f 0–3), which has a mean hydrated density of 1.05 g/ml (38). The HDL_1 fraction is present in small quantities in normal serum, and little is known about its chemical composition.

Barclay et al. (5, 6, 124) described two additional minor HDL groups whose densities are between those of HDL_1 and HDL_2. Their flotation rates are $S_{f(1.125)}$ 4–12 and $S_{f(1.125)}$ 12–20, and their hydrated densities are 1.079 and 1.071 g/ml, respectively. They are not always present in normal serum, the $S_{f(1.125)}$ 12–20 lipoproteins having been found in 47% of analyzed samples, and the $S_{f(1.125)}$ 4–12 lipoproteins in 86%. They have not been chemically characterized or separated in pure form. When present in plasma or serum, they are usually chemically analyzed together with HDL_2 or with HDL_{2+3} if the two main HDL classes are not separated.

In 1966 Alaupovic et al. (21) isolated and chemically characterized a new high-density lipoprotein that floats at solution densities between 1.210 and 1.250 g/ml and has a hydrated density of 1.155 g/ml. They called it very-high-density lipoprotein-1, or $VHDL_1$. Its lipid composition is discussed in Section VI.

On the basis of immunochemical and electrophoresis studies Levy and Fredrickson (122) concluded that alterations in the distribution of lipoproteins, especially HDL_2 and HDL_3, may occur during the preparative ultracentrifugation of serum. They concluded that HDL, or α-lipoproteins, may exist in two forms: α-LP_A, present in HDL, HDL_2, and HDL_3; and

α-LP_B, present only in HDL_3 and in lipoproteins with $d > 1.21$ g/ml. Only small amounts of α-LP_B are present in fresh plasma, and apparently LP_A is the native form in which these lipoproteins circulate (122). Containing relatively less lipid and having a greater density, α-LP_B was shown to be formed from α-LP_A by partial delipidation. It was concluded that repeated ultracentrifugation of α-LP_A was always associated with its partial transformation to α-LP_B. The HDL_2 peak obtained in the analytical ultracentrifuge consists only of LP_A, whereas the HDL_3 peak consists of α-LP_B and some LP_A. The authors speculated that LP_A is a "dimer," or a larger aggregate than α-LP_B, which represents a "monomer" form of HDL. The transformation from "dimer" LP_A to "monomer" α-LP_B is associated with loss of some lipids. Levy and Fredrickson (122) postulated that the HDL_2 and HDL_3 values obtained by preparative and analytical ultracentrifugation may be artifactual rather than real and therefore represent the transformation of α-LP_A to α-LP_B in human plasma.

Scanu and Granda (31), who confirmed the transformation of different HDL classes during recentrifugation, did not question the existence of HDL_2 and HDL_3 as two entities in normal blood. They observed that when purified HDL_2 or HDL_3 were respun for 48 hr, only 74% of HDL_2 and 72% of HDL_3 were recovered in native form. Their lipid contents differed from the remainder, which underwent some degree of degradation, during which part of the lipids were lost. However, the proteins of the degradation products were identical in terms of the amino acid and carbohydrate composition and N-terminal and COOH-terminal residues. The lipid-poor heavy lipoproteins recovered in the bottom 1 ml of the preparative tube after recentrifugation had the immunochemical characteristics of HDL protein. They were called very-high-density lipoproteins (VHDL). These were also detected immunochemically in the ultracentrifugal residue ($d > 1.21$ g/ml) after the separation of other HDL fractions and also in fresh serum adjusted directly to *d* 1.21 g/ml. The VHDL are analogous to, but probably not identical with, the $VHDL_1$ fraction of Alaupovic et al. (21).

Scanu and associates (31, 32, 125) showed that succinylation, acetylation, or treatment with sodium dodecyl sulfate (SDS) will reduce the protein moieties of HDL_2, HDL_3, and VHDL to subunits with average molecular weights of 27,500 (early estimated value 21,500). They estimated that HDL_2, HDL_3, and VHDL contain an average of six to seven, four to five, and two subunits respectively. This suggests that HDL_3 is derived from HDL_2 by the removal of lipid and the concomitant release of two protein units. The latter in turn contribute to the formation of VHDL. Whether such conversions represent ultracentrifugal artifacts or are operative physiologic processes *in vivo* is not clear.

The studies of Levy and Fredrickson (122) and Scanu and Granda (31) demonstrate that some changes in HDL_2 and HDL_3 may occur during the ultracentrifugal separation of HDL and can result in lower recoveries of these fractions. The work of Scanu and Granda (31, 125) also suggests a possible relationship between different HDL classes. The relationship between HDL_2 and HDL_3 is evidently more complicated. Differences in the antigenic behavior of HDL_2 and HDL_3 under certain conditions were explained by Scanu (31) as resulting from the presence of a lipid-poor protein in HDL_3.

Shore and Shore (126) have demonstrated that HDL_2 and HDL_3 contain comparable quantities of two types of polypeptide subunits with different amino acid sequences, but HDL_2 may have a third polypeptide type that is not present in HDL_3. Gofman (127), Barclay (6, 128), and their associates observed that in various physiologic and pathologic states either the HDL_2 or the HDL_3 fraction is selectively affected; this may indicate that HDL_2 and HDL_3 are indeed two entities.

B. Lipid Composition of HDL

Several investigators have studied the chemical composition of HDL_2 and HDL_3 together, as shown in Table XIX. (See also addendum at the end of this chapter, p. 574.) These lipoproteins are characterized by a high protein content, the protein-to-lipid ratio being usually 1.0 or slightly higher. The average results from six laboratories indicate that HDL are composed of 48.2% lipid and 51.8% protein.

The main components of the HDL lipid moieties are phospholipids, which comprise 42 to 51% of the total lipids (average 46%). High-density lipoproteins are also rich in cholesterol, mainly esterified. The actual values for cholesteryl esters range from 21 to 45% of the total lipids (average 32.4%). Some authors (19) emphasized the increase in the ratio of esterified to free cholesterol in HDL as compared with LDL. This has been supported by others, with some exceptions. The reported amounts of glycerides vary from 6 to 20% of the total HDL lipids. The highest value, 20%, was recently revised after improvement of the technique for lipoprotein separation. The new values are 7.0% for men and 6.2% for women (7). High-density lipoproteins also contain small amounts [2% (19) to 6% (107) of the total lipids] free fatty acids. Small amounts of other lipids—diglycerides, monoglycerides, hydrocarbons, and ceramide monohexosides—are present (19).

Three groups of investigators (19, 31, 129) who studied the lipid composition of HDL_2 and HDL_3 as separate fractions reported more lipid in HDL_2 than in HDL_3 (Table XIX). They also noted quantitative differences in the lipid compositions of HDL_2 and HDL_3. The latter have relatively more glycerides, free fatty acids, ceramide monohexosides, but less total, esterified, and free cholesterol. Hillyard et al. (129) found that HDL_3 had a relatively higher content of phospholipids than did HDL_2, but Skipski et al. (19) found the opposite to be true, as did Scanu and Granda (31). In general these three groups agree on the basic chemical differences between HDL_2 and HDL_3, with the exception of the total-phospholipid content. However, the investigators do not agree on the absolute values for the individual lipid classes and total proteins in HDL_2 and HDL_3.

Lindgren et al. (17) studied the chemical composition of a minor HDL class, HDL_1. They characterized HDL_1 as being high in lipid and low in protein (75 and 25% of the total lipoproteins, respectively). In this respect HDL_1 is more like LDL than HDL_2 or HDL_3. Lindgren and co-workers reported that the lipid moiety of HDL_1 contains high amounts of total cholesterol, mainly free. The relative amount of free cholesterol in HDL_1 was higher than it was in LDL or HDL_2 and HDL_3. The content of cholesteryl esters in HDL_1 was approximately the same as that reported by some authors for HDL_{2+3} [Lindgren et al. (17) reported lower values for cholesteryl esters in HDL_{2+3} than in HDL_1]. The amount of phospholipids in HDL_1 (20% of the total lipids) is much lower than those in other HDL classes and even lower than that in LDL. Since HDL_1 has a relatively high content of free fatty acids, it is similar to other HDL in this respect. Thus HDL_1 has a unique lipid composition, unlike other HDL and LDL. Further confirmation of the chemical composition of HDL_1 is necessary since the data of Lindgren et al. (17) were based on only two cases.

Table XX shows the phospholipid compositions of HDL_{2+3}, HDL_2, and HDL_3 analyzed separately. Lecithin constitutes 70 to 81% (average 73.6%) of the phospholipids in HDL_{2+3} according to reports from five different laboratories [the higher limit apparently also includes lysolecithin (113)], so the actual range of values for lecithin was narrower. The lysolecithin level was reported to be 3 to 11%. The high values for lysolecithin may be unrealistic, as in the case of LDL (see Section IV.B). According to most investigators, the sphingomyelin content varies from 12 to 14%, only Polonovski (114) having reported lower values in HDL_{2+3} (5–10%). The combined content of phosphatidylethanolamine and phosphatidylserine ranges from 4 to 9%, Polonovski reporting an average of 9%. However, there is no doubt that in some cases, when phosphatidylethanolamine and phosphatidylserine are analyzed together as "cephalins," phosphatidylinositol is also included in the "cephalin" group. If so, then the lower range (19) will increase 6%, since HDL_{2+3} contain 2% phosphatidylinositol. Small quantities (2%) of other non-nitrogen-containing phospholipids are present in HDL_{2+3} (19).

Skipski et al. (19) studied the phospholipid composition of HDL_2 and

Table XIX. Lipid Composition of High-Density Lipoproteins[a]

Component[f]	Source, Fraction, and References							
	Serum (129)[b]			Serum	Plasma	Serum (17, 38, 62, 63, 107)[c]		Plasma
	HDL_{2+3}[g]	HDL_2[h]	HDL_3[i]	HDL_{2+3} (64)[j]	HDL_{2+3} (105)[k]	HDL_1[l]	HDL_{2+3}[m]	HDL_{2+3} (108)[n]
Chemical composition, %:								
Total lipids, %	45.4	66.7	40.6	52.9	50.5	75.0	~50.0	
Proteins, %	54.6	33.3	59.4	47.1	49.5	25.0	~50.0	
Lipid Composition % of total lipids:								
Glycerides:								
Total	13.5	11.7	14.2	12.0	10.3	19.0	20.0	6.3
Cholesterol:								
Total	26.0	30.7	24.3	24.2	25.7	41.2	20.2	20.4
Free	6.8	10.0	5.6	4.1	5.7	21.0	6.0	7.9
Esterified	19.2	20.7	18.7	20.1	20.0	20.2	14.2	12.5
Cholesteryl esters	32.4	35.0	31.5	34.0	33.7	34.0	24.0	21.1
Free fatty acids						5.0	6.0	
Hydrocarbons								
Unidentified lipids								18.9
Total "neutral lipids"						79.0	56.0	
Glycolipids								
Phospholipids	47.3	43.4	48.8	49.7	49.3	20.0	44.0	45.8

Table XIX. (Continued)

	Source, Fraction, and References								
	Serum (31, 125)[d]			Serum HDL_{2+3} (7)[o]	Serum HDL_{2+3} (7)[p]	Serum HDL (21)[q]	Serum (19)[e]		
Component[f]	HDL_{2+3}	HDL_2	HDL_3				HDL_{2+3}[r]	HDL_2	HDL_3
Chemical composition, %:									
Total lipids, %	48.1	59.4	44.0				42.3	47.7	31.8
Proteins, %	51.9	40.6	56.0				57.7	52.3	68.2
Lipid Composition % of total lipids:									
Glycerides:									
Total	17.2	4.5	5.1	7.0	6.2	11.9	6.2	6.1	6.7
Triglycerides							4.5	4.6	4.4
Diglycerides							0.9	0.7	1.4
Monoglycerides							0.8	0.8	0.9
Cholesterol:									
Total	24.4	18.7	12.9			22.4	27.3	28.2	24.7
Free	6.5					8.1	6.7	7.4	4.6
Esterified	17.9					14.3	20.6	20.8	20.1
Cholesteryl esters	30.2			44.7	44.1	24.1	34.8	35.1	33.8
Free fatty acids						4.8	2.1	1.7	3.2
Hydrocarbons							0.9	0.9	0.8
Unidentified lipids							2.3	2.2	2.4
Total "neutral lipids"						48.9	53.0	53.4	51.5
Glycolipids							0.4	0.2	1.1
Phospholipids	46.1	36.2	26.2	43.1	43.4	51.1	41.8	42.4	40.9

[a] Unless otherwise indicated, the densities of the HDL fractions are as follows: HDL_{2+3}, 1.063–1.210 g/ml; HDL_2, 1.063–1.125 g/ml; HDL_3, 1.125 to 1.21 g/ml.

[b] Measured in the postabsorptive state.

[c] Fasting sample.

[d] Fasting males.

[e] Fasting females.

[f] Measured as percent of total lipids.

[g] Density 1.063–1.22 g/ml. Composition calculated on the basis of experimental data obtained for HDL_2 and HDL_3.

[h] Density 1.063–1.107 g/ml.

[i] Density 1.107–1.22 g/ml.

[j] Pooled and individual samples, predominantly nonfasting.

[k] Male subject.

[l] S_f 0–3 lipoprotein.

[m] Density 1.063–1.20 g/ml.

[n] Pooled samples. Values estimated by the author

[o] Nonfasting males.

[p] Nonfasting females.

[q] Fasting males and females. The HDL fraction had a density of 1.095–1.210 g/ml.

[r] Composition calculated on the basis of data obtained for HDL_2 and HDL_3.

Table XX. Phospholipid Composition of High-Density Lipoproteins

	Fraction and Reference[a]						
Component	HDL_{2+3}[b] (111)	HDL_{2+3}[c] (112)	HDL_{2+3}[d] (114)	HDL_{2+3}[e] (125)	HDL_{2+3}[f] (19)	HDL_2[g] (19)	HDL_3[h] (19)
Phospholipids in total-lipid extract, %		41.4		46.1	41.8	42.4	40.9
Phospholipid composition, % of total phospholipids:							
Lecithin	69.9	80.8	70–75	70.3	74.4	73.8	77.1
Lysolecithin	11.2		6–10	11.2	2.9	2.0	5.4
Sphingomyelin	13.6	11.8	5–10	12.6	13.2	14.5	9.2
Phosphatidyl-ethanolamine	} 5.2	} 7.4	} 7–10	} 5.9	3.1	3.3	2.5
Phosphatidyl-serine					0.8	0.9	0.6
Phosphatidyl-inositol					2.4	2.4	2.4
Polyglycero-phosphatides and phosphatidic acid					2.2	2.2	2.0
Unidentified phospholipids					0.9	0.9	0.8
Choline-containing phospholipids	94.7	92.6		94.1	90.5	90.3	91.7

[a] Serum samples unless otherwise indicated; HDL_{2+3} density 1.063–1.210 g/ml unless otherwise indicated.
[b] Fasting samples; HDL_{2+3} density > 1.063 g/ml.
[c] Samples collected during postabsorptive state; HDL_{2+3} density 1.075–1.203 g/ml.
[d] Plasma samples.
[e] Fasting males.
[f] Fasting females; calculated on the basis of HDL_2 and HDL_3 composition.
[g] Fasting females; HDL_2 density 1.063–1.125 g/ml.
[h] Fasting females; HDL_3 density 1.125–1.210 g/ml.

HDL_3 in detail and found that the latter contains more lecithin and lysolecithin than does HDL_2, which has relatively greater amounts of sphingomyelin. No essential differences were noted in the other phospholipid components of these two fractions.

C. Deficiency of HDL in Blood

Several cases of familial HDL deficiency were described by Fredrickson and co-workers (89, 130–133) and by Kahlke (134). This rare disease was also called hypo-α-lipoproteinemia, or Tangier disease (after Tangier Island in Chesapeake Bay, where the first cases were observed). Since it is generally described in Chapter 12, only the effect of the disease on lipid metabolism is discussed here. The most striking feature is the almost complete lack of plasma HDL. Preparative ultracentrifugation revealed the absence of the lipoproteins with *d* 1.063 to 1.210 g/ml. No stainable lipid material was seen in the α-region after paper-electrophoresis separation of lipoproteins. When the original samples were concentrated several times, small amounts of HDL were found, their level being approximately 2 to 8% of normal values. However, it was later discovered that the HDL from patients with Tangier disease differ somewhat antigenically from those of normal subjects (135).

The lipid pattern of the reticuloendothelial tissues (spleen, tonsils, lymph nodes, thymus, etc.) is altered: there is a twofold to threefold increase in total lipids in organs rich with reticuloendothelial tissues, due mainly to the accumulation of cholesteryl esters (20–100 times the normal level).

Also affected is the metabolism of chylomicrons, VLDL, and LDL. Small amounts of protein are always present in even very well washed chylomicrons (see Section II and Chapter 13). An HDL peptide was identified in chylomicron proteins (61, 136). It was postulated that HDL may stabilize chylomicrons, facilitate fat absorption, and promote chylomicron clearance. The presence of other peptides in chylomicrons was also demonstrated. The discovery that Tangier disease involves an HDL deficiency indicates that HDL are not essential for chylomicron formation. Patients with Tangier disease were found to have normal fat absorption from the intestine and to produce chylomicrons that behave physically like normal particles. However, the chemical composition of these chylomicrons appears to be altered, the cholesterol level being drastically decreased. The amounts of cholesteryl esters and free cholesterol are decreasd by a factor of 4 to 5. In some patients the removal of chylomicrons from the circulation is retarded. Apparently, though not essential for the formation of chylomicrons and their subsequent removal, HDL are involved in some way in the metabolism of chylomicrons.

Levy, Lees, and Fredrickson (137) observed that in normal subjects and in patients with hyperlipoproteinemia there is a reciprocal relationship between the concentrations of VLDL (pre-β-lipoproteins) and HDL (α-lipoproteins). For example, if the plasma-triglyceride concentration is increased two to three times because of increased VLDL in normal subjects fed a high-carbohydrate diet, the concentrations of HDL fall from 20 to 60%. Experimental heparin-induced lipolysis *in vivo* caused the decrease or disappearance of VLDL with simultaneous rise in HDL concentrations. When Levy et al. extracted pre-β-lipoproteins with ether and subjected the product to paper electrophoresis, two lipoprotein bands with the mobilities of α- and β-globulins were observed. No pre-β-lipoproteins were seen. The β-lipoproteins (LDL), by contrast, retained their mobility after identical treatment with ether. When pre-β-lipoproteins were extracted with ethanol–ether, paper electrophoresis showed an α-lipoprotein band and a band remaining at the origin, consistent with denatured β-lipoproteins. These experiments suggest that pre-β-lipoproteins contain in their complexes intact α- and β-lipoproteins.

A variety of antigen–antibody test systems showed that VLDL isolated in the native state cross-react only with antiserums to LDL. However, after the VLDL fraction was extracted with ether, which apparently removes some triglycerides and causes dissociation of the lipoprotein complex, the presence of HDL protein was demonstrated. Thus these tests indicate the presence of HDL and LDL proteins in VLDL. The hypothesis that VLDL are complexes of LDL, HDL, and triglycerides was proposed originally by Lindgren et al. (17) almost 15 years ago on the basis of the composition, mainly lipid, of the various lipoprotein classes.

In Tangier disease the alterations in the lipid composition of plasma, which is lacking in HDL, are more complicated than expected. Since HDL participates in the formation of VLDL, the latter are also absent. The plasma concentrations of triglycerides were abnormally high in patients on a regular diet. If patients were fed a high-carbohydrate diet for several days, the triglyceride concentration rose even higher (up to 600 mg/100 ml of serum). Such increases occurred in spite of the fact that these patients have no VLDL.

The only electrophoretically detectable plasma lipoproteins were in a single β-migration band on paper. This band widened and became more intensely stained when endogenous-glyceride concentrations increased. However, the forward boundary never reached the pre-β-lipoprotein range of migration. In the ultracentrifuge these components, with $d < 1.006$ g/ml, behave like VLDL.

Thus in patients with Tangier disease HDL and the usual VLDL are absent, and the LDL fraction accumulates high amounts of triglycerides, which result in their having the density properties of VLDL. As a consequence the concentrations of cholesterol and phospholipids are low, and the plasma triglycerides are elevated. The LDL ratio of lecithin to sphingomyelin is higher than it is in control subjects.

Fredrickson et al. (89) considered that the absence of HDL from plasma was probably responsible for the deposition of cholesteryl esters in reticuloendothelial tissues. There was no indication, however, that the reticuloendothelial tissues in patients with Tangier disease increased the biosynthesis of cholesterol or that such tissues engorged HDL. It is more likely that HDL enhance the stability of the circulating particles containing glycerides, cholesterol, and other lipids. When these lipoproteins are missing, the unstable particles are more susceptible to removal by phagocytosis. The cholesteryl esters probably represent the steadily increasing residue of such phagocytic uptake of lipid particles.

D. Abnormalities of HDL in Abetalipoproteinemia

Abetalipoproteinemia, a rare hereditary disease, is characterized by the absence from plasma of all lipoproteins with $d < 1.0635$ g/ml and by profound alterations in HDL. This disease is also known as acanthocytosis, or the Bassen–Kornzweig syndrome [after the physicians who reported the first two cases in 1950 (138)]. At least 20 cases have been described in the literature, and the general pathology has been reviewed by Farquhar and Ways (139) and Kahlke (140).

A typical manifestation is that most of the erythrocytes have irregular shapes with protruding "thorns" called acanthocytes ("akantha" in Greek means "thorn" or "spine"). The disease is called acanthocytosis by Singer, Fisher, and Perlstein (141). Abetalipoproteinemia is also characterized by malabsorption of fat (steatorrhea), degenerative neurological processes, and pigmentary degeneration of the retina.

The most consistent physiologic abnormality is the absence of several major systems for fat transport in the blood. No chylomicrons are found in the plasma or the lymphatic spaces of the intestines even after fatty meals or fat loading (142–145). When a patient received a fat load (1.4 ml of corn oil per kilogram of body weight) after 34 days on a fat-free diet, there was no visible turbidity in the plasma. There were no changes in cholesteryl ester or phospholipid levels. The levels of triglycerides were affected slightly: in the fasting sample the levels of triglycerides were 2.2 mg/100 ml plasma; 35, 95, 185, and 310 min after administration of corn oil, the levels were 2.4, 4.4, 2.0, and 1.8 mg/100 ml plasma, respectively (144). The lipid content (triglycerides) in the epithelium of the small intestines was 3.5 times higher than normal in the postabsorptive state (145). Evidently lipid transport from the mucosal into the lymphatic system had deteriorated because of the absence of β-lipoproteins, which are necessary for the normal formation of chylomicrons. As discussed in the preceding section, the absence of α-lipoproteins (Tangier disease) does not affect the formation of chylomicrons. However, in patients with abetalipoproteinemia the overall absorption of lipids (144), as determined by fat-balance studies, was 70 to 90% of ingested fat when the total fat intake was 13 to 36 g/day (139). This indicates that a quantitatively significant alternative pathway for fat transport operates in these patients. Some inconclusive evidence suggests that at least some of the long-chain fatty acids are transported to the liver via the portal vein, which normally transports only water-soluble short-chain fatty acids.

The total plasma lipid levels in abetalipoproteinemia were found to be lower [80–285 mg/100 ml (140)] than could be accounted for by the absence of all lipoproteins with $d < 1.0635$ g/ml. The decreases involve all lipid classes but are most notable in cholesterol (19–86 mg/100 ml) and the triglycerides (3–15 mg/100 ml); the total-phospholipid level is 23 to 90 mg/100 ml (140). These data were confirmed by Fredrickson, Levy, and Lindgren (133). There are also alterations in the amounts of lecithin and sphingomyelin, which Phillips (146) found to comprise 59.4 and 31.1%, respectively, of the total plasma phospholipids (average values in three patients) as compared with 68.3% and 20%, respectively, in normal individuals. These observations were confirmed in studies on three other patients by Ways and co-workers (147), who reported that the average values for lecithin and sphingomyelin were 48.8 and 37.2%, respectively, of the total plasma phospholipids. Analysis of the erythrocyte phospholipids also revealed a consistent and significant decrease in the relative and absolute amounts of lecithin and a corresponding increase in sphingomyelin concentration (146, 147). The values for erythrocyte plasmalogens were significantly decreased (147).

Lipoproteins with $d < 1.063$ g/ml are scarce or completely lacking in the plasma or serum of patients with abetalipoproteinemia, as indicated by ultracentrifugation (133, 147), paper electrophoresis (133, 148), and immunoelectrophoresis (147, 149). Dextran sulfate precipitation techniques revealed that the quantity of β-lipoproteins was 15 to 20 mg/100 ml plasma instead of the normal 120 to 570 mg/100 ml plasma (150). There is, however, the possibility that such small amounts of precipitate may result from the precipitation of globulins rather than β-lipoproteins. Furthermore, the possibility that abnormal β-lipoproteins are present cannot be excluded. Separation of serum lipoproteins by ultracentrifugation at d 1.063 g/ml demonstrated, at least in some cases, the presence of a small amount of material in the upper layer of the centrifuge tube (147). The amount was minimal and could have resulted from mixing in the tube during slicing. Ways et al. (147) recovered 0.004 to 0.06 mg/100 ml lipid phosphorus from the upper layers of the centrifuge tubes after the ultracentrifugation of serum from two patients (versus 3.0 to 3.5 mg/100 ml serum in normal subjects). The amounts of cholesterol detected were 0.8 to 2.2 mg/100 ml; serum samples obtained from normal individuals and analyzed simultaneously had values of 98 and 127 mg/ml.

Immunochemical studies demonstrated that serum from patients had no antigenic material to react with antiserum for LDL (147, 151, 152), even when the concentrations of lipoproteins were raised to 10 times the plasma levels (149). However, Lees (153) demonstrated that the plasma of patients with abetalipoproteinemia contains a lipid-free protein that is immunologically similar to the apoprotein of β-lipoproteins. Abetalipoproteinemia may result from a defect in the formation of the complete β-lipoprotein molecule rather than an inability to synthesize the apoprotein moiety of β-lipoproteins.

Levy, Fredrickson, and Laster (149) studied the sera of six patients with abetalipoproteinemia and showed by immunochemical methods that the small amounts of S_f 0–20 lipoproteins that floated at *d* 1.006 to 1.063 g/ml were actually α-lipoproteins (HDL). This abnormal shift in density was thought to result from excessive lipid loading of α-lipoproteins. When whole plasma or lipoprotein fractions with $d < 1.063$ and $d < 1.21$ g/ml, taken from patients with abetalipoproteinemia, were subjected to paper electrophoresis, only one lipoprotein band with the mobility of an α-component was revealed. This occurred even when large amounts of material were placed on the paper strip. Evidently abetalipoproteinemia is characterized by the complete absence of LDL, VLDL, and chylomicrons. The small amounts of lipoproteins that floated at $d < 1.0635$ g/ml were actually altered α-lipoproteins (HDL). In most cases of abetalipoproteinemia the concentrations of α-lipoproteins are below normal levels (133, 147, 151, 154). The following HDL values were reported: in a 17-month-old girl, 80 mg/100 ml serum (151); in a 21-year-old male, 145 mg/100 ml serum (133). The values for normal females and normal males are 437 ± 119 and 275 ± 72 mg/100 ml, respectively (133).

According to Jones and Ways (155) and others (140, 149), in abetalipoproteinemia only one HDL fraction, HDL_3 (*d* 1.110–1.21 g/ml), has substantially decreased in absolute and relative concentrations. The HDL_2 fraction (*d* 1.063–1.110 g/ml) is present in normal, or even increased, amounts (133). Levy et al. (149) considered that the best explanation for the alterations in HDL_2 and HDL_3 levels is an increase in the lipid carried by some of the available apoprotein. This could account for a reduction in the average density of the α-lipoproteins and consequently an unusual ultracentrifugal distribution pattern.

Table XXI shows the lipid and protein compositions of HDL_2 and HDL_3 in three patients with abetalipoproteinemia (7–10 years old) and in normal children and adults. The concentrations of lipid phosphorus, cholesterol, and protein were within the normal ranges in the HDL_2 fraction, but only one-half to one-third the normal levels in the HDL_3 fraction. Although all three patients had normal values for total cholesterol in HDL_2, the relative amounts of esterified cholesterol were below the normal range. From 53 to 57% of the cholesterol is esterified in patients, compared with 70% in normal children and 72 to 83% in normal adults. In patients with abetalipoproteinemia the ultracentrifugal residue ($d > 1.21$ g/ml) contained less phospholipids than did that of normal subjects. The content of total cholesterol in this lipoprotein fraction was close to normal.

The phospholipid composition of whole plasma and the individual lipo-

Table XXI. Composition of Plasma and Lipoproteins in Abetalipoproteinemia[a]

Fraction and Density (g/ml)	Normal Adults		Normal Children, Age 7–9[c]	Patients, Age 7–10[b]		
	Male	Female		J.D.	M.S.	J.G.
			Lipid Phosphorus (mg/100 ml plasma)			
Whole plasma	7.58–9.08	8.63–10.2	9.05			
LDL (<1.063)	3.18–4.28	2.86–3.89	2.99			0.11
HDL_2 (1.063–1.110)	0.53–1.08	0.70–2.40	1.05	0.94	1.10	0.75
HDL_3 (1.110–1.21)	2.02–2.54	2.25–3.11	3.08	0.69	0.79	0.90
Ultracentrifugal residue (>1.21)	0.52–0.78	0.59–0.70	1.01	0.16	0.19	0.24
			Total Cholesterol (mg/100 ml plasma)			
Whole plasma	174–262	220–230	216			
LDL (<1.063)	102–176	112–176	121			3
HDL_2 (1.063–1.110)	10–21	16–34	23	22	24	18
HDL_3 (1.110–1.21)	32–39	33–42	45	18	17	13
Ultracentrifugal residue (>1.21)	4–7	3–6	10	4	2	3
			Cholesteryl Esters (% of total cholesterol in fraction)			
HDL_2 (1.063–1.110)	82, 83	72	70	57	53	54
HDL_3 (1.110–1.21)	87, 87	87	72	70	70	63
			Triglycerides (mg/100 ml plasma)			
Whole plasma	108	37	74			
LDL (<1.063)	42, 83		48			
HDL_2 (1.063–1.110)	2, 2	3	4	1.9	1.2	0.9
HDL_3 (1.110–1.21)	3, 7	4	5	2.7	1.1	0.8
			Proteins (mg/100 ml plasma)			
HDL_2 (1.063–1.110)	18–40	66	30	40	33	20
HDL_3 (1.110–1.21)	125–148	138	146	44	47	55

[a] Data from Ref. 155.
[b] J.G.'s plasma was centrifuged initially at *d* 1.063 g/ml. The plasma from J.D. and M.S. was centrifuged first at *d* 1.110 g/ml. Hence the HDL_2 from J.D. and M.S. might include small amounts of material that floated in the supernatant at *d* 1.063 g/ml.
[c] Pooled sample.

protein classes are shown in Table XXII. As already mentioned, whole plasma from patients with abetalipoproteinemia contains more sphingomyelin and less lecithin than does the plasma of normal adults and children. In HDL_2 and HDL_3 isolated from the plasma of patients the concentration of sphingomyelin was 1.5 to 2 times higher than that in normal adults and children. The relative concentration of lecithin in HDL_2 and HDL_3 was lower than it was in normal subjects.

In the LDL fraction, which included all lipoproteins that floated at *d* 1.063 g/ml (and may not be real LDL, see p. 528), the same trend prevailed: increase in sphingomyelin and decrease in lecithin. However, as in the lipoproteins isolated from the serums of normal adults and children, the increase in the density of the lipoprotein classes (including the ultracentrifugal residue) was accompanied by a decrease in the relative amount

Table XXII. Phospholipid Compositions of Plasma Lipoproteins in Patients with Abetalipoproteinemia[a]

Fraction and Density (g/ml)	Normal Adults[b]	Normal Children, Age 7–9[c]	Patients, Age 7–10 J.D.	M.S.	J.G.
			Lecithin[d]		
Whole plasma	67	66	59	44	52
LDL (<1.063)	65	62		39	45
HDL_2 (1.063–1.110)	71	73	54	47	54
HDL_3 (1.110–1.21)	74	78	59	56	65
Ultracentrifugal residue (>1.21)	33	43	35	31	42
			Lysolecithin[d]		
Whole plasma	7	9	5	7	8
Ultracentrifugal residue (>1.21)	48	32	34	34	32
			Sphingomyelin[d]		
Whole plasma	21	20	30	48	31
LDL (<1.063)	27	30		54	46
HDL_2 (1.063–1.110)	21	22	35	47	39
HDL_3 (1.110–1.21)	17	16	31	38	30
Ultracentrifugal residue (>1.21)	10	14	16	21	23
			Phosphatidylethanolamine[d]		
Whole plasma	4	4	3	1	6
LDL (<1.063)	5	4		3	3
HDL_2 (1.063–1.110)	5	3	0.2	1	1
HDL_3 (1.110–1.21)	5	5	3	2	1
Ultracentrifugal residue (>1.21)	5	6	6	8	0

[a] Data from Ref. 155.
[b] Since no apparent differences were noted, the values from five normal males and two females were presented as averages.
[c] Pooled sample.
[d] % of total phospholipid in fraction.

of sphingomyelin and an increase in lecithin. The relative concentrations of phosphatidylethanolamine in HDL_2 and HDL_3 were lower in serum from the patients.

The fatty acid composition of plasma HDL is also affected in patients with abetalipoproteinemia. The lecithin fatty acids in HDL_2 and HDL_3 isolated from patients differed from those in normal serum mainly in a lower content of linoleic acid (in patients 6.5–12%, in normal subjects 20–34%). The content of oleic acid in lecithin was higher in the plasma of patients.

The sphingomyelin fatty acids in the plasma of three patients studied by Jones and Ways (155) had a high content of nervonic acid (24:1). Despite the lower level of HDL in patients with abetalipoproteinemia, not only the relative but also the absolute amounts of sphingomyelin nervonate were higher in the three patients studied. Accompanying this was both a relative and an absolute decrease in the following long-chain fatty acids: 22:0, 23:0, and 24:0.

Phosphatidylethanolamine fatty acids in normal subjects were characterized by a high content of polyunsaturated fatty acids 20:4 and 22:6. Patients with abetalipoproteinemia had less 20:4.

In normal subjects (155) the predominant fatty acid in cholesteryl esters was linoleic (over 50%). In patients with abetalipoproteinemia the linoleic acid level decreased to 24% even when the diet was supplemented with linoleic acid; accompanying this was an increase in cholesteryl palmitate and cholesteryl oleate.

The fatty acid abnormalities in the plasma of patients with abetalipoproteinemia are partly nonspecific and evidently result from steatorrhea. However, according to Jones and Ways (155), the low levels of HDL and the abnormalities in the distribution of phospholipids probably are specific to abetalipoproteinemia.

VI. ULTRACENTRIFUGAL RESIDUE

A. General Characteristics

After the ultracentrifugal removal of all major lipoproteins from plasma or serum at a solution density of 1.210 g/ml, all plasma proteins, including albumin, accumulate at the bottom of the tubes and are called the ultracentrifugal residue (17, 19, 63). It was logical to expect the presence of free fatty acids in the ultracentrifugal residue, since Kendall (156) in 1941 found that even crystalline serum albumin always contains small amounts of free fatty acids as impurities that could not be removed by recrystallization. The presence of fatty acids in serum albumin was confirmed by Cohn, Hughes, and Weare (157).

Havel, Eder, and Bragdon (158) observed also the presence of lipid phosphorus in the sedimented fraction after they centrifuged serum at *d* 1.21 g/ml. The phospholipid present in this sediment accounted for approximately 10 to 15% of the total serum phospholipids. Later Bragdon, Havel, and Boyle (64) concluded that this phosphorus was part of phosphopeptides rather than phospholipids and that in the fraction with $d > 1.21$ g/ml there were no lipids other than free fatty acids. On the other hand, in the ultracentrifugal residues isolated from the sera of humans, dogs, rabbits, rats, and chickens, Hillyard et al. (129) observed the presence of phospholipids and cholesterol in all fractions with $d > 1.21$ g/ml. Thus the presence of lipids other than free fatty acids in the ultracentrifugal residue was established.

At present the exact nature of the lipid–protein complexes in the ultracentrifugal residue is not known. It is still an open question whether the ultracentrifugal residue contains albumin–free fatty acid complexes along with one or two VHDL (very high density lipoproteins) fractions (21), or whether the presence of lipids other than free fatty acids, and perhaps lysolecithin, results from the transformation of HDL (d 1.063–1.210 g/ml) after ultracentrifugation (122).

A peculiar feature of the lipid composition of the whole ultracentrifugal residue is the high content of lysolecithin (159). The $VHDL_1$ fraction (d 1.210–1.250 g/ml) isolated by Alaupovic et al. (21) had a low content of lysolecithin. Most of the lysolecithin remained in the fraction with $d >$ 1.250 g/ml, which the authors named $VHDL_2$. This fraction also was characterized by a very high protein content. Its lipid moiety was characterized by a high content of free fatty acids (since it included the albumin–free fatty acid complex). Switzer and Eder (160) claimed that the lysolecithin of the ultracentrifugal residue was present in the form of an albumin–lysolecithin complex. They believed that this complex may be the form in which different tissues, including erythrocytes, are supplied with lysolecithin as a precursor of lecithin. This is a rather interesting working hypothesis.

On the other hand, the role of the albumin–free fatty acid complex present in the ultracentrifugal residue was recognized as the principal form in which fatty acids are transported from adipose tissue to various organs for metabolic and structural purposes (161).

B. Lipid Composition

Most data on the lipid composition of the ultracentrifugal residue were obtained on the whole residue, which is a heterogeneous fraction and is composed of various lipid–protein complexes as well as non-lipid-containing proteins.

Table XXIII shows the lipid compositions of the ultracentrifugal residues reported by various investigators.

The lipids in the total ultracentrifugal residue amount to 1.0 to 1.8%. The lipid-to-protein ratios in the ultracentrifugal residue have little sig-

Table XXIII. Lipid Composition of Serum Ultracentrifugal Residue[a]

	Reference						
		114[b]			21[c]		
Component	63[d]	mg %	%	19[e]	VHDL[f]	$VHDL_1$[g]	$VHDL_2$[h]
Total glycerides	9.0	3.5	(9.7)	10.2[i]	13.2	12.4	3.2
Cholesterol:							
Total	14.2	5.2	(14.2)	13.6	4.5	5.9	3.2
Free	13.0	0.7	(1.9)	3.3	1.6	0.9	1.3
Esterified	1.2	4.5	(12.3)	10.3	2.9	5.0	1.9
Cholesteryl esters	2.0	7.5	(20.7)	17.3	4.9	8.5	3.2
Free fatty acids	61.0	Not analyzed		29.0	34.6	1.5	38.7
Hydrocarbons				4.4			
Unidentified lipids		2.5	(6.9)	3.6			
Total "neutral lipids"	85.0			67.8	54.3	23.3	46.4
Glycolipids				1.5			
Phospholipids	17	13.5	(37.2)	26.8	45.5	76.7	53.5

[a] Lipoproteins with $d > 1.21$ g/ml. Lipid concentrations are in percentages of total lipids.
[b] Polonovski (114) did not determine the quantity of free fatty acids. Considering the high content of free fatty acids in these lipoproteins, it was impossible to present the data in percentage form (as all tables were composed). Therefore it was assumed that the free-fatty-acid content of this fraction is 32% [average of values from Alaupovic et al. (21) and Skipski et al. (19)], and the percentage composition of lipids was calculated. These figures are given in parentheses. The original figures (mg %) are given as the principal figures (without parentheses).
[c] Fasting subjects, male and female.
[d] Average data for two fasting patients, one with xanthoma tendinosum and one with xanthoma tuberosum.
[e] Fasting female. The ultracentrifugal residue was composed of 1% lipid, 99% protein.
[f] The VHDL fraction, d 1.210 g/ml, was composed of 1.82% lipid, 98.18% protein.
[g] The $VHDL_1$ fraction, d 1.210–1.250 g/ml, was composed of 37.6% lipid, 62.4% protein.
[h] The $VHDL_2$ fraction, $d > 1.250$ g/ml, was composed of 1.55% lipid, 98.45% protein.
[i] Glyceride composition in percentages of total lipids was triglycerides, 3.3%; diglycerides, 4.0%; monoglycerides, 2.9%.

nificance for its chemical characterization because of the heterogeneity of this fraction. However, these ratios have some physiologic significance; the total amount of plasma free fatty acids fluctuates greatly (19, 161, 162) and this apparently influences the amounts of free fatty acids associated with albumins and therefore the amounts of lipid in the ultracentrifugal residue.

Free fatty acids are the most abundant lipids in the ultracentrifugal residue, comprising 29 to 61% of the total lipids. Freeman et al. (63) reported 61% free fatty acids in two patients with xanthoma tendinosum and xanthoma tuberosum; this value may reflect a metabolic deviation under pathologic conditions. Two of the other values for the free-fatty-acid content of the ultracentrifugal residue, 35 and 29% of the total lipids (19, 21), are similar.

Of the total lipids in ultracentrifugal residues, 13 to 19% are glycerides; however, according to Skipski et al. (19), only one-third of them are triglycerides, the rest being diglycerides and monoglycerides. These authors observed this distribution of glycerides only in the ultracentrifugal residue, but small amounts of lower glycerides were observed in all lipoprotein classes studied.

The available information concerning the amount of cholesterol is conflicting. There is good agreement only in values reported by Polonovski (114) and Skipski et al. (19), who found that the ultracentrifugal residue contained 14% total cholesterol of which only 2 to 3% was free cholesterol. Freeman et al. (63) also reported 14% total cholesterol, but the predominant form was free, rather than esterified, cholesterol. Alaupovic et al. (21) reported a much lower value for total cholesterol (5%) in their VHDL. Most of this was esterified cholesterol.

There is no agreement among the values reported for phospholipids, which range from 17 to 46% of the total lipids.

Alaupovic et al. (21) separated the ultracentrifugal residue into two fractions: $VHDL_1$ (*d* 1.210–1.250 g/ml) and $VHDL_2$ ($d > 1.250$ g/ml). The lipid composition of the $VHDL_1$ fraction resembles that of the other high-density lipoproteins, HDL_2 and HDL_3. The amounts of most components in $VHDL_1$ follow the general trends observed in HDL_2 and HDL_3: 62% proteins and 38% lipids, phospholipids being the major lipid class (77%). The content of free fatty acids is low (2%). Values for lysolecithin are also low (3.5% of the total lipids) (Table XXIV). On the other hand, the $VHDL_2$ fraction of Alaupovic et al. (21) does not significantly differ in its chemical composition from the total ultracentrifugal residue (Tables XXIII and XXIV).

The ultracentrifugal residue is the richest lipoprotein fraction in the relative content of ceramide monohexosides and hydrocarbons (19). The average amount of hydrocarbons is 4.4% of the total lipids extracted from the ultracentrifugal residue, but the hydrocarbon content of the residue fluctuates greatly. In some samples of the ultracentrifugal residue isolated from the serums of normal subjects hydrocarbons comprised up to 10% of the total lipids.

Skipski et al. (19) studied the chemical composition of the hydrocarbons present in the ultracentrifugal residue. The hydrocarbons were isolated from the residue lipid extracts by silicic-acid-column chromatography. The infrared spectra of the isolated hydrocarbons showed the presence of only methyl and methylene groups, no other functional groups being observed. These crude hydrocarbon fractions were subjected to gas–liquid chromatography which revealed the presence of *n*-alkanes. These are distributed between carbon numbers C_{17} and C_{35}, with the largest peaks in the area between

C_{23} and C_{29}. Hydrogenation of the hydrocarbon fractions did not essentially alter the pattern of the gas–liquid chromatograms, which indicated that unsaturated hydrocarbons are either absent or present in very small amounts. The separation of *n*-alkanes from the other series of hydrocarbons by molecular sieves and subsequent gas–liquid chromatography demonstrated the same distribution in the *n*-alkane series with carbon numbers from C_{17} to C_{35} seen in gas chromatograms on crude hydrocarbon fractions. The amounts of *n*-alkanes in the hydrocarbon fractions ranged from 18 to 50%. The residual parts of hydrocarbon fractions, after the removal of *n*-alkanes, were subjected to gas–liquid chromatography and showed that the main peaks are distributed between C_{26} and C_{33}. Apparently they are different branched alkanes (*iso* and *anteiso*).

At present it is difficult to evaluate the significance of the presence of alkanes in blood in relation to physiologic or pathologic conditions. The presence of hydrocarbons (including the alkane series) in higher animals and humans has been known for several years (163–168). Probably, to some extent, *n*-alkanes are oxidized by animal tissues and then converted into fatty acids. When McCarthy (169) administered ^{14}C-labeled octadecane or hexadecane to goats, rats, and chickens, the radioactivity was recovered in fatty acids of the same chain lengths as the hydrocarbons administered and practically no radioactivity was recovered in isolated hydrocarbons. Hydrocarbons were present in all lipoprotein classes studied: in particulate fat ($S_f > 400$), VLDL, LDL, HDL_2, HDL_3, and the ultracentrifugal residue. The highest amount (in percentage) of hydrocarbons was in the ultracentrifugal residue, although appreciable amounts of hydrocarbons were found also in VLDL and in the particulate fat from fasting samples. Since several investigators (170, 171) showed that bovine-serum albumin has the capacity to bind long-chain hydrocarbons, it seemed logical to speculate that the hydrocarbons recovered from the ultracentrifugal residue were originally bound to albumin in the form of albumin–hydrocarbon complexes analogous to the albumin–free fatty acid complexes. In the cases of particulate fat and VLDL hydrocarbons might be simply associated with the lipid core. At present there is no substantial evidence that hydrocarbons are associated with albumins in the ultracentrifugal residue.

Several investigators (19, 21, 114, 159, 160) have studied the composition of phospholipids in the ultracentrifugal residue (Table XXIV). The most characteristic feature of the ultracentrifugal residue class is the high content of lysolecithin, which varies from 22 to 71% of the total phospholipids. The content of lecithin is lower than it is in the phospholipid fractions of other lipoproteins and ranges from 19 to 60%. The relative amounts of sphingomyelin are either equal to, or lower than, the amounts in HDL. Small quantities of phosphatidylethanolamine, phosphatidylserine, phosphatidylinositol, and some other phospholipids are also present.

Table XXIV. Phospholipid Composition of the Ultracentrifugal Residue[a]

	Reference						
					21[b]		
Component	159[b]	114[c]	160[d]	19[e]	VHDL[f]	$VHDL_1$[g]	$VHDL_2$[h]
Lecithin	25	30–40	18.5	47.4	59.5	71.6	28.1
Lysolecithin	56	50	70.8	34.5	21.8	3.5	64.1
Sphingomyelin	14	10	3.0	5.7	12.3	11.8	7.7
Phosphatidylethanolamine	6 (Phosphatidylethanolamine and Phosphatidylserine)	3–10 (Phosphatidylethanolamine and Phosphatidylserine)		4.2	1.7	2.9	
Phosphatidylserine				0.5			
Phosphatidylinositol			7.8 (Phosphatidylethanolamine through Unidentified phospholipids)	1.9	4.6	10.2	
Polyglycerophosphatides and phosphatidic acid				2.4			
Unidentified phospholipids				2.4			
Choline-containing phospholipids	94		92.3	87.6	93.6	86.9	99.9

[a] Lipoproteins with $d > 1.21$ g/ml. The phospholipid concentrations are in percentages of total phospholipids. Serum samples unless otherwise indicated.
[b] Fasting, male and female.
[c] The total-lipid extract contained 37.2% phospholipids.
[d] Plasma sample, nonfasting male.
[e] Fasting female. The total-lipid extract contained 26.8% phospholipids.
[f] The VHDL fraction, $d > 1.210$ g/ml, contained 45.5% phospholipids in the total-lipid extract.
[g] The $VHDL_1$ fraction, d 1.210–1.250 g/ml, contained 76.7% phospholipids in the total-lipid extract.
[h] The $VHDL_2$ fraction, $d > 1.250$ g/ml, contained 53.5% phospholipids in the total-lipid extract.

Alaupovic et al. (21) studied the phospholipid composition of two subfractions of the ultracentrifugal residue, $VHDL_1$ and $VHDL_2$. The former contains high amounts of lecithin and low amounts of lysolecithin. In general the lipid composition of $VHDL_1$ resembles rather closely the composition of HDL as reported by these authors (21). The $VHDL_2$ fraction has a very high content of lysolecithin (64% of phospholipids). It is possible that $VHDL_2$ basically represents an albumin–free fatty acid–lysolecithin complex (see below).

The presence of lysolecithin in serum and in the ultracentrifugal residue in particular requires some additional comments. Phillips (111, 159, 172) demonstrated the presence of lysolecithin in human serum and its distribution among the various lipoprotein classes. These observations raised the question of whether the lysolecithin in lipid extracts might be a degradation product of phosphatidylcholine (lecithin) or phosphatidal choline (plasmalogen) produced during extraction, purification, or chromatographic analysis. It is difficult to explain the presence in blood of a compound like lysolecithin, which has a high hemolytic activity.

However, Gjone, Berry, and Turner (173) confirmed its presence in normal human serum, at an average concentration of 8.9% of the lipid phosphorus. These authors showed that the concentration of lysolecithin was unchanged when purification of lipid extracts by water washing was omitted and remained constant in serum or lipid extracts processed within 2 hr or stored for a week at 4°C. No quantitative differences were observed in the phospholipid components when serum was compared with heparinized plasma from the same subject. Rechromatography of lecithin isolated from serum by silicic acid columns did not produce lysolecithin. All these control experiments made it unlikely that lysolecithin was formed during extraction, purification, or chromatography of the extracts. In addition, Gjone and Mendeloff (cited in Ref. 173) observed a marked elevation in serum lysolecithin in acute pancreatitis without a simultaneous increase in total phospholipid concentration. This suggests that lysolecithin is indeed a normal constituent of serum.

Newman, Liu, and Zilversmit (174) have accumulated evidence that lysolecithin is a normal component in the plasma of rats. Twenty hours after injection of ^{32}P-phosphate there was a considerable difference between the specific activities of lecithin and lysolecithin; lecithin has a higher specific activity than lysolecithin. If the latter were a simple *in vitro* breakdown product of lecithin, the specific activities of both compounds should have been the same unless there were a selective breakdown of part of the lecithin with a specific activity lower than that represented by the whole lecithin fraction. There is still a possibility that phosphatidal choline (plasmalogens) undergoes selective decomposition, with the formation of lysolecithin, since this type of phospholipid is very sensitive to acids. In order to test this possibility Newman et al. (174) analyzed rat serum for the presence of plasmalogens immediately after lipid extraction. Less than 3% of the plasma lipid phosphorus was represented by plasmalogens and therefore could not account for the presence of lysolecithin (17.5% of lipid phosphorus in rat serum).

Switzer and Eder (160) showed that lysolecithin isolated from rat plasma has a different fatty acid composition than lecithin isolated from the same plasma. Lysolecithin had the following fatty acid distribution: palmitic, 45.1%; stearic, 32.5%; linoleic, 12.9%; oleic, 4.6%; arachidonic, 3.3%; other, 1.6%. Lecithin, on the other hand, had the following fatty acid composition: palmitic, 35.7%; stearic, 21%; linoleic, 22%; oleic, 5.7%; arachidonic, 13.8%; other, 1.8%. None of these observations alone constitutes conclusive evidence for the existence of lysolecithin in circulating blood. However, combined evidence definitely shows that lysolecithin is a normal constituent of plasma and serum lipoproteins.

Switzer and Eder (160) further fractionated the ultracentrifugal residue by means of starch-block electrophoresis. They found that lysolecithin migrated with albumins, rather than with globulins. Gel filtration on Sephadex

G-200 of whole serum from rats and humans and also the ultracentrifugal residue demonstrated that most of the lysolecithin is bound to albumin. Confirmatory evidence that albumin is the carrier protein for lysolecithin in the ultracentrifugal residue from rat serum was obtained by ammonium sulfate precipitation of the proteins in this fraction. The albumin obtained yielded only a single band in agar-gel immunoelectrophoresis, and 98.3% of the phospholipids associated with this albumin was lysolecithin. These experiments essentially proved that the lysolecithin present in the ultracentrifugal residue is bound to albumin. The other phospholipids of this lipoprotein fraction are apparently associated with globulins.

At present it is not clear whether part of the ultracentrifugal residue represents a native *very*-high-density lipoprotein or HDL_2 and HDL_3 altered during ultracentrifugation (see Section V). Switzer and Eder (160) considered the possibility that all of the lysolecithin present in plasma is associated with albumin. They speculated that the small amounts of lysolecithin present in most lipoprotein classes might form from lecithin during the separation of lipoproteins by the activity of an acyltransferase in plasma (175). However, the fact that lysolecithin is more abundant in VLDL than it is in the LDL and HDL_2 fractions, which were separated first (19), speaks against this hypothesis.

Klopfenstein (176) investigated the ability of plasma albumin to bind lysolecithin. In a series of experiments employing microcalorimetry it was demonstrated that this phospholipid was bound exothermally (18,000 cal/mole) to bovine-serum albumin in a molar ratio of 1:1. The author interpreted this as the existence of one binding site for lysolecithin per albumin molecule.

C. Free Fatty Acids and the Albumin–Free Fatty Acid Complex

The presence of unesterified fatty acids in plasma was discovered almost 50 years ago by Szent-Gyorgyi and Tominaga (177) and later confirmed by Kelsey and Longenecker (178). Kendall (156) and Cohn et al. (157) attempted to purify human-serum albumin by crystallization. They observed that crystalline albumin contains fatty acids, which could be removed by extraction with organic solvents. It was deduced that *in vivo* plasma albumin exists as a complex with fatty acids. However, no physiologic significance was attributed to these observations until about 15 years ago, when several groups of investigators (162, 179–183) elucidated the physiologic role of plasma free fatty acids (FFA). The free fatty acids are the primary form in which lipids are transported from adipose tissue to most organs for their metabolic and structural utilization. The concentration of free fatty acids in plasma fluctuates with the physiologic status of the body. The hypothesis was formulated that free fatty acids represent the blood-lipid fraction that is immediately available to cells to meet their demands and that the release of free fatty acids into plasma is regulated by some physiologic mechanism. The decrease of the free-fatty-acid content in venous blood compared with the level in arterial blood, tested for several organs, shows that most of the organs "extract" free fatty acids from blood. Adipose tissue is the principal source of supply of new free fatty acids in blood. Since the levels of free fatty acids in plasma are relatively low (see below), they could play a significant metabolic role only if they had a high turnover rate. Indeed the plasma free fatty acids in humans and dogs were found to have a half-life in the range of 1.7 to 3.1 min, the turnover being 23 to 41% per minute (183).

Many factors of a physiologic nature as well as methods used for the determination of free fatty acids influence the so-called "normal" FFA values for plasma or serum (181, 184). According to Dole (162), the normal values for free fatty acids determined in the morning after a fast of 10 to 12 hr ranged from 0.315 to 1.210 meq/l (meq/l = milliequivalents of free fatty acids per liter of plasma or serum). Obese subjects tended to have higher concentrations of free fatty acids than did thinner subjects. With continued fasting the concentrations of plasma free fatty acids rose slowly. A mixed meal eaten after a period of fasting decreased the concentration. Consumption of fat alone did not increase the concentration to a greater extent than did fasting during the same period of time. Consumption of carbohydrates significantly decreased the concentration of plasma free fatty acids.

In the last decade numerous publications appeared dealing with the levels of free fatty acids in plasma and serum from normal subjects. Carlsten and associates (185) reported average fasting values for free fatty acids in arterial plasma as 0.79 ± 0.20 meq/l under resting and fasting conditions. According to Goldman (186) the average value for venous plasma under fasting conditions and moderate activity is 0.486 meq/l. Lieber et al. (187) studied the FFA levels in arterial plasma in a fully recovered patient after an overnight fast (no patients with liver disease or disturbance of lipid metabolism were used). The average calculated levels were 0.854 meq/l. Konttinen et al. (188) reported 0.588 ± 0.045 meq/l in the arterial plasma of young men in the basal state, whereas the venous value under the same conditions was 0.507 ± 0.045 meq/l. During physical exercise the levels of free fatty acids in arterial and venous plasma changed to 0.500 ± 0.047 and 0.418 ± 0.049 meq/l, respectively. Hollister and Wright (189) reported the fluctuations of plasma free fatty acids in hospitalized psychiatric patients who had regular working assignments. In the fasting condition the mean FFA level was 0.408 meq/l and decreased to 0.236 meq/l after breakfast; before dinner, and 2 hr after, the mean levels were 0.376 and 0.280 meq/l, respectively. Coefficients of variations for individual subjects were high, and replicability on successive tests, even when these were performed under basal conditions and separated by a 24-hr interval, was quite poor. The major source of variability was the actual fluctuation of the FFA concentration in blood rather than technical errors.

Castelli and co-workers (190) performed rather extensive measurements of serum FFA levels on prison volunteers (most of them 30–39 years old). The intersubject range in FFA concentration after an initial overnight fast (15 hr) was from 0.554 to 0.988 meq/l, with an overall mean of 0.679 meq/l. During the day the effects of different diets on the FFA levels were tested and then, after a second period of fasting (also 15 hr), the FFA levels were measured. After a second period of fasting the range was 0.602 to 1.068 meq/l, with an overall mean of 0.774 meq/l.

Castelli et al. (190) also tested the effects of various meals. Consumption of safflower oil gave the maximum FFA values, 1.286 ± 0.102 meq/l (9 hr after eating). Approximately the same values were observed after 24 hr of fasting (1.157 ± 0.096 meq/l). Consumption of proteins, 3 hr after a meal, somewhat decreased the FFA concentration (0.604 ± 0.040 meq/l), whereas for the same period of time a carbohydrate meal significantly decreased it to 0.413 ± 0.038 meq/l. Six hours after these meals had been consumed the FFA levels reached the control values (after a 15-hr fast).

Nestel (191) reported the mean concentration of free fatty acids in venous plasma as 0.420 meq/l after an overnight fast, whereas Carlson and Oro (192) found 0.72 meq/l in arterial plasma.

The majority of the mean values reported for plasma or serum FFA levels under fasting conditions in normal subjects range from 0.400 to 0.800 meq/l, although values for individual subjects might be slightly below or above this range. Probably the upper value in the range reported by Dole (162), 0.315 to 1.210 meq/l, is too high.

All of these measurements represent the total amounts of free fatty acids in plasma or serum. We have already seen that free fatty acids are present not only in the ultracentrifugal residue, mainly as the albumin–free fatty acid complex, but also in all other lipoprotein classes. According to Lindgren et al. (107) 33 to 54% of the total amount of free fatty acids present in serum is associated with the ultracentrifugal residue (albumin–free fatty acid complex). The other important carriers of free fatty acids are high-density lipoproteins. In general this picture of the FFA distribution in the various lipoprotein classes was confirmed by Skipski et al. (19) (Table XXV). In normal women who had fasted overnight, an average of 54% of free fatty acids was associated with the ultracentrifugal residue and 23%

Table XXV. Free-Fatty-Acid Distribution in Various Lipoprotein Classes[a]

	FFA Concentration	
Lipoprotein Class	In meq/l	Percent of Total Serum
Particulate fat ($S_{f(1.006)} > 400$)	0.0237	3.7
VLDL ($S_{f(1.006)}$ 0–400)	0.0422	6.7
LDL ($S_{f(1.063)}$ 0–20)	0.0801	12.7
HDL_2 (*d* 1.063–1.125 g/ml)	0.0863	13.7
HDL_3 (*d* 1.125–1.210 g/ml)	0.0560	8.9
Ultracentrifugal residue ($d > 1.210$ g/ml)	0.3430	54.3
Total in serum	0.6313	100.0

[a] Data from Ref. 19.

with the HDL class. Shafrir (193, 194) reported different results for the FFA distribution among lipoprotein classes. From 70.2 to 86.5% of the free fatty acids in serum from normal fasting subjects was associated with albumins, and only 13.5 to 29.8% was bound to all lipoproteins with $d < 1.210$ g/ml. The lipoproteins floating at *d* 1.019 g/ml contained 1.2 to 3.3%, whereas those floating at *d* 1.063 g/ml contained 4.6 to 9.3% of the serum free fatty acids. The HDL class contained 3.8 to 17.2% of serum free fatty acids. In serum from patients with hyperlipemia but normal albumin levels 17.7 to 31.8% was bound to lipoproteins other than the albumin–free fatty acid complex. In serum from patients with the nephrotic syndrome, with low albumin but normal FFA levels, 21.0 to 50.8% of the total free fatty acids was found in lipoproteins of $d < 1.210$ g/ml.

Goodman and Shafrir (195) questioned the validity of the measurements of FFA distributions among the various lipoprotein classes after their separation by ultracentrifugation in the presence of high salt concentrations. These authors believed that in the high-ionic-strength media employed for lipoprotein fractionations (19, 107, 127), the free fatty acids were displaced from serum albumin, resulting in a much greater percentage being associated with low- and high-density lipoproteins. Goodman (196) found three classes of binding sites on human-serum albumin with different affinities for fatty acids. The albumin molecules had 2 sites with high affinities, 5 with intermediate, and approximately 20 with low affinities. These observations were confirmed recently by Spector, John, and Fletcher (170), whose data were analyzed in terms of a model consisting of six high-energy binding sites and a large number of weak binding sites (estimated to be 63). The high-energy sites were resolved into two classes with different affinities, each containing three sites. All these observations were based on *in vitro* experiments with "pure" isolated serum albumins and should be extrapolated to *in vivo* conditions only with caution.

Goodman and Shafrir (195) studied the affinities of two lipoprotein classes for long-chain fatty acids in the presence of serum albumins. The lipoprotein fractions studied were those with $d < 1.019$ g/ml (roughly VLDL) and d 1.019 to 1.063 g/ml (most of LDL). The fatty acids were lauric, palmitic, stearic, oleic, or linoleic. Lipoproteins, albumins, and ^{14}C-labeled fatty acid salts were equilibrated and then separated by ultracentrifugation. Increased ionic strength was avoided by using deuterium oxide instead of salts to raise the density. The lipoprotein-to-albumin ratio used during the incubation was 10 to 15 times greater than the value for normal human serum. The concentration of fatty acids in each albumin and lipoprotein solution was determined by measuring the radioactivity. The data obtained were analyzed in terms of two classes of binding sites in each lipoprotein fraction. These two lipoprotein classes had four binding sites with affinities of the same order of magnitude (slightly stronger) than the strongest binding sites of serum albumin. There were approximately 150 weak binding sites also.

Goodman and Shafrir (195) concluded that only about 0.3% of free fatty acids is bound to each of these lipoproteins (VLDL and LDL) in circulating plasma. These conclusions derived from calculations based on the distribution of ^{14}C-labeled free fatty acids between albumin and the lipoprotein classes studied in *in vitro* experiments and the relative molar concentrations of those in plasma. Some preliminary experiments indicated that HDL bound about 5% of the circulating free fatty acids. The rest, about 94%, were bound to albumin. As the ionic strength of the solutions in which lipoproteins (d 1.019–1.063 g/ml), the fatty acid salt (palmitate), and albumin attained equilibrium was increased, the amount of palmitate bound to lipoproteins also was increased.

Goodman and Shafrir (195) concluded that when the actual amounts of free fatty acids associated with LDL and HDL exceeded the estimated values for the distribution of free fatty acids between the albumin–free fatty acid complex and other lipoproteins, these amounts were probably artifacts resulting from the high salt concentrations used in the separation of lipoproteins. These conclusions, although very provocative and possibly of physiologic significance, were based on data obtained from an isolated *in vitro* system. The assumption was made that free fatty acids are bound to the proteins in LDL.

Some of these conclusions were contradicted by other experiments performed by Shafrir (194) himself. He compared the fatty acid content of various lipoprotein fractions isolated by the conventional method of ultracentrifugation in the presence of high salt concentrations (potassium bromide) with those obtained by the use of deuterium oxide or deuterium oxide plus sucrose. In the latter case the separation of lipoproteins was performed at low ionic strengths, the suspected cause of the FFA redistribution between the albumin–free fatty acid complex and other lipoproteins being thus eliminated. The experiments were performed on the same serum. However, the results showed some small differences in FFA distribution in lipoproteins isolated by these two methods. Three experiments performed with serum from normal subjects gave the following amounts of free fatty acids associated with lipoproteins other than the albumin–free fatty acid complex, when lipoproteins were separated at a high salt concentration: 29.8, 16.8, and 15.8%. When these lipoproteins were isolated at low ionic strengths and hence FFA redistribution was excluded, the values were 21.0, 15.3, and 13.3%. These experiments showed that at least 13 to 21% of free fatty acids is associated with lipoproteins of $d < 1.210$ g/ml, but not 5.6% as concluded by Goodman and Shafrir (195) on the basis of model experiments.

Evidently *in vivo* a significant part of the plasma free fatty acids is associated with lipoproteins other than the albumin–free fatty acid complex. Unfortunately at present it is impossible to estimate, even approximately, the amount of free fatty acids associated with lipoproteins with $d < 1.210$ g/ml. Three groups of investigators [Lindgren et al. (107), Shafrir (193, 194), and Skipski et al. (19)] reported on the FFA distribution among various lipoproteins separated by conventional procedures at high salt concentrations. Thus all their values are subject to some error due to the "salt effect." In general there is good agreement between the data of Lindgren et al. (107) and those of Skipski et al. (19). However, the values for lipoprotein classes other than the albumin–free fatty acid complex reported by Shafrir (193, 194) are much lower than those found by the former authors (19, 107). It should be recalled that Shafrir (194) demonstrated that the "salt effect" is relatively small in this type of experiment.

Shafrir (194) also observed that patients with the nephrotic syndrome have a different FFA distribution among lipoproteins, although the total FFA level is not essentially altered. The amounts of free fatty acids associated with lipoproteins of $d < 1.21$ g/ml increased by a factor of 2 to 2.5.

The total serum free fatty acids bound to albumin averaged 35.7% in the patients, versus 77.6% in normal serum. The amount of albumin in the plasma of nephrotic patients was considerably decreased (from 3.45 to 1.31 g/100 ml of serum). In spite of the FFA redistribution among the various lipoprotein fractions, and the decreased amount in the form of the albumin–free fatty acid complex, there was an increase in the albumin–free fatty acid molar ratio. In normal subjects this ratio averaged 0.77 and in patients with the nephrotic syndrome, 1.07 (194). It was rather interesting that the shift of free fatty acids from the albumin complexes started before two of the binding sites with the highest affinities were saturated. This may be regarded as competition between the albumin and the lipoproteins for the available free fatty acids. Competition was indicated by the shift of free fatty acids in plasma with an increased lipoprotein-to-albumin ratio, as seen in nephrosis and also in hyperlipoproteinemia.

Accumulation of free fatty acids in the VLDL and LDL fractions of serum from patients with nephrosis caused some irregularities in their movements in the ascending boundary of free electrophoresis and in paper electrophoresis: β-lipoproteins were partially or totally displaced into the α_2-globulin zone. Gordon (197) also observed this displacement of β-lipoproteins in serum from patients with hyperlipoproteinemia after the injection of heparin and release of lipoprotein lipase. These displacements resulted from the accumulation of large amounts of free fatty acids in β-lipoproteins, thereby increasing their negative electrostatic surface charges.

Other metabolic disorders affect FFA levels in serum. In patients with controlled diabetes mellitus and under fasting conditions FFA levels were significantly above normal. Bierman, Dole, and Roberts (198) observed that in 20 patients with diabetes, without ketosis, the average serum FFA level was 0.849 ± 0.287 meq/l, whereas the serum FFA level of 40 fasting, nondiabetic, nonobese subjects averaged 0.572 ± 0.280 meq/l. In diabetics with ketonuria the average value was 1.311 ± 0.466 meq/l. Obese patients had a mean fasting value of 0.862 ± 0.214 meq/l, similar to that of the controlled diabetics, although none of the subjects had glycosuria.

Mehnert, Pelikan, and Zollner (199) confirmed the observations that diabetic patients have higher values for fasting levels of free fatty acids and stressed the relationship between fasting blood-sugar and FFA levels: when blood sugar was high, the FFA levels were high. In other words, the degree of disease or lack of control was reflected by the levels of both glucose and free fatty acids in blood. Administration of insulin (198) decreased both sugar and FFA levels in blood. Other hormones (epinephrine, glucagon) affected FFA levels in plasma. The regulation of FFA transport has been described in a review article by Fredrickson and Gordon (181).

VII. FATTY ACID COMPOSITIONS OF LIPIDS IN VARIOUS LIPOPROTEIN CLASSES AND THE FREE FATTY ACID COMPOSITION OF SERUM

A. Effect of Ingested Fat on the Fatty Acid Compositions of Various Lipoprotein Classes

In Section II it was shown that ingested fat to a great extent determines the fatty acid composition of chylomicron triglycerides. Ingested fat affects the fatty acid composition of other lipoprotein classes to a far lesser degree.

Bragdon and Karmen (71) studied the ratio of linoleic acid to oleic acid in several classes of lipoproteins isolated from the serum of a subject who had ingested a fat meal composed of corn oil. The ratio substantially increased in the VLDL fraction ($d < 1.019$ g/ml) and in the ultracentrifugal residue ($d > 1.21$ g/ml). The authors demonstrated that the alteration of the linoleic-to-oleic ratio in these lipoproteins did not result from the direct exchange of chylomicron fatty acids with these lipoproteins. When they incubated "corn oil chylomicrons" with separated lipoproteins, there were no alterations of the ratios in either VLDL or the ultracentrifugal residue. However, there was practically no change in the linoleic-to-oleic ratio in the LDL and HDL fractions in subjects fed corn oil.

Kayden et al. (72) also observed some effect of a single meal of corn or coconut oil on the fatty acid composition of VLDL (Table XXVI). However, this effect was moderate and more pronounced on the total lipids and triglyceride fractions than on the cholesteryl ester fraction isolated from VLDL. The LDL (*d* 1.019–1.063 g/ml) were the least affected by ingested fat. On the other hand, the fatty acid composition of HDL_{2+3} (*d* 1.063–1.21 g/ml) was affected by the ingested fat, but quantitatively less than that of VLDL.

In general the cholesteryl ester fraction of each lipoprotein class was much less affected than the triglyceride fraction. Moreover, the changes in all lipid fractions studied (total lipids, triglycerides, and cholesteryl esters) in VLDL, LDL, and HDL were neither so marked, nor was the amount of fat contained so high that it would be reasonable to conclude that these fractions carry a large portion of recently ingested fat even though the amount of ingested fat was much higher than that in normal meals. Thus the relative stability of the fatty acid composition of these lipoproteins indicates that their fats are synthesized primarily from lipid sources other than newly absorbed fat. After removal of chylomicrons, Dole et al. (68) observed even smaller effects of ingested fat on the fatty acid composition of

Table XXVI. Fatty Acid Composition of Total-Lipid Extracts of Human-Serum Lipoproteins and Their Triglycerides and Cholesteryl Esters[a,b]

	Composition (%) in								
	Total Lipids			Triglycerides			Cholesteryl Esters		
Fatty Acid	Fasting	After Corn Oil	After Coconut Oil	Fasting	After Corn Oil	After Coconut Oil	Fasting	After Corn Oil	After Coconut Oil
Lipoproteins with d < 1.019 *g/ml (VLDL)*[c]									
12:0	0	1	5	1	1	15	1	1	5
14:0	0	1	6	2	2	6	2	2	7
16:0	28	25	29	28	15	27	20	19	25
18:0	10	5	3	4	5	5	2	3	2
18:1	42	33	40	53	44	42	45	38	34
18:2	20	35	17	12	33	5	30	37	28
Lipoproteins with d *1.019–1.063 g/ml (LDL)*									
12:0	0	0	1	1	1	2	2	1	1
14:0	1	1	2	1	2	3	1	2	2
16:0	32	33	30	33	27	27	18	18	18
18:0	5	3	6	10	8	10	3	1	5
18:1	33	35	36	45	43	47	33	30	28
18:2	29	28	25	10	19	11	42	46	46
Lipoproteins with d *1.063–1.21 g/ml* (HDL_{2+3})									
12:0	0	0	0	2	0	6	6	1	4
14:0	1	1	5	2	2	6	3	4	3
16:0	37	32	31	30	24	28	19	20	16
18:0	8	8	8	8	4	5	4	3	1
18:1	33	30	30	46	39	42	28	29	31
18:2	21	29	20	12	31	13	40	43	45

[a] Data from Ref. 72.
[b] Postprandial samples were taken 8 hr after consumption of corn oil or coconut oil. Fatty acid composition of corn oil: 16:0, 11%; 18:1, 27%; 18:2, 61%. Coconut oil: 10:0, 9%; 12:0, 61%; 14:0, 20%; 16:0, 7%.
[c] Chylomicrons were removed.

plasma: triglycerides, cholesteryl esters, free fatty acids, and phospholipids.

B. Fatty Acid Compositions of Lipoprotein Classes After Mixed Diets

Since the effects of a fat meal on the fatty acid composition of the lipids in various lipoprotein classes are relatively moderate, the effects of a usual mixed diet will be even smaller. Therefore one can consider that individuals who eat a regular mixed diet will have a "normal" fatty acid composition in their serum lipoproteins. Table XXVII presents the fatty acid compositions of the total-lipid fractions of various lipoproteins as well as of the individual lipid classes (glycerides, cholesteryl esters, and phospholipids) that are most abundant in lipoproteins.

Lindgren and associates (63, 200, 201) studied the fatty acid composi-

Table XXVII. Fatty Acid Composition of Lipids in Various Lipoprotein Classes

	Composition (wt %)							
	Nonfasting Serum[a]				Fasting Plasma[b]			
Fatty Acid	Total Serum	VLDL[c]	LDL[d]	HDL_{2+3}[e]	Total Plasma	VLDL[f]	LDL[g]	HDL_{2+3}[h]
				Glycerides[i]				
Lower than 16:0	4.2	4.8	10.1	8.5	1.3	1.0	0.7	0.8
16:0	27.9	23.3	23.1	23.5	25.6	26.9	23.1	23.4
16:1	3.9	4.0	4.1	4.0	3.1	3.3	2.8	2.9
16:1–18:0	1.1	1.1	1.9	1.7	0.5	—	—	—
18:0	4.4	3.5	4.1	4.0	2.9	2.9	3.3	3.5
18:1	40.7	36.5	35.4	35.3	45.1	45.4	46.6	43.8
18:2	14.8	21.8	15.6	15.7	16.1	15.7	15.7	15.9
18:2–20:4	1.8	3.2	3.5	4.7	1.3	1.5	1.5	1.2
20:4	1.2	1.0	1.4	1.6	4.5	2.5	5.4	7.6
Higher	—	0.9	0.9	1.1	—	—	—	—
				Cholesteryl Esters				
Lower than 16:0	4.4	4.5	3.8	3.6	0.8	—	—	—
16:0	10.4	21.0	10.5	10.3	11.5	11.5	11.3	11.4
16:1	3.4	3.0	3.4	3.3	2.1	1.8	1.9	2.1
16:1–18:0	1.7	1.4	1.3	1.0	0.5	—	—	—
18:0	1.3	5.6	1.5	1.2	1.1	1.4	1.0	1.1
18:1	18.8	34.9	18.2	18.5	23.0	25.6	22.4	22.4

Fatty Acid	Composition (wt %)							
	Nonfasting Serum[a]				Fasting Plasma[b]			
	Total Serum	VLDL[c]	LDL[d]	HDL_{2+3}[e]	Total Plasma	VLDL[f]	LDL[g]	HDL_{2+3}[h]
18:2	50.4	25.3	50.7	51.0	53.5	51.8	54.9	54.8
18:2–20:4	3.0	2.5	3.8	3.0	1.2	0.8	0.7	0.6
20:4	6.1	1.8	5.6	6.3	6.8	6.1	6.9	6.3
Higher	0.6	—	1.6	1.9	—	—	—	—
				Phospholipids				
Lower than 16:0	3.3	3.6	4.2	3.9	0.8	—	—	—
16:0	30.5	33.2	30.1	29.6	34.0	33.8	36.0	31.8
16:1	1.3	1.5	1.4	1.6	0.5	0.5	0.5	0.4
16:1–18:0	1.0	1.9	1.5	1.8	0.5	—	—	—
18:0	13.9	19.0	15.1	15.5	14.3	14.7	14.3	14.5
18:1	12.1	13.4	12.1	12.6	11.9	12.2	11.6	12.3
18:2	20.7	16.0	19.3	18.9	20.4	20.3	18.9	20.6
18:2–20:4	4.3	4.1	4.4	4.7	4.0	4.1	4.6	3.9
20:4	9.9	4.9	7.5	9.5	14.0	13.6	13.2	15.7
Higher	3.0	2.5	4.4	1.9	—	—	—	—

[a] Data from Refs. 63, 200, and 201.
[b] Data from Ref. 110.
[c] $d < 1.006$ g/ml; S_f 20–10^5.
[d] d 1.006–1.070 g/ml; S_f 0–20.
[e] d 1.070–1.218 g/ml.
[f] $d < 1.019$ g/ml.
[g] d 1.019–1.063 g/ml.
[h] d 1.063–1.21 g/ml.
[i] "Glycerides" include triglyceride, diglyceride, and monoglyceride fatty acids and also free fatty acids present in lipoprotein classes.

tions of lipoprotein lipids isolated from the serum of nonfasting normal adults. Their VLDL fraction included all S_f 20–10^5 lipoproteins (d < 1.006 g/ml). Ultracentrifugal analysis of this fraction revealed only small amounts of S_f 400–10^5 lipoproteins. From the practical point of view the S_f 20–10^5 fraction can be considered to be nearly all S_f 20–400 lipoproteins (63).

Goodman and Shiratori (110) studied lipoproteins isolated from fasting adult men who had had a slightly reduced fat intake (30% of the total calories) for 1 week prior to the experiment. The VLDL fraction was isolated at d < 1.019 g/ml. Thus physicochemically and physiologically the lipoprotein fractions studied by Lindgren et al. (63, 200, 201) and Goodman and Shiratori (110) were not identical. In spite of this, the fatty acid compositions of the individual lipid species (e.g., glycerides, cholesteryl esters, and phospholipids) isolated from whole serum or plasma, or individual lipoprotein classes except VLDL were similar. The results of Goodman and Shiratori showed that each lipid class displayed a distinct and specific fatty acid pattern (Table XXVII). In the glyceride fraction, composed of triglycerides and small amounts of diglycerides and monoglycerides, the predominant fatty acids were oleic acid (18:1) and to a lesser extent palmitic (16:0) and linoleic (18:2) acids. In the cholesteryl esters the predominant fatty acids were linoleic acid and to a lesser extent oleic acid. The phospholipids, which were characterized by a high content of palmitic acid, also contained large quantities of linoleic, stearic (18:0), and arachidonic (20:4) acids.

The fatty acid compositions of the glycerides and cholesteryl esters in the VLDL fraction isolated from the sera of nonfasting subjects by Lindgren et al. (63, 200, 201) were significantly different from those of the VLDL fraction isolated from the plasma of fasting subjects by Goodman and Shiratori (110). Furthermore, in the nonfasting samples the VLDL glycerides contained a higher percentage of linoleic acid, and the VLDL cholesteryl esters contained relatively higher amounts of palmitic and oleic acids and a lower amount of linoleic acid than did the corresponding lipid classes in whole serum or in the other lipoprotein classes. Apparently these differences can be attributed to the effect of ingested food since the determinations were performed on nonfasting subjects (63, 200, 201).

Ingested food did not noticeably affect the lipid classes isolated from whole serum because the glycerides and cholesteryl esters present in whole serum are diluted by the glycerides and cholesteryl esters present in other lipoproteins. However, in separated VLDL the effects of diet are more obvious. The effects of diet on the fatty acid compositions of LDL and HDL lipids are not noticeable.

There is no information, so far, concerning the free-fatty-acid composi-

Table XXVIII. Free-Fatty-Acids Composition of Blood Plasma, Serum, and the Albumin–Free Fatty Acid Complex

	Composition (%)				
	Sample and References				
Fatty Acid	Fasting Plasma (68)	Nonfasting Serum (63, 200, 201)	Fasting Plasma (202)	Fasting Plasma (110)	Serum Cohn Fraction V[a] (203)
Lower than 16:0	2.6	7.6	5.4	1.9	<5.5
16:0	23.2	25.0	23.1	24.2	24.7
16:1	2.4	4.3	3.6	3.3	3.1
16:1–18:0	—	2.2	1.6	0.9	<1.0
18:0	12.9	10.0	14.3	13.2	1.5
18:1	32.6	26.0	35.2	45.0	33.1
18:2	14.5	15.9	8.1	9.0	20.0
18:2–20:4	1.3	4.1	4.3	1.4	3.4
20:4	4.7	2.0	—	1.3	5.0
Higher	—	3.7	4.5	—	<1.0

[a] Serum albumin.

tions of individual lipoprotein classes except the ultracentrifugal residue ($d > 1.21$ g/ml), although the compositions of whole serum and plasma have been studied extensively during the last 10 years. The results of some of these studies are presented in Table XXVIII. The predominant free fatty acids in whole plasma and serum are oleic and palmitic acids and, to a lesser extent, linoleic and stearic acids.

Saifer and Goldman (203) studied the fatty acid composition of the albumin–free fatty acid complex isolated by low-temperature ethanol fractionation (fraction V) according to the procedure of Cohn et al. (204). The free fatty acid composition of whole plasma or serum (i.e., all lipoprotein classes including the albumin–free fatty acid complex) is similar to that of the albumin–free fatty acid complex. The essential difference is in the content of stearic acid. Whereas stearic acid comprised an average 12.6% of the FFA fraction of whole plasma or serum, it comprised only 1.5% of the albumin–free fatty acid complex (203).

Dole et al. (68) have shown that the free-fatty-acid composition of total plasma is but slightly affected by a single fat meal. The pattern is similar to that of adipose tissue, whence the free fatty acids originate (10, 205). However, the amount of stearic acid in the plasma or serum free-fatty-acid

Table XXIX. Fatty Acid Composition of Phospholipids Isolated from Lipoproteins

	Composition[a]											
		Lecithin						Lysolecithin in $d < 1.20$ LP	Sphingomyelin			Phosphatidylethanolamine[b] in $d < 1.20$ LP
Fatty Acid	Whole Serum (112)	VLDL[c] (112)	LDL[d] (112)	HDL_{2+3}[e] (113)	$d < 1.20$ LP (113)	HDL_2[f] (155)	HDL_3[g] (155)	(113)	$d < 1.20$ LP (113)	HDL_2[f] (155)	HDL_3[g] (155)	(113)
Lower than 16:0					0.7	<1.0	<1.0	2.3	1.7	<1.0	<1.0	9.7
16:0	35.9	34.9	34.9	37.8	26.7	28.7	28.4	42.9	36.9	28.5	24.3	11.7
16:1	1.6	1.5	1.3	2.2	1.2	1.1	1.1	1.3	1.7			1.9
17:0					0.5	<1.0	<1.0	2.3	1.1	<1.0	<1.0	0.8
18:0	22.4	20.4	24.6	22.3	13.5	13.9	14.1	34.9	8.5	13.7	14.7	14.2
18:1	14.0	12.6	14.1	13.6	9.5	12.1	12.1	11.5	5.8	5.3	4.2	5.3
18:2	16.2	23.0	16.7	14.8	23.0	25.1	24.8	1.4	14.5	2.7	2.7	8.3
18:2–20:4					4.9	2.7	2.6	1.3	2.0	3.3	3.3	2.5
20:4	5.6	10.9	5.9	10.6	12.2	10.0	10.5		3.8	4.2	5.9	25.2
20:4–22:6					3.1	1.3	1.6	0.5	10.0	9.3	11.0	7.7
22:6					4.7	2.3	2.4		2.5			12.7
23:0								0.8	5.4	6.2	5.9	
24:0								1.4	3.0	7.4	8.1	
24:1									3.1	12.5	14.2	
24:2 and 25:0										0.9	1.2	
Unidentified	4.3	3.9	2.7	4.3								

[a] Expressed as mass percent of total methyl esters in sample (112, 113) except for the values of HDL_2 and HDL_3, which are expressed as moles per 100 moles of fatty acids (155). The reference numbers are shown below each fraction; LP = lipoproteins.
[b] Contains as impurities small amounts of phosphatidylserine and an unidentified compound.
[c] S_f 20–400.
[d] S_f 0–20.
[e] *d* 1.075–1.218 g/ml.
[f] *d* 1.063–1.110 g/ml.
[g] *d* 1.110–1.210 g/ml.

fraction was approximately double the quantity found in lipids extracted from adipose tissue; the amount of oleic acid was somewhat lower. Cornwell et al. (10, 205) attributed these differences to the discriminative utilization of these fatty acids in the peripheral tissues. In fact several investigators have demonstrated the preferential uptake of oleic acid by myocardial and skeletal muscles (206, 207).

A comparison of the free-fatty-acid composition of plasma or serum with that of the glycerides, cholesteryl esters, and phospholipids (Table XXVII) of whole plasma or serum or individual lipoprotein classes shows a close similarity in the pattern of free fatty acids and glycerides. Only stearic acid is significantly lower in the glycerides. This close resemblance between the compositions of free fatty acids and triglycerides is not surprising since the main source of circulating triglyceride fatty acids in the postabsorptive state is the circulating free fatty acids (208–210).

Table XXVII shows the fatty acid composition of the total phospholipid fractions present in various classes of lipoproteins and in whole plasma or serum. Unfortunately little is known concerning the fatty acid composition of individual phospholipid species in the different lipoprotein classes. Practically nothing is known concerning the presence of plasmalogens and ether bonds (alk-1-enyl and alkyl ethers of glycerol) in the various lipoprotein classes under normal and pathologic conditions.

In the early development of gas–liquid chromatography and its application to lipid analysis Nelson and Freeman (112) characterized the fatty acid pattern of some individual phospholipid species present in various lipoprotein classes. They studied the fatty acid compositions of lecithin in whole serum and in VLDL, LDL, and HDL_{2+3} from subjects in the postabsorptive state. The experiments were performed on two subjects, and the agreement between the two sets of values is poor. The authors themselves emphasized that these results must be regarded as preliminary, pending more detailed studies. The averages are given in Table XXIX. The fatty acid compositions of lecithin isolated from whole serum and individual lipoprotein classes are almost the same: palmitic and stearic acids together make up about 50% or more of the total fatty acids in all the lipoprotein classes. Two years later Nelson (113) investigated the fatty acid compositions of individual phospholipids in extracts of lipoproteins with $d < 1.20$ g/ml. He applied improved techniques for both the isolation of individual phospholipids and gas–liquid chromatography for the analysis of fatty acid esters. Unfortunately the author presented the fatty acid composition of individual phospholipids for VLDL, LDL, and HDL_{2+3} together as lipoproteins with $d < 1.20$ g/ml, but not for the individual lipoprotein classes. The new data showed that palmitic acid is the predominant fatty acid in lecithin, as observed earlier. However, the new techniques revealed that the second place is occupied by linoleic acid, rather than stearic acid, which is in third place.

Recently Jones and Ways (155) investigated the fatty acid composition of lecithin isolated from two HDL fractions, HDL_2 and HDL_3, and found it to be the same in both fractions. Five fatty acids are predominantly present in lecithin: palmitic, about 29%; linoleic, 25%; stearic, 14%; oleic, 12%; and arachidonic, 10%. Hence HDL lecithin is very similar in composition to the lecithin of the combined VLDL, LDL, and HDL fractions analyzed by Nelson (113). It seems that in all lipoprotein classes lecithin has a similar fatty acid composition. On the other hand, the fatty acid composition of lysolecithin isolated from lipoproteins with $d < 1.20$ g/ml distinctly differs from that of lecithin and is dominated by two saturated fatty acids, palmitic and stearic, which represent 78% of the fatty acids (113). Of the unsaturated fatty acids, only oleic acid is present in significant amounts (12%), the quantities of other unsaturated fatty acids being negligible.

Sphingomyelin isolated from lipoproteins with $d < 1.20$ g/ml is characterized by a high concentration of palmitic acid and long-chain fatty acids (20 or more carbon atoms). In general a similar pattern was observed by Jones and Ways (155) in sphingomyelin isolated from HDL_2 and HDL_3, which has, however, a higher content of long-chain fatty acids and much less linoleic acid. Phosphatidylethanolamine (which contains a small amount of phosphatidylserine and an unidentified compound) isolated by Nelson (113) from lipoproteins with $d < 1.20$ g/ml is characterized by a high content of arachidonic and other long-chain unsaturated fatty acids (22:4, 22:5, and 22:6, presented in Table XXIX as a group, 20:4–22:6).

The review of the fatty acid composition of the various phospholipids of plasma lipoproteins, although the information so far is fragmentary, shows that each phospholipid has its own pattern. It seems that in the various lipoprotein classes the pattern essentially does not change. However, further systematic studies are necessary.

C. Accumulation of an Atypical Fatty Acid in Blood Lipoproteins (Refsum's Disease)

An inborn error of metabolism called heredopathia atactica polyneuritiformis, or Refsum's disease, is characterized by the accumulation of a branched-chain fatty acid known as phytanic acid (3,7,11,15-tetramethylhexadecanoic acid) in plasma and many organs. This disease was first observed and described by the Norwegian physician S. Refsum approximately 25 years ago. Symptoms include night blindness, impairment of vision, cerebellar ataxia, muscle atrophy, retinitis pigmentosa, cardiac involvement, bone lesions, progressive degeneration of myelin, and dysfunction of the nervous system (212, 213). Detailed reviews of the clinical, pathophysiological, and biochemical aspects of this disease have been presented by Kahlke (211) and Steinberg et al. (212).

Klenk and Kahlke (213) first demonstrated the accumulation of phytanic acid in the serum and tissue lipids of a patient with Refsum's disease. The studies of Steinberg et al. (214, 215) showed that there is little or no endogenous biosynthesis of phytanic acid from mevalonate (the most logical precursor) in these patients. The other possible pathway for the formation of this compound is synthesis from phytol, which is the corresponding α,β-monounsaturated alcohol. The natural source of exogenous phytol is chlorophyll, which contains approximately 30% phytol. Phytol is readily converted to phytanic acid in animals, in patients with Refsum's disease, and in normal man (214, 216, 217).

The accumulation of phytanic acid in this disease is due to the patient's relative inability to oxidize it (218). Uniformly ^{14}C-labeled phytanic acid was injected intravenously as a complex with serum albumin into normal volunteers and patients. Respiratory $^{14}CO_2$ was collected, and the extent of phytanic acid oxidation was estimated. The oxidation rate in patients was less than 5% of that in normal subjects. This defect has also been observed in cultures of fibroblasts from the skin of patients, which oxidized phytanic acid-^{14}C at less than 1% of the rate observed in cultures of fibroblasts from normal skin.

Steinberg and co-workers (218–222) determined that the major metabolic pathway for phytanic acid degradation in normal rats and mice involves an unusual α-oxidation that yields pristanic acid (2,6,10,14-tetramethylpentadecanoic acid). Pristanic acid is further degraded by the usual way of successive β-oxidations, some intermediate products of which have been identified. Pristanic acid, the first product of phytanic acid degradation under normal conditions, is oxidized at the same rate in cultures of fibroblasts from patients with Refsum's disease and from normal subjects. These results indicate that the enzymatic defect in Refsum's disease is in the first step of the metabolic pathway for the oxidation of phytanic acid, α-oxidation.

Figure 3 shows the postulated pathway of phytanic acid oxidation under normal conditions and the nature of the block in Refsum's disease. The conclusion that the genetic defect lies in the very first step of phytanic acid oxidation is supported by the fact that in patients with Refsum's disease only phytanic acid is extensively accumulated, there being no accumulation of pristanic acid or any lower degradation products.

In patients with Refsum's disease phytanic acid usually accumulates in plasma or serum, as demonstrated by gas–liquid chromatography of the

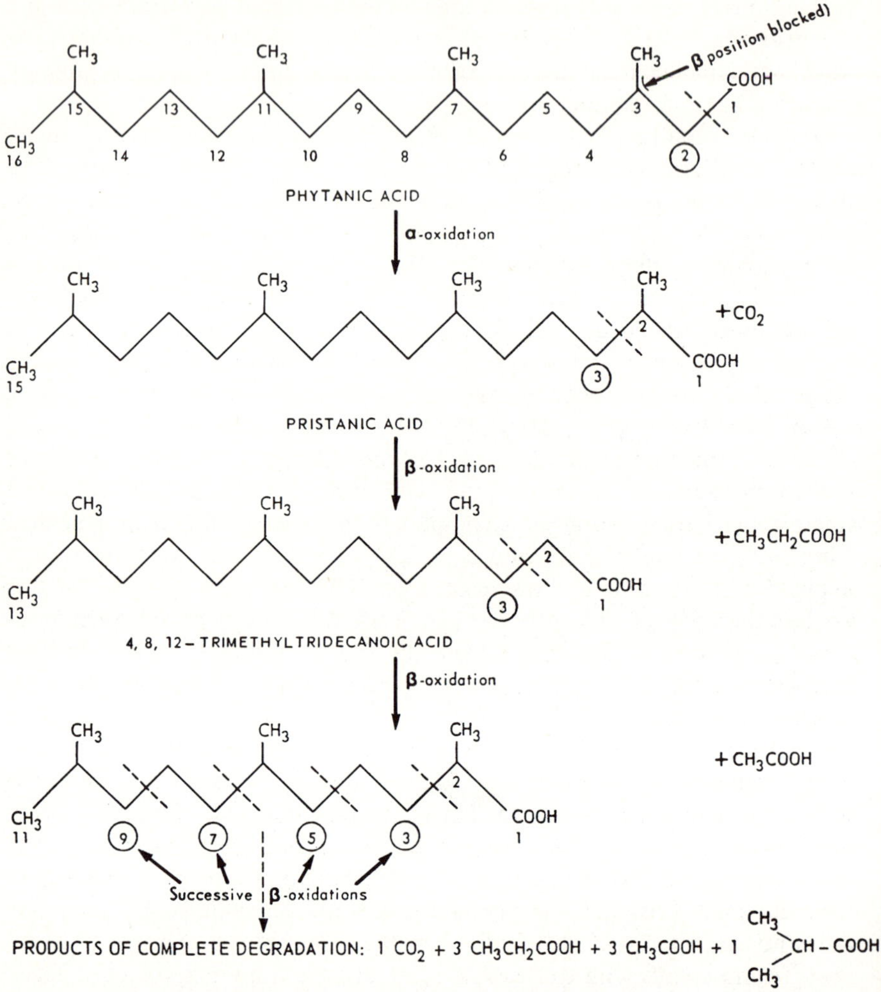

Fig. 3 The suggested pathway for the degradation of phytanic acid in mammals. (Reproduced from Ref. 212 with permission.)

total serum fatty acids. In patients phytanic acid constitutes 10 to 20% of the total plasma fatty acids, although in some cases the quantity was only 3 to 5% (211, 223). Table XXX shows several examples of the fatty acid composition of total plasma lipids in patients with Refsum's disease. In these selected cases the amount of phytanic acid varied from 7 to 23% of the total fatty acids. In the plasma of normal subjects phytanic acid occurs in traces or not at all (211, 223, 224).

Table XXX. Fatty Acid Composition of Plasma Lipids in Patients with Refsum's Disease[a]

Patient and Sex	Fraction	12:0	14:0	16:0	16:1	16: Branched (Phytanic Acid)	18:0	18:1	18:2	18:3	20:0	20:4	22:0	Unidentified
E.H.;F	Total lipids		1	21	6	20	4	23	21			5		
L.D.;F	Total lipids		1	21	5	21	5	21	20			5		
M.C.;F	Total lipids		1	21	3	7	7	24	31			5		
T.E.;F	Cholesteryl esters		2	8	8		1	22	53	1	1	3		1
	Triglycerides	1	5	22	6	15	5	27	9	5	1	2		2
	Free fatty acids	1	7	59		11	21							
	Lecithin[b]			38		7	47				8			
	Sphingomyelin[b]		2	45		7	17				9		21	
J.M.;M[c]	Total lipids		2	25	1	23	5	18	20			5		
	Cholesteryl esters		4	13	2	1	1	23	49			7		
	Triglycerides		3	23	1	51	2	17	4					
	Phospholipids		2	29	1	17	11	14	15			10		

[a] Data from Ref. 224 unless otherwise indicated (in % of total fatty acids.)
[b] Fatty acid analyses were performed after hydrogenation of samples.
[c] Data from Ref. 211. Values in wt. %.

Among the plasma-lipid classes most highly enriched by phytanic acid are the triglycerides. In patients studied by Sarouraud [reported by Kahlke (211)] phytanic acid constituted 51% of the fatty acids in the triglycerides isolated from serum. Plasma phospholipids contained about 25 to 50% of the phytanic acid present in triglycerides. Free fatty acids, diglycerides, and monoglycerides occupied an intermediate position between triglycerides and phospholipids. It is of interest that plasma cholesteryl esters contain only traces of phytanic acid, less than 1%, and frequently below the sensitivity of the test. The proportions of plasma-lipid fatty acids other than phytanic acid are usually more or less normal in patients with Refsum's disease (211, 223).

Kahlke and Wagner (225) studied the distribution of phytanic acid in lipoprotein classes. Lipoproteins from the plasma of patients with Refsum's disease were separated by dextran sulfate precipitation (226) into two fractions, called β- and α-lipoproteins. Apparently the β-lipoproteins included VLDL and LDL, whereas the α-lipoprotein fraction contained HDL as well as lipoproteins with $d > 1.21$ g/ml. Table XXXI shows the

Table XXXI. Fatty Acid Composition of Lipoproteins (LP) and Some of Their Lipid Fractions in Patients with Refsum's Disease[a]

	Composition (mass % of total fatty acids)									
	Normal Subjects			Patients with Refsum's Disease[b]						
							Triglycerides		Phospholipids	
Fatty acid	Whole Plasma	β-LP	α-LP	Whole Plasma	β-LP	α-LP	β-LP	α-LP	β-LP	α-LP
14:0	1.5	2.0	1.0	3.0	3.0	2.9	6.5	3.5	3.5	2.0
16:0	31.5	31.5	34.5	29.2	27.8	31.9	28.5	30.5	33.0	38.0
16:1	4.0	4.0	3.5	3.0	3.3	2.8	3.5	2.5	0.5	1.5
16:branched (phytanic acid)	—	—	—	5.8[c]	7.3[d]	4.1[e]	13.5	12.0	3.6	3.0
18:0	8.5	5.0	9.0	5.1	3.8	5.8	2.0	2.5	12.5	11.5
18:1	27.5	35.0	27.0	24.3	25.1	23.0	35.0	39.0	13.0	21.5
18:2	18.0	17.5	15.5	25.3	26.8	25.0	7.9	8.0	23.5	16.5
20:3	1.5	0.5	1.5	0.6	0.2	0.3	—	—	1.0	0.5
20:4	6.5	4.5	8.0	3.4	2.6	3.9	—	0.5	9.0	5.9

[a] Data from Ref. 225.
[b] Fatty acid concentrations in the total-lipid fraction of whole plasma, β-, and α-lipoproteins are averages of five patients. Fatty acid compositions in triglycerides and phospholipids represent results from one patient.
[c] Range 2.5–11.0.
[d] Range 4.0–13.0.
[e] Range 1.5–7.5.

fatty acid composition of β- and α-lipoproteins isolated from the plasma of patients with Refsum's disease and from normal subjects. A large proportion of phytanic acid was present in the β-lipoproteins, as expected, because of the larger amount of triglycerides in this lipoprotein fraction.

The triglycerides, as already mentioned, are the lipids that accumulate the greatest amount of phytanic acid.

The data in Table XXXI indicate that the amounts of phytanic acid in triglycerides isolated from β- and α-lipoproteins are similar and rather high, whereas the amounts of phytanic acid in the phospholipids of these lipoproteins are also similar, but low. Thus the difference in the lipid compositions of β- and α-lipoproteins determines the difference in the concentration of phytanic acid in these two lipoproteins.

Phytanic acid also accumulates in variable but considerable amounts in various tissues. According to O'Brien and MacBrinn (227, 228), the accumulation of phytanic acid in myelin tends to disrupt the packing of the hydrocarbon tails in the center of the bimolecular lipid leaflet due to steric hindrance imposed by its methyl groups and causes the demyelination of nerves. Many of the clinical manifestations of Refsum's disease can be explained on the basis of this hypothesis.

In general many abnormalities in Refsum's disease are not specific. Similar polyneuritic changes are seen in other lipidoses, in which phytanic acid does not play any role. However, analysis of serum lipids for phytanic acid plays a decisive role in the diagnosis of Refsum's disease.

VIII. COVALENTLY BOUND LIPIDS IN LIPOPROTEINS

All the lipids that were considered in the preceding sections are associated with proteins by forces weaker than covalent bonding. These comprise the main bulk of the lipids in lipoproteins and determine the "lipid composition" of blood plasma. These lipids are extractable by polar solvents. However, there are a few lipids in lipoproteins that cannot be removed even by very extensive organic-solvent extraction because they are firmly bound to proteins, apparently by covalent linkages.

Fisher and Gurin (35) observed the presence of such lipids in a mixture of VLDL, LDL, and HDL from human plasma (all lipoproteins with $d < 1.21$ g/ml) and in HDL from rat serum, the only lipoprotein fractions studied to date. Isolated lipoproteins were subjected to extensive extractions with diethyl ether, then with concentrated formic acid, followed by four precipitations of the proteins with diethyl ether. Thereafter the apoproteins were further extracted in a Soxhlet apparatus for 8 hr with an azeotropic mixture of chloroform and methanol. The authors observed that less than 0.001 micromole of fatty acids per 10 mg of protein was removed during the final hour of chloroform–methanol extraction. These extensively extracted apoproteins were hydrolyzed with 6 N HCl at 105°C for 16 hr. From 0.032 to 0.041 micromole of fatty acids was extracted from

10 mg of the apoproteins of human-serum lipoproteins with $d < 1.21$ g/ml. The fatty acids recovered were myristic, palmitic, and stearic. The apoprotein of the HDL hydrolysates of rat serum yielded only palmitic and stearic acids in a ratio of approximately 1 : 2. Only insignificant amounts of unsaturated fatty acids were present in either case.

The apoproteins of human lipoproteins ($d < 1.21$ g/ml) were digested with a mixture of trypsin and chymotrypsin. The polypeptides obtained after hydrolysis contained stearic and palmitic acids. Similar results were obtained with rat HDL apoproteins prelabeled with ^{14}C-palmitic acid, which was perfused through the liver. Radioactive palmitic acid was recovered from polypeptide hydrolysates.

Fisher and Gurin (35) indicated that these fatty acids or their derivatives are bound more firmly to the protein moieties of plasma lipoproteins than could be expected from electrostatic, polarization, and London–van der Waals forces. It is probable that they are bound to the proteins by covalent linkages.

The authors (35) also performed phosphorus analysis on the extensively extracted human lipoproteins and on the peptides of the apoproteins after partial enzymatic hydrolysis. The fraction containing fatty acids also contained phosphates. The ratio of phosphates to fatty acids in apoproteins ranges from 0.9 to 1.9. However, there was no proof that these phosphates are really parts of the lipid molecules bound to proteins.

The small amounts of lipids covalently bound to proteins may play an important role in the structural organization of lipoprotein molecules. The hydrocarbon chains of fatty acids, covalently bound to proteins, may substantially contribute to binding (by London–van der Waals forces) the hydrocarbon parts of lipids associated with proteins by noncovalent linkages. It is unlikely, however, that lipids covalently bound to proteins play significant physiologic roles in lipid transport (as a source of lipid supply).

IX. SECONDARY ALTERATIONS IN LIPID COMPOSITION IN SOME DISEASES

A. Introduction

Various diseases can affect the levels and compositions of plasma lipids. In most cases these alterations result from increases or decreases in some classes of lipoproteins (see Chapter 12). For example, an increase in the level of plasma LDL brings about increases not only in the total amount of lipids but also in the absolute and relative amounts of cholesterol since the LDL fraction is the major carrier of cholesterol. Parenthetically, this alteration in the lipid composition of blood (i.e., elevated cholesterol) can be a simple reflection of the LDL elevation. In many diseases involving changes in the lipid composition of plasma there are no alterations in the chemical compositions of lipoproteins or, more likely, there is no evidence of any alterations. In some diseases, however, alterations in the chemical compositions of lipoproteins do occur. In these diseases changes in the levels and relative compositions of plasma lipids reflect both alterations in lipoprotein composition and deviations from normal lipoprotein levels.

I have already discussed some hereditary diseases characterized by alterations in the lipid compositions of various lipoproteins. This section covers the nonhereditary diseases in which, as a consequence of the primary disease, there are secondary effects on lipid transport involving the chemical alterations of lipoproteins.

B. Liver Diseases: Obstructive Jaundice

Obstructive jaundice of varying etiology, whether intrahepatic or extrahepatic, is known to cause a marked alteration in plasma lipids. There is a significant increase in the levels of cholesterol, mainly unesterified, and phospholipids. Increase in the latter, which is relatively greater, results in an increased phospholipid-to-cholesterol ratio (229). Kunkel and Slater (230), who used zone electrophoresis to study lipoproteins, observed in biliary cirrhosis a marked reduction in α-lipoproteins with a concomitant increase in phospholipids in the lipoprotein fraction that has the mobility of β-globulins. Furman and co-workers (229, 231, 232), who used ultracentrifugation, noted a marked decrease or even complete lack of HDL in serum from patients with obstructive jaundice. The amounts of lipoproteins with $d > 1.21$ g/ml also decreased. On the other hand, the amounts of S_f 0–12 and S_f 12–20 lipoproteins were substantially increased. In most types of obstructive jaundice the $S_f > 20$ ($F_{1.21}$ 70–100) lipoproteins were usually missing.

Russ, Raymunt, and Barr (233) observed only traces of α-lipoproteins in the plasma of patients with primary biliary cirrhosis. The presence of normal LDL was inferred only from immunologic tests. However, these lipoproteins may account for only a small part of the enormous accumulation of plasma lipids. Most were combined with proteins to form atypical lipoproteins. The authors claim that the serum of a patient with primary biliary cirrhosis contained three different groups of abnormal β-lipoproteins, each of which migrates like β-globulin in moving-boundary electrophoresis. The protein-to-lipid ratio of these abnormal lipoproteins was much smaller than that of normal β-lipoproteins. Protein-to-lipid ratios for the three groups were 1:50, 1:80, and 1:7. These were markedly smaller than the ratios reported for normal LDL. The amounts of esterified cholesterol in these lipoproteins were low, and the total cholesterol-to-phospholipid ratios were lower than normal.

Switzer and Satenstein (234) further characterized these abnormal lipoproteins. However, only one species of abnormal lipoprotein was found in patients with extrahepatic biliary obstruction. The differences between the observations of these authors and Russ et al. (233) may reside in the methods applied by the two groups. Switzer and Satenstein (234) named the abnormal lipoprotein obstructive lipoprotein (OLP). It was present in considerable amounts in patients and was separated from serum by ultracentrifugation with the LDL ($d < 1.063$ g/ml). Separation of normal LDL from the OLP was performed by immunoprecipitation of normal LDL with the γ-globulins (antisera) prepared against lipoproteins with $d < 1.063$ g/ml from normal subjects. The reactive lipoproteins were precipitated, and the unreactive lipoproteins of $d < 1.063$ g/ml (OLP) stayed in the supernatant, from which they were recovered by polyanion precipitation. In the sera of patients more than half the lipoproteins with $d < 1.063$ g/ml were nonreactive lipoproteins, or OLP. Chemical analysis of OLP revealed a very high concentration of free cholesterol (26%) and phospholipids (61%), but only traces of cholesteryl esters and triglycerides. The protein levels, which varied from 13 to 5% were lower than those reported for normal LDL. Although these values were higher than those reported by Russ et al. (233) for two atypical lipoproteins, they were in the range of the third atypical lipoprotein.

The purified preparations of OLP did not react with antiserums to LDL prepared from normal serum, nor with antiserums to HDL. However, rabbits immunized with OLP produced specific antibodies that reacted with VLDL ($d < 1.006$ g/ml) in normal serum. The amino acid content of OLP resembles that of VLDL and differs significantly from those of LDL and HDL. These data are compatible with the hypothesis that OLP contains in its apoprotein an antigenic determinant similar to that present in lipoproteins with $d < 1.006$ g/ml. Switzer and Satenstein (234) were not certain whether OLP was abnormal because it contained a unique peptide or because its structure had undergone secondary alterations. Seidel, Alaupovic, and Furman (235) studied 61 patients with various forms of jaundice and confirmed the presence of an abnormal, or obstructive, lipoprotein in their plasma. However, in nonobstructive jaundice the authors observed no OLP, and the plasma concentrations of cholesterol and phospholipids were low or normal.

Seidel et al. (235) confirmed that in obstructive jaundice the lipoprotein pattern is characterized by a decreased concentration of HDL and increased concentration of "LDL" (d 1.006–1.063 g/ml). Their "LDL" fraction contained varying amounts of a specific lipoprotein, LP-X (apparently identical with OLP), which is immunochemically, electrophoretically, and chemically distinct from normal lipoproteins. Their terminology was based on the nature of the apolipoproteins LP-B for low-density lipoproteins with apoprotein B, LP-A for high-density lipoproteins with apoprotein A, and LP-X for specific lipoproteins with unknown apoprotein. The lipoprotein fraction with *d* 1.006 to 1.063 g/ml contained LP-X, LP-B, and small amounts of LP-A ($\sim$ 2%). The LP-A had a nearly normal chemical composition. The LP-X was responsible primarily for the unusual lipid composition of this lipoprotein fraction in patients with obstructive jaundice.

Table XXXII. Composition (%) of Lipoproteins in Patients with Obstructive Jaundice[a]

Lipoprotein Class and Density (g/ml)	Protein	Total Lipids	TG	CE	FC	PL	PL/Pr[b]
VLDL, *d* <1.006:							
Normal[c]	7.1	92.9	51.8	16.2	6.0	17.9	2.5
Patients	9.5	90.5	55.5	12.8	7.4	15.2	1.6
LDL, *d* 1.006–1.063:							
Normal[c]	20.7	79.3	9.3	39.4	7.5	23.1	1.1
Patients[d]							
Total	19.4	80.6	6.5	15.9	19.4	38.8	2.0
LP-B	26.4	73.6	5.9	27.3	13.9	26.5	0.9
LP-X	5.8	94.2	2.9	2.4	22.4	66.5	11.5
HDL, *d* 1.063–1.21:							
Normal[b]	47.7	52.3	4.6	18.5	2.3	26.9	0.6
Patients	43.7	56.3	2.3	11.0	4.5	38.0	0.9

[a] Data from Ref. 235. Abbreviations: TG, triglycerides; CE, cholesteryl esters; FC, free cholesterol; PL, phospholipids.
[b] Ratio of phospholipids to proteins.
[c] Values for normal subjects used by Seidel et al. (235) were taken from Ref. 64.
[d] This fraction was obtained by heparin precipitation and contains, therefore, only LP-B and LP-X.

Table XXXII shows the chemical composition of the whole "LDL" fraction and its two major lipoprotein constituents, as well as the composition of VLDL and HDL in patients with obstructive jaundice and in normal subjects. The compositions of VLDL and HDL were close to normal, with some increases in HDL phospholipids and decreases in HDL cholesteryl esters. The "LDL" fraction (total, including LP-B and LP-X from patients) was characterized by increases in phospholipids and free cholesterol, and decreases in cholesteryl esters, than those in normal subjects. The free-to-esterified cholesterol ratio and the phospholipid-to-protein ratio were substantially increased in patients with obstructive jaundice. The analysis of two major "LDL" subfractions showed that the composition of LP-B from patients differed only slightly from that of LDL in normal subjects, having a lower concentration of cholesteryl esters and more free cholesterol. On the other hand, LP-X was characterized by a very high content of phospholipids (66.5% of the total lipoprotein), a low content of protein (5.8%), a high content of free cholesterol (22.4%), and a low amount of cholesteryl esters (2.4%). In paper electrophoresis the unique LP-X migrated toward the anode with slightly less mobility than LP-B did.

The portion of "LDL" corresponding to LP-X varied rather extensively in different patients. Probably the concentration of LP-X depends on the degree or duration (or both) of biliary obstruction (235). The proteins of the "LDL" fraction represent 75 to 90% of whole-plasma-lipoprotein proteins, whereas the proteins of LP-X represent 20 to 60% of total-plasma-lipoprotein proteins. Its relatively low protein content made it obvious that under certain conditions LP-X is the major plasma lipoprotein in patients. It may carry up to 50% of plasma cholesterol and up to 80% of the phospholipids.

Seidel et al. (235) speculated on the origin of LP-X. Isselbacher and Budz (236) and Hatch et al. (237) reported that, along with LP-A and LP-B, the intestines synthesize an additional, as yet unidentified, lipoprotein. Alaupovic et al. (238) observed that the presence of apolipoprotein C in chyle coincides with the peak of triglyceride concentration. Seidel et al. (235) questioned whether LP-X is an intestinal lipoprotein similar to lipoproteins containing apoprotein C, which under normal conditions are rapidly catabolized in the liver and therefore escape detection.

C. The Nephrotic Syndrome

The nephrotic syndrome includes several kidney diseases characterized by (a) profuse proteinuria, (b) hypoalbuminemia, (c) hyperlipemia, and (d) generalized edema (239). Hyperlipemia very often is accompanied by lipiduria. However, these metabolic abnormalities are probably secondary to a primary kidney lesion of different etiology. Unfortunately there is some confusion in the use of the term "nephrotic syndrome," and hence I have retained the terminology used by the cited authors. The syndrome can be induced in experimental animals by the administration of antimetabolic agents or by injection of antikidney serum (239–241).

Hyperlipemia in patients with the nephrotic syndrome is characterized by high plasma levels of cholesterol, triglycerides, and phospholipids, the lipid level being usually much higher when the hypoalbuminemia is more pronounced (242). Baxter, Goodman, and Havel (242) studied 44 patients with nephrosis, or the nephrotic syndrome. The series were divided on the basis of the total cholesterol content in serum. Category A included those whose total cholesterol level was above 350 mg/100 ml serum; category B included those whose total cholesterol level was 300 mg/100 ml serum or lower. Each category was further subdivided according to the total amount of triglycerides in serum (in decreasing order). The appearance of the serum was also noted. The mean lipid composition of serum for each group of patients is presented in Table XXXIII.

Table XXXIII. Serum-Lipid Composition in Patients with Nephrosis[a]

Subjects	n[c]	Appearance of Serum	Lipid Composition (mg/100 ml serum)[b]						
			TL	TC	TG	PL	C/PL	C/TG	Alb[d]
Normal young adults			580	179	100	226	0.79	1.8	4.0
Patients:									
Group 1[e]	8	Very milky	5274	1112	2788	841	1.32	0.4	0.6
Group 2[e]	11	Milky	2403	659	882	545	1.21	0.8	1.0
Group 3[e]	19	Slightly milky	1734	574	409	475	1.19	1.5	1.1
Group 4[e]	20	Clear	1302	490	158	404	1.20	3.7	1.7
Group 5[f]	8	Clear	792	247	159	257	0.97	2.2	2.7
Group 6[f]	14	Clear	652	202	125	221	0.91	1.9	3.7

[a] Data from Ref. 242.
[b] Mean values. Abbreviations: TL, total lipids; TC, total cholesterol; TG, triglycerides; PL, phospholipids; C/PL, cholesterol-to-phospholipids ratio; C/TG, cholesterol-to-triglycerides ratio; Alb, albumin.
[c] Number of analyses.
[d] In grams per 100 milliliters of serum.
[e] Category with total cholesterol values of more than 350 mg/100 ml serum.
[f] Category with total cholesterol values of less than 350 mg/100 ml serum.

In severe nephrosis the levels of all lipids analyzed (total cholesterol, triglycerides, and phospholipids) were highly elevated, and the albumin level was decreased to one-seventh the normal value. Alteration of the ratios of total cholesterol to triglycerides, and total cholesterol to phospholipids, indicated either selective elevation of some lipoprotein classes or alterations in the chemical compositions of lipoprotein classes, or both. The lipid levels of patients with moderate proteinuria (group 5) and patients in periods of partial or complete remission (group 6) approached those of normal subjects. However, in a significant number of patients the levels of serum triglycerides were approximately normal and remained so in mild cases even when cholesterol and phospholipid levels were substantially elevated (243).

Nye and Waterhouse (244, 245) also observed an abnormality in the plasma-phospholipid pattern. The levels of lysolecithin and sphingomyelin were two to three times higher than normal, and the amounts of lecithin were approximately 50% below normal.

In patients with a severe nephrotic syndrome lipiduria occurs (240).

The following lipids have been identified in the urine: free cholesterol, cholesteryl esters, triglycerides, free fatty acids, and phospholipids (246, 247). Among the phospholipids, lecithin, phosphatidylethanolamine, and phosphatidylserine were found. Urinary lipid excretion varied widely among the 13 patients studied by Klahr, Tripathy, and Bolanos (247), and no quantitative correlation with serum level was observed. Total cholesterol excretion averaged 52 mg/24 hr compared with 3 mg/24 hr in normal subjects. The mean urinary excretion of phospholipids was 69 mg/24 hr in patients and 10 mg/24 hr in normal subjects. In patients the mean urinary excretion of triglycerides, which were not detected in normal subjects, was 23 mg/24 hr. A good correlation was observed between lipid excretion and glomerular permeability measured by albumin excretion and creatine clearance. The authors believe that most of the lipid in the urine enters the glomerular filtrate in the form of lipoproteins.

Several groups of investigators studied the plasma lipoproteins in patients with the nephrotic syndrome. Gitlin and associates (248) separated by ultracentrifugation the serum lipoproteins of six children with various degrees of the nephrotic syndrome. They observed an elevation of the S_f 10–200 lipoproteins. The amounts of HDL and S_f 3–9 lipoproteins (LDL) were normal or somewhat smaller than those in serum from normal children. Baxter et al. (242) investigated the levels and compositions of serum lipoproteins in four groups of patients with more severe forms of the nephrotic syndrome (total cholesterol content greater than 350 mg/100 ml). The lipid composition of their whole serum is shown in Table XXXIII. Concentrations of VLDL ($d < 1.019$ g/ml) were greatly elevated in the milky serums of group 1 (20–40 times), moderately increased in groups 2 and 3 (5–10 times), and only slightly above normal or normal in the clear serums of group 4. The extent of elevation was determined by chemical analysis rather than actual measurement of lipoprotein quantities in the analytical ultracentrifuge.

Low-density lipoproteins (d 1.019–1.063 g/ml) increased stepwise from group 1 (nearly normal levels) to group 4 (threefold increase). High-density lipoproteins (d 1.063–1.21 g/ml) were below normal in groups 1, 2, and 3, in which VLDL were substantially increased, and normal in group 4. In general, in more advanced or severe cases of the nephrotic syndrome, lipoproteins with $d < 1.019$ g/ml were very elevated, whereas in moderate cases, lipoproteins with d 1.019 to 1.063 g/ml were elevated and VLDL ($d < 1.019$ g/ml) were more or less normal.

Table XXXIV shows the mean compositions of lipoprotein classes isolated from the four groups of patients described above. In normal subjects lipoproteins of $d < 1.019$ g/ml had a total cholesterol-to-phospholipid ratio of 0.82, which in patients with the nephrotic syndrome was 1.05 to

Table XXXIV. Lipid Composition of Serum Lipoproteins in Patients with the Nephrotic Syndrome[a]

Component	Concentration (mg/100 ml serum)				
		Patients[b]			
	Normal	Group 1	Group 2	Group 3	Group 4
	Lipoproteins with d *<1.019 g/ml*				
Triglycerides	78	2901	831	334	114
Total cholesterol	23	894	377	220	63
Phospholipids	28	619	317	180	59
C/PL[c]	0.82	1.45	1.20	1.16	1.05
	Lipoproteins with d *1.019–1.063 g/ml*				
Total Lipids	265	270	480	764	793
Total Cholesterol	103	77	160	308	332
Phospholipids	74	84	127	217	218
Proteins	70	103	153	212	239
C/PL[c]	1.39	0.91	1.27	1.43	1.51
	Lipoproteins with d *1.063–1.21 g/ml*				
Total Lipids	190	91	102	119	220
Total Cholesterol	49	36	19	37	63
Phospholipids	101	58	37	66	92
Proteins	170	107	92	137	210
C/PL[c]	0.48	0.45	0.51	0.54	0.67

[a] Data from Ref. 242.
[b] Each group represents average values obtained on a minimum of five patients who had relatively similar values for total serum cholesterol.
[c] Ratio of total cholesterol to phospholipids.

1.45, indicating alterations in the lipid compositions of lipoprotein complexes. However, in the case of lipoproteins with $d < 1.019$ g/ml, because of their heterogeneity, alterations of the ratios may also indicate that some particular lipoprotein subfraction was selectively elevated and had changed this ratio. In most severe cases of the disease lipoproteins with d 1.019 to 1.063 g/ml had a subnormal cholesterol-to-phospholipid ratio, 0.91 (the normal ratio is 1.39), and in moderate cases this ratio approached normal values. In patients the total-lipid-to-protein ratio in this class of lipoproteins deviated from normal values. These observations indicate the change in the gross composition of lipoproteins with d 1.019 to 1.063 g/ml. The alteration in the lipid composition of HDL was relatively small, although significant.

Shafrir (194) showed that the proportion of free fatty acids bound to lipoproteins with $d < 1.21$ g/ml was considerably higher than that in normal serum, although the total amount was normal in patients. The average proportions of free fatty acids bound to albumin were 77.6 and 34.7% in normal subjects and patients with the primary nephrotic syndrome, respectively. In patients the remaining 65.3% was bound to lipoproteins with $d < 1.21$ g/ml. It seems that the amount of free fatty acids present in HDL was not essentially affected by the disease. However, the amounts bound to lipoproteins with $d < 1.019$ g/ml and lipoproteins with d 1.019 to 1.063 g/ml was increased by a factor of 2 to 3 or even more when lipemia was pronounced, and the amount of albumin was less than 1.0 g/100 ml of serum. The shift of free fatty acids from the albumin–free fatty acid complexes (lipoproteins with $d > 1.21$ g/ml) to lipoproteins with $d < 1.21$ g/ml apparently resulted from the decrease in the amount of plasma albumin. Indeed the molar ratio of free fatty acids to albumin in the patients averaged 1.13 versus 0.77 in normal controls.

As a result of the increased amounts of free fatty acids in lipoproteins with $d < 1.21$ g/ml in serum from patients, the moving-boundary-electrophoresis pattern of the lipoproteins showed irregularities in the α_2- and β-globulin regions. One or both of these fractions had abnormal mobility, and an additional component of intermediate mobility was recorded. Addition of free-fatty-acid-poor albumin to the nephrotic serum normalized the electrophoretic pattern of the lipoproteins.

Alterations in the lipid composition of lipoproteins in serum from patients with the nephrotic syndrome was observed also by Nye and Waterhouse (244, 245), who reported changes in the composition of phospholipids. The most pronounced changes occurred in lipoproteins with $d < 1.063$ g/ml (mainly 1.019–1.063 g/ml). In this fraction the relative and absolute amounts of lysolecithin and sphingomyelin were increased, and the amount of lecithin was decreased. Evidently there were no alterations in the HDL phospholipid composition ($d > 1.063$ g/ml) in patients with the syndrome.

Sodhi and Kalant (249) observed changes in the lipid composition of "LDL ($d < 1.063$ g/ml)," (VLDL + LDL) from which chylomicrons had been removed, in rats with a nephrotic syndrome experimentally induced by injection of anti-kidney serum. The amounts of cholesterol and proteins in the chylomicron and "LDL" fractions isolated from the nephrotic serum were from 10 to 20 times higher than those in serum from normal rats. However, the increase in cholesterol was proportionately much greater, resulting in a substantial increase in the cholesterol-to-protein ratio. In chylomicrons and "LDL ($d < 1.063$ g/ml)" isolated from normal rats the cholesterol-to-protein ratios were 1.4 and 4.7, respectively, whereas in lipoproteins isolated from nephrotic serum these ratios were 4.6 and 6.4, respectively. There was no change in the cholesterol-to-protein ratio in HDL isolated from the serum of nephrotic rats, which confirmed the observation that in human patients HDL are not affected significantly by this disease.

Sodhi and Kalant (250) demonstrated that in rats with experimental nephrosis the rates at which cholesterol enters and leaves the blood are increased. The hypercholesterolemia in rats with the nephrotic syndrome resulted mainly from a shift of the plasma–liver pool of cholesterol into vascular compartments (plasma). By using plasma lipoproteins labeled with ^{14}C-cholesterol, the authors (249) observed that the ratio of cholesterol transfer [exchange of cholesterol between "LDL ($d < 1.063$ g/ml)" and red blood cells] was markedly lower in rats with the nephrotic syndrome than it was in normal rats. The rate of cholesterol exchange between "LDL" and HDL in nephrotic rats was lower than it was in normal rats. On the other hand, HDL from normal and nephrotic rats had similar rates for cholesterol exchange with red blood cells.

These facts indicate that "LDL" from nephrotic rats bind cholesterol more strongly than do normal "LDL" and that HDL are not affected by the disease. The authors consider that in nephrotic rats the protein moiety of "LDL" has a stronger than normal affinity toward lipids because of a structural alteration, and that this leads to an alteration in the lipoprotein composition which causes the redistribution of cholesterol in the liver–plasma pool. This hypothesis is only one of several that attempt to explain the mechanism of lipemia in the nephrotic syndrome. For other possible mechanisms responsible for abnormalities of lipid metabolism in the nephrotic syndrome see Chapter 16.

X. SUMMARY

All lipids present in human plasma are bound to proteins, forming various classes of lipoproteins. Under normal conditions each class of lipoproteins has a specific pattern for its chemical composition. The lipid content of various lipoprotein classes varies from 99 to 98% in particulate fat to 1% or even less in the albumin–free fatty acid complex. With the decrease in lipid content and the corresponding increase in protein content, lipoprotein densities increase from 0.93 to 1.33 g/ml. Concomitant with the decrease in the lipid-to-protein ratio in lipoproteins (corresponding to an increase in density) are alterations in other physicochemical properties: molecular weights decrease in order of magnitude from 10^{10} to 10^4, the complexes diminish in size, and ultracentrifugal flotation rates are lowered. The various lipoprotein classes have different structural organizations and molecular shapes; and various types of proteins participate in lipoprotein formation. Each lipoprotein class represents a family of closely related compounds, rather than a single, firmly defined, chemical entity.

All lipoprotein classes, except possibly the albumin–free fatty acid complex, contain all types of lipids known to be present in plasma. The albumin–free fatty acid complex apparently has a specific lipid composition. Thus the differences in lipid composition between lipoprotein classes are, in most cases, quantitative rather than qualitative. The lipid compositions of the various lipoprotein classes are determined by their physiologic function in lipid transport in the organism and apparently by the requirement of stability in their molecular organization.

The majority of lipids are associated with proteins by forces weaker than covalent bonds and are therefore easily extracted by polar organic solvents. However, a small amount of lipid is apparently bound to protein by covalent bonds. Most likely the latter are significant for the structural organization of lipoprotein molecules rather than for lipid transport in the organism, as are the lipids that are more weakly bound to proteins, which constitute the primary transportable lipids in most instances.

The lipoproteins of the lowest density are particulate fats. Under normal physiologic conditions all or almost all particulate fat, usually called chylomicrons ($d < 1.006$ g/ml, $S_f > 400$), is of exogenous origin. Chylomicrons are composed largely of triglycerides (81–89%). The amount of protein varies from about 1 to 2.5%, depending on the source of the chylomicrons: chyle or blood (plasma or serum). Chylomicrons also contain 6 to 9% phospholipids, mainly lecithin and sphingomyelin, and small amounts of free and esterified cholesterol. The most polar components of chylomicrons —proteins, phospholipids, and free cholesterol—are concentrated exclusively on the surface, whereas triglycerides form the core.

The fatty acid composition of lymph chylomicrons mirrors that of ingested fat, providing the latter does not contain large amounts of short-chain fatty acids. Cholesteryl esters also resemble ingested fat in their fatty acid composition. However, the fatty acid composition of phospholipids isolated from chylomicrons is not affected by ingested fat.

Plasma or serum chylomicrons are heterogeneous. They consist of primary particles, for example, lymph chylomicrons slightly modified in the bloodstream, and secondary particles, which are more modified lymph chylomicrons. Both primary and secondary particles are composed predominantly of triglycerides. Whereas the triglyceride-fatty-acid pattern of primary particles resembles that of ingested fat, triglyceride fatty acids of secondary particles are a mixture of fatty acids from ingested fat and body fat.

Patients with carbohydrate-induced hyperlipoproteinemia may have endogenous particles in plasma. This particulate fat, although it consists mainly of triglycerides, has an elevated content of cholesterol and phospholipids compared with primary and secondary particles. Other disturbances in lipid transport or lipid metabolism may also cause the appearance of particulate fat that differs in lipid composition from particulate fat under normal physiologic conditions.

Very-low-density lipoproteins, or pre-β-lipoproteins ($d < 1.006$ g/ml, S_f 20–400) are characterized by a high content of triglycerides. This lipoprotein class contains about 8 to 10% proteins and 90 to 92% lipids. About 50% of the lipids are triglycerides, 20% total cholesterol, and 18% phospholipids. However, the rather poor agreement among the total cholesterol and phospholipid values reported by different investigators may be partially explained by the effects of sex differences. In VLDL the relative amount of free cholesterol compared with cholesteryl esters is much higher than that in total serum or other lipoproteins. The principal phospholipid is lecithin.

Low-density lipoproteins, or β-lipoproteins (d 1.006–1.063 g/ml, S_f 0–20) are characterized by a high content of cholesterol, both esterified and free. The total amount of proteins ranges from 20 to 25%, and the amount of lipids is 75 to 80%. According to the majority of investigators, cholesterol comprises about 40% of the lipids. The content of triglycerides is 10%, and the amount of phospholipids ranges from 28 to 30% of the total lipids. The most prominent phospholipids are lecithin and sphingomyelin. The relative content of sphingomyelin (25–26% of phospholipids in LDL) is higher than it is in any other lipoprotein class.

High-density lipoproteins, or α-lipoproteins are divided into two major classes: HDL_2 and HDL_3 (d 1.063–1.125 and 1.125–1.21 g/ml, respectively). High-density lipoproteins are composed of 52% protein and 48% lipids. Their lipid moiety is characterized by a high content of phospholipids, ranging from 42 to 51%, and a high content of total cholesterol. However, the amount of cholesterol is smaller than it is in LDL: 32 versus 40% of the total lipids. Most of the cholesterol is present as cholesteryl esters. A comparison of the chemical compositions of the two major classes shows that the HDL_2 fraction has less protein, non-phosphorus-containing glycerides, free fatty acids, and ceramide monohexosides; it also has more total cholesterol, as well as more esterified and free cholesterol.

The ultracentrifugal residue ($d > 1.21$ g/ml) appears to be a heterogeneous fraction consisting of very-high-density lipoproteins-1 ($VHDL_1$, d 1.21–1.25 g/ml), the albumin–free fatty acid complex, and lipid-free proteins with $d > 1.25$ g/ml. The presence of additional lipoprotein components is not excluded. The whole ultracentrifugal residue is characterized by a very high protein content, 98 to 99%, and a low lipid content, 1 to

2%. Free fatty acids constitute 29 to 61%, and phospholipids 17 to 46%, of the total lipids. In addition, there are significant amounts of cholesterol, both free and esterified; lower glycerides (diglycerides and monoglycerides); hydrocarbons of the alkane series; and ceramide monohexosides. The phospholipids are mainly lysolecithin (21–71%). The $VHDL_1$ fraction in general, has a chemical composition that is more or less similar to that of other high-density lipoproteins, with a low content of free fatty acids and lysolecithin.

The $VHDL_2$ fraction ($d > 1.25$ g/ml) contains most of the free fatty acids and lysolecithin (both of which are associated with plasma albumin) and small amounts of other lipids. It has not been established whether the other lipids found in this fraction represent impurities, degradation products of ultracentrifugation, or a third lipoprotein in the ultracentrifugal residue.

Apparently more than half the total free fatty acids present in plasma are associated with albumin; values reported range from 33 to 87%. The remaining free fatty acids are associated with other lipoproteins.

The total amount of free fatty acids in plasma varies greatly with physiologic and pathologic conditions. The majority of the mean values reported for plasma or serum free-fatty-acid levels, under fasting conditions and in normal subjects, range from 0.400 to 0.800 meq/l, although values for individual subjects are often slightly below or above this range.

Compared with its effects on the fatty acid composition of chylomicrons, a single fat meal affects the fatty acid composition of VLDL moderately, HDL slightly, and LDL not at all. These effects usually are noticeable only in the lipoprotein triglycerides, and hence it is possible to speak of a "normal" pattern for the free-fatty-acid composition of lipoproteins on a regular diet. Each lipid, in any lipoprotein class, has its own peculiar pattern of fatty acid composition. In triglycerides and lower glycerides the predominant fatty acids are, in order of decreasing amounts, oleic, palmitic, and linoleic. In cholesteryl esters the predominant fatty acids are linoleic, oleic, and palmitic. In phospholipids the most abundant fatty acids are palmitic, linoleic, and stearic. In the total free fatty acids of whole plasma and of the albumin–free fatty acid complex the predominant fatty acids are oleic and palmitic. Information on the fatty acid composition of individual phospholipids in the various lipoprotein classes is still fragmentary.

In the majority of the diseases that directly or indirectly involve an abnormality in lipid metabolism or lipid transport there are alterations in the levels of various plasma lipoproteins, reflecting changes in the lipid composition of the plasma. In most cases there are no changes per se in the lipid composition of the lipoproteins, but there are some diseases in which changes do occur.

Three rare hereditary diseases in which the chemical composition of lipoproteins is affected have been thoroughly investigated in the last decade. Tangier disease, or hypo-α-lipoproteinemia, is characterized by the complete absence of true HDL (α-lipoproteins) from plasma. Also absent are VLDL (pre-β-lipoproteins). The LDL fraction (β-lipoproteins) accumulates large amounts of triglycerides, and hence the amount of total serum triglycerides may reach 600 mg/100 ml serum. On the other hand, the plasma levels of cholesterol and phospholipids are subnormal.

Abetalipoproteinemia is characterized by the absence of true LDL, VLDL, and chylomicrons from plasma. The amount of HDL_3 is decreased, whereas that of HDL_2 is normal or even increased. The chemical compositions of both HDL_2 and HDL_3 are altered; the concentration of sphingomyelin is increased, and that of lecithin is decreased. In HDL_2, although the level of total cholesterol is normal, there is an alteration in the ratio of cholesteryl esters to free cholesterol, with an increase in the latter. The total amount of linoleic acid in all lipids investigated is significantly decreased.

Refsum's disease is characterized by the accumulation in lipids, including plasma lipoproteins, of a branched-chain fatty acid, phytanic acid (3,7,11,15-tetramethylhexadecanoic acid). In patients 10 to 20% of the total plasma-lipid fatty acids may be phytanic acid, which accumulates mainly in triglycerides, moderately in phospholipids, and is not present in cholesteryl esters. Therefore the chemical composition of the lipoprotein determines the amount of phytanic acid. Lipoproteins with $d < 1.063$ g/ml contain more phytanic acid than do those with $d > 1.063$ g/ml. In normal subjects there may be only traces of phytanic acid in serum lipoproteins.

Alterations in the lipid composition of lipoproteins may occur also when lipid metabolism or transport is affected secondarily by such primary diseases as obstructive jaundice and the nephrotic syndrome.

In obstructive jaundice the appearance of an abnormal lipoprotein, "obstructive lipoprotein," was noted in LDL (d 1.006–1.063 g/ml). This obstructive lipoprotein is immunologically different from either LDL or HDL, contains only small amounts of proteins (5–13%), and has 61 to 67% phospholipids and 22 to 26% free cholesterol. The concentrations of cholesteryl esters and triglycerides are extremely low in comparison with those in "normal" LDL. In certain conditions of obstructive jaundice the obstructive lipoprotein will carry most of the plasma lipids since the amounts of VLDL, true LDL, HDL, and the ultracentrifugal residue may be decreased drastically.

Severe cases of the nephrotic syndrome are manifested by hyperlipemia, with greatly increased amounts of cholesterol, triglycerides, and phospholipids. When the lipoprotein classes were separated, it was noted that the ratios of cholesterol to phospholipids and total lipids to proteins deviate from the normal. These deviations may indicate changes in the chemical composition of lipoproteins, especially in LDL. There are indications that the apoprotein of LDL has a stronger affinity for lipids, especially cholesterol, at least in rats with the nephrotic syndrome.

The relative amount of free fatty acids usually associated with albumin is decreased, and more of them are transported by lipoproteins with $d <$ 1.21 g/ml. However, the total amount of free fatty acids in plasma is usually in the normal range, and the redistribution occurs because of the decrease in plasma albumin. Lipoproteins with $d < 1.063$ g/ml have an abnormal phospholipid composition, with increased amounts of lysolecithin and sphingomyelin, and decreased amounts of lecithin.

Although a number of glycolipids are known to be present in serum, with the exception of ceramide monohexosides, their distribution in the lipoproteins is not known.

XI. ACKNOWLEDGMENTS

The author wishes to thank Drs. V. N. Schumaker and G. H. Adams for making available to him a prepublication copy of their valuable and useful review (Ref. 22); Dr. Marion Barclay for her assistance; Mrs. Dorman D. Israel for proofreading; and Mrs. Sophronia Myron for general assistance in the preparation of the final copy. The work was supported in part by research grant CA-08748 from the National Cancer Institute, U.S. Public Health Service.

ADDENDUM

New lipid in cancer patients. It was discovered recently by Skipski, Barclay, Archibald, Lynch, and Stock (251) that lipid extracts from HDL_2 and HDL_3 isolated from sera of patients with cancer contain a lipid-protein complex of the proteolipid type. This proteolipid is called neoproteolipid (251–253). The neoproteolipid is present only in serum high-density lipoproteins of these patients and not present in other lipoprotein classes. It is also absent from any lipoprotein classes of normal human beings or whole serum/plasma.

The neoproteolipid with chromatographic properties similar to that present in the lipid extracts from HDL_2 and HDL_3 of patients with cancer was isolated from a transplanted tumor of rats, the Walker carcinosarcoma 256, and called neoproteolipid-W (252–253). The neoproteolipid-W isolated from the rat tumor has the following composition (252): amino acids 8–9%, monosaccharides 40–45%, fatty acids 25–31%, sphingosines 12–

14%, cholesterol 1.0–1.5%, and phosphorus 0.25–0.28%. It seems that most, if not all the monosaccharides and sphingosines, are present in the form of glycosphingolipid. The neoproteolipid-W apparently is essentially a ceramide oligohexoside(s) and protein (or polypeptides) with a small content of other lipids (phospholipids, cholesterol). The authors consider that the presence of neoproteolipid in serum of patients with cancer and its absence in normal subjects may eventually be used as a tool for the detection of cancer ("cancer test"), or as a test for the efficacy of medical treatment.

REFERENCES

1. Folch-Pi, J., in *Brain Lipids and Lipoproteins, and the Leucodystrophies,* J. Folch-Pi and H. Bauer, Eds., Elsevier, Amsterdam, 1963, pp. 18–30.
2. Macheboeuf, M. A., *Bull. Soc. Chim. Biol.* **11**, 268–293, 485–503 (1929).
3. Macheboeuf, M., and P. Rebeyrotte, *Discussions Faraday Soc., Lipo-proteins,* No. 6, 62–70 (1949).
4. Oncley, J. L., and F. R. N. Gurd, in *Blood Cells and Plasma Proteins. Their State in Nature,* J. L. Tullis, Ed., Academic Press, New York, 1953, pp. 337–357.
5. Barclay, M., R. K. Barclay, O. Terebus-Kekish, E. B. Shah, and V. P. Skipski, *Clin. Chim. Acta* **8**, 721–726 (1963).
6. Barclay, M., G. C. Escher, R. J. Kaufman, O. Terebus-Kekish, E. M. Greene, and V. P. Skipski, *Clin. Chim. Acta* **10**, 39–47 (1964).
7. Ewing, A. M., N. K. Freeman, and F. T. Lindgren, *Adv. Lipid Res.* **3**, 25–62 (1965).
8. Dole, V. P., and J. T. Hamlin, III, *Physiol. Rev.* **42**, 674–701 (1962).
9. Walton, K. W., *J. Atheroscler. Res.* **7**, 533–536 (1967).
10. Cornwell, D. G., in *Lipids and Lipidoses,* G. Schettler, Ed., Springer-Verlag, New York, 1967, pp. 168–189.
11. Bierman, E. L., D. Porte, Jr., D. D. O'Hara, M. Schwartz, and F. C. Wood, Jr., *J. Clin. Invest.* **44**, 261–270 (1965).
12. Bierman, E. L., E. Gordis, and J. T. Hamlin, III, *J. Clin. Invest.* **41**, 2254–2260 (1962).
13. Gustafson, A., P. Alaupovic, and R. H. Furman, *Biochemistry* **4**, 596–605 (1965).
14. Gustafson, A., *Acta Med. Scand.* **179**, Suppl. 446 (1966).
15. Lees, R. S., and D. S. Fredrickson, *J. Clin. Invest.* **44**, 1968–1977 (1965).
16. Bierman, E. L., T. L. Hayes, J. N. Hawkins, A. M. Ewing, and F. T. Lindgren, *J. Lipid Res.* **7**, 65–72 (1966).
17. Lindgren, F. T., N. K. Freeman, A. V. Nichols, and J. W. Gofman, in *The Blood Lipids and the Clearing Factor* (Third International Conference on Biochemical Problems of Lipids, 1956), R. Ruyssen, Ed., Paleis der Academien, Brussels, 1957, pp. 224–242.
18. Scanu, A. M., *Adv. Lipid Res.* **3**, 63–138 (1965).
19. Skipski, V. P., M. Barclay, R. K. Barclay, V. A. Fetzer, J. J. Good, and F. M. Archibald, *Biochem. J.* **104**, 340–352 (1967).

20. Granda, J. L., and A. Scanu, *Biochemistry* **5**, 3301–3308 (1966).
21. Alaupovic, P., S. S. Sanbar, R. H. Furman, M. L. Sullivan, and S. L. Walraven, *Biochemistry* **5**, 4044–4053 (1966).
22. Schumaker, V. N., and G. H. Adams, *Ann. Rev. Biochem.* **38**, 113–136 (1969).
23. Cook, W. H., and W. G. Martin, *Can. J. Biochem. Physiol.* **40**, 1273–1285 (1962).
24. Hatch, F. T., and R. S. Lees, *Adv. Lipid Res.* **6**, 2–68 (1968); Nichols, A. V., in *Advances in Biological and Medical Physics,* Vol. 11, J. H. Lawrence and J. W. Gofman, Eds., Academic Press, New York, 1967, pp. 109–158.
25. Forte, G. M., A. V. Nichols, and R. M. Glaeser, *Chem. Phys. Lipids,* **2**, 326–408 (1968).
26. Hayes, T. L., N. K. Freeman, F. T. Lindgren, A. V. Nichols, and E. L. Bierman, in *Protides of the Biological Fluids,* (Proceedings of the 13th Colloquium), H. Peeters, Ed., Elsevier, Amsterdam, 1966, pp. 273–279.
27. Lossow, W. J., F. T. Lindgren, J. C. Murchio, G. R. Stevens, and L. C. Jensen, *J. Lipid Res.* **10**, 68–76 (1969).
28. Margolis, S., *J. Lipid Res.* **8**, 501–507 (1967).
29. Scanu, A., H. Pollard, and W. Reader, *J. Lipid Res.* **9**, 342–349 (1968).
30. Scanu, A., and R. Hirz, *Nature* **218**, 200–201 (1968).
31. Scanu, A., and J. L. Granda, *Biochemistry* **5**, 446–455 (1966).
32. Scanu, A., W. Reader, and C. Edelstein, *Biochem. Biophys. Acta* **160**, 32–45 (1968).
33. Entenman, C., *J. Amer. Oil Chem. Soc.* **38**, 534–538 (1961).
34. Hanahan, D. J., *Lipid Chemistry,* Wiley, New York, 1960.
35. Fisher, W. R., and S. Gurin, *Science* **143**, 362–363 (1964).
36. Gurd, F. R. N., in *Comprehensive Biochemistry,* Vol. 8, Part 2, M. Florkin and E. H. Stotz, Eds., Elsevier, Amsterdam, 1963, pp. 3–16, and in *Lipid Chemistry,* J. Hanahan, Ed., Wiley, New York, 1960, pp. 208–325.
37. Salem, L., *Can. J. Biochem. Biophys.* **40**, 1287–1298 (1962).
38. Lindgren, F. T., and A. V. Nichols, in *Plasma Proteins,* Vol. 2, F. W. Putnam, Ed., Academic Press, New York, 1960, pp. 1–58.
39. Cook, W. H., and W. G. Martin, *Biochim. Biophys. Acta* **56**, 362–365 (1962).
40. Vandenheuvel, F. A., *Can. J. Biochem. Physiol.* **40**, 1299–1326 (1962).
41. Day, C. E., and R. S. Levy, *J. Theor. Biol.* **23**, 287–399 (1969).
42. Scanu, A., *Proc. Natl. Acad. Sci. U.S.* **54**, 1699–1705 (1965).
43. Scanu, A., *J. Biol. Chem.* **242**, 711–719 (1967).
44. Scanu, A., and J. L. Granda, *Prog. Biochem. Pharmacol.* **4**, 153–158 (1968).
45. Scanu, A., and R. Hirz, *Proc. Natl. Acad. Sci. U.S.* **59**, 890–894 (1968).
46. Gotto, A. M., R. I. Levy, and D. S. Fredrickson, *Proc. Natl. Acad. Sci. U.S.* **60**, 1436–1441 (1968).
47. Gotto, A. M., R. I. Levy, A. S. Rosenthal, M. E. Birnbaumer, and D. S. Fredrickson, *Biochem. Biophys. Res. Commun.* **31**, 699–705 (1968).
48. Sodhi, H. S., and R. G. Gould, *J. Biol. Chem.* **242**, 1205–1210 (1967).
49. Avigan, J., *J. Biol. Chem.* **226**, 957–964 (1957).
50. Hamilton, R. I., *Proceedings of the Deuel Conference on Lipids,* Carmel, California, 1968, U.S. Public Health Service publication.
51. Tria, E., and A. M. Scanu, Eds., *Structural and Functional Aspects of Lipoproteins in Living Systems,* Academic Press, London and New York, 1969.
52. Gage, S. H., *Cornell Vet.* **10**, 154–155 (1920).
53. Gage, S. H., and P. A. Fish, *Amer. J. Anat.* **34**, 1–85 (1924).

54. Nestel, P. J., R. J. Havel, and A. Bezman, *J. Clin. Invest.* **41**, 1915–1921 (1962).
55. Bragdon, J. H., and R. S. Gordon, *J. Clin. Invest.* **37**, 574–578 (1958).
56. Rodbell, M., *J. Biol. Chem.* **235**, 1613–1620 (1960).
57. Olson, R. E., and J. W. Vestor, *Physiol. Rev.* **40**, 677–733 (1960).
58. Frazer, A. C., and H. C. Steward, *J. Physiol. (London)* **90**, 18–30 (1937).
59. Alaupovic, P., R. H. Furman, W. H. Falor, M. L. Sullivan, S. L. Walraven, and A. C. Olson, *Ann. N.Y. Acad. Sci.* **149**, 791–807 (1968).
60. Laurell, C. B., *Scand. J. Clin. Lab. Invest.* **6**, 22–24 (1954).
61. Scanu, A., and I. H. Page, *J. Exp. Med.* **109**, 239–256 (1959).
62. Lindgren, F. T., A. V. Nichols, T. L. Hayes, N. K. Freeman, and J. W. Gofman, *Ann. N.Y. Acad. Sci.* **72**, 826–844 (1959).
63. Freeman, N. K., F. T. Lindgren, and A. V. Nichols, in *Progress in the Chemistry of Fats and Other Lipids,* Vol. 6, R. T. Holman, W. O. Lundberg, and T. Malkin, Eds., Pergamon Press–Macmillan Co., New York, 1963, pp. 216–250.
64. Bragdon, J. H., R. J. Havel, and E. Boyle, *J. Lab. Clin. Med.* **48**, 36–42 (1956).
65. Wood, P., K. Imaichi, J. Knowles, G. Michaels, and L. Kinsell, *J. Lipid Res.* **5**, 225–231 (1964).
66. Jobst, H., and G. Schettler, in *The Blood Lipid and the Clearing Factor* (Third International Conference on Biochemical Problems of Lipids, 1956), R. Ruyssen, Ed., Paleis der Academien, Brussels, 1957, pp. 136–149.
67. Kayden, H. J., A. Karmen, A. E. Dumont, and J. Bragdon, *J. Clin. Invest.* **39**, 1001 (1960).
68. Dole, V. P., A. T. James, J. P. W. Webb, M. A. Rizack, and M. F. Sturman, *J. Clin. Invest.* **38**, 1544–1554 (1959).
69. Blomstrand, R., and O. Dahlbäck, *J. Clin. Invest.* **39**, 1185–1191 (1960).
70. Bragdon, J. H., and A. Karmen, *J. Lipid Res.* **1**, 167–170 (1960).
71. Bragdon, J. H., and A. Karmen, *J. Lipid Res.* **2**, 400–402 (1961).
72. Kayden, H. J., A. Karmen, and A. Dumont, *J. Clin. Invest.* **42**, 1373–1381 (1963).
73. Zilversmit, D. B., *J. Clin. Invest.* **44**, 1610–1622 (1965).
74. Gordis, E., *Proc. Soc. Exp. Biol. Med.* **110**, 657–661 (1962).
75. Albrink, M. J., *J. Clin. Invest.* **40**, 536–544 (1961).
76. Swahn, B., *Scand. J. Clin. Lab. Invest.* **5**, Suppl. 9, 1–114 (1953).
77. Nye, W. H. R., and G. Schultz, *Proc. Soc. Exp. Biol. Med.* **116**, 350–354 (1964).
78. Kay, R. E., and C. Entenman, *J. Biol. Chem.* **236**, 1006–1012 (1961).
79. Bierman, E. L., and D. E. Strandness, Jr., *Amer. J. Physiol.* **210**, 13–18 (1966).
80. Casley-Smith, J. R., *J. Cell. Biol.* **15**, 259–277 (1962).
81. Kay, D., and D. S. Robinson, *Quart. J. Exp. Physiol.* **47**, 258–261 (1962).
82. Salpeter, M. M., and D. B. Zilversmit, *J. Lipid Res.* **9**, 187–192 (1968).
83. Schoefl, G. I., *Proc. Roy. Soc. (London)* **B169**, 147–152 (1968).
84. Zilversmit, D. B., *Fed. Proc.* **26**, 1599–1605 (1967).
85. Zilversmit, D. B., *J. Lipid Res.* **9**, 180–186 (1968).
86. Huang, T. C., and A. Kuksis, *Lipids* **2**, 443–452 (1967).
87. Zilversmit, D. B., P. H. Sisco, Jr., and A. Yokoyama, *Biochim. Biophys. Acta* **125**, 129–135 (1966).
88. Pinter, G. G., and D. B. Zilversmit, *Biochim. Biophys. Acta* **59**, 116–127 (1962); Yokoyama, A., and D. B. Zilversmit, *J. Lipid Res.* **6**, 241–246 (1965).
89. Fredrickson, D. S., R. I. Levy, and R. S. Lees, *New Eng. J. Med.* **276**, 32–44, 94–103, 148–156, 215–226, 273–281 (1967).

90. Cornwell, D. G., F. A. Kruger, G. J. Hamwi, and J. B. Brown, *Amer. J. Clin. Nutr.* **9**, 41–54 (1961).
91. Carlson, L. A., and B. Olhagen, *Scand. J. Clin. Lab. Invest.* **6**, 70–73 (1954).
92. Ahrens, E. H., Jr., J. Hirsch, K. Oette, J. W. Farquhar, and Y. Stein, *Trans. Assoc. Amer. Physicians* **74**, 134–146 (1961).
93. Ahrens, E. H., Jr., and N. Spritz, in *Biochemical Problems of Lipids,* A. C. Frazer, Ed., Elsevier, Amsterdam, 1963, pp. 304–312.
94. Fredrickson, D. S., and R. S. Lees, in *The Metabolic Basis of Inherited Disease,* J. B. Stanbury, J. B. Wyngaarden, and D. S. Fredrickson, Eds., Blakiston–McGraw-Hill, New York, 1966, pp. 429–485.
95. Fredrickson, D. S., and R. S. Lees, *Circulation* **31**, 321–327 (1965).
96. Fredrickson, D. S., R. I. Levy, P. O. Kwiterovich, Jr., and A. Jover, in *Drugs Affecting Lipid Metabolism* (Proceedings Third International Symposium on Drugs Affecting Lipid Metabolism, Milan, Italy, 1968), W. L. Holmes, L. A. Carlson, and R. Paoletti, Eds., Plenum Press, New York, 1969, pp. 307–325.
97. Kinsell, L. W., G. Schlierf, W. Kahlke, and G. Schettler, in *Lipids and Lipidoses,* G. Schettler, Ed., Springer-Verlag, New York, 1967, pp. 446–489.
98. Lyon, I., M. S. Masri, and I. L. Chaikoff, *J. Biol. Chem.* **196**, 25–32 (1952).
99. Evans, J. D., and L. N. Norcia, *J. Lipid Res.* **5**, 395–401 (1964).
100. Quarfordt, S. H., R. I. Levy, A. Frank, and D. S. Fredrickson, *J. Clin. Invest.* **47**, 81a–82a (1968).
101. Lees, R. S., and F. T. Hatch, *J. Lab. Clin. Med.* **61**, 518–528 (1963).
102. Levy, R. I., R. S. Lees, and D. S. Fredrickson, *J. Clin. Invest.* **45**, 63–77 (1966).
103. Hatch, F. T., in *Serum Proteins and the Dysproteinemias,* F. W. Sunderman and F. W. Sunderman, Jr., Eds., Lippincott, Philadelphia, 1965, pp. 223–237.
104. Oncley, J. L., K. W. Walton, and D. G. Cornwell, *J. Amer. Chem. Soc.* **79**, 4666–4671 (1957).
105. Oncley, J. L., in *Brain Lipids and Lipoproteins, and the Leucodystrophies,* J. Folch-Pi and H. Bauer, Eds., Elsevier, Amsterdam, 1963, pp. 1–17.
106. Oncley, J. L., F. R. N. Gurd, and M. Melin, *J. Amer. Chem. Soc.* **72**, 458–464 (1950).
107. Lindgren, F. T., A. V. Nichols, and N. K. Freeman, *J. Phys. Chem.* **59**, 930–938 (1955).
108. Polonovski, J., *Rev. Athéroscler. (Arch. Malad. Coeur)* **1**, 60–68 (1959).
109. Polonovski, J., M. Ayrault-Jarrier, M. Petit, and D. Bard, *Ann. Biol. Clin.* **17**, 331–335 (1959).
110. Goodman, D. S., and T. Shiratori, *J. Lipid Res.* **5**, 307–313 (1964).
111. Phillips, G. B., *J. Clin. Invest.* **38**, 489–493 (1959).
112. Nelson, G. J., and N. K. Freeman, *J. Biol. Chem.* **235**, 578–583 (1960).
113. Nelson, G. J., *J. Lipid Res.* **3**, 71–79 (1962).
114. Polonovski, J., in *Collogues internationaux: digestion, absorption intestinale, et transport des glycerides chex les animaux superieurs,* Vol. 99, Centre National de la Récherche Scientifique, Paris, 1961, pp. 195–204.
115. Hazzard, W. R., F. T. Lindgren, and E. L. Bierman, *Biochim. Biophys. Acta* **202**, 517–525 (1970).
116. Kunkel, H. G., and R. Trautman, *J. Clin. Invest.* **35**, 641–648 (1956).
117. Lewis, L. A., A. A. Green, and I. H. Page, *Amer. J. Physiol.* **171**, 391–400 (1952).
118. Levy, R. S., A. C. Lynch, E. D. McGee, and J. W. Mehl, *J. Lipid Res.* **8**, 463–472 (1967).

119. Williams, J. H., M. Kuchmak, and R. F. Witter, *Lipids* **1**, 89–97 (1966).
120. Nye, W. H. R., C. Waterhouse, and G. V. Marinetti, *J. Clin. Invest.* **40**, 1194–1201 (1961).
121. Phillips, G. B., and J. T. Dodge, *J. Lipid Res.* **8**, 676–681 (1967).
122. Levy, R. I., and D. S. Fredrickson, *J. Clin. Invest.* **44**, 426–441 (1965).
123. Shore, B., and V. Shore, *Arch. Biophys. Biochem.* **71**, 1–10 (1957).
124. Barclay, M., O. Terebus-Kekish, V. P. Skipski, and R. K. Barclay, *Clin. Chim. Acta* **11**, 389–394 (1965).
125. Scanu, A., *J. Lipid Res.* **7**, 295–306 (1966).
126. Shore, B., and V. Shore, *Biochemistry* **7**, 2773–2777 (1968).
127. Gofman, J. W., O. deLalla, F. Glazier, N. K. Freeman, F. T. Lindgren, A. V. Nichols, B. Strisower, and A. R. Tamplin, *Plasma (Milan)* **2**, 413–484 (1954).
128. Barclay, M., R. K. Barclay, and V. P. Skipski, *Nature* **200**, 362–363 (1963).
129. Hillyard, L. A., C. Entenman, H. Feinberg, and I. L. Chaikoff, *J. Biol. Chem.* **214**, 79–90 (1955).
130. Fredrickson, D. S., in *The Metabolic Basis of Inherited Disease,* J. B. Stanbury, J. B. Wyngaarden, and D. S. Fredrickson, Eds., McGraw-Hill, New York, 1966, pp. 486–508.
131. Fredrickson, D. S., *J. Clin. Invest.* **43**, 228–236 (1964).
132. Fredrickson, D. S., and P. H. Altrocchi, in *Cerebral Sphingolipidoses,* S. M. Aronson and B. W. Volk, Eds., Academic Press, New York, 1962, pp. 343–357.
133. Fredrickson, D. S., R. I. Levy, and F. T. Lindgren, *J. Clin. Invest.* **47**, 2446–2457 (1968).
134. Kahlke, W., in *Lipids and Lipidoses,* G. Schettler, Ed., Springer-Verlag, New York, 1967, pp. 401–411.
135. Levy, R. I., and D. S. Fredrickson, *Circulation* **34**, Suppl. 3, 156 (1966).
136. Rodbell, M., and D. S. Fredrickson, *J. Biol. Chem.* **234**, 562–566 (1959).
137. Levy, R. I., R. S. Lees, and D. S. Fredrickson, *J. Clin. Invest.* **45**, 63–77 (1966).
138. Bassen, F. A., and A. L. Kornzweig, *Blood* **5**, 381–387 (1950).
139. Farquhar, J. W., and P. Ways, in *The Metabolic Basis of Inherited Disease,* 2nd ed., J. B. Stanbury, J. B. Wyngaarden, and D. S. Fredrickson, Eds., McGraw-Hill, New York, 1966, pp. 509–522.
140. Kahlke, W., in *Lipids and Lipidoses,* G. Schettler, Ed., Springer-Verlag, New York, 1967, pp. 382–400.
141. Singer, K., B. Fisher, and M. A. Perlstein, *Blood* **7**, 577–591 (1952).
142. Isselbacher, K. J., R. Scheig, G. R. Plotkin, and J. B. Caulifield, *Medicine (Baltimore)* **43**, 347–361 (1964).
143. Isselbacher, K. J., *Fed. Proc.* **24**, 16–22 (1965).
144. Ways, P. O., C. M. Parmentier, H. J. Kayden, J. W. Jones, D. R. Saunders, and C. E. Rubin, *J. Clin. Invest.* **46**, 35–46 (1967).
145. Ways, P., and C. Parmentier, *Clin. Res.* **11**, 77 (1963).
146. Phillips, G. B., *J. Lab. Clin. Med.* **59**, 357–363 (1962).
147. Ways, P., C. F. Reed, D. J. Hanahan, D. Dong, S. Palmer, M. Murphy, and G. Roberts, *J. Clin. Invest.* **42**, 1248–1260 (1963).
148. Wolff, O. H., *Ergebn. Med. Kinderheilk.* **23**, 190–201 (1965).
149. Levy, R. I., D. S. Fredrickson, and L. Laster, *J. Clin. Invest.* **45**, 531–541 (1966).
150. Becroft, D. M. O., J. M. Castello, and P. J. Scott, *Arch. Dis. Child.* **40**, 40–46 (1965).

151. Salt, H. B., O. H. Wolff, J. K. Lloyd, A. S. Fosbrooke, A. H. Cameron, and D. V. Hubble, *Lancet* **2**, 325–329 (1960).
152. Schwartz, J. F., L. P. Rowland, H. Eder, P. A. Marks, E. F. Osserman, E. Hirschberg, and H. Anderson, *Arch. Neurol.* **8**, 438–454 (1963).
153. Lees, R. S., *J. Lipid Res.* **8**, 396–405 (1967).
154. Lamy, M., J. Frezal, J. Polonovski, G. Druez, and J. Rey, *Pediatrics* **31**, 277–289 (1963).
155. Jones, J. W., and P. Ways, *J. Clin. Invest.* **46**, 1151–1161 (1967).
156. Kendall, F. E., *J. Biol. Chem.* **138**, 97–109 (1941).
157. Cohn, E. J., W. L. Hughes, Jr., and J. H. Weare, *J. Amer. Chem. Soc.* **69**, 1753–1761 (1947).
158. Havel, R. J., H. A. Eder, and J. H. Bragdon, *J. Clin. Invest.* **34**, 1345–1353 (1955).
159. Phillips, G. B., *Proc. Soc. Exp. Biol. Med.* **100**, 19–22 (1959).
160. Switzer, S., and H. A. Eder, *J. Lipid Res.* **6**, 506–511 (1965).
161. Fredrickson, D. S., and R. S. Gordon, Jr., *Physiol. Rev.* **38**, 585–630 (1958).
162. Dole, V. P., *J. Clin. Invest.* **35**, 150–154 (1956).
163. Nicholas, H. J., and K. J. Bombaugh, *Biochim. Biophys. Acta* **98**, 372–379 (1965).
164. Gazzarrini, F., and B. Nagy, *Arch. Biochem. Biophys.* **113**, 245–247 (1966).
165. Skipski, V. P., M. Barclay, F. M. Archibald, O. Terebus-Kekish, E. S. Reichman, and J. J. Good, *Life Sci.* **4**, 1673–1680 (1965).
166. Skipski, V. P., A. F. Smolowe, R. C. Sullivan, and M. Barclay, *Biochim. Biophys. Acta* **106**, 386–396 (1965).
167. Boitnott, J. K., and S. Margolis, *Bull. Johns Hopkins Hosp.* **118**, 414–422 (1966).
168. Rose, H. G., and A. F. Liber, *J. Lab. Clin. Med.* **68**, 475–483 (1966).
169. McCarthy, R. D., *Biochim. Biophys. Acta* **84**, 74–79 (1964).
170. Spector, A. A., K. John, and J. E. Fletcher, *J. Lipid Res.* **10**, 56–67 (1969).
171. Ray, A., J. A. Reynolds, H. Polet, and J. Steinhardt, *Biochemistry* **5**, 2606–2616 (1966).
172. Phillips, G. B., *Proc. Natl. Acad. Sci. U.S.* **43**, 566–570 (1957).
173. Gjone, E., J. F. Berry, and D. A. Turner, *J. Lipid Res.* **1**, 66–71 (1959).
174. Newman, H. A. I., C.-T. Liu, and D. B. Zilversmit, *J. Lipid Res.* **2**, 403–411 (1961).
175. Glomset, J. A., *Biochim. Biophys. Acta* **70**, 389–395 (1963).
176. Klopfenstein, W. E., *Biochim. Biophys. Acta* **181**, 323–325 (1969).
177. Szent-Gyorgyi, A., and T. Tominaga, *Biochem. Z.* **146**, 226–238 (1924).
178. Kelsey, F. E., and H. E. Longenecker, *J. Biol. Chem.* **139**, 727–740 (1941).
179. Gordon, R. S., Jr., and A. Cherkes, *J. Clin. Invest.* **35**, 206–212 (1956).
180. Gordon, R. S., Jr., A. Cherkes, and H. Gates, *J. Clin. Invest.* **36**, 810–815 (1956).
181. Fredrickson, D. S., and R. S. Gordon, Jr., *Physiol. Rev.* **38**, 585–630 (1958).
182. Fredrickson, D. S., and R. S. Gordon, Jr., in *Essential Fatty Acids* (Proceedings of the Fourth International Conference on Biochemical Problems of Lipids), H. M. Sinclair, Ed., Academic Press, New York, 1958, pp. 195–204.
183. Dole, V. P., and M. A. Rizack, *J. Lipid Res.* **2**, 90–91 (1961).
184. Svanborg, A., L. Svennerholm, J. VonDorrien, and M. R. Soomagi, *Clin. Chim. Acta* **3**, 443–449 (1958).

185. Carlsten, A., B. Hallgren, R. Jagenburg, A. Svanborg, and L. Werko, *Scand. J. Clin. Lab. Invest.* **14**, 185–191 (1962).
186. Goldman, J. K., *Proc. Soc. Exp. Biol.* **117**, 164–166 (1964).
187. Lieber, C. S., C. M. Leevy, S. W. Stein, W. S. George, G. R. Cherrick, W. H. Abelmann, and C. S. Davidson, *J. Lab. Clin. Med.* **59**, 826–832 (1962).
188. Konttinen, A., H. S. S. Sarajas, M. H. Frick, and M. Rajasalmi, *Ann. Med. Exp. Biol. Fenn.* **40**, 250–256 (1962).
189. Hollister, L. E., and A. Wright, *J. Atheroscler. Res.* **5**, 445–450 (1965).
190. Castelli, W. P., R. J. Nickerson, J. M. Newell, and D. D. Rutstein, *J. Atheroscler. Res.* **6**, 328–341 (1966).
191. Nestel, P. J., *J. Clin. Invest.* **43**, 77–82 (1964).
192. Carlson, L. A., and L. Orö, *Metabolism* **12**, 132–142 (1963).
193. Shafrir, E., *Fed. Proc.* **17**, 309 (1958).
194. Shafrir, E., *J. Clin. Invest.* **37**, 1775–1782 (1958).
195. Goodman, D. S., and E. Shafrir, *J. Amer. Chem. Soc.* **81**, 364–370 (1959).
196. Goodman, D. S., *J. Amer. Chem. Soc.* **80**, 3892–3898 (1958).
197. Gordon, R. S., Jr., *J. Clin. Invest.* **34**, 477–484 (1955).
198. Bierman, E. L., V. P. Dole, and T. N. Roberts, *Diabetes* **6**, 475–479 (1957).
199. Mehnert, H., L. Pelikan, and N. Zollner, *Klin. Wochenschr.* **39**, 888-891 (1961).
200. Lindgren, F. T., A. V. Nichols, and R. D. Wills, *Amer. J. Clin. Nutr.* **9**, 13–23 (1961).
201. Lindgren, F. T., and A. V. Nichols, *Ann. N.Y. Acad. Sci.,* **94**, Art. 1, 55–70 (1961).
202. Hallgren, B., and A. Svanborg, *Scand. J. Clin. Lab. Invest.* **14**, 179–184 (1962).
203. Saifer, A., and L. Goldman, *J. Lipid Res.* **2**, 268–270 (1961).
204. Cohn, E. J., F. R. N. Gurd, D. M. Surgenor, B. A. Barnes, R. K. Brown, G. Derouaux, J. M. Gillespie, F. W. Kahnt, W. F. Lever, C. H. Liu, D. Mittelman, R. F. Mouton, K. Schmid, and E. Uroma, *J. Amer. Chem. Soc.* **72**, 465–474 (1950).
205. Cornwell, D. G., F. A. Kruger, G. J. Hamwi, and J. B. Brown, *Metabolism* **11**, 840–849 (1962).
206. Rothlin, M. E., and R. J. Bing, *J. Clin. Invest.* **40**, 1380–1386 (1961).
207. Miller, H. I., M. Gold, and J. J. Spitzer, *Amer. J. Physiol.* **202**, 370–374 (1962).
208. Havel, R. J., *Metabolism* **10**, 1034 (1961).
209. Havel, R. J., J. M. Felts, and C. M. VanDuyne, *J. Lipid Res.* **3**, 297–308 (1962).
210. Norcia, L. N., and J. D. Evans, *Metabolism* **13**, 12–20 (1964).
211. Kahlke, W., in *Lipids and Lipidoses,* G. Schettler, Ed., Springer-Verlag, New York, 1967, pp. 352–381.
212. Steinberg, D., F. Q. Vroom, W. K. Engel, J. Cammermeyer, C. E. Mize, and J. Avigan, *Ann. Intern. Med.* **66**, 365–395 (1967).
213. Klenk, E., and W. Kahlke, *Z. Physiol. Chem.* **333**, 133–139 (1963).
214. Steinberg, D., J. Avigan, C. Mize, L. Eldjarn, K. Try, and S. Refsum, *Biochem. Biophys. Res. Commun.* **19**, 783–789 (1965).
215. Steinberg, D., C. Mize, J. Avigan, H. M. Fales, L. Eldjarn, K. Try, O. Stokke, and S. Refsum, *J. Clin. Invest.* **46**, 313–322 (1967).
216. Stoffel, W., and W. Kahlke, *Biochem. Biophys. Res. Commun.* **19**, 33–36 (1965).
217. Steinberg, D., J. Avigan, C. Mize, and J. Baxter, *Biochem. Biophys. Res. Commun.* **19**, 412–416 (1965).

218. Avigan, J., D. Steinberg, A. Gutman, C. E. Mize, and G. W. A. Milne, *Biochem. Biophys. Res. Commun.* **24**, 838–844 (1966).
219. Mize, C. E., D. Steinberg, J. Avigan, and H. M. Fales, *Biochem. Biophys. Res. Commun.* **25**, 359–365 (1966).
220. Steinberg, D., J. H. Herndon, Jr., B. W. Uhlendorf, J. Avigan, C. E. Mize, and H. M. Fales, *J. Clin. Invest.* **46**, 1120 (1967).
221. Steinberg, D., J. H. Herndon, Jr., B. W. Uhlendorf, C. E. Mize, J. Avigan, and G. W. A. Milne, *Science* **156**, 1740–1742 (1967).
222. Mize, C. E., J. Avigan, D. Steinberg, R. C. Pittman, H. M. Fales, and G. W. A. *Milne, Biochim. Biophys. Acta* **176**, 720–739 (1969).
223. Kahlke, W., *Klin. Wochenschr.* **41**, 783–784 (1963).
224. Kahlke, W., *Klin. Wochenschr.* **42**, 1011–1016 (1964).
225. Kahlke, W., and H. Wagner, in *Protides of the Biological Fluids* (Proceedings of the 13th Colloquium), H. Peeters, Ed., Elsevier, Amsterdam, 1966, pp. 351–354.
226. Sakagami, T., and D. B. Zilversmit, *J. Lipid Res.* **3**, 111–116 (1962).
227. O'Brien, J. S., *J. Theoret. Biol.* **15**, 307–324 (1967).
228. MacBrinn, M. C., and J. S. O'Brien, *J. Lipid Res.* **9**, 552–561 (1968).
229. Furman, R. H., L. L. Conrad, A. W. Fryer, B. S. Wamack, and E. L. McDearmon, *J. Clin. Invest.* **36**, 713–722 (1957).
230. Kunkel, H. G., and R. J. Slater, *J. Clin. Invest.* **31**, 677–684 (1952).
231. Furman, R. H., L. L. Conrad, and R. P. Howard, *Circulation,* **10**, 586 (1954).
232. Furman, R. H., R. P. Howard, K. Lakshmi, and L. N. Norcia, *Amer. J. Clin. Nutr.* **9**, 73–102 (1961).
233. Russ, E. M., J. Raymunt, and D. P. Barr, *J. Clin. Invest.* **35**, 133–144 (1956).
234. Switzer, S., and L. Satenstein, *J. Clin. Invest.* **46**, 1855–1866 (1967).
235. Seidel, D., P. Alaupovic, and R. H. Furman, *J. Clin. Invest.* **48**, 1211–1223 (1969).
236. Isselbacher, K. J., and D. M. Budz, *Nature,* **200**, 364–365 (1963).
237. Hatch, F. T., Y. Aso, L. M. Hagopian, and J. J. Rubenstein, *J. Biol. Chem.* **241**, 1655–1665 (1966).
238. Alaupovic, P., R. H. Furman, S. L. Walraven, W. H. Falor, and H. A. I. Newman, *Circulation* **36**, Suppl. II, 2 (1967).
239. Relman, A. S., in *Cecil and Loeb Textbook of Medicine,* 11th ed., P. B. Beeson and W. McDermott, Eds., Saunders, Philadelphia, 1963, pp. 832–837.
240. Schreiner, G. E., in *Diseases of the Kidney,* M. B. Strauss and L. G. Welt, Eds., Little, Brown, Boston, 1963, pp. 335–444.
241. Heymann, W., and H. Z. Lund, *Pediatrics* **7**, 691–706 (1951).
242. Baxter, J. H., H. C. Goodman, and R. J. Havel, *J. Clin. Invest.* **39**, 455–465 (1960).
243. Baxter, J. H., *Arch. Intern. Med.* **109**, 742–757 (1962).
244. Nye, W. H. R., and C. Waterhouse, *Clin. Res.* **8**, 244 (1960).
245. Nye, W. H. R., and C. Waterhouse, *J. Clin. Invest.* **40**, 1202–1207 (1961).
246. Zimmer, J. G., R. Dewey, C. Waterhouse, and R. Terry, *Ann. Intern. Med.* **54**, 205–214 (1961).
247. Klahr, S., K. Tripathy, and O. Bolanos, *J. Clin. Invest.* **46**, 1475–1481 (1967).
248. Gitlin, D., D. G. Cornwell, D. Nakasato, J. L. Oncley, W. L. Hughes, Jr., and C. A. Janeway, *J. Clin. Invest.* **37**, 172–184 (1958).
249. Sodhi, H. S., and N. Kalant, *Metabolism* **12**, 420–427 (1963).
250. Sodhi, H. S., and N. Kalant, *Metabolism* **12**, 414–419 (1963).

251. Skipski, V. P., M. Barclay, F. M. Archibald, T. P. Lynch, Jr., and C. C. Stock, *Proc. Soc. Exp. Biol. Med.* **136**, 1261–1264 (1971).
252. Skipski, V. P., F. M. Archibald, M. Barclay, and C. C. Stock, *Fed. Proc.* **30**, 1188 Abs. (1971).
253. Skipski, V. P., F. M. Archibald, C. R. Adler, A. W. Fine, M. Barclay, and C. C. Stock, *Res. Comm. Chem. Pathol. Pharmacol.* **3** (January 1972) (in press).

12. Lipoprotein Class Distribution in Normal and Diseased States

MARION BARCLAY

Division of Experimental Chemotherapy, Sloan-Kettering Institute for Cancer Research, Walker Laboratory, Rye, New York

I. INTRODUCTION

In this chapter an attempt has been made to bring together most of the present knowledge about serum-lipoprotein levels in subjects "clinically free from disease" and in patients in whom the fundamental disease may be directly related to lipid metabolism or may result in deranged lipid metabolism.

The normal, or "usually healthy," state has to be taken on faith in some instances. If persons who are now octogenarians had been the main subjects 30 or 40 years ago, the investigator would have felt more certain.

In many diseases, such as the hyperlipoproteinemias, there are overt signs pointing toward errors in lipid metabolism, but even with these, the fundamental biochemical problem may still be obscure.

Diseases involving organs known to be important in synthesis, enzyme and hormone production, detoxification, storage, and elimination, can result in serum-lipoprotein levels that are obviously not within the normal range.

When one compares serum levels in sick and healthy subjects, the magnitude of the overlap in ranges becomes important. Values or differences given for patients in the works cited are assumed to relate to satisfactorily matched controls.

At present there is growing evidence of "abnormal" lipoproteins in some diseases. However, it is possible that proteins and amino acids as well as the various lipids are involved.

Knowledge of lipid and lipoprotein metabolism in man and other species has grown as a genie since Walter Bloor and his colleagues rubbed the oil lamp.

II. SERUM-LIPOPROTEIN LEVELS IN SUBJECTS WITHOUT CLINICAL SYMPTOMS OF DISEASE

To describe the serum concentrations of any component in the "normal" human can be fraught with danger since it is impossible to know whether the subjects have occult lipid or lipoprotein abnormalities. Atheromatous plaques may be present at any age. Genetic propensities may play a role, and, of course, sex, diet, and exercise are influential factors.

The reviewer must assume that the investigators reporting lipoprotein values in normal subjects checked their clinical status, that in large populations the mean values are statistically reliable and meaningful, and that many humans are essentially free from diseases affecting lipoprotein metabolism. In addition to the health of the subject, there is the problem of measuring the lipoprotein components in the serum and correlating results obtained by different procedures.[1] This problem occurred even in the earliest reports.

[1] The material presented is derived from many sources. Several procedures were used to separate and quantify or to estimate the soluble serum lipoproteins. The details of these procedures are presented in Chapter 5 and are not repeated. However, to facilitate understanding and to offer some correlation between the different terms used by the authors cited, synonymous expressions are inserted after the terms of the authors as the topics are discussed [e.g., "β-lipoproteins (LDL, or lipoproteins $1.006 < d < 1.063$ g/ml)]. Some terms are described briefly *in situ,* in the tables where necessary, and in the text.

Most of the early work centered around low-density lipoproteins (LDL) in serum, described by Blix, Tiselius, and Svennson (1), who used moving-boundary electrophoresis to separate α- and β-globulins, with which most of the serum cholesterol is associated. Shortly thereafter Adair and Adair (2) reported a low-density protein that they separated by salting out. In 1947 Pedersen (3) used flotation (at a solution density of 1.04 g/ml) to isolate a "low-density" lipoprotein.

The fact that most of the cholesterol is associated with the low-density, or β-lipoprotein, fraction stimulated efforts to implicate these molecules with certain diseases, such as atherosclerosis. Although the Donner group, under the guidance of Gofman and Jones (4–7) perfected the ultracentrifugal separations, most early data were still based on lipoproteins with densities lower than 1.0635 g/ml.

Although probably the first successful isolation of a lipoprotein by Macheboeuf (8) in 1929 produced an α-lipoprotein (high-density lipoprotein), data were slow to evolve.

A. Children 2 to 14 Years Old

The dearth of data on serum-lipoprotein levels in normal children probably results from the comparative rarity of atherosclerosis and heart disease in young people. With the recent upsurge in associating lipoprotein abnormalities with diseases prevalent in children (hypolipoproteinemia and hyperlipoproteinemia), the levels in normal children should be known. Table I presents data compiled according to the methods used for isolating and measuring lipoproteins in the given age bracket.

The values obtained by a single procedure but from different laboratories are in good agreement. Children of this age do have fair amounts of very-low-density lipoproteins (VLDL), possibly the result of diet or a reflection of postprandial sampling. They have less of the low-density lipoproteins (LDL) than do adults, according to data obtained by ultracentrifugation, but, according to electrophoretic data, essentially similar ratios of β- to α-lipoproteins (66:33%) to those of many adults. The turbidimetric index for β-lipoproteins appears to be similar to that of adults (17).

B. Men and Women 14 to 65 Years Old

Many reports have come from the Donner Laboratory, where serum lipoproteins were originally separated and measured quantitatively by ultracentrifugal means. These normal values derived from Tamplin and Tandy (9) are presented because data from fasting and nonfasting subjects were included. In more recent work VLDL and LDL values were given sep-

Table I. Serum-Lipoprotein Levels in Normal Children 2 to 14 Years Old

Data Obtained by Ultracentrifugal Analyses[a] (mg/100 ml serum)

			VLDL		LDL				
Age	Sex	n[b]	S_f 100–400	S_f 20–100	S_f 10–20	S_f 0–10	HDL_2	HDL_3	Ref.
4	M	9	24	68	40	313			9
5	F	6	27	65	37	290			9
2	M	5	0	10	13	414			10
8	M	4	8	79	50	351	67	170	11

Data Obtained by Electrophoresis[c]

Age	Sex	n[b]	β-Lipoproteins[d]	α-Lipoproteins[d]	Ref.
			60–80	20–40	13
14	M	30	249[e]	139[e]	14
		13	66 (55–80)	33 (20–45)	15
3–12			70	28	16

Data Obtained by Other Procedures

Age	n[b]	β-Lipoprotein Index (Turbidimetric)[f]	Ref.
4–14	169	0.97	17

[a] VLDL, very-low-density lipoproteins (d <1.006 g/ml); LDL, low-density lipoproteins (d <1.063 g/ml); HDL_2, high-density lipoproteins-2 (d <1.125 g/ml); HDL_3, high-density lipoproteins-3 (d <1.21 g/ml). One Svedberg flotation unit (S_f) equals 1×10^{-13} cm/sec-dyne-g. The solution density 1.063 g/ml (5) essentially divides the LDL from the HDL. If a separate run at d 1.006 g/ml is not made, the S_f 0–20 fraction is usually LDL; the $d < 1.006$ g/ml fraction includes S_f 20–400 lipoproteins (VLDL). Lipoproteins with $d > 1.063$ g/ml may be HDL_2 or HDL_3 (12).

[b] Number of subjects.

[c] Electrophoresis on zonal media, paper, etc., moves lipoproteins in the following order: chylomicrons remain at origin; β-band; pre-β-band (α_2-band), if present; α_1-band.

[d] Concentrations are in percent of total, unless otherwise indicated.

[e] Concentration in mg/100 ml serum.

[f] Ratio of the β-lipoproteins found and the theoretical average value for healthy individuals.

arately (18), but no comments on the state of digestion were included. The averages of the means (Table II), which were calculated from the data of Tamplin and Tandy (9), serve only to simplify the presentation and not to offer further statistical evaluation.

The effects of fasting on the VLDL and LDL classes in males were not consistent in that only the S_f 100–400 lipoproteins were somewhat decreased. Since this class is rich in triglycerides (VLDL), it would be more affected by recent food intake than the S_f 0–100 lipoproteins.

In females the levels of S_f 20–100 and S_f 100–400 lipoproteins were lower after fasting, and the level of S_f 10–20 lipoproteins remained essentially the same. In both sexes the S_f 0–10 lipoproteins were increased in fasting subjects.

In males and females the levels of both LDL classes increased with age. In males the maximum values were attained by the fifties and sixties, but in females the maximum was not reached until the sixties. Both sexes had similar LDL values before age 25, after which males had significantly higher values until about age 50 (19).

The high-density lipoproteins HDL_1, HDL_2, and HDL_3 (hydrated densities 1.05, 1.075, and 1.145 g/ml, respectively) were first recorded in detail from clinically healthy adults by DeLalla, Elliott, and Gofman (20). In a large group (229 males and 227 females) the HDL_1 levels did not change with age. However, females under 40 had significantly less HDL_1 than did males. After age 40, there was no sex difference. The HDL_2 fraction was significantly higher in females from 20 to 60 years old. Beyond age 60, HDL_2 values were lower in females and about the same as in males. The HDL_3 fraction was higher in females in the 20- to 60-year period but did not differ as much as HDL_2.

Similar results were obtained by Barclay, Barclay, and Skipski (21), who calculated the concentrations of HDL_2 and HDL_3 after preparative separation at different densities. Women had significantly more HDL_2 than did men of the same ages, but women had somewhat less HDL_3 (Table III). The HDL_1 fraction does not show a sex difference.

Data were obtained as part of a cooperative study by several groups to ascertain any relationships among S_f 12–20 and S_f 20–100 lipoprotein levels, cholesterol levels, and atherosclerosis. Two groups, the Los Angeles Civil Service Study and the Framingham Heart Study (U.S. Public Health Service, National Heart Institute), had been organized previously to study cardiovascular diseases. Evaluations were made on 10,690 men and 3404 women. Lewis and co-workers (22), reporting on the data for S_f 12–20 and S_f 20–100 lipoproteins, concluded that the most sensitive fraction is S_f 20–100, especially in the age group 40 to 59. Men in all age groups had higher values than women. The graphs indicated no overlap in values. White

Table II. Mean Serum-Lipoprotein Levels in Fasting and Nonfasting Subjects 14 to 65 Years Old[a]

		VLDL[b]		LDL[b]	
Age	*n*[c]	S_f 100–400	S_f 20–100	S_f 10–20	S_f 0–10
		Fasting Males			
44	412	50	106	76	382
54	431	44	106	83	406
63	187	43	100	78	398
		Fasting Females			
44	105	23	64	70	352
54	68	30	83	93	388
63	28	43	105	106	426
		Nonfasting Males			
16	29	28	67	37	264
25	75	43	87	49	302
35	358	74	101	62	340
44	313	83	109	68	364
54	228	76	112	69	367
61	43	67	105	67	360
		Nonfasting Females			
17	32	14	52	38	271
24	86	16	49	42	283
35	452	26	64	54	304
44	399	39	78	70	346
54	269	52	99	90	363
62	43	67	132	102	369

[a] Averages of mean values, calculated from the data of Tamplin and Tandy (9).
[b] Concentrations in mg/100 ml serum.
[c] Number of samples.

subjects had significantly higher values for S_f 20–100 lipoproteins. The usual age trend was seen. In men the highest values were seen between 40 and 60 years of age, with a peak at ages 40 to 49 [also noted by Milch et al. (23) in controlled groups of men]. In women the highest values occurred later, at ages 45 to 65, with peaks at about the years 55 to 60. In this large population the S_f 20–100 class had the highest positive correlation with increased blood pressure (diastolic) and was higher in males. Furthermore, these values were highest in the heaviest subjects.

Tamplin and Tandy (9) reevaluated some of the data obtained by the Framingham study and the Los Angeles study. Their objectives were to record what variations in a serum-lipoprotein class can exist in and be-

Table III. Serum HDL Levels in Men and Women[a]

HDL Fraction	Women n^b	Women Concentration[c] (mg/100 ml)	Men n^b	Men Concentration[c] (mg/100 ml)
S_f 0–3 (HDL_1)[d]	132	37 ± 27	11	36 ± 32
S_f 12–20[e]	124	5 ± 7	10	4 ± 5
S_f 4–12[e]	124	14 ± 6	10	9 ± 11
S_f 0–4 (HDL_2)[e]	124	82 ± 21	9	36 ± 28
HDL_3[f]	116	125 ± 21	10	156 ± 41

[a] Data from Ref. 21.
[b] Number of samples.
[c] Mean ± standard deviation.
[d] Measured at 1.063-g/ml density, NaCl solution.
[e] Measured at 1.125-g/ml density, NaCl solution.
[f] Measured at 1.21-g/ml density, $NaNO_3$, D_2O solution.

tween large populations and to correlate these variations with those within an individual. There were over 10,000 subjects, men and women aged 30 to 70, and 15 children. Most samples were taken from nonfasting subjects. The subjects who came from different areas in the United States were variously employed. The trends for all the LDL classes in this large sampling were as follows:

1. *Standard S_f 0–12 Lipoproteins (LDL):*

Effect of Sex. Values were the same in both sexes before age 20. From age 20 to age 50 the mean values were significantly higher in the male. After the fifth decade, values were similar or equal in both sexes. From age 60 through age 70 the mean values were significantly higher in women.

Effect of Fasting or Not Fasting. The mean values for S_f 0–12 lipoproteins in samples from fasting subjects were higher, especially in the Los Angeles study, and there was much variation among samples from nonfasting subjects. The authors stated that "there is probably no real justification in a comparison of any of the nonfasting samples with the fasting samples. The obvious and ideal way to conduct this study would be to have both fasting and nonfasting samples on the same individuals" (9).

Effect on Individual Variation. The calculated biological variation for S_f 0–12 lipoproteins was significantly different between the two nonfasting groups, suggesting that *within* a group the variation may overwhelm the effects of fasting or not fasting, and, more importantly, there may be considerable variation in a single individual's serum-lipoprotein values.

2. *Standard S_f 12–20 Lipoproteins (LDL):*

Effect of Sex. The mean values for both sexes before age 20 were the same. From age 20 to age 50 mean values were significantly higher in the male. After the fifth decade, values were similar or equal in both sexes. From age 60 through age 70, the mean value was significantly higher in females.

The significant increases in standard S_f 0–12 and S_f 12–20 lipoproteins (the most abundant LDL fractions) in women during or after the fifth decade *suggest* the important role of estrogens in maintaining a serum LDL level that is compatible with "optimum good health" during the child-bearing period.[2]

3. Standard S_f 20–100 Lipoproteins (VLDL):

Effect of Sex. Before age 20 the mean values were higher in males than in females. This sex difference persisted until the sixth decade, after which the levels of S_f 20–100 lipoproteins were not higher in males (9, 22).

Effect of Fasting and Not Fasting. The mean values were lower in most samples taken from fasting persons (9, 21).

4. Standard S_f 100–400 Lipoproteins (VLDL):

Effect of Sex. Before age 20 the mean values were higher in males. This difference persisted until the sixth decade, after which the mean values were the same in both sexes.

Effect of Fasting and Not Fasting. The mean values were lower in the samples from fasting subjects in the Los Angeles Civil Service Study (9).

Consecutive data on individuals (10–20 samples on some) indicated intercorrelations or relationships between certain LDL classes: the S_f 0–12 and S_f 12–20 fractions were similarly affected, as were S_f 20–100 and S_f 100–400 lipoproteins, but the levels of these two groups did not rise or fall together. Whereas some correlation obtained between the S_f 12–20 and S_f 20–100 fractions, essentially no intercorrelation was found between S_f 0–20 and S_f 20–400 lipoproteins.

Tamplin and Tandy (9) stated that the ultracentrifuge photographs (presumably boundaries from the total fraction with $d < 1.063$ g/ml in serum) suggested two groups, or spectra, of LDL: S_f 0–20 and S_f 20–400; that is, the S_f 0–12 and S_f 12–20 fractions correlated as LDL with $d < 1.063$ and > 1.006 g/ml, and the S_f 20–100 and S_f 20–400 fractions correlated as VLDL with $d < 1.006$ g/ml. The lack of intercorrelation between S_f 0–20 and S_f 20–400 lipoproteins suggests that these two groups may have limited metabolic interdependence under *usual* conditions. In disease another situation may obtain. The concept of VLDL as distinct from LDL is included in the report (9).

My associates and I used separately prepared VLDL and LDL to mea-

[2] The physiologic and metabolic role of estrogen in relation to all the lipoproteins is detailed in Section V.

Table IV. Serum-Lipoprotein Levels in Normal Young Women Studied Serially for 12 Weeks[a]

Subject	VLDL (d <1.006 g/ml)[b]		LDL (d <1.063 g/ml)			HDL$_2$[d] (d <1.125 g/ml)	HDL$_3$[e] (d <1.121 g/ml)
	S_f 20–100	S_f 0–20	S_f 10–20	S_f 0–10	HDL$_1$[c]		
6	0.5 ± 1.3 (0–4)	14 ± 22 (0–69)	3 ± 2 (0–5)	278 ± 46 (174–340)	31 ± 15 (5–53)	125 ± 37 (57–176)	122 ± 17 (95–141)
8	0.4 ± 0.8 (0–2)	5 ± 7 (0–14)	2 ± 3 (0–10)	292 ± 38 (233–363)	37 ± 20 (10–67)	89 ± 22 (54–122)	121 ± 20 (93–149)
10	1.0 ± 3.0 (0–9)	10 ± 9 (0–28)	2 ± 3 (0–10)	358 ± 52 (300–443)	43 ± 20 (10–76)	26 ± 6 (15–35)	99 ± 21 (75–131)
11	6.0 ± 7.0 (0–22)	25 ± 12 (9–55)	41 ± 26 (0–75)	555 ± 31 (504–605)	39 ± 47 (0–143)	100 ± 19 (88–128)	133 ± 21 (87–144)
12	8.0 ± 6.0 (0–37)	10 ± 9 (0–23)	12 ± 12 (0–38)	387 ± 36 (339–436)	34 ± 28 (9–86)	168 ± 23 (137–215)	143 ± 22 (110–174)
15	0.4 ± 1.0 (0–2)	5 ± 3 (0–9)	27 ± 21 (5–56)	399 ± 63 (333–502)	20 ± 18 (5–48)	96 ± 22 (64–113)	110 ± 33 (62–151)
18	2.0 ± 4.0 (0–13)	10 ± 10 (0–28)	13 ± 25 (0–84)	421 ± 73 (346–506)	28 ± 20 (5–63)	89 ± 21 (51–118)	127 ± 21 (81–156)
16	6.0 ± 11.0 (0–35)	12 ± 13 (0–36)	11 ± 14 (0–46)	330 ± 76 (230–452)	48 ± 16 (19–62)	73 ± 16 (49–98)	152 ± 28 (97–178)
24	0.4 ± 1.0 (0–4)	3 ± 8 (0–27)	8 ± 9 (0–24)	405 ± 76 (228–460)	47 ± 31 (5–105)	27 ± 12 (15–45)	118 ± 22 (98–170)
25	0.5 ± 1.0 (0–2)	11 ± 8 (0–18)	6 ± 9 (0–19)	432 ± 105 (297–547)	48 ± 44 (9–57)	43 ± 14 (23–49)	107 ± 14 (88–119)
27	0 ± 0	3 ± 4 (0–12)	6 ± 7 (0–19)	309 ± 92 (140–484)	29 ± 28 (13–53)	47 ± 19 (23–88)	110 ± 23 (54–134)
4	1.8 ± 3.0 (0–9)	9 ± 13 (0–23)	14 ± 17 (5–38)	515 ± 143 (408–630)	35 ± 29 (10–87)	120 ± 20 (88–147)	124 ± 21 (98–159)
17	11.0 ± 6.0 (0–17)	14 ± 11 (0–27)	13 ± 14 (0–38)	323 ± 56 (262–387)	35 ± 9 (24–50)	113 ± 17 (88–132)	131 ± 20 (97–160)
9	11.0 ± 16.0 (0–48)	26 ± 29 (0–91)	24 ± 21 (4–64)	509 ± 115 (302–610)	36 ± 35 (0–95)	37 ± 47 (5–138)	124 ± 13 (109–143)

[a] Data from an unpublished study by M. Barclay et al. The samples were obtained after an overnight fast. The values (mg/100 ml serum) are means ± standard deviations; ranges are given in parentheses.

[b] These lipoproteins were separated preparatively in unaltered serum, then studied in the analytical ultracentrifuge. The S_f ranges started at 0 and went to 400. The S_f 0–20 fraction is probably comparable to S_f 20–100 lipoproteins (12, 25) when these are combined with LDL. The S_f 100–400 components were routinely absent in these fasting subjects. In normal subjects S_f ~400 lipoproteins may include the "secondary endogenous particles" described by Walton (26).

[c] HDL$_1$ can be calculated as S_f 0–3, usually a small shoulder below the large boundary, S_f 3–10, the bulk of LDL with d <1.063 g/ml. It has a hydrated density of 1.05, very near that of the solution in which these components are analyzed in the analytical ultracentrifuge. The S_f 0–10 values include HDL$_1$.

[d] The HDL$_2$ fraction was separated preparatively (from the infranatant of d <1.063 g/ml) at a solution d 1.125 g/ml, followed by calculation from the analytical-ultracentrifuge data.

[e] The HDL$_3$ fraction was separated preparatively (from the infranatant of d 1.125 g/ml) at solution d 1.21 g/ml, followed by calculation from the analytical-ultracentrifuge data.

sure the intersubject variability for the following two-component groups: S_f 0–10 and S_f 10–20 lipoproteins and the S_f 20–100 and S_f 100–400 fractions (24).[3] We recently completed a study on a normal population of 25- to 40-year-old premenopausal women who lived together, ate essentially the same diet, and had similar routines. For 12 consecutive weeks samples were taken after an overnight fast. The levels of some lipoproteins were remarkably constant throughout this period (Table IV).

Many subjects had zero values for the VLDL components. The S_f 100–400 lipoproteins were completely missing in all subjects. For the other classes occasionally a high value, like that in subject 9, resulted in higher standard deviations. This was also true of the LDL fractions, although the HDL_1 values varied the least within a subject.

In most subjects HDL_2 levels peaked at the ovulatory periods. As a result, there was more in-subject variability than there was for HDL_3 levels, which were fairly constant in most subjects.

Allen, Clark, and Wilson (27), who followed lipoprotein levels in 425 men for 14 years, concluded that few subjects actually had patterns similar to the one constructed from mean values. Variations among individuals were great and substantial for certain lipoproteins. The S_f 20–400 fraction showed the least, and S_f 0–12 lipoproteins the most, variation. Even HDL varied somewhat. This finding for S_f 20–400 lipoproteins does not agree with a report by Lewis et al. (22), who concluded that this fraction is the most sensitive to many factors.

If the samples measured by Allen and co-workers (27) were from fasting men, their results are similar to those reported in Table IV.

Table V presents data compiled from a study by Nichols (18). In these experiments the VLDL ($d < 1.006$ g/ml) were separated from LDL (which included HDL_1). Values for HDL_2 and HDL_3 are also given. Only results that quickly show "normal" values are included in this simplified table. The data compiled from a large number of samples, probably from nonfasting subjects, showed that all males had greater amounts of S_f 12–20 lipoproteins (LDL) and of both VLDL fractions. However, only men in the 16 to 29 age group had slightly lower values for S_f 0–12 lipoproteins than did women in the 30 to 49 age group. The HDL_1 levels were the same in both sexes. The most outstanding intersex difference was observed in the HDL_2 fraction, whose levels were consistently higher in women—an observation emphasized previously by Barclay et al. (21, 28), who used similar techniques.

The HDL_3 levels were similar in males and females, and somewhat higher than those reported by Barclay et al. (21), who found them to be higher in

[3] Some of our observations have not been published.

Table V. Serum-Lipoprotein Levels in Normal Men and Women[a]

Fraction and Density (g/ml)	Age (years)									
	16–29		30–39		30–49		40–49		50–65	
	M	F	M	F	M	F	M	F	M	F
VLDL (*d* <1.006):										
S_f 100–400	37	9	51	—	—	14	66	—	58	—
S_f 20–100	75	44	91	—	—	55	107	—	103	—
LDL (*d* <1.063):										
S_f 12–20	40	30	51	—	—	41	57	—	56	—
S_f 0–12	322	283	355	—	—	330	380	—	386	—
HDL_1 (*d* <1.063)	23	21	24	—	—	22	25	—	27	—
HDL_2 (*d* <1.125)	37	80	36	—	—	83	37	—	42	—
HDL_3 (*d* <1.21)	217	228	219	—	—	237	226	—	224	—

[a] Data from Ref. 18. Values in milligrams per 100 ml of serum.

men (see Table III). The data in Table V confirm and strengthen the values given by Tamplin and Tandy (9) on similar, but smaller, groups of subjects and infer that these relationships among the values for the sexes are reliable.

Nichols (18) pointed out some important aspects of lipoprotein distributions and interrelationships. Males with extremely high VLDL values usually had lower values for both HDL_2 and HDL_3, especially for HDL_2. The HDL_1 might be elevated. Males who had extremely high VLDL values had low LDL (S_f 0–12) values. The inverse relationship was observed in patients recovering from lipemia associated with diabetic acidosis: the LDL (S_f 0–12) levels rise as VLDL levels fall.

Nichols (18) also observed that S_f 0–12 lipoproteins (LDL) and HDL may decrease, and VLDL increase, in subjects on a high-carbohydrate, low-fat diet. The reduced intake of animal fat may be the primary cause (see Section IV).

In females Nichols noted an inverse relationship between VLDL and HDL_2 levels, but none between VLDL and LDL (S_f 0–12) levels in males. The HDL_1 levels were not elevated. Some healthy males may have a female-type pattern (i.e., low VLDL and LDL levels in conjunction with high HDL_2 levels).

Mills and associates (29–31) studied VLDL and LDL levels in large English, Neapolitan, and African populations. They concluded that a lipoprotein *pattern,* rather than the level of a single lipoprotein class, should serve as a base line against which abnormal values should be evaluated. They also indicated (and cautioned) that the "normal" pattern for one group should not be applied to another—this might be especially true for very different ethnic groups.

About the time (1949–1950) that ultracentrifugal separations were being perfected, the Harvard group (32–35) published data on their cold-ethanol, heavy metal precipitation procedures for isolating fraction I+III (with β-mobility in electrophoresis) and fraction IV+V+VI (with α_1-mobility).[4] After the fractions were separated, their cholesterol and phospholipid contents were determined and many of their physicochemical properties were established (34). It was determined that β-lipoproteins consist of approximately 31% cholesterol and 29% phospholipids, the remainder being protein or polypeptide (32).

The concentration of β-lipoproteins in normal pooled plasma (ACD) was about 5% of the total plasma protein. This agrees with the ultracentrifugal data of Gofman et al. (4). The α-lipoproteins were composed of approximately 12% cholesterol, 21% phospholipids, and 57% polypeptide (35).

About 70% of plasma cholesterol and 50% of plasma phospholipids were associated with β-lipoproteins, whereas 30% cholesterol and 50% phospholipids were associated with α-lipoproteins. From these compositions the investigators calculated the β- and α-lipoprotein levels.

Lever and co-workers (33) refined Cohn's method 10 (32) for use with smaller plasma samples. Their data and those from other laboratories are presented in Table VI, which shows good agreement among the values.

Table VI. Plasma Levels of Lipoproteins (LP) Isolated by Cold-Ethanol, Heavy-Metal Precipitation—Normal Men and Women[a]

Age	Men		Women		
(years)	α-LP	β-LP	α-LP	β-LP	Ref.
18–35	310	420	400	350	36
18–40	345	440			33
20–30			430	400	37
30–45			360	430	37
45–65	345	525	370	550	36

[a] Values in milligrams per 100 ml of plasma.

An important finding was that men of any age had more β-lipoproteins and less α-lipoproteins than women. In women 18 to 35 years old there were more α-lipoproteins than β-lipoproteins, but in women over 30 or near 45 the opposite was true. These proportional amounts agreed with the trends

[4] This procedure, known as Cohn's method 10, is described in Refs. 32 and 33.

in men and women when lipoproteins were separated and calculated by ultracentrifugal methods.

Wolff, Brignon, and Nicolas (38) used tris–EDTA–borate buffer on paper and reported the following relative amounts of lipoproteins from three different sources: β-lipoproteins, 70.4, 70.4, and 79.3%; α-lipoproteins, 29.6, 29.6, and 20.7%. The ranges of values for their normal subjects

Table VII. Proportions of α- and β-Lipoproteins (LP) in Serum from Normal Subjects[a]

Age		Concentration (%)	
(years)	Sex	α-LP	β-LP
17	M	30.9	58.9
22	M	43.6	51.7
24	M	41.0	54.2
		40.9	55.3
27	M	19.0	72.2
28	M	39.7	53.8
39	M	34.5	61.0
45	M	29.6	60.4
46	M	40.8	56.6
55	M	27.7	61.1
18	F	47.3	44.0
		59.9	34.2
		30.4	62.6
		28.1	64.0
19	F	20.5	71.8
		39.7	57.3
21	F	45.7	45.6
		48.6	47.1
22	F	47.5	43.2
		28.4	64.7
23	F	41.6	46.9
25	F	28.3	69.5
27	F	42.4	48.8
30	F	31.9	65.9
36	F	45.5	47.8
39	F	35.9	58.8
45	F	27.2	67.2
		42.9	47.2
46	F	38.6	58.6
47	F	25.3	73.1
49	F	21.9	60.7

[a] Data from Ref. 39.

were as follows: β-lipoproteins, 65.6 to 76.3%; α-lipoproteins, 23.7 to 33.3%; these were essentially the proportional amounts obtained by other procedures.

When lipoproteins were determined by electrophoresis, in general, proportional amounts were given. Normal serum from fasting subjects gave two prominent bands of stained lipids and one faintly stained band, as described in Chapter 5. When analyzed on a densitometer, the intensities of the stained bands can be converted to relative quantities, or percentages. Table VII shows some values reported by Edel (39).

Levy, Lees, and Fredrickson (40) used paper and starch electrophoresis to demonstrate the presence of a pre-β-lipoprotein, or α_2-lipoprotein, which they believed to be the same as VLDL ($d < 1.006$ g/ml). By manipulating the diet they concluded that a reciprocal relationship existed between the pre-β-lipoprotein (VLDL) and α_1-lipoprotein (HDL); this agrees with the conclusions drawn by Nichols (18) on the interrelationships between lipoprotein levels in normal subjects.

Cohen and Djordjevich (41) used starch-gel electrophoresis with different buffer systems and an improved staining procedure to obtain more distinct bands, especially of the α_1-lipoproteins. They observed three α_1-lipoprotein patterns in serum from fasting subjects. These differed in frequency in men and women. They designated the bands in the α_1-mobility regions as F (faintly stained), M (moderately stained), and S (strongly stained). In the serum-lipoprotein fraction routinely separated preparatively at d 1.063 to 1.21 g/ml they usually observed three components in 83% of 231 subjects. In some subjects they saw more than three components, as shown by the percentage distribution in Table VIII.

Among other things, these data provide additional evidence for heterogeneity as seen in HDL (28, 42, 43). The occurrence of several components in the fraction usually consisting of HDL_{2+3} can be observed in certain

Table VIII. α_1-Lipoprotein Patterns in Normal Subjects[a]

		Common Patterns (%)[b]			Uncommon patterns (%)[c]		
Sex	n[d]	F	M	S	F–M	M–S	U
Female	111	0	38	52	6	2	2
Male	120	18	42	16	8	8	8

[a] Data from Ref. 41.

[b] Key: F, faintly stained; M, moderately stained; S, strongly stained.

[c] F–M and M–S indicate that the patterns seen could not be classified as either F or M, or M or S, respectively; U refers to patterns not fitting any of the three common categories.

[d] Number of subjects.

pathologic conditions (see Sections VII and VIII) as well as in some normal subjects.

Another procedure for separating lipoproteins is based on the use of high-molecular-weight dextran sulfate to precipitate selectively β-lipoproteins (44). The following data are from Scott (45), who reported LDL levels in 1109 men and 745 women from an urban population in New Zealand. The subjects did not fast; most of the samples were from donors to the Transfusion Service; the oldest subjects, over 60, were from out-patient groups recovering from remediable conditions. To compare the New Zealand data with those from the United States some of Scott's results are presented in Table IX.

When the LDL results of Scott (45) are compared with those of Tamplin and Tandy (9) and Nichols (18) (some of which have been reproduced in Tables II and V), certain common trends are observed, as there are also with data obtained by other procedures described in this section. In men

Table IX. Serum LDL Levels in Men and Women in 10-Year Age Groups and in Total Population Samples[a]

Age (years)	Sex	n[b]	LDL Concentration (mg/100 ml serum)[c]
15–20	M	95	442 ± 123
21–30	M	205	476 ± 147
31–40	M	194	520 ± 173
41–50	M	241	567 ± 189
51–60	M	171	512 ± 193
61–70	M	130	478 ± 137
71 +	M	73	478 ± 120
	Total	1109	506 ± 169
15–20	F	95	414 ± 165
21–30	F	136	432 ± 160
31–40	F	124	430 ± 130
41–50	F	132	510 ± 163
51–60	F	98	560 ± 175
61–70	F	96	570 ± 142
71 +	F	64	580 ± 166
	Total	745	491 ± 156
	Total M + F	1854	500

[a] Data from Ref. 45. Nonfasting subjects. β-Lipoproteins precipitated by dextran sulfate.

[b] Number of subjects.

[c] Mean ± standard deviation. Mean values and 95% limits of ranges for the data are compared for calculations based on arithmetic distributions.

and women values increased with age; the maximum in men was attained in the fifties; and the increases in women often exceeded the values for the men in the fifth and sixth decades. Since no mention was made that any of the subjects in the New Zealand study were Maori, it is presumed that they were Caucasians. The diet would be quite different for the two ethnic groups.

By using the principle of immunochemical precipitation published by Burstein and Samaille (46) to estimate the amounts of β-lipoproteins (47), Allard and Goulet (48) compared several interesting and pertinent parameters in males (20–70 years old) with their serum levels of β-lipoproteins. Their results corroborated the age dependence of β-lipoprotein levels but also showed that β-lipoproteins tended to increase with weight gain, since they were higher in the more obese subjects. There was also a positive correlation with masculinity, but not with body structure (morphism). The measurements (millimeters of precipitate of β-lipoproteins in a calibrated column) followed the trend observed with more quantitative measurements: an increase in β-lipoproteins to ages 50 through 54 and then a decrease at age 65 or older.

The triglyceride-rich VLDL were measured by light scattering in a study by Stone and Thorp (49), who compared the subjects by sex, age, and weight. They found (Table X) that weight was a crucial factor. Although

Table X. Influence of Sex, Age, and Relative Body Weight on VLDL Light-Scattering Index (LSI) and Cholesterol Levels in 248 Normal Subjects[a]

	>10% Underweight		0–10% Underweight		0–10% Overweight		>10% Overweight	
Variable	20–49 yr	50–75 yr	20–49 yr	50–75 yr	20–49 yr	50–75 yr	20–49 yr	50–75 yr
Men								
Number of subjects	11	14	20	12	23	17	31	16
Median LSI units	77	88	104	111	132	136	154	138
LSI range	52–97	73–118	60–256	70–164	68–410	95–187	72–447	80–492
Mean total cholesterol, mg/100 ml serum	203	192	210	232	245	258	230	247
Women								
Number of subjects	10	6	12	7	6	10	31	22
Median LSI units	80	93	88	124	108	142	112	128
LSI range	64–145	50–126	68–141	96–167	95–187	89–172	68–348	64–292
Mean total cholesterol, mg/100 ml serum	199	261	212	253	218	246	234	257

[a] Data from Ref. 49.

the usual age and sex trends were present, young males who were (a) up to 10% overweight and (b) more than 10% overweight had significantly higher VLDL values than older males of normal weight. When samples from young males who were more than 10% underweight were compared with young males up to 10% underweight, the increase in light-scattering units in the heavier subjects was greater. Young females, though overweight, did not have the high values of older females.

The influence of sex was smaller in young subjects who were more than 10% underweight. Males up to 10% underweight and overweight had significantly higher values than did females of comparable age and weight. Only females who were more than 10% overweight had very high values.

In the older subjects the VLDL values were similar for both sexes, except that in the lower weight groups females had higher values than males, and in the higher weight groups males had higher values than the females.

C. Men and Women Over 65 Years Old

The reports cited give information about the levels of serum lipoproteins in subjects 17 to 65 years old. Several types of techniques are represented. For additional information review articles (12, 50) may be consulted. Serum-lipoprotein levels in normal subjects over 65 years of age are presented below.

Watkin and associates (51) presented lipoprotein values obtained by ultracentrifugal techniques. Duplicate samples of serum from 10 males were exchanged among the four laboratories involved in the cooperative study of lipoproteins and atherosclerosis (22). Most of the subjects were living in controlled environments and had similar activities and diets. Table XI presents their results as well as Ackermann's values for S_f 12–20 lipoproteins (52). A few subjects under 60 years old were included for comparison.

The data showed that the levels of S_f 35–100 lipoproteins were highest in men over 75 years old; the levels of S_f 20–35 lipoproteins were similar in all age groups; and the ranges for S_f 12–20 lipoproteins in men more than 70 years old were wide. The data of Watkin et al. and Ackermann are comparable.

Watkin and co-workers (51) also studied several subjects weekly, and their graphed data show considerable variation in all the lipoprotein classes except S_f 21–35. From statistical evaluation they concluded that when the levels were high, the fluctuations were greater.

In a group of elderly subjects 80 to 100 years old Eiber et al. (53) observed low levels of all the LDL and VLDL fractions. They considered that there was a "threshold" between 65 and 75 years of age, after which values gradually declined.

Table XI. Serum-Lipoprotein Levels in Males Predominantly over 65 Years Old[a]

Age (years)			Concentration (mg/100 ml serum)			
Mean	Range	*n*[b]	S_f 12–20	S_f 20–35	S_f 35–100	Ref.
33	26–41	6	33	19	35	51
53	47–58	5	28	16	24	51
53	47–59	11	39	21	33	51
55	53–58	10	45			52
65	61–69	12	43	18	31	51
65	60–68	13	42			52
69	63–76	6	26	15	26	51
72		25	29[c]			52
73		28	43[d]			52
74		27	42[e]			52
75	72–79	12	41	22	44	51
75	70–79	23	42			52
84	80–92	11	38	20	40	51
87	80–92	5	44	20	45	51
87	80–94	14	32			52

[a] Ultracentrifugal Separations.
[b] Number of samples.
[c] Range 16–50 mg/100 ml serum.
[d] Range 13–63 mg/100 ml serum.
[e] Range 22–60 mg/100 ml serum.

To compare the effects of sex in old age on serum-lipoprotein levels, Nikkilä and Niemi (54) obtained samples from 18 women (mean age 77) and 20 men (mean age 76). The subjects were all inmates of the Municipal Home of Helsinki and thus lived under standardized conditions. Serum lipoproteins were separated electrophoretically. The distribution of cholesterol and phospholipids in the α_1- and β-lipoproteins were the same for both sexes. However, women had higher lipid levels than men did. In women the lipid levels increased to about age 80, but in men the increase stopped at about age 65.

The β-lipoprotein data of Binet and associates (55) followed a similar pattern with respect to sex except that the "threshold" age was lower: 55 for men and 65 for women. Binet et al. concluded that β-lipoprotein levels diminish with increasing age in all healthy subjects.

Franzini, Turri, and Fumagalli (56) reported the lipid and protein levels in five groups of subjects, both women and men of advanced years. After reaching a peak at ages 50 to 59, the β-to-α-lipoprotein ratios declined steadily to ages 80 to 89. Women had slightly higher ratios after 70 years of age.

Table XII. Serum-Lipoprotein Levels in Pregnant and Nonpregnant Women of Similar Ages[a]

	VLDL ($d < 1.006$ g/ml)			LDL ($d < 1.063$ g/ml)			HDL_2 ($d < 1.125$ g/ml)			HDL_3 ($d < 1.21$ g/ml)
Subject	S_f 100–400	S_f 20–100	S_f 0–20	S_f 10–20	S_f 0–10	S_f 0–3[b]	S_f 12–20	S_f 4–12	S_f 0–4[c]	
					Pregnant					
24 weeks; age 22	54	122	97	15	535	173	0	0	102	213
30 weeks; age 27	11	107	101	30	568	230	0	24	88	250
					Nonpregnant					
Age 34[d]	0	3	12	16	389	45	6	16	111	126
Age 31[e]	2	3	5	1	339	45	7	13	141	126

[a] Data from an unpublished study by M. Barclay. Values in milligrams per 100 ml of serum.
[b] HDL_1.
[c] Main HDL_2 component floating at $d < 1.125$ g/ml (28).
[d] Six subjects from an institution studied each week for 12 weeks; values are means.
[e] Six subjects, single measurements; values are means.

Whereas certain lipoproteins have a high intrasubject variability, other components show surprisingly small differences among subjects of advanced years.

III. SERUM-LIPOPROTEIN LEVELS IN PREGNANCY, INFANCY, AND EARLY CHILDHOOD

A. Pregnancy

Since about 1845, when Becquerel and Rodier (57) noted lipemic serums in pregnant women, there have been numerous reports on lipids, especially cholesterol and phospholipids, in pregnancy, but not many concerned with lipoproteins.

As part of an extensive survey of lipoprotein levels in persons with a multitude of conditions, Gofman and associates (58) in 1954 included pregnancy. Blood samples were drawn during the second and third trimesters, and up to 9 months postpartum. During pregnancy the S_f 100–400, S_f 20–100 (VLDL), and S_f 12–20 and S_f 0–12 (LDL) lipoproteins increased significantly; HDL_1 (S_f 0–3 at $d < 1.063$ g/ml) did not increase; HDL_2 decreased, and HDL_3 increased slightly. Not until 9 months postpartum did S_f 100–400 lipoproteins decrease. It approached, but did not reach, the second-trimester levels. The 5-day and 6-month postpartum samples showed that S_f 20–100 and S_f 12–20 lipoproteins had decreased. The level of S_f 0–12 lipoproteins was still elevated at 6 months postpartum but was below the second-trimester levels by 9 months after delivery. The level of HDL_1 was not changed, but HDL_2 continued to decrease even at 9 months postpartum. The HDL_3 fraction continued to increase until 6 months after delivery but finally dropped at 9 months postpartum.

Table XII presents data from unpublished experiments of the reviewer. The lipoprotein data, although in more detail, are in accord with those of Gofman et al. (58). In general, compared with values for nonpregnant women, the triglyceride-rich VLDL were greatly elevated, the cholesterol-rich LDL were also elevated, the HDL_2 fraction was slightly decreased, and the HDL_3 fraction was greatly elevated.

Lewis (59) studied changes in the lipoprotein levels of two pregnant patients with hypercholesteremia who had been on vegetable-oil diets to control the elevated serum-cholesterol levels. The β-lipoproteins (S_f 3–12) were increased markedly, whereas the elevations in the S_f 12–20 fraction and α-lipoproteins (HDL) were less pronounced.

One of the earliest studies of the effects of normal pregnancy on the serum lipoproteins of primigravidas was that of Oliver and Boyd (60), who used paper electrophoresis. Blood was drawn from 12 women after a 3-hr fast. Samples were taken every 2 weeks, from the ninth week of pregnancy until 20 weeks postpartum. In order to approximate more closely the stage of pregnancy, the sample dates were judged retrospectively.

The levels of α- and β-lipoproteins were estimated by cholesterol distribution. A comparison was made on the basis of a 1:2 α-to-β ratio in nonpregnant women. By the 32nd week of pregnancy these lipoproteins had a 1:5 α-to-β ratio. The following α-to-β ratios were observed: 12th week, 25:75%; 32nd week, 16:84%; 20th postpartum week, 21:79% (α-to-β ratio in nonpregnant women, 34:66%). The authors pointed out that these changes were even greater because of the 20 to 25% increase in plasma volume. Between the 31st and 33rd weeks, the lipid pattern was similar to that frequently seen in patients with coronary sclerosis. The authors also speculated about some of the paradoxical hormone–lipid relationships—that is, high estrogen production but low serum α-lipoprotein levels.

The proportional amounts of lipoproteins Oliver and Boyd observed in the 32nd week of pregnancy were confirmed by the data in Table XII for pregnant subjects, who had high VLDL and LDL levels compared with HDL levels.

Scandrett (61) investigated the possible relationship between serum β-to-α-lipoprotein ratios in "normal" pregnancy and in patients with toxemias. The lipoprotein levels were estimated by paper electrophoresis (see Table XIII).

There were significant ($P < .01$) increases in the β-to-α-lipoprotein ratios as uncomplicated pregnancy advanced, and an even greater elevation in patients with preeclamptic complications. The elevations may have been the result of decreased α-lipoprotein levels since the concentration of cholesterol was decreased in these lipoproteins. There was a concomitant increase in β-lipoprotein cholesterol. Scandrett (61) noted that the increase was present largely in the pre-β-lipoprotein band (now recognized as VLDL). The β-to-α-lipoprotein ratios in women with essential hypertension and preeclampsia were similar.

In all sera obtained after the 26th week of pregnancy, Rejnek et al. (62) observed an atypical α_1-lipoprotein, which gave an abnormal immunoelectrophoretic picture. These serums, which had increased amounts of β-, α_2-, and α_1-globulins, inhibited proliferations of cell cultures. Serums taken before the 13th week contained no atypical α_1-lipoprotein and greatly stimulated the growth of HeLa cells, but after the 32nd week there was a marked inhibitory effect. Mitotic stimulation and inhibition followed the same schedule. Samples drawn 1 week postpartum contained no atypical α_1-lipoprotein and did not influence cell proliferation.

Table XIII. **β-to-α-Lipoprotein Ratios During Uncomplicated and Complicated Pregnancies**[a]

Condition	Duration of Pregnancy (weeks)	n[b]	β/α Ratio[c]
Normal	10–15	12	1.9 ± 0.15
	31–42	64	3.5 ± 1.32
Preeclampsia:			
Moderate	29–40	19	4.4
Severe	29–40	13	4.9
Average		32	4.6 ± 2.15
Essential hypertension	36–39	9	4.5 ± 1.01
Essential hypertension + preeclampsia	32–36	5	4.5

[a] Data from Ref. 61.
[b] Number of subjects.
[c] Mean ± standard deviation.

Whether the atypical α_1-lipoprotein is the inhibitor (or carrier of it) or is only associated with it is not known. There was a positive correlation between the stimulating effect and initial rapid fetal growth and differentiation, and between the inhibitory effect and a slowing down of differentiation and growth.

Roszkowski and co-workers (63) separated the proteins and lipoproteins in serums from 58 mothers of malformed infants, 31 of whom were premature. The data were compared with those for 48 women who delivered normal infants. The serums from women with malformed infants had slightly more β-lipoprotein, and in cases where the premature infant was abnormal both β- and α-lipoproteins were below normal levels. However, none of the differences was sufficient to provide clues to the malformations. The women had not taken drugs.

Blood samples drawn from 27 women immediately after delivery were studied by Russ, Eder, and Barr (64). The serum was separated into fractions IV+V+VI (α-lipoproteins) and fraction I+III (β-lipoproteins). Fraction I+III contained significantly ($P < .01$) more cholesterol and phospholipids ($P < .01$) than did those from a group of nonpregnant women of comparable age. In terms of ultracentrifugal separations this can be interpreted to mean that the LDL level was elevated. The cholesterol level in fraction IV+V+VI was the same in both groups, although the phospholipid levels were higher: 139 mg/100 ml serum in pregnant women versus 117 mg/100 ml serum in nonpregnant women.

Hydroxyapatite columns were used by Aurell and Cramér (65) to separate lipoproteins from the serums of 18 subjects during the 34th to 36th weeks of pregnancy and again 9 months postpartum. Although during pregnancy all lipid values were higher than the postpartum ones, the glycerides were elevated the most during pregnancy, with mean values of 1.89 millimoles/1 verus a postpartum value of 0.61 millimole/1. The LDL ($d < 1.019$ g/ml; $S_f > 12$) levels were greatly elevated. The authors reported an increase in cholesterol and glycerides in HDL fractions. There was no change in the phosphorus content. Two to three months after delivery there was a decrease in glycerides (VLDL) to "normal" levels. The decreases in lipids and (lipoproteins) occurred also in lactating women. Aurell and Cramér (65), as did Oliver and Boyd (60), discussed the lack of expected correlation between the hormonal levels during pregnancy and their expected (from data for nonpregnant women) effects on lipids and lipoproteins.

B. Infancy and Early Childhood

Table XIV presents data from three studies on lipoprotein levels in infancy and early childhood (10, 16, 66). Plasma from infants, averaging 7 months, was first separated as fractions I+III and IV+V+VI. Fraction I+III was then further separated at *d* 1.063 g/ml in the preparative ultra-

Table XIV. Plasma-Lipoprotein Levels in Infants to 3 Years of Age

	Age of Subjects		
Fraction	7 Months[a] (mg/100 ml plasma)	6–12 Months[b] (% of total)	1–3 Years[b] (% of total)
Fraction I+III:			
S_f 100–400	0		
S_f 20–100	10		
S_f 10–20	13		
S_f 0–10	414		
Fraction IV+V+VI:			
Cholesterol	41		
Phospholipids	98		
β-Lipoproteins		68.3	71.1
α-Lipoproteins		31.7	28.9

[a] Determined by Cohn's method 10 (32, 33) and analytical ultracentrifugation (10, 66).
[b] Determined by electrophoresis (16).

centrifuge. The lipoproteins with $d < 1.063$ g/ml were analyzed further in the ultracentrifuge. Infants and small children have little or no VLDL, but their levels of S_f 0–10 lipoproteins (LDL) and HDL are comparable to those of adults.

The total and proportional amounts of α- and β-lipoproteins in serum from premature infants are shown in Table XV, based on data obtained

Table XV. Serum Lipoproteins in Premature Infants on Different Formulas[a]

Lipoprotein Class	Fraction of Total[b] <3 Weeks old	Fraction of Total[b] 3–7 Weeks old
	Infants on Formula A[c]	
α-Lipoproteins	34 ± 3.2	35 ± 2.2
β-Lipoproteins	79 ± 10.0	77 ± 3.3
Total	113 ± 12.7	112 ± 4.4
	Infants on Formula B[d]	
α-Lipoproteins	28 ± 2.1	29 ± 2.0
β-Lipoproteins	64 ± 5.0	48 ± 2.9
Total	92 ± 3.5	77 ± 5.2

[a] Data from Ref. 67.
[b] Mean ± standard deviation.
[c] Results of 49 tests on 37 infants. Formula A contained 2.7 g % protein, 7.8 g % carbohydrate, 2.8 g % butterfat (cow's milk), and a 3:1 ratio of saturated to unsaturated fatty acids.
[d] Results of 32 tests on 24 infants. Formula B contained 1.5 g % protein, 7.0 g % carbohydrate, and 3.5 % fat, which was mainly of vegetable origin and had a 1:1 ratio of saturated to unsaturated fatty acids.

by György, Rose, and Chu (67). The infants on formula A had greater amounts of β-lipoproteins, especially, and only slightly more α-lipoproteins than infants on formula B. Apparently the lipoprotein patterns were quite diet dependent at this early age, and the β-lipoprotein, rather than α-lipoprotein, levels were influenced the most.

Infants given pooled human milk had low serum-cholesterol levels. They had poor weight gain until casein was added (67). Low serum-cholesterol levels were also observed in infants on cow's milk with 4.1 g % protein but low butterfat (1.5 g %). Both cholesterol and β-lipoproteins were low in infants fed cow's milk with 1.5 g % protein and 3.5 g % vegetable oil that had a high amount of polyunsaturated fatty acids.

The relative amounts of β- and α-lipoproteins in premature infants on formula A compare well with those in Table XIV (66) and those on formula B with slightly older children (15), who had 64 to 67% β-lipoproteins and 31 to 36% α-lipoproteins in their serums.

IV. DIETARY EFFECTS ON SERUM-LIPOPROTEIN LEVELS

The effects of dietary constituents on lipids and lipoproteins have been investigated in at least two important directions. When the lipoproteins as carriers for lipids were first recognized, interest in the relationship with heart disease was paramount. The studies were therefore concerned with whether the diets of certain groups of "normal" persons were related to the low incidence of heart disease among them. It followed, teleologically, that the information gained be applied to other subjects. These subjects, usually clinically normal volunteers, were willing to consume unusual and sometimes unpalatable mixtures of food. Another type of population has consisted of institutionalized mental patients, patients who had recovered from myocardial infarction, and persons who suffered from obesity.

Valuable information was gleaned from this first approach, even though the dietary regimen frequently was considered before the subject. Some leads in controlling blood lipids while maintaining adequate nutrition were useful.

The second approach, which includes studies on atherosclerosis and coronary heart disease, is more practical. It has been rather recently realized that hyperlipoproteinemia can arise from various causes, including intolerances to dietary constituents. The patient and type of hyperlipoproteinemia are the first concern, dietary control is second. Although many of these diseases are inherited (as inborn errors of metabolism), most of the worst symptoms can be alleviated, if only temporarily, by an intelligent dietary approach. Some of these are also discussed in Section IX.

There is essentially no true base-line diet, because of the variations in amounts and the different items of food consumed by even a close-knit group. There are, of course, some exceptions: cloistered living prescribes restricted diets because of rules.

A good "basic" diet maintains a weight that is commensurate with activity and good health. The total calories to supply energy to maintain that weight, according to Olson and Vester (68), should be derived, on the average, as follows: 15% from protein, 40% from fat, and 45% from carbohydrates. These proportions, which vary throughout the world with different consequences to the consumers, have been quite drastically altered in experimental and therapeutic diets.

When there is no evidence of malnutrition, the dietary components that affect blood lipids and lipoproteins most profoundly are the fats and carbohydrates. The effects from fats evidently reside in the nature of their constituent fatty acids. As determined by gas–liquid chromatography, the degree of saturation (or unsaturation) as well as carbon-chain length, and possibly even branching, are important. Fats from certain vegetable sources, such as coconut and palm oils, apparently increase serum lipoproteins, whereas those from sunflower-seed and corn oils lower them. This is also true of animal fats; those from fish oils have a hypolipoproteinemic effect. Therefore in citing certain diets the source of the fat is given, where possible.

A. Saturated and Unsaturated Fats

One of the first controlled experiments to test what effects, if any, are exerted on serum lipids by the nature of dietary fat was reported by Kinsell et al. in 1952 (69). These investigators substituted vegetable oils for animal fats, using isocaloric amounts and measured dietaries, and found that the serum-cholesterol level was greatly reduced. These observations were confirmed in many laboratories (70–74). The cholesterol associated with β-lipoproteins (S_f 0–12) was preferentially reduced (75, 76), whereas that in the S_f 12–100 fraction was reduced to a lesser extent. In patients with lipoidoses (10) a diet containing cotton-seed oil as the source of fat decreased the lipoproteins in some patients but not in others, depending on the disease (see Section VIII and Table XXIV). This suggested that, in addition to diet, other factors are involved: initial levels of lipoproteins as well as the type and severity of the disease.

Keys, Anderson, and Grande (77) derived a formula to predict the effects of fats (based on their degrees of saturation and proportion of total calories) on serum lipids and lipoproteins. The removal of saturated fat from the diet or the substitution of saturated fat by polyunsaturated fat was thought to have an important lipoprotein-lowering effect. In many instances the predictions were correct.

Nichols, Dobbin, and Gofman (76) noted that diets high in animal fat (not identified), in contrast to those high in vegetable fat, increased LDL levels. These observations also suggested a "fat-type" effect that could be demonstrated in relation to LDL levels. The nature of the fat did not affect VLDL levels, which were lowered (from a low-fat level) to the same extent regardless of the dietary fat.

Subjects on diets containing animal or vegetable fat had lower cholesterol (LDL) levels than did patients on vegetable-fat diets (71, 78–80). It was concluded that the nature of the fatty acids, mostly polyunsaturated in certain vegetable fats, decreases blood cholesterol (LDL) levels but does not increase triglycerides (VLDL), which do increase when low-fat diets of animal fat are given.

The lipid-lowering effects of polyunsaturated fat derived exclusively from menhaden body oil containing no essential fatty acids, given in isocaloric amounts as a substitute for corn oil, convinced Ahrens et al. (80) that essential fatty acids are not required to lower the levels of serum cholesterol (LDL). It is more the effect of polyunsaturation.

Corn-oil-formula feeding reduced cholesterol in β-lipoproteins (d 1.019–1.063 g/ml), and two other lipoprotein fractions (d 1.006–1.019 and $<$ 1.006 g/ml, respectively) were also reduced in a male patient with primary hyperglyceridemia and mild angina pectoris (81).

Subjects on low-fat, low-calorie diets had low serum triglycerides, which were significantly increased on a high-fat, high-calorie diet containing saturated fatty acids (82). The triglycerides (VLDL) remained elevated for 3 to 6 months even after a low-fat diet was instituted. The fatty acid composition of the triglycerides resembled that of the dietary fat. Thus the type and amount of fat may influence the rate of clearance of triglycerides and affect the residual triglycerides.

Bragdon and Karmen (83, 84), Kayden and co-workers (85), and recently Nichaman, Sweeley, and Olson (86) also showed that the fatty acid compositions of chylomicrons, LDL, and lipoproteins with $d > 1.21$ g/ml were similar to that of ingested fat. Nichaman et al. concluded that plasma-lipid fatty acid levels can be used to indicate past dietary intake in both normal and hyperlipemic subjects.

Hamwi and associates (87) observed that in controlled diabetics diets high in polyunsaturated fats normalized the serum lipoproteins, especially the S_f 10–400 fraction. In other studies it was determined by paper electrophoresis that infusion feeding of cotton-seed-oil emulsions increased β-lipoproteins and decreased α-lipoproteins (88, 89).

Studies on vegetarians have become increasingly popular because their diets (unless lactovegetarian) presumably contain more unsaturated fatty acids and less animal fat. Since most of these subjects have lived on this type of diet for many years, they are metabolically equilibrated to it. However, evaluation of the effects of vegetarian diets on lipoproteins is difficult because of doubtful control of variables that greatly influence the lipoprotein levels.

Several early studies showed that vegetarians had lower serum-cholesterol values than did persons consuming animal fats. Groen et al. (70) and Hardinge and Stare (90) observed this regardless of the amount of total fat eaten. The importance of these observations was obvious from the many controlled experiments that ensued to prove that it was the nature of the vegetable fat that was responsible.

Kirkeby (91) did an extensive survey on 293 healthy Norwegian men and women, 123 of whom were habitual vegetarians. Men on the vegetarian diet had somewhat less LDL (β-lipoproteins) than did those on usual Norwegian diets, which provide about 2700 calories (12% from protein, mostly from animal sources; 40% from fat; 48% from carbohydrates). The lactovegetarians ate a low-calorie diet (about 2400 calories, with only slightly less from fat, 36%), most of which was derived from soya and sunflower oil, with some cod-liver oil. The true vegetarians, or "vegans," ate no food from animal sources. Although their diet provided 53% of the total calories from carbohydrates, mostly starch, no lipemia occurred.

Lee and co-workers (92) studied another group of habitual vegetarians, 129 Buddhist monks and nuns. Their serum lipids were compared with those of U.S. Army personnel whose diets are certainly diverse. The Army diet provides 4500 calories (15% from protein, 42% from fat, and 43% from carbohydrates), and 29% of the fat is from animal sources. The vegetarian diet provided 2600 calories: 11% from protein of vegetable origin, 7% from fat (primarily from sesame and cotton-seed oils), and 82% from carbohydrates. Although the Buddhist monks are required to consume all their food, Army personnel are not. Age, general body condition, and activities were not great variables since the authors studied mainly officers. The Buddhists had 122 mg % of total cholesterol and 5.7 meq/l of triglycerides in serum, and the Army officers had 231 mg % of cholesterol and 12.3 meq/l of triglycerides. The incidence of coronary heart disease is reported to be very low in such a Buddhist population.

Some insidious nutritional problems may result from diets that are strictly vegetarian (no animal food) and from those that exclude meat and fish, but not milk and eggs. Of some importance is the quality of the protein. Some of these problems may affect lipid metabolism and lipoprotein levels in serum. Ellis (93, 94), who employed computer techniques to study the nutrient content of vegetarian diets, found a deficiency of vitamin B_{12} (levels below 140 pg/ml, whereas normal levels are between 140 and 900 pg/ml in omnivores) in some vegetarians. This, of course, could have serious metabolic consequences since severe deficiency causes pernicious anemia. Ellis reported that serum-cholesterol values in female vegans were within the normal range, but in male vegans they were lower than in males on omnivorous diets. He suggested (94) that the vegan diet be supplemented with vitamin B_{12} and used to prevent hypercholesteremia.

Animal fats, largely saturated unless from fish, contain a high concentration of cholesterol. They are more usually eaten than polyunsaturated vegetable fats, which contain little or no cholesterol. Several groups have studied the role of dietary or additive cholesterol in relation to animal and vegetable fats and their effects on serum lipids. Connor, Stone, and Hodges (95) used a basic 2500-calorie diet (period I) consisting of 100 g protein, 280 g carbohydrate, and 110 g fat, 40% of the total calories being derived from mixtures of fats containing only long-chain fatty acids. Total calories were increased or decreased by changing all ingredients proportionally, and 209 to 265 mg of sitosterols was included per day. Each diet was eaten for 4 weeks. The authors observed an 18% decrease in serum cholesterol on removal of the sterol (period II) from the diet, even when it contained relatively saturated fat from cocoa butter. In period III the diet contained no cholesterol, but the fats were 31.4% polyunsaturated and 18.6% saturated. The serum-lipid levels were the same as those in period II. Addition of 725 mg cholesterol increased serum cholesterol 16% in the presence of a diet high in polyunsaturated fat, as in period III. Thus on a cholesterol-free diet of polyunsaturated fats (iodine number 100) the levels of serum lipids were the same as those on a diet with no cholesterol but with relatively saturated fats, suggesting that dietary cholesterol per se influenced serum-cholesterol levels. The saturated fat with iodine number 64 was cocoa butter, which has been used in cholesterol-free diets by others to reduce serum cholesterol.

Connor et al. (95) were surprised that both cholesterol-free and polyunsaturated-fat diets did not further reduce serum-cholesterol levels. This may be explained by the fact that since the subjects had been on cholesterol-free diets for 8 weeks, the serum cholesterol was already at minimal levels. Coconut oil has mostly short-chain fatty acids, which are metabolized differently from the long-chain acids of corn oil. Cholesterol-free diets containing fats having both low (60–70) and high (95–100) iodine numbers did not affect serum-cholesterol values as predicted by the Keys formula (77), suggesting that other factors played a role.

In more recent experiments Connor et al. (96) reported that serum-cholesterol values in six normal men on formula diets were as follows: 222 mg % on cocoa-butter diets (iodine number 32), 177 mg % on corn-oil diets (iodine number 125), and 225 mg % on return to cocoa-butter diets. The fats provided 40% of the total calories, and each diet was fed for 3 weeks. Fecal steroid excretion increased from 744 mg/day when the subjects were on cocoa butter to 953 mg/day on corn-oil diets, and then dropped to 672 mg/day on return to cocoa-butter diets.

Effects of saturated (coconut oil or butter) or unsaturated (corn oil, safflower oil, or trilinolein) fats comprising 40% of total calories on steroid excretion and serum cholesterol were also studied by Spritz et al. (97, 98) and by Avigan and Steinberg (99), all of whom found that serum cholesterol is lower when unsaturated fats are eaten, confirming earlier reports. The lipids in the LDL, but not the HDL, fraction were decreased (98). Spritz et al. (97, 98) observed significantly increased steroid excretion when subjects were on sterol-containing fat diets, regardless of the degree of saturation in the dietary fats, but Avigan and Steinberg (99) found no consistent relation between fecal steroid excretion and dietary fats (coconut and/or corn oil). Several recent experiments suggest that these variations could be explained by differences in methodology, subjects, and diets.

Wood, Shioda, and Kinsell (100) suggest the "possibility of redistribution into other body pools as the mechanism by which polyunsaturated fat lowers plasma cholesterol." They have confirmed their previous work and that of Spritz et al. (97, 98), showing that increased fecal excretion of steroids occurs simultaneously with decreased serum cholesterol when polyunsaturated fats are fed.

B. High-Fat Diets

Ahrens (101) "force fed" formula diets in which up to 70% of the total calories were in the form of fat. When the amounts of unsaturated corn oil were increased from 40 to 70% of total calories, serum triglycerides, and thus VLDL, were reduced to low values. When the fat was saturated, the VLDL (S_f 12–400) were increased. Antonis and Bersohn (82) reported that such high-fat, high-calorie diets rich in monoenoic and saturated (butter) fatty acids produced significant rises in triglycerides (VLDL).

Meng et al. (88) infused a cotton-seed-oil emulsion into nine institutionalized patients. Each received 1.05 to 1.72 g/kg-day for 20 to 21 days. There were increases in serum total fatty acids in five patients, and increases in pre-β-lipoproteins (VLDL). The latter were not sustained. In these experiments, although cotton-seed oil was fed, there were no consistent elevations in LDL, measured as serum total cholesterol.

Scrimshaw and co-workers (102) reported that the S_f 0–12 and S_f 12–20 lipoproteins were not consistently affected by low- or high-fat diets from vegetable sources but were greatly increased by high-fat diets of animal origin. A survey of serum lipoproteins in people who habitually consume diets that are low in animal fat (and protein) and high in carbohydrate revealed lower values for S_f 12–20 and S_f 20–100 lipoproteins than are commonly observed in persons on more "usual" omnivorous diets.

It has been reported (7, 103) that several hours after a high-fat meal there is an acute increase in S_f 35–100 lipoproteins. When a low-fat (0.24 g/day) diet was changed to include more fat (49 g coconut oil per day), on an isocaloric basis, only a slight increase in LDL was observed in some subjects and essentially no change in VLDL (104).

Nichols et al. (76) confirmed to some extent the "slight" LDL increases resulting from diets in which vegetable fat was increased (104), but observed decreased VLDL levels.

Veleminsky and Mirejovska (105) reported that when obese subjects were given a high-fat meal, their serum contained greater amounts of β-lipoproteins and VLDL 6 hr after the fat loading than did the serum of lean persons; this suggests delayed clearance in the obese subjects.

Certain groups of people who live almost entirely on animal protein and fat have been studied (106). The men had somewhat less cholesterol in the VLDL ($d < 1.019$ g/ml) and LDL (d 1.019–1.063 g/ml) fractions than did men on more varied diets. There were no differences in lipoprotein levels between groups of women on the high-animal-fat and the more typical diets. Since little carbohydrate was included in the diets, the differences probably arose from decreased total calories.

Little, Shanoff, and Csima (107) compared the effects of habitual high-fat diets on lipoprotein levels in normal men and in those who had survived a myocardial infarction. The normal subjects responded differently to "hyperlipemic" foods in that there was a negative correlation between total dietary fat and amounts of S_f 0–20 (r — .060) and S_f 20–400 lipoproteins (r — .182). This contrasted significantly with a positive correlation (r .215) for S_f 0–20 and r .065 for (S_f 20–400) in the patients.

C. Low-Fat Diets

The percentage of carbohydrate calories is increased in most low-fat diets, unless total calories are reduced greatly and subjects lose weight. Unlike reducing total calories from carbohydrate sources, increasing them can raise the serum VLDL especially and have little or no effect on LDL.

It has been reported that when fat was decreased to 10% of total calories with no alterations in the type of fat or protein intake, there was a 90% (mg %) decrease in S_f 0–12 lipoproteins (76) and a 90% increase in S_f 12–400 lipoproteins (108). When the report was published (68), this seemed to represent no net change, but the change in distribution is presently considered to be important in view of the different metabolic roles now ascribed to LDL and VLDL.

Scrimshaw et al. (102) also observed increases in VLDL (S_f 12–100) and decreases in S_f 0–12 lipoproteins (LDL) in Central Americans and Costa Ricans who habitually eat low-saturated-fat diets that are relatively high in carbohydrate.

Subjects on low-fat, low-calorie diets lose, and do not regain, weight if they adhere to the diet. The levels of serum S_f 12–100 lipoproteins decrease (109). If the diet is low in fat but adequate in calories and does not cause weight loss, the S_f 12–100 levels still will decrease. This indicates a dietary fat effect that is separate from the calorie–weight effect. However, fat restriction per se does not lower S_f 12–100 lipoproteins in all subjects. The effect depends somewhat on the initial levels of this VLDL component.

Effects of fat (but not calorie) restriction were tested with patients consuming a rice-and-fruit diet for amelioration of symptoms of hypertension (110). Although there were only 3 g of fat per day in one of the test diets, the S_f 20–100 lipoproteins increased 100% after 4 to 18 weeks on the diet. Diets with more fat but similar in calories did not markedly reduce the lipoproteins. Hatch, Abell, and Kendall (110) pointed out that fat restriction implies increased carbohydrates if the diets are isocaloric. The carbohydrate is transformed to fat before utilization. This occurs at normal or high carbohydrate levels, regardless of the absence of fat or protein from the diet. Since storage of large amounts of carbohydrates is impractical, conversion to fat is practical when the food intake exceeds utilization requirements. Loss of weight can result from water loss (111), or water can be lost but not weight. The increase in VLDL (S_f 20–100), accompanied by lipemia, that was observed on the low-fat, high-carbohydrate rice-and-fruit diet could be the effect of high amounts of carbohydrates, rather than low amounts of fat. This diet, of course, is very unusual, and deficiencies of unrecognized essential nutrients cannot be ruled out.

Gofman, Tamplin, and Strisower (112) reported that a diet in which fat was lowered to 20 g daily but calories were maintained by carbohydrate, decreased VLDL in a healthy young man (whose initial levels were very high) from 1133 to 636 mg/100 ml serum in six weeks. The LDL fraction was not appreciably lowered in this subject, but it was in a patient who had xanthoma tendinosum with excessive LDL initially, the level changing from 1340 to 1235 mg/100 ml in eight weeks. On a similar diet men, but not women, had a highly significant increase in triglycerides (VLDL) (113).

When patients were transferred from a "regular" to an isocaloric diet containing essentially no fat (0.25 g/day), there were LDL decreases in all subjects (104). The VLDL fraction increased in most subjects, but the increments were smaller than those observed on the rice diet (110).

The levels of S_f 20–100 and S_f 100–400 lipoproteins were significantly elevated as a result of low fat intake (18 g/day) in comparison with the levels observed on either high-vegetable-fat (100 g/day) or high-animal-fat (103 g/day) diets (76). Thus diets low in triglycerides elevated the serum VLDL levels. The diets were high in carbohydrates (370–412 g/day) and isocaloric. The high-fat diets contained 203 to 219 g of carbohydrates per day.

If the fat in the low-fat diet was relatively unsaturated, the levels of S_f

0–12 lipoproteins were not changed, but there was a pronounced rise in S_f 12–400 VLDL (76). The VLDL fraction was increased regardless of whether the low-fat diet contained saturated or unsaturated fats when the carbohydrate was increased to isocaloric levels. This is undoubtedly the result of carbohydrate conversion to fat.

The levels of S_f 0–12 lipoproteins were lower when the low-fat diet contained unsaturated fat. In fact, regardless of the amount of fat in the diet (within 40% of the total calories) the S_f 0–12 lipoprotein levels were lower when the fat was unsaturated and higher when the fat was saturated.

D. Effects of Carbohydrates

Calories in isocaloric diets designed to test levels of carbohydrate intake are usually adjusted with fat rather than protein. Therefore in testing the effects of a high-carbohydrate diet on serum lipids the effects of low fat intake must be also considered, and vice versa.

Ingested carbohydrates influence lipid and lipoprotein metabolism. Monosaccharides and disaccharides especially provide ready energy. If taken in amounts exceeding energy requirements, they will be converted to fat and frequently to excess weight. High-carbohydrate diets usually result in elevated serum triglycerides, and hence VLDL (S_f 20–400) to transport them. The levels of S_f 0–10 lipoproteins (LDL) are not usually affected by carbohydrate intake but may be decreased if fat has been greatly reduced. The reverse situation is produced by low-carbohydrate diets.

The effects of the rice-and-fruit diet have been cited in the preceding section. This diet produces significant increases in VLDL.

Ahrens and associates (114) emphasized the phenomenon of carbohydrate-induced lipemia as differentiated from fat-induced lipemia. A patient on a diet in which 85% of the calories were from carbohydrates (0% from fat) had a greatly lipemic fasting serum. When placed on a diet in which 70% of the calories were supplied by fat and 15% by carbohydrates, the same patient had a clear fasting serum, regardless of whether corn oil or butter fat was fed. Ahrens proposed that carbohydrate-induced lipemia may be a common occurrence, especially in areas where high-calorie, carbohydrate-rich diets are consumed. According to Fredrickson and Lees (115), carbohydrate-induced hyperlipoproteinemia is described as type IV, with elevated or excessive VLDL, and may be associated with carbohydrate intolerance or a familial history of diabetes (or both). (For more details on the hyperlipoproteinemias see Section IX.)

Antonis and Bersohn (82) observed that both Caucasian and Bantu volunteers had elevated fasting VLDL (triglycerides) after consuming a diet with 70% of the calories derived from carbohydrates and 15% from fat. The peak values were not attained until about 5 weeks. They decreased slowly and did not reach normal levels for many weeks. This could result also from reducing fat calories from 40 to 15%.

There is some disagreement about the effect of the type of carbohydrate, starch or sucrose, on blood lipids. Yudkin (116, 117) and Kuo and Bassett (118), among others, have stated that sucrose, as a replacement for starch, will raise blood-lipid levels.

Akinyanju et al. (119) administered a basic diet of 3310 calories—48% from carbohydrates, 37% from fat, 11% from protein, and 4% from alcohol—to 10 male student volunteers. They were placed into two groups; one received the carbohydrate calories as sucrose, the other group ate cooked wheat starch. After the first experimental period the groups exchanged diets. Neither diet changed the "basal" level, 240 mg/100 ml, of serum cholesterol. Serum-triglyceride levels were changed: 2.29 meq/l on the sucrose diet decreased to 0.75 meq/l on the starch diet. If the sucrose diet was followed by the starch diet, there was no change in triglyceride levels. When the starch was changed to sucrose, triglyceride levels increased from 0.75 to 1.89 meq/l.

Subjects on the experimental sucrose diet (400 g/day) were found to have sugar in the urine; this did not occur when starch was eaten. All subjects gained weight during the first week. These subjects were eating what the authors described as an "atherogenic diet," which had less carbohydrate than other diets causing lipemia with large amounts of sucrose (110, 120–122).

Macdonald (123) continued to investigate the effects of the type of carbohydrate. Fructose and glucose labeled with ^{14}C were fed to both normal men and patients who had had a myocardial infarction. These subjects ate their regular diets and fasted before receiving the test sugar. Blood samples were taken before the test sugar and at several times after. Cholesterol levels were not affected. Fructose increased greatly the radioactive triglyceride in both groups, especially in the patients. The specific activity of triglyceride was increased only slightly by glucose, but again, more in the patients.

Macdonald (123) suggests different degrees of utilization, metabolic pathways, or both, for these two sugars in their roles as lipid precursors. Simple sugars should be reduced to a minimum in most diets, especially in sedentary individuals. However, complex carbohydrates are necessary to supply "bulk" to diets. Carbohydrates also play a role in adjusting the bacterial metabolism of sterols and bile acids in the gastrointestinal tract.

Bierman, Gordis, and Hamlin (124) studied the characteristics of the various types of fat particles produced in lipemia induced either by high-fat or high-carbohydrate diets. In normal subjects hyperlipoproteinemia (exogenous) from consuming a high-fat meal is usually transitory, and serum "clears" when the high-fat diet is replaced by a low-fat one. However, when hyperlipoproteinemia results from excessive carbohydrate (endogenous), it is less transitory and is usually associated with abnormality (125).

In fat-induced hyperlipoproteinemia Bierman et al. (124) observed "primary" particles, or lymph chylomicrons, and "secondary" particles, which originated in the liver and were derived from the primary particles. These had different electrophoretic (zone) properties, but all floated at *d* 1.006 g/ml and contained about 90% triglycerides. They belong to the VLDL class (126).

When high-carbohydrate, fat-free diets were fed (127), the resulting hyperlipoproteinemia came from a homogeneous group of fat particles. All subjects with sustained levels of hyperlipoproteinemia had an abnormal carbohydrate metabolism. In contrast to fat-induced particles, carbohydrate-induced particles are electrophoretically homogeneous, migrating as a single large peak between the β- and α_2-globulin regions. Fat-induced particles produce two peaks: "primary," with α_2-globulin mobility; and "secondary," with β-globulin mobility on nonabsorbing media.

When high-carbohydrate diets were given to normal subjects, plasma triglycerides (pre-β-lipoproteins, or VLDL) were two to three times higher than normal, and the concentration of α-lipoproteins (HDL) fell 20 to 60% (40). The cholesterol moiety of the lipoproteins was not affected. Administration of heparin, 10 units/kg, greatly reduced the pre-β-lipoproteins, whereas α-lipoproteins increased by about 28%. Heparin did not have this effect when normal levels of lipoproteins were present.

Low-carbohydrate diets reduced plasma triglycerides in patients with Tangier disease (who have abnormally high triglyceride levels). When isocaloric high-carbohydrate diets were fed, triglycerides increased to about 500 mg/100 ml, higher than in normal subjects on the same diets.

Patients homozygous for Tangier disease have elevated triglycerides (VLDL) when fed high-carbohydrate diets, but the lipoproteins did not move on paper with pre-β-lipoproteins; they moved with β-lipoprotein bands, which widened but did not reach, the pre-β-lipoprotein positions.

Diets with 85% carbohydrate and less than 1% fat were fed for 7 days to four normal subjects. As expected, the VLDL increased two to three times after synthesis and release of hepatic VLDL stimulated by the high carbohydrate intake. Ruderman and associates (128) reported increased protein and cholesterol as well as triglycerides, associated with the increased VLDL. The size of the VLDL particles increased (electron-microscope examination), presumably accounting for the rise in triglyceride released by the liver. Carbohydrate-induced lipemia also resulted in reduced protein and cholesterol in other lipoproteins (*d* 1.006–1.21 g/ml).

Hyperlipoproteinemia induced by high-carbohydrate diets is usually an inherited disorder. It is characterized by excessive VLDL and chylomicrons. This disorder may respond most effectively to reduction in carbohydrate intake. Jepson et al. (129) used this regimen (90 g carbohydrate and 226 g fat in a 2800-calorie diet) to reduce significantly plasma triglycerides.

E. Changes in Total Calorie Intake

1. Fasting for More than 24 hr. In serious fasting with no food triglycerides will be removed from adipose-tissue stores to provide energy. The levels of VLDL increase in order to transport the released free fatty acids or triglycerides.

After the second day of a 4-day fast, Rubin and Aladjem (130) noted pronounced increases in S_f 12–400 lipoproteins. Other lipoproteins (S_f 0–12) were only slightly increased. When sucrose (1 g/kg body wt) was administered at the end of the fasting period, measurements of lipoproteins after 3 hr showed no changes.

In a similar study Havel (131) observed a significant decrease in S_f 12–400 lipoproteins when 400 g of glucose was given to subjects who had fasted. Since VLDL play a significant role in the transport of fatty acids from endogenous sources, the decrease points to improved uptake of triglycerides by adipose tissue when this adequate amount of glucose was given.

2. Effect of Weight Loss from Reduced Calorie Intake. Weight loss in normal subjects usually occurs when the total calorie intake is reduced. A reduction in S_f 12–100 (109) and S_f 35–100 (111, 132) lipoproteins was reported when subjects were maintained on a reducing diet for up to 16 months. The lipoproteins were significantly reduced if there was a 12% weight loss. The greatest reductions (in the S_f 35–100 fraction) occurred in those who had the highest initial values. This suggested to the authors that caloric balance (in weight loss, usually a negative caloric balance) could influence the levels of serum lipoproteins. To test this point two individuals, after a 2-week equilibration, were force fed a highly-positive-caloric-balance diet of 5000 calories, high in carbohydrates, low in fat, for 30 days. During this regimen diuresis was pronounced, but weight gain still occurred. The S_f 35–100 lipoproteins increased greatly on this diet high in nonfat calories (111).

On a low-fat (27 g/day) low-calorie (969 calories per day) diet patients lost weight. Initial serum levels of S_f 0–20 lipoproteins were 465 mg/100 ml, and these decreased to 387 mg/100 ml after 2 months and 14-lb weight loss. The levels of S_f 20–400 decreased from 158 to 99 mg/100 ml (76).

Straus, Kositchek, and Wurm (133) reported reductions in β-to-α-lipoprotein ratios in most subjects on weight-reducing low-fat, low-calorie diets. The reduction derived from a decrease in β-lipoproteins (LDL).

3. Effect of Excessive Calorie Intake and Weight Gain. When otherwise healthy individuals ingest diets that contain excess calories (above the requirement commensurate with their work load) from either fat, carbohydrates, or both, they gain weight and can become obese. Obesity is usually estimated by the subject's weight compared with standard height–weight tables though it is more accurately determined by the percentage of deviation from normal or by measuring skin-fold thickness (134). What effect does obesity from overeating or improper eating have on serum lipoproteins? In an early study of obese subjects who usually ingested large quantities of fat Gofman and Jones (135) observed significantly higher levels of S_f 35–100 lipoproteins (68.3 mg/100 ml) than they did in subjects who were of normal weight (43.1 mg/100 ml). The S_f 12–20 lipoproteins were not so markedly increased in obese subjects. If obesity results from the excessive intake of carbohydrate calories, the S_f 20–400 lipoproteins may be elevated (112).

In general no direct relationship was reported between obesity and serum cholesterol (134, 135) or HDL (134) levels, but LDL (β-lipoprotein) levels were elevated (134). Skanse (136), however, reported that all obese women (otherwise normal), 16 to 74 years old, had less α-lipoprotein "lipids" in the serum (average 170 mg/100 ml) than did young controls, 18 to 35 years old (224 mg/100 ml). In obese women of all ages the α-lipoprotein levels were comparable to those of postmenopausal women, which suggested "early aging" to Skanse (136). Reasons for the obesity in these subjects were not given; probably simply overeating.

Rifkind, Begg, and Jackson (137) observed greatly elevated serum triglycerides and β-lipoproteins in obese men, and both low (79 mg/100 ml) and high (138 mg/100 ml) serum-triglyceride levels in obese women. They suggested that the causes of obesity (high fat *or* high carbohydrate intake) may have influenced the observed effects. In nearly all obese subjects VLDL (pre-β-lipoprotein) levels are elevated. In these the excess calories are probably derived from sugar. Other subjects who have excessive chylomicrons (not accompanied by excessive VLDL) may have delayed clearance of excessive dietary fat.

F. Changes in Quantity and Quality of Protein

The amino acid composition of a protein at any percentage level is a critical factor. Animal protein fulfills human requirements of essential amino acids and has the highest biologic value. If the protein intake drops to less than 10 to 15% of the total calories, there is danger of deficiency of methyl donors (choline and methionine), which are necessary for optimum fat metabolism. In addition, low levels of protein nitrogen result in a negative nitrogen balance and possibly weight loss.

Olson and associates (138, 139) equilibrated subjects on a diet containing 100 g of vegetable protein, 80 g of saturated fat, and 320 g of carbohydrate. They then substituted an isocaloric amount of carbohydrate for 75 g of protein, producing a diet with 4% protein, 30% fat, and 66% carbohydrate. The protein was deficient in methionine. There was a 44% decrease in serum cholesterol. This was reflected in a 25% decrease in S_f 0–12 lipoproteins and some decrease in the S_f 12–400 fraction. These changes did not stem from a negative nitrogen balance because the levels of both lipoprotein fractions were restored only after the administration of more protein than necessary to restore a positive nitrogen balance. Lipoproteins were also decreased if low levels of animal protein were fed. These experiments showed that both a source of labile methyl groups (choline) and adequate dietary protein of good biologic value were required to raise lipoproteins to pretreatment levels.

Decreased lipoprotein levels were reported by Furman, Howard, and Norcia (140), who substituted all the protein by isocaloric amounts of carbohydrates, though corn oil constituted 40% of the total calories.

In the protein-deficiency disease kwashiorkor both LDL and HDL levels are decreased (68), as they are in other starvation or near-starvation episodes. However, in these cases fat and calorie intakes are also insufficient.

Calatayud and co-workers (141) did not observe lower-than-usual levels of serum cholesterol or lipoproteins in a population of normal Trappist monks who had lived for many years on diets providing 500 g of carbohydrates, 25 g of fat (from eggs, dairy products, and corn or cottonseed oil), and 20 g of animal protein (milk, eggs, cheese).

Increased amounts of protein, like those the Eskimo consume, had no effect on serum-lipid levels, although they could have derived 47% of their calories from fat, 45% from protein, and only 8% from carbohydrates.

Olson and Vester (68) suggest that about 1 g of protein per kilogram of body weight (10% of total calories) is adequate in an otherwise balanced diet to maintain normal levels of about 200 mg % cholesterol in humans with sedentary habits.

G. Miscellaneous Substances in Diets

It seems to be established that serum cholesterol (LDL) is lowered by diets high in polyunsaturated fatty acids. The fats supplying these fatty acids are largely of vegetable origin, and it has been suggested that some component in the vegetable oil may contribute to the hypocholesteremic effect. Weiner, Walker, and Milch suggested that β-sitosterol reduces blood cholesterol and LDL under varying circumstances (142).[5]

Beveridge and associates (143, 144) tested this suggestion and observed a highly significant decrease in plasma cholesterol after β-sitosterol administration. Other investigators, however, do not agree that β-sitosterol is effective (80, 104). These differences may be complicated by the diets used, for example, restrictions in animal fat versus fat of any origin, low calorie intake versus other conditions that would also lower blood cholesterol. It seems reasonable to conclude that such factors play a minor role. Labecki (145) reported an *increase* in α-lipoproteins in subjects receiving moderate doses of safflower-seed oil, 4 mg of pyridoxine, and a lipotropic mixture: 1 g of choline, 1 g of *dl*-methionine, 750 mg of inositol, 18 μg of vitamin B_{12}, and 750 mg of desiccated liver per day (Methischol capsules, U.S. Vitamin Corporation, New York). Only 6 of 25 patients who had had myocardial infarctions showed a reduction in serum cholesterol as such. As already cited in Section IV.A, patients with lipidoses had reductions in plasma cholesterol on this type of diet (10), but not all had decreased S_f 0–10 lipoproteins.

Farquhar and Sokolow (146) studied the effects of both β-sitosterol and polyunsaturated fats from safflower oil for a period of 43 weeks. They observed a rapid decrease in β-lipoprotein cholesterol in the first period (8 weeks on β-sitosterol). Initial control levels of 233 mg/100 ml dropped to 186 mg/100 ml. During the next 8 weeks on safflower oil the latter value was not changed, but after an additional 6 weeks on the combination, the cholesterol decreased to 157 mg/100 ml. The combination was much more effective than either β-sitosterol or safflower-seed oil alone.

Carlson, Orö, and Östman (147) studied the lipotropic effects of nicotinic acid and recently reported on a long-time study. The addition of 1 g of nicotinic acid daily to a regular hospital diet lowered VLDL levels within 4 to 5 hr. From their previous studies in which nicotinic acid reduced

[5] β-sitosterol is a plant sterol that is believed to block the absorption of dietary cholesterol and the reabsorption of biliary cholesterol.

plasma levels of free fatty acids the authors postulated a reduced supply of free fatty acids in the liver for VLDL formation. Free fatty acids comprise 3.4% of the total VLDL lipids (148). A longer time elapsed before the LDL levels were decreased. The authors (147) suggested that the decrease in LDL resulted from lower quantities of available VLDL, assuming a conversion from VLDL to LDL.

Wilson and co-workers (149) recently reported that when corn-oil emulsion (or a lipid fraction of coconut oil containing octanoic and decanoic acids) was fed with 150 ml of ethanol, there was a marked lipemia (VLDL) after 6 hr, rising at 8 hr to 350% higher than fasting levels, and dropping off only after 10 hr. Neither fat alone nor ethanol alone caused this excessive increase in fasting VLDL. It was concluded that the great increase in VLDL was a function of fasting triglyceride concentrations, suggesting, for example, that patients with endogenous hyperlipoproteinemia would have exceptionally high VLDL after ingesting fat plus ethanol. Ethanol taken with fat greatly enhances serum VLDL (see also Section XIV.F).

To test the effect of calcium on serum-cholesterol levels Bhattacharyya and associates (150) measured serum cholesterol, phospholipids, and triglycerides, as well as fecal steroids, bile acids, and fatty acids. These authors concluded that the substitution of safflower oil for palm oil reduced serum cholesterol when the diet was either low or high in calcium. Since the amounts of dietary cholesterol were the same, this is a "fatty acid" effect. Subjects with initially high values for cholesterol had the greatest reductions. The substitution of safflower oil on either a high- or low-calcium intake caused an increase in fecal neutral steroid excretion, but no change in the excretion of bile acids.

The authors (150) observed no correlation between the changes in serum-cholesterol levels and the excretion of neutral steroids in individual subjects. They attributed variations in such data from different laboratories to experimental design, subjects used (whether normal or patients, and their ages), and the types of diets.

There were highly significant increases (3 g/day) in the fecal excretion of fatty acids when saturated fat (palm oil) replaced safflower oil in high-calcium diets. The results indicated that calcium interacts preferentially with saturated fatty acids in the intestine, forming insoluble calcium soaps, which are not absorbed. Increased calcium in the diet sharply decreased the digestability of the highly saturated fatty acids, but did not interfere with the absorption of cholesterol. Changes in the calcium content of the diet did not change steroid excretion.

The addition of calcium to the diet containing palm oil caused only a small decrease in serum-cholesterol levels, but a large increase in the fecal excretion of total fatty acids. Neutral-steroid excretion was significantly increased when safflower oil replaced palm oil: 71 and 47 mg/day on low- and high-calcium diets, respectively. Although the individual variation was high, these data imply that when polyunsaturated fatty acids lower serum-cholesterol levels, this is done through the mechanism of increased elimination of neutral steroids in feces.

Of the thousands of different dietary experiments that have been performed, the few reported here demonstrate the complexity of evaluating the results. There often appears to be little agreement regarding what effect(s) a certain diet really has. This results from many causes: choice of subjects, their health and activities, diets, time periods of study, analytical methods, interpretation of data, and so on.

From the "confusion" a few rather definite trends have emerged. The serum LDL fraction, with its high amount of cholesterol, is somewhat lower when subjects have a restricted fat intake, especially if the fat is primarily polyunsaturated, either from certain vegetable sources or fish. There is increased sterol excretion in the feces. Serum VLDL are decreased mainly by lowering the total calorie intake or at least maintaining a calorie intake that does not cause weight gain, using unsaturated fats, and restricting carbohydrate intake. Both LDL and VLDL decrease during weight loss with reduced, but balanced, food intake.

Serum LDL and VLDL are increased on high-fat diets, especially if saturated fats are eaten. The LDL fraction is not greatly increased on high-carbohydrate diets, which increase VLDL by virtue of the increased conversion of carbohydrates to fat and the necessity of transporting increased amounts of triglycerides.

If low-fat diets are isocaloric, the LDL fraction may decrease since its levels are not so affected by the concomitant increases in carbohydrates, which then increased VLDL.

Inadequate or low-quality protein will decrease all lipoproteins, including HDL, which seem quite stable in the face of changing dietaries that are not extreme.

Relative increases, and especially decreases in lipoproteins, seem to be very closely related to the initial levels and to metabolic conditions.

V. RELATIONSHIPS BETWEEN HORMONES AND SERUM-LIPOPROTEIN LEVELS

Different hormones affect serum-lipoprotein levels in a variety of ways. In most of the reported experiments the measurements were made before and after the administration of hormones. Although some subjects were not suffering from a defined disease, most of the subjects had clinical symptoms that indicated administration of the hormone(s) for relief.

A. Diabetes Mellitus

Some humans with diabetes mellitus and experimentally pancreatectomized dogs are known to have hyperlipemia. Inasmuch as crude extracts of pancreas and, later, insulin were found to abolish the lipemia along with the other diabetic symptoms, this defect in carbohydrate metabolism was linked to lipid metabolism (see also Sections IX and XI).

Early experiments in which serum-lipoprotein concentrations were measured involved patients with diabetes mellitus. The severity of the disease, its treatment and complications, especially atherosclerosis with age, had to be considered. For example, Lindgren and Nichols (12) reported that a patient in acidosis and coma can have extremely high levels (3739 mg/100 ml serum) of S_f° 100–400 and S_f° 20–100 lipoproteins (VLDL), with lower than normal levels of S_f° 0–20 lipoproteins (LDL) and not abnormal levels of HDL_{2+3}. After treatment, the VLDL and LDL values tended to become more normal, although the VLDL fraction remained elevated for a long time. Since the metabolism of lipoproteins is related in a highly sensitive way to carbohydrate metabolism, all lipoprotein values in patients with diabetes mellitus must be regarded with caution.

Bornstein (151) demonstrated early a possible relationship between serum lipoproteins and glucose metabolism. A substance that inhibited glucose uptake (*in vitro* by rat diaphragm) was associated with the plasma β-lipoproteins (fraction III-0) of diabetic rats. The inhibition was insulin reversible. Fraction III-0 obtained from the plasma of a patient 1 hr after injection of 100 units of insulin was inhibitory. This suggested that the factor appeared in blood, associated with β-lipoproteins, in response to hypoglycemia and participated in blood-sugar regulation as an antagonist of insulin.

Ejarque, Marble, and Tuller (152) studied a large group of diabetic patients with and without such complications as neuropathy, retinopathy, and nephropathy, single or combined. The β-lipoproteins were elevated when complications were present, but not in their absence. The quantities of α-lipoproteins were about the same in normal and diabetic subjects. Patients with vascular complications had somewhat lower amounts. Ditzel and Moinat (153) observed a positive correlation between the degree of intravascular erythrocyte aggregation and the amount of both total lipoproteins and the α- and β-lipoprotein fractions. The β-lipoproteins especially had wider bands on electrophoretic strips in patients with aggregation in all small blood vessels.

In 918 diabetic patients insulin treatment did not change the β-lipoprotein levels, but it did slightly reduce α-lipoprotein levels in patients in whom atherosclerosis and angiopathy were not demonstrated. Szücs and Csapó

(154) suggested that the lipoprotein levels reflect the severity, control, or lack of control of the disease. In general, as the blood-sugar level rose (155, 156), chylomicrons and β-lipoproteins were elevated, whereas α-lipoproteins decreased.

Normal serum-lipoprotein electrophoretic patterns were observed in 51 diabetic children with an average age of 11.7 years (157). They were receiving 46.4 units of insulin per day and were on controlled diets. No pre-β-lipoprotein (VLDL) band was observed. Bacon and Sanbar (157) suggested that the acceleration of atherosclerosis, usually associated with age and duration of disease in diabetics, "is not due to . . . hyperlipoproteinemia."

Vernet and Smith (158) observed no differences in the amount or frequency of the pre-β-lipoprotein (S_f 20–400) band in men and women, aged 24 to 66, with uncomplicated diabetes. They, too, suggested that this lipoprotein class was not implicated in the development of atherosclerosis or cardiovascular disease in diabetics. In diabetic women who had successful pregnancies the pre-β-lipoproteins increased to term, but decreased rapidly after delivery; in unsuccessful pregnancies they increased to a higher level during pregnancy and continued to increase for 2 weeks postpartum. These patients were not studied during a ketotic period. Only in severe and rapidly progressing cases was the VLDL level abnormally high.

The influence of diabetic acidosis on the *in vitro* formation of lipfanogens as related to lipoproteins was reported by Simms and Harmison (159).[6] The lipfanogens showed a positive correlation with the ultracentrifugal residue (albumin–free fatty acid complex) and also with S_f 20–400 lipoproteins. Untreated diabetics had a high level of free lipfanogens and a low antilipfanogen level, a condition favorable to fat deposition. After insulin administration the levels of lipfanogen and antilipfanogen were reversed.

B. Estrogens and Progesterone

1. Studies on Subjects without Serious Disease. It has been known that sex hormones and lipoproteins are interrelated since the incidence of atherosclerosis and coronary disease is higher in men than it is in premenopausal women. After quantitative methods for studying serum lipoproteins became available, Gofman and his group (4) started extensive surveys of serums from normal persons and from persons with a variety of diseases. A pronounced and unquestionable finding was that during the ages of 20 to 40 years men had more VLDL and LDL, and less HDL, than did women with normal ovarian function. Thus it was logical that the sex-hormone

[6] Lipfanogens are heat-stable, water-soluble lipoid substances, such as soaps and monoglyceryl esters of fatty acids.

effect be investigated. These studies could take two forms: (a) the classical experiments involving the injection of hormones into operated or whole animals to test their effects or (b) the administration of hormones to humans with symptoms requiring reinstatement of normal hormonal levels, as, for example, postmenopausal women with symptoms requiring relief.

In an early study Glass and co-workers (160) studied the effects of buccal estradiol in 50- to 70-year-old men with prostatic hypertrophy. The hormone, which was also given to nonmenstruating women, aged 42 to 65, was in some instances administered intramuscularly. The dosage levels were evidently not high enough to cause discomfort in most of the men and did control menopausal symptoms in the women. The authors observed no changes in the LDL (S_f 12–20 and S_f 20–100) at the estradiol levels used: 0.25, 0.5, and 0.75 mg, increasing by the month. In one male receiving 0.75 mg daily for about 4 months there were increases in S_f 12–20 lipoproteins. A follow-up study by these authors (161) revealed similar results with physiologic doses of estradiol. Berezin and Von Studnitz (162) administered 0.05 mg of ethinylestradiol daily to seven women, aged 18 to 36, with amenorrhea. The α-lipoprotein levels increased in all cases, as they did in five postmenopausal women, aged 46 to 62, who received 0.3 to 0.5 mg of diethylstilbestrol daily. The values for serum cholesterol were more variable, and increases or decreases were somewhat dependent on pretreatment levels.

Robinson, Cohen, and Higano (163) reported that the daily administration of 5 mg of Enovid [which consists of 17-α-ethinylestradiol 3-methyl ether and 17-α-ethinyl-19-nortestosterone (norethindrone)] increased α-lipoproteins and decreased β-lipoproteins in postmenopausal women. They also observed a decrease in α-lipoproteins and an increase in β-lipoproteins when ovariectomies were performed before the natural menopause.

The complete spectrum of serum lipoproteins, separated and calculated by ultracentrifugal means (164) was studied for 12 consecutive weeks in normal women living under conditions that provided the same diet and activities. At ovulation HDL_2 ($d < 1.125$ g/ml) was the only fraction that consistently increased. The values rose on the seventh day of the menstrual cycle, reached a peak at the fourteenth day (ovulation), and then decreased. In most cases the LDL levels did not change appreciably.

Oliver and Boyd (165) had earlier reported that during the menstrual cycle normal women show fluctuations in the serum levels of both cholesterol and phospholipids, but the increases appeared later than the fourteenth day. When ovulation was expected, both cholesterol and phospholipids dropped and the ratio of total cholesterol to phospholipids reached its lowest value, possibly because the cholesterol decreased more than the phospholipids.

Kroman and co-workers (166) measured the plasma levels of estrone, estriol, and 17-β-estradiol in asymptomatic women, 29 to 39 years old, and related them to the days in the menstrual cycle and the proportions of α- and β-lipoproteins. In the controls the concentrations of 17-β-estradiol in plasma generally tended to be highest near the fourteenth day of the menstrual cycle, as was the proportion of α-lipoproteins.

2. Studies on Subjects with Serious Disease. Most of the subjects with serious disease to whom estrogens were administered in a study by Russ, Eder, and Barr (167, 168) were males who had survived myocardial infarctions. Ethinylestradiol (1.0 mg/day) was given orally. Initially these patients had abnormally high β-to-α-lipoprotein ratios (fractions I+III to fractions IV+V+VI), which were changed toward an increase in α-lipoproteins and a lower ratio. Although the administration of ethinylestradiol to patients with hypercholesteremic xanthomatosis or nephrosis caused an improvement in the ratio, normal patterns were not restored.

Oliver and Boyd (169) observed similar results with more graduated doses of the hormone, which resulted in increased phospholipids (α-lipoproteins) and decreased cholesterol in the β-lipoprotein fraction, estimated by zone electrophoresis.

A long-term (1–5 years) study was made by Danemann, Pick, and Katz (170) on 46 men who had suffered myocardial infarctions. Most were given 10 mg of Premarin (conjugated estrone sulfate) daily. Lipoproteins (α-to-β ratios) were estimated by zone electrophoresis and by ultracentrifugal analysis by the method of Green, Lewis, and Page (171). Estrogen increased the α-to-β-lipoprotein ratio in about 4 weeks after therapy began, and the ratio decreased in about the same time after cessation of treatment. The results obtained by the two methods were essentially in agreement.

A similar long-term (7 years) study on the effects of estradiol on 275 men, all under 50 years, who had survived previous myocardial infarctions was done by Stamler et al. (172). On a regimen of 10 mg of oral estradiol daily, the serum α-lipoproteins and phospholipids rose while the β-lipoproteins and cholesterol (and cholesterol-to-phospholipid ratios) fell so that the pattern was "more feminine." The men who received the estrogens had longer survival times. The authors concluded that estrogens caused a long-term, and sustained, increase in α-lipoprotein levels and exerted a significant antiatherogenic effect.

Plasma lipoproteins were measured before and after removal of the ovaries for temporary palliation of advanced mammary carcinoma. The type of metastatic lesion and the response of the patient could be related to the changes in lipoprotein levels. In general all lipoproteins increased, but especially the LDL S_f 0–10 fraction in patients with soft-tissue (brain) metastases. When there was a favorable response (some regression of lesions, especially bone healing), both the α- and β-lipoproteins (S_f 10–20 fraction) increased. Those with soft-tissue disease who responded favorably also had increases in α-lipoproteins and decreases in the S_f 20–100 VLDL fraction (173).

C. Testicular Hormones

1. Studies on Subjects without Serious Disease. Berezin and Von Studnitz (174) studied the effects of androgens (methylandrostenediol, buccally, 25–50 mg/day) in women with the following conditions: premenopausal with regular cycles, menstruating irregularly or anovulatory, postmenopausal symptoms, and after surgical castration. The α-lipoproteins decreased similarly in nearly all the subjects.

Furman and Howard (175) reported that androsterone, a metabolic product of testosterone (80–240 mg/day intramuscularly) administered for 16 to 28 days to nonhyperlipemic subjects with normal thyroid function and normal serum-cholesterol values decreased α-lipoproteins. In the less abnormal subjects the β-lipoproteins changed little after androsterone treatment.

2. Studies on Subjects with Serious Disease. Furman and Howard (175) studied the effects of androsterone on patients with decreased thyroid function and increased serum lipids. Androsterone (usually low in patients with hypothyroidism) markedly reduced the VLDL fraction ($d < 1.019$ g/ml) not only in patients with severe hypothyroidism but also in others with milder disease. The levels of lipoproteins with $d > 1.019$ and < 1.063 g/ml (LDL) were not regularly changed.

This hormone also reduced α-lipoproteins (phospholipids) in all but one subject studied by Oliver and Boyd (176). Androsterone, like testosterone, lowered α-lipoproteins consistently and produced a less pronounced effect on β-lipoproteins. The effects were consistent with those observed in patients during and after episodes of myocardial infarction in whom the "α-to-β-lipoprotein ratio fell from 13.87 to 6.94." In patients with a variety of diseases cholesterol and phospholipids were consistently decreased in Fraction IV+V+VI and increased in Fraction I+III after administration of methyltestosterone (167, 168).

D. Combined Estrogens and Androgens

When methyltestosterone was administered to patients surviving a myocardial infarction, their previously abnormal lipoprotein patterns were exaggerated; the simultaneous administration of estrogen did not counteract the effects of testosterone. When testosterone was discontinued and estrogen continued, a normal lipoprotein pattern was seen: Fraction IV+V+VI increased and Fraction I+III decreased. If testosterone was superimposed during estrogen therapy, the effects of the androgen nullified those of the estrogen, and the lipoprotein picture was reversed. Removal of the androgen again permitted the favorable effects of only 0.25 mg of ethinylestradiol to reappear (167).

This "mutually antagonistic" effect of estrogens and androgens was reported also by Oliver and Boyd (176), Cramér (177), and Furman et al. (178) when dioxydiethylstilbestrol and methyltestosterone were used.

Aurell and Cramér (179) assessed the effects of long-term (1 year) administration of an oral contraceptive on serum lipoproteins. They used a preparation containing 50 μg of 17-ethinylestradiol and 4 mg of 17-α-ethinyl-19-nortestosterone acetate (norethindrone) per tablet. One tablet daily was given from the fifth to the twenty-fifth day of the cycle, followed by a 7-day period of no drug. The LDL and HDL fractions were separated by hydroxyapatite chromatography (180).

The LDL components were an average of 36% higher than the initial values, whereas the HDL levels were not regularly changed. The levels of all lipoproteins were similar to those in serum from postmenopausal women. The authors suggested that the effects may have resulted either from the androgenlike behavior of norethindrone or that prolonged administration had inhibited the normal ovarian function. A possible disposition to coronary disease can be a serious problem and should be considered in view of the well-documented relationships between abnormal lipoprotein levels and heart disease (181). The fact that the HDL levels were not greatly affected may be of crucial importance in maintaining an optimum concentration of serum phospholipids.

Wynn, Doar, and co-workers recently reported the effects of oral contraceptives on both lipoprotein (182) and carbohydrate metabolism (183). A variety of estrogen–progestogen combinations were used. The possible relationship between occlusive vascular disease and atherosclerosis and elevated serum lipoproteins prompted the study. There is also relative impairment of glucose tolerance in women taking oral contraceptives. This could eventually influence lipid metabolism.

Table XVI shows the results of their experiments. There were 41 women in group A, tested before and during therapy, and 13 women in group B, tested initially during therapy and after therapy was discontinued. The data show that oral contraceptives resulted in significantly elevated serum lipids and lipoproteins. An exception was the S_f 12–20 lipoprotein fraction. The changes in group B were less pronounced. Two unusual observations were

Table XVI. Effects of Oral Contraceptives on Serum Lipid and Lipoprotein Levels in Women[a]

Lipid or Lipoprotein Class	Group[c]	Serum Level (mg/100 ml)[b] Off Therapy	On Therapy	*P*
Serum triglycerides	A + B	76.7 ± 31.1	116.2 ± 44.8	<.001
	A	70.5 ± 26.2	106.0 ± 34.7	<.001
	B	96.2 ± 38.1	148.4 ± 58.1	<.01
Serum cholesterol	A + B	181.2 ± 41.0	194.3 ± 35.8	<.01
	A	175.6 ± 36.1	185.3 ± 31.8	<.05
	B	198.8 ± 51.2	223.8 ± 33.8	<.05
S_f 0–12	A + B	232.0 ± 75	269.0 ± 64	<.001
	A	216.0 ± 59	266.0 ± 63	<.001
	B	298.0 ± 63	281.0 ± 68	N.S.
S_f 12–20	A + B	34.0 ± 21	37.0 ± 17	N.S.
	A	30.0 ± 18	35.0 ± 15	N.S.
	B	44.0 ± 26	42.0 ± 23	N.S.
S_f 20–100	A + B	32.0 ± 28	50.0 ± 34	<.001
	A	25.0 ± 21	48.0 ± 31	<.001
	B	51.0 ± 37	57.0 ± 41	N.S.
S_f 100–400	A + B	5.0 ± 12	13.0 ± 22	<.01
	A	3.0 ± 5	9.0 ± 12	<.001
	B	17.0 ± 22	26.0 ± 38	N.S.
$S_f\ \overline{0–12}$	A + B	7.5 ± 0.8	6.7 ± 0.8	<.001
	A	7.6 ± 0.8	6.8 ± 0.8	<.001
	B	7.0 ± 0.5	6.4 ± 0.8	<.01
Atherogenic index	A + B	36 ± 15	45 ± 15	<.001
	A	32 ± 11	43 ± 13	<.001
	B	49 ± 18	49 ± 20	N.S.

[a] Data from Ref. 182.
[b] Mean ± standard deviation.
[c] Group A: 41 women, tested before and during therapy; group B: 13 women tested during and after therapy.

that both the flotation and the quantity of the modal component ($S_f\ \overline{0–12}$) were reduced.

E. Thyroid Hormones

Administration of 180 mg of desiccated thyroid decreased LDL, but not VLDL, levels (184, 185). This decrease was maintained over the period of treatment when 600 mg were given (186). An increase in the dosage to 180, 240, or 300 mg/day decreased most of the LDL and VLDL for about 3.5 months during treatment and 27 weeks after treatment stopped. The S_f 0–12 lipoprotein levels fell with all dosages but remained low only when 300 mg were given daily. Both LDL and VLDL increased after thyroid medication was stopped. The S_f 12–20 lipoproteins, which remained low at all dosage levels, did not rise above control levels, as did the S_f 0–12 fraction. When 180 mg were given daily, the lower density S_f 20–100 and S_f 100–400 lipoproteins did not decrease, but when 240 mg were given, they decreased and remained low during the 300-mg period. Both fractions rose to prethyroid levels after treatment stopped. There was only a small weight loss during the 180-mg regimen.

By using a turbidimetric β-lipoprotein index, Ledvina, Coufalová, and Souček (187) studied patients with various thyroid conditions that lead to unfavorable symptoms. Hypothyroidism and thyroidectomy (without symptoms of hypofunction) increased the index (increased β-lipoproteins), but untreated hyperthyroidism decreased the index. In patients with simple goiter and eufunction, the index was decreased slightly. The influence of nutritional status, especially in cases of hyperthyroidism, when cachexia may occur, was considered by these authors in connection with decreases in β-lipoproteins.

3,5,3′-Triiodothyronine decreased the β-lipoproteins in nonhyperlipemic subjects. In patients with hyperlipemia this compound greatly reduced the VLDL fraction, and this effect seemed to be independent of severe hyperthyroidism (175).

Even in schizophrenic, hospitalized patients with no apparent thyroid abnormalities, thyroid reduced the LDL as it did in patients with untreated hyperthyroidism. Thus an important relationship was indicated between this hormone and LDL metabolism. This was established further by the increases in β-lipoproteins that have been observed in patients with hypothyroidism and thyroidectomy, which in turn might be related to atherosclerosis or coronary disease (184, 185).

F. Other Hormones

During the successful treatment of the severe cutaneous disease pemphigus vulgaris with adrenocorticotropic hormone or cortisone, Lever, Hurley, and Blaney (188) observed that the α-lipoproteins increased to abnormally high levels in all patients, although they returned to normal after therapy was discontinued. These hormones did not change the β-lipoprotein levels, but there were pronounced increases in both cholesterol and phospholipids.

Adlersberg and co-workers (189, 190) observed increases in all lipids and lipoproteins in subjects treated with cortisone, and Soffer et al. (191) observed hypercholesteremia early in Cushing's syndrome. Bossak, Wang, and Adlersberg (192) studied the effects of corticoids. Their series consisted of normal men and women, aged 18 to 45, as controls, patients with a variety of diseases who were receiving cortisone acetate for treatment, and two patients with Cushing's syndrome involving adrenal hyperplasia. These authors observed a predominance of β-globulins, but no effects on the pattern of plasma lipids or lipoproteins.

The effects of oxandrolone (17-β-hydroxy-17-α-methyl-2-oxa-5-α-andro stan-3-one) on serum lipoproteins seem to be unique. It is effective in lowering lipoproteins only in carbohydrate-induced elevated endogenous VLDL (hypertriglyceridemia, types III and V).[7] In patients with elevated LDL (type II) or elevated chylomicron levels (fat-induced, type I) the drug may cause even greater elevations.

Sachs and Wolfman (193) postulated that oxandrolone inhibited the excessive synthesis of (or synthesis of excessive) triglycerides and thus there was a decrease in chylomicrons and VLDL. In the case of the fat-induced hyperchylomicronemia (type I) the drug increased the serum triglycerides, and the authors believe, as did Havel and Gordon (194), that in this disorder there is a defective mechanism for the removal of exogenous chylomicrons rather than increased chylomicron synthesis.

VI. THE HYPOLIPOPROTEINEMIAS

There are two primary hereditary hypolipoproteinemias: (a) that in which β-lipoproteins (LDL) are essentially absent and (b) that in which α-lipoproteins (HDL) are essentially absent.

A. Abetalipoproteinemia

In 1950 Bassen and Kornzweig (195) described the disease now known as abetalipoproteinemia, or the Bassen–Kornzweig syndrome, in a patient with generalized degeneration of the central nervous system. The red cells were abnormal in appearance, with crenated surfaces, which suggested to Singer, Fisher, and Perlstein (196) another name for this disease, acanthocytosis. Salt et al. (197) reported the lack of β-lipoproteins in the serum of a 17-month-old child whose parents and paternal grandfather had about one-half the normal level of β-lipoproteins.

The lack of, or very low levels of, β-lipoproteins in this disease was

[7] See Section IX.

Table XVII. Serum Lipoproteins in Abetalipoproteinemia[a]

	Serum Level (mg/100 ml)				
	α-Lipo-	β-Lipoproteins		β/α	
Subjects	proteins[b]	PE[b]	DSP[c]	Ratio	Ref.
Patients	80	0		0	197
			20		203
			15		203
	110	0		0	204
Normal subjects	150–280	300–580		1.5–3.0	197
			120–570 (0–10 yr)		197
			250–780 (30–40 yr)		203

[a] Reprinted with permission from Ref. 202.
[b] Determined as lipid by paper electrophoresis.
[c] Determined by dextran sulfate precipitation.

verified by Lamy et al. (198–201), who described it as a "new example of an inborn error of metabolism." There may be some β-lipoproteins present, but they may be abnormal. Table XVII, from Kahlke (202), shows the absence of β-lipoproteins in these subjects.

Kuo and Bassett (205) studied the lipoproteins in the mother and siblings of a patient. The mother had increased α-lipoproteins and S_f 0–12 LDL. The patient had decreased HDL_3 and S_f 0–400 lipoproteins. These were decreased also in the patient's three siblings.

Greatly diminished levels of β-lipoproteins (*d* 1.019–1.063 g/ml) were reported by Eder (206), Lamy et al. (198–201), and Schwartz et al. (207).

When four patients with abetalipoproteinemia were given sufficiently high amounts of carbohydrates to cause elevated VLDL (increased glycerides) in normal subjects, the VLDL did not appear in their serums (208). By immunochemical techniques Levy, Fredrickson, and Laster (208) were unable to show the presence of β-lipoproteins, which were electrophoretically defined in six patients. They also observed α-lipoproteins that had a lower density (25% floated at $d < 1.063$ g/ml and over 50% at *d* 1.063–1.1 g/ml). The authors attributed this to excessive amounts of lipids in otherwise normal α-lipoproteins. The protein moieties and amino acid compositions of the α-lipoproteins were normal.

It was concluded that the protein moieties essential for the synthesis of β-lipoproteins are either not synthesized or not made available. Recently Lees (209) suggested that the proteins are synthesized, but the β-lipoproteins are not (210).

Jones and Ways (211), who measured the most prominent lipids in lipoprotein fractions, reported that not only was there no $d < 1.063$ g/ml lipoprotein but also a greatly reduced amount of HDL_3 ($d < 1.21$ g/ml). The HDL_2 fraction was not abnormally low.

Abetalipoproteinemia is inherited as an autosomal recessive trait (199, 200). Frequently there are indications of abnormal lipid metabolism in relatives, as cited above, but as frequently there are not. Lloyd (212) has recently presented a concise and clear survey of this disease.

Cases of hypobetalipoproteinemia have been reported (205, 213), but evidently it is a rare disease unless it results from other primary diseases such as nephrosis or biliary cirrhosis. The mutations involved presumably differ from those that cause abetalipoproteinemia. In contrast to abetalipoproteinemia, a small amount of β-lipoproteins is synthesized in hypobetalipoproteinemia. There is some absorption of fat, and chylomicrons are formed.

There is a nonspecific precipitin in serum from patients with abetalipoproteinemia. Murray and Blumberg (214) consider the immunochemical evidence insufficient to classify the precipitin as an antibody, but there is a reaction between the LDL in normals and at least two components in serum from patients with this disease. The relationship to the LDL deficiency is still obscure.

B. Tangier Disease

A disease in which there is a deficiency or complete lack of serum HDL was described by Fredrickson and associates in 1961 (215). The syndrome was called Tangier disease (after an island in Chesapeake Bay, in which the first cases were observed), and many of its characteristics were defined. For the present purpose, an important aspect is that little or no α-lipoproteins appear in the serum from these patients. However, if the serum was concentrated, small amounts of α-lipoproteins could be detected immunochemically. Whether or not the α-lipoproteins are antigenically identical with normal α-lipoproteins (216) was not definitely decided (217).

According to Fredrickson et al. (125) the β-lipoproteins, although present on electrophoresis strips, were also abnormal in that they were mostly molecules with $d < 1.006$ g/ml, the usual density of the VLDL fraction. There was great storage of cholesterol, especially in the reticuloendothelial tissues. The stoichiometric relationship between phospholipids and cholesterol, deemed advantageous for optimum solubility of cholesterol, may be broken in this syndrome.

The genetics of the disease also involve proportional amounts of "Tangier α-lipoproteins" and normal α-lipoproteins. There were low α-lipoprotein levels in each parent and in one of each pair of grandparents of the patients. The trait is believed to be a Mendelian autosomal recessive (218). Table XVIII illustrates the genetic aspect determined at that time from concentrations of α-lipoproteins in serum.

Table XVIII. Phenotypes in Offspring in Whom the Phenotypes of Both Parents Were Defined[a]

		Offspring HDL Phenotypes			
Parent HDL Phenotypes	No.	Total No.	Normal (AA)	Low (Aa)	Absent (aa)
Normal × normal (AA × AA)	5	16	15	1	0
Normal × low (AA × Aa)	5	19	9	10	0
Low × low (Aa × Aa)	4	10	2	4	4

[a] Reprinted with permission from Ref. 218.

Patients who were homozygous for Tangier disease had no HDL when serum was examined by ultracentrifugal means (219). The S_f 20–100 and S_f 100–400 lipoproteins had abnormally high values. There were more chylomicrons than in control groups, but the chylomicrons had less cholesterol than "normal" ones. The phospholipids were normal. Kahlke (217) speculated that if the HDL peptide is missing from chylomicrons synthesized by patients with Tangier disease, "it may not be necessary for chylomicron formation in contrast to the β-lipoprotein peptides, the absence of which (in abetalipoproteinemia) results in an inability of chylomicron formation or release."

The absence of the pre-β-lipoprotein (VLDL) band in electrophoresis was explained on the basis of previous experiments (203), in which the α-lipoproteins were believed to be involved, usually, in determining the mobility of VLDL. Since there was little or no α-lipoprotein, the lipoproteins that had β-globulin mobility on paper had lower densities than usual and thus appeared as VLDL in separations based on density.

Table XIX, taken from Fredrickson (220), shows the low values for

Table XIX. Cholesterol and Phospholipid Content of Whole Plasma and Various Lipoprotein Classes in Tangier Disease[a]

					Lipoproteins (mg/100 ml plasma)[b]							
			Whole Plasma		$d < 1.019$		d 1.019–1.063		d 1.063–1.21		$d > 1.21$	
Patient	Sex	Age (years)	C	PL	C	PL	C	PL	C	PL	C	PL
E.L.	F	7	84	113	53	55	31	42	<1	5	<1	11
Pe. Lo.	F	8	107	137	14	33	92	91	1	2	<1	11
Pa. Lo.	F	12	67	96	12	37	54	44	1	3	<1	12
Controls	F	23–29	187	237	19	24	108	78	54	134	<2	21
T.L.	M	6	93	127	35	57	56	56	2	2	<1	12
G.N.	M	45	30	68	19	44	11	15	1	2	<1	7
L.N.	M	48	50	104	33	70	13	23	1	3	<1	8
Controls	M	21–28	171	215	26	31	97	69	43	111	<2	21

[a] Reproduced, with minor alterations, from *The Metabolic Basis of Inherited Disease,* 2nd ed., J. B. Stanbury, J. B. Wyngaarden, and D. S. Fredrickson, Eds., Blakiston Division, McGraw-Hill, New York, 1966, p. 486, by permission of the copyright owner, McGraw-Hill Book Co.

[b] Abbreviations: C, cholesterol; PL, phospholipids. The various lipoprotein classes are indicated by the densities at which they were separated.

cholesterol in whole plasma and in most of the lipoprotein fractions separated according to the method of Havel, Eder, and Bragdon (221). The cholesterol and phospholipids used to estimate the quantity of lipoprotein in the fractions were not below the normal values in the $d < 1.019$ g/ml fraction, in contrast to the other fractions. In a recent report (219) elevations in S_f 0–400 lipoproteins were seen in a patient heterozygous for Tangier disease. The observation tends to confirm the above data, as the $d < 1.019$ g/ml sample would include some of this fraction.

In the patient heterozygous for Tangier disease with a single abnormal gene there was some HDL in serum studied in the analytical ultracentrifuge (219). As mentioned, there was an elevation in S_f 0–400 lipoproteins, but the increase in chylomicrons was about one-half of that seen in homozygous patients. Fredrickson, Levy, and Lindgren (219) believed that since the results from both procedures were comparable, paper-electrophoresis estimations may be used with confidence. However, paper electrophoresis did not reveal a band for VLDL (S_f 0-400) or for chylomicrons (218) (see also Section IX).

Neurological abnormalities are frequently seen in such familial diseases involving lipids. Engel et al. (222) reported that two patients with Tangier disease also had recurrent peripheral neurological symptoms with muscle weakness. Thorough neurological examination of five other patients with α-lipoprotein deficiency revealed no involvement of the nervous system. However, the authors advised that determinations of lipoproteins (especially α-lipoproteins, cholesterol, and triglycerides) be included in clinical surveys of patients with peripheral neuropathy.

A patient with α-lipoprotein deficiency had cholesteryl ester deposits in sternal marrow and rectal mucosa along with increased triglycerides in β-lipoproteins and a widespread loss of pain and temperature sensation. Kocen et al. (223) emphasized the greatly increased triglycerides in all lipoprotein fractions. They speculated that a function of HDL may be concerned with regulating the lipid compositions of all the lipoproteins. There was increased lecithin and decreased sphingomyelin in the erythrocyte lipids (224).

VII. EFFECTS OF CANCER ON SERUM-LIPOPROTEIN LEVELS

When methods for the study of lipoproteins became available, their concentrations were investigated in many diseases. Especially was this so in diseases whose etiologies were largely unknown or where the cause might be suspected but the biochemistry involved was still not well known.

In 1955 the first paper appeared suggesting that cancer might be related in some way to lipoprotein metabolism (37). The small-scale ethanol fractionation procedure of Lever and co-workers (33), a modification of method 10 of Cohn et al. (32), was used and, in addition, lipoproteins corresponding to fraction I+III were separated at *d* 1.063 g/ml, and the $d < 1.063$ g/ml lipoproteins were measured in the analytical ultracentrifuge. Many of the factors that could influence serum-lipoprotein levels were recognized and had to be ruled out with special care. The subjects, young women with advanced carcinoma of the breast, were in the 30- to 45-year age group, still menstruating, had received no hormone therapy or other drugs known to affect lipoproteins, and had no thyroid, hepatic, biliary, or renal involvement. They were of average weight and ate a normal diet.

In these early studies Barclay et al. (37), who measured α- and β-lipoproteins by their cholesterol and phospholipid contents, observed significantly lower amounts of α-lipoproteins. There were significantly higher amounts of S_f 10–20 and S_f 20–100 LDL (including some VLDL) in patients with cancer.

Since many of the patients had metastases to osseous tissue, Kaufman et al. (225) compared the data from these patients with patients without osseous metastases. The decreased α-lipoproteins and increased levels of S_f 10–20 and S_f 20–100 LDL were accentuated in those with osseous metastases.

Miller and Erf (226) observed an increase in β-lipoproteins in patients with cancer. When patients with prostatic cancer were given estrogens, the favorable effects were associated with a decrease in β-lipoproteins and an increase in α-lipoproteins. After the successful surgical removal of a breast carcinoma, the serum α-lipoprotein levels increased above those seen in normal controls.

Miller and Erf also noted an accentuation of abnormal levels with progression of malignancy. This was also observed and reported in detail in 1956 and 1959 by Barclay and co-workers (227, 228). The phospholipids in fraction IV+V+VI decreased in 88 subjects in the following order: normal values in controls, lower values in patients with benign lesions, still lower values in patients with primary operable disease, and much lower values in patients with advanced inoperable disease. The S_f 10–20 and S_f 20–100 LDL increased in comparable order, and the S_f 20–100 class increased the most.

In eight of the patients studied before and after radical mastectomy, there was an increase in α-lipoproteins, as observed also by Miller and Erf (226). After bilateral ovariectomy as a possible palliative procedure in advanced mammary carcinoma, α-lipoprotein phospholipids increased in all patients regardless of the types of metastases or whether or not the disease was considered to be in regression. The response of lipoprotein levels was related to their values before surgery and to the clinical response; for example, if a patient had very low α-lipoprotein levels and had a good response to surgery, the postcastration α-lipoprotein levels were higher.

That decreased α-lipoprotein levels were not peculiar to patients with breast cancer was indicated when Wolffram (229) observed decreased proportional amounts of α-lipoproteins in women with genital cancer of various types.

Several reports on the effects of myeloma on lipoproteins have been published. Burstein and Fine (230), using precipitation procedures, observed a low level (about one-half the normal amounts) of β-lipoproteins, and Neufeld, Halpenny, and Morton (231) described a patient with "a very rare type" of β-2-lipoprotein myelomatosis. The S_f 0–12 lipoproteins were increased to the greatest extent, and the S_f 20–400 lipoproteins were also increased.

In some cases there were associations between myelomatosis, xanthomatosis, and hyperlipemia. The case reported by Cohen et al. (232) was cited as the first with a definite familial aspect. The hyperlipemia was induced by carbohydrates. There was an unusual amount of the carbohydrate-induced lipid in the fraction with d 1.006–1.019 g/ml, but not in the $d <$ 1.006 g/ml fraction. A factor in the patient's serum caused alterations in the lipoproteins and proteins in normal serum in mixing experiments. The factor may be associated with HDL.

A serum-lipoprotein-altering factor was isolated and characterized by Spikes, Cohen, and Djordjevich (233) from the serum of a patient with myeloma and hyperlipemia. The active factor, "paraprotein," which was present mainly in the ultracentrifugal residue ($d > 1.21$ g/ml) altered β-lipoprotein behavior in starch-gel electrophoresis. After mixing the factor with whole serum, the β-lipoproteins were not detectable in the gel, and staining of β_1-globulins and some haptoglobins was reduced. Most of the protein and lipoprotein remained at the origin.

This factor was not observed in serum from normal persons or from those with normolipemic myeloma or familial hypercholesteremia. Only hyperlipemic (lactescent) serums produced a similar alteration in the migration of β-lipoproteins. In these serums the factor was in the fraction containing VLDL ($d < 1.006$ g/ml) and was not in the fraction with $d > 1.21$ g/ml, as it was in patients with both hyperlipemia and myeloma. Experiments with latex particles and polyvinylpyrrolidone suggested that the activity of the factor did not result from a simple particle-size phenomenon.

Spikes et al. (233) suggested that the myeloma proteins may have a "peculiar reactivity" with the β-lipoproteins, but the nature of this *in vitro* alteration and its role in the combination of myeloma with hyperlipemia are not yet clear.

An association of β-lipoproteins with cancer was reported by Tremblay and Welfling (234). The β-lipoproteins, when administered intramuscularly, reduced intractable hyperthermia in a patient with Hodgkin's disease.

By paper-electrophoresis and immunochemical methods, Ohya (235) determined the β-to-α-lipoprotein ratios in patients with cancer. It was above normal (average 2.08) in patients with lung and breast cancer. The author reported a cancer-specific antigen in the β-lipoproteins from patients with various types of cancer. With similar techniques, Nanava and Tsintsadze (236) reported greatly elevated β-lipoproteins and slightly increased α-lipoproteins in patients with breast cancer. (This can be explained by the fact that "α-lipoproteins" are composed of both HDL_2 and HDL_3. The latter comprises the greater part and is not influenced by cancer, as will be seen).

Losticky, Rijnek, and Bednarik (237) observed an abnormal immunoelectrophoretic precipitation line for α_1-lipoproteins in serum from women with malignant tumors. In 124 cases of advanced inoperable or metastatic cancer the α-lipoproteins and α-phospholipid values were very low (238a).

By using entirely ultracentrifugal procedures (28, 42), Barclay et al. (24) measured values for VLDL, LDL, HDL_2, and HDL_3 ($d < 1.006$, < 1.063, < 1.125, and < 1.21 g/ml, respectively) in 20 young normal subjects and in 9 young women with advanced cancer of the breast. Ten of the normal subjects lived in a convent, so that their diet and activities were similar. Serums from these women were analyzed each week for 12 weeks. Serums from other normal women were analyzed once or twice. The normal subjects were classified according to whether or not there had been cancer in a blood relative (especially in direct line or siblings; there had to be at least two uncles or aunts). In this category most subjects reported maternal relatives with cancer, of whom 75% had carcinoma of the breast. The data were analyzed statistically by comparing pairs of weekly samples and pairs of single samples. Only the lipoprotein values that were statistically different are included in Table XX.

Table XX. Serum-Lipoprotein Levels in Normal Subjects and in Patients with Carcinoma of the Breast[a]

Subject and History	Serum Level (mg/100 ml) VLDL	Serum Level (mg/100 ml) HDL_2
Normal:		
Negative family history of cancer	12	126[b]
Positive family history of cancer	10	48
Patients	100[b]	51

[a] Data from Refs. 24 and 238b.

[b] These values are significantly higher than comparable values for which $P < .001$.

Table XXI. Serum Lipoproteins in Normal Women Related to Incidence of Cancer in Their Immediate Families[a]

			Serum Level (mg/100 ml)[b]			Family Members with Cancer		
						Period		
Subject	Age	n[c]	VLDL ($d < 1.006$ g/ml)	HDL_2 ($d < 1.125$ g/ml)	HDL_3 ($d < 1.21$ g/ml)	I	II	III
Positive Incidence of Cancer in Family								
DP-8	25	10	5 ± 5 (0–14)	89 ± 22 (54–107)	121 ± 20 (93–149)	None	Father	......[d]
MM-10	25	10	10 ± 5 (0–28)	26 ± 6 (15–35)	99 ± 21 (75–131)	None	None	Sister
HM-16	29	9	18 ± 11 (0–36)	73 ± 16 (49–89)	152 ± 27 (97–178)	Maternal grandmother, mother, 5 maternal aunts	......	Two first cousins
KM-24	31	10	3 ± 5 (0–27)	27 ± 11 (15–45)	118 ± 22 (98–170)	Father, mother, uncle	Brother, sister	Subject
KL-25	44	4	11 ± 4 (0–11)	43 ± 13 (23–49)	107 ± 14 (88–119)	Two maternal aunts, one uncle	......	Subject
GG-27	38	9	3 ± 4 (0–12)	42 ± 19 (23–63)	110 ± 23 (54–134)	Mother, father	......	......
HR-21	39	1	0	88	142	Mother	......	Brother
Little or No Incidence of Cancer in Family								
JM-4	25	9	9 ± 10 (0–23)	120 ± 20 (88–147)	124 ± 21 (98–159)	Maternal uncle	......	......
FF-15	41	5	5 ± 2 (0–9)	96 ± 21 (64–113)	110 ± 33 (62–151)	Maternal aunt	......	......
MR-6	25	8	14 ± 10 (0–18)	135 ± 36 (108–176)	122 ± 16 (95–141)	None	None	None
BM-11	43	10	25 ± 10 (0–55)	104 ± 19 (79–128)	133 ± 21 (87–152)	None	None	None
CM-12	37	10	10 ± 9 (0–37)	168 ± 23 (137–215)	143 ± 22 (110–174)	Paternal aunt	......	......
DJ-18	34	10	10 ± 2 (0–28)	93 ± 21 (69–118)	127 ± 20 (81–156)	None	None	None

[a] Data from Refs. 24 and 238b.
[b] Mean ± standard deviation; the ranges are shown in parentheses.
[c] Number of samples.
[d] Broken line: no additional family members reported to have cancer.

The normal subjects were followed by physical examinations and questionnaires at two additional periods since the initial observation (period I). Table XXI presents the serum values for VLDL, HDL_2, and HDL_3, obtained at the time of the first survey, period I. These are followed by information accrued 5 years later (period II) and 10 years later (period III) concerning the incidence of cancer in the subjects' blood relatives (238b). The table separates the subjects who reported a positive family history as defined above from those who reported an essentially negative family history for cancer. Of the clinically normal women with positive family histories, the majority reported an incidence of cancer in closely related family members at period I. Two with no cancer in their families at period I reported relatives with cancer in periods II and III. Two of the subjects, KM-24 and KL-25, themselves developed cancer. All of the subjects had values for HDL_2 below the lowest value of the subjects listed in the lower group on Table XXI who reported very little or no incidence of cancer in their families. The other components were unremarkable.

Normal men with and without positive histories of cancer in their families are listed in the upper part of Table XXII. None of those with positive histories had values for HDL_2 above the lowest in the group who reported no cancer in their immediate families. All the men with positive histories

Table XXII. Serum Lipoproteins in Normal Men Related to Incidence of Cancer in Their Immediate Families[a]

	Serum Level (mg/100 ml)			
Subject	Total VLDL, ($d < 1.006$ g/ml)	S_f 100–400 ($d < 1.006$ g/ml)	HDL_2 ($d < 1.125$ g/ml)	HDL_3 ($d < 1.21$ g/ml)
Positive Incidence of Cancer in Family				
1-La	264	5	27	157
2-Um	73	0	39	212
3-Ge	247	28	16	91
4-Mo	99	4	46	124
5-Br	296	4	17	115
6-Gr	200	72	10	153
Little or No Incidence of Cancer in Family				
1-Gr	40	0	117	112
2-Ba	43	0	80	187
3-Ho	42	0	122	160
4-Mac	46	0	70	131

[a] Data from Ref. 238b.

had higher values for VLDL than those without positive histories. The HDL_3 values were the same in both groups.

Subjects 5-Br and 6-Gr, who had positive family histories, subsequently developed cancer and, like the two women, KM-24 and KL-25 in Table XXI (positive histories), had low values for HDL_2 in serum. These two men also had greatly elevated VLDL, as did 1-La and 3-Ge. Whereas this relationship between VLDL and HDL_2 was not observed in the normal women, it did occur in women with advanced carcinoma of the breast (24, 238b).

Because of the recent emphasis on hereditary dyscrasias in lipid metabolism, (consult Sections VI, VIII, and IX) the higher incidence of very low values for HDL_2 in subjects with a positive family history for cancer is provocative.

A new proteolipid, designated neoproteolipid, was observed first in serum HDL fractions, especially HDL_2, only in patients with cancer (238c). It is present in serum from both men and women, with different kinds of cancer. It is not detectable in serum from normal men or women. Neoproteolipid has been isolated from the serum of rats with tumors and from the tumor tissue, which supplies a ready source, enabling chemical characterization of this unusual proteolipid.

Higazi et al. (239) studied lipoproteins (separated by paper electrophoresis) in 44 cases of various types of leukemia. Patients with acute myeloid leukemia had an increase in total lipids. They had the highest values for β-lipoproteins and high values for "non-mobile" (chylomicrons?) lipids. In monocytic leukemia the picture was similar. In acute lymphatic and in chronic lymphocytic leukemias, the values for α-lipoproteins were lowest.

Low α-lipoprotein values (36.8 versus 117–185 mg % in other patients) were observed also as a marked decrease or absence of HDL_2 in children with acute leukemia (11).

Aside from the generally elevated VLDL and very low HDL_2 in most children with cancer, LDL were greatly elevated only in a patient with Hodgkin's disease. In acute leukemia, Hodgkin's disease, and lymphangiomatosis the main component that floats at solution d 1.125 g/ml (HDL_2) was absent or not within the resolution limits of the optics of the analytical ultracentrifuge. However, these patients had one or two faster moving lipoproteins in this fraction (28, 42). These were present in only one other child (with malignant reticuloendotheliosis), who also had the principal HDL_2 component. These observations are reminiscent of "Tangier α-lipoproteins" (40).

In Table XXIII the proportional amounts of LDL and HDL in children with cancer and normal children are compared with those in children who had no malignancies but were subjected to surgical stress. It appears that

Table XXIII. Low-Density and High-Density Serum Lipoproteins in Children

		LDL (%)		HDL (%)		
Subjects	*n*[a]	Range	Average	Range	Average	Ref.
With cancer	7	74–90	82	10–26	18	11[b]
Normal	3	60–71	67	29–40	33	11[b]
Without cancer, under stress (surgery):	13					
Preoperative		55–73	64	27–45	36	15
Postoperative:						
24 hr		59–77	69	23–41	31	15
4 days		60–80	67	20–40	33	15

[a] Number of subjects.
[b] Ultracentrifugal data converted to percentages to compare with the electrophoretic data of Giugiaro et al. (15).

stress per se did not alter the ratios and that children with cancer had greatly elevated LDL and greatly decreased HDL.

Kellen (240) emphasized the increased levels of β-lipoproteins in cancer patients. He considered these the most important because of their immunologic involvement. β-lipoproteins and (VLDL) were precipitated by turbidimetric methods in 169 different patients and in some patients before and after treatment with chemotherapeutic agents.

Kellen observed the greatest elevations in β-lipoproteins in patients with breast cancer, sarcomatosis, lung cancer, Hodgkin's disease, rectal carcinoma, uterine carcinoma, and ovarian carcinoma, in decreasing order. No correlations between nutritional status or metastases were observed. Kellen (240) concluded that "a definitive trend for normal or increased β-lipoprotein levels seems to be present in different tumours, in relation to their respective localization."

The lowest "β-lipoprotein index" in patients with ovarian carcinoma was at variance with the data observed in the reviewer's unpublished experiments, but the differences in techniques must be considered. Patients with ovarian carcinoma had LDL values ($d < 1.063$ g/ml) that were equal to or higher ($\sim$ 600 mg/100 ml serum) than those in most patients with carcinoma of the breast. Their VLDL ($d < 1.006$ g/ml) values were also high, about 100 mg/100 ml fasting serum. A patient with Hodgkin's disease had equally high LDL values. In agreement with Kellen (240), serum from most patients, when studied by ultracentrifugal techniques, also had very elevated LDL and VLDL (over 500 and 200 mg/100 ml, respectively).

VIII. SERUM-LIPOPROTEIN LEVELS IN THE LIPIDOSES

In the lipidoses, which involve abnormal lipid metabolism, there are unusually large accumulations of certain complex lipids in nervous tissue or other tissues. This major class has been recently discussed in detail by Schettler and Kahlke (241). The subclasses discussed herein are dependent on the type of complex lipid deposited. The serum-lipoprotein data are given where known.

A. Gangliosidoses (Amaurotic Family Idiocy)

1. Infantile Amaurotic Family Idiocy (Tay–Sachs Disease). The complex lipid that accumulates in nervous tissue in Tay–Sachs disease is a ganglioside (*N*-acetylneuraminic-acid-containing glycosphingoside) that occurs normally only in trace amounts.

One of the first accounts of the measurements of lipoproteins in a child with Tay–Sachs disease was that of Dargeon et al. (66). The serum lipoproteins were measured in a fasting sample from a 5-month-old child who was still on a regular infant formula. All the LDL (S_f 0–20) and probably VLDL (S_f 20–400) were elevated, but the value for S_f 20–100 lipoproteins was six times as great as it was in control babies. The HDL level (as measured by total phospholipids) was lower than it was in control babies.

This child was given a new dietary regimen. It included vegetable fat and polyunsaturated fatty acids with additional choline or methionine or both. After 4.5 months the patient's serum lipoproteins were again measured. Total cholesterol and phospholipids decreased, and, most important, the S_f 100–400 lipoproteins decreased 100%; S_f 20–100, 61%; S_f 10–20, 24%; and S_f 0–10, 49%. However, the values for both S_f 10–20 and S_f 20–100 lipoproteins remained above those of the control babies who were eating the usual infant formula. The patient survived an attack of acute tracheobronchitis at 15 months but became progressively weaker and died at 21 months (see part C of this section for complete tabulation of data).

The child's parents knew of no consanguinity, but because a sibling had evidence of a lipid disorder, their serum lipoproteins were studied. The mother had higher amounts of the S_f 20–100 lipoproteins and less α-lipoprotein than other comparable normal young women. Although the father had more cholesterol in his plasma than the average male, the values for both parents fell within normal ranges.

O'Brien and Okada (242) have recently reported the genetic deficiency of the enzyme hexosaminidase A as the key defect in Tay–Sachs disease. Lack of this enzyme results in an accumulation of a glycolipid in the brain. This enzyme was absent from all tissues in patients with Tay–Sachs disease. O'Brien (243) states that lysosomal hydrolase enzymes are deficient in three other recently discovered gangliosidoses. Both hexosaminidase A and B were absent in two patients. The disease phenotypically resembles Tay–Sachs disease. It is now considered that there are five different gangliosidoses, involving storage of different gangliosides and producing different clinical symptoms.

2. Juvenile Amaurotic Family Idiocy. There is no evidence of stored lipid in juvenile amaurotic family idiocy. The serum lipids have been reported to be within normal limits (241). No reports on serum lipoproteins were found in the literature.

3. Adult Amaurotic Family Idiocy (Kufs–Hallervorden Syndrome). Adult amaurotic family idiocy, unlike the other types, does not result in blindness and may run a chronic course, with patients surviving for decades. There are no data at present on serum lipids and lipoproteins or on stored lipids in fresh tissue.

B. Cerebrosidosis (Gaucher's Disease)

Gaucher's disease is characterized by hepatosplenomegaly and the appearance of cerebroside-containing cells (Gaucher cells) in the reticuloendothelial system. The cerebroside is of the glucose type. Gangliosides also accumulate. Svennerholm (244) believes the metabolism of brain gangliosides to be abnormal.

In 1951 Uzman (245) reported the isolation of a lipoprotein from the spleen. This material contained 62% lipid and 38% protein. Apparently part of the lipid was glycolipid since a galactose content of 20% was found.

When serum from a patient with Gaucher's disease was fractionated by the method of Lever et al. (33), a modification of Cohn's method 10 (32), subnormal levels of both α- and β-lipoprotein cholesterol and α-lipoprotein phospholipids were found. The β-lipoproteins had a greater concentration of phospholipids than did those of control subjects (10). The β-lipoproteins were separated into the different ultracentrifugal classes (see Table XXIV). Except for the S_f 0–10 lipoproteins, a low-fat diet resulted in elevated values for the various S_f-classes. This is in marked contrast to the results observed in patients with Tay–Sachs and Niemann–Pick diseases.

Recent data on two male patients with "chronic" Gaucher's disease

Table XXIV. Physical and Chemical Measurements of Lipoproteins in Three Types of Lipoidoses Before and After a Therapeutic Diet[a]

Subjects	LDL Ch	S_f Class					Total Ch (Σ S_f classes)	HDL	
		0–10	10–20	20–100	100–400	Total		Ch	PL
Controls	144	414	13	10	0	437	144	41	98
Tay–Sachs:									
Before diet	176	452	33	61	6	552	182	42	86
After diet	98	232	25	24	0	281	93	35	76
Niemann–Pick:									
Before diet	230	625	197	292	49	1163	384	18	69
After diet	176	651	101	169	0	921	304	~2	93
Gaucher's:									
Before diet	128	302	38	33	0	373	123	21	51
After diet	118	271	68	68	0	407	134	~3	37

[a] Data from Ref. 10. All values in mg %. Abbreviations: Ch, cholesterol; PL, phospholipids.

(Barclay, unpublished observations) were obtained by ultracentrifugal methods. The younger, age 11, had high VLDL values, which, however, were not out of line with those from control children. He had quite low LDL values and very low values for the HDL_2 and HDL_3 fractions. The older patient, age 23 years, whose VLDL values were higher than those of normal men, also had low HDL_2 and HDL_3 levels. The LDL values were low, but not abnormal. In both patients the majority of the lipoproteins floating at *d* 1.125 g/ml were less dense than usually seen. In the older patient there were two boundaries in addition to the usual HDL_2.

The low LDL values coincide with the observation that in Gaucher's disease the serum cholesterol is low (10). The low HDL values agree with the hypoproteinemia noted by Groen (246).

When a patient with Gaucher's disease was put on a low-fat diet (see Table XXIV), there was a reduction in the cholesterol associated with α-lipoproteins but not with the total S_f-classes of β-lipoproteins. The phospholipids were decreased, but the VLDL fraction was increased (10).

C. Sphingomyelin Lipidosis (Niemann–Pick Disease)

In Niemann–Pick disease sphingomyelin is deposited in the endothelial, mesenchymal, and parenchymal cells of nearly all organs and tissues. There is hepatosplenomegaly and neurological symptoms, which usually appear in infancy. Most children survive only for a short time. In recent years, probably because of more definitive diagnoses, the disease has also been noted in adults.

Pansky and Lee (247) used electrophoretic techniques to study the lipoprotein levels in the serum of a 16-month-old boy. They observed an intensely stained β-lipoprotein band, some staining in the α_2-lipoprotein (pre-β-lipoprotein, or VLDL) band, and only a faintly stained α_1-lipoprotein band. Cortisone treatment exaggerated these abnormal results.

Similar results were observed in a 4-month-old child by Barclay et al. (10), who separated plasma into fractions I + III (β-lipoproteins) and fractions IV + V + VI (α-lipoproteins). Serum cholesterol and phospholipids were elevated as a reflection of the substantial increase in β-lipoproteins. The levels of the β-lipoprotein S_f-fractions were much higher than the levels observed not only in controls but also in patients with Tay–Sachs and Gaucher's diseases (see Table XXIV).

A low-fat diet reduced β-lipoprotein levels in the patient with Niemann–Pick disease, except for the S_f 0–10 fraction (the bulk of the LDL). The α-lipoproteins, as estimated by both cholesterol and phospholipids, were quite low. The α-lipoprotein phospholipids increased toward normal levels after a low-fat diet.

Fredrickson (220) reported abnormally high triglycerides (VLDL) and low HDL values, which confirmed earlier data (10) on serum lipoproteins in this disease.

D. Glycolipid Lipidosis (Fabry's Disease)

In Fabry's disease two or more neutral glycolipids accumulate in tissues. These may be ceramide trihexosides or dihexosides (kidney). Blood lipid and lipoprotein levels may be normal, but elevated β-lipoproteins have been reported (248).

E. Phytanic Acid Lipidosis (Refsum's Disease)

In Refsum's disease total serum lipids and cholesterol may be low, but not abnormally so. Lipoprotein levels, studied by electrophoresis, were reported to be not abnormal (249). Large quantities (10–20%) of phytanic acid (3,7,11,15-tetramethylhexadecanoic acid) were noted in serum from patients with full-blown disease. There was twice as much in the β-lipoproteins as in the α-lipoproteins separated by dextran sulfate precipitation (250). Since phytanic acid may comprise 30% of the fatty acid moiety of triglycerides, this observation was not surprising. If VLDL had been separated, most of the phytanic acid would probably have been in these lipoproteins. The concentration of phytanic acid in triglycerides and phospholipids was the same in each lipoprotein fraction.

IX. THE HYPERLIPOPROTEINEMIAS

Hyperlipoproteinemia results from greater than usual concentrations of lipoproteins in the blood. The nature of these lipoproteins depends on the biochemical defect, which may involve enzymatic hydrolysis, synthesis, or deposition and removal from the blood. To qualify as a hyperlipoproteinemia in this sense the abnormality should be essential, or idiopathic, and not secondary to another disease.

Each syndrome has some symptoms peculiar to itself, which aid the physician in diagnosis and treatment. These include xanthoma, both tuberous and tendinous, ocular signs, glucose intolerance, fat intolerance, and reactions to heparin. There is usually some incidence of the condition in the family of the patient.

The kinds of lipoprotein molecules that are excessive in the serum can supply clues. Simple observation of a blood sample can show lipemia, and the extent of chylomicronemia will be more obvious after the serum has stood in the cold overnight. These signs, with our present knowledge, would indicate excessive amounts of chylomicrons. However, abnormally high LDL levels and even slightly elevated VLDL levels might not cause serum to be lipemic and thus would be undetected unless some tests were applied to measure the concentrations of these lipoproteins in serum.

In a sample from a patient who has fasted overnight the levels of the various lipoproteins should be compared with each other and also with the levels in a normal fasting subject. It is important to use a fasting sample because in many hyperlipoproteinemias recent food intake distorts the picture.

For historical reviews and some details about metabolism, transport, incidence, sex relationships, and genetic predisposition to the hyperlipoproteinemias the reader is referred to Fredrickson, Levy, and Lees (125), Kinsell et al. (251), and Schettler, Kahlke, and Schlierf (252).

In Chapter 5 two principal techniques for studying serum or plasma lipoproteins are detailed: ultracentrifugal separation based on density, and electrophoresis based on electrical charges on the molecules. In hyperlipoproteinemias there may be alterations in lipoprotein compositions such that there is not complete agreement between results obtained by the two procedures [see type III of Fredrickson and Lees (115)].

These diseases are classified here mainly according to lipoproteins separated by ultracentrifugation (and ultimately determined by chemical composition, which, if it is changed, may represent the abnormality). Data obtained by other procedures, especially electrophoresis, are also given.

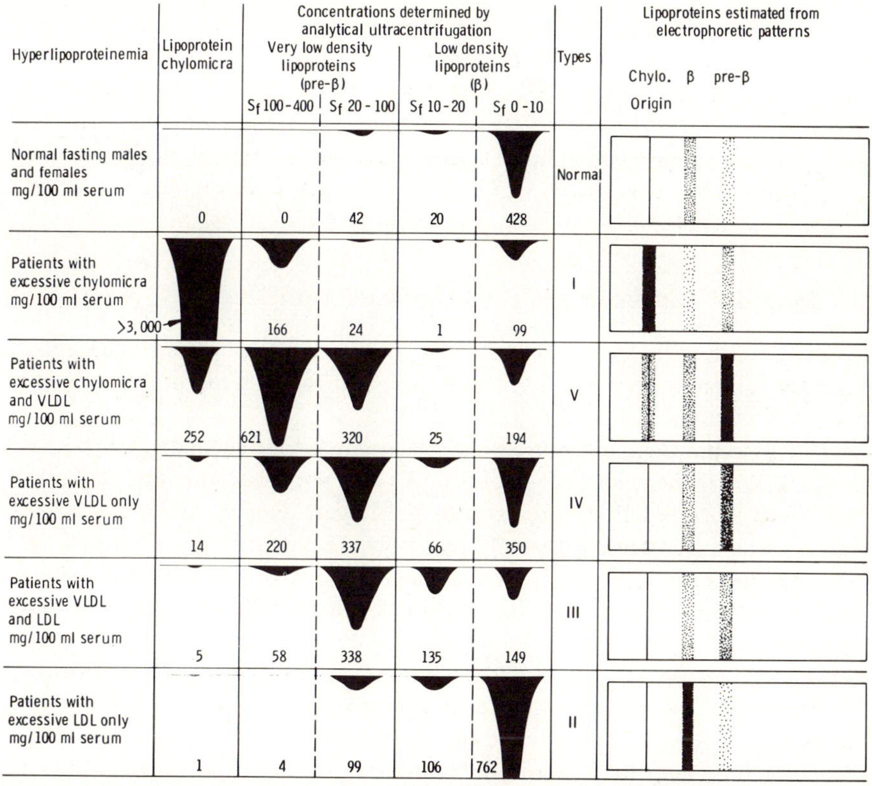

Fig. 1 Ultracentrifuge values and electrophoretic patterns of lipoproteins in whole serum or plasma from normal subjects and patients with hyperlipoproteinemias.
Left: Lipoproteins separated according to density properties. Chylomicrons, by centrifugation for 1 hr at 10,000 to 15,000 rpm; VLDL, S_f 100–400 and S_f 20–100, by ultracentrifugation (Beckman-Spinco) for 19 hr at 40,000 rpm in #40 rotor at density of serum, approximately 1.006 g/ml; LDL, S_f 10–20 and S_f 0–10, by ultracentrifugation as above at solution *d* 1.0635 g/ml. Solid lines separate these fraction; broken lines, their subclasses. The number in each block represents mg per 100 ml serum, for normal fasting men and women, averaged, from Ref. 24; for patients with hyperlipoproteinemias, from Ref. 219. Scale factor for peak heights: 1 mm = about 25 mg lipoprotein.
Right: Lipoproteins separated by paper electrophoresis in barbital buffer plus albumin (257). Chylomicrons remain at the origin; β-lipoproteins are comparable to LDL (S_f 0–20); pre-β-lipoproteins are comparable to VLDL (S_f 20–400).

Types refer to serum lipoproteins of the patients as described in the far-left column (115). No data are given for HDL (α-lipoproteins).

Figure 1 shows the lipoprotein fractions separated by these two procedures. Whereas the lipoproteins are well separated and their amounts may be calculated from the ultracentrifugal procedures, even when the total lipid content is extremely elevated, the "well-defined" bands drawn in the figure for paper electrophoresis may trail and be indistinguishable. This is especially true when both VLDL and LDL are excessive and a "broad β-band" is formed.

A. Excessive Chylomicrons, or Exogenous Particles

This condition is also known as fat-induced hyperlipemia, alimentary hyperglyceridemia, hyperchylomicronemia, and type I hyperlipoproteinemia of Fredrickson and Lees (115).

The chylomicrons, or particles, elevated in fat-induced disease contain 85 to 90% triglyceride, 8% cholesterol, 4% phospholipid, and 1% protein. They represent lipoproteins with the lowest density, 0.94, $S_f > 400$. They are derived from digested (hydrolyzed) dietary fat, absorbed and resynthesized (protein added) in the intestinal mucosa, and carried through the lymphatic vessels to the thoracic duct, through which they pour into the blood.

The triglyceride fatty acids are essentially those, or resemble those, of the dietary fat, whereas cholesterol and phospholipids are added from endogenous pools. The entry of these exogenous chylomicrons (lipoprotein particles) into the blood results in temporary lipemia that lasts 2 to 8 hr after a fat meal in the normal subject but may persist much longer in patients with hyperlipoproteinemia. The time varies even in normal subjects, since the type of diet, nutritional state, and activity can be influential.

The concentration of chylomicrons in blood represents the net between income and expenditure. The expenditure may be the critical factor (193, 194) since a pile-up will result if it fails. There are several routes and destinations for the chylomicrons. Adipose tissue is a main and logical one since it is a most flexible storage area. But the storage is not simple and must be preceded by other metabolic processes wherein may reside the abnormality. Of some import are the roles of glucose and enzymes (clearing factor, or lipoprotein lipase). Chylomicrons are, of course, used for energy and may also be removed by the liver under both normal and pathologic conditions.

Exogenous chylomicrons cannot be conveniently measured quantitatively in the ultracentrifuge because of their exceptionally low density, but they can be easily removed from serum by centrifugation for 1 hr at about 15,000 rpm. They produce a wide band at the origin when small amounts of serum or plasma are separated by paper electrophoresis. This behavior served as the basis for the definition of the type I hyperlipoproteinemia of Fredrickson and Lees (115). In patients suspected of having the syndrome the serum after a 14- to 16-hr fast is turbid, or "milky." If a high-fat test meal takes an unusually long time to clear, abnormal postheparin lipolytic activity can be suspected.

This relatively rare disease is seen most frequently in infants and children who are intolerant to dietary fat. Essentially, fat-free or restricted-fat diets (not high in carbohydrates) with adequate protein frequently ameliorate the symptoms, but it is not definitely known what role reduced calorie intake plays. There is evidence that an enzymatic deficiency is present (194, 251, 253, 254) since postheparin lipolytic activity has been reported to be low. It has also been demonstrated to be low in nonlipemic family members (118, 255). There is normal glucose tolerance. The amounts of chylomicrons present may be seen in Fig. 1 [averaged from patients (219)].

Investigations designed to show that the chylomicrons in this syndrome are structurally abnormal have not produced conclusive results. Of interest, however, are the experiments of Bierman et al. (124, 126, 127) showing the different kinds of particles in the fat-induced and carbohydrate-induced hyperlipoproteinemias (see Section IV of this chapter and Tables I, VIII, and XIII in Chapter 11).

Kinsell and co-workers (256) described a number of patients with hyperglyceridemia. They were classified into several groups: (a) those who were unable to "remove" or metabolize absorbed polyunsaturated fat but not dietary saturated fat; (b) those who could not tolerate large amounts of polyunsaturated fat; (c) those who maintained elevated glyceride levels under any dietary regimen as well as fasting; and (d) those whose glyceride levels rose on a very-high-carbohydrate diet [low fat, as described by Ahrens et al. (114)]. Some of these are described below.

B. Excessive Chylomicrons and VLDL

Excessive chylomicrons and VLDL are seen simultaneously in some cases, described as type V hyperlipoproteinemia. The LDL and HDL levels are usually decreased. The VLDL are endogenous in origin, but the excessive chylomicrons arise from alimentary fat. However, the basic defect resides in the synthesis or removal of endogenous VLDL. Sachs and Wolfman (193) speculated that excessive synthesis is prevalent. The serum is lipemic or creamy, depending on the magnitude of VLDL excess and the presence of chylomicrons. The VLDL ($d < 1.006$ g/ml) can be separated and measured in the ultracentrifuge; their flotation is S_f 20–400. They move in front of the usual β-lipoproteins in paper electrophoresis and form a band in the procedure of Lees and Hatch (257), using 1% albumin in the buffer. Types III, IV, and V show this pre-β-lipoprotein band along with bands of varying intensity for the other lipoproteins.

The VLDL may be increased by both fat and carbohydrate ingestion. As stated, both VLDL and chylomicrons are elevated in these patients with the exception of those on a very low calorie intake, which must be adjusted to the individual.

Kruger et al. (258) studied serum-lipoprotein metabolism by using ^{131}I-labeled triolein. In two patients, who probably qualified for the category of excessive VLDL and chylomicrons, they observed greatly elevated chylomicrons and S_f 10–400 lipoproteins. The elevations were sustained for 24 hr after a labeled-triolein test meal. The levels of S_f 3–9 lipoproteins (LDL) were low, and those of the HDL fraction even lower.

Furman, Howard, and Alaupovic (253) tested the effect of chronic heparin administration on serum lipids and lipoproteins in normal and heparin-responsive and heparin-unresponsive hyperglyceridemic subjects. Patients responsive to heparin had greatly decreased VLDL levels and increased β-lipoprotein ($1.019 < d < 1.063$ g/ml) levels. In a control subject HDL levels increased also, but the increase in LDL levels was not as great.

A patient unresponsive to heparin did not have decreased VLDL after administration of the drug. There was actually an increase in lipoproteins with $d < 1.019$ g/ml, termed low-density β-lipoproteins. The HDL and β-lipoprotein ($1.019 < d < 1.063$ g/ml) levels did not change. This patient had an inherited abnormality that was not immediately associated with lipoprotein lipase deficiency. No xanthomas were present. This subject's disease was described as "dietary-fat-induced" and could be ameliorated by a restricted-fat diet.

In a heparin-responsive subject there were indications of inherited defects in lipid metabolism. There were xanthomas on elbows, knees, and toes. This subject and a sibling were considered to have a dietary-carbohydrate-induced type of disease.

Another heparin-responsive subject had no family history of hyperlipemia but had suffered a cerebral vascular accident. There were no xanthomas. The hyperglyceridemia was increased by a high-carbohydrate, low-fat diet.

Furman et al. (259) investigated the ability of these and other patients and normal subjects to utilize labeled serum α-lipoproteins. The shorter half-time radioactivity in the serum from subjects with hyperglyceridemia indicated that they had a more rapid α-lipoprotein turnover. It was lowest in patients with initially low levels of α-lipoproteins. The greatest radioactivity (α-LP-^{131}I) was in the VLDL in the subjects with excessive chylomicrons, especially after a fat meal. This suggested to the authors that

α-lipoprotein had a greater tendency to be associated with exogenous rather than endogenous triglyceride.

C. Excessive VLDL Only (Carbohydrate Induced)

Most patients with elevated serum VLDL have an abnormal carbohydrate metabolism or a predisposition to abnormality. It has been suggested, but not proved, that such patients are more sensitive to dietary sucrose than to polysaccharides (118). The excessive VLDL may be carbohydrate induced even though the subject is on a very-low-fat diet (isocaloric with high carbohydrate). This disease is defined as type IV hyperlipoproteinemia by Fredrickson and Lees (115). Only pre-β-lipoproteins (VLDL) seem to be elevated.

Kinsell et al. (251, 256) reported that VLDL were greatly elevated in a subject on a high-carbohydrate, low-fat diet. When the carbohydrate intake was reduced and peanut oil was substituted for the carbohydrates (even above the previous caloric level), the VLDL values fell.

On a high-carbohydrate, low-fat diet the VLDL (pre-β-lipoproteins) and/or particles, if present, may also be endogenous in origin. There is some indication that they differ in chemical composition from those in normal subjects on regular diets: Levy et al. (40) found that in 11 normal subjects made lipemic by a high-carbohydrate diet there was an increase in the pre-β-lipoprotein band and a marked decrease in the α-lipoprotein band. Their observations "suggested that α-lipoproteins were incorporated into pre-β-lipoproteins as the latter appeared in plasma with rising glyceride concentrations."

Injection of sodium heparin, 10 units per kilogram of body weight, into normal subjects at the peak of carbohydrate-induced lipemia caused the pre-β-lipoprotein band to diminish to extinction, and the α-lipoprotein cholesterol to increase. There were also increases in α-lipoproteins in paper electrophoresis. Injection of heparin into normal subjects who were on a regular diet and had no pre-β-lipoprotein band, caused no changes.

Attempts to delipidize chylomicrons and VLDL resulted in two "proteins" that may be the building blocks of these proteins: one with β-mobility and one with α-mobility. The VLDL fraction ($d < 1.006$ g/ml) from patients with type I (excessive chylomicrons), type IV (excessive VLDL only, carbohydrate induced), and type V (excessive chylomicrons plus VLDL) hyperlipoproteinemia also produced two bands after ethanol–ether delipidation. Serum from these patients showed a distinct pre-β-lipoprotein band associated with low α-lipoproteins. Levy et al. (40) proposed that pre-β-lipoproteins elevated in patients with type III, IV, and V hyperlipoproteinemia are a complex of β- and α-lipoproteins and concluded that "a reciprocal relationship between pre-β- and α-lipoproteins was demonstrated."

Plasma triglycerides were elevated in patients with Tangier disease who had essentially no α-lipoproteins and were on a regular diet (40). On a low-carbohydrate diet the triglycerides decreased, and on an isocaloric high-carbohydrate diet the triglycerides rose to high levels (300–600 mg/100 ml). Triglycerides did not increase to these levels in normal persons on a high-carbohydrate diet.

In patients homozygous for Tangier disease a high-carbohydrate diet did not result in elevated pre-β-lipoproteins, although there was lipemia. The β-band, however, widened and became more intensely stained. Normally much of this β-migrating band would have moved to the pre-β area in paper electrophoresis.

A male patient with an "acquired deficiency in α-lipoprotein" resulting from a hepatoma had greatly decreased levels of α-lipoproteins (cholesterol less than 6 mg/100 ml serum, compared with a normal minimum of 32 mg/100 ml). This patient was not given a high-carbohydrate diet. In at least six fasting samples the plasma-triglyceride concentrations were above 200 mg/100 ml. Paper electrophoresis of plasma showed only a densely stained β-lipoprotein band but no pre-β- or α-lipoprotein bands; "these 'VLDL' had beta mobility on paper electrophoresis" (40).

Type IV, the major hyperlipoproteinemia, is characterized by greatly elevated VLDL (S_f 20–400; $d < 1.006$ g/ml) which were accented by a sharp, darkly stained band in the pre-β-position in paper electrophoresis. Fredrickson and Lees (115) described type IV as the "hallmark of endogenous lipemia"—glycerides usually synthesized in the liver pile up in plasma (220). The syndrome may be related to emotional stress, alcohol consumption, or caloric excess, as well as abnormal carbohydrate metabolism. It may be related to abnormal glucose tolerance and is frequently associated with a family history of diabetes.

A relationship between increased or excessive VLDL levels and coronary artery disease, especially in young men, has been recently established (see Section XI). Such patients may have type IV hyperlipoproteinemia.

When present, xanthomas are frequently eruptive (260), and there may be xanthoma palmare.

Both excessive glyceride release and decreased glyceride removal were suggested as possible mechanisms and the association with carbohydrate metabolism must be emphasized. This disease, with elevated VLDL, was seen as a result of several primary diseases: diabetes, pancreatitis, alcoholism, and hypothyroidism; these should be ruled out before a firm diagnosis of carbohydrate-induced excessive VLDL is made.

D. Excessive VLDL and LDL

In one major class of hyperlipoproteinemia, described as type III by Fredrickson and Lees (115), both VLDL and LDL are elevated. The lipoproteins may be elevated by high-carbohydrate diets. Such patients have tendinous, rather than tuberous, xanthomas and a turbid serum. These are cases in which a study of lipoproteins is essential since two types are elevated; VLDL containing primarily triglycerides and LDL with large amounts of cholesterol. There is a suggestion that some of the lipoproteins that move in the β-zone have unusually high amounts of triglycerides and phospholipids since their densities may be below 1.006 g/ml rather than below 1.063 g/ml.

In line with this observation is that of Bobbitt and Levy (261), who studied the protein moieties of the S_f 10–400 lipoproteins of lipemic plasma from which chylomicrons had been removed. Proteins from the S_f 10–400 fraction were delipidized by exhaustive extraction with cold ether. One major protein component of the protein residue of the S_f 0–400 lipoproteins from lipemic plasma, appeared to be identical with the S_f 0–10 lipoproteins from nonlipemic plasma. This component was also present in the protein residue of chylomicrons. Its abundancy increased with the degree of lipemia. Bobbitt and Levy suggested that "under the conditions in which the liver is required to form large amounts of lipoprotein, some of the protein which normally is found in S_f 0–10 lipoproteins is incorporated into S_f 10–400 lipoproteins and chylomicrons," imparting to S_f 10–400 lipoproteins the mobility of the S_f 0–10 fraction (β-lipoproteins) in paper electrophoresis.

A specific feature of excessive VLDL and LDL (type III) hyperlipoproteinemia is the presence of xanthomas on the palms of the hands as well as in other areas. Baes et al. (260) reported tuberous xanthomas, which may be eruptive, and a preponderance of tendinous xanthomas. From the occurrence of the different xanthomas, Baes suggested that type III is intermediate between type II (excessive LDL) and type IV (excessive VLDL only) hyperlipoproteinemia. The lesions appear after age 25, rather than at an early age as in excessive LDL (type II). Peripheral vascular disease is common. The inheritability of type III is pronounced, but type II was not observed in any relative. However, some relatives with type IV may be seen (220).

Gofman and associates (262) reported increased levels of S_f 20–100 and S_f 100–400 lipoproteins in patients described as having idiopathic hyperlipemia. The elevations in these components would suggest increases in pre-β-lipoproteins (VLDL) or type III (and IV and V) hyperlipoproteinemia.

In studies with patients described as having idiopathic hyperlipemia, Sohar, Bossak, and Adlersberg (263) observed a much wider electrophoretic "β-lipoprotein band" than that seen in patients with hypercholesteremia. Considering the techniques used at that time, the "β-lipoprotein band" probably contained unseparated pre-β-lipoproteins. These authors used serum from two patients before and after a low-fat diet. The lipid levels decreased, but the lipoprotein pattern remained characteristically abnormal.

An attempt has been made to present the hyperglyceridemias, or hyperlipoproteinemias, as follows:

1. The syndrome in which exogenous chylomicrons are greatly elevated (fat induced, rare, mostly infantile, with glucose tolerance, and probably resulting from enzyme deficiencies).
2. The syndrome in which both endogenous (or exogenous if fat induced) chylomicrons and VLDL (triglycerides) are elevated (may be induced by both fat and carbohydrates and may result from enzyme deficiency; patients have glucose intolerance; the syndrome produced solely by carbohydrate intolerance is very rare).
3. The syndrome in which only VLDL are elevated (carbohydrate inducible, with glucose intolerance and no apparent enzyme deficiency).
4. The syndrome in which both VLDL and LDL are elevated (glucose intolerance and no evidence of enzyme deficiency).

This leads toward the next category, in which only the LDL levels are usually elevated.

E. Excessive LDL Only

Other names for this condition are primary hypercholesteremia, idiopathic hypercholesteremia, idiopathic hypercholesteremic xanthomatosis, possibly xanthoma tuberosum and xanthoma tendinosum, hyperbetalipoproteinemia, and type II hyperlipoproteinemia.

A review by Schettler, Kahlke, and Schlierf (252) described the history, sex incidence, and familial occurrence. In contrast to the other hyperlipoproteinemias described here, the serum is clear in this syndrome. The main defects in lipid biochemistry are elevations in cholesterol and phospholipid levels, a high cholesterol-to-phospholipid ratio, and a *significant* increase in LDL (β-lipoproteins); serum-glyceride levels are normal. Smith (264) determined that 85 to 90% of the serum cholesterol was present in S_f 0–12 fraction in patients with hypercholesteremic xanthomatosis. Usually the LDL must be *greatly* elevated since there is a rather wide range of "normal" values. Xanthomas, predominantly tendinous and frequently extensive, and xanthelasmas on the eyelids and corneal arcus are clinical signs that are helpful in diagnosis. The disease is accompanied by, or predisposes to, atherosclerosis and its complications, which may occur almost from birth (252).

McGinley, Jones, and Gofman (265) studied the serum lipoproteins in 14 patients with tuberous and tendinous xanthoma, but no overt evidence of other diseases. They were considered to have the primary inherited lipid abnormality, although only three patients had a familial history of xanthoma. The patients, 10 females and 4 males, ranged in age from 2 to 25 years. Most had some evidence of coronary artery disease, and the majority had excessive amounts of S_f 10–20 lipoproteins. The S_f 40–100 lipoprotein levels were variable and the S_f 0–10 lipoproteins were often decreased in the patients with the most severe defects. The authors noted a correlation between greatly increased S_f 10–20 and S_f 20–40 lipoproteins, decreased S_f 0–10 lipoproteins, and the severity of the disease. In patients with tendinous xanthomas S_f 0–20 lipoproteins were increased and S_f 20–400 lipoprotein levels were normal or low; in patients with tuberous xanthomas S_f 0–10 lipoprotein levels were low, the S_f 10–20 and S_f 20–40 fractions were greatly increased, and the levels of S_f 40–100 lipoproteins were variable.

Biggs and Colman (266) essentially confirmed these data but added that S_f 100–400 lipoproteins were greatly increased in patients with tuberous xanthoma.

Gofman and associates (267) compared lipoprotein levels in 12 patients with tuberous xanthomas and in 12 patients who had no xanthomas but did have elevated serum-cholesterol values. The cholesterol values were essentially the same in both groups, but the patients with xanthomas had three times the amount of S_f 12–20 lipoproteins. Gofman et al. (262) reported markedly increased values for S_f 0–12 and S_f 12–20 lipoproteins in patients with idiopathic hypercholesteremia.

Schettler and co-workers (252) used ultracentrifugation, fractional precipitation, and starch electrophoresis to obtain a lipoprotein pattern typical for familial hypercholesteremia (excessive LDL). The observations of Gofman et al. (262) were confirmed. The β-lipoproteins contained much greater amounts of cholesterol and phospholipids than usual. Investigators using different procedures have observed greatly elevated cholesterol and phospholipids in the β-lipoprotein fractions isolated from the serum and plasma of patients with this disease (268, 269).

Wheeler and Sprague (270) and Lever, Herbst, and Lyons (268) measured serum lipoproteins in patients characterized as having "primary hypercholesteremic xanthomatosis." They observed no elevations in the

S_f 12–20 fraction. Experiments reported by Sohar et al. (263) were done with filter paper on which they observed an increased β-lipoprotein band and a decreased α-lipoprotein band, with a slight increase in stainable lipid remaining at the origin.

In 1965 Beaumont, Swynghedauw, and Beaumont (271) typed the familial hypercholesteremias as H.F.X.$_1$. There were great elevations in S_f 0–12 lipoproteins (LDL), which had over four times more cholesterol and over three times more protein than usual. The protein moiety was considered "abnormal." In type H.F.X.$_2$, the S_f 0–12 lipoproteins were not increased, but S_f 12–400 lipoproteins were (hyperglyceridemia with excessive VLDL). There was an abnormal tolerance for vitamin A. Patients with the first type, H.F.X.$_1$, were also described by Laudat et al. (272) as having a clear serum, no elevations in triglycerides, and tendinous xanthomas.

It should be evident that patients with excessive VLDL are frequently confused with patients with excessive LDL or with patients who have excessive VLDL and LDL, as described by type III hyperlipoproteinemia (115). Fredrickson and Lees (115) typed the "hypercholesteremia syndrome" as type II, in which only the β-lipoprotein band is predominant. The VLDL fraction may be slightly to moderately increased (273), and the α-lipoprotein levels are low. Xanthomas are usual.

Baes et al. (260) classified the various forms of xanthomas, which are important common denominators in primary hyperlipoproteinemia of the various types described by Fredrickson and Lees. In type II hyperlipoproteinemia mostly tendinous xanthomas are seen. There might be tuberous xanthomas, but not of the eruptive type. Xanthoma palmare is not seen.

Four patients with familial idiopathic hypercholesteremia were studied by Scott and Winterbourn (274) in an experiment designed to track the serum LDL into location in the xanthoma deposits. The LDL peptide was labeled with ^{125}I and injected intravenously into patients in whom xanthomas were growing rapidly. Some xanthomatous areas were protected from friction by a device over the elbows (essentially an immobilizing cast over the affected area). Within 72 hr there was an accumulation of LDL in these tissues, especially in the unprotected lesions, which apparently were more irritated and were therefore more rapidly metabolizing.

Excessive LDL, or type II hyperlipoproteinemia, is exquisitely sensitive to genetic relationships since severe disease occurs in the progeny of two affected parents. It is a recognized autosomal dominant trait (251, 252).

Numerous authors suggested that excessive LDL was the major lipoprotein abnormality involved in accelerated atherosclerotic vascular disease, a thesis propounded by Gofman and associates (262).

The elevated LDL can be lowered by a low-fat, high-carbohydrate diet *without* significantly raising VLDL. A patient, especially a young patient, can be managed on a low-cholesterol diet with a minimum of saturated fatty acids, although polyunsaturated fats are preferred. However, in most patients with familial excessive LDL (type II) these lipoproteins remain above normal levels. This point was also observed by Sohar et al. (263) in a patient with excessive VLDL.

When heparin was administered to patients with "essential hypercholesteremia," S_f 0–10 lipoproteins increased, S_f 12–20 lipoproteins decreased, and S_f 30–70 (VLDL?) disappeared. When paper electrophoresis was used, Lever et al. (268) observed a shift from β-lipoproteins to α_2-lipoproteins (VLDL) and no change in α_1-lipoproteins. The authors did not observe these heparin effects in normal subjects (275).

Beaumont (276) cited two reports of men with hyperlipemia described as autoimmune. The condition was suspected to arise from abnormal β-lipoproteins, which apparently migrated poorly on paper and in agar. Most of them moved in the ultracentrifuge with densities between 1.006 and 1.019 g/ml. In one patient there was a small quantity of lipoproteins with d 1.019–1.063 g/ml and no lipoprotein with $d < 1.006$ g/ml even when the serum-triglyceride levels were high or after a fat meal. A large part of the antigenically reactive β-lipoproteins were heavier than normal β-lipoproteins and floated only at d 1.080 g/ml.

Some hypercholesteremic patients (LDL > 1000 mg/100 ml serum) who were refractory to the accepted cholesterol-lowering drugs underwent surgery to produce ileal bypass. The object of this procedure was to lower the very excessive LDL. There were reductions in S_f 0–12 LDL. If the complications can be overwhelmed, the procedure may have possibilities, especially in young patients (277).

Gjone and Norum (278), who discussed the relationships between corneal opacity (arcus) and hyperlipoproteinemia, suggested that pronounced corneal opacity should be regarded as a characteristic of the deficiency of the Sperry enzyme (plasma lecithin:cholesterol acyltransferase) described by Glomset (279) and Glomset and Kaplan (280). Gjone and Norum reported, however, the presence of corneal opacity in a patient with normal plasma levels of total cholesterol and triglycerides. They suggested that the formation of corneal arcus may involve factors other than hyperlipemia or hyperlipoproteinemia. They recommended that plasma-lipoprotein patterns be determined in patients with premature arcus and that "deficiency in plasma-cholesterol esterification should be borne in mind."

Paper electrophoresis was proposed as a comparatively simple procedure for diagnosing the hyperlipoproteinemias (115). If the lipemia is extensive, or if both VLDL and LDL (type III) are elevated, or if the elevations in lipoproteins are only slight, this procedure has limitations. Pries et al. (281) concluded that differentiations of certain types (II from III and IV) can be made by measuring triglycerides. The concentrations of triglycerides and cholesterol (as percentages of the lipids) are more precise for type II. They stated that paper electrophoresis alone "permits differentiation between Types II, III, and IV in only a limited percentage of the cases, but complete misinterpretation was also infrequent." Levy and Fredrickson (273) suggest, as they did previously, that type III may require ultracentrifugal separations, and in type I excess chylomicrons will rise to the top if plasma is kept cold overnight. In his survey of 214 patients Schatz (282) had 44 patients whose disease was not classifiable by these procedures.

The suggestion is made here that chylomicrons can be easily removed from plasma by centrifugation for 1 hr at 10,000 to 15,000 rpm in a high-speed centrifuge (not necessarily an ultracentrifuge). The infranatant fluid can then be centrifuged overnight at 40,000 rpm to yield VLDL. After removal of VLDL and centrifugation at *d* 1.063 g/ml, the LDL can be collected. If analytical ultracentrifugation is not possible, paper electrophoresis can be used to identify the separated lipoproteins (reasonably purified) and to obtain an estimate of their amounts in relation to the normal.

X. EFFECTS OF PSYCHOLOGICAL STRESS ON SERUM-LIPOPROTEIN LEVELS

In an early paper Fisk, Berry, and Chanutin (283) studied serum from 68 patients with neurologic disturbances and 18 with psychoses. The authors used ultracentrifugation for separating and analyzing the lipoproteins (S_f 0–70). They reported that "the distribution and concentration of plasma lipoproteins are not affected in patients with neurologic or psychotic disorders."

The VLDL have been shown to increase after emotional stress. Grundy and Griffin (284) measured the levels of S_f 0–12 (cholesterol-rich) and S_f 12–400 (VLDL, triglyceride-rich) lipoproteins in medical students at the time of their examinations. The S_f 0–12 lipoprotein levels did not change, but the S_f 12–400 fraction increased greatly.

Čěněk and Fialová-Přecechtělová (285) studied serum lipoproteins in 25 medical students, 8 women and 17 men, 24 to 26 years old, 4 weeks before, and just after, the final state examinations. Paper electrophoresis showed that the β-lipoproteins increased in 12 men and 4 women. The α-lipoproteins decreased in 17 subjects.

Wolf and co-workers (286) recorded changes in total-cholesterol and triglyceride levels in several patients with diseases known to influence lipid metabolism. The diet and activities of the subjects were regulated, and each served as his own control. Measurements were made before and after a "stress interview." Total cholesterol increased in all subjects, and triglycerides increased in some. In most cases the changes occurred within 60 min.

Page, Moinuddin, and Lewis (287) studied the effects of performing surgery ("surgeons under moderate mental stress and some physical strain") and playing in a highly competitive bridge tournament (severe stress). All samples were postprandial, and dietary data were obtained. The authors concluded that mental stress of 4- to 8-hr duration did not alter the serum-lipoprotein levels in normal subjects. The results ". . . do not support the concept that short-term stress necessarily contributes to atherogenesis by the mechanism of temporary serum lipid elevations. The possible long-term effects of nervous overactivity on lipid metabolism were not considered."

Pupita, Rappelli, and Bazzoli (288) reported that in most of the normal students they observed the total lipids, cholesterol, and especially triglycerides increased because of mental stress. Phospholipids, however, decreased in all subjects.

Free fatty acids and triglycerides rose in the serums of 33 men subjected to such stresses as noise, intense light, and urgency (time shortage to perform a task). When nicotinic acid was given, triglyceride levels fell below the prestress values and caused a decrease in cholesterol as well. Carlson, Levi, and Orö (289) suggested that the triglyceride increase (with no accompanying change in cholesterol) indicated an increase in VLDL.

Carlson et al. postulated that stress stimulated mobilization of free fatty acids from adipose tissue. The free fatty acids were incorporated into triglycerides, with resulting increases in the VLDL. The VLDL decreases observed after nicotinic acid administration are explained "by an inhibition of the sympathoadreno-medullary-mediated mobilization of free fatty acids from adipose tissue." The authors suggested that the infinitely greater and more prolonged stress situations in "real life" should be considered in view of the increased triglycerides in patients with coronary heart disease.

XI. RELATIONSHIPS BETWEEN ATHEROSCLEROSIS, ITS COMPLICATIONS, AND SERUM-LIPOPROTEIN LEVELS

Brunner, Manelis, and Altman (290), who studied a large group of men and women living in kibbutzim, noted in patients with heart disease a substantial decrease in the cholesterol usually associated with serum α-lipoproteins. They made the assumption "that the first step in the development of atherogenic lipid patterns is a re-distribution of the serum cholesterol from the alpha- to the beta-lipoproteins, and only the next step is an increase of total serum cholesterol, occurring mainly in the beta-lipoproteins."

There is logic for this. Many diseases known to predispose to atherosclerosis and its complications (coronary occlusion leading to myocardial infarction, cerebral occlusion leading to strokes, and peripheral occlusion leading to various problems, including gangrene) appear to be linked with abnormal lipid metabolism.

Atherosclerotic plaques contain substantial amounts of cholesterol and its esters as well as phospholipids, triglycerides, and fatty acids. Therefore an elevated level ($>$ 300 mg%) of cholesterol in serum was deemed a predisposing factor even before it was known that lipoproteins are the principal carriers of cholesterol.

The analytical techniques pioneered by the Donner Laboratory (5) led to extensive reports on the relationship between atherosclerosis and the concentrations of the various classes of serum lipoproteins.

In their early studies Gofman et al. (5) noted several important points. The most abundant lipoprotein with $d < 1.063$ g/ml had a flotation of S_f 3–8, was about 25% protein, carried a major fraction of serum cholesterol, was present in all samples, and was quite constant regardless of recent food intake. It then appeared not to be implicated in atherosclerosis. A species, or class, that contained more lipid and less protein and moved somewhat faster [S_f 40–70 or $S_f > 70$ (VLDL)] was influenced by food intake. An intermediary class, S_f 10–20 lipoproteins, which contained 30% cholesterol by weight and little protein, was thought not to be influenced by immediately preceding food intake but to be implicated in atherosclerosis.

These investigators concentrated on the S_f 10–20 fraction and observed that it was significantly higher in males than in females, between 20 and 40 years of age. After 40 years the sex difference was minimized. It was present in nearly every patient who had survived a myocardial infarction. Other lipoprotein classes did not show this relationship. There was little or no relationship between serum-cholesterol levels and the presence of measurable S_f 10–20 lipoproteins. However, in patients with more than 300 mg % cholesterol, in diabetics, and in survivors of myocardial infarctions, an increased amount of serum cholesterol was bound in S_f 10–20 lipoproteins. In addition many persons with normal cholesterol levels may transport more in the S_f 10–20 fraction than do hypercholesteremic subjects. Such "normal" persons may be likely candidates for atherosclerosis (6).

In a group of patients with angina pectoris and coronary insufficiency but no evidence of myocardial infarction (with either normal electrocardiographic tracings or minor changes in the ST-T waves) 90% had high values for S_f 10–20 lipoproteins (6).

A diet restricted in fat and cholesterol, taken faithfully for over 3 months, tended to reduce the amount of S_f 10–20 lipoproteins in serum.

Jones et al. (7) stated that the positive correlation of elevated S_f 10–20 lipoprotein levels with the incidence of myocardial infarction was two to four times as great as that of serum-cholesterol levels with myocardial infarction. Therefore these lipoprotein molecules were associated with atherosclerosis, and their levels could predict which subjects were candidates for severe atherosclerosis. Subsequent examination of patients indicated that early recurrence of an infarct was associated with elevated S_f 10–20 lipoprotein levels, and an increased level indicates a poor prognosis. True dietary restriction was suggested as a protective measure against a recurrence (87).

Further experiments on the association among the various LDL ($d <$ 1.063 g/ml) fractions indicated that not only the S_f 10–20 but also the S_f 35–100 fraction showed a strong relationship to a predilection for atherosclerosis as evidenced by clinical episodes. The intermediate S_f 20–35 fraction was less associated. The implication of the S_f 35–100 class, which can be lowered readily by dietary fat restriction, was important from the ameliorative aspect. Now the levels of both S_f 10–20 lipoproteins (more stable and not greatly influenced by diet) and S_f 35–100 lipoproteins (more variable and affected by diet) were considered to be important parameters in relation to atherosclerosis (135). Since both classes were related to obesity, which in turn is associated with atherosclerotic cardiovascular disease, the control of obesity was deemed imperative for prophylactic and therapeutic reasons (135).

It is of interest that Stone and Thorp (49) observed that underweight subjects had somewhat lower VLDL values.

Observations on the various serum-lipoprotein classes in numerous subjects led to the formulation of a possible atherogenic index (A.I.) based on the concentrations (mg %) of two classes: S_f 0–12 and S_f 12–400 lipoproteins. These spectra have been widened to include essentially all of the LDL ($1.006 < d < 1.063$ g/ml) and possibly the VLDL ($d < 1.006$ g/ml) as presently considered. The values were corrected for Johnston–Ogston effects (291) and the self-slowing of flotation rates when concentration of lipoproteins increases. The term "standard" was used to precede the S_f-spectrum (292) and has more recently been symbolized by $S_f°$. The standard S_f 12–400 lipoproteins were considered to be nearly twice (1.75) as important as standard S_f 0–12 lipoproteins in association with atherosclerosis. Therefore each standard S_f 12–400 lipoprotein value was multiplied by 1.75 in the formula (293) once the ultracentrifugal data were obtained. Many parameters were investigated, and the A.I. was observed to provide a useful measure.

Whereas an A.I. value below 50 was deemed desirable, a value over 90 was considered a hazard, and suitable prevention in the form of diet management, etc., was advised (293). The Gofman group considered that other important factors were a high diastolic blood pressure (292) and cigarette smoking, especially in young men (294).

In 1959 Gofman published a comprehensive review (295) in which he considered all the parameters that affect lipoprotein levels and their relationships to coronary heart disease. This book can still be consulted profitably.

Krăsno and co-workers (296) recorded values for the various LDL classes (total lipoproteins with $d < 1.063$ g/ml) in 81 patients who survived, and 55 patients who did not survive, a myocardial infarction. The survivors ranged in age from 35 to 77 years, and the nonsurvivors were from 31 to 59 years old. All the patients over age 60 survived.

As the S_f 0–20 class transported most of the serum cholesterol while the S_f 20–400 class was largely triglycerides, these data suggested that both the S_f 0–12 and S_f 100–400 lipoproteins served to differentiate nonsurvivors from survivors. Both lipoprotein classes, but especially the S_f 100–400 lipoproteins, were significantly more elevated in the nonsurvivors. The VLDL (S_f 20–400) were elevated in 46% of the survivors and in 64% of the nonsurvivors. Because of the high triglyceride content of VLDL, a different dietary regimen was indicated.

The LDL (S_f 0–12) were elevated in 76% of the survivors and in 90% of the nonsurvivors; therefore the quantities of S_f 0–20 lipoproteins should also be determined. Both fractions were abnormally high in 60% of the nonsurvivors and 35% of the survivors. Each class seemed to be unrelated to the other with respect to the outcome for the patients. There was an unquestioned association between elevated or abnormal serum lipids (lipoproteins) and atherosclerotic heart disease. Krăsno et al. (296) suggested that both LDL (S_f 0–12) and VLDL (S_f 20–400) should be measured routinely.

Spain, Bradess, and Greenblatt (297) carried out postmortem studies on 157 apparently healthy persons who had died violently and on several patients who died suddenly from coronary occlusion. They were classified according to somatotypes and degree of disease. Subjects with evidence of other diseases were excluded. The lipoprotein values were judged against normal values obtained on about 1000 cases (5). The correlation between serum LDL values and degree of aortic and coronary atherosclerosis was 84%. The ectomorphic male had the lowest correlation, and the mesomorphic male had the highest.

A. Lipoproteins Separated by Zone Electrophoresis

Because the techniques are simpler and the equipment less costly, many investigators employed zone electrophoresis on various media to pursue the theory of the association of blood-lipoprotein levels with atherosclerosis and its possible consequences.

Oliver and Boyd (298) separated α- and β-lipoproteins and estimated the cholesterol in each. Compared with their normal subjects, patients with coronary sclerosis had more cholesterol in the β-lipoproteins and less in the α-lipoproteins. Such comparative quantitative studies were made by numerous investigators, and the results in patients with coronary disease were the same: a wider lipid-staining band in the area of the β-lipoproteins, and a correspondingly narrower band in the α-lipoprotein area (39, 290, 299–301).

Adlersberg, Drachman, and Schaefer (302) and Gottfried et al. (300) observed that the elevated β-lipoprotein levels measured soon after an infarct became lower as the time after the infarct increased, presumably during recovery. The question is whether these patients had abnormal lipoprotein distributions some time before or just preceding the infarct, or did the episode cause them. In line with this was the report by Miettinen (303), who studied the effects of myocardial infarction on the distribution of cholesterol and phospholipids in the lipoprotein fractions. This author reported notable decreases in both cholesterol and phospholipid in α-lipoproteins and only slight decreases in β-lipoproteins in samples taken 3 to 10 days after the episode. He was unable to conclude whether the changes derived from the infarction or from the anticoagulants given. In any case the data indicated a marked decrease in α-lipoproteins.

Many investigators have reported an increase in cholesterol associated with atherosclerosis and cardiovascular disease whether determined as such, in connection with lipoproteins from fractions I + III and IV + V + VI or α and β-lipoproteins from zone electrophoresis. Because the molar ratio of phospholipids to free cholesterol appears to be constant, Chapin and Proger (304), following the suggestion of Hoffman and others (305, 306) proposed that phospholipids tend to keep "cholesterol in solution in plasma and that relative increases of cholesterol may result in instability of the lipid solution." They therefore emphasized studies of changes in phospholipids in lipoproteins separated by paper electrophoresis.

Subjects with known cardiovascular disease had relatively less lipid and phospholipids in the α-lipoproteins than did normal subjects. Although the total lipid content of the β-lipoproteins was greatly increased, the slight increase in the phospholipid moiety was out of proportion. This indicated to Chapin and Proger (304) a disturbed lipid distribution in atherosclerosis, signifying decreased stability in the whole lipid–lipoprotein system in blood.

Allard and Choquette (307) described a zone-electrophoresis procedure for prestained human serum—a procedure that was designed to be standardized, rapid, and routine. Since they observed a markedly lower concentration of α-lipoproteins in patients with coronary disease versus the healthy male controls, they considered the concentration of α-lipoproteins to be a better characterization of coronary disease than total cholesterol values and as good as total triglyceride values, as suggested by Albrink (308). One of the points in this thesis was the lack of variability (r —.042) in the concentration of α-lipoprotein in serum in contrast to cholesterol, which had a high variability (r .646). The lack of variability in α-lipoproteins in normal persons has been noted by others (309) and by Barclay (unpublished observation). The LDL (carrying the bulk of cholesterol) and the VLDL (carrying the bulk of triglycerides) fractions are more subject to dietary factors than the HDL fraction. Even though the subjects fast, long-term previous dietary habits should be considered but may be ruled out if the subjects have similar backgrounds.

The report of Allard and Choquette (307) should be considered in the search for the biochemical abnormality in atherosclerosis and its attendant diseases. Autopsies were performed on two girls aged 7 and 19, in both of whom the cholesterol levels were below the "critical value" but the concentrations of α-lipoproteins were extremely low for young females. In both cases there was evidence of atherosclerosis.

Brunner and associates (290, 310) found that there was a redistribution of cholesterol from α-lipoproteins to β-lipoproteins in 82% of all male patients and 78% of all female patients with ischemic heart disease. The cholesterol content in α-lipoproteins was less than 20%. The levels of serum total cholesterol were not markedly affected. Female controls matched by serum-cholesterol levels had higher concentrations of cholesterol in α-lipoproteins than did males, and the healthy men had higher concentrations than did male patients with coronary disease.

Patients with occlusive arterial disease of the legs had very high β-to-α-lipoprotein ratios: 4.6 versus 2.7 in symptomless controls. In patients with myocardial infarction the ratio was 3.1 versus 2.9 in sedentary controls (311).

The studies of Albrink (308) point up the importance of investigating the whole lipoprotein spectrum (although she concentrated on lipoproteins with $d < 1.063$ g/ml). She compared the serum levels of triglycerides and cholesterol and related this to coronary artery disease and age. A concentration of 5.45 meq/l (triglyceride fatty acids) was used as the boundary between normal subjects and those with disease. Of the coronary patients, 80% had values in excess of this. In over one-third of the normal men with high triglycerides, there was a family history of coronary artery disease and diabetes. Albrink believes that triglycerides are more commonly involved in coronary artery disease than cholesterol, but a very high cholesterol level is obviously significant. She considers that cholesterol and triglycerides should be determined chemically in fasting samples rather than by statistical manipulation of several lipoprotein classes. Furthermore, she suggested that the response to a fatty meal is a better indication of the lipid defect in coronary artery disease than fasting triglycerides or other lipid parameters.

Several investigators who used zone electrophoresis to separate serum lipoproteins noted changes in the form of additional areas that appeared with lipid stains. Smith (312) and Schettler et al. (313) reported a pre-β-lipoprotein[8] fraction that seemed to be associated with myocardial infarction, and Toro et al. (314) noted an increase in α_2-lipoproteins[9] in men. Toro et al. investigated the increase in the α_2-lipoprotein area in 300 men, aged 35 to 83, who were examined for routine checkups because of a history of disease. Of the 38 men who had an α_2-lipoprotein (cholesterol), only three were asymptomatic. Of the remainder, over 20% had histories of definite myocardial infarctions and other diseases known to affect lipid metabolism. Only three were asymptomatic. Thirty-four had α_2-lipoprotein levels of 16 to 20%, and of these, 17 had histories of cardiovascular disease. Of the 228 men whose α_2-lipoprotein (cholesterol) levels were less than 16%, only three had histories of disease. In the three groups the average ages were similar: 56, 55, and the most "normal," 62 years.

Toro et al. (314) concluded that elevated α_2-lipoprotein levels together with decreased α_1-lipoprotein (HDL) levels could be associated with history of myocardial infarction or other cardiovascular diseases. It is not known whether the abnormal or unusual distribution was present (and if so, for how long) before evidence of cardiovascular disease appeared. In contrast to the results of other investigators, the abnormal distributions did not disappear in many patients with time (up to 2 years) after the incident.

Chulkova and Travina (315) also reported increases in α_2-lipoprotein levels in patients with cardiovascular disease. These corresponded to the severity of damage to the myocardium. The α_2-lipoproteins were increased also in patients with diseases associated directly with the heart, such as sclerosis and coronary insufficiency. The β-lipoproteins were also increased in most of these patients.

The appearance of the pre-β-lipoprotein was noted by Ruszkowski (316) in 39 patients with atherosclerosis, but not in healthy persons. After heparin injection the pre-β-lipoprotein area disappeared and α_1-lipoproteins increased.

[8] The α_1-fraction appears next to albumin, whereas α_2 and β_1, or pre-β, are between α_1 and the usually large area for β_2.

[9] The α_2-fraction (d 1.006–1.019, S_f 12–20) travels with α_2-globulins. It is usually included in "β-lipoproteins" and is not seen in normal serum. It is not really VLDL ($d < 1.006$) but can be associated with them, depending on the techniques used.

Hatch (317) observed a paper-electrophoresis pattern showing decreased α_1-lipoproteins and a greatly increased pre-β-lipoprotein area, the latter representing VLDL (S_f 20–400), in young (34 and 43 years old) men with coronary heart disease. The pre-β-lipoprotein area appeared whenever the triglyceride levels were above normal. Since there is some cholesterol in VLDL, serum cholesterol was also elevated, but not as much as the triglycerides. The subjects were 10 young men, aged 27 to 42, who had recently recovered from myocardial infarctions. The similarities among them included being overweight and a family history of coronary heart disease in many. Most were heavy smokers. Although few had high serum-cholesterol levels, all but one had high serum triglycerides. A meal of 100 g of fat was not cleared within 9 hr in 50% of the men. However, by 12 hr the fasting triglyceride level was attained.

Hatch (317) postulated that the VLDL levels participated in the development of early atherosclerosis and the abnormal fasting levels did not represent a "holdover" from the alimentary fat intake of the previous day. There was also the possibility that routine overnutrition with either carbohydrate or fat led to increased VLDL. There was an abnormal response to a glucose-tolerance test in several of the patients. This was corroborated in a report by Demerdash et al. (318), who observed an abnormally slow rate of glucose utilization in young patients with coronary disease. Above age 50 this was not seen. There was no correlation between the utilization of glucose and the β-to-α-lipoprotein ratio determined electrophoretically. One or the other, or both, were observed in all patients below age 50. These authors, like Hatch (317), concluded that abnormal carbohydrate or lipoprotein metabolism may act independently to accelerate premature coronary atherosclerosis. In older patients coronary disease may occur in the absence of either abnormality.

That serum-triglyceride (or VLDL) levels may surpass other parameters as guides to lipid metabolism in relation to atherosclerosis was suggested also by Kroman and co-workers (319), who presented a detailed statistical analysis of the relationships between serum cholesterol, triglycerides, and lipoproteins in control subjects and those with proved coronary artery disease.

Banerjee and Deb (320) also observed in agar electrophoresis a "split β-lipoprotein," which may compare with pre-β-lipoprotein in patients with coronary artery disease.

In a study by Blankenhorn and co-workers (181) eight males and seven females (two in the twenties and one in the fifties, and all the rest in the thirties and forties) were hospitalized for 2 weeks and given a complete battery of metabolic tests combined with angiography. These patients either had or were suspected of having coronary atherosclerosis and were possible candidates for myocardial revascularization. Acute studies of cardiac metabolism were made. The basic problem was whether the cause in each case could be discerned and treated. In addition to blood lipids, numerous enzymes, and protein-bound iodine, lipoproteins were estimated by electrophoresis on cellulose acetate strips. In some of the patients the concentration (%) of pre-β-lipoproteins was used to evaluate changes induced by diet.

With the electrophoresis technique described, the pre-β-lipoprotein had about the same mobility as α_2-globulin. It has a more rapid migration than pre-β-lipoprotein has on filter paper, with a much sharper band, and better separation of the pre-β-fraction from β-lipoproteins.

Ten of the fifteen patients had coronary atherosclerosis, and of these, five had excessive carbohydrate-induced VLDL (type IV hyperlipoproteinemia). These patients had greatly increased triglycerides by the seventh day of the 85% carbohydrate diet. Two patients who had excessive LDL (type II hyperlipoproteinemia) had xanthomas and family histories of hypercholesteremia. In both the cholesterol levels were higher than 330 mg/100 ml and the triglyceride levels were lower than 260 mg/100 ml of serum, a value considered within the normal range in Blankenhorn's laboratory, where a previous study of 96 normal twin pairs had shown 28 individuals with triglyceride levels of 200 to 400 mg/100 ml (321). Two of the 15 patients had diabetes mellitus with excessive chylomicrons and VLDL (type V hyperlipoproteinemia). Fat-tolerance tests before and after a high-carbohydrate diet showed delayed clearance.

Five of the fifteen patients had no coronary atherosclerosis, but chest pain in three was the result of myocardial disease. One of these patients had previously had bilateral internal mammary artery transplants, which were still functioning; there was no visible narrowing of the coronary arterial vessels. She responded normally to exercise testing but had continued postoperative chest pain. She definitely had excessive VLDL (type IV hyperlipoproteinemia) characterized by rising triglyceride levels after a high-carbohydrate diet and a prominent pre-β-lipoprotein band.

After the 85% carbohydrate diet, the rise in triglyceride levels in six patients with excessive VLDL (type IV) varied from 73 to 18% by the seventh day. The remaining patients showed almost constant or decreased triglyceride levels.

Blankenhorn et al. (181) concluded that the response of the VLDL or serum-triglyceride levels to a high-carbohydrate diet could be an important guide in diagnosing coronary artery disease, especially in younger patients.

Engelberg (322) has suggested that investigators are attributing virtues to lipoprotein phenotyping beyond those that can apply to diagnosing and managing patients with atherosclerosis and its sequelae. Slack's (323, 324) answers are of equal interest: "Serum cholesterol and triglyceride levels may well be important in the aetiology of atheroma, but it is perhaps the duration of the hyperlipidaemia and the identity of the lipoprotein involved that are crucial to prognosis. Information about these two factors is best obtained, though as yet incompletely, by identification of the specific types of hyperlipoproteinaemia as characterized by electrophoresis or ultracentrifugation."

B. Lipoproteins Separated by Precipitation or Columns

In a careful evaluation of data current at the time, Barr, Russ, and Eder (325, 326) concluded that the value ranges for total cholesterol, cholesterol-to-phospholipid ratios, and S_f 10–20 lipoproteins in survivors of myocardial infarction were too similar to those observed in presumably normal adults. However, the phospholipid and especially the cholesterol distribution among the lipoproteins was sufficiently different between the two groups. Subjects, both animals and man, who are most likely to have a low order of atherosclerosis have the greatest amounts of α-lipoproteins (separated as fraction IV+V+VI), whereas survivors of myocardial infarction, dogs and rabbits with experimentally induced atherosclerosis, and nephrotics have the smallest amounts.

Cramér (327) used a heparin–phenol precipitation technique (328) to follow the β-lipoprotein cholesterol-to-phospholipid ratio in patients with myocardial infarctions for periods ranging from a few hours to about 8 months after the incident. Within a few hours and even by the second day after an acute episode, the ratio was significantly above normal values. By the third week the ratio decreased below normal values and remained depressed even after the eighth month. The absolute amount of β-lipoproteins, however, was greatly elevated throughout the period. Since the combined administration of estrogen and androgen caused a depression of the ratio due to a sharp increase in phospholipids, the authors suggested that during the abnormal lipemic states following an acute episode the chemical composition of the β-lipoproteins was different from that found during the normal state.

Cramér followed this report by a study of serum β-lipoproteins and their lipids and proteins in 55- to 65-year-old male survivors of myocardial infarction (329). He used hydroxyapatite columns to measure lipoprotein protein. His purpose was to determine whether the high β-lipoprotein cholesterol-to-protein ratio of normal elderly males occurs in survivors of myocardial infarction and whether the chemical composition of the β-lipoproteins changed. Results showed an elevation of β-lipoprotein protein in the patients, but no elevation in the lipids. Both the cholesterol-to-protein and the cholesterol-to-phospholipid ratios were lower.

De Oliveira (309) studied 292 apparently normal individuals and 156 patients with coronary heart disease. He worked with the β- and α-lipoprotein fractions of serum and used a modification of the flocculation method of Burstein and Berlinski (330). His normal values for different ages and sexes were similar to those determined by other procedures. The comment was made that the α-lipoproteins were relatively unchanged throughout life. In patients with coronary heart disease he observed decreases in the cholesterol fraction of α-lipoproteins and increases in both β-lipoproteins and their cholesterol moiety, regardless of sex and age. The abnormalities were more pronounced in women over 50 years old. In the normal subjects the serum β-lipoproteins showed a sharp rise in the 41- to 50-year age group—the ages at which atherogenesis may reach its maximum.

In 1949 Ahrens and Kunkel (306) suggested "that phospholipids may act as colloidal cholesterol stabilizers, and their lack may favor cholesterol deposition. It may be that a relative increase in the plasma phospholipids can modify or even prevent the atherosclerotic process, and conversely a decrease in plasma phospholipids may accentuate this process."

Since this idea was propounded and reiterated by others (304, 305), the etiology of atherosclerosis and coronary heart disease in patients without evidence of such diseases as diabetes, in which the incidence of association is quite high, has been earnestly and vigorously sought.

At first cholesterol increase in serum was emphasized and then increases in certain of the LDL, which transport the largest quantities of cholesterol. These observations led to the implication of the lower-density, triglyceride-rich lipoproteins, VLDL.

Many investigators observed decreased α-lipoproteins in patients with heart disease. The crucial factor may be the proportion of β-lipoproteins (LDL) to α-lipoproteins (HDL) or the proportion of VLDL (including chylomicrons) to α-lipoproteins. Gordon (331) proposes chylomicron formation and levels as important clues.

Schrade and Böhle (301) suggested that "hyperlipidemia in atherosclerotic patients is only one component of a complex disturbance of the regulatory mechanisms. The disturbance is not conditioned by the atherosclerosis, and is therefore not a symptom of atherosclerosis. Thus, investigation of the blood is *not* a method by which atherosclerosis can be diagnosed. Hyperlipidemia and other anomalies reflect aberrations of metabolic regulation rather than the atherosclerotic disease process."

These biochemical anomalies occur more often in patients with this disease, but other conditions should be considered. Brunner et al. (290) observed that physical activity was a factor. There are, of course, others: genetics, sex, body build, diet, and age. Results from investigations of blood lipoproteins may not diagnose atherosclerosis and coronary artery disease, but they can serve as clues to associated derangements and often suggest treatment.

Cholesterol *is* deposited in arteries. It may be that the conditions for its optimum solubility were abnormal from birth or became that way for other reasons—that is, decreased HDL with subsequent decreases in phospholipids "to stabilize" in some men of all ages and after estrogen levels drop in women.

XII. SERUM-LIPOPROTEIN LEVELS IN DISEASES INVOLVING THE LIVER

Diseases of the liver can have many etiologies and manifestations. The symptoms can arise from (a) hepatocellular damage or (b) obstruction of the flow of bile, whether hepatic or extrahepatic, into the intestine. In both conditions lipid or lipoprotein metabolism is affected.

When hepatocellular damage, whether acute or chronic, has occurred, the normal functions of the liver are impaired. Two of the diseases that cause hepatocellular (parenchymal) damage have been studied extensively: hepatitis and cirrhosis (Laennec's disease).

A. Hepatitis

Snavely et al. (332) in 1952 reported VLDL increases in patients with hepatitis, and Pierce, Kimmel, and Burns (333) reported increases in LDL (S_f 12–20). Pierce and Gofman (334) observed very high levels of S_f 10–20 lipoproteins in two male patients, 17 and 21 years old, "in contrast to the rarity of such high levels in normal persons in the same age group." Eder et al. (335), who used the cold-ethanol fractionation procedure on serum from male and female patients, aged 20 to 73 years, reported deviations in fraction IV+V+VI (α-lipoproteins), estimated by cholesterol and phospholipid compositions. In most of the patients with acute hepatitis the cholesterol and phospholipid values were within the normal range in fraction I+III (β-lipoproteins). The values for the components of fraction IV+V+VI were below the ranges of the control subjects. The ratios of free to esterified cholesterol were increased in both fractions.

There was also an indication of a low degree of synthesis of an "abnormal lipoprotein" in fraction IV+V+VI, which had the electrophoretic and ultracentrifugal properties of β-lipoproteins. Fraction I+III from patients had a lower cholesterol-to-phospholipid ratio than did fraction I+III from normal subjects. Any abnormal ratios tended to revert to normal as the disease became less acute and recovery was foreseen. In electrophoresis

Eder et al. (335) observed all the stainable lipid in the β-lipoprotein area and essentially none in the α-lipoprotein area.

Popova (336) reported a considerable increase in the percentage of β-lipoproteins and a decrease in α-lipoproteins in acute hepatitis; again a normalization occurred with recovery.

Furman and Conrad (337), who used the ultracentrifugal technique of Green et al. (171), observed that patients with homologous serum hepatitis frequently had high values for VLDL (—$S_{f(1.21)}$ 70–100), a phenomenon not usually observed in patients with liver diseases.

B. Portal Cirrhosis

In patients with portal cirrhosis Pierce and Gofman (334) observed elevations in LDL (S_f 0–20). Eder and co-workers (335) did not observe a consistent rise or fall in the lipids of 36 patients (men and women, ages 16–69) with this disease, nor did they observe evidence of the "abnormal lipoproteins" present in large amounts in acute hepatitis and biliary cirrhosis.

C. Biliary Cirrhosis

In primary biliary cirrhosis (cholangiolitic or Hanot's disease) there is degeneration of the liver cells, with proliferation of connective tissue and reduced liver function. Electrophoretic separations of serum from patients with this disease enabled Kunkel and Ahrens (338) to observe pronounced increases in the β-globulin fractions. The high serum-lipid values indicated increased β-lipoproteins.

Eder et al. (335) studied seven females (6 months to 8 years of age) with primary biliary cirrhosis. Their cholesterol (mostly free) levels were above normal, and the cholesterol had accumulated in fraction IV+V+VI. There was a marked increase in plasma phospholipids in fraction I+III. From these unusual ratios and the electrophoretic behavior these authors concluded that in primary biliary cirrhosis, as well as in acute hepatitis, large amounts of the abnormal lipoproteins were synthesized. Their synthesis was unrelated to cellular impairment and function in early biliary cirrhosis, as opposed to hepatitis, in which function and synthesis are usually temporarily impaired. Concurrent with the synthesis and accumulation of these abnormal lipoproteins there appears to be a depression of the α-lipoproteins. There were five female children, 18 months to 7 years old, with secondary biliary cirrhosis. Increases in cholesterol may indicate elevated β-lipoprotein (fraction I+III) levels, and the free-cholesterol level was abnormally high.

Russ, Raymunt, and Barr (339) carried out physiochemical and immunochemical studies on the abnormal lipoproteins observed in primary biliary cirrhosis. Only traces of α-lipoproteins were seen, and the β-lipoprotein fractions were abnormal.

These abnormal lipoproteins were studied in more detail by Switzer (340), who used serum from patients with biliary obstruction and separated the lipoproteins by ultracentrifugal density-gradient techniques. Switzer termed this abnormal lipoprotein the "obstructive lipoprotein." It was present in large amounts in lipoproteins with $d < 1.063$ g/ml (LDL) and was unreactive immunologically to antiserums to which normal lipoproteins react. It had a high content of free cholesterol and phospholipids, and an unusually low protein content. Switzer believed that "obstructive lipoprotein" is the principal serum lipoprotein in patients with biliary cirrhosis and obstructive jaundice. When extrahepatic obstruction is relieved, the abnormal LDL rapidly disappears.

Mills, Alaupovic, and their associates (341, 342) have separated the abnormal lipoprotein from the serums of patients with obstructive jaundice. It has a flotation rate of 15.9 in sodium chloride at d 1.063 g/ml and appears as a single boundary. It should be pointed out that some of these patients had cancer of the pancreas (see Section XIV.F).

Dangerfield and Hurworth (343) observed that when serum from patients with biliary cirrhosis was frozen, a "cryolabile lipoprotein" in the β-lipoprotein spectrum was detectable. They did not observe this particular phenomenon in most normal serums nor in the serums of patients with other diseases associated with serum-lipid abnormalities. They considered this unstable lipoprotein to have an unusually high phospholipid content.

Further observations on the abnormal lipoprotein of biliary cirrhosis and obstructive jaundice were made by Burstein and Caroli (344), who ascribed β_1-mobility to it and noted that it was precipitated by sulfated polysaccharides, but not by antibodies against normal β-lipoproteins.

Furman and Conrad (337) studied postabsorptive serum from 28 patients with obstructive jaundice of varied etiology. They reported that lipoproteins with $d > 1.063$ g/ml (HDL; $-S_{f(1.21)}$ 0–12) were markedly reduced or even absent. Two patients with pericholangiolitic biliary cirrhosis did not have abnormally low HDL levels. Furman and Conrad therefore worked out a factor for the lowest normal limit to which data from their patients could be related. The factor, 2.63 (the ratio of lipoprotein to cholesterol), was the lowest value calculated for the normal subjects. Most of the patients had values well below 2.63. When the cause of obstructive jaundice was removed, the HDL levels increased toward normal. Increases in the LDL (S_f 0–12) were noted in these patients.

D. Acute and Chronic Forms of Fatty Liver

Fatty liver may result from excessive fat intake, intoxicants like ethanol and carbon tetrachloride, chronic infections, and certain metabolic disorders. In certain dietary deficiencies, such as pellagra, fatty liver may result from lack of lipotropic factors like choline. There are usually marked elevations of VLDL in a lactescent serum (345). The LDL fraction may also be elevated somewhat, and when serum is studied electrophoretically, elevations in the β-lipoproteins are seen.

Since alcoholism can result in fatty liver and other liver abnormalities, a separate mention of its effect on the liver and the lipoprotein levels is made. As Switzer (345) emphasizes, there are two types of syndrome: in one the serum is very lipemic and VLDL very elevated; in the other, more chronic, form the serum may be clear, VLDL not elevated, but LDL greatly increased. The first type can be produced experimentally, and the effects are transitory even though some fatty infiltration has occurred. There is essentially no cirrhosis. In the second, damage to the liver may be extensive, and the secretion of bile may be impaired. If the disease progresses, lipoprotein synthesis will ultimately be impaired, resulting in hypolipoproteinemia.

XIII. SERUM-LIPOPROTEIN LEVELS IN DISEASES INVOLVING THE KIDNEY

In 1953 Lewis and Page (346) reported that α- and β-lipoprotein levels in patients with early hypertension were not unlike those in normal persons. If the hypertension became more severe or malignant, the α_2- and β-lipoproteins increased. Patients with severe renal disease had greatly increased values for S_f 10–20 lipoproteins, and in glomerulonephritis the less dense lipoproteins (VLDL) were greatly increased.

Gofman et al. (262) observed increases in all classes—S_f 0–400 lipoproteins, LDL, and VLDL—in patients with nephrosis. Additional evidence for abnormal lipoprotein metabolism in this disease was reported by Gitlin and co-workers (347), who observed an increase in VLDL (S_f 10–400) and a decrease in LDL (S_f 3–9). They suggested that the rate of VLDL conversion to LDL decreased in patients with nephrosis.

Baxter, Goodman, and Havel (348) conducted a thorough study of 44 hospitalized patients with uncomplicated nephrosis. They concluded that the severity of the disease (manifested by a milky serum) influences the lipoprotein levels. This was observed also by Lewis and Page (346). The VLDL ($d < 1.019$ g/ml) values were much above normal levels and LDL levels were below normal when the disease was severe. In mild or moderate cases, however, LDL (d 1.019–1.063 g/ml) were elevated while VLDL remained at normal levels. In other words, the VLDL and LDL levels were in inverse relationship, depending on the severity of the disease. Baxter et al. (348), like Gitlin et al. (347), suggested the possibility of metabolic interactions between VLDL and LDL. The HDL level, which was also low in severe disease, did not reflect the degree of disease, although it was slightly higher, and even above normal values, in least severe disease.

Kalugina (349) measured the serum lipoproteins in 50 patients with arterial hypertension associated with atherosclerosis. Forty of the patients had stage II disease (less severe); ten had stage III disease (more severe). There was some correlation between age and β-lipoprotein levels. In patients 46 to 56 years of age β-lipoprotein values averaged 74.4%; in patients 57 to 68 years of age the values averaged 79%.

In patients who had had hypertension for 16 to 20 years the β-lipoprotein levels reached 82 to 87%. Overweight patients had higher levels (80%) than thinner patients (74–78%, except in two cases with pronounced atherosclerosis in whom the values rose to 88%).

Treatment of the disease consisted of rest, low-salt and low-fat diets, hypotensive drugs, anticoagulants (Dicoumarin or Neodicoumarin), and cardiotonics. Kalugina concluded that the alterations in β-lipoprotein levels showed the extent to which lipid metabolism was affected by this disease and that after a patient developed stage III disease treatment was less effective in reducing β-lipoprotein levels.

Somewhat different observations concerning α-lipoprotein levels were reported more recently by Lewis and co-workers (350). They studied the levels of these lipoproteins in 64 patients who had renal transplants. Before the transplants, when the existing kidneys were faulty, the α-lipoprotein values were very low, as they were in patients maintained by chronic dialysis after nephrectomy. The values rose after successful transplants and again fell if the transplanted kidneys were rejected. These authors observed little change in β-lipoprotein bands in paper electrophoresis.

Bryla (351) also reported electrophoretic analyses of serum from 49 patients with various kidney abnormalities. The author suggested electrophoretic examination of serum for the differential diagnosis of various types of kidney diseases (e.g., glomerulonephritis versus nephrosis). The α_1-lipoprotein (HDL) levels are lower in glomerulonephritis. Large quantities of α-lipoproteins are present in the urine in nephrosis and in the Kimmelstiel–Wilson syndrome, which might explain why the serum levels are so low. The fact that α-lipoproteins pass into the urine whereas β-lipoproteins stay in the serum may be related to the considerable differences in the sizes of their molecules.

XIV. SERUM-LIPOPROTEIN LEVELS IN MISCELLANEOUS DISEASES AND SOME OTHER ASPECTS OF LIPOPROTEIN METABOLISM

A. Infectious Mononucleosis

Rubin (352) reported the levels of S_f 0–12 and S_f 12–20 lipoproteins (LDL) and S_f 20–100 and S_f 100–400 lipoproteins (VLDL) in 36 university students with infectious mononucleosis and 14 students below age 35 with various illnesses other than infectious mononucleosis or hepatitis and a thymol turbidity of 5.5 units or greater. Two HDL categories were measured: HDL_2, $1.063 < d < 1.125$ g/ml, and HDL_3, $1.125 < d < 1.199$ g/ml, termed L and T, respectively. The subjects were tested during the illness and for 1 year thereafter.

The S_f 0–12 (LDL) fraction was below normal values at the outset of the disease and gradually returned to normal. The S_f 12–20 fraction was increased, and both S_f 20–100 and S_f 100–400 (VLDL) were significantly elevated and remained so until the seventh or eighth week. By the ninth week most lipoprotein values had returned to normal levels.

The HDL_2 fraction was decreased, and the HDL_3 fraction was greatly decreased and remained low until about the seventh week, when it rose rapidly. In females the HDL levels were decreased more than in males.

The author points out the similarities in pathology between infectious hepatitis and infectious mononucleosis; at the onset of jaundice it is difficult to distinguish between the two diseases. However, the serum-lipoprotein levels are different: in infectious mononucleosis lipoproteins with S_f-values less than 12 are decreased and those with S_f-values greater than 12 are increased; the reverse occurs in infectious hepatitis. The HDL changes are in the same direction: decreased in both diseases.

B. Mongolism

Simon and associates (353) measured serum-lipoprotein class S_f 12–20 (an LDL subfraction) in 24 mongoloid children 5 to 15 years old and in 17 mentally deficient children of the same ages. Dietary factors were ruled out. The mongoloid children had the highest values for S_f 12–20 lipoproteins. The mentally deficient children also had higher values than normal children, who had less than 11 mg % S_f 12–20 lipoproteins in their serums.

In an older age category the same relationship occurred, but in the 26 to 50 age group the differences were not obvious, possibly because of the fewer numbers of mongoloid patients who survive this long. At autopsy patients with mongolism do not show evidence of an unusual number of atherosclerotic plaques.

C. Hemophilia

Barkhan (354) studied the serum from men, 21 to 68 years old, with moderate to severe hemophilia. Lipoproteins were separated by paper electrophoresis, and the cholesterol in α- and β-lipoproteins was determined. The total serum cholesterol was significantly lower than that in a group of healthy men, but the percentage of cholesterol in the β-lipoproteins was about the same. The author suggested that the low total cholesterol could be related to frequent episodes of blood loss, general poor health, and poor dietary intake.

D. Muscular Dystrophy

Table XXV is adapted from Oppenheimer and Milhorat's (355) study of lipoproteins (estimated by paper electrophoresis) in children and adults with muscular dystrophy and related diseases. The table includes a column designated "O" lipoproteins, about which the authors make the following comment: "The values for the 'O' band, which trails the β-band and is not

Table XXV. Paper Electrophoresis of Lipoproteins in Muscle Diseases[a]

Condition	n[b]	Relative Concentration (% of total ± S.D.)		
		α-Lipoprotein	β-Lipoprotein	"O" Lipoprotein[c]
		Children		
Normal	9	42.3 ± 5.5	43.8 ± 6.1	13.9 ± 5.5
Perthes' disease	3	30.6 ± 6.1	44.7 ± 8.6	24.7 ± 13.6
Scoliosis	6	33.1 ± 7.3	44.3 ± 8.4	22.6 ± 8.9
Pseudohypertrophic muscular dystrophy	16	35.7 ± 7.2[d]	44.1 ± 6.8	20.2 ± 7.5
		Adults		
Normal	10	33.2 ± 7.6	43.2 ± 4.2	23.6 ± 7.5
Myositis	8	28.2 ± 6.8	46.8 ± 10.4	25.0 ± 11.7
Myotonia dystrophica	3	28.2 ± 10.2	56.0 ± 2.5[e]	15.8 ± 8.7
Amyotrophic lateral sclerosis	3	35.7 ± 4.7	39.7 ± 1.7	24.5 ± 3.9

[a] Data from Ref. 355.
[b] Number of subjects.
[c] Lipids "trailing" after β-band.
[d] $P < .02$.
[e] $P < .01$.

always sharply separated from the latter, scattered considerably and indicated no definite trend." However, when the data from the groups of children were listed together in the table, it could be seen that normal children had less lipid in the trailing region ("O" lipoproteins). These may be comparable to chylomicrons, which are not present in large amounts in normal fasting children. Neither the time of the previous meal nor the ages of the children were indicated in the original report (355). Nonfasting children can have large amounts of chylomicrons.

The adult patients were not qualified as to age nor sex, both of which are important in comparing serum-lipoprotein levels. The β-lipoproteins were highest in patients with myotonia dystrophica, but it should be noted that the "O" value was the lowest in this group.

E. Chronic Inflammatory Conditions

Nordh (356) studied two groups of patients with and without chronic oral inflammatory conditions. The lipoproteins were separated by paper electrophoresis. There were no differences in the percentages of α- and β-lipoproteins between the two groups or in comparison with a normal group.

F. Pancreatitis

The β-to-α-lipoprotein ratio is greatly elevated in men with pancreatitis. "It may be probable that these elevations are closely connected with hyperlipemia in pancreatitis." Fujita (357) discussed the possible mechanism on the basis of experiments with dogs in which pancreatitis was induced. He speculated that the greatly elevated β-lipoprotein values resulted from a metabolic defect in the removal of chylomicrons from the blood because of the lack of the necessary protein moiety.

Greenberger et al. (358) studied serum lipid and lipoprotein changes in 25 patients with acute pancreatitis. In only three of these were there elevated serum triglycerides, as high as 11,150 mg/100 ml, and cholesterol, 1410 mg/100 ml. These are the extremes; the ranges were 142 to 11,150 mg/100 ml for triglycerides and 163 to 1410 mg/100 ml for cholesterol. One subject had a "milky serum," suggesting excessive chylomicrons as well. Paper electrophoresis showed marked trailing and even extension of stained lipid into the zone of α-lipoproteins.

After considering the effects of alcoholism (the three subjects with lipemia were alcoholics), the authors suggested that these three had an underlying defect in lipid metabolism. It was aggravated by the pancreatitis.

They consider the alcoholism a contributory factor only. This was based on the statement that ingestion of even large amounts of ethanol would not raise the triglyceride levels much above 1000 mg/100 ml. Recent reports (see Section IV.G. and Ref. 149) show that ethanol and fat ingested together will cause triglycerides to increase 350% *above* fasting levels in normal subjects. In these patients with pancreatitis the presence of excess triglycerides in serum (with either overproduction or underremoval being the underlying defect) coupled with the ethanol could have resulted in the excessive lipemia.

G. Chronic Enterocolitis

Budyanskii (359) studied patients with chronic enterocolitis of several months' to even 15 years' duration. The α- and β-lipoproteins were not greatly changed in patients with damaged small intestines. He found that pathological conditions in the large intestines affected the lipoproteins similarly.

H. Rheumatoid Arthritis

The effects of rheumatoid arthritis, in various stages of severity, on the β-to-α-lipoprotein ratio were studied by Cervini and Nuti (360), in 15 men and 20 women. In most of the subjects the ratios were quite low. There was, however, a wide range of values: 1.2 to 4.1. The authors do not state whether this resulted from decreased β- or increased α-lipoproteins.

I. Infectious Diseases

Hartmann and Schneider (361) investigated the serum-lipoprotein levels in patients inoculated with malaria for experimental purposes. These patients had had six to nine attacks of elevated temperature. The authors noted a decrease in α-lipoproteins, especially by the sixth attack, but little variation in the amount of β-lipoproteins.

J. Clotting Mechanisms

Lipoproteins have been implicated in the clotting process, especially in relation to their possible role in the formation of atherosclerotic plaques and thrombi. Antiplasmin activity was separated from human plasma by Siegel, Barclay, and Cliffton (362) by the Cohn fractionation technique and further characterized by starch electrophoresis. Fraction III-0 (largely β-lipoproteins) contained the most activity, but fraction IV-1 (α-lipoproteins) proved a better source of plasminogen-free antiplasmin. The active material had the mobility of α_2-lipoproteins in starch electrophoresis. This material was insoluble in trichloroacetic acid and lacked antitrypsin activity.

Recently Riding and Ellis (363) confirmed Siegel's report by showing antiplasmin activity in fraction III-0 and in IV-1. These authors discussed the relationship between rising cholesterol (β-lipoproteins) and the β-lipoprotein-antiplasmin activity with the progress of gestation in pregnant women. They speculated that there is a link among the antiplasmin activity in β-lipoproteins, thrombogenesis, and the lipogenic hypothesis for the pathogenesis of atherosclerosis.

The β-lipoproteins were precipitated from serum by dextran sulfate, and α-lipoproteins and chylomicrons were also obtained by precipitation procedures. Skrzydlewski and Niewiarowski (364) observed that all the antiplasmin activity was associated with the β-lipoprotein fraction. The α-lipoproteins and chylomicrons did not inhibit plasmin. About 10% of the total plasma antiplasmin activity was associated with β-lipoproteins.

In patients with puerperal fever who were lipemic there was a close correlation between β-lipoprotein levels and fibrinolysis time. The inhibition of fibrinolysis in patients with atherosclerosis depended only partly on β-lipoprotein levels, although the β-lipoprotein concentration in serum and β-lipoprotein-antiplasmin activities correlated well in both groups of patients.

K. Interactions with Bacterial Endotoxins

Skarnes (365) employed immunodiffusion techniques and proposed a role for serum α_1-lipoproteins (HDL): its interaction with bacterial endotoxin in a plasma-detoxifying system in which calcium-ion concentration was decreased. The author proposed this as an important host mechanism, gradually brought into function, with decreasing calcium-ion concentration, to interact with and detoxify bacterial endotoxins *in vivo*. Esterase activity was also attributed to the α_1-lipoproteins, the presence of which was detected by positive staining with Sudan Black.

L. Enzyme Associations

Important information is emerging regarding the relationships between lipids and lipoproteins and enzymes. A few examples only are cited.

Transaminase activity was associated with serum β-lipoproteins in a report by Mermall and McDonald (366). The lipoproteins were isolated by both ultracentrifugation and heparin precipitation. When 10-KHz ultrasound was applied to the β-lipoproteins, at pH conditions below 7.00, the glutamic–oxalacetic transaminase activity was released. There was a reciprocal relationship between salt concentration (saline) and the rate of enzyme release.

Blood groups A and AB are more closely associated with serum lipids than groups B and O. This is also true for one of the acid-phosphatase isoenzymes. Preliminary results by Beckman (367) suggest that when intestinal alkaline phosphatase loses its sialic acid, it will combine with lipids.

The greatest specific activity of two principal marker enzymes in the plasma membranes isolated from rat-liver cells (368), 5′-nucleotidase and Na^{+}–K^{+}–Mg^{2+}–ATPase, are associated with one of the HDL ($d < 1.125$, but not necessarily HDL_2) separated from these membranes (Barclay et al., unpublished observations).

XV. SUMMARY

From the observations compiled in this review several characteristics of lipoproteins appear. Since these lipid–protein complexes have different chemical compositions and probably sites of synthesis, it is logical to expect them to be affected differently by various diseases.

The "normal" absolute quantities and relative amounts can vary from person to person, and hence for the most part statistically significant deviations are required to assign a cause-and-effect relationship to disease. This is especially true with the very-low-density and the low-density lipoproteins. Their amounts are more readily changed temporarily by less abnormal physiologic processes, such as exogenous supply of lipids or carbohydrates. The key is the temporary change. In the normal subject these lipoproteins soon return to basic levels, but if some metabolic aberration is present, the rate of clearance from the serum can be greatly delayed.

The amounts of the high-density lipoproteins are usually quite stable. They are changed, for the most part, only by biochemical changes or adjustments, such as hormonal ones, or by some as yet unclarified error in metabolism, dramatically exemplified in Tangier disease.

In normal subjects serum-lipoprotein levels are related to sex, age, diet, body weight, exercise, and possibly even genetic determinants. Men have higher serum levels of VLDL and LDL and lower levels of HDL_2 than do women of the same age group, 16 to 50 years. The VLDL and LDL levels tend to increase with age in both sexes, with maximum values for men in the fifth and sixth decades and for women in the sixth decade. The HDL_1 levels are lower in women until age 40. From then on they do not change with age in either sex. The HDL_2 fraction is significantly higher in women from 20 to 60 years old, after which the values decline and approach those for men. Both VLDL and LDL levels decline in subjects over 80 years old, but may remain at higher levels in women. The variability in values declines with increasing age. The HDL_3 levels, which tend to be more peculiar to the subject, do not change greatly with age in men. They may be higher or lower in women.

The effects of fasting are also variable. They depend somewhat on previous diet, original weight, exercise, and genetic factors. In men S_f 100–400 lipoproteins (VLDL) decrease and in women both S_f 20–100 and S_f 100–400 lipoproteins decrease after fasting overnight. (Usually normal fasting young women have no S_f 100–400 lipoproteins in their serums.) Fasting may cause a rise in S_f 0–10 lipoproteins (LDL) in both sexes.

Most values in normal subjects fluctuate to some degree. The most variable are the VLDL components. The LDL fraction is fairly constant, and the HDL_1 and HDL_3 fractions vary the least. In normal women before the menopause HDL_2 fluctuates with the production of estrogens; the levels rise at ovulation.

Certain interrelationships become obvious when many subjects are studied: the LDL (S_f 0–12 and S_f 12–20) and VLDL (S_f 20–100 and S_f 100–400), as subgroups of the so-called low-density lipoproteins, or β-lipoproteins, are not affected to the same degree by many factors. These, or just the VLDL subgroup, may be very high concurrently with low values for the HDL (α-lipoproteins) or just HDL_2. In some men with extremely high VLDL levels there are usually low values for LDL, HDL_2, and HDL_3.

Normal subjects from different ethnic groups can have "normal" levels of serum lipoproteins that are not alike. When comparisons with patients are made, the ethnic background and the diets are factors to consider.

For the most part, the proportional amounts of major lipoprotein groups in an individual and in a population average are similar whether measured by density (ultracentrifugally), electric charge (electrophoretically), or other physicochemical properties (fractional precipitation). However, certain procedures permit detailed studies of subgroups that may be of critical importance in relating serum lipoproteins to disease and thus are advantageous in that more precise data can be obtained.

Pregnant women have elevated values for serum VLDL and LDL, frequently associated with decreased HDL_2 but increased HDL_3. The elevations in VLDL and LDL can be sustained for several months postpartum (about 9 months). In pregnancies complicated by eclampsia or hypertension or both the abnormal levels are exaggerated. Although they have very little VLDL, infants have amounts of LDL and HDL that are similar to those of older children and even to young adults. Diet, largely milk, is an important factor.

Diet can be a critical determinant in adjusting serum levels of lipoproteins with $d < 1.063$. The ideal diet supplies only enough calories to maintain a "normal" weight and sufficient energy for the individual commensurate with his work load. Of these calories, about 15% should be supplied by a good protein of high biologic value, 40% by fat, primarily polyunsaturated, and 45% by carbohydrates supplied by as little sucrose as practicable. Essential components, such as vitamins and minerals, water, and bulk, should be supplied. On this diet a normal fasting subject's serum will have average amounts of lipoproteins. Other factors, such as hormonal balance, especially in older women, may cause increases in VLDL and LDL and decreases in HDL, but these need not be abnormal.

If this diet is eaten in amounts providing excessive calories, the subject will gain weight and VLDL and LDL may increase. There are some reports that in the obese subject HDL will be decreased.

If this diet is eaten in amounts providing insufficient calories for the energy expended, and the subject loses about 10% weight, VLDL, especially, will be reduced, and so will LDL.

The magnitude of the increases (on a high-calorie intake) and decreases (on a low-calorie intake) in lipoproteins will often depend on the levels before dietary changes were made.

Alterations in the proportional amounts of constituents in this basic diet will do the following: if the fat contains large amounts of saturated fatty acids, LDL will increase (VLDL are not so sensitive to type of fatty acid); LDL will decrease if fat with polyunsaturated fatty acids is substituted isocalorically. If total fat calories, especially from saturated fatty acids, are increased above 40%, LDL and VLDL are usually increased, but in some extreme diets VLDL reductions have been reported; carbohydrates in excess of 45% of total calories usually increase VLDL but have little effect on LDL (the relationships between carbohydrates and fat levels in *isocaloric* diets must always be considered); decreases in fat below 40% calories will usually decrease LDL, but VLDL may increase (if carbohydrate intake is increased); S_f 0–12 LDL are lower if the fat is unsaturated; decreases in carbohydrates usually lower VLDL. Reduction of protein to quite suboptimal levels (4%) interposes other variables, such as amino acid deficiencies and negative nitrogen balance, which in themselves can affect lipoprotein metabolism; both LDL and VLDL (and HDL) are decreased.

In patients with "primary" hyperlipoproteinemias diets must be selected to cope with the specific problem: low fat (preferably with low saturated-fatty-acid content, and little carbohydrate) for excessive chylomicrons (type I), low fat for excessive LDL (type II), low carbohydrate for excessive VLDL (type IV), and both low for excessive VLDL plus chylomicrons (type V) and for excessive VLDL plus LDL (type III).

Since coronary artery disease has been observed more frequently in young men than in young women, and since atherosclerotic plaques are largely deposited lipid, an association between serum-lipoprotein levels and hormones seems logical. Extensive surveys were made to link certain of the LDL classes with the incidence of heart disease. More recently sustained elevations in the VLDL have been considered by some authors to be more closely related to the etiology of coronary artery disease. Dietary control and weight loss are emphasized.

Ovarian hormones have been used as therapy. The rationale is that they lower the VLDL and LDL and raise the HDL, thereby producing a more feminine pattern and hopefully lowering the incidence or the rate of lipid deposition on the arterial wall.

In opposition to estrogens, administration of testicular hormones causes substantial rises in VLDL and LDL, and decreases in HDL in serum. In combination studies testicular hormones overwhelm the effects of estrogens.

Patients with thyroid diseases have abnormal levels of lipoproteins in serum. Administration of 180 mg of thyroid decreases LDL, but 300 mg is required to reduce VLDL levels. These effects are transitory.

Adrenocorticotropic hormone or cortisone causes increases in HDL, but in some instances do not affect LDL.

When insulin production is inadequate, severe disturbances in carbohydrate metabolism occur. Concurrently there are disturbances in lipoprotein metabolism, as seen frequently in the hyperlipoproteinemias, many of which are carbohydrate induced. In diabetic acidosis both VLDL and LDL are greatly elevated, and VLDL remains so for a longer period after treatment. The HDL are not changed, but insulin lowers HDL.

In addition to diet and hormones, certain drugs have been used to alter the levels of serum lipoproteins. Parenteral heparin causes a rapid reduction in VLDL and an increase in LDL. Long-term heparin treatment keeps both VLDL and LDL depressed. New drugs designed to lower blood cholesterol (cholestyramine) and both cholesterol and triglycerides. LDL and VLDL (clofibrate) are being tried for the hyperlipoproteinemias. Atromid also decreases VLDL, with some reduction in LDL and increase in HDL. Oxandrolone lowers lipoproteins in carbohydrate-induced hyperlipoproteinemia.

The widespread use of oral contraceptives has prompted experiments recently of their effect on serum lipoproteins. Long-term ingestion of oral contraceptives results in significant increases in LDL (except possibly the S_f 12–20 subfraction) and in VLDL. These are elevated especially during use of the drug; the values are not so elevated after therapy has been discontinued. Sustained elevation of these lipoproteins should be considered in view of their relationship with occlusive vascular disease and/or coronary heart disease.

There can be pronounced increases in serum lipoproteins in the group of diseases characterized as hyperlipoproteinemias. The types of lipoproteins that are excessively high depend on the fundamental metabolic error. When excessive chylomicrons are present, especially in infants, the disease may result from failure to utilize exogenous fat. When both chylomicrons and VLDL are excessive, the error is more complex: the VLDL arise from an endogenous error, frequently in carbohydrate metabolism, coupled with an intolerance of exogenous lipid or a deficiency in clearing-factor lipase. In other syndromes only VLDL are excessive, largely carbohydrate induced. The VLDL may have an "abnormal" chemical composition.

In a syndrome in which both VLDL and LDL (cholesterol-rich) are excessive both triglycerides and cholesterol are elevated. The protein moiety of the lipoproteins may be altered. Palmar xanthomas and coronary or peripheral atherosclerosis are hallmarks. The disease is usually hereditary. An abnormality in which only LDL are excessive is also seen. In this syndrome both cholesterol and phospholipids are elevated. These lipid elevations are usually accompanied by xanthomas, either tendinous or tuberous, depending somewhat on which lipoprotein is excessive and why. The excessive LDL are usually accompanied by severe atherosclerosis. A similar lipoprotein pattern is induced by a high-saturated-fat diet and may be associated with atherosclerosis. Xanthomas are probably present only in the hereditary form.

The lipidoses are a class of lipid diseases characterized by the deposition of different types of complex lipid in tissues. In Tay–Sachs and Niemann–Pick diseases there are elevations in VLDL and LDL, usually accompanied by low HDL. Recent studies point to a deficiency in an enzyme, hexosaminidase A, in Tay–Sachs disease.

There are several diseases in which the lipoprotein abnormality, congenital in some, appears to reside in a defect in synthesis. The final result is that these patients have essentially none of a particular lipoprotein in their serum. At present two types are prominent: the Bassen–Kornzweig syndrome, in which abetalipoproteinemia occurs, and Tangier disease, in which essentially no HDL are detectable in serum.

In most patients with cancer the HDL_2 fraction is significantly lower than it is in control subjects. In addition there are concurrent elevations in VLDL in many patients. Clinically normal subjects who have cancer in close blood relatives (first degree) may have decreased values for HDL_2, but the concurrent increase in VLDL occurs only in men. Some of these subjects develop cancer.

Probably the most important association of serum lipoproteins with disease is with atherosclerosis and coronary artery disease. If there are basic metabolic defects, they are not clearly defined. The disease is especially prevalent in men. The serum-lipoprotein levels are frequently abnormally high and are undoubtedly related in some way to the hormonal differences between men and women. The incidence of atherosclerosis and coronary artery disease increases in women after the menopause.

Early studies related S_f 10–20 lipoproteins with coronary artery disease and atherosclerosis. Dietary restriction of fats and cholesterol were advocated. Further studies implicated the lipoproteins with less density (S_f 35–100). Recent emphasis is on the undesirability of elevated VLDL (S_f 100–400) coupled with decreased HDL, which transports most of the serum phospholipids believed to "facilitate the solubility" of cholesterol. Another concept is that in patients with heart disease or those likely to suffer from it there is a redistribution of cholesterol from the α-lipoproteins (HDL) to the β-lipoproteins (LDL), resulting in less stable lipoprotein complexes.

An important approach is the study of the entire lipoprotein spectra to evaluate the status of the subject's serum-lipoprotein levels. The response of these levels to high-fat and high-carbohydrate test meals or diets may be informative, since carbohydrate metabolism may be involved as well as lipid metabolism.

Biliary obstruction, hepatocellular damage, or both, can result in failure to provide bile salts to the intestine for lipid emulsification prior to absorption. Consequently, since most lipoproteins are synthesized in the liver, either or both conditions may lead to grossly abnormal levels of serum lipoproteins.

Patients with hepatitis have high levels of VLDL and often LDL, with decreased HDL. "Abnormal lipoproteins" may be synthesized—abnormal in the sense of unexpected behavior in electrophoresis and ultracentrifugation. These may also be synthesized in primary biliary cirrhosis. In this disease the α-lipoproteins may be reduced to traces and the β-lipoproteins (LDL and VLDL) rise. In obstructive jaundice a similar pattern occurs.

In acute fatty liver VLDL may be greatly elevated, resulting in lipemic serum. In the more chronic form the serum may be clear, the VLDL not elevated, and the LDL greatly elevated. In this form there may be extensive damage to the liver and impaired secretion of bile.

In the nephrotic syndrome the VLDL are greatly elevated, whereas LDL (S_f 3–9) may be decreased. The HDL are usually quite low, and in nephrosis can pass into the urine. The degrees of increase or decrease in the serum lipoproteins depend on the severity of the disease.

Serum levels of VLDL are elevated in infectious mononucleosis and pancreatitis; LDL are elevated in mongolism, in some diseases involving muscles, and in pancreatitis. The HDL are decreased in infectious mononucleosis and infectious hepatitis.

Lipoproteins play a role in blood clotting, as suggested early from observations of the effects of heparin on both clotting and serum-lipid levels. Antiplasmin activity is associated with both major classes of lipoproteins, but predominantly with β-lipoproteins. The association of lipoproteins with enzyme activities is becoming more obvious as data are obtained.

Appreciation of the importance of lipoprotein macromolecules in metabolism has increased tremendously since attention was first called to them about 25 to 30 years ago. Great strides forward were made after suitable techniques for their isolation and characterization were devised in the early 1950s. Since that time many of the mysteries of lipid transport and metabolism have been solved. Their importance in health is obvious. But their roles in disease may be vital from many points of view: basic metabolic defect (etiology), specific properties, such as the serum levels of the different classes, which can aid or even clinch diagnosis; and most important, possible prevention (especially of coronary heart disease) or alleviation of symptoms and, it is to be hoped, cures in some cases. Lipoproteins have come of age!

XVI. ACKNOWLEDGMENTS

The author is most grateful to Mrs. Dorman D. Israel for devoted and valuable assistance throughout the entire preparation of this chapter; to Mrs. Leonard Chase for organizing the original literature sources; to Mrs. Walter Newhouse for editorial review; to Dr. Ralph K. Barclay for valuable advice and practical assistance; to the Sisters of Mercy, Philadelphia, Pennsylvania for supplying samples, and to Mr. Edward M. Greene for arranging questionnaires and conferences with the members of this order; to my co-worker, Mrs. Olga Terebus-Kekish, for translating many Polish and Russian articles and relieving the author of many tasks during the preparation of this chapter; and to Elsie Buck Martin, without whose inspiration the chapter could not have been written. The work was supported in part by research grants CY-3192, CY-3215, and CA-08748 from the National Cancer Institute, U.S. Public Health Service.

REFERENCES

1. Blix, G., A. Tiselius, and H. Svennson, *J. Biol. Chem.* **137**, 485–494 (1941).
2. Adair, G. S., and M. E. Adair, *J. Physiol.* **102**, 17P (1943–1944).
3. Pedersen, K. O., *J. Phys. Colloid Chem.* **51**, 156–163 (1947).
4. Gofman, J. W., F. Lindgren, and H. Elliott, *J. Biol. Chem.* **179**, 973–979 (1949).
5. Gofman, J., F. Lindgren, H. Elliott, W. Mantz, J. Hewitt, B. Strisower, V. Herring, and T. P. Lyon, *Science* **111**, 166–186 (1960).

6. Gofman, J. W., H. B. Jones, F. T. Lindgren, T. P. Lyon, H. A. Elliott, and B. Strisower, *Circulation* **2**, 161–178 (1950).
7. Jones, H. B., J. W. Gofman, F. T. Lindgren, T. P. Lyon, D. M. Graham, B. Strisower, and A. V. Nichols, *Amer. J. Med.* **11**, 358–380 (1951).
8. Macheboeuf, M. A., *Bull. Soc. Chim. Biol.* **11**, 268–293 (1929).
9. Tamplin, A. R., and R. K. Tandy, *J. Appl. Physiol.* **15**, 145–148 (1960).
10. Barclay, M., D. N. Calathes, and H. W. Dargeon, *J. Dis. Children* **97**, Part II, 719–729 (1959).
11. Barclay, M., H. W. Dargeon, E. M. Greene, O. Terebus-Kekish, and V. P. Skipski, *Clin. Chim. Acta* **24**, 225–231 (1969).
12. Lindgren, F. T., and A. V. Nichols, in *The Plasma Proteins,* Vol. 2, F. W. Putnam, Ed., Academic Press, New York, 1960, pp. 2–52.
13. Caspani, R., M. Negri, and C. Sticca, *Minerva Pediat.* **5**, 198–201 (1953).
14. Pantelakis, S. N., and S. A. Doxiadis, *Arch. Dis. Childhood* **42**, 328–331 (1967).
15. Giugiaro, A., A. Ponzone, and S. Baratono, *Minerva Pediat.* **18**, 262–269 (1966).
16. Angelopoulos, B., D. Karalis, A. Tsoukantas, E. Eleftheriadou, and E. Danopoulos, *Med. Pharmacol. Exp.* **14**, 517–527 (1966).
17. Ledvina, M., *Sb. Ved. Pr. Lek. Fak. Karlovy Univ. Hradci Kralove* **9**, 329–334 (1966).
18. Nichols, A. V., in *Advances in Biological and Medical Physics,* Vol. 11, J. H. Lawrence and J. W. Gofman, Eds., Academic Press, New York, 1967, pp. 109–158.
19. Glazier, F. W., A. R. Tamplin, B. Strisower, O. F. deLalla, J. W. Gofman, T. R. Dawber, and E. Phillips, *J. Gerontol.* **9**, 395–403 (1954).
20. DeLalla, O. F., H. A. Elliott, and J. W. Gofman, *Amer. J. Physiol.* **179**, 333–337 (1954).
21. Barclay, M., R. K. Barclay, and V. P. Skipski, *Nature* **200**, 362–363 (1963).
22. Lewis, L. A., F. Olmsted, I. H. Page, E. Y. Lawry, G. V. Mann, F. J. Stare, M. Hanig, M. A. Lauffer, T. Gordon, and F. E. Moore, *Circulation* **16**, 227–245 (1957).
23. Milch, L. J., R. F. Redmond, and H. I. Chinn, *J. Aviation Med.* **23**, 589–593 (1952).
24. Barclay, M., G. C. Escher, R. J. Kaufman, O. Terebus-Kekish, E. M. Greene, and V. P. Skipski, *Clin. Chim. Acta* **10**, 39–47 (1964).
25. Lindgren, F. T., A. V. Nichols, T. L. Hayes, N. K. Freeman, and J. W. Gofman, *Ann. N.Y. Acad. Sci.* **72**, 826–844 (1959).
26. Walton, K. W., *J. Atheroscler. Res.* **7**, 533–536 (1967).
27. Allen, M. F., D. A. Clark, and F. H. Wilson, Jr., *U.S. Air Force School Aerospace Med.,* SAM-TR67-101, pp. 1–9 (October 1967).
28. Barclay, M., R. K. Barclay, O. Terebus-Kekish, E. B. Shah, and V. P. Skipski, *Clin. Chim. Acta* **8**, 721–726 (1963).
29. Mills, G. L., and P. A. Wilkinson, *Clin. Chim. Acta* **8**, 701–709 (1963).
30. Mills, G. L., C. E. Taylaur, and P. A. Wilkinson, *Clin. Chim. Acta* **14**, 273–275 (1966).
31. Mancini, M., and G. L. Mills, *Clin. Chim. Acta* **17**, 163–170 (1967).
32. Cohn, E. J., F. R. N. Gurd, D. M. Surgenor, B. A. Barnes, R. K. Brown, G. Derouaux, J. M. Gillespie, F. W. Kahnt, W. F. Lever, C. H. Liu, D. Mittelman, R. F. Mouton, K. Schmid, and E. Uroma, *J. Amer. Chem. Soc.* **72**, 465–474 (1950).

33. Lever, W. F., F. R. N. Gurd, E. Uroma, R. K. Brown, B. A. Barnes, K. Schmid, and E. L. Schultz, *J. Clin. Invest.* **30**, 99–111 (1951).
34. Gurd, F. R. N., J. L. Oncley, J. T. Edsall, and E. J. Cohn, *Discussions Faraday Soc.*, No. 6, 70–74 (1949).
35. Oncley, J. L., in *The Harvey Lectures,* Academic Press, New York, Series L, 1954–1955, pp. 71–91.
36. Russ, E. M., H. A. Eder, and D. P. Barr, *Amer. J. Med.* **11**, 468–493 (1951).
37. Barclay, M., G. E. Cogin, G. C. Escher, R. J. Kaufman, E. D. Kidder, and M. L. Petermann, *Cancer* **8**, 253–260 (1955).
38. Wolff, R., J. J. Brignon, and J. P. Nicolas, *Ann. Biol. Clin. (Paris)* **21**, 15–28 (1963).
39. Edel, H., *Z. Kreislaufforsch.* **51**, 556–573 (1962).
40. Levy, R. I., R. S. Lees, and D. S. Fredrickson, *J. Clin. Invest.* **45**, 63–77 (1966).
41. Cohen, L., and L. Djordjevich, *Lipids* **3**, 420–424 (1968).
42. Barclay, M., O. Terebus-Kekish, V. P. Skipski, and R. K. Barclay, *Clin. Chim. Acta* **11**, 389–394 (1965).
43. Levy, R. I., and D. S. Fredrickson, *J. Clin. Invest.* **44**, 426–441 (1965).
44. Stokes, R. P., A. Jacobsson, and K. W. Walton, *J. Atheroscler. Res.* **7**, 187–196 (1967).
45. Scott, P. J., *Clin. Chim. Acta* **15**, 449–456 (1967).
46. Burstein, M., and J. Samaille, *Rev. Fr. Etud. Clin. Biol.* **3**, 780–781 (1958).
47. Heiskell, C. L., R. T. Fisk, W. H. Florsheim, G. Tachia, Jr., and C. M. Carpenter, *Amer. J. Clin. Pathol.* **35**, 222–226 (1961).
48. Allard, C., and C. Goulet, *Can. Med. Assoc. J.* **97**, 1321–1328 (1967).
49. Stone, M. C., and J. M. Thorp, *Clin. Chim. Acta* **14**, 812–830 (1966).
50. Altman, P. L., in *Blood and Other Body Fluids,* Vol. 1, D. Dittmer, Ed., Federation of American Society for Experimental Biology, Washington, D.C., 1961, pp. 65–72.
51. Watkin, D. M., E. Y. Lawry, G. V. Mann, and M. Halperin, *J. Clin. Invest.* **33**, 874–883 (1954).
52. Ackermann, P. G., H. J. Buehler, G. Toro, and W. B. Kountz, *Proc. Soc. Exp. Biol. Med.* **88**, 447–448 (1955).
53. Eiber, H. B., A. A. Goldbloom, L. J. Boyd, I. Chapman, and O. Deutschberger, *Bull. N.Y. Acad. Med.* **30**, 719–720 (1954).
54. Nikkilä, E. A., and T. Niemi, *Scand. J. Clin. Lab. Invest.* **9**, 109–115 (1957).
55. Binet, L., F. Bourlière, H. Cendron, and M. M. Burstein, *Compt. Rend., Ser. D,* **252**, 2797–2799 (1961).
56. Franzini, C., C. Turri, and E. Fumagalli, *Minerva Med.* **54**, 2001–2011 (1963).
57. Becquerel, A., and A. Rodier, *Untersuchungen über die Zusammensetzung des Blutes,* Erlangen, 1845.
58. Gofman, J. W., O. deLalla, F. Glazier, N. K. Freeman, F. T. Lindgren, A. V. Nichols, B. Strisower, and A. R. Tamplin, *Plasma (Milan)* **2**, 413–484 (1954).
59. Lewis, L. A., *Ann. N.Y. Acad. Sci.* **94**, 320–335 (1961).
60. Oliver, M. F., and G. S. Boyd, *Clin. Sci.* **14**, 15–23 (1955).
61. Scandrett, F. J., *J. Obstet. Gynaecol. Brit. Commonw.* **66**, 270–276 (1959).
62. Rejnek, J., T. Bednarik, E. Rerabkova, and A. Dolezal, *Clin. Chim. Acta* **8**, 108–115 (1963).
63. Roszkowski, I., I. Chojnowska, J. Iwańska, and L. Myszkowski, *Ginek. Pol.* **39**, 521–523 (1968).
64. Russ, E. M., H. A. Eder, and D. P. Barr, *J. Clin. Invest.* **33**, 1662–1669 (1954).
65. Aurell, M., and K. Cramér, *Clin. Chim. Acta* **13**, 278–284 (1966).

66. Dargeon, H. W., M. Barclay, D. N. Calathes, and M. J. Brownell, *J. Pediat.* **52**, 48–53 (1958).
67. György, P., C. S. Rose, and E. H. Chu, *Amer. J. Dis. Child.* **106**, 165–169 (1963).
68. Olson, R. E., and J. W. Vester, *Physiol. Rev.* **40**, 677–733 (1960).
69. Kinsell, L. W., J. Partridge, L. Boling, S. Margen, and G. Michaels, *J. Clin. Endocrinol. Metab.* **12**, 909–913 (1952).
70. Groen, J., B. K. Tjiong, C. E. Kamminga, and A. F. Willebrands, *Voeding* **13**, 556–587 (1952).
71. Ahrens, E. H., Jr., D. H. Blankenhorn, and T. T. Tsaltas, *Proc. Soc. Exp. Biol. Med.* **86**, 872–878 (1954).
72. Keys, A., J. T. Anderson, and F. Grande, *Lancet* **i**, 66–68 (1957).
73. Malmros, H., and G. Wigand, *Lancet* **ii**, 1–7 (1957).
74. Beveridge, J. M. R., W. F. Connell, G. A. Mayer, J. B. Firstbrook, and M. S. DeWolfe, *J. Nutr.* **56**, 311–320 (1955).
75. Bronte-Stewart, B., A. Antonis, L. Eales, and J. F. Brock, *Lancet* **i**, 521 (1956).
76. Nichols, A. V., V. Dobbin, and J. W. Gofman, *Geriatrics* **12**, 7–17 (1957).
77. Keys, A., J. T. Anderson, and F. Grande, *Lancet* **i**, 787 (1957).
78. Kinsell, L. W., G. Michaels, L. T. DeWind, J. Partridge, and L. Boling, *Calif. Med.* **78**, 5–10 (1953).
79. Ahrens, E. H., Jr., J. Hirsch, W. Insull, Jr., T. T. Tsaltas, R. Blomstrand, and M. L. Peterson, *Lancet* **i**, 943–953 (1957).
80. Ahrens, E. H., Jr., W. Insull, Jr., J. Hirsch, W. Stoffel, M. L. Peterson, J. W. Farquhar, T. Miller, and H. J. Thomasson, *Lancet* **i**, 115–119 (1959).
81. Furman, R. H., R. P. Howard, K. Lakshmi, and L. N. Norcia, *Amer. J. Clin. Nutr.* **9**, 73–102 (1961).
82. Antonis, A., and I. Bersohn, *Lancet* **i**, 3–9 (1961).
83. Bragdon, J. H., and A. Karmen, *J. Lipid Res.* **1**, 167–170 (1960).
84. Bragdon, J. H., and A. Karmen, *J. Lipid Res.* **2**, 400–402 (1961).
85. Kayden, H. J., A. Karmen, and A. Dumont, *J. Clin. Invest.* **42**, 1373–1381 (1963).
86. Nichaman, M. Z., C. C. Sweeley, and R. E. Olson, *Amer. J. Clin. Nutr.* **20**, 1057–1069 (1967).
87. Hamwi, G. J., O. Garcia, F. A. Kruger, G. Gwinup, and D. G. Cornwell, *Metabolism* **11**, 850–862 (1962).
88. Meng, H. C., J. S. Kaley, and J. L. Shapiro, *Metabolism* **11**, 315–328 (1962).
89. Pezold, F. A., in *Protides of the Biological Fluids,* Vol. 10, H. Peeters, Ed., Elsevier Publ. Co., Amsterdam, 1963, pp. 142–145.
90. Hardinge, M. G., and F. J. Stare, *J. Clin. Nutr.* **2**, 83–88 (1954).
91. Kirkeby, K., *Acta Med. Scand.* Suppl. **179**, 7–84 (1966).
92. Lee, K. T., D. N. Kim, Y. S. Han, and F. Goodale, *Arch. Environ. Health* **4**, 4–10 (1962).
93. Ellis, F. R., *Proc. Nutr. Soc.* **26**, 205–212 (1967).
94. Ellis, F. R., *Lancet* **i**, 304 (1970).
95. Connor, W. E., D. B. Stone, and R. E. Hodges, *J. Clin. Invest.* **43**, 1691–1696 (1964).
96. Connor, W. E., D. T. Witiak, D. B. Stone, and M. L. Armstrong, *Circulation* (Suppl. II) **35,36**, II–7 (1967).
97. Spritz, N., E. H. Ahrens, Jr., and S. Grundy, *J. Clin. Invest.* **44**, 1482–1493 (1965).
98. Spritz, N., and M. A. Mishkel, *J. Clin. Invest.* **48**, 78–86 (1969).

99. Avigan, J., and D. Steinberg, *J. Clin. Invest.* **44**, 1845–1856 (1965).
100. Wood, P. D. S., R. Shioda, and L. W. Kinsell, *Lancet* **ii**, 604–607 (1966).
101. Ahrens, E. H., Jr., *Amer. J. Med.* **23**, 928–952 (1957).
102. Scrimshaw, N. S., M. Trulson, C. Tejada, D. M. Hegsted, and F. J. Stare, *Circulation* **15**, 805–813 (1957).
103. Harlan, W. R., and D. E. Beischer, *Amer. Heart J.* **66**, 61–67 (1963).
104. Wilkinson, C. F., Jr., E. Boyle, R. S. Jackson, and M. R. Benjamin, *Metabolism* **4**, 302–309 (1955).
105. Veleminsky, J., and E. Mirejovska, *Vnitrni Lek.* **10**, 871–875 (1964).
106. Bosch, V., *Acta Cient. Venez.* **18**, 159–161 (1967).
107. Little, J. A., H. M. Shanoff, and A. Csima, *Amer. J. Clin. Nutr.* **20**, 133–138 (1967).
108. Olson, R. E., paper presented at the Annual Meeting of the American Medical Association, June 1959, Atlantic City, N.J.
109. Gofman, J. W., *Bull. N.Y. Acad. Med.* **28**, 279–293 (1952).
110. Hatch, F. T., L. L. Abell, and F. E. Kendall, *Amer. J. Med.* **19**, 48–60 (1955).
111. Walker, W. J., E. Y. Lawry, D. E. Love, G. V. Mann, S. A. Levine, and F. J. Stare, *Amer. J. Med.* **14**, 654–664 (1953).
112. Gofman, J. W., A. Tamplin, and B. Strisower, *J. Amer. Diet. Assoc.* **30**, 317–326 (1954).
113. Beveridge, J. M. R., S. N. Jagannathan, and W. F. Connell, *Can. J. Biochem.* **42**, 999–1003 (1964).
114. Ahrens, E. H., Jr., J. Hirsch, K. Oette, J. W. Farquhar, and Y. Stein, *Trans. Assoc. Amer. Physicians,* **74**, 134–146 (1961).
115. Fredrickson, D. S., and R. S. Lees, *Circulation* **31**, 321–327 (1965).
116. Yudkin, J., *Lancet* **i**, 1335 (1963).
117. Yudkin, J., *Lancet* **i**, 418 (1970).
118. Kuo, P. T., and D. R. Bassett, *Ann. Intern. Med.* **62**, 1199–1212 (1965).
119. Akinyanju, P. A., R. U. Qureshi, A. J. Salter, and J. Yudkin, *Nature* **218**, 975–977 (1968).
120. Kuo, P. T., L. Feng, N. N. Cohen, W. T. Fitts, and L. D. Miller, *Amer. J. Clin. Nutr.* **20**, 116–125 (1967).
121. Macdonald, I., and D. M. Braithwaite, *Clin. Sci. (London)* **27**, 23–30 (1964).
122. Macdonald, I., *Clin. Sci. (London)* **29**, 193–197 (1965).
123. Macdonald, I., *Amer. J. Clin. Nutr.* **21**, 1366–1373 (1968).
124. Bierman, E. L., E. Gordis, and J. T. Hamlin, III, *J. Clin. Invest.* **41**, 2254–2260 (1962).
125. Fredrickson, D. S., R. I. Levy, and R. S. Lees, *New Engl. J. Med.* **276**, 34–43, 94–103, 148–155, 215–224, 273–281 (1967).
126. Bierman, E. L., T. L. Hayes, J. N. Hawkins, A. M. Ewing, and F. T. Lindgren, *J. Lipid Res.* **7**, 65–72 (1966).
127. Bierman, E. L., D. Porte, Jr., D. D. O'Hara, M. Schwartz, and F. C. Wood, Jr., *J. Clin. Invest.* **44**, 261–270 (1965).
128. Ruderman, N., A. Jones, R. Krauss, and E. Shafrir, *Clin. Res.* **17**, 261 (1969).
129. Jepson, E. M., M. F. I. Fahmy, P. E. Torrens, J. D. Billimoria, and N. F. Maclagan, *Lancet* **ii**, 1315–1319 (1969).
130. Rubin, L., and F. Aladjem, *Amer. J. Physiol.,* **178**, 263–266 (1954).
131. Havel, R. J., *J. Clin. Invest.* **36**, 855–859 (1957).
132. Walker, W. J., *Ann. Intern. Med.* **39**, 705–716 (1953).
133. Straus, R., R. J. Kositchek, and M. Wurm, *J. Amer. Geriat. Soc.* **10**, 954–968 (1962).

134. Keys, A., J. T. Anderson, F. Fidanza, M. H. Keys, and B. Swahn, *Clin. Chem.* **1**, 34–52 (1955).
135. Gofman, J. W., and H. B. Jones, *Circulation* **5**, 514–517 (1952).
136. Skanse, B., *Acta Endocrinol.* **25**, 445–451 (1957).
137. Rifkind, B. M., T. Begg, and I. D. Jackson, *Proc. Roy. Soc. Med.* **59**, 1277–1278 (1966).
138. Olson, R. E., J. W. Vester, D. Gursey, N. Davis, and D. Longman, *Amer. J. Clin. Nutr.* **6**, 310–324 (1958).
139. Olson, R. E., J. W. Vester, D. Gursey, and D. Longman, *J. Clin. Invest.* **36**, 917–918 (1957).
140. Furman, R. H., R. P. Howard, and L. N. Norcia, *Clin. Res.* **6(2)**, 262–263 (1958).
141. Calatayud, J. B., C. A. Caceres, G. A. Kelser, Jr., and H. H. Orvis, *Amer. J. Clin. Nutr.* **12**, 368–373 (1963).
142. Weiner, N., W. J. Walker, and L. J. Milch, *Amer. J. Med. Sci.* **235**, 405–409 (1958).
143. Beveridge, J. M. R., W. F. Connell, and G. A. Mayer, *Can. J. Biochem. Physiol.* **35**, 257–270 (1957).
144. Beveridge, J. M. R., W. F. Connell, G. A. Mayer, and H. L. Haust, *Can. J. Biochem. Physiol.* **36**, 895–911 (1958).
145. Labecki, T. D., I. B. Bright, W. W. Lake, and C. Thompson, *Proc. Soc. Exp. Biol. Med.* **97**, 260–263 (1958).
146. Farquhar, J. W., and M. Sokolow, *Circulation* **17**, 890–899 (1958).
147. Carlson, L. A., L. Orö, and J. Östman, *J. Atheroscler. Res.* **8**, 667–677 (1968).
148. Skipski, V. P., M. Barclay, R. K. Barclay, V. A. Fetzer, J. J. Good, and F. M. Archibald, *Biochem. J.* **104**, 340–352 (1967).
149. Wilson, D. E., P. H. Schreibman, A. C. Brewster, and R. A. Arky, *J. Lab. Clin. Med.* **75**, 264–274 (1970).
150. Bhattacharyya, A. K., C. Thera, J. T. Anderson, F. Grande, and A. Keys, *Amer. J. Clin. Nutr.* **22**, 1161–1174 (1969).
151. Bornstein, J., *J. Biol. Chem.* **205**, 513–519 (1953).
152. Fjarque, P., A. Marble, and E. F. Tuller, *Amer. J. Med.* **27**, 221–230 (1959).
153. Ditzel, J., and P. Moinat, *J. Lab. Clin. Med.* **54**, 843–859 (1959).
154. Szücs, S., and G. Csapó, *Amer. J. Med. Sci.* **246**, 100/710-103/713 (1963).
155. Szücs, S., and G. Csapó, *Orv. Hetil.* **105**, 2 (1964).
156. Szücs, S., G. Csapó, and K. I. László, *Orv. Hetil.* **105**, 928 (1964).
157. Bacon, G. E., and S. S. Sanbar, *Univ. Mich. Med. Cent. J.* **34**, 84–87 (1968).
158. Vernet, A., and E. B. Smith, *Diabetes* **10**, 345–350 (1961).
159. Simms, H. S., and C. R. Harmison, *Angiology* **17**, 872–881 (1966).
160. Glass, S. J., H. Engelberg, R. Marcus, H. B. Jones, and J. Gofman, *Metabolism* **2**, 133–136 (1953).
161. Engelberg, H., and S. J. Glass, *Metabolism* **4**, 298–301 (1955).
162. Berezin, D., and W. von Studnitz, *Acta Endocrinol.* **25**, 427–434 (1957).
163. Robinson, R. W., W. D. Cohen, and N. Higano, *Amer. J. Med. Sci.* **244**, 736–743 (1962).
164. Barclay, M., R. K. Barclay, V. P. Skipski, O. Terebus-Kekish, C. H. Mueller, E. Shah, and W. L. Elkins, *Biochem. J.* **96**, 205–209 (1965).
165. Oliver, M. F., and G. S. Boyd, *Clin. Sci.* **11–12**, 217–222 (1952–1953).
166. Kroman, H. S., S. R. Bender, A. N. Brest, and M. L. Moskovitz, *J. Atheroscler. Res.* **6**, 247–255 (1966).
167. Russ, E. M., H. A. Eder, and D. P. Barr, *Amer. J. Med.* **19**, 4–24 (1955).

168. Eder, H. A., in *Recent Progress in Hormone Research,* G. Pincus, Ed., Academic Press, New York, 1958, pp. 405–425.
169. Oliver, M. F., and G. S. Boyd, *Lancet* **ii,** 1273 (1956).
170. Danemann, H. A., R. Pick, and L. N. Katz, *J. Lab. Clin. Med.* **55**, 682–688 (1960).
171. Green, A. A., L. A. Lewis, and I. H. Page, *Fed. Proc.* **10**, 191 (1951).
172. Stamler, J., L. N. Katz, R. Pick, L. A. Lewis, I. H. Page, A. Pick, B. M. Kaplan, D. M. Berkson, and D. Century, in *Drugs Affecting Lipid Metabolism,* S. Garattini and R. Paoletti, Eds., Elsevier, Amsterdam, 1962, pp. 432–453.
173. Barclay, M., R. J. Kaufman, D. W. Sved, E. D. Kidder, G. C. Escher, and M. L. Petermann, *Cancer* **10**, 1076–1085 (1957).
174. Berezin, D., and W. von Studnitz, *Acta Endocrinol.* **25**, 435–444 (1957).
175. Furman, R. H., and R. P. Howard, *Metabolism* **11**, 76–93 (1962).
176. Oliver, M. F., and G. S. Boyd, *Circulation* **13**, 82–91 (1956).
177. Cramér, K., *Acta Med. Scand.* **171**, 429–434 (1962).
178. Furman, R. H., R. P. Howard, L. N. Norcia, and E. C. Keaty, *Amer. J. Med.* 24, 80–97 (1958).
179. Aurell, M., K. Cramér, and G. Rybo, *Lancet* **i**, 291–293 (1966).
180. Hjertén, S., *Biochim. Biophys. Acta* **31**, 216–235 (1959).
181. Blankenhorn, D. H., H. P. Chin, and F. Y. K. Lau, *Ann. Intern. Med.* **69**, 21–33 (1968).
182. Wynn, V., J. W. H. Doar, G. L. Mills, and T. Stokes, *Lancet* **ii**, 756–760 (1969).
183. Wynn, V., and J. W. H. Doar, *Lancet* **ii**, 761–766 (1969).
184. Strisower, B., J. W. Gofman, E. Galioni, J. H. Rubinger, G. W. O'Brien, and A. Simon, *J. Clin. Endocrinol. Metab.* **15**, 73–80 (1955).
185. Strisower, B., J. W. Gofman, E. F. Galioni, J. H. Rubinger, J. Pouteau, and P. Guzvich, *Lancet* **i**, 120–123 (1957).
186. Strisower, B., J. W. Gofman, E. Galioni, A. A. Almada, and A. Simon, *Metabolism* **3**, 218–227 (1954).
187. Ledvina, M., S. Coufalová, and V. Souček, *Clin. Chim. Acta* **5**, 818–823 (1960).
188. Lever, W. F., N. A. Hurley, and A. E. Blaney, *J. Invest. Dermatol.* **19**, 55–70 (1952).
189. Adlersberg, D., L. E. Schaefer, and R. Dritch, *Proc. Soc. Exp. Biol. Med.* **74**, 877–879 (1950).
190. Adlersberg, D., L. E. Schaefer, and S. R. Drachman, *J. Clin. Endocrinol.* **11**, 67–83 (1951).
191. Soffer, L. J., J. Eisenberg, A. Iannaccone, and J. L. Gabrilove, in *Ciba Foundation Colloquia on Endocrinology,* G. E. W. Wolstenholme and M. P. Cameron, Eds., Little, Brown, Boston, 1955, pp. 487–530.
192. Bossak, E. T., C. I. Wang, and D. Adlersberg, *J. Clin. Endocrinol. Metab.* **16**, 613–621 (1956).
193. Sachs, B. A., and L. Wolfman, *Metabolism* **17**, 400–409 (1968).
194. Havel, R. J., and R. S. Gordon, Jr., *J. Clin. Invest.* **39**, 1777 (1960).
195. Bassen, F. A., and A. L. Kornzweig, *Blood* **5**, 381–387 (1950).
196. Singer, K., B. Fisher, and M. A. Perlstein, *Blood* **7**, 577–591 (1952).
197. Salt, H. D., O. H. Wolff, J. K. Lloyd, A. S. Fosbrooke, A. H. Cameron, and D. V. Hubble, *Lancet* **ii**, 325–329 (1960).
198. Lamy, M., J. Frézal, J. Polonovski, and J. Rey, *Presse Méd.* **69**, 1511–1514 (1961).
199. Lamy, M., J. Frézal, and J. Rey, *Folia Hered. Pathol.* **10**, 275–284 (1961).

200. Frézal, J., J. Rey, J. Polonovski, G. Lévy, and M. Lamy, *Rev. Fr. Etud. Clin. Biol.* **6**, 677–683 (1961).
201. Druez, G., M. Lamy, J. Frézal, J. Polonovski, and J. Rey, *Presse Méd.* **69**, 1546–1548 (1961).
202. Kahlke, W., in *Lipids and Lipidoses,* G. Schettler, Ed., Springer-Verlag, New York, 1967, pp. 382–400.
203. Becroft, D. M. O., J. M. Castello, and P. J. Scott, *Arch. Dis. Child.* **40**, 40–46 (1965).
204. Forsyth, C. C., J. K. Lloyd, and A. S. Fosbrooke, *Arch. Dis. Child.* **40**, 47–51 (1965).
205. Kuo, P. T., and D. R. Bassett, *Circulation* **26**, 660 (1962).
206. Eder, H., *Amer. Practitioner* **13**, 225–238 (1962).
207. Schwartz, J. F., L. P. Rowland, H. A. Eder, P. A. Marks, E. Osserman, E. Hirschberg, and H. Anderson, *Arch. Neurol.* **8**, 438–454 (1963).
208. Levy, R. I., D. S. Fredrickson, and L. Laster, *J. Clin. Invest.* **45**, 531–541 (1966).
209. Lees, R. S., *J. Lipid Res.* **8**, 396–405 (1967).
210. Lloyd, J. K., *Arch. Dis. Child.* **43**, 393–403 (1968).
211. Jones, J. W., and P. Ways, *J. Clin. Invest.* **46**, 1151–1161 (1967).
212. Lloyd, J. K., *Postgrad. Med. J.* **43**, 691–694 (1967).
213. Lewis, L. A., A. L. Robertson, Jr., H. Mars, and G. H. Williams, Jr., *Circulation* (Suppl. III) **34**, 19 (1966).
214. Murray, R. F., Jr., and B. S. Blumberg, *Nature* **208**, 357–359 (1965).
215. Fredrickson, D. S., P. H. Altrocchi, L. V. Avioli, D. S. Goodman, and H. C. Goodman, *Ann. Intern. Med.* **55**, 1016–1031 (1961).
216. Levy, R. I., and D. S. Fredrickson, *Circulation* (Suppl. III) **33–34**, 156–157 (1966).
217. Kahlke, W., in *Lipids and Lipidoses,* G. Schettler, Ed., Springer-Verlag, New York, 1967, pp. 401–411.
218. Fredrickson, D. S., *J. Clin. Invest.* **43**, 228–236 (1964).
219. Fredrickson, D. S., R. I. Levy, and F. T. Lindgren, *J. Clin. Invest.* **47**, 2446–2457 (1968).
220. Fredrickson, D. S., in *The Metabolic Basis of Inherited Disease,* J. B. Stanbury, J. B. Wyngaarden, and D. S. Fredrickson, Eds., McGraw-Hill, New York, 2nd ed., 1966, pp. 486–508.
221. Havel, R. J., H. A. Eder, and J. H. Bragdon, *J. Clin. Invest.* **34**, 1345–1353 (1955).
222. Engel, W. K., J. D. Dorman, R. I. Levy, and D. S. Fredrickson, *Arch. Neurol.* **17**, 1–9 (1967).
223. Kocen, R. S., J. K. Lloyd, P. T. Lascelles, A. S. Fosbrooke, and D. Williams, *Lancet* **i**, 1341–1345 (1967).
224. Shacklady, M. M., E. M. Djardjouras, and J. K. Lloyd, *Lancet* **ii**, 151–153 (1968).
225. Kaufman, R. J., M. Barclay, E. D. Kidder, G. C. Escher, and M. L. Petermann, *Cancer* **8**, 888–889 (1955).
226. Miller, B. J., and L. Erf, *Surg. Gynecol. Obstet. Int. Astr. Surg.* **102**, 487–491 (1956).
227. Barclay, M., R. J. Kaufman, E. D. Kidder, D. Calathes, G. C. Escher, and M. L. Petermann, *Proc. Amer. Assoc. Cancer Res.* **2**, 93 (1956).

228. Barclay, M., D. N. Calathes, J. C. DiLorenzo, A. Helper, and R. J. Kaufman, *Cancer* **12**, 1163–1170 (1959).
229. Wolffram, E., *Zentralbl. Gynäkol.* **81**, 805–818 (1959).
230. Burstein, M., and J. M. Fine, *Rev. Hematol.* **14**, 380–383 (1959).
231. Neufeld, A. H., G. W. Halpenny, and H. S. Morton, *Can. J. Biochem.* **42**, 1499–1508 (1964).
232. Cohen, L., R. K. Blaisdell, J. Djordjevich, V. Ormiste, and L. Dobrilovic, *Amer. J. Med.* **40**, 299–317 (1966).
233. Spikes, J. L., Jr., L. Cohen, and J. Djordjevich, *Clin. Chim. Acta* **20**, 413–421 (1968).
234. Tremblay, E. C., and P. Welfling, *Proc. Congr. Intern. Soc. Blood Transfus.*, Karger, Basel–New York, 1965, pp. 224–228.
235. Ohya, A., *Juzen Igakkai Zasshi* **64**, 387–408 (1960).
236. Nanava, I. G., and T. M. Tsintsadze, *Nauch.-Issled. Inst. Onkol. Gruz. SSR* **1**, 139–145 (1961).
237. Losticky, C., J. Rejnek, and T. Bednarik, *Cas. Lek. Cesk.* **101**, 1291-1294 (1962).
238a. Toyoda, N., *Hirosaki Med. J.*, Abstract, *Excerpta Med. Cancer* **12**, 5 (1964).
238b. Barclay, M., V. P. Skipski, O. Terebus-Kekish, E. M. Greene, R. J. Kaufman, and C. C. Stock, *Cancer Res.* **30**, 2420–2430 (1970)..
238c. Skipski, V. P., M. Barclay, F. M. Archibald, T. P. Lynch, Jr., and C. C. Stock, *Proc. Soc. Exp. Biol. Med.* **136**, 1261–1264 (1971).
239. Higazi, A. M., A. A. Ata, Y. M. Abdel-Rahman, A. Malek, and K. Mansour, *J. Egypt. Med. Assoc.* **49**, 679–689 (1966).
240. Kellen, J., *Neoplasma* **15**, 139–143 (1968).
241. Schettler, G., and W. Kahlke, in *Lipids and Lipidoses,* G. Schettler, Ed., Springer-Verlag, New York, 1967, pp. 213–259.
242. O'Brien, J. S., and S. Okada, *Chem. Eng. News,* September 8, p. 39 (1969).
243. O'Brien, J. S., *Lancet* **ii**, 805 (1969).
244. Svennerholm, L., *Biochem. J.* **98**, 20P (1966).
245. Uzman, L. L., *Arch. Pathol.* **51**, 329–339 (1951).
246. Groen, J. J., *Israel J. Med. Sci.* **1**, 507–510 (1965).
247. Pansky, B., and R. Lee, *J. Pediat.* **51**, 290–299 (1957).
248. Sweeley, C. C., and B. Klionsky, in *The Metabolic Basis of Inherited Disease,* J. B. Stanbury, J. B. Wyngaarden, and D. S. Fredrickson, Eds., McGraw-Hill, New York, 2nd ed., 1966, pp. 618–632.
249. Kahlke, W., in *Lipids and Lipidoses,* G. Schettler, Ed., Springer-Verlag, New York, 1967, pp. 401–411.
250. Kahlke, W., and H. Wagener, in *Protides of the Biological Fluids,* Vol. 13, H. Peeters, Ed., Elsevier, Amsterdam, 1966, pp. 351–354.
251. Kinsell, L. W., G. Schlierf, W. Kahlke, and G. Schettler, in *Lipids and Lipidoses,* Vol. 1, G. Schettler, Ed., Springer-Verlag, New York, 1967, pp. 446–489.
252. Schettler, G., W. Kahlke, and G. Schlierf, in *Lipids and Lipidoses,* G. Schettler, Ed., Springer-Verlag, New York, 1967, pp. 412–445.
253. Furman, R. H., R. P. Howard, and P. Alaupovic, *Metabolism* **11**, 879–892 (1962).
254. Gustafson, A., *Acta Med. Scand.* (Suppl. 446) **179**, 1–44 (1966).
255. Knittle, J. L., and E. H. Ahrens, Jr., *J. Clin. Invest.* **43**, 485–495 (1964).
256. Kinsell, L. W., G. D. Michaels, G. Walker, S. Splitter, and G. Fukayama, *Metabolism* **11**, 863–878 (1962).
257. Lees, R. S., and F. T. Hatch, *J. Lab. Clin. Med.* **61**, 518–528 (1963).

258. Kruger, F. A.. D. G. Cornwell, G. J. Hamwi, and J. B. Brown, *Amer. J. Clin. Nutr.* **8**, 44–49 (1960).
259. Furman, R. H., S. S. Sanbar, P. Alaupovic, R. H. Bradford, and R. P. Howard, *J. Lab. Clin. Med.* **63**, 193–204 (1964).
260. Baes, H., M. K. Polano, C. Pries, and C. M. van Gent, *Dermatologica* **136**, 300–303 (1968).
261. Bobbitt, J. L., and R. S. Levy, *Biochemistry* **4**, 1282–1288 (1965).
262. Gofman, J. W., L. Rubin, J. P. McGinley, and H. B. Jones, *Amer. J. Med.* **17**, 514–520 (1954).
263. Sohar, E., E. T. Bossak, and D. Adlersberg, *J. Lab. Clin. Med.* **49**, 716–722 (1957).
264. Smith, E. B., *Lancet* **ii**, 530–534 (1962).
265. McGinley, J., H. Jones, and J. Gofman, *J. Invest. Dermatol.* **19**, 71–82 (1952).
266. Biggs, M. W., and D. Colman, *Circulation* **7**, 393–402 (1953).
267. Gofman, J. W., H. B. Jones, T. P. Lyon, F. Lindgren, B. Strisower, D. Colman, and V. Herring, *Circulation* **5**, 119–134 (1952).
268. Lever, W. F., F. S. M. Herbst, and M. E. Lyons, *Arch. Dermatol.* **71**, 158–171 (1955).
269. Guravich, J. L., *Amer. J. Med.* **26**, 8–29 (1959).
270. Wheeler, E. O., and H. B. Sprague, *J. Clin. Invest.* **32**, 611 (1953).
271. Beaumont, J. L., B. Swynghedauw, and V. Beaumont, *Rev. Fr. Etud. Clin. Biol.* **10**, 221–224 (1965).
272. Laudat, P., M. Lefeure, H. Saltiel, and J. DeGennes, *J. Atheroscler. Res.* **6**, 192–195 (1966).
273. Levy, R. I., and D. S. Fredrickson, *Amer. J. Cardiol.* **22**, 576–583 (1968).
274. Scott, P. J., and C. C. Winterbourn, *J. Atheroscler. Res.* **7**, 207–223 (1967).
275. Lever, W. F., F. S. Herbst, and N. A. Hurley, *Arch. Dermatol.* **71**, 150–157 (1955).
276. Beaumont, J. L., *Progr. Biochem. Pharmacol.* **4**, 110–121 (1968).
277. Strisower, E. H., R. M. Kradjian, A. V. Nichols, E. Coggiola, and J. Tsai, *J. Atheroscler. Res.* **8**, 525–534 (1968).
278. Gjone, E., and K. R. Norum, *Lancet* **ii**, 359 (1968).
279. Glomset, J. A., *Biochim. Biophys. Acta* **70**, 389–395 (1963).
280. Glomset, J. A., and D. M. Kaplan, *Biochim. Biophys. Acta* **98**, 41–46 (1965).
281. Pries, C., C. M. VanGent, H. Baes, M. K. Polano, H. A. M. Hulsman, and A. Querido, *Clin. Chim. Acta* **19**, 181–190 (1968).
282. Schatz, I. J., *J. Amer. Med. Assoc.* **210**, 701–704 (1969).
283. Fisk, A. A., E. R. Berry, and A. Chanutin, *J. Lab. Clin. Med.* **39**, 202–210 (1952).
284. Grundy, S. M., and A. C. Griffin, *J. Amer. Med. Assoc.* **171**, 1794–1796 (1959).
285. Cěněk, F., and V. Fialová-Přecechtělová, *Acta Univ. Carolinae Med.* **3**, 221–226 (1960).
286. Wolf, S., W. R. McCabe, J. Yamamoto, C. A. Adsett, and W. W. Schottstaedt, *Circulation* **26**, 379–387 (1962).
287. Page, I. H., M. Moinuddin, and L. A. Lewis, *J. Atheroscler. Res.* **2**, 62–67 (1962).
288. Pupita, F., A. Rappelli, and G. Bazzoli, *Boll. Soc. Ital. Biol. Sper.* **39**, 378–380 (1963).
289. Carlson, L. A., L. Levi, and L. Orö, *J. Clin. Invest.* **47**, 1795–1805 (1968).
290. Brunner, D., G. Manelis, and S. Altman, *Pathol. Microbiol.* **30**, 648–652 (1967).

291. Johnston, J., and A. Ogston, *Trans. Faraday Soc.* **42**, 789–799 (1946).
292. Gofman, J. W., F. Glazier, A. Tamplin, B. Strisower, and O. deLalla, *Physiol. Rev.* **34**, 589–607 (1954).
293. Gofman, J. W., B. Strisower, O. deLalla, A. Tamplin, H. B. Jones, and F. Lindgren, *Mod. Med.,* June 15, 119–140 (1953).
294. Gofman, J. W., F. T. Lindgren, B. Strisower, O. deLalla, F. Glazier, and A. Tamplin, *Geriatrics* **10**, 349–354 (1955).
295. Gofman, J. W., *Coronary Heart Disease,* Thomas, Springfield, Ill., 1959.
296. Krăsno, L. R., G. J. Kidera, A. R. Lack, H. P. Johnson, and L. Nathanson, *Aerospace Med.* **34**, 821–824 (1963).
297. Spain, D. M., V. A. Bradess, and I. J. Greenblatt, *Amer. J. Med. Sci.* **229**, 294–301 (1955).
298. Oliver, M. F., and G. S. Boyd, *Brit. Heart J.* **17**, 299–302 (1955).
299. Rosenberg, I. N., E. Young, and S. Proger, *Amer. J. Med.* **16**, 818–821 (1954).
300. Gottfried, S. P., R. H. Pope, N. J. Friedman, I. B. Akerson, and S. DiMauro, *Amer. J. Med. Sci.* **229**, 34–40 (1955).
301. Schrade, W., and E. Böhle, *J. Atheroscler. Res.* **2**, 161–170 (1962).
302. Adlersberg, D., S. R. Drachman, and L. E. Schaefer, *Circulation* **4**, 465 (1951).
303. Miettinen, M., *Ann. Med. Intern. Fenn.* **46**, 69–76 (1957).
304. Chapin, M. A., and S. Proger, *J. Lab. Clin. Med.* **53**, 39–52 (1959).
305. Hoffman, W. S., in *The Biochemistry of Clinical Medicine,* Year Book Publishers, Chicago, 1954, p. 109.
306. Ahrens, E. H., Jr., and H. G. Kunkel, *J. Exp. Med.* **90**, 409–416 (1949).
307. Allard, C., and G. Choquette, *Can. J. Biochem. Physiol.* **40**, 1515–1527 (1962).
308. Albrink, M. J., *Arch. Intern. Med.* **109**, 345–359 (1962).
309. De Oliveira, J. M., *Amer. Heart J.* **67**, 177–183 (1964).
310. Brunner, D., and K. Loebl, *Progr. Biochem. Pharmacol.* **4**, 140 (1968).
311. Nestel, P. J., *Circulation* **21**, 522–525 (1960).
312. Smith, E. B., *Lancet* **273**, 910–914 (1957).
313. Schettler, G., F. Dietrich, M. Eggstein, and H. Jobst, *Klin. Wochenschr.* **35**, 268–275 (1957).
314. Toro, G., P. G. Ackermann, W. B. Kountz, and J. Toro, *Proc. Soc. Exp. Biol. Med.* **101**, 34–37 (1959).
315. Chulkova, M. S., and O. V. Travina, *Vrach. Trud. Ekspert. pri Vnutr. Boloz'nyakh,* Moscow, *Sbornik,* 1960, pp. 167–176.
316. Ruszkowski, M., *Poznan. Tow. Przyj. Nauk, Wydz. Lek.* **22**, 21–29 (1961).
317. Hatch, F. T., in *Serum Proteins and the Dysproteinemias,* F. W. Sunderman and F. W. Sunderman, Jr., Eds., Lippincott, Philadelphia, 1964, pp. 422–429.
318. Demerdash, H., H. E. Edeen, S. Hamza, S. Hanna, E. M. Abdelwahab, M. Attia, L. Basta, and A. Eissa, *J. Egypt. Med. Assoc.* **50**, 466–476 (1967).
319. Kroman, H., J. Nodine, S. Bender, and A. Brest, *Amer. J. Med. Sci.* **248**, 571–580 (1964).
320. Banerjee, M. D., and A. K. Deb, *J. Assoc. Physicians India* **13**, 935–938 (1965).
321. Jensen, J., D. H. Blankenhorn, H. P. Chin, P. Sturgeon, and A. G. Ware, *J. Lipid Res.* **6**, 193–205 (1965).
322. Engelberg, H., *Lancet* **i**, 303–304 (1970).
323. Slack, J., *Lancet* **i**, 304 (1970).
324. Slack, J., *Lancet* **ii**, 1380–1382 (1969).
325. Barr, D. P., E. M. Russ, and H. A. Eder, *Trans. Assoc. Amer. Physicians* (Philadelphia) **65**, 102–111 (1952).

326. Barr, D. P., *Circulation* **8**, 641–654 (1953).
327. Cramér, K., *J. Atheroscler. Res.* **1**, 317–334 (1961).
328. Scanu, A., L. A. Lewis, and I. H. Page, *J. Lab .Clin. Med.* **51**, 325–332 (1958).
329. Cramér, K., *Acta Med. Scand.* **174**, 421–424 (1963).
330. Burstein, M., and M. Berlinski, *Rev. Fr. Etud. Clin. Biol.* **5**, 193–196 (1960).
331. Gordon, I., *J. Atheroscler. Res.* **3**, 1–9 (1963).
332. Snavely, J. R., W. H. Goldwater, M. L. Randolph, and W. G. Unglaub, *J. Clin. Invest. (Proc.)* **31**, 664 (1952).
333. Pierce, F. T., Jr., J. R. Kimmel, and T. W. Burns, *Metabolism* **3**, 228–239 (1954).
334. Pierce, F. T., and J. W. Gofman, *Circulation* **4**, 25–29 (1951).
335. Eder, H. A., E. M. Russ, R. A. R. Pritchett, M. M. Wilber, and D. P. Barr, *J. Clin. Invest.* **34**, 1147–1162 (1955).
336. Popova, N. L., *Klin. Med. (Moscow)* **40**, 71–75 (1962).
337. Furman, R. H., and L. L. Conrad, *J. Clin. Invest.* **36**, 713–722 (1957).
338. Kunkel, H. G., and E. H. Ahrens, Jr., *J. Clin. Invest.* **28**, 1575–1579 (1949).
339. Russ, E. M., J. Raymunt, and D. P. Barr, *J. Clin. Invest.* **35**, 133–144 (1956).
340. Switzer, S., *J. Clin. Invest.* **46**, 1855–1866 (1967).
341. Mills, G. L., D. Seidel, and P. Alaupovic, *Clin. Chim. Acta* **26**, 239–244 (1969).
342. Alaupovic, P., D. Seidel, W. J. McConathy, and R. H. Furman, *Fed. Eur. Biol. Soc. Letters* **4**, 113–116 (1969).
343. Dangerfield, W. G., and E. Hurworth, *Clin. Chim. Acta* **7**, 292–296 (1962).
344. Burstein, M., and J. Caroli, *Rev. Fr. Etud. Clin. Biol.* **12**, 898–901 (1967).
345. Switzer, S., *Gastroenterology* **53**, 790–793 (1967).
346. Lewis, L. A., and I. H. Page, *Circulation* **7**, 707–717 (1953).
347. Gitlin, D., D. G. Cornwell, D. Nakasato, J. L. Oncley, W. L. Hughes, Jr., and C. A. Janeway, *J. Clin. Invest.* **37**, 172–184 (1958).
348. Baxter, J. H., H. C. Goodman, and R. J. Havel, *J. Clin. Invest.* **39**, 455–465 (1960).
349. Kalugina, G. V., *Ter. Ark.* **34**, 53–57 (1962) [*Fed. Proc. Transl. Suppl.* **22**, 67–68 (1963)].
350. Lewis, L. A., V. Zuehlke, S. Nakamoto, W. J. Kolff, and I. H. Page, *New Engl. J. Med.* **275**, 1097–1100 (1966).
351. Bryla, R., *Pol. Tyg. Lek.* **23**, 7–9 (1968).
352. Rubin, L., *Amer. J. Med.* **17**, 521–527 (1954).
353. Simon, A., C. Ludwig, J. W. Gofman, and G. H. Crook, *Amer. J. Psychiat.* **3**, 139–145 (1954).
354. Barkhan, P., *Lancet* **i**, 773–774 (1958).
355. Oppenheimer, H., and A. T. Milhorat, *Ann. N.Y. Acad. Sci.* **94**, 308–319 (1961).
356. Nordh, F., *Odontol. Revy* **15**, 112–129 (1964).
357. Fujita, A., *Nagoya J. Med. Sci.* **29**, 1–15 (1966).
358. Greenberger, N. J., F. T. Hatch, G. D. Drummey, and K. J. Isselbacher, *Medicine,* Vol. 45, No. 2, Williams and Wilkins, New York, 1966, pp. 161–174.
359. Budyanskii, M. B., *Patol. Klin. Sist. Krovi,* 190–195 (1961).
360. Cervini, C., and M. Nuti, *Rass. Ital. Gastro-Enterol.* **11**, 3–10 (1962).
361. Hartmann, L., and J. Schneider, *Ann. Soc. Belg. Med. Trop.* **4**, 503–510 (1963).
362. Siegel, M., M. Barclay, and E. E. Cliffton, *Amer. Chem. Soc. Abstr.,* 72C–73C (Sept. 1956).
363. Riding, I. M., and D. Ellis, *J. Atheroscler. Res.* **4**, 189–193 (1964).

364. Skrzydlewski, Z., and S. Niewiarowski, *Thromb. Diath. Haemorrh.* **17**, 482–490 (1967).
365. Skarnes, R. C., *J. Bacteriol.* **95**, 2031–2034 (1968).
366. Mermall, H. L., and H. J. McDonald, *Amer. Chem. Soc. Abstr.*, 52C (Sept. 1964).
367. Beckman, L., *Lancet* **ii**, 799 (1969).
368. Barclay, M., R. K. Barclay, E. S. Essner, V. P. Skipski, and O. Terebus-Kekish, *Science* **156**, 665–667 (1967).

13. Fat Absorption and Chylomicron Formation

WILFRED J. SIMMONDS

Department of Physiology, University of Western Australia, Nedlands

I. INTRODUCTION

Chylomicrons are usually defined as the lipid particles found in intestinal and thoracic-duct lymph during fat absorption. Most, but not all, of the lipid is of dietary origin, and the major constituent is triglyceride. Thus chylomicron formation and the absorption of fat and other lipids have to be discussed together.

In the last few years there have been excellent reviews tracing the successive steps in lipid absorption, from physical and chemical changes while in the lumen through final transport from the absorptive cells by lymph and the portal bloodstream (1–4). It is too soon to attempt another systematic account of evidence so recently reviewed. The approach in this chapter is more limited and less systematic. It starts with a brief description of the chylomicrons as they are found in lymph and then follows up some of the questions on lipid absorption that arise from the general composition and properties of this end product. The history of the chylomicron is followed only to the point at which thoracic duct lymph mixes with the venous blood. Here fresh chylomicrons mingle with others that have become modified during their residence in the blood stream and with endogenous particles originating chiefly or entirely in the liver—and other chapters take up the story.

II. GENERAL FEATURES OF CHYLOMICRONS IN LYMPH

The lipid particles in intestinal or thoracic-duct lymph form a stable emulsion that can be stored for months at 4°C or repeatedly creamed by centrifugation and redispersed with minimal "oiling out." The size and distribution of the particles are not easy to measure directly. The majority of particles are too small for accurate measurement by light microscopy with dark field or phase contrast. The preparation of samples for electron microscopy may alter the particle size. Elegant and detailed indirect measurements have been made by Zilversmit's group (5–7), who used centrifugation through a density gradient. The calculations were checked by the use of polystyrene spheres of known diameter. Their results showed a continuous spectrum of particles merging at the low end into particles usually classed as very-low-density lipoproteins (VLDL). In rats 50% of absorbed fat was carried in particles 200 mμ in diameter or smaller and 90% in particles less than 400 mμ in diameter. Less than 0.1% of the particles had diameters greater than 500 mμ. The number of particles increased exponentially with decreasing size, so that there were large numbers of very small particles, which, however, contained in the aggregate only a small proportion of the mass of fat.

The particles consist mainly of triglycerides (∼ 95% of the total lipids), the remainder being phospholipids and cholesterol, free and esterified (8). There are only traces of free fatty acids and partial glycerides. Protein constitutes probably 1% or less of the mass, estimates of the amount varying considerably with the method of isolating the chylomicrons from lymph. There is good evidence that protein, all the phospholipids, and much of the cholesterol form the surface layer, whereas the oily core contains nearly all the triglycerides and cholesteryl esters, and a minor part of the free cholesterol. The particles are negatively charged at the pH of lymph.

From this introductory account of the end product isolated from the lymph—70- to 400-mμ-diameter particles composed mainly of triglycerides and a little cholesteryl ester coated with phospholipids, protein, and free cholesterol—arise the questions that are the main concern of this chapter. How important are nondietary components? How does lipid pass from the lumen into the absorptive epithelium, and how do intracellular lipid particles form? How do the particles escape from the epithelial cell, and are they modified during progress through tissue fluid and lymph? What factors determine how much of the absorbed lipid is carried away in chylomicrons, and how much is transported in lipoproteins other than lymph chylomicrons and by the portal bloodstream?

III. NONDIETARY (ENDOGENOUS) COMPONENTS OF CHYLOMICRONS AND OTHER LIPOPROTEINS

Intestinal lymph from fasting animals contains lipid, even particulate lipid. The nondietary lipid output increases during fat absorption, and much of the increase is found in chylomicrons. The sources of this material and its role in modulating the composition of the chylomicron are relevant to much of what follows in this chapter. It seems justifiable, therefore, to consider the nondietary contribution in some detail. A concise and authoritative treatment has been given by Bierman (9).

Nondietary (endogenous) and dietary lipid molecules or their components may become mixed in three sites before they reach the lymph.

1. In the intestinal lumen endogenous lipid is added in secretions, particularly bile, or by shed cells.
2. In the absorptive epithelium lipid may be synthesized de novo, or bloodborne components may be utilized in addition to the mixture absorbed from the lumen. Endogenous lipid may mix in metabolic pools in various chemical forms—for example, as free fatty acids or as lower glycerides—and thereafter be treated as indistinguishable from similar molecular species of dietary origin.
3. In the tissue fluids lipoproteins that have escaped from blood capillaries mingle with the lipid leaving the absorptive cells.

Within the lymphatic system there is a further admixture of extravascular plasma lipoprotein from regions other than the intestine, the most important being the contribution of hepatic lymph to the cisterna chyli when the ab-

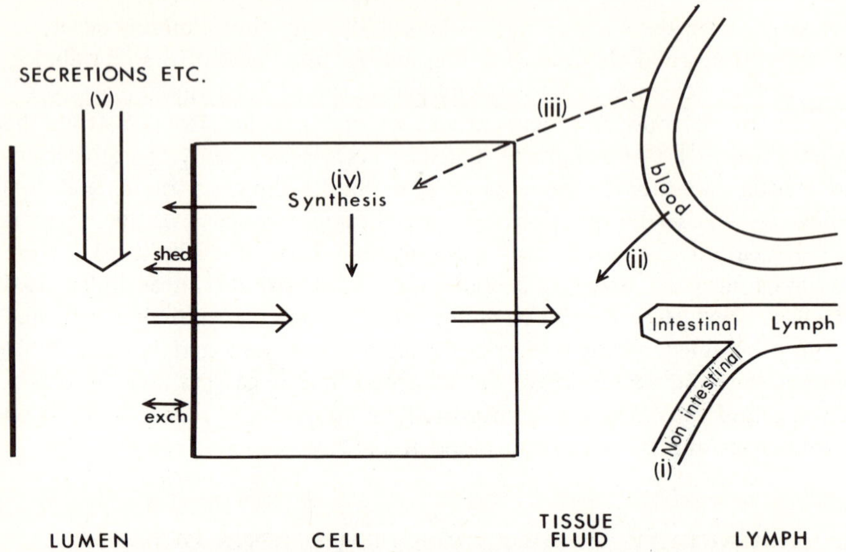

Fig. 1 Sources of endogenous lipid in thoracic-duct lymph. Plasma lipoproteins that have passed into tissue fluid, especially in the liver, may reach the thoracic duct in nonintestinal lymph (i), mingling with those from intestinal tissue fluid (ii), which pass into intestinal lymph. Nonlipid precursors or free fatty acids may pass from the bloodstream to the mucosal cell (iii). The pool of endogenous lipid in the mucosal cell consists of material synthesized from bloodborne components (iv) and of nondietary lipid absorbed from the lumen (v). Digestive secretions, especially bile, shed cells, and some products of mucosal synthesis contribute to the endogenous pool in the lumen. In isotopic experiments exchange ("exch,") of unlabeled endogenous components with labeled exogenous components may have to be taken into account.

dominal thoracic duct is cannulated. Finally, exchanges of certain lipids may take place between particulate and soluble lipoproteins during passage through tissue fluids and lymphatics. The sites of mixing are summarized in Fig. 1.

A. Sources of Endogenous Fatty Acids in Triglycerides

1. Mixed Lymph. Most of the lymph from a thoracic-duct cannula comes from the intestine and the liver, whether the cannula is placed a little above the cisterna chyli, as in rats, or in the thorax or neck, as in larger animals (10a). This is probably true also for man, though there is no direct evidence. The relative volume of intestinal and hepatic lymph varies, probably with species, anesthesia, and other factors, but the intestinal contribution seems to be greater. It accounts for 70 to 90% of the flow in unanesthetized rats (11–13). More important for the present discussion, most of the lipid in thoracic-duct lymph seems to come from the intestine. In rats that were fasting or on a fat-free diet, the output of lipid in thoracic-duct lymph was reduced by about 90% when the intestinal lymph was drained separately (14). As a minor reservation it should be remembered that there may be connections between hepatic and intestinal ducts. Evidence to exclude these, by injection of Evans Blue into liver tissue, is seldom presented in experiments involving separate cannulation. The soluble-lipoprotein contribution of liver lymph may be somewhat greater in other species than it is in rats, but it seems unlikely, for reasons given below, that significant amounts of particulate lipid are added. The endogenous-lipid output increases in thoracic-duct and intestinal lymph during fat absorption, but there is little or no change in hepatic lymph (15, 16).

2. Extravascular Plasma Protein. The formation of tissue fluid is accompanied by the leakage through the capillary wall of some protein and lipoprotein, which are then returned to the bloodstream via the lymphatics. In the course of a day this extravascular circulation of plasma protein is considerable, amounting to 50% or more of the intravascular plasma protein. Most of it occurs through the intestinal and hepatic lymph ducts (10b). The amount of endogenous plasma lipid added in this way to intestinal and thoracic-duct lymph is not easy to quantitate. A number of considerations suggest that it is not a major part, at least not of the endogenous triglycerides.

Baxter (14) found in rats on a fat-free diet that the lipid concentration in the $d > 1.006$ g/ml fraction of lymph lipoproteins (α- and β-lipoproteins) was less than that in serum, whereas the triglyceride-rich $d < 1.006$ g/ml fraction was in very much higher concentration than it was in serum and also accounted for 80% of the total lipids. This suggests that most of the VLDL and chylomicron fraction in thoracic-duct lymph cannot originate from the bloodstream. Grotte, Juhlin, and Sandberg (17) found that spherical particles of polymethylmethacrylate up to 70 mμ in diameter (of the same order as VLDL) passed from plasma into liver lymph, but with considerable "sieving," so that the lymph-to-plasma ratio equilibrated at about 0.2, compared with 0.8 or more for albumin molecules. Morris and Courtice (18) showed that very few chylomicrons normally passed into hepatic lymph, although considerable leakage occurred with hepatic venous congestion. Since intestinal capillaries are less permeable than liver sinusoids (16), it seems unlikely that endogenous, triglyceride-rich particles in fasting intestinal lymph come from blood plasma.

It is difficult to evaluate what proportion of the soluble lipoproteins in thoracic-duct lymph comes from plasma. Lipoproteins pass with other plasma proteins through the capillary wall, but β-lipoproteins, in particular, escape much less readily than the smaller protein molecules. Evidence considered later (Section V.C.) suggests that much of the β-lipoproteins in fasting thoracic-duct lymph may be synthesized in the intestine. Hence, although recycling of plasma lipoproteins accounts for all of the smaller hepatic contribution to fasting thoracic-duct lymph, it probably accounts only for some of the intestinal contribution. Fat absorption increases the turnover of tissue fluid, extravascular protein, and lymph from the intestine and also increases the endogenous-lipid output. But nearly all the increase in triglycerides and much of the increase in phospholipids and cholesterol, both exogenous and endogenous, occur in the chylomicron fraction. Thus it seems unlikely that increased recycling of plasma lipoproteins is a major source of the increased endogenous-lipid output.

3. Epithelial Contribution. There is evidence that the intestinal epithelium, like other tissues, can extract free fatty acids from the circulating plasma (19). So far there is nothing to suggest that this is a major source of endogenous fatty acids for chylomicron triglycerides. Baxter (14) calculated that in rats the intestinal epithelium would have to extract about 4% of the circulating free fatty acids per hour to make 3 mg of triglycerides, which is rather less than the hourly fasting output. Only about 4% of ^{14}C-palmitic acid was incorporated into lymph lipids within 24 hr after intravenous injection and hardly any within the first 4 hr. Very little radioactivity was recovered from the intestinal mucosa shortly after intravenous injection. Verdino, Blank, and Privett (20) showed that in fasting rats the fatty acid spectrum of lymph triglycerides was affected by the composition of fat in the diet on which they had been reared. However, the fatty acid composition of biliary phospholipids is similarly affected (21). Evidence given below suggests that such an alteration of the intraluminal, endogenous pool could mediate an effect on lymph lipids. Synthesis de novo has been demonstrated by the incorporation of ^{14}C-acetate into triglycerides in everted sacs of the small intestine. The intestinal epithelium does not appear to be particularly active in this respect, nor is the process notably accelerated by absorption of long-chain fat (22). In rats in which the body water was labeled with tritium it was estimated that less than 2% of the fatty acids in fasting lymph were synthesized in the epithelium of the small intestine (23).

4. Intraluminal Sources. During fasting all of the esterified fatty acid in lymph is endogenous, and there is evidence that a large fraction of it comes from bile in the intestinal lumen. In fasting rats the output in thoracic-duct lymph is reduced by 50% or more when the common bile duct is drained (14). Return of bile salts to the intestinal lumen in normal concentrations and at a rate exceeding the normal enterohepatic recirculation restores only a small part of the missing endogenous fat in the lymph (24). Thus the decrease following bile fistula is not due mainly to deficiency of bile salts leading to malabsorption of endogenous fat from the lumen or to altered metabolism of the intestinal epithelium. When bile is entering the intestine, the fatty acid pattern of lymph quite closely resembles the fatty acid pattern of biliary phospholipids (14, 25). When bile is diverted, the decrease in output in lymph occurs predominantly in the fatty acids that are the major constituents of bile (24). These findings suggest that digestion and absorption of biliary phospholipids contribute a major part of the fatty acid pool from which the ester fat of fasting lymph is derived, at least in rats.

After fat feeding, an endogenous contribution to lymph triglycerides is demonstrable by differences in the fatty acid distributions of dietary and lymph fat (26, 27). The amount and composition of the endogenous fatty acid mixture have been determined by labeling the dietary fat (27–29). Often a single dose of labeled fat has been given, and the total lymph collected during the ensuing 24 hr has been analyzed. This does not show clearly how much the endogenous turnover is increased by fat absorption, whether the increase varies with the rate of absorption, nor whether the endogenous fatty acid mixture varies. Similar values for 24-hr outputs of endogenous fatty acids have been reported after consumption of different amounts of dietary fat—for example, outputs of 80 to 160 mg (27), about 150 mg (30), and about 100 mg (31). But the total endogenous output includes a basal turnover that continues in the absence of dietary fat. Due to differing estimates of this contribution, the effect of fat absorption seemingly varied from small to very large in the studies quoted.

Serial collections of lymph before and after a single dose of labeled fat allow repeated estimates of the output of unlabeled endogenous fatty acids while the output of labeled dietary fatty acids rises and falls. Several studies in rats (31, 32) showed that fat absorption increased the endogenous-triglyceride-fatty-acid output, but the increase was little affected by the quantity of fat ingested or the lymphatic output of exogenous triglyceride fatty acids. The endogenous mixture was always much the same, with palmitic (16:0), oleic (18:1), and linoleic (18:2) acids making up about 80% of the total. The endogenous mixture was also similar in composition after feeding trierucin or erucic acid (22:1) (33). In similar experiments in man the endogenous output was greater after ingestion of 22 g of triglycerides than it was after ingestion of 6 g of mixed fatty acids (34), and the concentration of endogenous triglyceride fatty acids rose and fell during the course of absorption (35). Further work will be needed to show whether there are differences between rat and man.

Steady-state experiments would seem preferable to the usual single dose of fat. In rats steady intraduodenal perfusion of labeled fat establishes after some hours a steady output of both unlabeled endogenous and labeled exogenous fat in the lymph (36). It is then more easy to relate endogenous turnover to such factors as the rate of fat absorption or absence of biliary lipids than is possible during the rapidly changing conditions after a gastric test meal.

B. Phospholipids

In fasting thoracic-duct lymph phospholipids comprise about 20 wt % of the total lipids (14, 37) and are apparently found mainly in the soluble-lipoprotein fraction (38). Some of this basal endogenous output is contributed by intact plasma-lipoprotein molecules that have passed from hepatic and intestinal capillaries into tissue fluid and lymph (39). It is likely that this contribution is higher than that for triglycerides, which is mainly in particles and large β-lipoprotein molecules, but we do not know how much of the basal phospholipid output is synthesized from the mucosal endogenous fatty acid pool.

During fat absorption the output of phospholipids increases with increasing triglyceride output in thoracic-duct lymph (37, 40). The increase is presumably of intestinal origin since hepatic lymph is unchanged (15). The total phospholipid output is relatively limited [e.g., two to three times the fasting value (41)] but there is evidence that it occurs almost entirely in the chylomicron fraction whereas the output in the chylomicron-free fraction is unchanged (38).

Thus the increase in phospholipid output is related to the increased formation of chylomicrons. However, there is a marked difference between the sources of fatty acids for the triglyceride core and for the phospholipid shell. The majority of the fatty acids for chylomicron triglycerides seem to be drawn from a pool to which diet makes a dominating contribution during fat absorption. There is little discrimination, overall, between the fatty acids used for synthesis (27, 42), though the intramolecular distribution of fatty acids between the 1- and 2-positions does not follow a completely random pattern (20, 43). In the synthesis of chylomicron phospholipids, on the other hand, the majority of the fatty acid chains are endogenous. There is a marked preference for stearic acid—as shown by its higher relative specific activity in lymph phospholipids—when a mixture of labeled fatty acids is fed (44, 45). There is also a positional specificity for saturated fatty acids in the 1-position and unsaturated fatty acids in the 2-position (46, 47). However, differences in the dietary fatty acid mixture are still reflected to some extent in chylomicron phospholipids (45).

These differences between chylomicron triglycerides and phospholipids raise a question that is also briefly discussed later: To what extent are triglycerides and phospholipids assembled from a common free-fatty-acid pool, and to what extent do the two lipid species come from different, partly assembled molecules with a predominantly exogenous or endogenous fatty acid content? For example, absorbed 1-monoglycerides would come predominantly from dietary triglycerides. In chylomicron triglycerides synthesized from this source the mixture of endogenous and exogenous free fatty acids in the intestinal epithelium would affect the composition of only two-thirds of the chains. A similar process could operate in lecithin synthesis, involving absorbed lysolecithin in this instance. In man, 1-lysolecithin is the predominant (60–100%) form of phospholipids in the contents of the small intestine (48) and forms a considerable part, 14 to 36%, though not the majority, in the digesta in rats (49). Some of the 1-lysolecithin is absorbed intact (38, 49, 50) and appears in chylomicrons (38). Any lecithin synthesized in this way after a test meal of triglycerides or free fatty acids without dietary lecithin will draw only a fatty acid from the 2-position from the mixed pool of intracellular fatty acids. The fatty acids in the 1-position, 50% of the total, would be exclusively endogenous and probably come mainly from biliary phospholipids. Even on a mixed diet containing some phospholipids the endogenous biliary contribution to the intestinal contents would need to be taken into account.

Whyte, Goodman, and Karmen (47) fed a labeled fatty acid mixture to rats and measured the distribution of endogenous and exogenous fatty acids separately in the 1- and 2-positions of chylomicron phospholipids. A notable feature was the high ratio of endogenous to exogenous palmitic acid in the 1-position. To account for this distribution Whyte et al. calculated that about 40% of the lecithin precursor molecules would need to enter the pool with endogenous palmitic acid already in the 1-position. They were careful not to imply that this was the only possible explanation nor to select from the possible sources of partly formed endogenous precursors. Nevertheless, it is tempting to relate their results for endogenous palmitic acid to the high proportion of palmitic acid in biliary lecithin. It would be interesting to see if the same preponderance of endogenous chains in the palmitic acid in the 1-position would be found if similar experiments were done on rats with bile fistulas but with adequate replacement of bile salts.

Lysolecithin from the lumen may be acylated to form chylomicron phospholipid. Yet labeled exogenous lecithin or lysolecithin increased the specific activity but not the total output of lecithin in lymph (38, 51, 52), although this varies with triglyceride output; that is, it seems as though the total amount of phospholipids during fat absorption is determined by chylomicron formation, whereas the proportion of exogenous and endogenous fatty acids may be modified by the fatty acids and lysolecithin available from dietary and nondietary sources.

C. Cholesterol and Cholesteryl Esters

The greater part of the cholesterol in thoracic-duct lymph is esterified. Any discussion of nondietary lymph cholesterol must therefore deal with both cholesterol and fatty acid moieties of the esters as well as with the interrelationship between free and esterified cholesterol. These topics involve complex problems in cholesterol absorption, exchange, and metabolism—topics that have been recently reviewed (4, 53, 54). Only a few points relevant to later sections of this chapter are mentioned.

In fasting or on a fat-free diet some free and esterified cholesterol is contributed to thoracic-duct lymph as plasma lipoprotein that has escaped into the tissue fluids of the liver and the intestine. Two sets of observations suggest that this contribution may not be large. Baxter (14) found that the total lipid output in the lymph of fasting nephrotic rats with high serum lipids was the same as in normal rats. Windmueller and Levy (55) fed orotic acid to rats. This inhibited the synthesis and release of β-lipoproteins by the liver, and reduced plasma phospholipid and cholesterol concentrations to about 30% of normal, but the output of phospholipids and cholesterol in lymph was still 65 to 70% of normal.

Apart from the cholesteryl esters added by the recycling of plasma lipoproteins, the fatty acid moiety is added in the mucosa since only free cholesterol is absorbed from the intestinal lumen (4). Like phospholipid, the cholesterol-esterifying mechanism draws selectively on the mucosal pool or pools of fatty acids. Whereas stearic acid is selected for phospholipids, oleic acid is favored for incorporation into cholesteryl esters (27, 42). Otherwise the fatty acid composition reflects in part the pool of exogenous fatty acids, during fat absorption. The endogenous contribution is greater than it is in the case of triglyceride esterification but less than that for phospholipids (45).

Although lymph cholesterol is mainly esterified, it is derived from a pool consisting predominantly of free cholesterol. The size of the pool relative to endogenous output in lymph is much larger for free cholesterol than it is for the fatty acid precursors of triglycerides and other esters. In fasting rats the mucosal cholesterol pool turns over once or twice a day (56).

The intestine makes a major contribution to endogenous lymph cholesterol in two ways: by nondietary cholesterol absorbed from the lumen and by cholesterol synthesized de novo. Virtually no cholesterol is absorbed in the absence of bile salts. Hence the low lymph output in fasting bile-fistula rats, less than 50% of normal, suggests a large luminal contribution (4). In man biliary cholesterol might account for most of the fasting pool in the lumen (57). In rats the biliary excretion of 1–2 mg/day (58, 59) seems to be too small to account for the decrease in lymphatic output (5 mg/day or more) after bile fistula (4). At present, however, one cannot draw up a valid balance sheet, even for rats. Uncertainties include the effects of chronic biliary and lymphatic fistula on biliary cholesterol excretion and on mucosal synthesis of cholesterol and its transfer to lymph.

Cholesterol synthesized in the mucosa makes a significant contribution to the endogenous output in lymph (60). The relationship of newly synthesized cholesterol to chylomicron formation is puzzling. Lipid is absorbed and chylomicrons are elaborated mainly in the jejunum, whereas synthesis occurs mainly in the ileum. Moreover the crypts, not the villi, appear to be the site of synthesis (61). In the absence of bile salts from the lumen synthesis may be increased (61), but esterification and transfer to the lymph are greatly depressed (62). A preliminary report suggests that about half the cholesterol in fasting thoracic-duct lymph is present in very small particles (VLDL) and a small amount in chylomicrons. The particulate fraction of cholesterol disappears after bile fistula (63).

Much of the cholesterol, both free and esterified, in the chylomicrons is endogenous. The endogenous turnover increases with chylomicron formation when a fatty meal free of dietary cholesterol is fed (64). Absorbed dietary cholesterol is carried, mainly esterified, in chylomicrons. There may be species differences in transport, since Zilversmit, Courtice, and Frazer (65) found a higher proportion of cholesterol in very-low-density lipoproteins in the thoracic-duct lymph of rabbits than in those of dogs and rats. Assessment of the role of specific lipoprotein fractions in lymph is complicated by exchanges and net transfer of free cholesterol between soluble and particulate fractions (66). These are discussed in a later section.

IV. LIPID TRANSFER FROM THE INTESTINAL LUMEN

As shown in the preceding section, the intestinal contents supply a major part of the endogenous lipids as well as the dietary components from which chylomicrons are formed. Much of the lipid in the intestinal lumen is insoluble, as oily globules or emulsified particles. This oily phase can be separated from a water-clear phase by high-speed centrifugation (57).

When bile salts are absent or below the critical micellar concentration, the water-clear phase contains very little lipid. Triglycerides, diglycerides, cholesteryl esters, and free cholesterol are so insoluble that their aqueous concentrations are negligible. There will be traces of more polar lipid like monoglycerides. At the usual slightly acid pH of the upper intestinal contents the solubility of long-chain fatty acids is also very low, but there may be substantial amounts of short- and medium-chain fatty acids if these are present in dietary triglycerides.

When bile salts are above the critical micellar concentration, considerable amounts of fatty acids and monoglycerides are cosolubilized as mixed bile salt–lipid micelles, and smaller amounts of less polar lipids, chiefly free cholesterol and fat-soluble vitamins, are taken up into the mixed micelles. Only traces of bulky, nonpolar, or slightly polar molecules, such as triglyceride, diglyceride, and cholesteryl ester, are solubilized (67, 68). Several excellent reviews of the role of bile salts in micelle formation and other aspects of the biophysics of lipids in aqueous systems have been published (69–71).

A. Physical State of Absorbed Lipid

The principal components of the lipid mixture entering the absorptive cell are free fatty acids, 2-monoglycerides, 1-lysolecithin, and free cholesterol (3, 4, 38), all of which may be incorporated into micelles. There is good evidence that to be absorbed at a significant rate a lipid must either be solubilized in micelles or have an appreciable aqueous solubility in the absence of micelles. The lucid and authoritative reviews by Hofmann (2, 71) on the role of micelles in lipid transfer from the lumen leave little to be added here, other than a few points on the role of particles and of nonmicellar lipids in aqueous dispersion.

It seems that lipid is absorbed only in vary small amounts as insoluble particles. A small absorption of nonlipid, inert, solid particles has been demonstrated in some experiments (72, 73), but not in others (74, 75). As regards liquid droplets, absorption of small amounts of aliphatic and cyclic hydrocarbons has been repeatedly demonstrated (76, 77), and substantial absorption has been claimed to occur from fine emulsions (78, 79). On the other hand, silicone oil (80) and glyceryl triethers (81, 82) are not appreciably absorbed, nor is finely emulsified triglyceride if bile salts and pancreatic juice are excluded (83). In these experiments (81–83) there was no appreciable uptake from the lumen, so that it could not be argued that appreciable amounts were taken up into cells but not incorporated into chylomicrons or otherwise moved through the cells. Observations with light and electron microscopes have suggested to many workers that there was uptake of finely emulsified particles by micropinocytosis (84). However, the same intracellular pictures have been produced by incubating everted sacs of the small intestine (85) or perfusing the intestine *in situ* (86) with particle-free micellar solutions.

The digestion of fat should promote emulsification, since monoglycerides and free fatty acids stabilize emulsions with bile salts (78). And yet, even when particulate absorption was the preferred hypothesis, it was surprising how little real information was available on the intestinal emulsion. There is still no quantitative data on particle-size distribution or other aspects of emulsification in normal or abnormal conditions. Such information would be useful since the volume of oil and the size of particles may indirectly play a part in absorption. The volume of oil affects the partition of lipid between oil and micelles (87). It is not known whether this is a determinant of rate and efficiency of absorption or whether the mere presence of some micellar lipid is sufficient. The size of emulsified particles might limit the rate of supply of lipid molecules to the aqueous phase (Fig. 2).

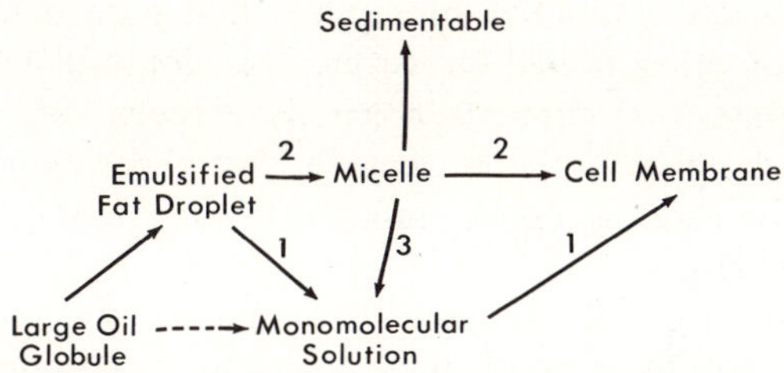

Fig. 2 Transfer of lipid from lumen to cell membrane. Lipid molecules may be transferred from droplet to micelle and then to cell membrane while still in the micellar aggregate (pathway 2, 2). Alternatively micellar solubilization may facilitate diffusion of individual lipid molecules (pathway 2, 3, 1). In the absence of micelles molecules probably must diffuse from particles to monomolecular solution and so to cell membrane (pathway 1, 1) since uptake of whole emulsified droplets is slight. Although transfer is shown in one direction only, a two-way flux can be demonstrated isotopically. Loss of monoglyceride and fatty acid from mixed micelles, by rapid absorption, may lead to precipitation of cholesterol, "sedimentable," under some circumstances (107). (Reproduced from Ref. 88 by permission.)

The interdependence of digestion, emulsification, and solubilization makes such questions difficult to study (88). Physicochemically the digestion of lipid may perhaps be looked on as device for converting nonpolar molecules into polar products, so promoting their incorporation into bile-salt micelles.

In the absence of micelles, since uptake of emulsified particles is negligible, there remains only diffusion from the oily phase through the aqueous medium (pathway 1, 1, Fig. 2). Calculations suggest that fatty acids could be absorbed by diffusion alone (89, 90). Under rather artificial circumstances (finely emulsified and in low dosage) labeled long-chain fatty acids were absorbed into thoracic duct lymph in rats as rapidly when a micellar phase was minimal or absent as they were when the same lipid mixture was entirely micellar. Under normal dietary conditions an association between malabsorption of long-chain fatty acids and defective micelle formation has been repeatedly demonstrated (71). Medium-chain fatty acids are much more soluble, and their absorption is not appreciably affected by the absence of a micellar phase (91). Thus, for fatty acids, absorption by a nonmicellar pathway (pathway 1, 1, Fig. 2) seems to vary with solubility in the aqueous nonmicellar phase.

Monoglycerides form hydrated liquid crystals in water but do not dissolve to an appreciable extent. In the absence of a micellar phase monoglycerides or analogous glycerol monoethers appear to be absorbed to a lesser extent than free fatty acids (92; also unpublished results by R. G. H. Morgan and A. F. Hofmann, and from the author's laboratory).

Lysolecithin is itself a soluble amphiphile, that is, a detergent and micellar solubilizer of other lipids. However, it is doubtful whether its concentration in the intestinal contents normally exceeds the critical micellar concentration for long before it is removed by absorption or hydrolysis. There is no data on rates of uptake relative to fatty acids, in the presence or absence of bile salts.

Cholesterol is so insoluble in water (93) that only micellar transport to the cell membrane would seem adequate to sustain absorption. *In vivo*, absorption is virtually nil in the absence of bile salts (94, 95).

Thus the importance of a micellar phase for absorption varies with the type of lipid molecule, from cholesterol, which is almost entirely dependent on micellar solubilization, to medium-chain fatty acids, which are virtually independent of it. Throughout the absorptive period much of the absorbable lipid will be in the oily phase, and there must be a continuous and rapid transfer of molecules from oil to isotropic phase and thence to the cell membrane (Fig. 2). Very little is known of the rates of interphase lipid exchange in the lumen or of possible rate-limiting steps. The residence in micelles must be very short for bile-salt molecules, and there is some indication that even lipids may exchange very rapidly. Benzene molecules were found to have a lifetime of 0.1 msec in sodium lauryl sulfate micelles (96). Whether this applies to the physiological micellar solutes and whether there are differences among fatty acids, monoglycerides, and cholesterol is unknown. Nor is it known whether the particle size of droplets in the oil phase significantly affects lipid transfer to the aqueous medium or to micelles.

B. Penetration of Cell Membrane

How lipid finally enters the cell is still unknown. Broadly speaking, there are two possibilities: entry by diffusion of individual molecules or penetration by molecular "packages." The particulate hypothesis, in which the packages would be finely emulsified droplets, is no longer generally accepted, but there is still the possibility of lipid penetration in small molecular aggregates, as more or less intact micelles.

Micellar penetration and diffusion are not, of course, mutually exclusive. As noted in the preceding section, absorption of long-chain fatty acids and monoglycerides continues in the absence of micelles. Nor does increased absorption with micellar solubilization necessarily imply micellar penetration of the cell membrane. Micelles might act as a reservoir of lipid in relatively high concentration and close to the cell membrane, to replace molecules diffusing from the intervening aqueous film into the cell membrane (pathway 3, 1, Fig. 2).

The most direct evidence of micellar penetration would be visualization by electron microscopy. Particles of micellar dimensions have been observed on or in the membranes of the microvilli in some studies (97–101), but not in others (75, 85). Considering the lability of micellar aggregates, it seems unlikely that they would retain their identity during processing for electron microscopy. However, Ashworth and Lawrence (102) fixed and embedded on filter paper a micellar solution of monoglycerides and fatty acids in bile salts. They saw osmiophilic particles, 3 to 20 μ in diameter. Similar particles were seen between the microvilli and in the "fuzz" coating them, in sections from rats that were absorbing fat (103). Nevertheless, it seems unlikely in the present state of the art that penetration of the cell membrane by intact micelles can be demonstrated morphologically.

A priori, it is difficult to conceive of labile molecular aggregates like micelles remaining intact during passage through a cell membrane, and the tide of evidence is now running against the notion of engulfment by pino cytosis (104). It would be particularly difficult to reconcile penetration of whole micelles with the well-documented findings that uptake of lipid and uptake of bile salts occur predominantly from different regions of the small intestine. Glycine conjugates can be absorbed proximally to some extent (105); taurine conjugates cannot (106, 107). The bulk of the bile salts is absorbed in the distal ileum (108). Under normal circumstances a large proportion of lipid absorption occurs proximally. When a micellar solution of monoolein and cholesterol in purified bile salts was perfused through the upper small intestine in man, a steady state of absorption of isotopic and chemically measured lipid was reached. Monoolein and the fatty acids released from it were rapidly absorbed, cholesterol was absorbed more slowly, and bile salts (taurine conjugates) were not absorbed at all (107). Thus different lipids were taken up at different rates from the same micellar solution.

Even if intact micelles do not penetrate the cell membrane, they might accelerate lipid transfer by "collision" with the membrane, followed by rearrangement of the micellar aggregate at the surface. If the microvilli in life are covered with a surface coat (109), adsorption of micelles to this coating could be followed by diffusion of lipid through an unstirred aqueous film before the cell membrane was reached. The end result, a partition of lipid between micelle and cell membrane, might well be the same as for "collision," although the mechanism of lipid transfer would be different at a molecular level. In model systems micelles accelerate the diffusion of non-polar solute through an aqueous layer that is not penetrated by intact micelles (110, 111).

In principle uptake of lipid may be separated from subsequent metabolic incorporation by exposure of intestine *in vitro* to low temperature (0°C) or metabolic inhibitors. Under these conditions progressive uptake of isotopic fatty acids occurs at a rate similar to that of metabolically active intestinal rings or segments, but without esterification (112, 113). Uptake is faster from micellar solutions in bile salts (112). The progressive uptake of lipid indicates that it is actually penetrating the cell membrane, although it has been suggested that it is merely adsorbed to the surface (101). Strauss (85) has shown in elegant electron-microscope and biochemical studies that fatty acids and monoglycerides taken up at 0°C can be utilized subsequently at 37°C for incorporation into ester fat and assembly into particles. In some studies labeled monoglycerides and fatty acids were taken up in the proportions found in the micellar phase (112) but not in others (114). Interpretation of *in vitro* studies may not be straightforward, for a number of reasons:

1. When small segments or rings are used, the absorptive cells are exposed to the incubation medium on both sides. Conceivably abnormal concentrations of bile salts in the "tissue fluids" and exposure of basal aspects of the cell to micellar lipid might affect uptake and reesterification.
2. The *in vitro* preparation is a closed system and uptake may be determined mainly by partition of lipid between incubation medium and cell membrane. For example, cholesterol ethers with a high partition ratio between oil and bile salt micelles were taken up *in vitro* to a greater extent than cholesterol, which is much more soluble in micelles, whereas cholesterol ethers of long-chain fatty alcohols are virtually unabsorbable *in vivo* (115). *In vivo* the system is an open one, with absorbed products being continually removed from the cell membrane to be resynthesized, assembled into intracellular particles, and extruded as chylomicrons. *In vitro* usually little or no extrusion of chylomicrons occurs.
3. The *in vitro* preparation is functioning at a rate well below that *in vivo*. Uptake and incorporation *in vivo* may well be limited by factors that are not limiting *in vitro*.

4. Usually only isotopic distribution is measured. Isotopic uptake measures only influx. Though often expressed as millimicromoles of fatty acids per unit weight of sac or segment, this is strictly valid only if the specific activity of the incubation medium remains virtually unaltered. Such a condition is not realized when the volume of incubate is small. Efflux of fatty acids (113) and cholesterol (116) has been demonstrated concurrently with influx. The rate of net uptake (mass) of lipid is seldom determined. In one study it was found that there was a net release of free fatty acids to the medium during uptake and incorporation of isotope (117).

5. Finally, although incorporation of isotopic fatty acids into glycerides is usually a one-way process (i.e., lipolysis is small), the overall rate of fat resynthesis is not measured directly by isotopic incorporation. The latter measures the turnover of isotope in the precursor pool. Changes in the rate of isotope incorporation may reflect changes in the rate of labeling of the pool or alterations in pool size without changes in the absolute rate of reesterification. This could be true even when incorporation is expressed as a percentage of isotope uptake.

Some of the above comments anticipate points raised in later discussion (e.g., on the intracellular role of bile salts), but it seemed preferable to collate in one section a number of reservations concerning *in vitro* preparations as models for lipid absorption. The passage of absorbed lipid from cell membrane to intracellular sites of synthesis and chylomicron assembly is considered in Section V.B.

V. THE INTRACELLULAR LIPID PARTICLE

The intracellular metabolic phase of lipid absorption has been admirably reviewed (3, 4) and here is sketched only in outline. The cited reviews should be consulted for references to the literature. Attention here is concentrated mainly on the unresolved problems of the site and mode of assembly of intracellular particles and the possible intracellular origin of the lipoprotein coating of the formed lymph chylomicron. Such problems will probably be solved by exploiting combinations of morphological, biochemical, and physicochemical techniques (104).

A. Reesterification

There are two distinct metabolic pathways for triglyceride synthesis. On the one hand, 2-monoglyceride can be acylated successively to 1,2-diglyceride and triglyceride. On the other hand, L-α-glycerophosphate can be acylated to phosphatidic acid, which is dephosphorylated to 1,2-diglyceride and then acylated to triglyceride. It was at first thought that glycerokinase was absent from intestinal mucosa so that L-α-glycerophosphate would be generated by glycolysis. It was later shown that free glycerol could be phosphorylated. However, intestinal glycerokinase seems unlikely to be important normally since (a) triglyceride digestion yields mainly 2-monoglyceride, with very little free glycerol, (b) free glycerol absorbed from the lumen is rapidly translocated to the portal bloodstream, and (c) absorbed 2-monoglyceride is reacylated to triglyceride rather than hydrolyzed by intestinal monoglyceride lipase to glycerol and free fatty acids.

Johnston (3) has set out very clearly the evidence that the monoglyceride pathway is the main source of triglyceride. The arguments from experiments *in vitro* and *in vivo,* in man and in animals, are not recapitulated here. As he points out, monoglyceride lipase could provide additional fatty acids when there is a relative excess of monoglyceride. When there is a relative excess of fatty acids, they could be utilized via the α-glycerophosphate pathway. Thus the relative importance of the monoglyceride and α-glycerophosphate pathways could be affected by the relative supply of 2-monoglyceride and free fatty acids, although the α-glycerophosphate pathway is less efficient, in the sense of having a higher Michaelis constant for the incorporation of free fatty acids (3). There could therefore be a link between mode and rate of absorption and intracellular metabolism. When only free fatty acids are supplied, by feeding in lymph-fistula experiments or in the incubate with segments *in vitro,* triglyceride synthesis will be almost entirely via α-glycerophosphate. Consequently there might be rate-limiting factors, such as supply of glucose for glycolysis, that would not operate when a normal mixture of monoglyceride and fatty acids is absorbed. It was mentioned in the preceding section that monoglyceride absorption is probably depressed more than fatty acid absorption when bile-salt concentrations are below the critical micellar concentration. Could this in turn affect the mode and efficiency of triglyceride resynthesis?

Discussion of the details of phospholipid synthesis is outside the scope of this chapter. Evidence for absorption of α-lysolecithin and its appearance with α-chains intact as chylomicron lecithin (38, 49, 50) is mentioned in Section III.B. This work shows that there are two pathways for the incorporation of fatty acids into lecithin, which forms 75% of chylomicron phospholipids (8). One pathway involves the reacylation of 1-lysolecithin derived from dietary and endogenous (biliary) lecithin, and the other diverges from the α-glycerophosphate pathway for triglyceride after the addition of two fatty acid chains. It is probably too early to evaluate the factors that determine the preponderance of one or another mode of synthesis. Perhaps 40% of the lecithin molecules may be asembled from preformed lysolecithin (47, 118).

Two points have been already mentioned but merit reemphasis. First, the amount of chylomicron phospholipid varies with the amount of fat in the lymph, and not with the alimentary load of phospholipids. Thus it seems that phospholipid synthesis is stimulated in some way by chylomicron formation. Second, the fatty acid pool utilized for phospholipid synthesis is probably partly different from the pool for triglyceride synthesis. This is indicated by the high proportion of endogenous chains in phospholipids. A separation of precursor pools was clearly shown by experiments (119) in which 1,2-diglyceride on the monoglyceride pathway to triglyceride synthesis did not mix with 1,2-diglyceride on the α-glycerophosphate pathway that contributes to both phospholipid and triglyceride synthesis.

Cholesterol leaves the epithelial cells predominantly as cholesteryl ester (4). The proportion of endogenous fatty acid chains is higher than that for triglycerides but lower than that for phospholipids. There is a preference for oleic acid, both exogenous and endogenous (27). The esterifying mechanism, unlike that for glycerides, does not require fatty acyl–coenzyme A complexes (120, 121). Although the cholesteryl-ester pool in the mucosa is smaller than the free-cholesterol pool, it turns over more rapidly and its specific activity during the absorption of labeled cholesterol approaches closely the specific activity of chylomicron cholesteryl esters (122). This has suggested that esterification of cholesterol occurs late in the assembly of chylomicrons, possibly just before extrusion from the cell. However, the nature and site of cholesteryl ester synthetase and its relation to the cholesterol esterase of pancreatic juice are not well understood (4, 53).

Whether bile salts do or do not have an intracellular role in lipid absorption is still debatable (71, 88). *In vitro* conjugated bile salts promote the incorporation of labeled fatty acid into triglyceride by intestinal rings (123), but it is not clear whether the effect is intracellular or due to accelerated uptake by micellar solubilization (113, 124, 125). Some of the uncertainties in evaluating *in vitro* results are discussed in Section IV. B. *In vivo* evidence for defective triglyceride resynthesis has been found during studies of lymphatic absorption in bile-fistula rats in several laboratories (126–128), but equally convincing evidence against such a defect has come from the author's laboratory (129).

There is no unequivocal evidence that bile salts play an intracellular role in cholesterol esterification. Bile salts are virtually indispensable for cholesterol absorption, but this could be explained by the need for micellar solubilization. Homogenates of mucosa from bile-fistula rats are deficient in cholesterol-esterifying activity, which is restored by intestinal perfusion with bile (95). Since there is relatively little cholesterol-esterifying activity associated with the brush border (130, 131), an intracellular effect is suggested.

In contrast to a possible stimulation of cholesterol esterification, an inhibitory effect of conjugated bile salts on cholesterol synthesis from ^{14}C-acetate has been demonstrated (132). Since synthesis occurs principally in the ileum, where bile salts are actively transported, an intracellular effect is less difficult to understand than in the case of cholesterol absorption and esterification in the proximal small intestine. A possibility that has not been explored for triglyceride synthesis or cholesterol esterification is that bile salts at the surface of the brush border might activate an intracellular mechanism, analogous to the effects of some hormones on adenyl cyclase activity.

The inhibitory effects of unconjugated bile acids on many intracellular processes have been well documented (123, 133, 134). These and other contaminants have complicated results in studies on conjugated bile salts *in vitro*. There is some evidence for effects in the distal ileum of rats under normal circumstances. It is uncertain whether intracellular effects or deficient micellar formation are more important in pathological states, such as the blind-loop syndrome, in which there are high intraluminal concentrations of unconjugated bile salts (135, 136).

B. Assembly

Most of the absorbed lipid enters the cell membrane in a state of very fine subdivision, as single molecules or possibly as the lipid cores of micellar aggregates. Although there have been claims that lipid aggregates of micellar dimensions can be seen on their way through the cell membrane, the possibility of artifact cannot be excluded. As already mentioned, opinion has swung against the idea that a major fraction of lipid enters as large particles by pinocytosis.

During fat absorption there is a rapid increase in particulate lipid in the cells, but the majority of the droplets are enclosed, singly or in clusters, by membranes of the endoplasmic reticulum and are thus separated from the cytoplasmic matrix. There is then the problem of how lipid is transported from the brush border through the cytoplasmic matrix of the terminal-web region and across an intracellular membrane before assembly into particles. Palay and Karlin (84) made the point that the few vesicles seen in the terminal-web region could transport quite a lot of fat as particles from the caveolae between the microvilli if they represented a numerically small but rapidly moving fraction. The elegant studies of Strauss (104), however, strongly support diffusion of fatty acid molecules through the cytoplasmic matrix before synthesis of triglyceride and assembly in particles. The publication of his autoradiographic studies will be of great interest. As reported in his review, these showed isotopic fatty acid throughout the cytoplasmic matrix after incubation of tissue slices at 0°C, a temperature that inhibits reesterification, but not uptake. When reesterification was slow (at 10°C) or in the early stage of incubation at 37°C, there was evidence that small, discrete droplets in the vesicles of the endoplasmic reticulum were preceded by a form of lipid that aggregated as large solitary droplets in the cytoplasmic matrix. Later there seemed to be about the same absolute amount of lipid in solitary, cytoplasmic droplets but much more as droplets in the endoplasmic reticulum. The detailed autoradiographic findings will be important since there are statistical problems in evaluating the distribution of developed grains and technical problems due to losses or shift of lipid during processing.

Although there is evidence that fatty acid is transferred in molecular dispersion through the cytoplasmic matrix, the mode of transport is unknown. Transfer may be facilitated by the formation of fatty acyl–coenzyme A derivatives. These essential intermediates for glyceride resynthesis have a detergent structure, with the paraffinic chain attached to a strongly hydrophilic head group, and are water soluble (137). To mediate transport, the synthesizing enzyme, fatty acid thiokinase, would need to be either in the cell sap or deep in the brush-border membrane. It seems, however, that most of the activity is microsomal (i.e., on endoplasmic reticulum membranes).

The mode of transport may differ for different lipids. Nearly all the free cholesterol is bound to the membrane both in fasting and during absorption of exogenous cholesterol (138, 139). The cholesterol content of brush-border and intracellular membranes increases during cholesterol absorption. Changes in specific activity show accumulation of exogenous labeled molecules first in the brush-border and later in the intracellular membranes (131). The transfer of cholesterol between membranes may be mediated by lipoprotein (139). Current studies of exchange and net transfer of cholesterol between red-cell membranes and plasma lipoproteins (140, 141) could suggest useful analogies for experiments on intracellular transport.

Although it is uncertain how the components get there, the major site of triglyceride synthesis seems to be the membranes of the endoplasmic reticulum. Most of the activity of the enzymes concerned is recoverable in the microsomal fraction of mucosal homogenates, though a soluble, high-molecular-weight factor may be involved in the steps following phosphatidic acid on the α-glycerophosphate pathway (142). A multienzyme complex synthesizing triglyceride from monoglyceride has been identified by Rao and Johnston (143, 144) in the microsomal fraction and purified about 70 times. The concurrent purification of a functional group of enzymes and cofactors gives strong evidence for localization. For single enzymes there is always the possibility that a fraction that is apparently of minor importance in the disrupted cellular homogenate could be of major significance in the integrated activity of the whole cell.

The morphological evidence points to assembly of the lipid cores of chylomicrons within the vesicles and cisterns of the endoplasmic reticulum (104). The initiation of the process is very rapid. The speed with which radioactive fatty acid is taken up and incorporated into triglyceride is matched by the speed with which lipid droplets can be observed to accumulate in the apical endoplasmic reticulum and by the rapidity of labeling of the droplets in autoradiographs (145, 146).

It is not known whether there is a progressive maturation of the "prechylomicron" from the apical vesicles to the sites of exit laterally into the intercellular spaces. An attempt has been made after feeding labeled lipids to separate the small apical vesicles with their contained lipid particles from the larger and presumed deeper membrane-bound particles (147), by gentle homogenization and gradient centrifugation. There was more triglyceride relative to fatty acid in the larger vesicles. Free cholesterol was predominantly bound to the membrane in all fractions, and there were no differences in the proportion of labeled cholesteryl ester, which was low. Radioautography has suggested that outlying vesicles of the Golgi apparatus are an important site of triglyceride and phospholipid synthesis and particle assembly (148). Electron-microscopic appearances have been variously interpreted as suggesting an active role of the Golgi complex in particle formation (84) or, on the contrary, as indicating that the Golgi complex lies off the main thoroughfare of particle formation and flow (75).

It is not known whether the surface constituents—cholesterol, phospholipid, and protein—are added piecemeal as the droplets pass through the endoplasmic reticulum or whether a coating is added at some specific site (see Section V.C). Cardell, Badenhausen, and Porter (75) noted appearances suggesting that rough endoplasmic reticulum progressively transformed to smooth membranes during fat absorption. They raised the possibility that this might serve to transfer protein, which was synthesized by membrane-bound ribosomes, to lipid particles, which were predominantly enclosed by smooth membranes. Brindley and Hubscher (142) found that most of the activity for the synthesis of triglyceride from monoglyceride and a number of the enzymes for phospholipid synthesis were associated with rough-surface vesicles.

C. Lipoprotein Coating

The chylomicrons in lymph have a coating of polar lipid and protein. Because polar lipid molecules would spontaneously concentrate at the surface and because lipid droplets acquire a protein coating *in vitro* by adsorption (149), it is difficult to be sure whether the chylomicron "membrane" has been added within the absorptive cell or acquired during passage through tissue fluid and lymph. At present the evidence, though not conclusive, favors an intracellular origin, with some extracellular modifications by lipid exchange and extra protein adsorption. There are three main lines of evidence, as follows:

1. Differences in lipid and protein composition between the chylomicron surface and the soluble lipoproteins in lymph (Section VI.B).
2. Data suggesting that the intestinal mucosa is active in lipoprotein synthesis.
3. Evidence that chylomicron formation is defective when intestinal synthesis of lipoprotein is disturbed.

The intestinal epithelium is probably a major source of lipoprotein in the VLDL and chylomicron fractions of lymph. *In vitro* intestinal slices can incorporate radioactive amino acids into lipoproteins, and *in vivo* the specific activity is highest in the chylomicron and VLDL fractions (150–152). Such evidence is not unequivocal. *In vitro,* for example, it is difficult to exclude possible contamination of lipoproteins and chylomicrons with small amounts of highly radioactive nonlipoprotein material. *In vivo* the source of radioactive lipoprotein in lymph from thoracic duct fistulas could be liver lymph, which is mixed with intestinal lymph. However, in acute experiments low-density lipoprotein in lymph was labeled after intravenous administration of ^{14}C-lysine in hepatectomized dogs, whereas the plasma LDL fraction was not (153). Even stronger evidence has come from rats on a diet containing sufficient orotic acid to suppress β-lipoprotein synthesis and endogenous-particle (VLDL) formation by the liver (23, 55). Immunochemically measured β-lipoprotein in thoracic duct and intestinal lymph remained abundant, and chylomicrons appeared in high concentration after a fat meal. On a fat-free diet the lymphatic output of triglycerides and total fatty acids was unchanged. The composition and output of very-low-density lipoproteins in lymph was the same as in controls, as was VLDL labeling after intravenous injection of 4,5-^{3}H-leucine. The plasma β-lipoprotein and triglyceride concentrations, on the other hand, were less than 5% of those in control rats. Thus intestinal synthesis of β-lipoproteins might serve the transport of particulate lipid from epithelium to lymph in the same way that liver synthesis of β-lipoproteins is thought to serve the transport from liver cell to plasma. Only the latter was suppressed by orotic acid. Since plasma concentrations of β-lipoproteins and triglycerides were very low even when lymph returned to the bloodstream, intestinal synthesis did not seem to make a large contribution to plasma levels. It is possible that clearance of lymph lipoproteins from plasma may be accelerated by treatment with orotic acid. It has not yet been shown whether intestinal synthesis of lipoprotein occurs in absorptive cells or in the crypts.

Evidence that intestinal synthesis of β-lipoproteins is essential for the formation of chylomicrons and their passage out of the cell comes mainly from two sources: (a) disordered lipid absorption in abetalipoproteinemia in man, in contrast to normal absorption in α-lipoprotein deficiency (Tangier disease); (b) the effect of inhibitors of protein synthesis in rats.

In abetalipoproteinemia the virtual absence of β-lipoproteins from the circulating plasma (154) is associated with apparent failure to transfer particulate lipid from liver cell to plasma and from intestinal epithelium to tissue fluid and lymph. Thus plasma triglycerides are very low, and there is no triglyceridemia on a high-carbohydrate diet (154), although the triglyceride content of the liver is high (155). There is no postprandial lipemia, although mucosal triglycerides may be high on a fat-containing diet (156). The electron microscope appearances are consistent with defective "packaging" of lipid for export (157). After a fatty meal in such patients lipid droplets are seen in the endoplasmic reticulum as usual, though they are less numerous and possibly more diverse in size. The striking feature is the absence from intercellular spaces of chylomicrons and of the osmiophilic "dust," which may represent small lipoprotein particles (158), possibly VLDL. The other significant abnormality is the presence of large, solitary droplets, many of them appearing to lie in distended vesicles of the endoplasmic reticulum. These are most prominent at a considerable time, even days, after the last fatty meal.

The whole picture would be consistent with some mucosal triglyceride synthesis but failure to extrude the resultant fat particles. Although radioactive fatty acid was readily incorporated into triglyceride (155), little increase in triglyceride content occurred after quite a large dose of corn oil (156), suggesting that triglyceride synthesis was depressed. Despite the absence of chylomicron formation, a large proportion of dietary fat is still absorbed, indicating increased absorption by a nonlymphatic pathway, presumably as free fatty acid via the portal blood. There are no data on cholesterol absorption.

The effects of protein-synthesis inhibitors on fat absorption have also been interpreted on the basis of defective lipoprotein synthesis. In rats treated with puromycin or cycloheximide (159) a large dose of corn oil intragastrically gave very little increase in plasma triglycerides in 6 hr. Histologically the intestinal epithelium was loaded with fat droplets. Incorporation of radioactive fatty acid into triglyceride was normal. Incorporation of labeled amino acids into chylomicron protein and other lipoproteins was not measured in these experiments, but in a previous investigation (151) was found to be depressed in intestinal slices from puromycin-treated rats. Ethionine decreased incorporation of radioactive amino acid into mucosal protein (unfractionated) in female rats and in its effects on fat absorption was similar to puromycin (160).

These experiments with protein inhibitors have been frequently quoted as a model for the intestinal defect in abetalipoproteinemia. However, it is important to bear in mind that the inhibitors have complex physiological effects *in vivo*. Some of these were acknowledged but still not fully taken into account in the original experiments. Recent work emphasizes that there is still insufficient evidence of an essential role of protein synthesis in the release of chylomicrons (161). Caution seems warranted for the following reasons:

1. Decreased absorption of an oral dose of fat in rats was attributable to impaired gastric emptying after puromycin administration. The reduced amount of fat that entered the small intestine was efficiently absorbed (161).
2. When the effects on gastric emptying were bypassed by steady intra-duodenal infusion of fat emulsion, puromycin did not affect lymph-triglyceride concentration or chylomicron composition. However, the usual increase in lymph flow during fat absorption did not occur, and so there was a concomitant impairment in hourly triglyceride output (161). Some inhibitors greatly reduced lymph formation, even in fasting animals, with correspondingly greater effects on fat output during absorption. The effects were not attributable to hypotension (162).
3. Changes in plasma triglycerides give an unreliable index of fat absorption since endogenous (hepatic) secretion is impaired by the inhibitors used (163).
4. Deficient incorporation of labeled amino acid by mucosa *in vitro* need not mean a serious decrease in mucosal protein synthesis *in vivo* (163). When actinomycin had depressed incorporation by 75%, chylomicron release into lymph remained normal (162).

To sum up: there is evidence that the intestinal mucosa can synthesize lipoprotein, including chylomicron protein, though it is not yet definitely proved that this occurs in absorptive cells. Chylomicron formation and release are virtually absent in abetalipoproteinemia. Formal proof that intestinal lipoprotein synthesis is defective in this disease awaits an ethically justifiable opportunity to study intestinal or thoracic duct lymph. In experimental animals the use of protein-synthesis inhibitors has not yet given satisfactory evidence that mucosal synthesis of proteins is essential for chylomicron release. The hypothesis remains an attractive one. Perhaps further evidence may come from analysis of lipid particles isolated from mucosal cells that are actively absorbing fat. Just possibly, animals recovering from mitotic inhibitors may provide a model for "blocked" release (164).

D. Extrusion of Particles

How lipid particles leave the absorptive cells is not known. Since the classical studies of Palay and Karlin (84) it has been generally accepted that most of the droplets pass into the lateral intercellular spaces. The absence of a membranous coating and the general similarity in size of droplets outside the cell and just inside the lateral plasmalemma in profiles of the endoplasmic reticulum have suggested that intracellular membranes and plasmalemma may fuse to form pits from which free droplets may be discharged. Very few pits containing droplets have been observed, however. Cardell et al. (75) observed pits in the lateral plasmalemma coated with an electron-dense lining material similar to that in the Golgi complex. They felt that there was little evidence to link these structures with extrusion of chylomicrons. Mention has also been made in the preceding section (157, 158) of appearances suggesting that lipoproteins smaller than chylomicrons may also leave the cell via the lateral plasmalemma. Such tantalizing hints can only serve to spur the search for experimental models of the mucosal disorder in abetalipoproteinemia.

VI. TRANSPORT FROM CELL

Throughout the preceding sections it has been implied, first, that most of the absorbed lipid is transported by lymph and, second, that absorbed lipid in lymph is carried mainly in chylomicrons. These generalizations must be qualified in a number of particular instances which are considered in this final section.

A. Lymphatic and Vascular Pathways

It is well known that the proportion of absorbed fatty acids that is transported by lymph varies with the chain length. Fatty acids with a chain of eight carbon atoms or less are not transported in lymph to an appreciable extent (91, 165, 166). A small proportion of 10-carbon-atom fatty acids, about half of the absorbed 12-carbon-atom fatty acids, and 80% or more of fatty acids with 14 or more carbon atoms normally pass into thoracic-duct lymph (51, 167, 168). These differences can be correlated with the degree to which the fatty acid is incorporated into chylomicron triglycerides. For example, mixing tripelargonin (C_9) with long-chain triglyceride led to some incorporation of medium-chain fatty acid into mixed triglyceride and so to an appreciable recovery in lymph (169).

It is probable that a number of factors operate to determine the low incorporation of short- and medium-chain fatty acids into chylomicron triglycerides. The most important is presumably the low activity of fatty acid thiokinase, and possibly of other enzymes of the esterifying system, for fatty acids with 12 or fewer carbon atoms (137, 170, 171). The high activity of mucosal lipase against medium-chain triglyceride and monoglyceride could play a part (172, 173). Rapid transit through the intestinal cell might also be important (91). The high absorptive capacity of the small intestine for medium-chain triglyceride (91), its rapid intraluminal hydrolysis, its independence of bile salts for absorption, and independence of chylomicron formation and lymphatics for transport have been exploited in the treatment of a variety of malabsorptive states. An excellent symposium on laboratory and clinical aspects has been recently published (174).

Nearly all the fatty acids that are incorporated into triglycerides pass into lymph, presumably because triglycerides are transported mainly in particles and a little in β-lipoproteins, to both of which the blood capillary is almost impermeable. The relatively high permeability of lymphatics to particles has been ascribed to passage through loose junctions between endothelial cells (84). It has been suggested that the loosely apposed cells may have a flap-valve action so that chylomicrons pass in but do not readily leak out again (158). The role of caveolae and vesicle transport across the cytoplasm is uncertain. An apparent exception to lymphatic transport occurs in the chick, in which particulate lipid seems to pass directly into the portal bloodstream (175). This merits further anatomical and biochemical study.

Absorbed long-chain monoglycerides and fatty acids are not completely recovered in lymph. Incomplete recovery does not appear to be due to catabolism by the intestinal epithelium. With a satisfactory fistula of the thoracic duct in an unanesthetized rat the discrepancy is often small and does not conclusively prove that an appreciable amount is transported by an alternative pathway. Accessory lymphaticovenous communications to the portal vein and inferior vena cava (176) could bypass the lymphatic cannula. Opening up of such anastomoses could explain the frequently poor lymphatic recoveries after a partial obstruction of the cannula by clot, even if free flow is reestablished before the absorptive period.

The experiments of Hyun, Vahouney, and Treadwell (177) provide good evidence that some absorbed long-chain fatty acids escape reesterification and are transported by the portal bloodstream. They found no trace of ^{3}H-cholesterol in portal venous blood after feeding a dose that should have rendered detectable any significant lymphaticovenous connections, whereas in the same unanesthetized lymph-fistula rats ^{14}C-oleic acid was present in portal blood, about 50% of it as unesterified fatty acid. In two other animals with thoracic-duct and portal-vein cannulas the concentration of ^{14}C-oleic acid in the portal vein was 1.5 and 3.2 times that in the inferior vena cava. The authors considered that up to 15% (30 mg) of absorbed oleic acid might be transported by the portal bloodstream in 8 hr.

The branched long-chain fatty acids (2,2-dimethylstearic and 2,2-dimethylnonadecanoic acids) are esterified to a lesser extent during absorption than are long, straight-chain fatty acids, and pass into the lymph to a lesser extent (178, 179). This suggests that there might be some compensatory increase in vascular transport when chylomicron formation or reesterification is defective. The relatively small degree of malabsorption of fat in abetalipoproteinemia has already been mentioned as suggestive of such a process. In lymph-fistula rats small amounts of $^{14}CO_2$ are recovered in expired air after feeding isotopic long-chain fatty acids. Treatment with puromycin decreased absorption into lymph but increased $^{14}CO_2$ excretion (180).

The suggestion that bile salts act intracellularly to promote reesterification has already been discussed. If reesterification were defective in bile-fistula animals, an abnormally high proportion of absorbed fatty acids might pass unesterified into the portal blood and a correspondingly low proportion as ester fat into the lymph. Detailed studies by Dawson and his colleagues (127, 128) supported and amplified earlier observations (126) suggesting that this was indeed so. A low percentage of absorbed labeled oleic acid was recovered in lymph. A high proportion—in fact a very high proportion—of lymph radioactivity was in the free-fatty-acid fraction. There was a higher concentration of labeled oleic acid in portal venous blood than there was in aortic blood, but no difference was observed in control rats without bile fistulas.

On the other hand, Morgan (129) showed in steady-state experiments that a high output of esterified fatty acids in lymph was sustained in bile-fistula rats whether bile salts were absent or were returned to the lumen, provided that fatty acid was given in fine dispersion. Chemically measured free fatty acids were not increased in the lymph during fat absorption (181). A postoperative depression of lymphatic absorption complicated studies carried out in the first 24 to 36 hr after establishing bile and lymphatic fistulas (182). It seems unlikely that agreement will be reached on a specific intracellular effect of bile salts until further evidence is available.

B. Fat Absorption and Lymph Flow

It is well known that fat absorption is accompanied by increased flow of thoracic-duct lymph. This is due to an increase in the intestinal, and not the hepatic, contribution (183). When a single large dose of long-chain fat is given to lymph-fistula rats, the increase may be very large, with peak lymph flows equivalent to about 40% of the circulating plasma volume in a 1-hr collection. An unusual feature is the absence of any notable alteration in protein concentration (166, 183). This makes it unlikely that the increased flow is due to fluid absorbed from digestive secretions or from the meal. An increase in lymph flow due to fluid absorption is accompanied by a decrease in protein concentration in lymph due to dilution of tissue fluid with protein-free absorbed fluid (183, 184). Moreover, the effect is specific for fat and is not found with comparable amounts of a fat-free meal or pure carbohydrate or protein (166, 183, 184), which should also stimulate digestive secretions. Nor does the effect seem to be attributable to increased intestinal motility affecting the formation and propulsion of lymph. In the rat, in which the villi do not pump, intestinal motility can be at least greatly diminished during fat absorption without decrease in lymph flow or fat output (185, 186).

The increase in flow is related to the rate of fat absorption, is sustained during steady absorption, and is less for lipid rich in medium-chain triglycerides, for example, coconut oil (187). This indicates that the increased flow is in some way related to the rate of intracellular processing of lipid that is destined for the lymph. The most likely mechanism seems to be a humoral agent released during fat absorption and acting on the microcirculation. The gut is rich in vasoactive material, but no specific release during fat absorption has been observed. Cholinergic agents increase fasting lymph flow (185, 188), but anticholinergics do not diminish the increase during fat absorption. Fasting lymph flow is increased by 5-hydroxytryptamine, but the protein concentration falls, unlike the effect of fat absorption (185, 189). Kinins have not been tested. Impure preparations of the duodenal hormones secretin and pancreozymin-cholecystokinin increase lymph flow, but pure preparations do not (190, 191). The magnitude of the effect with large doses of fat implies a potent vasoactive mechanism. A continued search for a humoral mediator could be rewarding, at least pharmacologically.

There is no clear evidence that the rate of lymph flow in itself limits fat absorption. When fluid intake is varied during steady fat absorption, the output of fat in the lymph soon returns to the same steady level, the concentration of fat varying inversely with the lymph flow. When fluid intake is steady, a decrease in lymph flow can provide a useful experimental indication of diminished mucosal circulation, which may precede diminished absorption (162, 192, 193).

C. Chylomicrons and Other Transport Particles in Lymph

Baxter (14) found 80% of fasting lymph lipid in the $d < 1.006$ g/ml fraction. Karmen, Whyte, and Goodman (27) found only 10 to 20% of lymph lipid in chylomicrons, in rats receiving only glucose–saline. Taken together these findings suggest that most of the lipid is present in very small particles (VLDL) when only a small amount of fat is being transported. Results similar to those for total lipids have also been reported for cholesterol (63).

After fat feeding there is a shift to larger transport particles, so that nearly all the triglycerides and most of the cholesterol are found in chylomicrons (194). Moreover, as the load of absorbed fat increases, there appears to be a shift toward larger particles within the chylomicron fraction (166, 183). This was substantiated by detailed electron-microscopy measurements by Fraser, Cliff, and Courtice (195). The larger particles have a lower percentage of phospholipids (5), but the surface area per phospholipid molecule is the same for larger chylomicrons, with a lower surface-to-volume ratio, as it is for smaller chylomicrons, with a higher surface-to-volume ratio (195). It will be recalled (Section III.B) that the phospholipid content of lymph increases proportionately less than the triglyceride content during fat absorption. The increasing size of particles may possibly be dictated by limited availability of phospholipids and associated proteins to stabilize the surface of the particles.

There is little information on other factors that may determine the size of lipid-transport particles in lymph. It was claimed that butter ingestion produced unusually large chylomicrons (196), but later studies have not confirmed this (7). It has been reported that after ingestion of saturated fatty acids more cholesterol is carried in the lymph VLDL fraction than there is after ingestion of unsaturated fatty acids (63). The size of particles that transport cholesterol and other lipids to the bloodstream may be of physiological importance. It has been shown that large chylomicrons are cleared from the circulation more rapidly than are small ones (197), and chylomicrons are cleared more rapidly than very-low-density lipoproteins (63).

It has not been established whether the size of lipid particles is fixed at the time they leave the cell or whether small particles merge to become larger ones in tissue fluid and lymph (6). As already mentioned, the final size may be determined by the proportion of polar lipids, particularly phospholipids, to nonpolar lipids, mainly triglycerides; however, the protein of the surface coating could also be an important factor.

Not only the size but also the chemical composition of the chylomicrons may change after extrusion from the cell. Indirect evidence (Section V.C) suggests that the particles have a lipoprotein coating when they leave the cell. This is also supported by resemblances (e.g., a high content of nonpolar amino acids) between intracellular lipoprotein and chylomicron protein (152). Zilversmit (7, 8) showed that the class distribution of phospholipids and their fatty acid spectra in pelleted chylomicron "membranes" were different from those of chylomicron-free lymph. However, Huang and Kuksis (198), who washed their chylomicron fraction fewer times, did not find marked differences in phospholipid composition. Methodologically the problem is a difficult one. Some washing is needed to remove adsorbed material, but too much washing may remove polar lipids or lipoproteins "native" to the chylomicron. After leaving the cell, the chylomicrons may exchange polar lipids with soluble lipoproteins, and the content of individual lipids may change. Chylomicrons, particularly in a dilute emulsion, take up free cholesterol from soluble lipoproteins and transfer phospholipids to them (66). Comparisons of intracellular lipid particles and chylomicrons are needed during rapid but steady absorption with fast transit of particles from cells to lymph. Although technically difficult, such comparisons may help to show how closely the lipid-transport particles in lymph resemble their intracellular precursors.

VII. SUMMARY

Lymph chylomicrons are lipid particles mostly between 70 and 400 mμ in diameter; their core is composed mainly of triglycerides and a small amount of cholesteryl esters and is coated with phospholipids, protein, and free cholesterol. Though they are predominantly a vehicle for absorbed dietary lipid, small numbers are found in fasting lymph together with smaller particles (VLDL) and soluble lipoproteins. This nondietary (endogenous) lymph lipid increases during fat absorption, when it is found chiefly in chylomicrons.

A major portion of endogenous lymph lipid comes from nondietary components (particularly biliary lipid) absorbed from the intestinal lumen. Synthesis from nonlipid constituents in the intestinal cell is a significant source of endogenous cholesterol, but probably not of fatty acids. The endogenous-fatty-acid contribution varies among lipid classes, being greatest for phospholipids, smaller for cholesteryl esters, and smallest for triglycerides. The implications of this and of differences in the endogenous-fatty-acid spectrum are examined.

Lipid is transferred from the intestinal lumen to the absorptive cell mainly in very fine aqueous dispersion, in monomolecular solution, or in mixed bile-salt micelles. The importance of micellar solubilization varies with the type of lipid molecule, from cholesterol, which is almost entirely dependent, to medium-chain fatty acids, which are virtually independent of bile salts for absorption. Micellar solubilization may promote uptake of lipid by diffusion without actual penetration of the cell membrane by micellar aggregates. Such a mechanism would be consistent with most of the available data.

Within the absorptive cell much of the triglyceride is generated by reesterification of absorbed monoglyceride, and a significant proportion of chylomicron lecithin may come from absorbed 1-lysolecithin. Thus the precursor pools for chylomicron lipid include partly assembled molecules in which the proportion of dietary and endogenous components are different from the free-fatty-acid pool used in the α-glycerophosphate pathway. The rate of reesterification and the pathway taken might be modified by the nature of the lipid mixture taken up from the lumen as well as by the rate of uptake.

The details of intracellular assembly of chylomicrons and their extrusion from the cell are still obscure. Evidence favors the view that absorbed lipid is transported from the brush border through the cytoplasm before it is reesterified on or in the membranes of the endoplasmic reticulum and then coalesces as particles within the cisternae. There is accumulating evidence pointing to the synthesis of β-lipoproteins by the intestinal mucosa and suggesting its participation in the final coating and extrusion of chylomicrons.

Particulate lipids are transported almost exclusively by lymph, probably entering lymphatic capillaries between loosely apposed endothelial cells. Absorbed lipids (such as medium-chain fatty acids) that are not reesterified or incorporated into particles are removed by the portal bloodstream. It is possible that the normally small proportion of unesterified long-chain fatty acids removed by the vascular pathway is increased when reesterification and chylomicron formation are defective. There is conflicting evidence on whether such changes occur after bile fistulas and on whether bile salts normally promote reesterification intracellularly.

Fat absorption is accompanied by an increase in lymph flow, the mechanism of which is still unknown. Decreased formation and flow of intestinal lymph may give a useful experimental index of disturbances in the microcirculation but is probably not in itself a significant limiting factor in absorption.

The size of lipid-transport particles in lymph increases with the absorbed fat load and possibly with other factors. This could modify the fate of particles after they reach the bloodstream. The particles extruded into tissue fluid might alter in size or composition before their final collection in lymph. Adsorption of protein and exchange and net transfer of phospholipids and cholesterol between chylomicrons and soluble lipoproteins have been demonstrated *in vitro*. Technically difficult comparisons have yet to be made between the fully assembled intracellular particles, those freshly extruded into tissue fluid, and the chylomicrons in lymph flowing in the intestinal lymphatics.

VIII. ACKNOWLEDGMENTS

It is a pleasure to acknowledge the stimulus and encouragement derived from personal collaboration and correspondence with Dr. A. F. Hofmann, the support of Dr. E. H. Ahrens, Jr., during a year spent in his laboratories at the Rockefeller University, the original work of many associates in this laboratory or now overseas, and helpful criticism of the manuscript by Drs. R. G. H. Morgan and N. Hoffman. Research support by the Australian University Research Grants Committee, National Health and Medical Research Council of Australia, University of Western Australia Medical School Research Funds, and the Commonwealth Fund of New York is gratefully acknowledged.

REFERENCES

1. Senior, J. R., *J. Lipid Res.* **5**, 495–521 (1964).
2. Hofmann, A. F., *Gastroenterology* **50**, 56–64 (1966).
3. Johnston, J. M., in *Handbook of Physiology,* Sect. 6, Vol. III, American Physiological Society, Washington, D.C., 1968, pp. 1353–1375.
4. Treadwell, C. R., and G. V. Vahouny, in *Handbook of Physiology,* Sec. 6, Vol. III, American Physiological Society, Washington, D.C., 1968, pp. 1407–1438.
5. Yokoyama, A., and D. B. Zilversmit, *J. Lipid Res.* **6**, 241–246 (1965).
6. Zilversmit, D. B., P. H. Sisco, and A. Yokoyama, *Biochim. Biophys. Acta* **125**, 129–135 (1966).
7. Zilversmit, D. B., *Fed. Proc.* **26**, 1599–1605 (1967).
8. Zilversmit, D. B., *J. Clin. Invest.* **44**, 1610–1622 (1965).
9. Bierman, E. L., in *Handbook of Physiology,* Sect. 5, American Physiological Society, Washington, D.C., 1965, pp. 509–518.
10. Yoffey, J. M., and F. C. Courtice, *Lymphatics, Lymph and Lymphoid Tissue,* Edward Arnold, London, 1956: (a) p. 124; (b) p. 87.
11. Bollman, J. L., J. C. Cain, and J. H. Grindlay, *J. Lab. Clin. Med.* **33**, 1349–1352 (1948).

12. Benson, J. A., Jr., K. S. Kim, and J. L. Bollman, *Amer. J. Physiol.* **182**, 217–220 (1955).
13. Mann, J. D., and G. M. Higgins, *Blood* **5**, 177–190 (1950).
14. Baxter, J. H., *J. Lipid Res.* **7**, 158–166 (1966).
15. Bollman, J. L., E. V. Flock, J. C. Cain, and J. H. Grindlay, *Amer. J. Physiol.* **163**, 41–47 (1950).
16. Morris, B., *Quart. J. Exp. Physiol.* **41**, 318–325 (1956).
17. Grotte, G., L. Juhlin, and N. Sandberg, *Acta Physiol Scand.* **50**, 287–293 (1960).
18. Morris, B., and F. C. Courtice, *Quart. J. Exp. Physiol.* **41**, 341–348 (1956).
19. Havel, R. J., and A. Goldfien, *J. Lipid Res.* **2**, 389–395 (1961).
20. Verdino, B., M. L. Blank, and O. S. Privett, *J. Lipid Res.* **6**, 356–362 (1965).
21. Glenn, J. L., F. Christensen, and H. Dam, *Biochim. Biophys. Acta* **84**, 753–755 (1964).
22. Reeve, J., and J. J. Franks, *Amer. J. Physiol.* **214**, 1425–1428 (1968).
23. Windmueller, H. G., and R. I. Levy, *Circulation* **36**, 43 (1967).
24. Shrivastava, B. K., T. G. Redgrave, and W. J. Simmonds, *Quart. J. Exp. Physiol.* **52**, 305–312 (1967).
25. Balint, J. A., E. C. Kyriakides, H. L. Spitzer, and E. S. Morrison, *J. Lipid Res.* **6**, 96–99 (1965).
26. Kayden, H. J., A. Karmen, and A. Dumont, *J. Clin. Invest.* **42**, 1373–1381 (1963).
27. Karmen, A., M. Whyte, and D. S. Goodman, *J. Lipid Res.* **4**, 312–321 (1963).
28. Borgström, B., *Acta Physiol. Scand.* **25**, 291–314 (1952).
29. Blomstrand, R., and E. H. Ahrens, Jr., *J. Biol. Chem.* **233**, 321–326 (1958).
30. Mattson, F. H., and R. A. Volpenhein, *J. Biol. Chem.* **239**, 2772–2777 (1964).
31. Savary, P., and M. J. Constantin, *Biochim. Biophys. Acta* **144**, 549–555 (1967).
32. Boucrut, P., and J. Clement, *Biochim. Biophys. Acta* **164**, 558–565 (1968).
33. Savary, P., and M. J. Constantin, *Biochim. Biophys. Acta* **125**, 118–128 (1966).
34. Blomstrand, R., J. Gurtler, and B. Werner, *J. Clin. Invest.* **44**, 1766–1777 (1965).
35. Blomstrand, R., in *The Fate of Dietary Lipids* (Deuel Conference, 1967), G. Cowgill and L. W. Kinsell, Eds., U.S. Public Health Service Publication, U.S. Government Printing Office, Washington, D.C., 1967, pp. 99–123.
36. Simmonds, W. J., T. G. Redgrave, and R. L. S. Willix, *J. Clin. Invest.* **47**, 1015–1025 (1968).
37. Rampone, A. J., *Amer. J. Physiol.* **199**, 1015–1020 (1960).
38. Scow, R. O., Y. Stein, and O. Stein, *J. Biol. Chem.* **242**, 4919–4924 (1967).
39. Reinhardt, W. O., M. C. Fishler, and I. L. Chaikoff, *J. Biol. Chem.* **152**, 79–82 (1944).
40. Morris, B., *Aust. J. Exp. Biol. Med. Sci.* **32**, 763–782 (1954).
41. Byers, S. O., and M. Friedman, *Amer. J. Physiol.* **191**, 87–89 (1957).
42. Blomstrand, R., J. Gurtler, and B. Werner, *Acta Chem. Scand.* **18**, 1019–1021 (1964).
43. Blomstrand, R., *Acta Chem. Scand.* **19**, 1778–1780 (1965).
44. Blomstrand, R., O. Dahlback, and E. Linder, *Proc. Soc. Exp. Biol. Med.* **100**, 768–771 (1959).
45. Whyte, M., A. Karmen, and D. S. Goodman, *J. Lipid Res.* **4**, 322–329 (1963).
46. Blomstrand, R., and O. Dahlback, *J. Clin. Invest.* **39**, 1185–1191 (1960).
47. Whyte, M., D. S. Goodman, and A. Karmen, *J. Lipid Res.* **6**, 233–240 (1965).
48. Borgström, B., *Acta Chem. Scand.* **11**, 749–751 (1957).

49. Saunders, D. R., C. M. Parmentier, and P. O. Ways, *Gastroenterology* **54**, 382–391 (1968).
50. Nilsson, A., and B. Borgström, *Biochim. Biophys. Acta* **137**, 240–254 (1967).
51. Blomstrand, R., N. A. Thorn, and E. H. Ahrens, Jr., *Amer. J. Med.* **24**, 958–966 (1958).
52. Bragdon, J. H., *J. Lab. Clin. Med.* **52**, 564–570 (1958).
53. Goodman, D. S., *Physiol. Rev.* **45**, 747–839 (1965).
54. Chevallier, F., in *Advances in Lipid Research,* Vol. 5, R. Paoletti and D. Kritchevsky, Eds., Academic Press, New York, 1967, pp. 209–239.
55. Windmueller, H. G., and R. I. Levy, *J. Biol. Chem.* **243**, 4878–4884 (1968).
56. Swell, L. E., E. C. Trout, R. Hopper, H. Field, Jr., and C. R. Treadwell, *Ann. N.Y. Acad. Sci.* **72**, 813–825 (1959).
57. Borgström, B., *J. Clin. Invest.* **39**, 809–815 (1960).
58. Friedman, M., S. O. Byers, and F. Michaelis, *Amer. J. Physiol.* **162**, 575–578 (1950).
59. Light, H. G., C. Witmer, and H. M. Vars, *Amer. J. Physiol.* **197**, 1330–1332 (1959).
60. Wilson, J. D., *J. Clin. Invest.* **47**, 175–187 (1968).
61. Dietschy, J. M., and M. D. Siperstein, *J. Clin. Invest.* **44**, 1311–1327 (1965).
62. Wilson, J. D., and R. T. Reinke, *J. Lipid Res.* **9**, 85–92 (1968).
63. Ockner, R. K., and K. J. Isselbacher, *J. Clin. Invest.* **47**, 73a (1968).
64. Vahouny, G. V., I. Fawal, and C. R. Treadwell, *Amer. J. Physiol.* **188**, 342–346 (1957).
65. Zilversmit, D. B., F. C. Courtice, and R. Fraser, *J. Atheroscler. Res.* **7**, 319–329 (1967).
66. Minari, O., and D. B. Zilversmit, *J. Lipid Res.* **4**, 424–436 (1963).
67. Hofmann, A. F., and B. Borgström, *Fed. Proc.* **21**, 43–50 (1962).
68. Hofmann, A. F., and B. Borgström, *J. Clin. Invest.* **43**, 247–257 (1964).
69. Hofmann, A. F., and D. M. Small, *Ann. Rev. Med.* **18**, 333–376 (1967).
70. Small, D. M., *J. Amer. Oil Chem. Soc.* **45**, 108–119 (1968).
71. Hofmann, A. F., in *Handbook of Physiology,* Sect. 6, Vol. IV, American Physiological Society, Washington, D.C., 1968, pp. 2507–2533.
72. Sanders, E., and C. T. Ashworth, *Exp. Cell Res.* **22**, 137–145 (1961).
73. Payne, J. M., B. F. Sansom, R. J. Garner, A. R. Thomson, and B. J. Miles, *Nature* **188**, 586–587 (1960).
74. Juhlin, L., *Acta Physiol. Scand.* **47**, 365–369 (1959).
75. Cardell, R. R., Jr., S. Badenhausen, and K. R. Porter, *J. Cell Biol.* **34**, 123–155 (1967).
76. Shoshkes, M., R. P. Geyer, and F. J. Stare, *J. Lab. Clin. Med.* **35**, 968–975 (1950).
77. Savary, P., and M. J. Constantin, *Biochim. Biophys. Acta* **137**, 264–276 (1967).
78. Frazer, A. C., J. H. Schulman, and H. C. Stewart, *J. Physiol. (London)* **103**, 306–316 (1944).
79. Molander, D. W., *Yale J. Biol. Med.* **21**, 201–210 (1948).
80. Paul, J., and W. F. R. Pover, *Brit. J. Ind. Med.* **17**, 149–154 (1960).
81. Spener, F., F. Paltauf, and A. Holasek, *Biochim. Biophys. Acta* **152**, 368–371 (1968).
82. Morgan, R. G. H., and A. F. Hofmann, *Clin. Res.* **16**, 448 (1968).
83. Masarei, J., and W. J. Simmonds, *Gut* **7**, 114–118 (1966).
84. Palay, S. L., and L. J. Karlin, *J. Biophys. Biochem. Cytol.* **5**, 373–384 (1959).

85. Strauss, E. W., *J. Lipid Res.* **7**, 307–323 (1966).
86. Redgrave, T. G., *Quart. J. Exp. Physiol.* **52**, 130–138 (1967).
87. Borgström, B., *J. Lipid Res.* **8**, 598–608 (1967).
88. Simmonds, W. J., *Amer. J. Clin. Nutr.* **22**, 266–272 (1969).
89. Davson, H., and J. F. Danielli, *The Permeability of Natural Membranes,* Cambridge University Press, London, 1952, pp. 121–124.
90. Hogben, C. A. M., *Gastroenterology* **50**, 51–55 (1966).
91. Clark, S. B., and P. R. Holt, *J. Clin. Invest.* **47**, 612–623 (1968).
92. Morgan, R. G. H., and B. Borgström, *Quart. J. Exp. Physiol.* **54**, 228–243 (1969).
93. Bourges, M., D. M. Small, and D. G. Dervichian, *Biochim. Biophys. Acta* **144**, 189–201 (1967).
94. Siperstein, M. D., I. L. Chaikoff, and W. O. Reinhardt, *J. Biol. Chem.* **198**, 111–114 (1952).
95. Borja, C. R., G. V. Vahouny, and C. R. Treadwell, *Amer. J. Physiol.* **206**, 223–228 (1964).
96. Nakagawa, T., and K. Tori, *Kolloid-Z.* **194**, 143–147 (1964).
97. Lacy, D., and A. B. Taylor, *Amer. J. Anat.* **110**, 155–186 (1962).
98. Sjostrand, F., *J. Ultrastruct. Res.* **8**, 517–541 (1963).
99. Shiner, M., *Gut* **7**, 107–113 (1966).
100. Rostgaard, J., and R. J. Barrnett, *Anat. Record* **152**, 325–350 (1965).
101. Dermer, G. B., *J. Ultrastruct. Res.* **21**, 1–8 (1968).
102. Ashworth, C. T., and J. F. Lawrence, *J. Lipid Res.* **7**, 465–472 (1966).
103. Ashworth, C. T., and J. M. Johnston, *J. Lipid Res.* **4**, 454–460 (1963).
104. Strauss, E. W., in *Handbook of Physiology,* Sect. 6, Vol. III, American Physiological Society, Washington, D.C., 1968, pp. 1377–1406.
105. Hislop, I. G., A. F. Hofmann, and L. J. Schoenfield, *J. Clin. Invest.* **46**, 1070 (1967).
106. Borgström, B., G. Lundh, and A. F. Hofmann, *Gastroenterology* **45**, 229–238 (1963).
107. Simmonds, W. J., A. F. Hofmann, and E. Theodor, *J. Clin. Invest.* **46**, 874–890 (1967).
108. Weiner, I. M., and L. Lack, in *Handbook of Physiology,* Vol. III, American Physiological Society, Washington, D.C., 1968, pp. 1439–1455.
109. Ito, S., *J. Cell Biol.* **27**, 475–491 (1965).
110. Dean, R. B., and J. R. Vinograd, *J. Phys. Chem.* **46**, 1091–1098 (1942).
111. Mysels, K., in *Pesticidal Formulations Research,* J. W. van Valkenburg, Ed., Advances in Chemistry Series 86, American Chemical Society, Washington, D.C., 1969, pp. 24–38.
112. Johnston, J. M., and B. Borgström, *Acta Chem. Scand.* **17**, 905 (1963).
113. Porte, D., Jr., and C. Entenman, *Amer. J. Physiol.* **208**, 607–614 (1965).
114. Thornton, A. G., G. V. Vahouny, and C. R. Treadwell, *Proc. Soc. Exp. Biol. Med.* **127**, 629–632 (1968).
115. Feldman, E. B., and B. Borgström, *Biochim. Biophys. Acta* **125**, 148–156 (1966).
116. Feldman, E. B., *Biochim. Biophys. Acta* **150**, 727–729 (1968).
117. Porte, D., and C. Entenman, U.S. Navy Radiol. Def. Lab. Tech. Rept. No. 526, 1961.
118. Stein, Y., in *The Fate of Dietary Lipids* (1967 Deuel Conference), G. Cowgill and L. W. Kinsell, Eds., U.S. Public Health Service Publication, U.S. Government Printing Office, Washington, D.C., 1967, pp. 54–58.

119. Johnston, J. M., G. A. Rao, and P. A. Lowe, *Biochim. Biophys. Acta* **137**, 578–580 (1967).
120. Murthy, S. K., and J. Ganguly, *Biochem. J.* **83**, 460–469 (1962).
121. Lossow, W. J., R. H. Migliorini, N. Brot, and I. L. Chaikoff, *J. Lipid Res.* **5**, 198–202 (1964).
122. Swell, L., E. C. Trout, Jr., J. R. Hopper, H. Field, Jr., and C. R. Treadwell, *J. Biol. Chem.* **232**, 1–8 (1958).
123. Dawson, A. M., and K. J. Isselbacher, *J. Clin. Invest.* **39**, 730–740 (1960).
124. Johnston, J. M., and B. Borgström, *Biochim. Biophys. Acta* **84**, 412–423 (1964).
125. Philippon, F., and F. Kern, Jr., *Clin. Res.* **16**, 290 (1968).
126. Borgström, B., *Acta Physiol. Scand.* **28**, 279–286 (1953).
127. Saunders, D. R., and A. M. Dawson, *Gut* **4**, 254–260 (1963).
128. Gallagher, N., J. Webb, and A. M. Dawson, *Clin. Sci.* **29**, 73–82 (1965).
129. Morgan, R. G. H., *Quart. J. Exp. Physiol.* **49**, 457–465 (1964).
130. Gallo, L. L., and C. R. Treadwell, *Proc. Soc. Exp. Biol. Med.* **114**, 69–72 (1963).
131. David, J. S. K., P. Malathi, and J. Ganguly, *Biochem. J.* **98**, 662–668 (1966).
132. Dietschy, J. M., *J. Clin. Invest.* **47**, 286–300 (1968).
133. Pope, J. L., T. M. Parkinson, and J. A. Olson, *Biochim. Biophys. Acta* **130**, 218–232 (1966).
134. Dietschy, J. M., *Fed. Proc.* **26**, 1589–1598 (1967).
135. Kim, Y. S., N. Spritz, M. Blum, J. Terz, and P. Sherlock, *J. Clin. Invest.* **45**, 956–962 (1966).
136. Donaldson, R. M., Jr., *Ann. Int. Med.* **64**, 948–952 (1966).
137. Senior, J. R., and K. J. Isselbacher, *Biochim. Biophys. Acta* **44**, 399–400 (1960).
138. Glover, J., and C. Green, *Biochem. J.* **67**, 308–316 (1957).
139. Green, C., *Biochem. J.* **90**, 543–547 (1964).
140. Bruckdorfer, K. R., and C. Green, *Biochem. J.* **104**, 270–277 (1967).
141. Cooper, R. A., and J. H. Jandl, *J. Clin. Invest.* **47**, 809–822 (1968).
142. Brindley, D. N., and G. Hubscher, *Biochim. Biophys. Acta* **106**, 495–509 (1965).
143. Rao, G. A., and J. M. Johnston, *Biochim. Biophys. Acta* **125**, 465–473 (1966).
144. Rao, G. A., and J. M. Johnston, *Biochim. Biophys. Acta* **144**, 25–33 (1967).
145. Jersild, R. A., Jr., *J. Cell Biol.* **31**, 413–427 (1966).
146. Jersild, R. A., Jr., *Anat. Record* **160**, 217–230 (1968).
147. Sjostrand, F. S., and B. Borgström, *J. Ultrastruct. Res.* **20**, 140–160 (1967).
148. Dermer, G. B., *J. Ultrastruct. Res.* **22**, 312–325 (1968).
149. Elkes, J. J., A. C. Frazer, J. H. Schulman, and H. C. Stewart, *Proc. Royal Soc. (London)* **A184**, 102–115 (1945).
150. Rodbell, M., D. S. Fredrickson, and K. Ono, *J. Biol. Chem.* **234**, 567–571 (1959).
151. Isselbacher, K. J., and D. M. Budz, *Nature* **200**, 364–365 (1963).
152. Hatch, F. T., A. Yoshiro, L. M. Hagopian, and J. J. Rubenstein, *J. Biol. Chem.* **241**, 1655–1665 (1966).
153. Roheim, P. S., L. I. Gidez, and H. A. Eder, *J. Clin. Invest.* **45**, 297–300 (1966).
154. Levy, R. I., D. S. Fredrickson, and L. Laster, *J. Clin. Invest.* **45**, 531–541 (1966).
155. Isselbacher, K. J., R. Scheig, G. R. Plotkin, and J. B. Caulfield, *Medicine* **43**, 347–361 (1964).
156. Ways, P. O., C. M. Parmentier, H. J. Kayden, J. W. Jones, D. R. Saunders, and C. E. Rubin, *J. Clin. Invest.* **46**, 35–46 (1967).
157. Dobbins, W. O., *Gastroenterology* **50**, 195–210 (1966).

158. Casley-Smith, J. R., *J. Cell Biol.* **15**, 259–277 (1962).
159. Sabesin, S. M., and K. J. Isselbacher, *Science* **147**, 1149–1151 (1965).
160. Hyams, D. E., S. M. Sabesin, N. J. Greenberger, and K. J. Isselbacher, *Biochim. Biophys. Acta* **125**, 166–173 (1966).
161. Redgrave, T. G., and Zilversmit, D. B., *Amer. J. Physiol.* **217**, 336–340 (1969).
162. Redgrave, T. G., *Proc. Soc. Exp. Biol. Med.* **130**, 776–780 (1969).
163. Schlunk, F. F., D. S. Longenecker, and B. Lombardi, *Biochim. Biophys. Acta* **158**, 425–434 (1968).
164. Redgrave, T. G., and W. J. Simmonds, *Gastroenterology* **52**, 54–66 (1967).
165. Hughes, R. H., and E. J. Wimmer, *J. Biol. Chem.* **108**, 141–144 (1935).
166. Simmonds, W. J., *Aust. J. Exp. Biol. Sci.* **33**, 305–314 (1955).
167. Bergstrom, S., B. Borgström, A. Carlsten, and M. Rottenberg, *Acta Chem. Scand.* **4**, 1142–1143 (1950).
168. Bloom, B., I. L. Chaikoff, and W. O. Reinhardt, *Amer. J. Physiol.* **166**, 451–455 (1951).
169. Lee, D. S., S. A. Hashim, and T. B. van Itallie, *Amer. J. Physiol.* **214**, 294–297 (1968).
170. Gelb, A. M., and J. I. Kessler, *Amer. J. Physiol.* **204**, 821–824 (1963).
171. Brindley, D. N., and G. Hubscher, *Biochim. Biophys. Acta* **125**, 92–105 (1966).
172. Playoust, M. R., and K. J. Isselbacher, *J. Clin. Invest.* **43**, 878–885 (1964).
173. Senior, J. R., and K. J. Isselbacher, *J. Clin. Invest.* **42**, 187–195 (1963).
174. Senior, J. R., Ed., *Medium Chain Triglycerides,* University of Pennsylvania, Philadelphia, 1968.
175. Noyan, A., W. J. Lossow, N. Brot, and I. L. Chaikoff, *J. Lipid Res.* **5**, 538–541 (1964).
176. Job, T. T., *Amer. J. Anat.* **24**, 467–491 (1918).
177. Hyun, S. A., G. V. Vahouny, and C. R. Treadwell, *Biochim. Biophys. Acta* **137**, 296–305 (1967).
178. Borgstrom, B., and N. Tryding, *Acta Physiol. Scand.* **37**, 127–133 (1956).
179. Blomstrand, R., N. Tryding, and G. Westoo, *Acta Physiol. Scand.* **37**, 91–96 (1956).
180. Kayden, H. J., and M. Medick, *Biochim. Biophys. Acta* **176**, 37–43 (1969).
181. Morgan, R. G. H., Ph.D. thesis, University of Western Australia, 1964.
182. Morgan, R. G. H., *Quart. J. Exp. Physiol.* **51**, 33–41 (1966).
183. Borgström, B., and C.-B. Laurell, *Acta Physiol. Scand.* **29**, 264–280 (1953).
184. Simmonds, W. J., *Aust. J. Exp. Biol. Med. Sci.* **32**, 285–300 (1954).
185. Simmonds, W. J., *Quart. J. Exp. Physiol.* **42**, 205–221 (1957).
186. Bennett, S. P., Shepherd, and W. J. Simmonds, *Aust. J. Exp. Biol. Med. Sci.* **40**, 225–231 (1962).
187. Shepherd, P., and W. J. Simmonds, *Aust. J. Exp. Biol. Med. Sci.* **37**, 1–9 (1959).
188. Beznak, A. B. L., *Quart. J. Exp. Physiol.* **26**, 253–263 (1937).
189. Shim, W. T. K., E. L. Pollak, and T. Drapanas, *Amer. J. Physiol.* **201**, 81–84 (1961).
190. Razin, E., M. G. Feldman, and D. A. Dreiling, *J. Surg. Res.* **2**, 320–331 (1962).
191. Bartos, V., V. Brzek, and J. Groh, *Amer. J. Med. Sci.* **252**, 31–38 (1966).
192. Woolley, G., and W. J. Simmonds, *Aust. J. Exp. Biol. Med. Sci.* **37**, 125–132 (1959).
193. Woolley, G., *Aust. J. Exp. Biol. Med. Sci.* **39**, 583–594 (1961).
194. Zilversmit, D. B., *Proc. Soc. Exp. Biol. Med.* **128**, 1116–1121 (1968).

195. Fraser, R., W. J. Cliff, and F. C. Courtice, *Quart. J. Exp. Physiol.* **53**, 390–398 (1968).
196. Jones, R., W. A. Thomas, and R. F. Scott, *Exp. Molec. Path.* **1**, 65–83 (1962).
197. Quarfordt, S. H., and D. S. Goodman, *Biochim. Biophys. Acta* **116**, 382–385 (1966).
198. Huang, T. C., and A. Kuksis, *Lipids* **2**, 443–452 (1967).

14. Plasma Lecithin:Cholesterol Acyltransferase

JOHN A. GLOMSET

Department of Medicine and Regional Primate Research Center, University of Washington, Seattle

I. INTRODUCTION

It has been recognized for many years that the blood plasma of many species contains an enzyme that can esterify cholesterol. This enzyme can easily be demonstrated by incubating plasma at 37°C and measuring the decrease in unesterified cholesterol. Alternatively plasma can be incubated with radioactive cholesterol, and the formation of radioactive cholesteryl esters can be followed. For many years after its discovery the plasma-cholesterol-esterifying enzyme was believed to be a cholesterol esterase. However, it is now known to be an acyltransferase that mainly transfers fatty acids from the lecithin to the cholesterol of plasma lipoproteins (lecithin: cholesterol acyltransferase, or LCAT). There is good evidence that the enzyme is a specific component of plasma, that it reacts preferentially with plasma high-density lipoproteins (HDL), and that it is an important source of plasma cholesteryl esters. Finally, although the enzyme's broader physiological role has not been established conclusively, there is some particularly suggestive evidence that its principal function is to diminish the unesterified cholesterol and the lecithin of plasma lipoproteins and plasma membranes. Some of this evidence has been provided by the recent discovery of an inborn error of metabolism characterized by the absence of plasma LCAT activity. Patients with this disease have very high levels of plasma unesterified cholesterol and lecithin, and very low levels of plasma cholesteryl esters and lysolecithin. Their erythrocytes contain nearly twice the normal amount of unesterified cholesterol and lecithin, and there is evidence that this unesterified cholesterol may be increased in other tissues as well. Finally, the patients have corneal opacity, anemia, and proteinuria, and these clinical abnormalities appear to be associated with an accumulation of lipid in the cornea, bone marrow, and kidney.

Much of the early work on the LCAT reaction has been reviewed recently (1). Therefore it is summarized only briefly here, and the review should be consulted for further details. The purpose of this chapter is to discuss the available evidence concerning the physiology of the LCAT reaction and to emphasize present concepts concerning the reaction's function even though some are still highly speculative.

II. REACTION MECHANISM

A. Lipid Reactants

When Sperry (2) first discovered that cholesterol becomes esterified during the incubation of human plasma, he thought that the reaction was caused by a plasma cholesterol esterase and suggested that the fatty acids involved were derived from the hydrolytic breakdown of lecithin by a plasma lipase. Later, however, he and Stoyanoff (3) concluded that the cholesterol-esterifying enzymes that they had found in human, monkey, and dog serums differed from the cholesteryl-ester-hydrolyzing enzyme present only in dog serum. Nevertheless, this observation apparently was not appreciated by many subsequent investigators, because the impression lingered (4–6) that a plasma cholesterol esterase and a plasma lecithinase are involved in the esterification reaction, and it was not until 1962 that the reaction was shown to be catalyzed by a transacylase (7, 8). At that time the reaction mechanism shown in Fig. 1 was proposed, mainly on the basis of the following evidence:

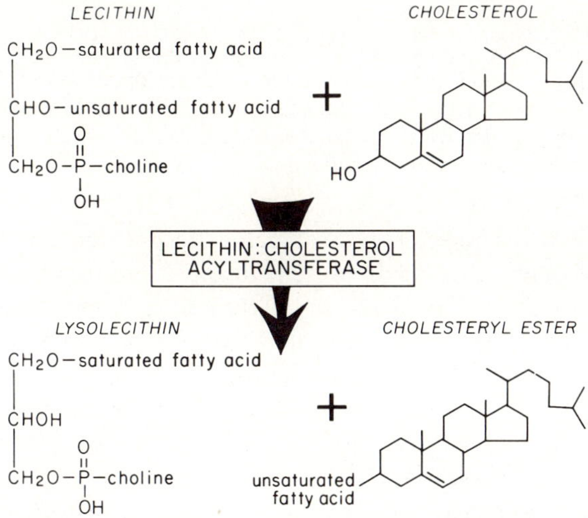

Fig. 1 Principal reaction catalyzed by plasma lecithin:cholesterol acyltransferase.

1. Labeled cholesteryl esters are formed when plasma is incubated either with radioactive cholesterol or with lecithin that contains radioactive unsaturated fatty acids, but not when plasma is incubated with radioactive free fatty acids (7). This indicates that the reaction is caused by a transacylase.
2. Unesterified cholesterol and lecithin decrease at nearly equimolar rates during the incubation of plasma. This suggests that lecithin is the principal acyl donor and that approximately one fatty acyl group is transferred per molecule.
3. More than 80% of the fatty acid transferred is unsaturated (8). This provides further evidence that essentially one fatty acid is transferred per lecithin molecule and indicates that most of the fatty acids originate from the 2-position (9).

It should be noted that Fig. 1 in no way represents the complete reaction mechanism. For example, it does not explain why 10 to 15% of the fatty

Table I. Comparison of Fatty Acids Transferred to Cholesterol with Fatty Acids of the 2-Position of Lecithin[a]

Fatty Acid	Cholesteryl Esters (% radioactivity)	Lecithin (mole % fatty acids released by venom)
Δ:0	12.3	3.5
Δ:1	20.6	14.5
Δ:2	56.6	56.5
Δ:⩾4	10.5	25.4

[a] In this experiment human plasma free of low-density lipoproteins (LDL) was incubated with ^{14}C-cholesterol for 6 hr, and the distribution of radioactivity in the cholesteryl esters was compared with the fatty acid composition of the fatty acid released from the lipoprotein lecithin by *Crotalus adamanteus* venom. (From Ref. 1.)

acid transferred to cholesterol is saturated despite the much smaller proportion of saturated fatty acids present in the 2-position of lecithin (Table I). Further, it does not explain why saturated and monounsaturated fatty acids in preference to tetraunsaturated fatty acids are transferred to the cholesterol of human-plasma lipoproteins.

One possibility is that human-plasma LCAT preferentially transfers saturated and monounsaturated fatty acids from the 2-position. This would contrast with the apparent specificity of rat-plasma LCAT, which transfers arachidonic acid in nearly the same proportion as it is present in the 2-position of rat-plasma lecithin (8, 10). However, it is also possible that other types of intermolecular transfer are involved. For example, early experiments (7) showed that small amounts of cholesteryl ^{14}C-palmitate are formed during the incubation of plasma with emulsified ^{14}C-tripalmitin. Later Shah, Lossow, and Chaikoff (11) confirmed and extended these observations and suggested that the enzyme first transfers labeled palmitoyl groups from the triglyceride to lecithin and then from the lecithin to cholesterol. Another possibility not yet excluded is that the fatty acids in the 1-position of lecithin are transferred directly or indirectly to cholesterol. Thus the amount of lysolecithin that can be demonstrated after the incubation of plasma is always less than would be predicted from the mechanism shown in Fig. 1 (12; Fig. 2) and glycerylphosphorylcholine accumulates (13). Although the presence of a lysolecithinase in plasma might explain both observations, the possible involvement of LCAT deserves further exploration.

B. Lipoprotein Substrates

A second and particularly important feature of the reaction not shown in Fig. 1 concerns the influence of lipoprotein structure on the character of the LCAT reaction. In view of their amphipathic properties, both lecithin and unesterified cholesterol would be expected to be located on the surfaces of plasma lipoproteins, and the LCAT reaction presumably occurs there as well. In contrast, the lysolecithin (and probably also the cholesteryl ester) to a large extent leaves the lipoprotein surface. Figure 2 shows that

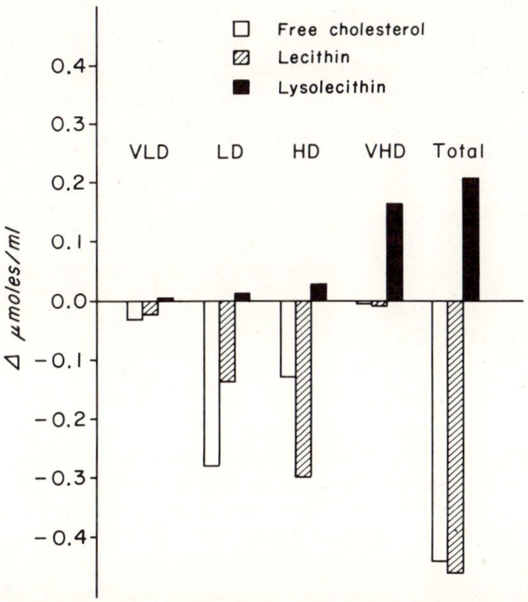

Fig. 2 Changes in lipoprotein cholesterol and phospholipids during incubation of plasma. Aliquots of human plasma were incubated with and without *p* hydroxymercuribenzoate and subsequently fractionated by preparative ultracentrifugation. The figure shows the differences in the distribution of unesterified cholesterol, lecithin, and lysolecithin in the active compared with the blocked plasma. VLD = lipoproteins of $d < 1.006$ g/ml; LD = lipoproteins of *d* 1.006–1.063 g/ml; HD = lipoproteins of *d* 1.063–1.21 g/ml; VHD = lipoproteins of $d > 1.21$ g/ml. (From Ref. 12.)

most of the lysolecithin formed during a 24-hr incubation of human plasma becomes associated with the $d > 1.21$ g/ml proteins; and the experiments of Switzer and Eder (14) suggest that the lysolecithin-binding protein in this fraction is albumin. As for the bulky, nonpolar cholesteryl esters, their physical properties make it likely that they would be displaced away from the lipoprotein surface to some position in the interior of the molecule. Consequently the fact that the LCAT reaction causes a net formation of cholesteryl esters at the expense of unesterified cholesterol and lecithin may be due to changes in the positions of the reactants after attack by the enzyme.

It is also possible that the location of specific molecules of lecithin and unesterified cholesterol affects the specificity of the LCAT reaction. Thus the relative lack of transfer of tetraunsaturated fatty acids from the lecithin to the cholesterol of human-plasma lipoproteins might depend on the specific position of arachidonoyl lecithin on lipoproteins.

That lipoprotein structure is an important determinant of the character of the LCAT reaction is directly indicated by the fact that not all plasma lipoproteins react equally well with the enzyme. This can be demonstrated by separately incubating human-plasma lipoprotein fractions with partially purified (essentially lipid-free) LCAT. The results of an experiment of this type are shown in Table II. Clearly, during the 24-hr incubation period

Table II. Incubation of Human-Plasma Lipoproteins with LCAT[a]

Lipoprotein Class	Unesterified Cholesterol (micromoles/ml)		
	0 hr	24 hr	P[b]
HDL	0.260	0.065	<.001
LDL	0.365	0.320	<.05
VLDL	0.758	0.747	N.S.

[a] The VLDL, LDL, and HDL fractions were prepared by ultracentrifugation and incubated with partially purified (essentially lipid-free) LCAT for 24 hr at 37°C. The concentration of LCAT was approximately equal to that in fresh human plasma. (Modified from Ref. 15.)
[b] Student's "*t*" test.

employed in this experiment, the high-density lipoproteins (HDL) reacted most extensively, whereas the low-density lipoproteins (LDL) reacted to a lesser degree, and the very-low-density lipoproteins (VLDL) did not react significantly. It should be noted that this type of experiment provides only an approximation and not an exact comparison of the ability of these lipoproteins to act as substrates. First, the table shows the relative extent, rather than the initial rate, of esterification. Second, exact comparison is difficult because of the problem of rigorously defining the substrate lipoproteins. The lipoprotein fractions obtained in the ultracentrifuge are classes of molecules rather than single lipoproteins, and each class is heterogeneous not only with respect to density and molecular weight, but also with respect to composition. Moreover, as suggested above, even the individual lecithin and unesterified cholesterol molecules of a single lipoprotein may not all be equally accessible to the enzyme.

The problem of lipoprotein heterogeneity is particularly relevant in the case of the HDL. Not only are the HDL a heterogeneous class of lipoproteins, but individual HDL subfractions react differentially with LCAT. The compositional heterogeneity of the HDL class has been demonstrated by ultracentrifugation (16) and by gel filtration (17). In both cases the results suggest that the HDL are composed not of three subfractions (HDL_1, HDL_2, and HDL_3), as commonly inferred from data obtained in the analytical ultracentrifuge (18), but rather of a large population of molecules. Figures 3 and 4 show the type of separation obtained when human-plasma

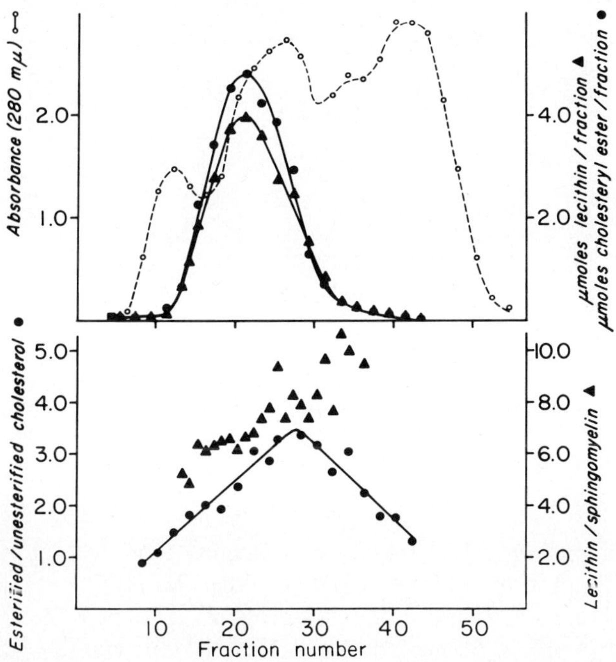

Fig. 3 Subfractionation of human-plasma $d > 1.063$ g/ml proteins on Sephadex G-200. The relative position of the HDL compared with the other plasma proteins is indicated in the top section of the figure. The lower section shows the relative lipid composition of the subfractions that comprise the HDL peak. (From Ref. 17.)

HDL are filtered through columns of Sephadex G-200. In both experiments the VLDL and LDL fractions were removed from human plasma by chromatography on hydroxyapatite before filtering the remaining plasma proteins through the gel. In both figures the position of the HDL fraction relative to that of the other plasma proteins is shown and the lipid compositions of the several HDL subfractions are compared. The compositions of these HDL subfractions clearly vary in a complex way as a function of elution

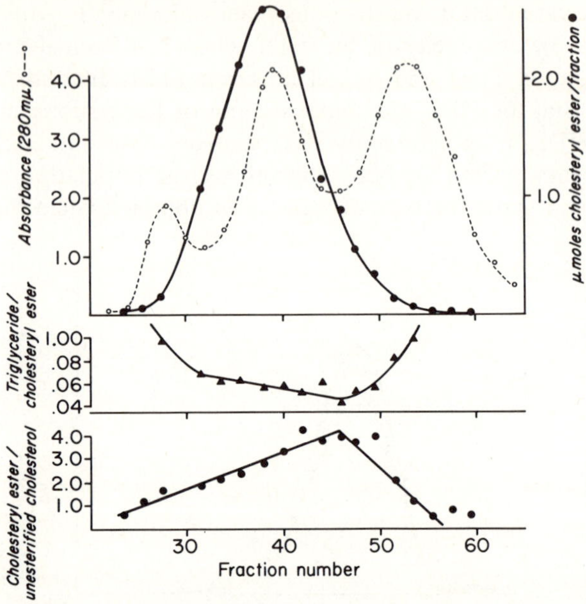

Fig. 4 Subfractionation of $d > 1.063$ g/ml proteins of human plasma on Sephadex G-200. Plasma from a human female fed a high-carbohydrate diet for 4 days before starting the fractionation. The procedure was the same as that followed in the experiment shown in Fig. 3, except that triglycerides were measured instead of phospholipids. (W. King and J. A. Glomset, unpublished experiments.)

volume and, presumably, of molecular weight. Moreover, it is difficult to explain this variation except by assuming that the HDL peak is composed of a large number of individual lipoproteins. The possible basis of this heterogeneity will be discussed later. What is important here is that the individual HDL molecules react differentially with LCAT, as demonstrated by the gel-filtration experiment shown in Fig. 5. In this experiment human whole blood was incubated with ^{14}C-cholesterol for 1 hr before the plasma was separated, the VLDL and LDL fractions were removed, and the remaining proteins were subfractionated on Sephadex. The lower part of the figure shows the specific activity of the cholesteryl esters in the HDL subfractions. The HDL of lower apparent molecular weight—that is, those corresponding to the subfractions with the highest lecithin-to-sphingomyelin ratios in Fig. 3—have cholesteryl esters with the highest specific activity, and the most probable explanation of this is that they have reacted preferentially with LCAT.

Why HDL, and particularly the smaller HDL subfractions, are preferred substrates of LCAT is not known with certainty. However, both the rela-

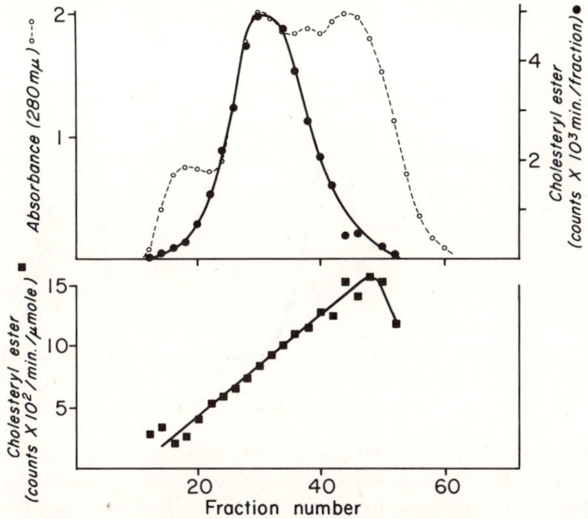

Fig. 5 Incorporation of ^{14}C-cholesterol into the cholesteryl esters of human-plasma HDL. Whole blood was incubated with ^{14}C-cholesterol for 1 hr, and the plasma $d > 1.063$ g/ml proteins were subsequently fractionated on Sephadex G-200. The upper section of the figure shows the position of the HDL peak relative to the other plasma proteins. The lower section shows the specific activity of the HDL subfraction cholesteryl esters. (From Ref. 17.)

tive content of lecithin compared with unesterified cholesterol and the relative content of HDL apoprotein may be important. Nichols and Gong (19) have concluded from model experiments that LCAT reacts more favorably with lipid–protein aggregates that contain lecithin and unesterified cholesterol in a ratio of 3:1 than with aggregates that contain the same lipids in a ratio of 1:1. Presumably the lecithin, unesterified cholesterol, and apoprotein make up specific sites on the lipoprotein surface that have a special affinity for LCAT. Some evidence in support of this has been provided by recent studies of the binding of LCAT to lipoproteins. These studies were performed with human-plasma HDL that had been coupled to agarose gel activated with cyanogen bromide (20); LCAT reacts with these agarose-coupled HDL molecules, and LCAT that has been partially purified also binds to them. This can be shown by passing a solution of enzyme through a column of HDL–agarose and comparing the activity in the effluent to that in the effluent from control columns containing agarose alone. The experiment in Fig. 6 shows an example of this. Two separate control columns were employed: one with agarose gel alone, and one with agarose gel that had been pretreated with cyanogen bromide and then washed in the same way as the HDL–agarose. Equal aliquots of partially purified human-plasma

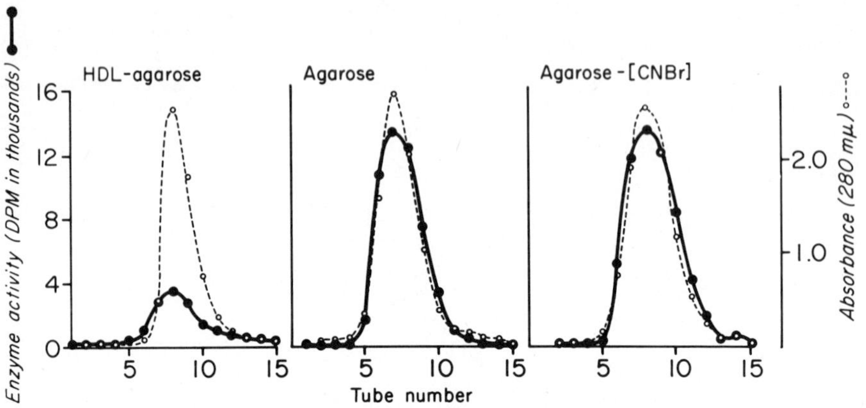

Fig. 6 Adsorption of LCAT on HDL–agarose. Aliquots of partially purified LCAT were passed through columns of HDL–agarose, untreated agarose, and agarose that had been treated with cyanogen bromide. LCAT activity and absorbance measurements in the effluent from the three columns indicate specific adsorption of LCAT on HDL. (From Ref. 20.)

LCAT were passed through each column, and approximately equal amounts of protein were recovered in the effluents. However, *considerably less LCAT was recovered from the HDL–agarose column* than from the control columns. This must have been caused by selective adsorption of the enzyme to the HDL–agarose, because LCAT activity subsequently could be eluted from the HDL–agarose column, but not from the two control columns.[1]

Another procedure has been used to compare the binding of LCAT to different soluble lipoproteins (Y. Akanuma and J. A. Glomset, unpublished experiments). In this procedure LCAT is incubated with a suspension of HDL–agarose in tris buffer, and the bound and free enzymes are subsequently separated by low-speed centrifugation. When soluble HDL are included in the incubation mixture, the amount of enzyme bound to the HDL–agarose is inversely proportional to the amount of free HDL in the solution. In other words, the bound and free HDL compete for the enzyme. Then, if other free lipoproteins, such as VLDL or LDL, are included, their affinity for LCAT can be investigated by determining whether a similar, inverse relation exists. Experiments of this type have demonstrated that LCAT binds preferentially to HDL, suggesting that the special reactivity

[1] Raz, Kummerow, and Nishida (21) were unable to demonstrate the binding of LCAT to HDL, but they employed the crude plasma protein fraction of $d > 1.21$ g/ml and separated LCAT and HDL by prolonged centrifugation at a density of 1.21 g/ml; this probably disrupted any HDL–LCAT complexes present.

of HDL with LCAT is related to the ability of these lipoproteins to form reactive complexes with the enzyme. Furthermore, additional experiments that have been performed suggest that HDL apoprotein is involved in this complex formation. In these experiments LCAT was incubated with agarose that had been coupled to HDL apoprotein, and binding of the enzyme to the apoprotein alone was demonstrated.

III. PROPERTIES OF THE ENZYME

A. Assay

The most widely used assay (22) for the enzyme is convenient but limited. It is based on the fact that the enzyme forms labeled cholesteryl esters when incubated with lipoproteins containing radioactive unesterified cholesterol. A lipoprotein substrate is formed by heating plasma at 56 to 60°C for 30 min and then equilibrating it with radioactive cholesterol. A small volume of the enzyme solution to be tested is added to the substrate, and the mixture is incubated for 3 to 6 hr. Subsequently the reaction is stopped by adding several volumes of chloroform–methanol, the lipids are extracted and chromatographed on thin-layer plates of silica gel, and the radioactive cholesteryl ester is measured.

This simple procedure is adequate for such purposes as following enzyme activity during chromatographic separations. However, for more accurate work the specific activity of the unesterified cholesterol in the mixture must be determined and used to calculate the amount of cholesteryl ester formed. Even under these conditions the validity of the measurement depends on the degree of equilibration of the radioactive cholesterol with the unesterified cholesterol of the substrate lipoproteins, and Rose (23) has shown that this can be very complex. Also, heated plasma is far from an ideal substrate because it is neither well defined nor reproducible. As already mentioned, the plasma lipoproteins react differentially with the enzyme, and both the absolute and the relative amounts of the various lipoprotein subfractions can vary. Clearly a stable artificial substrate would be preferable to heated plasma. However, even when artificial mixtures of lecithin and unesterified cholesterol are used, as in the experiments of Nichols and Gong (19), the amount of endogenous lipoprotein and apoprotein in the final incubation mixture is a critical variable.

At times investigators have "assayed" LCAT simply by incubating fresh nonradioactive plasma at 37°C and measuring the change in cholesterol. This "assay" does not effectively measure absolute levels of enzyme activity independently of substrate. Nevertheless, measurements of the initial rate of the LCAT reaction by this approach probably provide the best approximation of the rate of cholesterol esterification by the reaction *in vivo*. If this approach is to be used, it is important that all measurements be made during a time when the reaction follows essentially zero-order kinetics [1–3 hr in the case of human plasma (24), but not necessarily for the same period in the plasma of other species]. Measurements made after longer periods of incubation (in much of the early work incubations were carried out for 24 hr or more) provide information that is more difficult to interpret and is related largely to the substrate rather than to the enzyme.

B. Purification and Physical Properties

Two principal methods are available for the purification of LCAT. One (Y. Akanuma, C. Mitchell, and J. A. Glomset, unpublished results), based on a chromatographic method described earlier (25), utilizes human plasma as starting material and employs the following steps in sequence: chromatography on diethylaminoethyl (DEAE) cellulose, precipitation with ammonium sulfate, preparative ultracentrifugation at a density of 1.25 g/ml, chromatography on hydroxyapatite, and affinity chromatography on HDL–Sepharose. This procedure makes use of the fact that bile salt solutions release bound LCAT from HDL–Sepharose (Fig. 7). It yields a preparation that is about 1200 times purified in comparison to the starting plasma. A second, considerably simpler, method has been used by Ho and Nichols

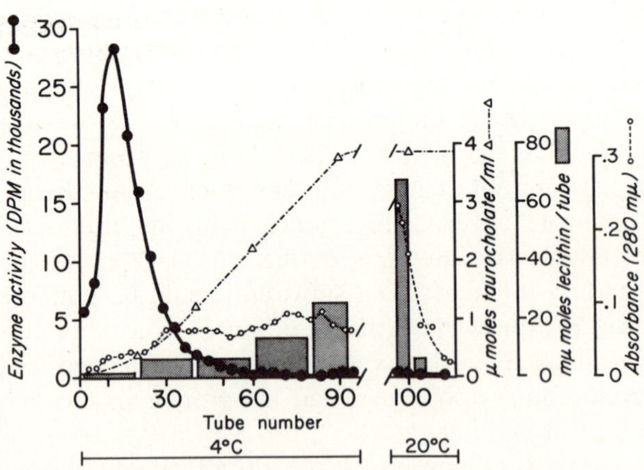

Fig. 7 Elution of LCAT from HDL–agarose. Partially purified LCAT was adsorbed on HDL–agarose and subsequently eluted by means of a sodium taurocholate gradient. Measurements of lecithin in the effluent indicate disruption of the HDL. (From Ref. 20.)

(26). In this method plasma is centrifuged at a density of 1.21 g/ml to remove most of the lipoproteins, and the infranatant is subsequently adsorbed to a sonicated dispersion of lecithin. Desorption in the presence of taurocholate yields a preparation reported to be about 500 times purified.[2]

Relatively little is known about the physical properties of the enzyme. Not only are the most highly purified preparations of the enzyme still contaminated with other proteins, but in addition the fact that LCAT tends to form complexes with HDL presents a problem. Thus when human serum is fractionated by zone electrophoresis (Fig. 8), the LCAT activity over-

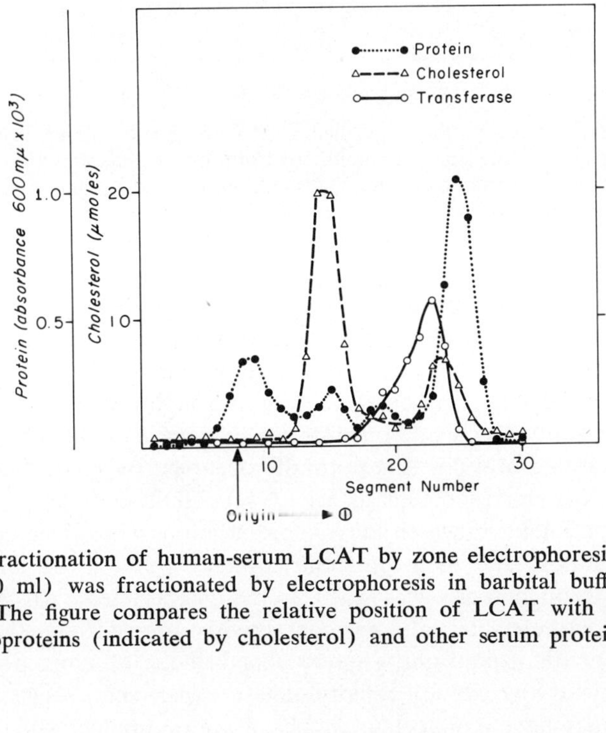

Fig. 8 Fractionation of human-serum LCAT by zone electrophoresis. Fresh human serum (20 ml) was fractionated by electrophoresis in barbital buffer, pH 8.6, on Pevikon. The figure compares the relative position of LCAT with that of the α_1 and β-lipoproteins (indicated by cholesterol) and other serum proteins. (From Ref. 25.)

laps the position of the α_1-lipoproteins. However, as much as two-thirds of the enzyme activity is lost, and the possibility has not been excluded that the detected activity is mainly that of a stable HDL–LCAT complex; that is, the free enzyme may migrate in a different position but quickly lose its

[2] Recently a third method for purifying LCAT has been reported (C. J. Fielding and P. E. Fielding, *FEBS Letters,* Vol. 15, page 355, 1971). This method, which employs desorption of the enzyme from native HDL, yields a highly purified enzyme preparation and should permit definitive studies of the enzyme's physical properties.

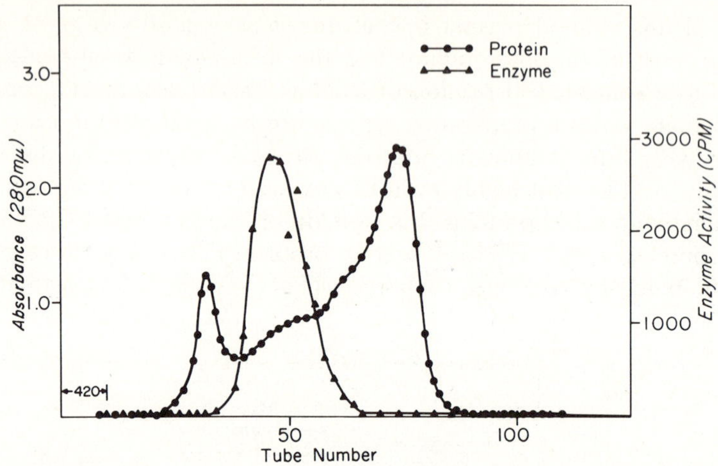

Fig. 9 Fractionation of partially purified LCAT by gel filtration. Human-plasma LCAT previously purified approximately eightfold by chromatography on DEAE-cellulose was filtered through Sephadex G-200. Aliquots of the effluent were analyzed for LCAT activity and for protein. (From Ref. 25.)

activity when separated from stabilizing plasma proteins. A similar phenomenon also may occur on gel filtration. In the experiment shown in Fig. 9 a plasma fraction that had been purified approximately eightfold by chromatography on DEAE-cellulose was filtered through a column of Sephadex G-200. Again, only about one-third of the enzyme activity was recovered, and it was detected in a position normally occupied by HDL (see Fig. 3). That this activity corresponded to an LCAT–HDL complex is suggested by further experiments in which enzyme preparations were chromatographed on DEAE-cellulose and then ultracentrifuged to remove the HDL before being passed through Sephadex G-200. In these experiments (J. A. Glomset and W. King, unpublished) the enzyme activity emerged later than the activity shown in Fig. 9 and only slightly ahead of the albumin peak. Moreover, the enzyme lost activity rapidly. These experiments suggest that the free enzyme may have a molecular weight of approximately 100,000. However, attempts to further define the molecular weight have been deferred pending further purification studies because of the possibility that the enzyme may still be in aggregate form.

C. Distribution in Tissues

Most enzymes that can be detected in plasma are not specific plasma enzymes (27). They catalyze reactions that involve intracellular, rather than extracellular, substrates; they are present in much greater concentrations in tissues than in the plasma; and they have no apparent physiological function in plasma. On the other hand, a few enzymes are specific for plasma, and LCAT is apparently one of these. As already mentioned, it acts primarily on the plasma HDL and LDL; Table III shows that it is present in considerably greater concentrations in rat plasma than in rat tissues; and evidence discussed later indicates that it is an important source of plasma cholesteryl esters in several species *in vivo*. The data in Table III were obtained from experiments in which rat tissues were perfused with

Table III. The Relative Cholesterol-Esterifying Activity of Rat Tissues[a]

Tissue	Relative Activity	Tissue	Relative Activity
Plasma	1.00	Blood cells	0.02
Liver	0.18	Heart	0.12
Intestinal mucosa	0.20	Lung	0.11
Spleen	0.09	Skin	0.04
Kidney	0.11	Brain	0.24
Adrenal[b]	0.18	Muscle	0.04
Testes	0.08	Adipose tissue	0.13

[a] Rat tissues were perfused with 0.25 *M* sucrose *in situ*, homogenized, and incubated with heated, radioactive substrate. The activity per gram wet weight of each tissue was compared with that of 1 ml of plasma. (From Ref. 28.)
[b] Assayed in the presence of 0.01 *M* ethylenediaminetetraacetic acid.

cold 0.25 *M* sucrose *in situ*, homogenized, and incubated in heated plasma that contained radioactive cholesterol. The activity of the homogenates was compared with that of plasma from the same rats; and control experiments were performed to correct for possible inhibitory effects by the tissues. Clearly, rat plasma contains a considerably higher concentration of LCAT than any of the tissues. Moreover, the relative amount of LCAT activity in the plasma–interstitial fluid pool may be even greater than suggested by the table, because the perfusion probably was not completely effective and because other types of cholesterol-esterifying enzymes could have contributed to the tissue activity.

The low activity of the liver homogenates is particularly noteworthy because of the evidence (see Section IV.B) that LCAT may be formed in the liver. Akiyama, Minari, and Sakagami (29) have studied the liver enzyme in some detail. In contrast to the ATP-dependent and coenzyme A–dependent cholesterol-esterifying enzyme in microsomes (30), it is present in the soluble fraction. It forms labeled cholesteryl esters from radioactive lecithin or "cephalin," and, like the plasma enzyme, it is inhibited by *N*-ethylmaleimide. However, under the incubation conditions employed by Akiyama et al., the pH optimum of the reaction was 6.5, rather than 7.3 as in plasma. Therefore it is not entirely certain that the liver enzyme is identical with the plasma enzyme, although the possibility has not been ruled out that the soluble-liver-enzyme activity may simply reflect contamination by LCAT present in the space of Disse.

D. Distribution in Species

It is known that LCAT activity is present in the plasma of many species, but the relative levels of activity in different species have never been systematically compared. The enzyme is present in the plasma of not only humans, monkeys, dogs, and rats, but also rabbits (31, 32), calves and sheep (J. A. Glomset, unpublished experiments), and chickens (33). Recently Puppione (34) studied the plasma of some marine animals (harbor seals, a walrus pup, and a killer whale) and found evidence of only minimal LCAT activity. His results suggest that comparative studies of the distribution of LCAT in different species might provide valuable insight into the physiology of the reaction.

IV. REGULATION OF THE REACTION

A. Regulation *in vitro*

The rate of the LCAT reaction *in vitro* is influenced by several factors. One of these is pH. As indicated above, the pH optimum of the reaction in rat plasma is 7.3 (29). Furthermore, the pH optimum of the human-plasma enzyme also lies in the range 7 to 8 (2, 25). This is significant in view of the likelihood that the reaction is physiologically important *in vivo* (see Section V.A). The reaction also is affected by ionic strength. It is faster in physiological saline than in more dilute salt solution, and it is inhibited by higher concentrations of salt (21, 25). Finally, although LCAT seems to be a sulfhydryl enzyme (see below) and readily becomes oxidized when partially purified, the addition of mercaptoethanol to fresh plasma does not increase the rate of the reaction (J. A. Glomset, unpublished results). This suggests that the physiological antioxidant effect of albumin and other components of plasma is sufficient to maintain the enzyme in the active, reduced state *in vivo*.

Among the other factors that influence the LCAT reaction *in vitro* are some that clearly affect the enzyme directly. As already mentioned, heating at 56 to 60°C for 30 min irreversibly inactivates LCAT without appreciably altering the capacity of the plasma lipoproteins to act as substrates. Furthermore, LCAT is also inactivated by lowering the pH of plasma below 6.0 (J. A. Glomset, unpublished experiments) and by such reagents as *p*-hydroxymercuribenzoate, iodoacetate, or *N*-ethylmaleimide (1). Of these reagents, the first has the advantage that it can be removed from the enzyme by adding an excess of mercaptoethanol or some related sulfhydryl compound. This suggests that a sulfhydryl group plays an important role in maintaining the enzyme's active configuration, or that it is a part of the enzyme's active center. Other reagents that inactivate the enzyme are diisopropyl fluorophosphate (35), paraoxon (36), and urea in high concentration (25).

The LCAT reaction can be stimulated or inhibited *in vitro* by factors that modify the plasma-lipoprotein substrates. The *extent* of the reaction (the total amount of cholesteryl ester formed during a prolonged incubation) can be increased by adding lecithin (37) or by adding extracts of group A streptococci (38). The increase caused by lecithin is probably due to increased substrate availability, although more subtle changes in lipoprotein structure may also be involved. The effect of the streptococcal extracts seems to be due to a selective enzymic alteration of HDL (38). Unfortunately, relatively little is known about the nature of this alteration except that cholesteryl esters are released from the lipoprotein. Without question, the enzymic alteration involved deserves further study. Among the factors that inhibit the LCAT reaction *in vitro* are 4 to 6 m*M* concentrations of bile salts (39). In these concentrations bile salts disrupt HDL (Fig. 7). Phospholipases have a similar effect (11, 40). Also thymol (4), saponin (41), and phlorizin (4) probably inhibit the reaction by interacting with lipoproteins. Finally, ions exert both stimulatory and inhibitory effects, although neither is well understood. Polyvalent anions like phosphate or sulfate stimulate the reaction, whereas Mg^{2+} and Ca^{2+} inhibit it (25).

B. Regulation *in vivo*

Relatively little is known about the factors that regulate the LCAT reaction *in vivo,* nor have any activators or inhibitors of the reaction as yet been identified in plasma. The rate of the reaction probably depends mainly on the level of enzyme activity in plasma and on the level and composition of the plasma lipoprotein substrates. Unfortunately, few investigators have analyzed the influence of such factors as physiological conditions and diet on the levels of *both* LCAT *and* its substrates. Nevertheless, some studies deserve mention.

Wagner and Poindexter (42) and Gherondache (43) studied the influence of age on the esterification of cholesterol during the incubation of human plasma and concluded that plasma-cholesterol-esterifying activity decreases with age. However, they measured the extent, rather than the initial rate, of the esterification reaction. Consequently their studies do not provide evidence of the effect of age on either the level of LCAT activity in plasma or the possible rate of the reaction *in vivo*. All they indicate is that either the enzyme or the substrate or both are affected by age. Therefore further studies need to be done, particularly in view of the known influence of age on both the level of cholesterol and the ratio of cholesterol to cholesteryl esters in human plasma (44).

Sex appears to exert a variable influence on the plasma-cholesterol-esterification reaction in different species. No certain influence has been demonstrated in humans, although only Gherondache's study (43) bears on this question. His results indicate that the absolute amount of cholesterol esterified during a 48-hr incubation does not differ in males and females. In rats, however, a sex difference may exist. Aftergood and Alfin-Slater (45) incubated the serums of male and female rats for 5 hr and found that significantly less cholesterol became esterified in the former, whereas no sex differences were present in the serums of immature rats. Aftergood and Alfin-Slater did not attempt to determine whether the sex difference in the serums of the mature rats was due to a difference in the level of LCAT or in the level or composition of the lipoprotein substrates, but the latter may have been the case because more arachidonic acid was present in the serum phospholipids and cholesteryl esters of the females than of the males, even though the total-serum-cholesterol levels did not differ significantly.

In a related subsequent study Aftergood, Hernandez, and Alfin-Slater (46) administered Enovid, a mixture of estrogenic and progestational compounds, to female rats and found evidence of a further increase in the rate of plasma-cholesterol esterification. The mixture of sex hormones decreased the total plasma cholesterol and also the relative amount of cholesteryl ester, but when plasma from the treated rats was incubated for 4 hr, a much larger proportion of the cholesterol became esterified. Again, this type of study does not differentiate between effects on the level of enzyme activity and effects on the substrates, and it provides no information about the rate of the reaction *in vivo*. Therefore it clearly should be extended, particularly in view of the findings of Sugano, Chinen, and Wada (33) on the influence of sex on the rate of cholesterol esterification in chickens. The Japanese authors found that the rate of esterification is greater in male chickens than in laying hens, and suggested that this may be related to differences in HDL.

Several studies of the effect of diet on the LCAT reaction have been reported. By far the most thorough of these is that of Sugano and Portman (47), who found that LCAT activity is increased in essential-fatty-acid-deficient rats. Their study illustrates the fact that the overall rate of the LCAT reaction can depend on the lipoprotein substrates as well as on the level of LCAT activity. They showed that more cholesterol becomes esterified during a 5-hr incubation in plasma from deficient rats than in plasma from control rats. They also assayed LCAT directly by incubating aliquots of fresh plasma with radioactive, heated substrate prepared from either deficient or control rats. They found that the activity was high in the deficient rats, irrespective of the substrate, and also that the lipoproteins from the deficient rats were better substrates. Finally, they studied the rate of plasma-cholesterol esterification *in vivo* and found that it also was greater in the deficient rats.

Wells and Hogan (48) have studied the effect of other types of dietary deficiency on plasma-cholesterol esterification in rats. Enzyme activity, measured by a radioactive-substrate method similar to that mentioned earlier, was increased by diets deficient in pantothenic acid or choline and decreased by a diet deficient in inositol. Finally, Swell and Law (49) have reported that the rate of the LCAT reaction is increased in fasting rats, although they did not establish whether the faster rate is caused by altered enzyme or by altered substrate levels.

The study of Wells and Rongone (31) suggests that plasma-cholesterol esterification also may be affected by the amount of cholesterol in the diet. They fed rabbits cholesterol, produced the usual hypercholesteremia, measured LCAT activity by a radioactive-substrate method, and concluded that the enzyme activity increases as a function of the plasma unesterified cholesterol. However, they apparently based their calculations on the assumption that the unesterified cholesterol of their enzyme samples equilibrated instantaneously with the radioactive cholesterol of the substrate; and this is unlikely. Therefore the effect of hypercholesteremia on LCAT levels in rabbits needs further evaluation, particularly since Shapiro, Jastremsky, and Kritchevsky (50) incubated the serum of cholesterol-fed rabbits, rats, and chickens and found that the changes in unesterified cholesterol were *less extensive* than those that occurred in serum from control animals. The whole question deserves further study in view of the fact that both Monger and Nestel (51) and Takahashi and Muto (52) have found that plasma LCAT activity is positively correlated with the level of plasma unesterified cholesterol in man.

It is difficult to visualize the mechanisms that underlie the above effects because so little is known about the factors that affect the synthesis and secretion of LCAT and its principal substrates, the HDL. About all that is known at present is that both LCAT and HDL are synthesized in the liver. The first evidence implicating the liver as a site of LCAT synthesis was obtained independently by Turner and Pratt (53) and by Castro Mendoza and Jimenez Diaz (54). Both groups incubated human plasma for 24 hr or more, employed the relative decrease in unesterified cholesterol as a measure of enzyme activity, and concluded that the latter is decreased in patients with liver disease. The Spanish authors also performed animal experiments that suggested that the level of LCAT activity in plasma decreases with progressive liver damage. They ligated the bile ducts of dogs and rats, incubated the plasma from these animals, and found that the percent decrease in unesterified cholesterol caused by the enzyme at first was normal or increased, but later decreased, apparently as a function of liver damage. (The enzyme activity decreased in parallel with a drop in the absolute level of cholesteryl ester in the starting plasma.)

Because they did not measure LCAT activity independently of substrate, the results of Turner and Pratt and of Castro Mendoza and Jimenez Diaz must be qualified. Nevertheless, they are in general agreement with several more recent studies (52, 55–57) including some in which radioactive-substrate assays were employed to measure LCAT activity. Furthermore, other studies also have pointed to a relation between the liver and the enzyme. Brot, Lossow, and Chaikoff (58) showed that the LCAT activity of rat plasma is sharply reduced by removal of the liver, gastrointestinal tract, pancreas, and spleen, and inferred from this that the liver is probably involved in LCAT synthesis. Also, known hepatotoxins like ethionine (59) and carbon tetrachloride (60) reduce LCAT activity in plasma. Finally, several groups (61–63) have been able to demonstrate the release of LCAT by the perfused rat liver.

V. ROLE OF THE REACTION

The physiological role of the LCAT reaction has not been conclusively established. However, enough is known to justify an attempt to put the reaction into metabolic perspective. In the following discussion the role of the reaction is viewed from three different vantage points. First, the reaction's importance as a source of plasma cholesteryl esters is considered. Second, its effect on the composition and properties of plasma lipoproteins is evaluated. Finally, its possible effects on tissues are discussed.

A. Formation of Plasma Cholesteryl Esters

The relative importance of the LCAT reaction as a physiological source of plasma cholesteryl esters is difficult to evaluate. In attempting to assess its importance in a given species several factors must be taken into account. One of these is the initial rate of the reaction *in vitro*. Another, of equal importance, is the rate of formation of plasma cholesteryl esters *in vivo*. This has been measured in only a few species. Where a substantial difference exists between the rates of plasma-cholesteryl-ester formation *in vitro* and *in vivo,* it is reasonable to implicate the cholesterol-esterifying enzymes of the intestine and the liver (64). There is good evidence that in the rat both are involved in the formation of the cholesteryl esters of the $d < 1.063$ g/ml fraction. Indeed, in no species has the role of the intestinal enzyme in the formation of chylomicron cholesteryl esters been questioned. This enzyme is stimulated by bile acids, and preferentially forms cholesteryl oleate and palmitate from the appropriate unesterified fatty acids. Although most of the chylomicron cholesteryl esters circulate only briefly before being taken up and hydrolyzed by the liver, some apparently transfer to other lipoproteins and remain in plasma. The intestinal mucosal cells also form some VLDL (65), so that these cells must also be considered a potential source of VLDL cholesteryl esters in most species.

The role of the cholesterol-esterifying enzyme(s) of the liver may be more variable. An enzyme system present in rat-liver microsomes has been extensively studied (64). Cholesterol esterification by this system requires both ATP and coenzyme A, and preferentially forms cholesteryl oleate and cholesteryl palmitate. There is good evidence (66) that this enzyme is the predominant source of VLDL cholesteryl esters in rats fed cholesterol. As the VLDL are metabolized, some of the cholesteryl esters probably transfer to higher density lipoproteins and the VLDL themselves are probably converted to LDL. Therefore the rat-liver enzyme is probably of considerable importance as a general source of plasma-lipoprotein cholesteryl esters. A similar enzyme may be important in other species as well. However, there is no evidence that it is important or even present in the human liver.

In practical terms the following approach is useful in evaluating the relative importance of the plasma enzyme in any given species. First, the initial rate of the LCAT reaction *in vitro* should be compared with the rate of plasma-cholesterol esterification *in vivo* under the same dietary conditions. Second, the relative importance of LCAT, compared with the intestinal and liver enzymes, can be evaluated by comparing the fatty acid composition of the cholesteryl esters formed by the LCAT reaction with that of the cholesteryl esters of fresh plasma, and by comparing the relative incorporation of radioactive cholesterol into lipoprotein cholesteryl esters *in vitro* and *in vivo*. The results of this approach indicate that the LCAT reaction is the principal source of plasma cholesteryl esters in man. Thus the initial rate of the reaction of the plasma of young adults is about 0.1 micromoles per milliliter of plasma per hour *in vitro* (8), and Nestel and Monger (67) arrived at essentially the same value in their studies of

Table IV. Cholesteryl Esters Formed During the Incubation of Human Plasma *in vitro*[a]

Relative Saturation	Radioactivity Distribution (%)	Mass Distribution (μmole %)
Δ 0	13.3	13.3
Δ 1	19.4	21.8
Δ 2	56.8	55.0
Δ 4	10.6	9.9

[a] Human-plasma proteins with $d > 1.063$ g/ml were incubated for 1 hr with ^{14}C-cholesterol. Then LCAT activity was blocked, and the incubation was continued for 2 hr. Finally, the distribution of radioactivity among the cholesteryl esters was compared with the distribution of mass. (From Ref. 15.)

the rate of plasma-cholesteryl-ester formation in human subjects *in vivo*. Second, the fatty acid composition of the cholesteryl esters formed by the LCAT reaction *in vitro* is essentially identical with that of the cholesteryl esters of fresh plasma (Table IV). Finally, the pattern of incorporation of labeled cholesterol into plasma-lipoprotein cholesteryl esters is similar *in vitro* and *in vivo*. In both cases the cholesteryl esters of the HDL initially have a much higher specific activity than those of either the VLDL, which have the next highest specific activity, or the LDL, which have the lowest specific activity (Figs. 10 and 11). Furthermore, the individual cholesteryl esters of each separate lipoprotein class have essentially identical specific activities whether labeled *in vitro* or *in vivo*, and this suggests that they are formed by a single source.

Although fewer comparisons have been made in lower primates, the data

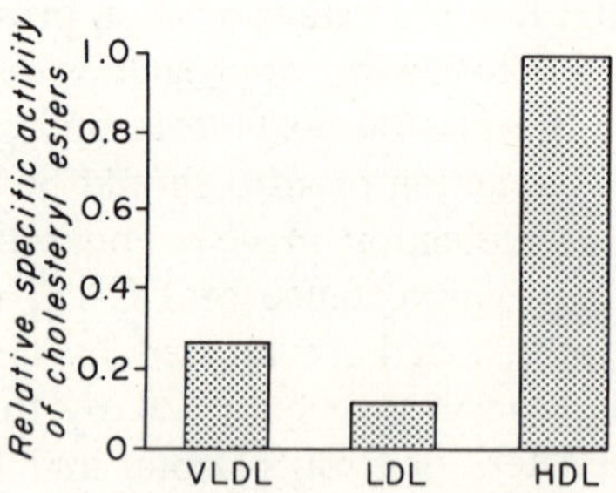

Fig. 10 Incorporation of ^{14}C-cholesteral into human-plasma-lipoprotein cholesteryl esters *in vitro*. Human plasma was incubated for 1 hr with radioactive cholesterol, the plasma lipoproteins were subfractionated by preparative ultracentrifugation, and the specific activity of the lipoprotein cholesteryl esters was determined. (Data from Ref. 15.)

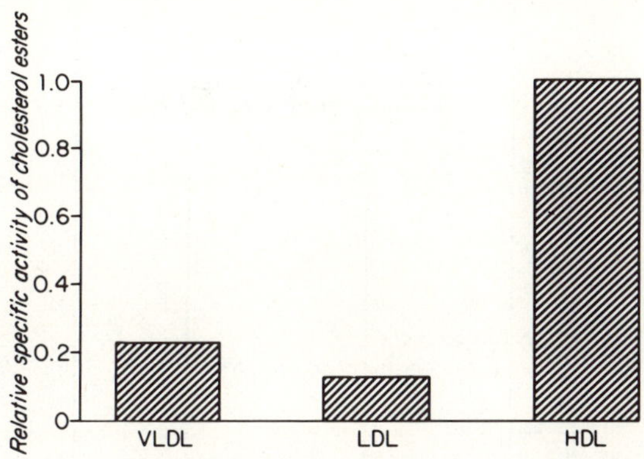

Fig. 11 Incorporation of ^{14}C-mevalonate into human-plasma-lipoprotein cholesteryl esters *in vivo*. A fasting male was injected with radioactive mevalonate. Approximately 2 hr later blood was withdrawn, the plasma lipoproteins were subfractionated by preparative ultracentrifugation, and the specific activity of the lipoprotein cholesteryl esters was determined. (Redrawn from data in Ref. 68.)

suggest that the LCAT reaction is also an important source of plasma cholesteryl esters in monkeys and baboons. Sugano and Portman (69) found that in the cebus monkey the rate of cholesteryl ester formation *in vitro* (estimated from the incorporation of radioactive cholesterol) was 0.24 micromole per milliliter of plasma per hour, whereas the rate of plasma-cholesteryl-ester formation *in vivo* was in approximately the same range (0.17 micromole/ml-hr). They also found that LCAT forms very nearly the same amount of cholesteryl linoleate, but slightly less oleate and slightly more palmitate and arachidonate than are present in fresh plasma (Fig. 12). The relative specific activities of the HDL, VLDL, and LDL cholesteryl esters of lower primates labeled *in vitro* and *in vivo* have not been compared. However, a comparative study of the labeling of the HDL subfraction cholesteryl esters has been carried out in baboons (17), and the results obtained *in vitro* were very similar to those obtained *in vivo*.

Figure 13 shows the results of an *in vitro* labeling experiment. Baboon blood was incubated with radioactive cholesterol for 1 hr at 37°C; the plasma was then separated, VLDL and LDL were removed by chromatography on hydroxyapatite, and the remaining plasma proteins were filtered through a column of Sephadex G-200. As in the gel-filtration experiments with human plasma discussed in Section II.B, the upper part of the figure shows the position of the HDL relative to that of the other plasma proteins, and the lower part shows the specific activity of the HDL cholesteryl esters. The specific activity pattern is clearly similar to that obtained in the *in vivo* experiment shown in Fig. 14, in which a baboon was injected with radio-

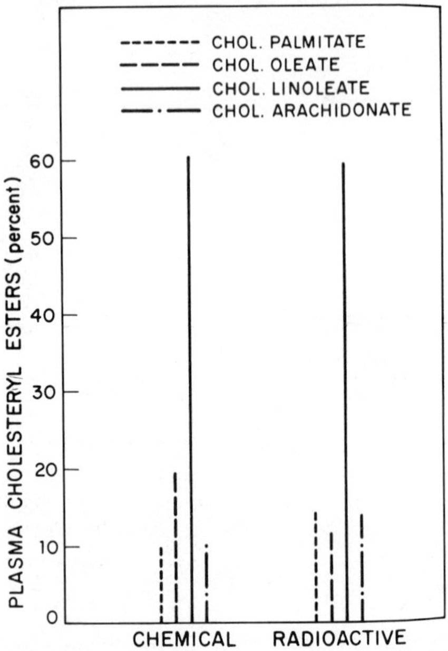

Fig. 12 *In vitro* formation of cholesteryl esters in the plasma of the cebus monkey. Plasma was incubated with ^{14}C-cholesterol, and the distributions of radioactivity and chemical mass in cholesteryl esters were compared. (From Ref. 69.)

active mevalonate. In this experiment blood was withdrawn 1 hr after injection of the labeled precursor, and plasma free of VLDL and LDL was again prepared and filtered through a column of Sephadex G-200. The similarity between the results of the two experiments is excellent evidence of the importance of LCAT in forming HDL cholesteryl esters in the baboon *in vivo*.

In the rat the LCAT reaction appears to be the source of some, but not all, of the plasma cholesteryl esters. Sugano and Portman (69) found that the rate of cholesteryl ester formation in fed rats *in vitro* and *in vivo* is 0.08 and 0.16 micromole per milliliter of plasma per hour, respectively. Furthermore, they found that the LCAT reaction forms more cholesteryl arachidonate and less cholesteryl oleate and palmitate than are present in fresh plasma. Finally, such *in vivo* studies as those of Goodman and Shiratori (71) and Gidez, Roheim, and Eder (66) have shown that the VLDL cholesteryl esters of fed rats are more rapidly labeled than the HDL or LDL cholesteryl esters, and that the cholesteryl palmitate and cholesteryl oleate of the VLDL fraction have considerably higher specific activities than does cholesteryl arachidonate. Taken together, the above experiments strongly suggest that rat-plasma cholesteryl esters are formed by more than one reaction and, furthermore, that the source of most of the VLDL cho-

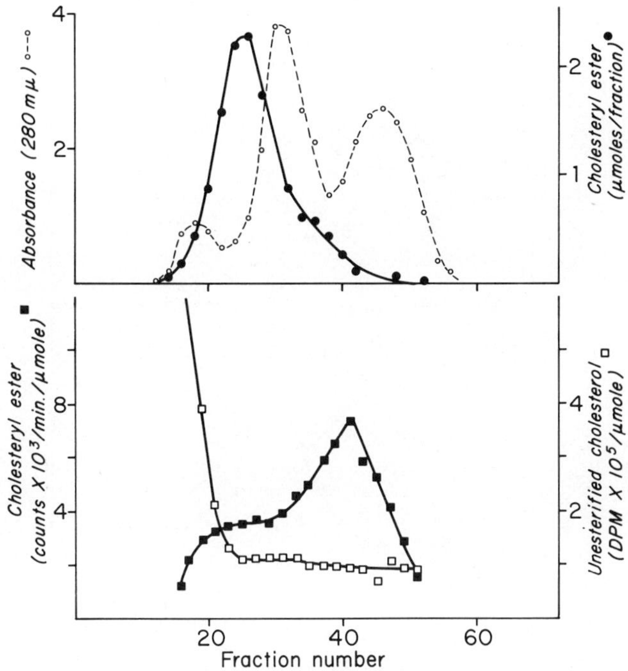

Fig. 13 Incorporation of ^{14}C-cholesterol into baboon-plasma HDL cholesteryl esters *in vitro*. Whole baboon blood was incubated with ^{14}C-cholesterol for 75 min, VLDL and LDL were removed from the plasma, and the remaining plasma proteins were subfractionated on Sephadex G-200. The lower part of the figure shows the specific activity of the esterified and unesterified cholesterol in the HDL subfractions. (From Ref. 70.)

lesteryl esters is the liver microsomal reaction, whereas most of the HDL cholesteryl esters are formed by the LCAT reaction in plasma.

As already indicated, the plasma of some mammals, such as the harbor seal, walrus, whale, and dolphin (34), contains only very low levels of LCAT activity. This also appears to be true of the cow and the sheep (J. A. Glomset, unpublished experiments). Nevertheless, there are not sufficient data to permit an evaluation of the relative role of the LCAT reaction in these species, particularly because so little is known about cholesterol esterification *in vivo*. The same applies to the chicken (33).

B. Influence on the Composition and Properties of Lipoproteins

A major goal of lipoprotein physiology is to determine the full sequence of events from the moment of lipoprotein secretion to the moment of their removal from plasma; and a major goal in the study of the LCAT reaction

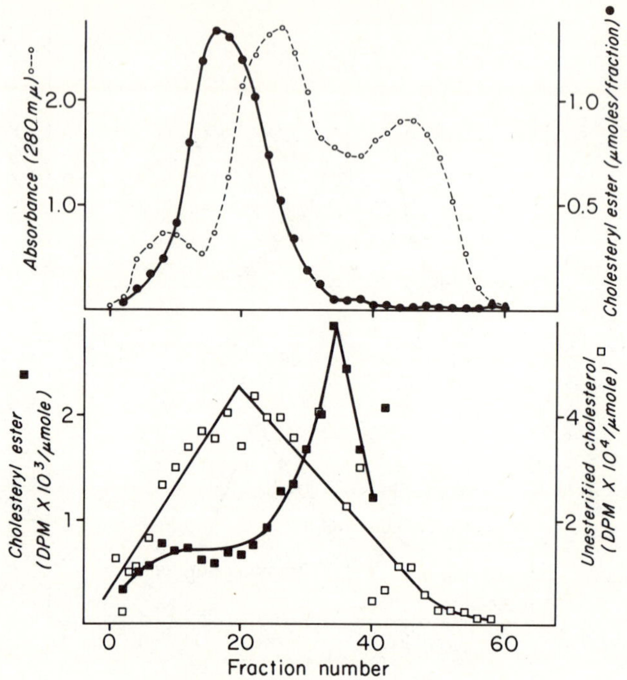

Fig. 14 Incorporation of ^{14}C-mevalonate into baboon-plasma HDL cholesteryl esters *in vivo*. A male baboon was injected with ^{14}C-mevalonate, and 1 hr later plasma was obtained and subfractionated as in the experiment shown in Fig. 13. The lower part of the figure again shows the specific activity of the esterified and unesterified cholesterol in the HDL subfractions. (From Ref. 70.)

is to understand its significance in the perspective of this sequence. That the reaction's role is important, particularly in man, is indicated by the evidence concerning plasma-cholesteryl-ester formation just discussed. This evidence implies that newly secreted lipoproteins contain few, if any, cholesteryl esters and that they also differ in other respects from the cholesteryl-ester-containing lipoproteins commonly recognized in plasma. However, it is difficult to understand the sequence of changes that newly secreted lipoproteins undergo on appearing in plasma. In the first place, the number of different lipoproteins secreted into plasma has not been conclusively established, nor is the exact composition of these lipoproteins at the moment of secretion known. Second, newly secreted lipoproteins probably begin to undergo changes as soon as they enter the plasma. They probably change in polar lipid composition, as suggested by the studies of Minari and Zilversmit (72), who mixed chylomicrons from dog lymph with plasma and ob-

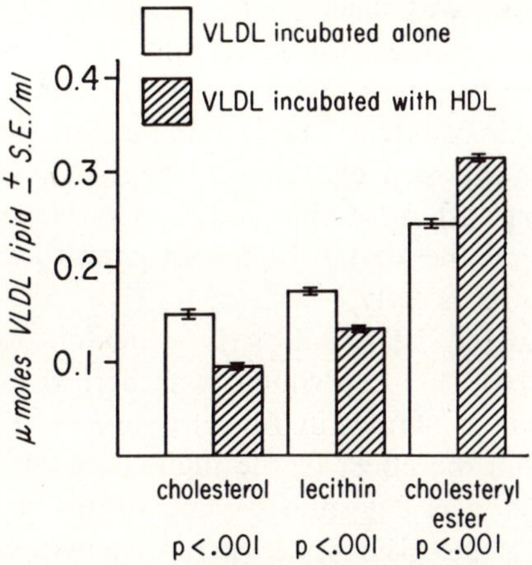

Fig. 15 Nonenzymic transfer of lipid between human VLDL and HDL. The $d > 1.063$ g/ml proteins of human plasma were preincubated for 18 hr. Then LCAT was blocked by adding *p*-chloromercuriphenylsulfonate, VLDL were added, and the incubation was continued for another 18 hr. Finally, the VLDL were removed by adsorption on hydroxyapatite and analyzed. (From Ref. 76.)

served a rapid and apparently nonenzymic loss of lecithin to the plasma and an uptake of unesterified cholesterol from the plasma.[3] Although analogous changes have not yet been demonstrated in the case of other plasma lipoproteins, it is very likely that they occur and that they depend on the difference between the competitive lipoprotein environment within the blood and those at the intracellular sites of lipoprotein formation.

Another change that newly secreted chylomicrons and very-low-density lipoproteins undergo probably involves tissue-bound lipoprotein lipase. There is evidence (74, 75) that this enzyme not only converts triglyceride-rich lipoproteins into higher density molecules by catalyzing the breakdown of their triglyceride but also attacks their lecithin.

Another fact that adds to the complexity of intravascular plasma-lipoprotein metabolism is that the LCAT reaction causes *indirect* as well as direct changes in the composition of plasma lipoproteins. Indeed, these indirect changes may form the basis of the physiological function of the enzyme. They depend on nonenzymic redistributions of lipids among lipoproteins that have reacted differentially with LCAT; and they can be demonstrated convincingly by experiments such as that shown in Fig. 15 (76). In this experiment human-plasma HDL were incubated with LCAT for several

[3] Bierman and Strandness (73) have shown that a change in electrophoretic mobility also occurs under similar conditions.

hours. Then the enzyme was inactivated, VLDL were added, and the incubation was continued. Finally, the HDL and VLDL were separated, and the VLDL lipids were compared with the lipids of VLDL that had been incubated in the absence of HDL. The results indicate that the preincubated HDL decrease the unesterified cholesterol, lecithin, and triglycerides, and increase the cholesteryl esters of the VLDL. Consequently, by acting on the HDL, LCAT affects the VLDL indirectly even though, as indicated in Table II, it cannot do so directly.

That LCAT also affects LDL indirectly is demonstrated by the experiment shown in Fig. 16. This experiment was performed in the same way as the VLDL experiment shown in Fig. 15, except that LDL were substituted for VLDL, and the effect of the incubation on the composition of the preincubated HDL was determined. The results indicate that the unesterified cholesterol of the HDL increased, and, though not shown in this experiment, other results indicate that HDL lecithin also increases under similar circumstances. However, no net change in HDL (or LDL) cholesteryl esters occurred, in contrast to the VLDL experiments.

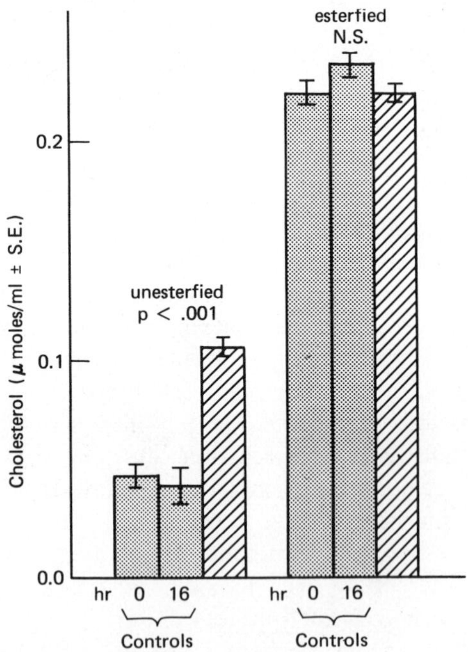

Fig. 16 Nonenzymic transfer of lipid between human LDL and HDL. An experiment analogous to that shown in Fig. 15 was performed, except that LDL were substituted for the VLDL and the HDL were analyzed after the second incubation. (From Ref. 76.)

These redistribution experiments appear to explain the changes previously observed (12) when whole plasma was incubated. Thus in the experiment shown in Fig. 2 aliquots of human plasma were incubated for 24 hr in the presence or absence of active LCAT. The lipoproteins were then fractionated by ultracentrifugation, and their cholesterol and phospholipid compositions were compared. Although the LCAT reaction caused equimolar changes in *total* unesterified cholesterol and lecithin, the changes within each major lipoprotein class were dissimilar. These results can be explained by assuming a direct, preferential action of LCAT on HDL and a lesser, direct action of the enzyme on LDL, coupled with nonenzymic transfers of unesterified cholesterol and lecithin from the VLDL and LDL to the HDL. These nonenzymic transfers partially compensate for the decreases in HDL unesterified cholesterol and lecithin directly caused by the LCAT reaction. It should be noted that in this experiment the nonenzymic transfers were such that the *proportions* of the total unesterified cholesterol and lecithin associated with each separate lipoprotein class were not appreciably altered by the LCAT reaction, even though the *amounts* of these lipids present were greatly reduced.

A similar type of nonenzymic transfer of lipid occurs between erythrocyte plasma membranes and plasma lipoproteins as first demonstrated by Murphy (77). He incubated normal human erythrocytes in preincubated human serum and showed that a loss of erythrocyte cholesterol to the serum occurred. Furthermore, he showed that at low hematocrit levels enough unesterified cholesterol was removed from the erythrocytes to seriously increase their osmotic fragility. These experiments have been confirmed, and the HDL have been shown to be particularly effective in removing erythrocyte cholesterol (J. A. Glomset and W. King, unpublished experiments). In fact, if the more reactive HDL subfractions obtained by gel filtration are incubated in the presence of LCAT and erythrocyte ghosts, the total HDL cholesterol can increase by 100% or more (Table V).

Not enough is known about the structure of either lipoproteins or plasma membranes to permit more than the following provisional explanation of these nonenzymic redistributions: The lipids of plasma lipoproteins and plasma membranes are mainly, if not solely, associated with protein or lipid through hydrophobic bonds. To some extent these bonds (particularly those that involve unesterified cholesterol) are disrupted reversibly during collisions among lipoproteins and plasma membranes. At such times, the surface lipids can exchange among individual lipoproteins and between lipoproteins and erythrocyte membranes, as has been observed in the case of unesterified cholesterol and lecithin (77–81). In a sense, the apoproteins of the various lipoproteins and plasma membranes compete for common pools of lipid during these collisions. As already indicated, this competition can lead to net transfers of lipid in the case of newly secreted lipoproteins

Table V. Changes in HDL Cholesterol During Incubation with Erythrocyte Membranes in the Presence and Absence of LCAT[a]

		Concentration (nanomoles/ml)	
Sample	Time (hr)	Unesterified Cholesterol	Cholesteryl Esters
HDL + membranes + LCAT	0	21	54
	16	53	112
	Δ	+32	+58
HDL + membranes	0	23	60
	16	51	58
	Δ	+28	− 2

[a] Human-plasma HDL were subfractionated on Sephadex G-200. The lipoproteins at the "tail" of the HDL peak were concentrated and incubated for 16 hr with erythrocyte membranes in tris–HCl buffer in the presence and absence of active LCAT. (J. A. Glomset and W. King, unpublished experiments.)

that have not yet reached equilibrium with the plasma pools. Finally, net transfers also occur when the equilibrium is disturbed by the preferential action of LCAT on HDL. These concepts appear to be particularly applicable to unesterified cholesterol. They are evidently less applicable to lecithin, because no significant net transfer of lecithin from erythrocyte membranes to plasma lipoproteins have been observed (77).

The basis for the redistribution of cholesteryl esters and triglycerides between VLDL and HDL appears to be more complicated. Until recently, neither of these nonpolar lipids was believed to exchange readily among lipoproteins (64). Both are presumably located in the interior, rather than on the surface, of lipoproteins, and intermolecular collisions would not be expected to promote exchange effectively. Nevertheless, Nichols and his colleagues (82, 83) have demonstrated that HDL cholesteryl esters *do* transfer to VLDL in the presence of LCAT, and that this transfer is accompanied by a back transfer of VLDL triglycerides to the HDL. Their observations suggest that the LCAT reaction has a special effect on lipoproteins and that this causes the redistribution. Although the nature of this effect remains to be clarified, one possibility is that LCAT forms cholesteryl esters on the surfaces of the HDL, and these surface esters transfer more readily than those that have undergone rearrangements within HDL molecules. More likely still is the possibility that indirect changes in VLDL surface unesterified cholesterol and lecithin caused by the LCAT reaction promote the transfer of nonpolar molecules during intermolecular collisions between HDL and VLDL.

Even in the absence of changes not related to the LCAT reaction, the continuous direct and indirect effects of the enzyme on lipoproteins, continuously being secreted into plasma, would be expected to result in complex populations of lipoproteins. Lipoproteins that have circulated in the plasma for some time would be expected to contain less lecithin and more cholesteryl esters than lipoproteins that have recently entered the circulation. Also, they would be expected to contain less unesterified cholesterol, although how much less is difficult to predict because of the secondary uptake of plasma-membrane unesterified cholesterol by lipoproteins after their reaction with LCAT. Furthermore, it is possible that lipoproteins undergo changes in physical properties on reacting with LCAT. The results of metabolic experiments with human and baboon plasma HDL led my colleagues and me (17) to propose that recently secreted HDL are of lower molecular weight than most of the HDL typically found in plasma and that reaction with LCAT gradually causes these HDL to form larger aggregates. We suggested that changes in surface lecithin and unesterified cholesterol might cause aggregation and thus reduce the relative surface area. Moreover, it is now apparent that the LCAT reaction can also cause a net increase in total cholesterol, and this would be expected to influence the size of the HDL molecules. Finally, Nichols and his colleagues (84) have obtained evidence that suggests that HDL molecules undergo physical changes independently of the LCAT reaction. They showed that HDL from serum incubated with or without *p*-hydroxymercuribenzoate lose protein and float at increased rates compared with HDL from control serum.

Although the simultaneous occurrence of the several changes discussed above makes understanding of lipoprotein metabolism difficult, the following provisional and highly speculative sketch of the role of the LCAT reaction in the intravascular metabolism of plasma lipoproteins may be useful:

Both VLDL and some HDL are secreted directly into plasma. The VLDL immediately begin to lose triglyceride to peripheral tissues, decrease in size, and increase in density. At the same time they may lose lecithin due to attack by lipoprotein lipase and possibly by exchange with other lipoproteins and plasma membranes. Finally, they lose both lecithin and unesterified cholesterol through LCAT-induced transfer to HDL, and they lose triglyceride to, and gain cholesteryl ester from, the HDL.

These changes gradually convert VLDL to LDL and possibly HDL. The LDL continue to change by LCAT-induced nonenzymic transfer of unesterified cholesterol and lecithin, and in addition react directly with LCAT. The LCAT reaction causes a slow increase in LDL cholesteryl ester content during the several days that the LDL circulate in the plasma (85). This cholesteryl ester, derived partly from the transfer of HDL cholesteryl ester to VLDL and partly from the direct attack of LCAT on the LDL, becomes the predominant lipid component of the LDL. The HDL that are secreted directly into the plasma are at first smaller than most of the HDL in a typical plasma sample. They contain relatively little cholesterol and very little, if any, cholesteryl ester. They correspond to the lipoproteins near the "tail" of the HDL peak in Figs. 3, 4, and 5. As they circulate in the plasma, they lose lecithin, particularly by reacting with LCAT, and this lecithin is only partially replenished by net transfer from the VLDL and LDL. The HDL also lose unesterified cholesterol, but in contrast to lecithin this unesterified cholesterol is more completely replenished by net transfer from VLDL, LDL, and plasma membranes. Even though some of the cholesteryl esters formed by the LCAT reaction subsequently transfer to the VLDL and presumably the liver (86), the net effect of the LCAT reaction on HDL is to increase their content of cholesterol and their molecular size.

At present very little is known about the HDL that may be formed during the metabolic breakdown of VLDL. The VLDL can be degraded into higher density lipoproteins by the action of postheparin lipoprotein lipase (74), but the only evidence that this occurs physiologically is the fact that the VLDL contain peptides in common with the HDL and particularly the lower density HDL (see Chapter 15) and the fact that an inverse relation exists between the concentrations of VLDL and HDL in plasma (87). However, the plasma of patients with familial LCAT deficiency contains an HDL subfraction of unusually large molecular size that conceivably may be derived from the VLDL (see SectionVI).

C. Influence on Tissues

Why a large proportion of the plasma cholesteryl esters should be formed by a specific enzyme *within the plasma* is worth considering. Even though the reaction is slow in comparison with many intracellular reactions, the more than 2 g of cholesterol esterified in human plasma each day is appreciable compared with the 300 to 500 mg of cholesterol absorbed from the diet (88) and the ~1.5 g of cholesterol and bile acids excreted (89). Indeed, more than 2 g of cholesteryl esters may be formed by the LCAT reaction if significant amounts of both the enzyme and HDL are present in interstitial fluid as in the case of albumin (90) and 7-S γ-globulin (91).

One possible reason why cholesteryl esters are formed in the plasma may be that they have some important, but unknown, function per se. For example, several years ago it was suggested (92) that plasma cholesteryl esters play a role in the transport of polyunsaturated fatty acids. However, what little evidence there is suggests that the plasma lecithin, which is the primary source of the cholesteryl ester unsaturated fatty acids, is synthesized mainly in the liver (93) and that the plasma cholesteryl esters are ultimately catabolized by the liver (86). Therefore a function of LCAT in fatty acid transport seems unlikely.

Another possible function of the LCAT reaction might be to provide lysolecithin for utilization in peripheral tissues. Most, if not all, tissues contain enzymes that can reacylate lysolecithin (94), and it is possible that a large proportion of the lecithin of peripheral tissues is formed in this way. This possibility needs further exploration.

A third possible function of the LCAT reaction could be to regulate the level of cholesterol in peripheral tissues. As indicated earlier, LCAT indirectly diminishes the unesterified cholesterol of erythrocyte membranes *in vitro* by first reducing the unesterified cholesterol of the HDL. If this type of phenomenon occurs *in vivo,* as seems likely, then it probably occurs in the case of other plasma membranes as well. This possibility is supported by the fact that the unesterified cholesterol of many tissues is able to exchange with that of plasma lipoproteins (95–97). Also, LCAT activity is present in peripheral lymph (1) and hence probably in interstitial fluid. Both facts suggest that LCAT acts on plasma lipoproteins in interstitial fluid, a necessary condition for the removal of unesterified cholesterol from the plasma membranes of peripheral cells. Figure 17 shows how the action of LCAT on HDL might promote the transfer of cholesterol from peripheral cells to the liver. That such a mechanism could be of physiological importance is suggested by the following line of reasoning:

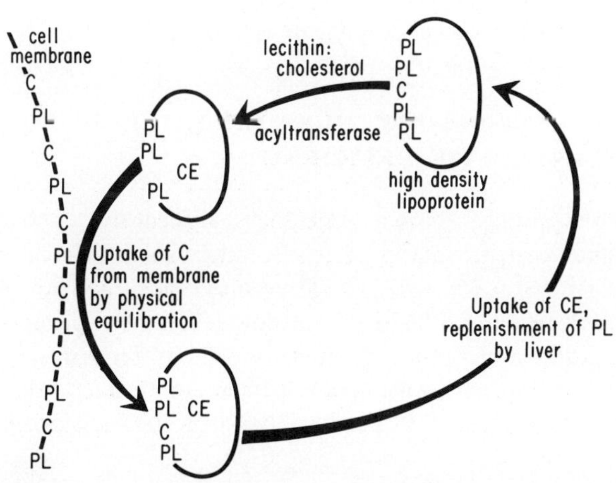

Fig. 17 Postulated role of LCAT reaction in transporting cholesterol from peripheral tissues to the liver: LCAT reacts with HDL to form cholesteryl esters (CE) from unesterified cholesterol (C) and lecithin (PL); the HDL subsequently pick up unesterified cholesterol from cell membranes and release cholesteryl esters to the liver. (From Ref. 1.)

1. There is a need for a mechanism of transporting cholesterol from peripheral tissues to the liver because most tissues can synthesize cholesterol, whereas the liver is the principal organ that catabolizes and excretes it.
2. It seems likely that plasma lipoproteins can enter the interstitial fluid, collide with the membranes of peripheral cells, and return to the plasma.
3. There is good evidence that the liver is active in removing plasma lipoproteins from the circulation (86).

Although this postulate has recently received considerable support from studies of patients with familial LCAT deficiency (see Section VI), several details of the postulated metabolic sequence remain to be clarified. For example, it is not at all clear that the unesterified cholesterol removed from plasma membranes is formed mainly by biosynthesis within the cell. Another possibility is that much of it comes from the plasma itself. Thus, Schumaker and Adams (98) have suggested that a relative excess of VLDL unesterified cholesterol and lecithin develops as triglycerides are removed by lipoprotein lipase. In the absence of LCAT this "excess" cholesterol would be expected to distribute among the other plasma lipoproteins and the plasma membranes in equilibrium with them and possibly even "bud off" to form myelin figures (see discussion of abnormal lipoproteins in familial LCAT deficiency in Section VI). Consequently it would be this cholesterol that is normally removed by the LCAT reaction. A second detail of the postulated cholesterol-transport sequence that is unclear concerns the uptake of the lipoprotein cholesteryl esters by the liver. The mechanism by which is is accomplished is unknown.

VI. FAMILIAL PLASMA LECITHIN:CHOLESTEROL ACYLTRANSFERASE DEFICIENCY

Patients with familial LCAT deficiency, a recently discovered disease (99, 100) have corneal opacity, anemia, and proteinuria as well as very little or no plasma LCAT activity. They also have high levels of plasma unesterified cholesterol and lecithin, and low levels of cholesteryl esters and lysolecithin in addition to other plasma-lipoprotein abnormalities. Although the primary defect in the disease has not been conclusively identified, many of these pathological features seem to depend on the lack of plasma LCAT activity.

A. Plasma Lipids and Lipoproteins

The high levels of plasma unesterified cholesterol and lecithin, and the low levels of cholesteryl esters and lysolecithin (Table VI) are consistent

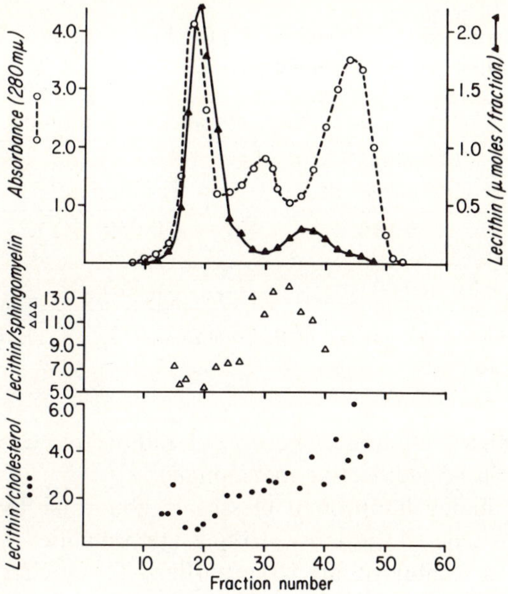

Fig. 18 Gel filtration on Sephadex G-200 of the $d > 1.063$ g/ml proteins from a patient with familial LCAT deficiency. Compare with Figs. 3 and 4 (From Ref. 105.)

with the evidence that LCAT forms most of the plasma cholesteryl esters in man. The few cholesteryl esters that *are* present in the patients' plasma are probably derived from chylomicrons because they occur mainly in the $d < 1.006$ g/ml lipoproteins (Tables VII and VIII); because like the chylomicrons of human thoracic-duct lymph (101), they contain large proportions of cholesteryl oleate and palmitate (Table IX); and because

Table VI. Concentration of the Principal Plasma Lipids in Three Patients with Familial LCAT Deficiency[a]

	Cholesterol			Phospholipids			
				Lecithin		Lysolecithin	
Patient	Total (mg %)	Unesterified (mg %)	Esterified (% total)	μg P/ml	% total P	μg P/ml	% total P
A.R.	350	340	2.9	136	85	2.1	1.3
I.S.	505	468	7.3	270	83	5.9	1.8
M.R.	166	150	9.6	69	83	1.7	2.0

[a] From Ref. 99.

Table VII. Distribution of Principal Lipids in the Plasma Lipoproteins of a Patient with Familial LCAT Deficiency[a]

Lipoprotein Class	Concentration (micromoles/ml)		
	Total Cholesterol	Lecithin	Triglycerides
VLDL	0.138	0.060	0.161
LDL	1.586	0.867	0.599
HDL	0.601	0.512	0.056

[a] Plasma lipoproteins from patient M.R. fractionated by preparative ultracentrifugation. (From Ref. 76.)

they become labeled after the *ingestion* of radioactive cholesterol, but not after the *injection* of radioactive mevalonate.

Each of the major lipoprotein classes is abnormal by several criteria (76, 102, 103). One of the most striking abnormalities is the presence in the LDL fraction of abnormally large particles. They contain variable, but unusually large, proportions of unesterified cholesterol and lecithin, appear to be made up of whorls of myelin figures on examination in the electron microscope, and have diameters in the range of 900 to 1200 Å. Another striking abnormality involves the patients' HDL. Originally HDL were thought to be absent from the patients' plasma because α_1-lipoproteins were absent in cellulose-acetate-strip electrophoresis. However, HDL were later demonstrated by preparative ultracentrifugation (Table VII). These HDL are abnormal in size, composition, and appearance upon electron microscopy (102, 103). However, they react with antiserum to normal human HDL (104) and with LCAT. A major, large-molecular-weight, subfraction and a minor, smaller-molecular-weight, subfraction are present (Fig. 18).

Table VIII. Lipid Ratios in the Plasma Lipoproteins of a Patient with Familial LCAT Deficiency[a]

Lipoprotein Class	Lipid Ratios[b]		
	Le/Sph	Le/C	CE/C
VLDL	12.00	0.67	0.55
LDL	6.62	0.68	0.24
HDL	6.02	0.89	0.04

[a] Plasma lipoproteins from patient M.R. fractionated by preparative ultracentrifugation. Same experiment as that shown in Table VII. (From Ref. 76.)

[b] Abbreviations: Le, lecithin; Sph, sphingomyelin; C, cholesterol; CE, cholesteryl esters.

Table IX. Comparison of Plasma Cholesteryl Esters of a Patient with Familial LCAT Deficiency with Those of a Normal Human[a]

	Esters (%)					
Subject	16:0	16:1	18:0	18:1	18:2	20:4
Patient (M.R.)	23.3	5.3	8.7	40.2	15.5	1.0
Normal human	12.4	6.1	2.4	18.4	47.8	5.3

[a] From Ref. 99.

Upon electrophoresis the major subfraction migrates as an α_2-globulin, whereas the minor subfraction migrates in the prealbumin region.

The patients' VLDL also are abnormal in electrophoretic mobility. They migrate as β-lipoproteins rather than as pre-β-lipoproteins (see Chapter 5). It is conceivable that this abnormal electrophoretic mobility is caused by reduced levels of one or more of the VLDL peptides. If this is the case, both the VLDL abnormality and the very low level of HDL peptide in the plasma might be related to reduced synthesis of these peptides.

Whether all of the abnormalities of the patients' lipoprotein can be explained on the basis of the LCAT deficiency remains to be demonstrated but appears likely. Some of the abnormalities may be late, secondary changes, however. Thus all but one of the patients have hyperlipemia, and the patient who is not hyperlipemic also is the youngest.

B. Erythrocytes and Anemia

The patients' erythrocytes are abnormal both in shape and in composition, and this probably is directly caused by the LCAT deficiency. Smears of the patients' erythrocytes show "target cells" similar to those of patients with obstructive jaundice. Moreover, as in obstructive jaundice (106, 107) the erythrocytes contain abnormally large amounts of unesterified cholesterol and lecithin (Table X). Both lipids are present in nearly twice the normal amount, although the total amount of phospholipids per erythrocyte is not elevated. These erythrocyte abnormalities are evidently secondary to the patients' plasma-lipoprotein abnormalities because both the proportion of "target cells" and the cholesterol content of the erythrocytes can be diminished *in vitro* by incubating the patients' erythrocytes in normal plasma (109) or *in vivo* by transfusing the patients with normal plasma (110). These induced changes support the concept, already discussed, that plasma lipoproteins and plasma membranes compete for a common pool of unesterified cholesterol and that LCAT plays an important role in regulating the size of this pool. The fact that the lecithin of the patients' erythrocytes

Table X. Erythrocyte Lipids in Patients with Familial LCAT Deficiency and in Normal Humans[a]

Subjects	Concentration per Cell (10^{-10} mg) Total Cholesterol	Total Lipid Phosphorus	Phospholipid Distribution (% of total lipid phosphorus)[b] PE	PS	PI	PC	Sph	LL
Normal controls ($n = 10$):								
Mean	1.11	1.00	29.0	14.0	1.6	27.4	25.9	2.1
±S.D.	0.11	0.07	2.2	1.7	0.4	1.5	1.7	1.1
Patients:								
A.R.	1.72	1.02	19.9	14.8	1.9	46.2	15.9	1.3
I.S.	1.77	1.06	19.8	12.5	0.7	49.6	16.7	0.7
M.R.	2.00	0.96	21.2	11.9	0.9	51.4	14.3	0.9

[a] Data from Ref. 108.
[b] Abbreviations: PE, phosphatidylethanolamine; PS, phosphatidylserine; PI, phosphatidylinositol; PC, phosphatidylcholine (lecithin); Sph, sphingomyelin; LL, lysolecithin.

is also increased suggests that plasma lipoproteins and plasma membranes also compete for phospholipids. However, the situation evidently differs from the case of cholesterol. Although more lecithin is present per cell, the total phospholipid content per cell is not increased. Second, no changes in the phospholipids of the patients' erythrocytes were noted in the *in vitro* and *in vivo* experiments in which changes in erythrocyte cholesterol occurred. Finally, in his experiments with normal erythrocytes, Murphy (77) noted no change in erythrocyte phospholipid content under conditions where the unesterified cholesterol content decreased. Nevertheless, the fact that the patients' erythrocyte lecithin is high, whereas their erythrocyte sphingomyelin and phosphatidylethanolamine are low, suggests that the phospholipid-binding sites on the membranes are not entirely specific and that a certain amount of slow interchange among phospholipid molecules can occur. On the other hand the binding sites for phosphatidylserine may be specific, because the patients' erythrocyte phosphatidylserine is not abnormal.

Whether the patients' anemia is directly related to their erythrocyte abnormalities is uncertain. However, it seems to be caused by a combination of increased destruction and decreased formation of erythrocytes; and the fact that foam cells have been noted in the patients' bone marrow suggests that lipid accumulating there may be interfering in some way with erythrogenesis.

C. Proteinuria

The most serious clinical problem associated with familial LCAT deficiency involves the kidneys. Proteinuria has been observed in all of the patients, and in two of the patients the proteinuria has been severe enough to cause edema. The kidney function of one of these patients deteriorated to the point of renal failure and death at the age of 41, and the second patient is currently being treated by dialysis. As in the case of the patients' anemia, the cause of their proteinuria is unknown. However, foam cells have been demonstrated in the patients' glomerular tufts, and this evidence of the accumulation of lipid (presumably cholesterol) again suggests that the renal dysfunction is secondary to a lipid abnormality. It seems worth considering the possibility that the fundamental lipid abnormality in both the kidneys and the bone marrow is related to the presence of the abnormal LDL found in the patients' plasma. Accumulation of these particles in the tissues with time might eventually cause secondary damage.

VII. SUMMARY

The plasma-cholesterol-esterification reaction is catalyzed by an acyltransferase that mainly transfers fatty acids from the lecithin to the cholesterol of plasma lipoproteins. Although the lecithin:cholesterol acyltransferase acts primarily on high-density lipoproteins, it acts also on low-density lipoproteins. Moreover, it appears to influence indirectly the lipid composition of very-low-density lipoproteins and of plasma membranes. In man the acyltransferase reaction appears to be the principal source of the plasma cholesteryl esters, but its relative role in forming the plasma cholesteryl esters of other species varies. In the rat plasma cholesteryl esters appear to be formed both in the liver and in the plasma, and the relative role of the acyltransferase apparently depends on the nutritional state of the animal.

Although the significance of the plasma reaction is still not understood, the reaction's indirect effect on very low density lipoproteins and plasma membranes may be of primary importance. By reducing the unesterified cholesterol of plasma lipoproteins, the enzyme promotes a nonenzymic transfer of unesterified cholesterol from erythrocyte, and probably other cell membranes to the plasma. Because of this effect, the reaction may play a role in the transport of cholesterol from peripheral tissue to the liver.

Support for this postulate has been provided recently by the discovery of several individuals in three Scandinavian families who are apparently unable to synthesize or secrete lecithin:cholesterol acyltransferase. These patients have increased amounts of unesterified cholesterol and lecithin in their plasma, in their erythrocyte membranes, and probably in the plasma membranes of other cells. In addition foam cells have been detected in their bone marrow and kidneys, and these foam cells are probably related to the patients' anemia and proteinuria.

REFERENCES

1. Glomset, J. A., *J. Lipid Res.* **9**, 155–167 (1968).
2. Sperry, W. M., *J. Biol. Chem.* **111**, 467–478 (1935).
3. Sperry, W. M., and V. A. Stoyanoff, *J. Biol. Chem.* **126**, 77–89 (1938).
4. LeBreton, E., and J. Pantaléon, *Arch. Sci. Physiol.* **1**, 199–215 (1947).
5. Klein, W., *Z. Physiol. Chem.* **254**, 1–17 (1937).
6. Etienne, J., and J. Polonovski, *Bull. Soc. Chim. Biol.* **41**, 805–812 (1959).
7. Glomset, J. A., F. Parker, M. Tjaden, and R. H. Williams, *Biochim. Biophys. Acta* **58**, 398–406 (1962).
8. Glomset, J. A., *Biochim. Biophys. Acta* **65**, 128–135 (1962).
9. Hanahan, D., R. Watts, and D. Pappajohn, *J. Lipid Res.* **1**, 421–432 (1960).
10. Portman, O. W., and M. Sugano, *Arch. Biochem. Biophys.* **105**, 532–540 (1964).
11. Shah, S. N., W. J. Lossow, and I. L. Chaikoff, *Biochim. Biophys. Acta* **84**, 176–181 (1964).
12. Glomset, J., *Biochim. Biophys. Acta* **70**, 389–395 (1963).
13. Etienne, J., and J. Polonovski, *Bull. Soc. Chim. Biol.* **41**, 813–819 (1959).
14. Switzer, S., and H. A. Eder, *J. Lipid Res.* **6**, 506–511 (1965).
15. Akanuma, Y., and J. Glomset, *J. Lipid Res.* **9**, 620–626 (1968).
16. Oncley, J. L., and S. E. Allerton, *Vox Sang. (Basel)* **6**, 201–203 (1961).
17. Glomset, J., E. Janssen, R. Kennedy, and J. Dobbins, *J. Lipid Res.* **7**, 639–648 (1966).
18. Lindgren, F. T., and A. V. Nichols, in *The Plasma Proteins,* Vol. 2, F. Putnam, Ed., Academic Press, New York, 1960, pp. 2–58.
19. Nichols, A. V., and E. L. Gong, *Biochim. Biophys. Acta* **231**, 175–184 (1971).
20. Akanuma, Y., and J. Glomset, *Biochem. Biophys. Res. Commun.* **32**, 639–643 (1968).
21. Raz, A., F. Kummerow, and T. Nishida, *Biochim. Biophys. Acta* **176**, 591–599 (1969).
22. Glomset, J., in *Methods of Enzymology,* Vol. 15, R. Clayton, Ed., Academic Press, New York, 1969, pp. 543–548.
23. Rose, H., *Biochim. Biophys. Acta* **152**, 728–741 (1968).
24. Stokke, K. T., and K. R. Norum, *Scand. J. Clin. Lab. Invest.* **27**, 21–28 (1971).
25. Glomset, J., and J. Wright, *Biochim. Biophys. Acta* **89**, 266–276 (1964).
26. Ho, W. K. K., and A. V. Nichols, *Biochim. Biophys. Acta* **231**, 185–193 (1971).
27. Hess, B., *Enzymes in Blood Plasma,* Academic Press, New York, 1963, p. 5.
28. Glomset, J., and D. Kaplan, *Biochim. Biophys. Acta* **98**, 41–46 (1965).
29. Akiyama, M., O. Minari, and T. Sakagami, *Biochim. Biophys. Acta* **137**, 525–532 (1967).
30. Goodman, D. S., D. Deykin, and T. Shiratori, *J. Biol. Chem.* **239**, 1335–1345 (1964).
31. Wells, I. C., and E. L. Rongone, *Proc. Soc. Exp. Biol. Med.* **130**, 661–664 (1969).
32. Stefanovich, V., *Biochem. J.* **115**, 555–561 (1969).
33. Sugano, M., I. Chinen, and M. Wada, *J. Biochem.* **58**, 285–292 (1965).
34. Puppione, D. L., *A Physical and Chemical Characterization of the Serum Lipoproteins of Marine Mammals.* Dissertation, University of California at Berkeley, 1969.

35. Rowen, R., and J. Martin, *Biochim. Biophys. Acta* **70**, 396–404 (1963).
36. Vogel, W., and E. Bierman, *J. Lipid Res.* **8**, 46–53 (1967).
37. Wagner, A., *Quart. Bull. Northw. Univ. Med. School* **33**, 282–284 (1960).
38. Rowen, R. J., *Exp. Med.* **114**, 807–823 (1961).
39. Sperry, W. M., and V. A. Stoyanoff, *J. Biol. Chem.* **117**, 525–532 (1937).
40. Rowen, R., *Biochim. Biophys. Acta* **84**, 761–764 (1964).
41. Tayeau, F., and R. Nivet, *Compt. Rend.* **240**, 567–569 (1955).
42. Wagner, A., and C. A. Poindexter, *J. Lab. Clin. Med.* **40**, 321–323 (1952).
43. Gherondache, C. N., *J. Clin. Endocrinol. Metab.* **23**, 1024–1028 (1963).
44. Lopez-S., A., W. A. Krehl, and R. E. Hodges, *Amer. J. Clin. Nutr.* **20**, 808–815 (1967).
45. Aftergood, L., and R. B. Alfin-Slater, *J. Lipid Res.* **8**, 126–130 (1967).
46. Aftergood, L., H. J. Hernandez, and R. B. Alfin-Slater, *J. Lipid Res.* **9**, 447–452 (1968).
47. Sugano, M., and O. W. Portman, *Arch. Biochem. Biophys.* **109**, 302–315 (1965).
48. Wells, I. C., and J. M. Hogan, *J. Nutr.* **95**, 55–62 (1968).
49. Swell, L., and M. L. Law, *Proc. Soc. Exp. Biol. Med.* **129**, 363–366 (1968).
50. Shapiro, I. L., J. A. Jastremsky, and D. Kritchevsky, *Lipids* **3**, 381–383 (1968).
51. Monger, E. A., and P. J. Nestel, *Clin. Chim. Acta* **15**, 269–273 (1967).
52. Takahashi, Y., and Y. Muto, *Jap. J. Gastroenterol.* **65**, 1139–1142 (1968).
53. Turner, K. B., and V. Pratt, *Proc. Soc. Exp. Biol. Med.* **71**, 633–637 (1949).
54. Castro Mendoza, H., and C. Jimenez Diaz, *Bull. Inst. Med. Res. (Madrid)* **2**, 81–93 (1949).
55. Jones, D. P., F. R. Sosa, J. Shartsis, P. T. Shah, E. Skromak, and W. T. Beher, *J. Clin. Invest.* **50**, 259–265 (1971).
56. Simon, J. B., and R. Scheig, *New Engl. J. Med.* **283**, 841–846 (1970).
57. Gjone, E., and K. R. Norum, *Acta Med. Scand.* **187**, 153–161 (1970).
58. Brot, N., W. J. Lossow, and I. L. Chaikoff, *J. Lipid Res.* **3**, 413–415 (1962).
59. Lossow, W. J., S. N. Shah, N. Brot, and I. L. Chaikoff, *Biochim. Biophys. Acta* **70**, 593–595 (1963).
60. Sugano, M., K. Hori, and M. Wada, *Arch. Biochem. Biophys.* **129**, 588–596 (1969).
61. Simon, J. B., and J. L. Boyer, *Biochim. Biophys. Acta* **218**, 549–551 (1970).
62. Marsh, J. B., and E. Kashub, *Fed. Proc.* **29**, No. 2, 673 (1970).
63. Osuga, T., and O. W. Portman, *Amer. J. Physiol.* **220**, 735–741 (1971).
64. Goodman, D. S., *Physiol. Rev.* **45**, 747–839 (1965).
65. Windmueller, H. G., *J. Biol. Chem.* **243**, 4878–4884 (1968).
66. Gidez, L. I., P. S. Roheim, and H. A. Eder, *J. Lipid Res.* **8**, 7–15 (1967).
67. Nestel, P. J., and E. A. Monger, *J. Clin. Invest.* **46**, 967–974 (1967).
68. Goodman, D. S., *J. Clin. Invest.* **43**, 2026 (1964).
69. Sugano, M., and O. W. Portman, *Arch. Biochem. Biophys.* **107**, 341–351 (1964).
70. Glomset, J. A., E. Janssen, R. Kennedy, and J. Dobbins, *J. Lipid Res.* **7**, 638 (1966).
71. Goodman, D. S., and T. Shiratori, *J. Lipid Res.* **5**, 578–586 (1964).
72. Minari, O., and D. B. Zilversmit, *J. Lipid Res.* **4**, 424–436 (1963).
73. Bierman, E., and D. Strandness, *Amer. J. Physiol.* **210**, 13–18 (1966).
74. Nichols, A. V., E. H. Strisower, F. T. Lindgren, G. L. Adamson, and E. L. Coggiola, *Clin. Chim. Acta* **20**, 277–283 (1968).
75. Vogel, W., and E. Bierman, *Proc. Soc. Exp. Biol. Med.* **127**, 77–80 (1968).

76. Glomset, J. A., K. R. Norum, and W. King, *J. Clin. Invest.* **49**, 1827–1837 (1970).
77. Murphy, J. R., *J. Lab. Clin. Med.* **60**, 86–109 (1962).
78. Eder, H. A., *Amer. J. Med.* **23**, 269–282 (1957).
79. Roheim, P. S., D. E. Haft, L. I. Gidez, A. White, and H. A. Eder, *J. Clin. Invest.* **42**, 1277–1285 (1963).
80. Gould, R. G., G. V. LeRoy, G. T. Okita, J. J. Kabora, P. Keegan, and D. M. Bergenstal, *J. Lab. Clin. Med.* **46**, 372–384 (1955).
81. Reed, C. F., *J. Clin. Invest.* **47**, 749–760 (1968).
82. Rehnborg, C. S., and A. V. Nichols, *Biochim. Biophys. Acta* **84**, 596–603 (1964).
83. Nichols, A. V., and L. Smith, *J. Lipid Res.* **6**, 206–210 (1965).
84. Nichols, A. V., E. L. Coggiola, L. C. Jensen, and E. H. Yokoyama, *Biochim. Biophys. Acta* **168**, 87–94 (1968).
85. Volwiler, W., P. Goldsworthy, M. MacMartin, P. Wood, I. Mackay, and K. Fremont-Smith, *J. Clin. Invest.* **34**, 1369–1374 (1955).
86. Friedman, M., and S. O. Byers, *J. Clin. Invest.* **34**, 1369–1374 (1955).
87. Nichols, A. V., *Advances in Biological and Medical Physics,* Vol. 11, J. H. Lawrence and J. W. Gofman, Eds., Academic Press, New York, 1967, pp. 109–158.
88. Wilson, J., and C. Lindsey, *J. Clin. Invest.* **44**, 1805–1814 (1965).
89. Bergström, S., H. Danielsson, and B. Samuelsson, *Lipid Metabolism,* K. Bloch, Ed., Wiley, New York, 1960, p. 328.
90. Berson, S., R. Yalow, S. Schreiber, and J. Post, *J. Clin. Invest.* **32**, 746–768 (1953).
91. Solomon, A., T. Waldman, and J. Fahey, *J. Lab. Clin. Med.* **62**, 1–17 (1963).
92. Klein, P. D., *Amer. J. Clin. Nutr.* **8**, 104–111 (1960).
93. Goldman, D., I. Chaikoff, W. Reinhardt, C. Entenman, and W. Dauben, *J. Biol. Chem.* **184**, 727–733 (1950).
94. Lands, W., and P. Hart, *J. Biol. Chem.* **240**, 1905–1911 (1965).
95. Avigan, J., D. Steinberg, and M. Berman, *J. Lipid Res.* **3**, 216–221 (1962).
96. Chobanian, A. V., B. A. Burrow, and W. Hollander, *J. Clin. Invest.* **41**, 1738–1744 (1962).
97. Field, H., Jr., L. Swell, P. E. Schools, Jr., and C. R. Treadwell, *Circulation* **22**, 547–558 (1960).
98. Schumaker, V., and G. Adams, *J. Theoret. Biol.* **26**, 89–91 (1970).
99. Norum, K. R., and E. Gjone, *Scand. J. Clin. Lab. Invest.* **20**, 231–243 (1967).
100. Gjone, E., and K. R. Norum, *Acta Med. Scand.* **183**, 107–112 (1968).
101. Blomstrand, R., Gurtler, J., and B. Werner, *Acta Med. Scand.* **18**, 1019 (1964).
102. Norum, K. R., J. A. Glomset, A. V. Nichols, and G. M. Forte, *J. Clin Invest.* **50**, 1131–1140 (1971).
103. Forte, G. M., K. R. Norum, J. A. Glomset, and A. V. Nichols, *J. Clin. Invest.* **50**, 1141–1148 (1971).
104. Torsvik, H., *Scand. J. Clin. Lab. Invest.* **24**, 187–196 (1969).
105. Norum, K. R., J. A. Glomset, and E. Gjone, in *Metabolic Basis of Inherited Disease,* 3rd ed., J. B. Stanbury, J. B. Wyngaarden, and D. S. Fredrickson, Eds., Blakiston–McGraw-Hill, New York, in press.
106. Cooper, R., and J. Jandl, *J. Clin. Invest.* **47**, 809–822 (1968).
107. Nye, W., and G. Marinetti, *J. Clin. Invest.* **44**, 1081 (1965).

108. Gjone, E., H. Torsvik, and K. Norum, *Scand. J. Clin. Lab. Invest.* **21**, 327 (1968).
109. Norum, K., and E. Gjone, *Scand. J. Clin. Lab. Invest.* **22**, 94–98 (1968).
110. Norum, K., and E. Gjone, *Scand. J. Clin. Lab. Invest.* **22**, 287–290 (1968).

15. The Apolipoproteins: Their Structure and Functional Roles in Human-Serum Lipoproteins

VIRGIE G. SHORE and BERNARD SHORE

Bio-Medical Division, Ernest O. Lawrence Livermore Laboratory, Livermore, California

I. INTRODUCTION

Nearly all of the plasma lipids are associated with specific proteins in the form of soluble lipoproteins. These lipoproteins comprise a broad spectrum of macromolecules and micelles varying in size, hydrated density, and in the content of protein, carbohydrate, phospholipids, triglycerides, cholesteryl esters, free cholesterol, and other lipids (1–6). The structures of the protein moieties of the lipoproteins undoubtedly will prove to be important determinants of the composition and structure of the lipoproteins, of their physical and chemical properties, and of their biochemical and physiological functions. Since 1967 more than a dozen different polypeptide components of human-serum lipoproteins have been isolated and characterized chemically and physically, suggesting that the serum lipoproteins are more diverse with respect to structure and function than had previously been suspected.

Almost all studies of the composition, structure, function, and metabolism of the serum lipoproteins have been done on four major density fractions. On the basis of hydrated density, human-serum lipoproteins are normally distributed among the high-density lipoproteins (HDL, *d* 1.063–1.20 g/ml), the low-density lipoproteins (LDL, *d* 1.006–1.063 g/ml), the very low-density lipoproteins (VLDL, *d* 0.94–1.006 g/ml), and the chylomicrons ($d < 0.94$ g/ml) plus a few minor fractions (1, 3, 5, 6). In addition, a small fraction of the plasma lipids is transported as complexes with proteins usually not considered among the plasma lipoproteins. These include albumin, which binds fatty acids (7) and lysolecithin (8); retinol-binding protein, which transports vitamin A (9); and transcholesterin, which may be a system of proteins that combine with cholesterol and are found in the α-globulin fraction of lipoprotein-free serum (10). In the electrophoresis of plasma on paper or agarose (11) the major lipoprotein classes are seen as α (HDL), β (LDL), pre-β (VLDL), and chylomicron bands whose mobilities are determined primarily by their protein moieties (12).

The lipoproteins are often defined in terms of the S_f-rate, the rate of flotation under unit centrifugal field in an NaCl solution of *d* 1.063 g/ml at 26°C (1). The S_f values, which are a function of lipoprotein size, shape, and density, are in the range of 0–20 for LDL, 20–400 for VLDL, and > 400 for chylomicrons; HDL sediment, so S_f values are not used to describe this fraction. The various density classes of lipoproteins are often isolated from serum by ultracentrifugation in solutions of appropriate densities or in density gradients (1, 3, 11). In preparative methods in which the solvent density is uniform at the beginning of each ultracentrifugation step, the density of the serum or plasma is increased in steps for each of the density fractions by the addition of sodium chloride, potassium bromide, deuterium oxide, or other substances (11, 13). At solvent densities greater than the lipoprotein density, the lipoproteins float at rates depending on their densities, sizes, and shapes. Two other centrifugal methods of lipoprotein isolation, isopycnic equilibrium (14) and continuous-flow zonal centrifugation (15), involve the use of density gradients.

Other purification procedures include the specific precipitation of LDL and VLDL by high-molecular-weight polyanions like heparin (16) and dextran sulfate (17) and the aggregation of VLDL by the polycation polyvinylpyrrolidone (18).

Each of the major density classes of lipoproteins characteristically differs from the others in the kinds of proteins and the proportions of the various lipids it contains as well as in size and hydrated density. However, heterogeneity of size and density does exist within a given lipoprotein class (3, 13), possibly due to variable amounts of some lipids (e.g., triglycerides) bound to a basic protein–lipid core, to the presence in varying proportions of different lipoprotein species of similar density, and to the existence of several kinds of lipoprotein subunits that combine in different proportions and in different numbers to form the lipoprotein molecules or micelles. The extent to which each of these factors contributes to heterogeneity within the lipoprotein fractions is largely unknown, but heterogeneity of the protein moiety exists in all the major density classes. Isolation and characterization of the polypeptide components of the lipoprotein fractions indicate that molecular heterogeneity with respect to polypeptide composition exists in all the lipoprotein fractions and that VLDL contains some polypeptides in common with LDL and others in common with HDL. However, fractionation of the lipoproteins themselves on the basis of their protein moiety, rather than density, is necessary for further clarification of lipoprotein heterogeneity.

Although the normal plasma-lipoprotein concentrations and distributions among the various density classes fall within fairly well-known ranges (1, 3), variations characteristic of diet and physiological conditions like age and sex are also known (1). In addition to abnormalities in plasma-lipoprotein concentrations and distributions as a function of hydrated density, atypical lipoprotein species have also been observed.

Some abnormalities in plasma lipoproteins associated with a disease state may result from a great increase of a lipoprotein species that is normally present in small amounts rather than a primary defect in the lipoproteins. However, some abnormalities will undoubtedly prove to be the consequence of variations in the primary structure of the polypeptide components of the lipoproteins.

The studies of Fredrickson and co-workers (19, 20) on serum-lipoprotein distributions and concentrations in more than 1000 subjects suggest that there are at least five abnormal genotypes expressed primarily as hyperlipoproteinemia. Other genetic defects affecting serum lipoproteins are Tangier disease, which is characterized by an HDL deficiency (20), and abetalipoproteinemia, which is characterized by the absence of LDL (β-lipoproteins), VLDL, and chylomicrons (20–24) as well as by abnormalities in HDL concentration and composition (25). In patients with obstructive jaundice the characteristic elevation of plasma-lipoprotein levels (26) is due to the presence of an LDL species of abnormal composition and properties (27–30). Another abnormal or unusual lipoprotein (possibly a genetic variant of β-lipoprotein, or LDL), which differs in charge and density from the known plasma lipoproteins, has been found in a healthy child (31). In addition, a number of structural variants, or allotypes, have been detected by serological tests with anti-β-lipoprotein antiserums (32–34).

The Lp(a) genetic variant of human-serum β-lipoproteins was detected by Berg (35) and has been separated from serum by several investigators. Wiegandt, Lipp, and Wendt (36) observed that its density was between 1.050 and 1.125 g/ml, that it was electrophoretically homogeneous, and that both it and its lipid-free protein moiety exhibited the immunological properties of β-lipoproteins in addition to its Lp(a+) activity. Schultz, Shreffler, and Harvie (37), who isolated and partially purified the Lp(a) lipoprotein by density-gradient centrifugation, estimated its density to be about 1.07 g/ml at 20°C and its uncorrected flotation rate $S_{f\ (1.21, 20°)}$ to be about 24S. Immunological techniques indicated Lp(a) lipoprotein to be absent from all subfractions of serum from Lp(a—) individuals. The frequency of Lp(a+) individuals was 0.50 in their study, compared with 0.33 found by Berg and others in Caucasian populations.

Another example of heterogeneity due to genetic polymorphism is the LDL variant called Ag by its discoverers, Allison and Blumberg (32). More recent studies (38) indicate that it does not represent a unique density class. The structural basis for the variants is unknown, but very likely they will be found by studies of the amino acid and carbohydrate composition and the amino acid sequences of the polypeptide components of the lipoproteins. However, glycolipids also could be antigenic determinants. Giblett (34) suggested that the actual gene products of the Ag system could be enzymes capable of mediating the synthesis of Ag antigenic sites, but she considered this possibility unlikely. If the carbohydrate moiety is the antigenic determinant of Ag, analogous to the blood-group carbohydrate antigens, it would not be the direct gene product.

Far less immunochemical evidence is available on the occurrence of polymorphism or genetic variants among HDL and VLDL, but their existence would not be surprising. Perhaps structural studies on polypeptide moieties isolated from various lipoprotein fractions, both normal and abnormal, will indicate the occurrence of some genetic variants in the lipoproteins. Such studies should enhance our understanding of the factors underlying many of the abnormalities in lipoprotein metabolism, the various types of hyperlipemia, and the deficiencies in lipoproteins associated with Tangier disease and abetalipoproteinemia. The studies of lipoprotein abnormalities have already contributed much to our knowledge of the functions and metabolism of the serum lipoproteins.

Among the best known functions of the serum lipoproteins are those of lipid transport (7, 39, 40). The transport processes are undoubtedly involved in maintaining the steady-state concentrations of lipids in plasma, tissues, cell membranes, and other subcellular structures and in transferring lipids in water-soluble form from sites of synthesis and absorption to those of storage and utilization. The amount of lipids transported daily in the normal adult is estimated to be 70 to 150 g of exogenous triglycerides by chylomicrons, 25 to 50 g of endogenous triglycerides by VLDL, 1 g of cholesterol by all lipoprotein fractions, and 50 to 150 g of free fatty acids by albumin (40). By contrast, the serum lipids amount to about 0.5 g/100 ml in the normal human (6).

The processes of lipid transport may involve both simple exchanges and enzyme-catalyzed transfers of lipids. These lipids are associated by noncovalent forces with specific proteins or glycoproteins, or both, in water-soluble complexes, the lipoproteins, and apparently are continuously exchanged among the various serum-lipoprotein fractions and with erythrocyte lipids (3, 39, 41). Triglycerides, lecithin, and cholesterol undergo extensive exchange, both *in vitro* and *in vivo,* possibly during collisions of the lipoproteins. The cholesteryl esters of LDL and HDL appear to be exchangeable for the triglycerides of VLDL (42), although cholesteryl esters have not been observed to undergo exchange among the various lipoproteins (43). In man about 60% of erythrocyte lecithin and about 30% of erythrocyte sphingomyelin is exchangeable (44). The 12-hr fractional turnover was about 13% of the membrane lecithin pool and about 14% for sphingomyelin, and was due entirely to the exchange of the whole molecule with the corresponding plasma compound. The erythrocyte-membrane cholesterol also exchanges rapidly with the cholesterol of plasma at 37°C (45). Transfer of lipids from one density class to another in the form of polypeptide-lipid complexes probably occurs also.

Certain of the apolipoproteins have activator and regulator functions in enzyme systems involved in metabolism of the plasma lipids. The plasma enzyme lecithin:cholesterol acyltransferase is the major source of cholesteryl esters in plasma, probably has a major role in cholesterol transport and homeostasis in the body, and could be involved in tissue utilization of lecithin transported by lipoproteins (46–48). The enzyme catalyzes transfer of an acyl group from lecithin to cholesterol in lipoproteins. It requires for activity a protein cofactor present in HDL (49). Other apolipoproteins have activator and inhibitor functions for the lipoprotein lipase enzyme system necessary for removal of and tissue utilization of the triglycerides of chylomicrons and VLDL (50–52).

It is not yet clear to what extent protein heterogeneity in a given density fraction (e.g., VLDL or HDL) is associated with a multiplicity of physiological functions. HDL is involved in both cholesterol ester and trigylceride metabolism by different mechanisms. All the density classes may be interrelated in one or more aspects of the transport and utilization of the plasma lipids. This appears to be so in triglyceride metabolism. It is also clear that the lipoprotein peptides have specific functions in enzyme systems, in addition to other possible roles in the structure and properties of the lipoproteins. However, the reason for the considerable variety of polypeptides found in each density class of lipoproteins is largely unknown, and only a few functions of some apolipoproteins are known. Some of the polypeptides may serve primarily as specific binders for lipids, and others may confer water solubility on the lipid–protein complexes. It is also possible that polypeptide constituents of the lipoproteins may be the determinants of receptor sites in cells and tissues. In any case the compositions and structures of the polypeptide moieties of lipoproteins are of greatest interest because they can be related to the functions and properties of the lipoproteins. Studies on the polypeptides of the various lipoprotein classes bear directly on possible structural and metabolic relationships among the serum lipoproteins.

II. HIGH-DENSITY LIPOPROTEINS

The high-density lipoproteins have the highest percentage of protein and the smallest particle sizes among the major lipoprotein classes (1, 3, 5, 39). However, approximately 30 to 40% of the serum lipids is found in HDL because their concentration is relatively high in normal human plasma: approximately 260 and 330 mg/100 ml in males and females, respectively (1, 3, 39). Cholesteryl esters and phospholipids are the predominant lipids in HDL; triglycerides, unesterified cholesterol, fatty acids, ceramide monohexosides, and other lipids are present in small amounts (6). Small amounts of carbohydrates—hexosamine, methylpentose, hexoses, and sialic acid—are covalently attached to the protein moiety (53).

The HDL fraction is not continuously distributed over the entire density range but contains two overlapping subgroups, HDL_2 and HDL_3, the latter being usually predominant (1). The proportion of HDL_2 to HDL_3 is considerably affected by various physiological and pathological conditions and is related to estrogen production (6). In abetalipoproteinemia HDL_3 is reduced, but HDL_2 is present in normal amounts (25). The protein moiety accounts for approximately 53 to 56 wt % of HDL_3 (54, 55), which has an average molecular weight of 150,000 to 180,000 (54, 56) and is made up of several subunits, usually three or four, according to electron micrographs (57, 58). The protein moiety accounts for about 33% (V. G. Shore and B. Shore, unpublished observation) to 40% (54) of the larger, less dense HDL_2 molecules, which have a molecular weight of about 340,000 to 380,000 (54, 56) and usually contain five or six subunits (57).

Although two major proteins and a half a dozen or so minor ones are present in HDL, until recently the human-serum HDL fraction was generally thought to be a single species of lipoprotein with one kind of protein subunit and variable amounts of lipids (1, 3, 5, 53–55). The amino acid compositions of the proteins were very similar, if not identical, in HDL subfractions differing in density (1, 54), but some differences in composition were observed (1, 59). Results of early end-group analyses of the protein were consistent with one polypeptide subunit containing carboxyl-terminal threonine and amino-terminal aspartic acid (1, 60). Moving-boundary electrophoresis of HDL subfractions indicated one component in all fractions that migrated with identical (61) or very similar mobilities (62). Unfractionated HDL and its subfractions gave one broad band each after starch-gel electrophoresis and staining for protein, and mobility differences among the fractions were thought to depend on the lipid content of the fractions (53). The lipid-free proteins (α-protein) of HDL and subfractions were separated by vertical starch-gel electrophoresis into several components, which, however, reacted identically to anti-HDL or anti-α-protein serums (53). Other investigators (63) found that HDL gave multiple bands in starch-gel electrophoresis when lauric acid was added to improve the resolution, but no definite conclusion was reached about the basis for the heterogeneity.

Immunodiffusion and immunoelectrophoresis experiments from a number of laboratories have led to an equivocal view about the possible heterogeneity of the HDL fraction and its protein moiety. From one of the earliest immunochemical studies, Aladjem, Lieberman, and Gofman (64) concluded that the HDL fraction contains several antigenic components. Several other groups of investigators (53, 61, 65–68) have observed two antigenic forms of HDL protein and HDL. Some investigators (65, 68) have concluded that HDL can be altered serologically during purification or on standing and that one of the two antigenic forms was an artifact from HDL, since fresh plasma contained only one. Scanu (53) concluded that the antigenic polymorphism of HDL, HDL_2, and HDL_3 proteins was probably related to the presence in solution of monomeric and polymeric forms having different reactivities against anti-HDL and anti-α-protein serums. He found a single antigenic determinant after dissociation by a detergent or after acetylation of the protein. Other investigators (69) found that HDL protein (lipid-free) gave a single line of precipitation on double diffusion against anti-HDL serum, in spite of the fact that they were able to fractionate the protein into two different components.

More recently, disk electrophoresis of HDL_2 and HDL_3 at pH 8.8 in polyacrylamide gels (7.5%) containing 8 *M* urea indicated the presence of two major components that stained for protein with Amido Schwarz in both HDL_2 and HDL_3, and minor components that were more abundant in HDL_2 than in HDL_3 (70, 71). The lipoproteins were not resolved into bands in 7.5% gels that did not contain urea or the detergent (V. G. Shore and B. Shore, unpublished observation). The disk-electrophoresis patterns of the lipid-free HDL_3 and HDL_2 proteins in 12.5% acrylamide gels containing 8 *M* urea or Triton X-100 were very similar to those obtained from the lipoproteins (72 and unpublished observation). Rudman, Garcia, and Howard (69) also observed two major components in disk electrophoresis of HDL protein at pH 8.8 and 4 in 7.5% acrylamide gels containing 5 *M* urea.

The disk-electrophoresis experiments suggest polymorphism or the presence of different protein components in HDL protein, but it cannot be concluded from these results that the HDL fraction is a mixture of different lipoprotein species that contain one or the other of the proteins. Urea and detergents effect partial or complete delipidation of the lipoprotein, in addition to dissociating the protein into its polypeptide components.

The protein moieties of HDL and its subfractions are readily obtained in essentially complete yield in lipid-free, water-soluble form by extracting the lipids with mixtures of diethyl ether and ethanol (53, 55). Alternatively the lipids can be removed by gel filtration on a Sephadex LH-20 column in a medium of 2-butanol–acetic acid–water (4:1:5, v/v) (69).

In the absence of dissociating agents like detergents, urea, or alkali, the lipid-free protein of HDL or its subfractions readily forms polymers. Dissociation is also favored by acetylation of the protein (53). In an early study by sedimentation and diffusion the protein was observed to have a sedimentation coefficient of 4.1S and a molecular weight of 75,000 (73). Later sedimentation-velocity experiments with the lipid-free protein in dilute salt solution indicated two components with sedimentation coefficients of 2.3 to 2.6S and 4.2 to 4.6S (74); the detergent sodium dodecyl sulfate (SDS) dissociated the component with the higher sedimentation coefficient.

The HDL_3 protein in the presence of the detergent (3:1, w/w) usually showed a high degree of homogeneity with respect to molecular weight—about 30,000 in sedimentation-equilibrium experiments. In guanidine hydrochloride solutions the protein exhibited heterogeneity in molecular weight (55). Other studies on the unfractionated protein moiety of HDL by the Archibald method involving measurements during the approach to sedimentation equilibrium have yielded molecular-weight values of 28,000 for the protein in the presence of SDS (5), 22,300 $\pm$ 1500 and 23,000 $\pm$ 2400 for HDL_2 and HDL_3 proteins, respectively, in the presence of SDS, and 22,800 $\pm$ 2200 and 22,000 $\pm$ 2000 for the acetylated proteins of HDL_2 and HDL_3, respectively, in pH 8.6 tris buffer of ionic strength 0.1 (53). The succinylated protein of HDL and its subfractions at concentrations between 0.01 and 0.02% had a molecular weight of 25,800 ± 1000 by sedimentation equilibrium and was not dissociated further by increasing the pH to 12.5 or by reduction or alkylation (75). Now that the polypeptide components have been isolated, it can be concluded from these studies that the lipid-free protein of HDL is not readily dissociated into its polypeptide constituents. The higher molecular-weight values, 28,000 to 30,000, probably correspond to dimers of HDL polypeptides.

That HDL protein is a mixture of polypeptides differing markedly in composition was established by isolation of its components (69, 70–72, 76) after the heterogeneity was indicated by carboxyl-terminal analysis and polyacrylamide-gel electrophoresis (70). Reinvestigation of carboxyl-terminal amino acids of HDL disclosed that glutamine, as well as the previously recognized threonine, was a major carboxyl-terminal group of HDL_2 and HDL_3. It was the amino acid most rapidly released by carboxypeptidase action on HDL protein, and glutamic acid γ-hydrazide, a product of hydrazinolysis of peptides with carboxyl-terminal glutamine, was identified in HDL-protein hydrazinolysate by chromatography of the di-dinitrophenyl derivative (70). The sum of carboxyl-terminal threonine and glutamine was approximately 2 moles per 30,000 g of protein. The molar ratio of the peptides with these carboxyl termini usually appears not to be 1:1 and is not constant among different HDL preparations.

The polypeptides were isolated from HDL_3 (70, 72) and HDL_2 (71) by chromatography of the lipid-free proteins in 8 *M* urea on diethylaminoethyl (DEAE) cellulose; they were eluted with tris–HCl buffers in 8 *M* urea at pH 8 and 8°C. One of the peptides, which contained the carboxyl-terminal sequence R–Thr–Gln, contained no histidine, arginine, tryptophan, or cysteine (72). Its amino acid composition is as follows: Lys_{15}, Cys_2, Asp_5, Thr_{11}, Ser_{11}, Glu_{26}, Pro_7, Gly_6, Ala_9, Val_{10}, Met_2, Ile_2, Leu_{14}, Tyr_6, Phe_7; the total number of residues is 133, and the molecular weight from amino acid composition is 14,900. The molecular weight from the yield of carboxyl-terminal glutamine after digestion by carboxypeptidase was approximately 14,000 (70). From sedimentation-equilibrium data on the polypeptide R–Thr–Gln in urea or guanidine hydrochloride solutions, Shore and Shore (72) calculated the molecular weight to be between 14,000 and 15,000. Scanu and co-workers (76) obtained an apparent molecular-weight value of 17,200 to 17,600 from sedimentation equilibrium in 8 *M* urea of a fraction from gel filtration of HDL protein in 8 *M* urea which corresponds in amino acid composition to R–Gln. The peptide is obtained in two fractions (polymorphic forms) of identical amino acid composition by DEAE-cellulose chromatography. It contains a carbohydrate moiety of undetermined composition and a blocked amino terminal group.

The other major HDL polypeptide contained no isoleucine, cystine, or cysteine. Its amino acid composition is Lys_{10}, His_3, Arg_9, Asp_{13}, Thr_5, Ser_8, Glu_{24}, Pro_5, Gly_6, Ala_{10}, Val_7, Met_2, Leu_{20}, Tyr_4, Phe_3, Trp_4; the number of amino acid residues per molecule is 133, and the molecular weight from amino acid composition is 15,500 (72). By the Edman method, the sequence of part of the molecule from the amino-terminal was found to be as follows: Asp-Glu-Pro-Pro-Gln-Ser-Pro-Trp-Asp-Arg-Val-Lys-Asp-Leu-Ala-Thr-Val-Tyr-Val-Asp-Val-Leu-Arg-Asp-Ser-Gly-Arg-Asp-Tyr-Val-Ser-Gln-Phe-Glu-Gly-Arg-Ala-Leu-Gly-Gln- (V. G. Shore and B. Shore, unpublished observation). Sedimentation-equilibrium experiments on the polypeptide either in dilute salt solution containing sodium dodecyl sulfate or in urea solution indicated heterogeneity with respect to molecular weight and weight-average molecular weights of approximately 20,000; in guanidine hydrochloride solutions the molecular weight of the peptide, possibly a dimer in this solvent, was about 31,000 (72). The polypeptide appears to occur in at least three polymorphic forms, of which two are major components of HDL protein. They are very similar in size and composition; they are separated by chromatography on DEAE-cellulose columns, but not by disk electrophoresis at pH 8.8 in polyacrylamide gels containing 8 *M* urea (71). This peptide is thought to contain carboxyl-terminal threonine (70), but it has also been reported that glutamine is carboxyl-terminal (77). Carboxyl-terminal glutamine was found in two different HDL proteins (71). However, the yield of glutamine from carboxypeptidase digests was inadequate for glutamine to be the sole carboxyl-terminal amino acid of the major HDL peptides regraded by the enzyme; furthermore, threonine is a major product of hydrazinolysis of HDL protein (70). Heterogeneity at the carboxyl-terminal, as found by Wuu and co-workers (78) in the polypeptide porcine neurophysin I, is also possible in the HDL protein.

More recently these polypeptide components of HDL have been obtained in lipid-free or almost lipid-free form by column chromatography of the lipoprotein in 8 *M* urea on DEAE-cellulose under the same conditions that are used for fractionation of the lipid-free protein (V. G. Shore and B. Shore, unpublished observations). These preparations were homogeneous with respect to molecular weight in dilute tris buffer in sedimentation-equilibrium experiments. The molecular weights, calculated by using values for partial specific volume obtained from amino acid composition (the carbohydrate content was ignored), were 15,800 and 13,800, respectively, for R–Thr and R–Gln.

Several other groups of investigators also have established the heterogeneity of human-serum HDL protein. In one instance Scanu and co-workers (76) separated HDL_2 protein, previously dialyzed at 27°C for 48 hr against 8 *M* urea containing 10^{-2} *M* tris buffer (pH 8.6) and 10^{-3} *M* ethylenediaminetetraacetic acid (EDTA), into four fractions by chromatography in Sephadex G-200 columns equilibrated at 27°C with the eluting buffer, a mixture of 10^{-2} *M* tris buffer (pH 8.6), 10^{-3} *M* EDTA, and 8 *M* urea.

In another study Rudman and co-workers (69) obtained three protein fractions from HDL by gel filtration of the protein moiety on a Sephadex G-200 column in 1.0 *N* acetic acid at 25°C. Either gel-filtration procedure gave two major fractions that resembled in amino acid composition the polypeptides R–Gln and R–Thr isolated by DEAE-cellulose chromatography by Shore and Shore (72). End-group analyses were not carried out on the fractions obtained by gel filtration. Rudman and co-workers obtained a third and minor fraction that in composition appeared very similar to, if not identical with, their largest fraction (R–Thr ?). Rudman and co-workers (69) considered that their procedure gave the two polypeptide components of HDL in pure form, but criteria other than homogeneity in polyacrylamide-gel electrophoresis would be useful. The amino acid compositions published by Scanu et al. (76) and by Rudman et al. (69) indicate that gel filtration alone does not yield the proteins in pure form. Unlike Shore and Shore (72), Rudman et al. (69) found both histidine and arginine (3.6–3.8 and 9.0–9.8 residues per 10^3 amino acid residues, respectively) in their fraction, which resembled R–Gln in composition.

The polypeptides R–Thr–Gln and R–Thr were the major protein components in about a dozen different samples of HDL_2 and HDL_3 from apparently healthy young adults of both sexes (70, 71). In addition to the major components, DEAE-cellulose chromatography of the lipid-free protein of HDL in urea yields five or more components present in variable but minor amounts (71 and unpublished observation). The less dense HDL_2 subfraction in general appears to contain more of the minor components than does the higher density subfraction (71). Some of the minor HDL polypeptides, or polypeptides of very similar if not identical composition, have been found in other lipoprotein fractions; in VLDL they comprise a considerably larger percentage, as much as 60%, of the total protein (71); in HDL_1 (*d* 1.050–1.063 g/ml), they usually occur to a greater extent than in HDL; in LDL they are trace components that appear more in the density 1.007–1.019 g/ml fraction than in the major LDL component of density 1.029–1.041 g/ml.

The amino acid compositions of some HDL protein fractions from DEAE-cellulose chromatography are shown in Table I. In addition, HDL protein contains variable but small amounts of the VLDL polypeptides whose amino acid compositions are presented in Section IV.

The roles of the various polypeptides in HDL structure are of consider-

Table I. Amino Acid Composition of HDL Polypeptides

	Quantity (moles/10^3 moles amino acids)				
	Major Components		Minor Components		
Amino Acid	R–Gln	R–Thr	1	2	3
Lysine	116	79	101	100	77
Histidine	0	22	13	7	14
Arginine	0	67	65	13	51
Aspartic acid	41	95	87	53	83
Threonine	81	38	38	65	47
Serine	81	62	108	114	69
Glutamic acid	198	183	156	186	186
Proline	52	38	24	46	42
Glycine	43	45	55	78	47
Alanine	67	76	79	76	83
Cystine (½ residue)	15	0	0	15	0
Cysteine	0	0	0	0	0
Valine	76	52	32	65	60
Methionine	15	15	14	8	14
Isoleucine	15	0	30	14	7
Leucine	102	149	111	91	139
Tyrosine	46	28	25	28	28
Phenylalanine	51	23	38	41	28
Tryptophan	0	29	25	0	28

able interest in relation to the biochemical and physiological processes of lipid transport. The major polypeptides R–Thr and R–Gln, which differ so strikingly in composition, might be expected to have different affinities for HDL lipids. It is very likely that both R–Gln and R–Thr occur in the same molecule. However, molecular species of HDL and HDL_1 containing R–Thr but not R–Gln also occur. The proportion of the two peptides varies among different individuals and among different density subfractions of HDL. In one individual, whose plasma lipoproteins distribution showed a specific elevation in HDL_1 (79), the HDL_1 and HDL contained, relatively, very little of the glycopeptide R–Gln (80). Thus much of her HDL, which was relatively enriched in the less dense HDL_2 subfraction, contained one but not the other of the major HDL polypeptides. From immunochemcial experiments, Albers and Aladjem (81) concluded that about 90% of HDL_2 and HDL_3 molecules contain both peptides and that about 10% of the molecules contain R–Thr but not R–Gln.

The proportion of the two major polypeptides in HDL appears to be important in cholesteryl ester formation by lecithin:cholesterol acyltransferase. C. Fielding and co-workers (private communication) found that the isolated, lipid-free R–Thr markedly activated cholesteryl ester formation by the purified enzyme in the presence of sonically dispersed lipids and that R–Gln depressed the activation by R–Thr.

An HDL_3 molecule of molecular weight 170,000 would contain about six to eight polypeptides of molecular weight 14,000 to 15,000, and an HDL_2 molecule of molecular weight 360,000 would contain about eight to ten polypeptides. The electron-microscope studies of Forte and co-workers (57, 58) with negative-staining techniques show that an HDL_3 molecule is made up of three to four subunits and that an HDL_2 molecule usually contains five to six subunits, although as few as three are occasionally seen. The average diameter of an HDL_2 molecule was 95 Å (range 60–140 Å), with 77% of the molecular diameters falling between 70 and 100 Å; the average diameter for an HDL_3 molecule was 65 Å (range 45–100 Å), with 78% of the diameters being between 60 and 80 Å. Estimation of subunit dimensions from electron micrographs was difficult because of the resolution limits of the technique, but Forte and co-workers estimated the subunit molecular weights to be 60,000 for HDL_3 and slightly less for HDL_2. The number of subunits seen in electron micrographs is roughly one-half the number of polypeptide subunits estimated from the molecular weight and protein content of the lipoproteins, and the molecular weight of the polypeptides.

It has been suggested by Gotto and Shore (82) that the polypeptide R–Gln may be more intimately involved in interactions with the lipids than is the polypeptide R–Thr, since helical segments of most proteins are located at the surface and away from the hydrophobic interior. From amino acid composition, R–Thr could be expected to be almost completely helical, whereas R–Gln could contain 40 to 50% helix. The prediction was qualitatively supported by measurements of the optical rotatory dispersion and circular-dichroism spectra of the two polypeptides (82). Both polypeptides, as well as HDL, exhibit negative troughs at 208 and 222 nm in their circular-dichroism spectra, which are characteristic of the α-helix. From the CD spectra of the lipid-free polypeptides, the α-helix contents of R–Thr and R–Gln were estimated to be 51 to 65% and 32 to 35%, respectively; they are probably higher in the presence of lipids, in the intact lipoprotein (80, 82).

Considerable conformational differences between LDL and HDL have been observed (4, 82–84); HDL is the more helical and may contain 60 to 70% helical structure, which is to a large extent retained in the lipid-free protein. Reversible thermal transitions in conformation, followed by circular-dichroism measurements and ultraviolet spectroscopy, appeared greater in apo-HDL_2 than in HDL_2 (85). From nuclear-magnetic-resonance studies of HDL_2 and HDL_3, Chapman and co-workers (86) concluded that the presence of protein exerts little constraining effect on the proton resonance of lipoprotein lipids. The lipids appeared to be in a magnetically isotropic environment, with considerable molecular freedom. Gotto and Kon (87) observed in electron-spin-resonance experiments that lipid appreciably constrains nitroxide tumbling in the spin-labeled protein moiety, an effect that was greater in HDL than in LDL. There appeared to be two distinct kinds of substituted amino acid sites on both HDL and LDL. At one the spin label was strongly immobilized, probably due to a lipid–protein interaction. Removal of lipids from the protein decreased the intensity of the effect.

Other studies that relate to the interaction of protein and lipids in HDL are those of Hayashi, Lindgren, and Nichols (88) and Nichols and co-workers (private communication). In the former diethyl ether was found to extract very little lipid from HDL but to change its physical characteristics markedly. Before treatment the HDL fraction contained mainly HDL_3 with some HDL_2; it was 52% protein. After extraction of the lipoprotein in aqueous solution with ether, which removed about 2% of the total lipids, there was a marked reduction in HDL_3 and an increase in HDL_2. Considerable amounts of the starting material were found in the LDL fraction and in a fraction with $d > 1.20$ g/ml. The LDL product was 79% lipid by weight and was estimated to have a molecular weight of 1.1×10^6; the HDL product was 61% lipid and had a molecular weight of 5.2×10^5. The other product contained only 1% lipid and had a molecular weight of 4.3×10^4.

A. V. Nichols and co-workers (private communication) produced a similar effect by dehydrating HDL in ammonium acetate at pH 7.4 and then redissolving the lipoprotein; they identified the products in terms of polypeptide moieties as well as the densities of the fractions. They, like Hayashi and co-workers, observed a much broader density spectrum in the analytical centrifuge in the redissolved HDL than in the starting material. They obtained lower density fractions, including some of S_f 20–400 and a fraction with $d > 1.21$ g/ml. The HDL component was higher in phospholipids, and the VLDL component was rich in cholesteryl ester, not triglycerides. The densest fraction, which contained a small amount of phospholipids, was found to be the HDL polypeptide R–Thr; the least dense fraction (S_f 20–400) was found to contain the minor HDL polypeptide components that are also normally present in VLDL; the LDL fraction (d 1.006–1.063 g/ml) contained R–Gln and small amounts of the minor polypeptide components; HDL with d 1.063 to 1.21 g/ml contained almost exclusively R–Gln.

The cholesterol-rich VLDL particles produced by the rehydration procedure were seen in electron micrographs as spherical particles with an average diameter of 1000 Å (range 250–2000 Å). The LDL contained approximately spherical particles, with diameters of 140 to 190 Å, which tended to aggregate. The HDL counterpart was made up of rodlike structures, about 40 to 300 Å long, which tended to associate along their long axes.

From these experiments, the following three conclusions can be drawn about the HDL polypeptides:

1. The minor polypeptide components of HDL have a considerable affinity for lipids, especially cholesteryl esters.
2. The polypeptide R–Gln has a stronger affinity for lipids than does R–Thr and binds phospholipids.
3. The polypeptide R–Thr is not a strong binder of lipids, at least not when competing with R–Gln and the polypeptides found in common between HDL and VLDL.

It is interesting that the last two observations bear out the prediction based on the conformation studies of Gotto and Shore (82) regarding the relative affinities of R–Gln and R–Thr for lipids.

The role of the minor polypeptide constituents in the structure of HDL is even less certain. Some of them, or their lipid complexes, may undergo exchange between the HDL and VLDL fractions. It is probable that some of the minor HDL polypeptides are derived from VLDL by the action of specific lipases involved in the utilization of the VLDL triglycerides; the lipolysis of VLDL has been found to yield products in the density ranges of LDL and HDL (89, 90). It is possible that these peptides or their lipid-peptide complexes are released from their site of synthesis into the HDL fraction of plasma directly, without a VLDL intermediate. Gotto and co-workers (91) found these peptides in plasma in abetalipoproteinemia, in which LDL and VLDL were absent. Havel and co-workers (92) suggest that nascent VLDL does not contain these peptides, but acquires them from HDL on entering the plasma. Thus HDL would be a source of VLDL peptides (including the activator for lipoprotein lipase), which would be returned to the HDL fraction during lipolysis of the VLDL triglycerides. Whether they represent minor HDL species distinct from HDL containing R–Gln and R–Thr, or whether lipid complexes of the minor polypeptides associate with HDL molecules to give larger, less dense HDL molecules, remains to be seen.

To answer some of the questions about the roles of the various polypeptides in HDL structure it will be necessary to fractionate the lipoproteins themselves (rather than the protein) on the basis of polypeptide content and to isolate lipoprotein subunits. Application of the usual fractionation techniques to lipoproteins is complicated by the fact that lipids can be removed and redistributed during the process. Perhaps a fractionation of the lipoprotein based on reaction with a specific antibody to one or another of the polypeptides isolated from the protein might circumvent some of the problems associated with the usual physical and chemical techniques. Studies of the polypeptides associated with HDL in abnormal physiological states or in genetic disorders affecting HDL also may give clues to HDL structure.

III. LOW-DENSITY LIPOPROTEINS

Studies on the proteins of LDL and other lipoprotein classes—together with physical, chemical, and immunological studies on the lipoproteins themselves—have confirmed that the normal-human-plasma LDL isolated on the basis of density are for the most part a distinct lipoprotein species not related to HDL by common polypeptides or molecular substructure. Like HDL, however, LDL are rich in cholesteryl esters and phospholipids, and account for a large fraction of the total serum lipids (1, 6). Triglycerides account for about 8% of LDL lipids (1); smaller amounts of other lipids, including glycolipids (6), are also present. The average concentration of LDL is approximately 400 and 340 mg/100 ml in normal males and females, respectively (1), and of this about 22% is glycoprotein. The carbohydrate moiety amounts to 4 to 5% of the glycoprotein, which contains mannose and galactose (2.7–3.2%), fucose ($\sim$ 0.3%), glucosamine (1.2%), and *N*-acetylneuraminic acid (0.4–1.5%) (93, 94).

Heterogeneity of the LDL fraction in size, hydrated density, and composition has been reported by several investigators (1, 3, 95–97). In a recent investigation Oncley (3, 97) applied an ultracentrifuge method devised by Baldwin and Williams (98) to the evaluation of size and density distributions among lipoproteins. The considerable heterogeneity of LDL so demonstrated appeared as a single bivariate normal distribution when sedimentation-distribution functions were interpreted in terms of size and density variations; size and density were inversely related; that is, the less dense, the larger the molecule.

Molecular-weight measurements have given values ranging from about 2×10^6 to about 3.5×10^6. The latter value was estimated by Margolis (99) from elution volumes of agarose-gel columns. Light-scattering measurements by Bjorklund and Katz (100) indicated molecular weights of about 2.8×10^6. Sedimentation-velocity methods have given values between 2×10^6 and 3×10^6. Oncley (101) reported a molecular weight of 2.3×10^6 for spherical particles with a hydrated density of 1.032 g/ml. Adams and Schumaker (102) have reported a value of 2.38×10^6 on the basis of a density of 1.030 g/ml, a frictional ratio (f/f_0) of 1.05, and a hydration 10%. Earlier they had obtained values in the range 2.43×10^6 to 2.98×10^6 (96). Lindgren and co-workers (103) obtained molecular-weight values of 2.16×10^6 for males and 2.29×10^6 for females.

From sedimentation-equilibrium data, Scanu, Pollard, and co-workers (104, 105) obtained molecular weights of 2.1×10^6 to 2.3×10^6 for both LDL (*d* 1.019–1.063 g/ml) and its succinylated derivative. Graphical analysis of their sedimentation-equilibrium data suggests considerable homogeneity, since the molecular weight was the same at all values of r^2, where r is the distance from the center of rotation. However, variations in molecular weight might have been offset by variations in partial specific volume in the sedimentation-equilibrium distribution of these molecules. If increases in molecular weight in this lipoprotein species are associated with increased lipid content, as indicated by the work of Oncley (3), the sedimentation-equilibrium distribution of molecular species would not be a reliable indicator of the variability in molecular weight.

In electron micrographs of negatively stained lipoproteins LDL appear as spherical structures with a mean diameter of about 216 Å. Gotto and co-workers (106, 107) observed considerable uniformity in particle size for an LDL fraction precipitated by heparin and manganese. Forte and co-workers (58) observed a somewhat broader size range (170–260 Å) for a fraction with *d* 1.006 to 1.063 g/ml (S_f 0–20), a mean diameter of 216 Å, and a high degree of deformability. They calculated a molecular weight of 3.29×10^6 from the mean diameter and the density, 1.035 g/ml. Hamilton's (108) electron micrographs of LDL are very similar to those of Gotto et al. and Forte et al. He noted that the particle size was more uniform than it was in other lipoprotein fractions, but that LDL molecules varied in diameter from 150 to 250 Å. The LDL structures appeared granular with no discernible subunits in the electron micrographs from all three laboratories.

However, in their electron micrographs of negatively stained LDL (*d* 1.019–1.063, 22% protein), Pollard, Scanu, and Taylor (105) saw LDL as a population of spherical particles with an average diameter of 193 Å and a visible substructure suggesting a dodecahedral arrangement of subunits with characteristic twofold, threefold, and fivefold rotation axes as well as five and six edges. Assuming a density of 1.37 g/ml for the LDL subunits, they obtained a subunit molecular weight of 30,000. From the average diameter of 193 Å and a density of 1.040 g/ml, they obtained a molecular weight of 2.2×10^6 to 2.3×10^6 for LDL. From these results Pollard et al. proposed a model of LDL containing 20 protein subunits, each with a molecular weight of 25,000 to 30,000, at the vertices of a dodecahedron with a diameter of about 193 Å. The protein subunits were thought to be most likely globular.

Pollard and co-workers consider the model to be compatible with the one proposed by Oncley et al. (109) for LDL structure if the phospholipids occupy the faces of the dodecahedron formed by the protein subunits and the neutral lipids are in the interior of the shell. After removal of the neutral lipids, LDL appeared as small subunits arranged in strings of variable length up to 500 Å. Lipid-free LDL protein appeared as beaded strings and spherical structures with diameters of 50 to 150 Å (105). In the electron micrographs of Gotto and co-workers (107) the lipid-free protein appeared as long fibrillar chains and fibrous structures.

Several other physicochemical techniques—including optical rotatory dispersion, circular dichroism, infrared spectroscopy, nuclear magnetic resonance, and electron spin resonance—have been used for structural studies of LDL protein and its interaction with lipids in the molecule. The nuclear-magnetic-resonance studies of Steim, Edner, and Bargoot (110) do not indicate any extensive ($>$ 5–10%) hydrophobic association of lipid and protein in either LDL or HDL molecules. The spectra of both lipoproteins at 35°C were similar and resembled those of the sonically dispersed lipids in water. The apparent mobility of the cholesterol molecules was interpreted as indicative of solubilization in phospholipid micelles. From their electron spin resonance studies, Gotto and Kon (87) concluded that lipid exerts a constraint on one of two types of nitroxide-labeled protein sites in LDL, but the effect is less pronounced than it is in HDL.

Despite these similarities, LDL and HDL proteins are very different in physical and chemical properties. The protein of LDL, unlike that of HDL, contains a considerable quantity of antiparallel-chain β-structure and a lesser amount of disordered or helical content, or both; this is apparent from the infrared and circular-dichroism spectra (107, 111). The circular-dichroism spectrum of LDL has a major negative trough at 215 to 218 nm, which is associated with β-structure, and a shoulder at 208 to 210 nm, possibly indicative of some helical or disordered structure or both. The infrared spectrum of LDL in deuterium oxide exhibited absorption bands characteristically found with compounds containing β- and helical or disordered structures. The soluble, lipid-free LDL protein retained essentially the spectral characteristics of the lipoprotein, although an approximate 25% increase in the content of disordered structure was noted (107).

These findings on LDL conformation have been confirmed by other investigators, who also found that the proportions of the different structures in LDL were dependent on temperature (112, 113) and on the density of the LDL fraction (113). The protein contained more pleated-sheet, or

β, structure at higher temperatures and in LDL of lower density (higher lipid content). Kobozev and Troitskii (114) had previously observed a considerable reversible temperature dependence in their optical-rotatory-dispersion studies of LDL structure. It was interpreted as indicating a loose interrelationship between the peptide chains and increased freedom of rotation around the α-carbon. The temperature dependence was nonlinear and reflected, it was suggested, conversion from a given conformation to another with change in temperature. Their data gave a positive value for b_0 in the Moffitt–Yang (115) method of analysis. Kobozev and Troitskii concluded that the considerable optical activity of LDL appeared to be due to an unfolded, metastable conformation rather than a helical one, which, under physiological conditions, was predisposed to denaturation.

Although a number of genetic variants of LDL have been observed (32–34), the human-serum LDL fraction is usually thought of as normally made up almost entirely of a single lipoprotein species. Several investigators (1, 3, 5, 116, 117) have provided immunochemical evidence for LDL homogeneity, and antibodies to β-lipoprotein have been isolated (118). However, Aladjem's (119) immunoelectrophoretic studies indicated that LDL S_f 6 and S_f 13 subfractions, which were similar to each other, each contained six or eight components. The S_f 6 lipoproteins were fairly homogeneous electrophoretically, but S_f 17 and $S_f > 17$ lipoproteins contained a fast component, a component with intermediate mobility, and a third component (probably chylomicrons) that remained at the origin (119). Normally, LDL and HDL are antigenically unrelated; LDL and VLDL have antigenic determinants in common, but VLDL has additional components not present in LDL.

As in the case of HDL, more than one experimental approach appears necessary to answer questions regarding the extent of heterogeneity in LDL. Some of the differences noted above may result from the presence in the major LDL species of more than one kind of polypeptide subunit, which are now known to be present in LDL protein (71, 120, 121). However, it appears certain that lipoproteins in the lower and higher density regions, at least, of the LDL range may be made up of more than one lipoprotein species. The higher density fraction, S_f 0–3, or HDL_1, may contain mostly HDL-type molecules or largely β-lipoprotein-type molecules, or both, judging from the amino acid compositions of the fractions and the content of HDL polypeptides, which was established by polyacrylamide-gel electrophoresis and fractionation on the ion exchanger DEAE-cellulose (80). Puppione et al. (79) have also observed from electron micrographs that in substructure HDL_1 may largely resemble HDL in some individuals and LDL in others. In hyperthyroidism, β-lipoprotein is found in the HDL density range (D. Seidel, personal communication). Peptides that are major components of VLDL and minor components of HDL are also present in HDL_1 (S_f 0–3) and, to a lesser extent, in LDL of density 1.007–1.019 g/ml (S_f 12–20). In Lp(a)-positive individuals (33–37), HDL_1 and HDL_2 contain the Lp(a) lipoprotein, which has a density of 1.05–1.12 g/ml (122). The lipoprotein contains a sialic acid rich-glycopeptide in addition to the protein of LDL of Lp(a)-negative individuals, has pre-beta mobility, and appears to have a molecular weight of approximately 5×10^6; its lipid composition is similar to that of LDL (122). The molecular basis for the LDL variant, the Ag system, is not known, but it is a complex system found in LDL and VLDL (32–34, 38).

Characterization of the polypeptide moieties of LDL has only recently been initiated, mainly because of difficulties in preparing a lipid-free protein fraction in a water-soluble form amenable to study. The LDL, although only 22% protein and almost 50% hydrophobic lipids—cholesteryl esters and triglycerides—are very soluble in water and in concentrated salt solutions. The lipid-free protein readily aggregates, especially at concentrations higher than about 2 mg/ml or in the presence of salts. The protein tends to form insoluble gels in the absence of lipids or detergents and appears to undergo surface denaturation readily since insoluble films are often formed at surfaces. The solubility of the protein is increased by sodium dodecyl sulfate or sodium decyl sulfate (106, 123), by succinylation (104), and by maleylation (120).

Several procedures have been used to prepare the soluble, almost lipid-free protein. Scanu and co-workers (104) extracted LDL containing sodium dodecyl sulfate with ethanol–diethyl ether (3:1) at −10°C. A second extraction with ether was followed by an ether wash and drying of the protein under nitrogen. The protein was dissolved in pH 8.6 tris buffer (μ = 0.1) containing 0.2 *M* sodium dodecyl sulfate. Most of the detergent was then removed by dialysis or by ion-exchange chromatography. Concentrated urea was sometimes used to facilitate the solubilization of the protein (105). Gotto and co-workers (106) found that sodium decyl sulfate is more suitable than sodium dodecyl sulfate because it is more soluble in water and can be removed completely by dialysis. In some cases they succinylated the lipoprotein before delipidation and obtained a soluble, succinylated protein. Detergent was found to be unnecessary during the delipidation process. Simons and Helenius (120) maleylated the lipoprotein before extraction by the Scanu method.

Alternatively the protein moiety of LDL has been prepared in soluble form by extraction of the neutral lipids with diethyl ether from a dilute solution of the lipoprotein (~ 1–2 mg protein /ml) in the presence of salt. After removal of the salt by dialysis, the phospholipids are removed by extraction with mixtures of ether and ethanol (71).

A procedure for removing much of the LDL lipid without organic solvents has been reported by Gotto and co-workers (124). They found that after centrifugation of a mixture of the lipoprotein and sodium decyl sulfate, essentially all the protein was recovered in a fraction that sedimented at *d* 1.063 g/ml. About 50% of the phospholipids and 50% of the free cholesterol were retained with the protein, and the remainder of the lipids floated to the top on centrifugation. More recently, Helenius and Simons (125) reported that the lipid can be removed from LDL protein by four different detergents: sodium deoxycholate, the nonionic detergent Nonidet P40, cetyltrimethylammonium bromide, and sodium dodecyl sulfate. The protein was separated from the lipid-detergent micelles by gel filtration in the presence of the detergent. The detergent was removed from the protein by gel filtration in solvent containing no detergent. Sodium deoxycholate and Nonidet P40 did not—but sodium dodecyl sulfate and cetyltrimethylammonium bromide did—change the immunological properties of LDL protein.

Sedimentation-velocity and sedimentation-equilibrium experiments on the lipid-free protein of LDL clearly show that the protein moiety of the lipoprotein molecule is made up of a number, perhaps 20 or more, of subunits. However, because of the difficulty of obtaining completely dissociated protein, these studies alone permit only limited conclusions about the minimum subunit size and the possible existence of subunits of different molecular weights. Gotto and co-workers (106) observed that, although both LDL and its succinylated derivative sedimented with a single boundary, the succinylated protein exhibited heterogeneity in the presence and in the absence of the sodium decyl sulfate. They always found two schlieren peaks, but the sedimentation rates of the slower and faster components varied among different preparations. In the presence of 20 m*M* sodium dodecyl sulfate, $S^\circ_{20,\,w}$ values of 4.2 and 5.6 were observed for the two components. In another experiment $S^\circ_{20,\,w}$ values for the slower component were 3.3 in the presence of the detergent and 6.0 in its absence.

From sedimentation-equilibrium experiments on the protein of LDL in 8 *M* urea at pH 11.5 by the Yphantis high-speed method, Pollard and co-workers (105) concluded that LDL may contain protein subunits as small as 27,500 in molecular weight. This value is a minimum one obtained near the meniscus, and considerable heterogeneity in molecular weight was observed. The authors believed that aggregation was the main factor contributing to the observed heterogeneity, but the possibility of different proteins with unequal molecular weights cannot be ruled out.

Kane and co-workers (121) found on gel filtration of the maleylated β-protein in 6 *M* guanidine HCl that as much as 25% of the total protein was eluted in a fraction of approximate molecular weight 26,000. In 6 *M* urea, over 75% of the maleylated protein was eluted in two fractions: a major but heterogeneous one of about 25,000 molecular weight and a minor one of about 5,000 to 10,000 molecular weight (Shore and Shore, unpublished observation).

Amino- and carboxyl-terminal amino acid analyses have been of limited value in characterizing the polypeptides of LDL protein. Very likely the major end groups of LDL protein have not yet been reported. Amino-terminal glutamic acid and carboxyl-terminal serine are present (1), but the amounts are far too small to account for subunits with molecular weights of 30,000. In addition, LDL yielded very small amounts of amino-terminal serine, threonine, and aspartic acid (1).

The LDL protein is made up of several different polypeptides, as shown by recent studies involving fractionation of the protein by gel filtration and ion-exchange chromatography. After removing most of the lipids from maleylated LDL, Simons and Helenius (120) obtained two fractions by gel filtration of the maleylated protein in Sephadex G-200 equilibrated with 0.1% sodium dodecyl sulfate in 0.1 *M* tris buffer at pH 9. The two fractions differed in amino acid composition, but one of them resembled the unfractionated protein. Rabbit antibodies to the maleylated protein gave two precipitin lines with the maleylated protein. Kane and co-workers (121) also obtained two fractions of different amino acid composition by gel filtration. Both groups of investigators presented evidence for the existence of protein subunits with molecular weights of less than 30,000. The smaller fraction obtained by Kane and co-workers was relatively rich in serine, glutamic acid, glycine, and cystine and low in methionine in comparison with the unfractionated protein. Its composition and those of the unfractionated protein and several fractions obtained by ion-exchange chromatography of the protein in 7 *M* urea are given in Table II. The composition of the Lp(a) variant of LDL is also given. There is much work yet to be done on isolation and characterization of the LDL polypeptides.

Besides the several major polypeptide components of normal LDL, abnormal LDL may contain significant amounts of other components normally present in very small amounts or not at all. The marked elevation of serum cholesterol that is characteristic of biliary obstruction is associated with an LDL species of atypical composition (27–30). Switzer (29) showed that it does not react with antibodies to normal LDL or with antiserums to HDL; antibodies to the obstructive lipoprotein did not react with any lipoprotein fraction from normal serum. The lipoprotein was contained in the *d* 1.019 to 1.063 g/ml fraction of LDL; it was high in free cholesterol (26%) and phospholipids (61%) but had only traces of cholesteryl esters and triglycerides, and much less protein (5%) than is normally found in

Table II. Amino Acid Composition of LDL Proteins

	Quantity (moles/10^3 moles amino acids)					
Amino Acid	UP[a]	Lp(a)[b]	A[c]	1[d]	2[d]	3[d]
Lysine	75	63	72	68	70	79
Histidine	22	21	20	24	17	22
Arginine	33	40	39	18	35	28
Aspartic acid	103	99	82	69	89	108
Threonine	65	68	67	46	64	60
Serine	91	78	104	197	89	111
Glutamic acid	129	118	138	156	133	120
Proline	36	54	38	20	55	33
Glycine	48	75	104	166	69	64
Alanine	65	83	75	77	69	64
Cystine (1/2 residue)	7	18	29		14	9
Valine	54	60	48	40	57	59
Methionine	21	16	1	9	21	15
Isoleucine	50	44	37	26	45	50
Leucine	108	85	90	43	108	99
Tyrosine	34	35	30	18	28	26
Phenylalanine	49	35	26	18	38	48
Tryptophan	7	9				

[a] Unfractionated protein.
[b] Unfractionated Lp(a) protein (122).
[c] Fraction II (MW 26,000) from gel filtration of maleylated protein in 6*M* guanidine hydrochloride (121).
[d] Fractions from DEAE-cellulose chromatography of protein in 8*M* urea (B. Shore and V. Shore, unpublished data).

LDL (29). The amino acid composition of the protein resembled that of VLDL (29).

More recently, Alaupovic and co-workers (126) presented evidence that the protein moiety of the lipoprotein, which they designated LP-X, contains albumin (~ 40%) and a protein designated apolipoprotein C (~ 60%), which is found also in VLDL. Although LP-X did not react with antialbumin serums, the partially delipidated product did. The nonalbumin component had the carboxyl-terminal sequence R–Val–Ala–Ala and was immunochemically identical with apolipoprotein C from VLDL (126). The average S_f-rate of LP-X in an NaCl solution of *d* 1.063 g/ml was 15.9S (127).

The studies of Hamilton and co-workers (128) indicate that the abnormal lipoprotein associated with bilary obstruction is a vesicle, the wall of which is a bilayer of cholesterol and lecithin in equimolar amounts. The lecithin head groups are about 45 Å apart, and the fatty acid chains and cholesterol ring structure are at the center. In electron micrographs, the negatively stained particle appears to be a disk of about 100 by 500 Å.

Other abnormalities in LDL are associated with genetic deficiencies resulting in abetalipoproteinemia (21, 22, 24) and the type II and type III hyperlipoproteinemias (40). Abnormal LDL proteins are suspected to occur in abetalipoproteinemia and type III hyperlipoproteinemia, but the problem is not yet solved. Elucidation of the molecular defects associated with these abnormalities should greatly increase our knowledge of the structural and metabolic interrelationships between LDL and VLDL. Many studies indicate that such interrelationships exist (1–3, 5, 39). The triglyceride-transport systems for moving VLDL from the liver and the intestine, and for moving chylomicrons from the intestinal mucosa, require LDL for their formation and secretion (1, 3, 5), and there is evidence that LDL protein is a component of VLDL (1, 3, 5, 117, 123).

In persons afflicted with abetalipoproteinemia (absence or deficiency of plasma LDL) VLDL and chylomicrons are also absent from plasma (20, 23, 39, 40, 129, 130), and triglycerides accumulate in the liver and intestinal mucosa (24, 40). The involvement of LDL in the formation of VLDL and chylomicrons is indicated also by comparative studies of normal rats and rats fed orotic acid (131–133); these studies provided evidence for the synthesis of LDL and VLDL in the intestine as well as the liver. Infusion of LDL into abetalipoproteinemic patients does not reverse the defects in glyceride transport and does not result in the formation of VLDL and chylomicrons (129). The half-time of 2.3 days for the removal of infused LDL from an abetalipoproteinemic patient was normal (129). The serum of abetalipoproteinemic patients contains no immunologically cross-reacting species, as might be expected if a genetic mutation were causing the production of abnormal LDL protein (23, 134). Deficiency of LDL protein at the tissue site of LDL formation is still possible.

In type III hyperlipoproteinemia, which has also been described as xanthoma tuberosum because of the characteristic cutaneous lipid deposits (26, 40), the normal major component of LDL is decreased in concentration and LDL of lower density and VLDL are increased (20, 40). It has been suggested that the decreased triglyceride removal from plasma in type III hyperlipoproteinemia may be the result of an abnormal LDL protein–lipid complex (40).

Type II hyperlipoproteinemia, or familial hyperbetalipoproteinemia, is associated with a decreased LDL turnover rate, possibly as a result of a mutation affecting the rate of catabolism of either cholesterol or LDL (40), although the metabolic error is unknown. The amino acid compositions of the LDL protein moieties from two type II individuals did not differ from that of normal LDL, according to Pinon and Laudat (135). However, further studies, including amino acid sequence studies, are needed to establish the presence or absence of small structural differences in the LDL proteins of normal and type II individuals or others in which a variant is suspected.

IV. VERY-LOW-DENSITY LIPOPROTEINS

The very-low-density lipoproteins (S_f 20–400; *d* 0.94–1.006 g/ml) of human plasma are largely lipid, with a glycoprotein moiety amounting to 5 to 12% of their mass (1, 3, 6, 11). The major lipids are triglycerides (50–60%), phospholipids (20–25%), and cholesteryl esters (18–26%). In electron micrographs by Forte and co-workers (58), negatively stained VLDL appear as large, electron-transparent spheres with no apparent fine structure. Electron microscopy indicates a wide range, 230 to 700 Å, of particle diameters (39, 58), but there is some uncertainty in size estimation due to possible flattening or spreading of the particles during the procedure.

Other studies also have indicated heterogeneity of VLDL (1, 11, 13); in a recent one Oncley and Harvie (3) applied the Baldwin and Williams ultracentrifugal test (98) for analysis of the distribution of size and density. For VLDL they found two bimodal normal distributions, one around a diameter of 269 Å and a density of 0.992, and the second around a diameter of 402 Å and a density of 0.965. One distribution contained particles in the S_f range 12 to 60 and accounted for about 36% of the VLDL preparation. The remainder of the VLDL preparation (64% by weight) fell within the second distribution, which contained particles in the S_f range 30 to 600. The test also indicated an inverse relationship between size and density, as has been concluded from the composition of various VLDL subfractions (1, 13). In general, as particle size increases, so does the percentage of triglyceride content (1). The simplest explanation for the existence of two overlapping VLDL distributions, Oncley and Harvie suggest, is that they contain different apolipoproteins.

Although it is known that VLDL contain a number of different polypeptides, the extent and nature of heterogeneity in VLDL species as a result of different protein moieties is largely unknown. Normally VLDL migrate as a single band, the pre-β-lipoproteins in paper or agarose electrophoresis and exhibit heterogeneity only after partial removal of lipids (11, 12). Ether-extracted VLDL gave β (LDL) and α (HDL) bands in paper electrophoresis and, unlike intact VLDL, reacted with antibodies to HDL as well as those to LDL (12). Gustafson and co-workers (117) found that

Pevikon zone electrophoresis partially resolves the phospholipid–protein residues of VLDL into three immunochemically distinct components, two of which correspond to HDL and LDL proteins, respectively, and one of which contains amino-terminal serine and threonine. The ratio of phospholipid to protein in the latter complex (2.4:1) was considerably higher than the ratios in the HDL and LDL components (0.9:1 and 0.7:1). The proportion of the three components varied considerably among six VLDL preparations, although the LDL component was always a major one (48–78%). Serine, threonine, glutamic acid, and aspartic acid are the amino-terminal amino acids found in VLDL protein (1, 89, 117, 136–138); they are also found in variable proportions among different VLDL fractions. There is no evidence that any of the three phospholipid–protein complexes is derived from a distinct species of VLDL, but variations among different VLDL preparations in the proportions of the three phospholipid–protein complexes and of the four end groups are evidence that VLDL vary in protein composition.

Several studies have indicated that VLDL are related structurally and metabolically to both HDL and LDL. Formation and secretion of VLDL require LDL, but not HDL (39, 130). Lipolysis of VLDL triglycerides by parenteral administration of heparin (12, 90) or *in vitro* by heparin-activated lipases (89) gives lipoprotein products in the LDL and HDL density classes. Immunochemically VLDL protein is related to both LDL and HDL proteins (12, 117). Amino-terminal groups are found in common between VLDL and LDL and between VLDL and HDL (1, 60, 89, 117, 136–138). "Fingerprint" maps from high-voltage electrophoresis of the pepsin digests and trypsin digests of the protein moieties indicated that HDL and LDL proteins are present in VLDL (117). However, when these studies were done, it was generally thought that HDL and LDL each contained a single protein rather than, as is now known to be the case, a complex mixture of polypeptides.

The metabolic and structural relationships between VLDL and LDL and between VLDL and HDL based on common polypeptides are not yet completely known. However, such components are partially identified by isolation and characterization of polypeptides of VLDL protein, together with the results of similar studies on HDL and LDL proteins. Ultimately complete identification and characterization of all the polypeptide components of the various lipoprotein classes in normal and abnormal serum should provide a much more complete knowledge of interrelationships among the various lipoprotein classes. Isolation of VLDL species characterized in terms of polypeptide constituents as well as density and lipid composition is very important for the elucidation of the roles of the various polypeptides in lipoprotein structure, metabolism, and function.

Several different polypeptide components of VLDL protein have been isolated by two groups of investigators: Brown, Levy, and Fredrickson (139, 140) and Shore and Shore (71, 141). The major HDL polypeptides R–Thr and R–Gln were not isolated from VLDL protein in either study, although the experimental procedure used in the latter study yields these polypeptides when applied to HDL protein (70, 71). The proteins common to HDL and VLDL are not the major HDL proteins, but several, possibly five, polypeptides are major protein components in VLDL and minor ones in HDL. Since in plasma the total amount of HDL protein is much greater than the total amount of VLDL protein, the HDL and VLDL fractions may contain comparable amounts of these peptides. Besides the VLDL peptides shown in Table III, VLDL frequently contains smaller

Table III. Amino Acid Composition of VLDL Polypeptides

	Concentration (moles/10^3 moles amino acids)					
Amino Acid	R–Ser	R–X_1	R–X_2	R–Glu	R–Ala	R–X_3
Lysine	154	61	49	68	76	67
Histidine	0	15	11	4	15	28
Arginine	54	30	106	18	29	14
Aspartic acid	90	74	48	68	88	70
Threonine	45	52	39	102	65	41
Serine	126	141	60	118	139	203
Glutamic acid	159	183	228	180	130	188
Proline	12	30	29	44	27	21
Glycine	32	161	59	36	40	186
Alanine	54	71	106	85	123	70
Valine	35	46	67	54	73	29
Cystine (½ residue)	0	0	0	0	0	7
Methionine	15	8	23	23	24	7
Isoleucine	48	25	12	12	0	14
Leucine	104	63	108	94	65	36
Tyrosine	0	16	14	48	25	7
Phenylalanine	48	25	14	25	47	14
Tryptophan	24		28	23	34	0

amounts of other polypeptides (71, 141, and V. Shore, unpublished observation) and proteins in common with LDL.

The amino acid compositions of some VLDL polypeptides isolated by column chromatography of the lipid-free protein on DEAE-cellulose are shown in Table III. All of the polypeptides except possibly R–Ser contain carbohydrate moieties as indicated by reaction with Schiff's reagent after periodate ovidation (V. G. Shore and B. Shore, unpublished observation). Several of the polypeptides exhibit polymorphism. In the case of R–Ala differences in sialic acid content occur (140); in the case of the polypeptide with the high arginine content, the reason is not yet known, although the amino acid composition of the two fractions appears to be identical; in other cases (e.g., in R–Ala and the polypeptide with the high serine, glutamic acid, and glycine content, small differences in amino acid composition may occur (71).

The complete amino acid sequence of the VLDL polypeptide R–Ala was determined by Brewer and co-workers (142). It is: Ser-Glu-Ala-Glu-Asp-Ala-Ser-Leu-Leu-Ser-Phe-Met-Gln-Gly-Tyr-Met-Lys-His-Ala-Thr-Lys-Thr-Ala-Lys-Asp-Ala-Leu-Ser-Ser-Val-Gln-Ser-Gln-Gln-Val-Ala-Ala-Gln-Gln-Arg-Gly-Trp-Val-Thr-Asp-Gly-Phe-Ser-Ser-Leu-Lys-Asp-Tyr-Trp-Ser-Thr-Val-Lys-Asp-Lys-Phe-Ser-Glu-Phe-Trp-Asp-Leu-Asp-Pro-Glu-Val-Arg-Pro-Thr-Ser-Ala-Val-Ala-Ala. It has a single carbohydrate moiety (galactose:galactosamine:neuraminic acid = 1:1:1 or 2 moles/mole of polypeptide) attached to threonine, residue 74.

All of the polypeptides isolated from VLDL appear to have molecular weights of less than 10,000 (71, 140, and unpublished observations), according to data from sedimentation-equilibrium experiments and the yield of end groups from the purified polypeptides. However, as might be predicted from the considerable differences in amino acid composition evident in Table III, the circular-dichroism spectra of these polypeptides indicate considerable conformational differences among them (V. G. Shore and B. Shore, unpublished observations). The polypeptides R–Ala and R–Glu are random coils with only small amounts, if any, of helical structure, whereas the polypeptide with the highest arginine content (R–X_2 of Table II) yields a circular-dichroism spectrum, with negative troughs at 208 and 222 nm, that is associated with α-helical structures, and the molar ellipticity values indicate a helical content of 70% or more. The polypeptide R-Ser of Table III is approximately 45 to 50% α-helix. All these estimates were made on the lipid-free polypeptides in water at pH 7. The conformations may be somewhat different in the native lipoprotein.

The differences in composition and physical properties among the VLDL polypeptides suggest that they may have specific and complementary roles in VLDL structure and function. However, the reasons for such a variety of peptides in VLDL and for variations in the proportions of these peptides among different preparations of VLDL are not known. No VLDL with an absolute deficiency in any of these peptides has been prepared from normal or hyperlipemic plasmas, but VLDL are clearly heterogeneous in their content of these peptides (V. Shore, unpublished observations). In most VLDL (from fasting persons), the peptide R-Ala is the predominant peptide. In some, R-Ser and the peptide with highest arginine content (Table III), are the predominant VLDL peptides. Several of the peptides may be involved in triglyceride metabolism, but specific roles for only one or two peptides have been demonstrated. The peptide R-Glu is a very potent activator of lipoprotein lipases from cows' milk (50), human post-heparin plasma (143), and rat adipose tissue (51); the peptide R-Ala at higher concentrations inhibits lipolysis (50, 143). Contrary to the findings of these studies, Ganesan and co-workers (52) reported that the peptide R-Val (R-Ser of Table III) is more active than R-Glu as activator of a lipoprotein lipase purified from post-heparin plasma. On lipolysis, the protein moiety of VLDL is partitioned between LDL and HDL; to LDL goes the β-protein component, and to HDL go most of the peptides of Table III (144–146). Havel and co-workers (92) proposed that HDL constitutes a reservoir from which these peptides (the activator proteins) are transferred to newly secreted triglyceride-rich lipoproteins and to which they are returned after the triglycerides have been removed by action of lipoprotein lipase.

V. CHYLOMICRONS

Chylomicrons, the relatively large, triglyceride-rich particles produced in the intestine from ingested fat, contain approximately 2% protein (3, 11, 39). In electron micrographs (39, 58, 147) chylomicrons appear as spheres ranging in diameter from about 1000 to 11,000 Å, with the majority of the plasma particles after fat ingestion having diameters of 1500 to 4000 Å. No substructure was indicated in these studies, but chylomicrons appear to contain an outer layer of material consisting of protein, cholesterol, and triglycerides in a monolayer of phospholipids (148–150). The percentages of protein and phospolipids increase with decreasing particle size, but the amount of protein per particle appears to decrease with decreasing size (147).

In 1959, Rodbell and Fredrickson (136) reported the finding of three proteins in both dog and human chylomicrons. One of the proteins appeared to be identical with the major HDL protein in paper-electrophoresis mobility, in amino-terminal aspartic acid content, and in "fingerprint" patterns from paper-electrophoresis chromatography of the tryptic digests. In human chylomicrons a second component contained amino-terminal serine and was thought to be a protein found throughout the density spectrum. The third human component, which was present in smaller amounts, was thought to be the protein with amino-terminal threonine. Plasma chylomicrons contained much more of the third component than did lymph chylomicrons, suggesting that this protein can be added after the entry of chylomicrons into the blood. The investigation of Rodbell and Fredrickson did not indicate the presence of LDL protein in chylomicrons. However, other evidence suggests that it is present. No chylomicrons are formed in the absence of LDL (130), and in the immunochemical studies of Alaupovic and co-workers (151) chyle chylomicrons gave a precipitin reaction with anti-LDL, anti-HDL, and anti-VLDL serums.

The amino acid composition of chylomicrons has been less extensively investigated than that of other lipoprotein classes. However, the results from a single hydrolysate of plasma-chylomicron protein from fasting males indicate it to be significantly different from other apolipoproteins in composition (152); it resembled HDL more than LDL and VLDL. Isoleucine content was much lower than it was in VLDL and LDL proteins, and about twice as high as it was in HDL protein. The chylomicron protein contained much more cystine than did any of the other proteins. Isolation of its polypeptide components has not yet been reported, but none of the polypeptides isolated from the other lipoprotein classes could account for the chylomicron cystine observed by Levy and co-workers (152). Further studies on the composition of chylomicron proteins in lymph and in plasma, and the isolation and characterization of the polypeptide components, are clearly important for understanding the function of chylomicrons and their interrelationships with other lipoproteins in lymph and plasma.

VI. CONCLUSIONS

Studies on the protein moieties of the plasma lipoproteins have furthered our understanding of structural and metabolic interrelationships among the lipoproteins and the role of apolipoproteins in the enzyme systems by which the lipids are metabolized. However, these studies also show a much greater complexity of the lipoproteins than was generally believed 4 or 5 years ago.

Each of the major density classes of lipoproteins contains a half a dozen or more different polypeptide moieties, many of which have not been characterized with respect to biochemical or physiological function. Some of the polypeptides may be multifunctional—important both for the structure and properties of the lipoprotein and for activation or inhibition (regulation) of enzyme systems by which the lipid moieties are metabolized. Although thermodynamically favored lipid-lipid interactions are undoubtedly important for lipoprotein structure and properties, the proteins probably are the major determinants of lipoprotein substructure. The protein-lipid interactions are not well understood, but the polypeptides vary in their affinities for phospholipids and other lipids. Some peptides may be important in lipid exchange, either by molecular exchange of lipids or by exchange of lipid-peptide complexes, among different lipoprotein molecules or between lipoproteins and cell membranes.

Perhaps a reason for the lack of a preponderance of hydrophobic residues in the unfractionated apolipoproteins is that the latter play a dual role in binding the water-insoluble lipids and in conferring water solubility on the protein–lipid complexes. Each apolipoprotein contains polypeptide components whose amino acid compositions differ strikingly among themselves as well as from the major polypeptides of other lipoprotein classes. The polypeptides also differ considerably in tertiary structure, as indicated by physicochemical studies of their conformations. Some may interact more extensively with the lipids, and others may be relatively hydrophilic in nature. The conformational differences, together with those in composition, indicate that the lipid-binding properties of apolipoproteins very likely will be elucidated in terms of amino acid sequences that are unique to specific polypeptides and are the major determinants of secondary structure. Thus the extent of exposure of nonpopular groups, determined by the conformation as well as the proportion of hydrophobic amino acids, will be important for the interaction of polypeptides with lipids. Sequence studies might also reveal both hydrophobic and hydrophilic regions in one polypeptide molecule. Whereas the proteins effect the water solubility of the lipids, the lipids appear to increase the solubility of the proteins. Perhaps lipids resemble detergents in preventing intermolecular interactions leading to aggregation of the polypeptides.

In addition to protein heterogeneity in each major density class, the lipoproteins themselves appear to be heterogeneous with respect to protein moiety. Not all HDL (or VLDL) molecules have identical polypeptide composition. This heterogeneity is further complicated by that due to the existence of polymorphism among several of the apolipoproteins. Heterogeneity of the lipoproteins is related undoubtedly to their metabolism and possibly to their sites of syntheses. Each of the major lipoprotein classes probably is involved in more than one aspect of lipid metabolism. For example, HDL plays a major role in cholesterol ester formation in plasma and in cholesterol homeostasis in the body. One of the major HDL polypeptides activates and the other inhibits the enzyme lecithin:cholesterol acyltransferase. However, HDL also appears to have an important part in the lipoprotein lipase system by which the triglycerides of VLDL and chylomicrons are utilized. In this role, the minor polypeptides of HDL are involved, one as activator of the lipase and another as inhibitor. HDL may act as an acceptor for these lipid-peptide complexes derived from lipolysis of VLDL and as a source of these peptides for newly released VLDL and chylomicrons. LDL also is a product of VLDL lipolysis. Thus it appears that all the major density classes may be interrelated in several major aspects of lipid metabolism, but in each case through different protein and lipid components.

VII. ACKNOWLEDGMENTS

We wish to thank Dr. Valeska Evertsbusch for her suggestions on the manuscript. This review was written under the auspices of the U.S. Atomic Energy Commission.

REFERENCES

1. Nichols, A. V., *Adv. Biol. Med. Phys.* **11**, 109–158 (1967).
2. Schumaker, V. N., and G. H. Adams, *Ann. Rev. Biochem.* **38**, 113–136 (1969).
3. Oncley, J. L., and N. R. Harvie, *Proc. Natl. Acad. Sci. U.S.* **64**, 1107–1118 (1969).
4. Gotto, A. M., R. I. Levy, and D. S. Fredrickson, *Physiol. Rev.*, in press.
5. Alaupovic, P., *Progr. Biochem. Pharmacol.* **4**, 91–109 (1968).
6. Skipski, V. P., M. Barclay, R. K. Barclay, V. A. Fetzer, J. J. Good, and F. M. Archibald, *Biochem. J.* **104**, 340–352 (1967).
7. Fredrickson, D. S., R. I. Levy, and R. S. Lees, *New Engl. J. Med.* **276**, 34–44 (1967).
8. Switzer, S., and H. A. Eder, *J. Lipid Res.* **6**, 506–511 (1965).
9. Kanai, M., A. Raz, and D. S. Goodman, *J. Clin. Invest.* **47**, 2025–2044 (1968).
10. Ling, N. S., and T. Krasteff, *Proc. Natl. Acad. Sci. U.S.* **60**, 928–935 (1968).
11. Hatch, F. T., and R. S. Lees, *Adv. Lipid Res.* **6**, 1–68 (1968).
12. Levy, R. I., R. S. Lees, and D. S. Fredrickson, *J. Clin. Invest.* **45**, 63–77 (1966).
13. Ewing, A. M., N. K. Freeman, and F. T. Lindgren, *Adv. Lipid Res.* **3**, 25–61 (1965).
14. Oncley, J. L., and S. E. Allerton, *Vox Sang.* **6**, 201–203 (1961).
15. Wilcox, H. G., D. C. Davis, and M. Heimberg, *Biochim. Biophys. Acta* **187**, 147–150 (1969).
16. Havel, R. J., H. A. Eder, and J. H. Bragdon, *J. Clin. Invest.* **34**, 1345–1353 (1955).
17. Oncley, J. L., K. W. Walton, and D. G. Cornwell, *J. Amer. Chem. Soc.* **179**, 4666–4671 (1957).
18. Gordis, E., *Proc. Soc. Exp. Biol. Med.* **110**, 657–661 (1962).
19. Fredrickson, D. S., R. S. Lees, and R. I. Levy, *Progr. Biochem. Pharmacol.* **3**, 343–352 (1967).
20. Fredrickson, D. S., R. I. Levy, and F. T. Lindgren, *J. Clin. Invest.* **47**, 2446–2457 (1968).
21. Levy, R. I., and D. S. Fredrickson, *Circulation* **34**, III-156–157 (1966) (abstract).
22. Salt, H. B., O. H. Wolff, J. K. Lloyd, A. S. Fosbrooke, A. H. Cameron, and D. V. Hubble, *Lancet* **ii**, 325–329 (1960).

23. Levy, R. I., D. S. Fredrickson, and L. Laster, *J. Clin. Invest.* **45**, 531–541 (1966).
24. Mars, H., L. A. Lewis, A. L. Robertson, Jr., A. Butkus, and G. H. Williams, Jr., *Amer. J. Med.* **46**, 886–900 (1969).
25. Jones, J. W., and P. Ways, *J. Clin. Invest.* **46**, 1151–1161 (1967).
26. Gofman, J. W., O. deLalla, F. Glazier, N. K. Freeman, F. T. Lindgren, A. V. Nichols, B. Strisower, and A. R. Tamplin, *Plasma* (*Milan*) **2**, 413–484 (1954).
27. Eder, H. A., E. M. Russ, R. A. Rees Pritchett, M. M. Wilber, and D. P. Barr, *J. Clin. Invest.* **34**, 1147–1162 (1955).
28. Russ, E. M., J. Raymunt, and D. P. Barr, *J. Clin. Invest.* **35**, 133–144 (1956).
29. Switzer, S., *J. Clin. Invest.* **46**, 1855–1866 (1967).
30. Seidel, D., P. Alaupovic, and R. H. Furman, *J. Clin. Invest.* **48**, 1211–1223 (1969).
31. Sodhi, H. S., *Metabolism* (*Clin. Exp.*) **18**, 852–859 (1969).
32. Allison, A. C., and B. S. Blumberg, *Progr. Med. Genet.* **4**, 176–201 (1965).
33. Prokop, O., and G. Uhlenbruck, *Human Blood and Serum Groups,* McLaren and Sons, London, 1969, pp. 669–679.
34. Giblett, E. R., *Genetic Markers in Human Blood,* Blackwell Scientific Publications, Oxford and Edinburgh, 1969, pp. 176–191.
35. Berg, K., *Acta Pathol. Microbiol. Scand.* **59**, 369–382 (1963).
36. Wiegandt, H., K. Lipp, and G. G. Wendt, *Hoppe-Seyler's Z. Physiol. Chem.* **349**, 489–494 (1968).
37. Schultz, J. S., D. C. Shreffler, and N. R. Harvie, *Proc. Natl. Acad. Sci. U.S.* **61**, 963–970 (1968).
38. Rittner, C., *Vox Sang.* **12**, 225–226 (1967).
39. Nichols, A. V., *Proc. Natl. Acad. Sci. U.S.* **64**, 1128–1137 (1969).
40. Fredrickson, D. S., *Proc. Natl. Acad. Sci. U.S.* **64**, 1138–1146 (1969).
41. Gurd, F. R. N., in *Lipide Chemistry,* D. J. Hanahan, Ed., Wiley, New York, 1960, pp. 282–284.
42. Nichols, A. V., and L. Smith, *J. Lipid Res.* **6**, 206–210 (1965).
43. Goodman, D. S., *J. Clin. Invest.* **43**, 2026–2036 (1964).
44. Reed, C. F., *J. Clin. Invest.* **47**, 749–760 (1968).
45. Gould, R. G., *Amer. J. Med.* **11**, 209–227 (1951).
46. Torsvik, H., E. Gjone, and K. R. Norum, *Acta Med. Scand.* **183**, 387–391 (1968).
47. Glomset, J. A., *J. Lipid Res.* **9**, 155–167 (1968).
48. Glomset, J. A., K. R. Norum, and W. King, *J. Clin. Invest.* **49**, 1827–1837 (1970).
49. Fielding, C. J., and P. E. Fielding, *Fed. Eur. Biochem. Soc. Letters* **15**, 355–358 (1971).
50. Havel, R. J., V. G. Shore, B. Shore, and D. M. Bier, *Circ. Res.* **27**, 595–600 (1970).
51. LaRosa, J. C., R. I. Levy, P. Herbert, S. E. Lux, and D. S. Fredrickson, *Biochem. Biophys. Res. Commun.* **41**, 57–62 (1970).
52. Ganesan, D., R. H. Bradford, P. Alaupovic, and W. J. McConathy, *Fed. Eur. Biochem. Soc. Letters* **15**, 205–208 (1971).
53. Scanu, A., *J. Lipid Res.* **7**, 295–306 (1966).
54. Scanu, A., and J. L. Granda, *Biochemistry* **5**, 446–455 (1966).
55. Shore, V., and B. Shore, *Biochemistry* **6**, 1962–1967 (1967).
56. Hazelwood, R. N., *J. Amer. Chem. Soc.* **80**, 2152–2156 (1955).

57. Forte, G. M., A. V. Nichols, and R. M. Glaeser, *Biophys. Soc. Annu. Meet. Abstr.* **9**, A-111 (1969).
58. Forte, G. M., A. V. Nichols, and R. M. Glaeser, *Chem. Phys. Lipids* **2**, 396–408 (1968).
59. Shore, B., and V. Shore, *Fed. Proc.* **25**, Part I, 705 (1966) (abstract).
60. Shore, B., *Arch. Biochem. Biophys.* **71**, 1–10 (1957).
61. Scanu, A., and W. L. Hughes, *J. Clin. Invest.* **41**, 1681–1689 (1962).
62. Shore, B., and V. Shore, *Biochem. Biophys. Res. Commun.* **1**, 228–231 (1959).
63. Cohen, L., and J. Djordjevich, *Lipids* **3**, 420–424 (1968).
64. Aladjem, F., M. Lieberman, and J. W. Gofman, *J. Exp. Med.* **105**, 49–67 (1957).
65. DeLalla, L., L. Levine, and R. K. Brown, *J. Exp. Med.* **106**, 261–271 (1957).
66. Ayrault-Jarrier, M., G. Lévy, and J. Polonovski, *Bull. Soc. Chim. Biol.* **45**, 703–713 (1963).
67. Burstein, M., and J. M. Fine, *Rev. Fr. Etud. Clin. Biol.* **9**, 105–108 (1964).
68. Levy, R. I., and D. S. Fredrickson, *J. Clin. Invest.* **44**, 426–441 (1965).
69. Rudman, D., L. A. Garcia, and C. H. Howard, *J. Clin. Invest.* **49**, 365–372 (1970).
70. Shore, B., and V. Shore, *Biochemistry* **7**, 2773–2777 (1968).
71. Shore, B., and V. Shore, *Biochemistry* **8**, 4510–4516 (1969).
72. Shore, V., and B. Shore, *Biochemistry* **7**, 3396–3403 (1968).
73. Scanu, A., L. A. Lewis, and F. M. Bumpus, *Arch. Biochem. Biophys.* **74**, 390–397 (1958).
74. Shore, V., and B. Shore, *Biochem. Biophys. Res. Commun.* **9**, 455–460 (1962).
75. Scanu, A., *J. Clin. Invest.* **46**, 1113 (1967).
76. Scanu, A., J. Toth, C. Edelstein, S. Koga, and E. Stiller, *Biochemistry* **8**, 3309–3316 (1969).
77. Kostner, G., and P. Alaupovic, *Fed. Eur. Biochem. Soc. Letters* **15**, 320–324 (1971).
78. Wuu, T. C., S. Crumm, and M. Saffran, *J. Biol. Chem.* **246**, 6043–6063 (1971).
79. Puppione, D. L., G. M. Forte, A. V. Nichols, and E. H. Strisower, *Biochim. Biophys. Acta* **202**, 392–395 (1970).
80. Shore, B., and V. Shore, *Proceedings of the 1970 Meeting of the European Society for Atherosclerosis,* J. Polonovski, Ed., Masson et Cie, Paris, in press.
81. Albers, J. J., and F. Aladjem, *Biochemistry* **10**, 3436–3442 (1971).
82. Gotto, A. M., and B. Shore, *Nature* **224**, 69–70 (1969).
83. Scanu, A. M., *Proc. Natl. Acad. Sci. U.S.* **54**, 1699–1705 (1965).
84. Scanu, A. M., and R. Hirz, *Proc. Natl. Acad. Sci. U.S.* **59**, 890–894 (1968).
85. Scanu, A. M., *Biochim. Biophys. Acta* **181**, 268–274 (1969).
86. Chapman, D., R. B. Leslie, R. Hirz, and A. M. Scanu, *Nature* **221**, 260–261 (1969).
87. Gotto, A. M., and H. Kon, *Biochem. Biophys. Res. Commun.* **37**, 444–450 (1969).
88. Hayashi, S., F. T. Lindgren, and A. Nichols, *J. Amer. Chem. Soc.* **81**, 3793–3798 (1959).
89. Shore, B., and V. Shore, *J. Atheroscler. Res.* **2**, 104–114 (1962).
90. Nichols, A. V., E. H. Strisower, F. T. Lindgren, G. L. Adamson, and E. L. Coggiola, *Clin. Chim. Acta* **20**, 277–283 (1968).
91. Gotto, A. M., R. I. Levy, K. John, and D. S. Frederickson, *New Engl. J. Med.* **284**, 813–818 (1971).

92. Havel, R. J., M. L. Kashyap, and J. P. Kane, *Circulation* **44**, II–9 (1971) (abstract).
93. Ayrault-Jarrier, M., R. I. Cheftel, and J. Polonovski, *Bull. Soc. Chim. Biol* **43**, 811–816 (1961).
94. Marshall, W. E., and F. A. Kummerow, *Arch. Biochem. Biophys.* **98**, 271–273 (1962).
95. Adams, G. H., and V. N. Schumaker, *Nature* **202**, 490–491 (1964).
96. Adams, G. H., and V. N. Schumaker, *Ann. N.Y. Acad. Sci.* **164**, 130–146 (1969).
97. Oncley, J. L., *Biopolymers* **7**, 119–132 (1969).
98. Baldwin, R. L., and J. W. Williams, *J. Amer. Chem. Soc.* **72**, 4325 (1950).
99. Margolis, S., *J. Lipid Res.* **8**, 501–507 (1967).
100. Bjorklund, R., and S. Katz, *J. Amer. Chem. Soc.* **78**, 2122–2126 (1956).
101. Oncley, J. L., *Vox Sang.* **5**, 91–92 (1960).
102. Adams, G. H., and V. N. Schumaker, *Anal. Biochem.* **29**, 117–129 (1969).
103. Lindgren, F. T., L. C. Jensen, R. D. Wills, and N. K. Freeman, *Lipids* **4**, 337–344 (1969).
104. Scanu, A., H. Pollard, and W. Reader, *J. Lipid Res.* **9**, 342–349 (1968).
105. Pollard, H., A. M. Scanu, and E. W. Taylor, *Proc. Natl. Acad. Sci. U.S.* **64**, 304–310 (1969).
106. Gotto, A. M., R. I. Levy, and D. S. Fredrickson, *Lipids* **3**, 463–470 (1968).
107. Gotto, A. M., R. I. Levy, A. S. Rosenthal, M. E. Birnbaumer, and D. S. Fredrickson, *Biochem. Biophys. Res. Commun.* **31**, 699–705 (1968).
108. Hamilton, R. L., in *The Turnover of Lipids and Lipoproteins, Proceedings of the 1968 Deuel Conference on Lipids,* G. Cowgill, D. L. Estrich, and P. D. Wood, Eds., U.S. Government Printing Office, Washington, D.C., 1969, pp. 3–28.
109. Oncley, J. L., F. R. N. Gurd, and M. Melin, *J. Amer. Chem. Soc.* **72**, 458–464 (1950).
110. Steim, J. M., O. D. Edner, and F. G. Bargoot, *Science* **162**, 909–911 (1968).
111. Gotto, A. M., R. I. Levy, and D. S. Fredrickson, *Proc. Natl. Acad. Sci. U.S.* **60**, 1436–1441 (1968).
112. Scanu, A., H. Pollard, R. Hirz, and K. Kothary, *Proc. Natl. Acad. Sci. U.S.* **62**, 171–178 (1969).
113. Dearborn, D. G., and D. B. Wetlaufer, *Proc. Natl. Acad. Sci. U.S.* **62**, 179–185 (1969).
114. Kobozev, G. V., and G. V. Troitskii, *Mol. Biol.* **1**, 202–213 (1967).
115. Moffitt, W., and J. T. Yang, *Proc. Natl. Acad. Sci. U.S.* **42**, 596–603 (1956).
116. Scanu, A., L. A. Lewis, and I. H. Page, *J. Exp. Med.* **108**, 185–196 (1958).
117. Gustafson, A., P. Alaupovic, and R. H. Furman, *Biochemistry* **5**, 632–640 (1966).
118. Kostner, G., and A. Holasek, *Biochim. Biophys. Acta* **188**, 157–159 (1969).
119. Aladjem, F., *Nature* **209**, 1003–1005 (1966).
120. Simons, K., and A. Helenius, *Scand. J. Clin. Lab. Invest.* **23**, Suppl. 108, 33 (1969) (abstract).
121. Kane, J. P., E. G. Richards, and R. J. Havel, *Proc. Natl. Acad. Sci. U.S.* **66**, 1075–1082 (1970).
122. Simons, K., C. Enhholm, O. Renkonen, and B. Bloth, *Acta. Pathol. Microbiol. Scand.* **78B**, 459–466 (1970).
123. Granda, J. L., and A. Scanu, *Biochemistry* **5**, 3301–3308 (1966).

124. Gotto, A. M., R. I. Levy, F. T. Lindgren, and D. S. Frederickson, *Biochim. Biophys. Acta* **176**, 667–669 (1969).
125. Helenius, A., and K. Simons, *Biochemistry* **10**, 2542–2547 (1971).
126. Alaupovic, P., D. Seidel, W. J. McConathy, and R. H. Furman, *Fed. Eur. Biochem. Soc. Letters* **4**, 113–116 (1969).
127. Mills, G. L., D. Seidel, and P. Alaupovic, *Clin. Chim. Acta* **26**, 239–244 (1969).
128. Hamilton, R. L., R. J. Havel, J. P. Kane, A. E. Blaurock, and T. Sata, *Science* **172**, 475–478 (1971).
129. Lees, R. S., and E. H. Ahrens, Jr., *New Engl. J. Med.* **280**, 1261–1266 (1969).
130. Fredrickson, D. S., R. I. Levy, and R. S. Lees, *New Engl. J. Med.* **276**, 94–103 (1967).
131. Sabesin, S. M., and K. J. Isselbacher, *Science* **147**, 1149–1151 (1965).
132. Windmueller, H. G., and R. I. Levy, *J. Biol. Chem.* **242**, 2246–2254 (1967).
133. Windmueller, H. G., and R. I. Levy, *J. Biol. Chem.* **243**, 4878–4884 (1968).
134. Gotto, A. M., R. I. Levy, M. E. Birnbaumer, and D. S. Fredrickson, *Nature* **223**, 835–837 (1969).
135. Pinon, J.-C., and P. Laudat, *Biochim. Biophys. Acta* **187**, 144–146 (1969).
136. Rodbell, M. R., and D. S. Fredrickson, *J. Biol. Chem.* **234**, 562–566 (1959).
137. Bobbit, J. L., and R. S. Levy, *Biochemistry* **4**, 1282–1288 (1965).
138. Rodbell, M., *Science* **127**, 701–702 (1958).
139. Brown, W. V., R. I. Levy, and D. S. Fredrickson, *J. Biol. Chem.* **244**, 5687–5694 (1969).
140. Brown, W. V., R. I. Levy, and D. S. Fredrickson, *Fed. Proc.* **29**, 327 (1970) (abstract).
141. Shore, B., and V. Shore, in *Proceedings of the Second International Symposium on Athersclerosis,* R. Jones, Ed., Springer-Verlag, Heidelberg, 1970, pp. 144–150.
142. Brewer, H. B. Jr., R. Shulman, P. Herbert, R. Ronan, and K. Wehrly, *Adv. Exp. Med. Biol.,* in press.
143. Brown, W. V., and M. L. Baginsky, *Circulation* **44**, II–9 (1971) (abstract).
144. LaRosa, J. C., R. I. Levy, W. V. Brown, and D. S. Fredrickson, *Amer. J. Physiol.* **220**, 785–791 (1971).
145. Eisenberg, S., D. W. Bilheimer, F. T. Lindgren, and R. I. Levy, *Circulation* **44**, II–9 (1971) (abstract).
146. Gulbrandsen, C. L., R. B. Wilson, and R. S. Lees, *Circulation* **44**, II–9 (1971) (abstract).
147. Lossow, W. J., F. T. Lindgren, J. C. Murchio, G. R. Stevens, and L. C. Jensen, *J. Lipid Res.* **10**, 68–76 (1969).
148. Zilversmit, D. B., *J. Clin. Invest.* **44**, 1610–1622 (1965).
149. Zilversmit, D. B., *J. Lipid Res.* **9**, 180–186 (1968).
150. Salpeter, M. M., and D. B. Zilversmit, *J. Lipid Res.* **9**, 187–192 (1968).
151. Alaupovic, P., R. H. Furman, W. H. Falor, M. L. Sullivan, S. L. Walraven, and A. C. Olson, *Ann. N.Y. Acad. Sci.* **149**, 791–807 (1968).
152. Levy, R. S., A. C. Lynch, E. D. McGee, and J. W. Mehl, *J. Lipid Res.* **8**, 463–472 (1967).

16. Serum-Lipoprotein Synthesis and Metabolism

SIMEON MARGOLIS and DAVID CAPUZZI

Departments of Medicine and Physiological Chemistry, The Johns Hopkins University, Baltimore, Maryland

I. INTRODUCTION

The biosynthesis and metabolism of serum lipoproteins are important from both a basic and a medical point of view. Transport of triglycerides from the liver as very-low-density lipoproteins (VLDL) and from the intestine as chylomicrons and VLDL, is the major recognized function of these lipoproteins. Clear definition of triglyceride transport is central to an understanding of lipid metabolism. An increased rate of lipoprotein synthesis or a diminished rate of removal leads to elevated levels of serum lipoproteins (hyperlipoproteinemia) and their constituent lipids (hyperlipemia). The accumulation of evidence linking hyperlipemia with atherosclerosis in both animals (1–3) and man (4–7) has greatly stimulated interest in the factors that control serum-lipoprotein concentrations.

The sources of fatty acids for the triglycerides transported from the liver, bound primarily to VLDL, vary with the feeding status of the animal. In the postprandial period fatty acids are derived mainly by hydrolysis of chylomicron triglycerides and by de novo hepatic synthesis from carbohydrates. Serum free fatty acids (FFA) released from adipose-tissue stores provide the major source of triglyceride fatty acids in the postabsorptive state (8). The VLDL and chylomicron triglycerides may be stored in adipose tissue (9–11) or utilized directly by peripheral tissues, such as muscle (11–16), as an energy source. Both types of triglyceride utilization require the presence of lipoprotein lipase to split the circulating triglycerides to their constituent fatty acids and glycerol.

It has been suggested that optimal triglyceride removal from VLDL also requires the enzyme lecithin:cholesterol acyltransferase (LCAT) to continually "remodel" the partially delipidated VLDL so that lipoprotein lipase activity can proceed at a maximal rate (17, 18). The high-density lipoproteins (HDL) may interact with VLDL (19) and chylomicrons (20), and have been demonstrated to activate the hydrolysis of artificial triglyceride emulsions by lipoprotein lipase (21–23). It is unlikely, however, that HDL are required for lipoprotein-lipase activity *in vivo* because VLDL, and possibly chylomicrons, contain the major activator peptide, R–Glu, as an integral part of the molecule (24). The HDL may serve to activate LCAT (17) and provide substrate for its action (25). In the process of lipoprotein-lipase activity and LCAT remodeling some of the VLDL polypeptides may be released either as free apoproteins or as polypeptide–lipid complexes that have the density properties of HDL.

This complex series of reactions may finally convert VLDL to low-density lipoproteins (LDL) (26). In this scheme LDL appear in serum solely as an intermediate product in the catabolism of VLDL. It is not known whether LDL carry out any specific functions. Nor is it clear whether LDL per se are secreted by the liver. One could postulate that synthesis of B peptide proceeds at a fairly uniform rate and that the relative proportions of LDL and VLDL released by the liver are determined primarily by the load of triglycerides available for transport. When hepatic triglyceride synthesis is rapid, VLDL are actively secreted, whereas little or no LDL is released. At times when relatively small amounts of VLDL are secreted, under conditions of minimal hepatic triglyceride synthesis, large amounts of LDL may be released. Alternatively, the liver may secrete only VLDL and HDL. All the circulating LDL would then be derived from the partial catabolism of VLDL.

Several additional functions have been attributed to the serum lipoproteins. Because of the accumulation of cholesteryl esters in the tissues of patients with HDL deficiency (Tangier disease) it has been suggested that HDL are required for the transport of cholesterol from peripheral tissues to its site of degradation and excretion in the liver (25, 27). In addition, the serum lipoproteins clearly function to transport carotenoids and fat-soluble vitamins (28).

Because of their major lipid component, the regulation of lipoprotein synthesis and removal is more complicated than that of other serum proteins. Thus the rate of synthesis may be altered by factors that influence the availability of lipids, formation of the peptide portion of the lipoprotein, coupling of lipid to peptide, or secretion of the completed lipoprotein. Similarly the turnover of serum lipoproteins involves removal from serum of both the lipid and the protein portions of the molecule and is complicated by the ready exchange of certain lipids between the serum lipoproteins and the tissues (28). For these reasons the synthesis and metabolism of serum lipoproteins more nearly resemble those of the cellular elements of the blood than those of the other serum proteins.

A number of excellent reviews can be recommended for further information on lipoprotein biosynthesis (17, 29) and metabolism (17, 30), plasma triglyceride (30–32) and cholesterol (33) turnover, the role of chylomicrons in the regulation of cholesterol synthesis by the liver (34), and the various disorders of fat transport (27, 35–37).

II. BIOSYNTHESIS

The biosynthesis of serum lipoproteins is not simply a specialized case of the more general process of protein synthesis, the stepwise details of which are largely understood. Far less is known about protein synthesis in mammals than in bacteria, and few studies have been done on the synthesis of specific proteins in mammalian tissues. Furthermore, human- and rat-serum lipoproteins contain small amounts of carbohydrates (38), covalently bound to the apopeptide, in addition to the large complement of noncovalently bound lipid. The carbohydrate component may be a determinant of the lipid-binding capacity of the molecule, or may be required for its secretion from the hepatic cell, as has been suggested for other secreted proteins (39). Whereas lipoprotein triglycerides represent transport cargo, part of the lipid moiety—the phospholipids and perhaps cholesterol—is undoubtedly required to stabilize the structure of the complex aggregate and to facilitate its solubility in plasma. Another major lipid component—cholesteryl ester—is apparently largely formed from cholesterol and phospholipid fatty acids by the action of LCAT while the lipoproteins are in the bloodstream (25).

Failures in the biosynthesis of these lipoproteins lead both to a fall in their serum levels and to deposition of lipids at the normal biosynthetic sites. Interruption of VLDL synthesis or secretion by the liver results in triglyceride accumulation, or fatty liver (40, 41). Fatty liver may be produced experimentally by a variety of agents that inhibit protein synthesis (41–44), or increase the transport of free fatty acids to the liver or the synthesis of fat by the liver beyond the capacity of this organ to export lipids bound to serum lipoproteins (45). Similarly inhibitors of intestinal protein synthesis impair chylomicron formation; the resultant defect in triglyceride transport leads to accumulation of lipid droplets in the mucosal cell (46). In man inherited defects in VLDL synthesis cause lipid deposition in the liver and the intestinal mucosa (35, 47). These observations emphasize the crucial role of VLDL in the process of lipid transport from hepatic parenchymal and intestinal mucosal cells. Thus information on the biosynthesis of serum lipoproteins is essential for a proper understanding of the accumulation of excessive lipid in both plasma and cells. Conversely, genetic defects in man have provided important clues to a better recognition of the transport role of the lipoproteins.

A. Sites of Biosynthesis

In vivo experiments in hepatectomized and eviscerated dogs showed that the liver is the major site for the synthesis of all serum lipoproteins other than chylomicrons (48). *In vitro* studies with rat livers demonstrated lipoprotein synthesis by perfused liver (49, 50), slices (50, 51), isolated cells (52–54), and broken-cell preparations (55, 56). Studies on isolated liver cells indicate that the hepatic parenchymal cell is the cell type responsible for the synthesis of $d < 1.063$ g/ml lipoproteins (52).

There is growing evidence that the intestinal mucosa synthesizes HDL and VLDL both in the fasting state and during lipid absorption. In hepatectomized dogs amino acid incorporation into serum lipoproteins was almost obliterated by removal of the intestine (48). The major lipoprotein present in the mesenteric lymph of fasting rats was VLDL (57). The intestinal origin of these lipoproteins was demonstrated by administration of cholestyramine and by diversion of bile flow, which resulted in virtual disappearance of VLDL-size particles from the mucosal cells. In fed rats the amount of VLDL present in mesenteric lymph depended on the fatty acid composition of the administered lipids. A larger proportion of both triglycerides and cholesterol was transported by VLDL than by chylomicrons during the absorption of saturated fatty acids; this observation may partially explain the cholesterol-lowering effect of unsaturated fatty acids. Particles with the physical properties of VLDL were isolated from the intestinal mucosa of fasting human volunteers (58). Both VLDL and LDL are present in the intestinal lymph of rats fed orotic acid (59), although the livers of such rats are incapable of secreting LDL or VLDL (60).

Intestinal slices from lipid-fed rats incorporated labeled leucine into chylomicrons and into the lipoprotein fraction with *d* 1.006 to 1.21 g/ml (61). No immunochemical data or peptide maps were given to further identify the labeled proteins. Isolated mucosal cells of rat intestine incorporated amino acids into VLDL, but there was poor correlation between the peptide maps of the synthesized lipoproteins and those of rat-serum VLDL (62). Furthermore, the lipoproteins were obtained from cell homogenates and were not released into the incubation medium.

On a fat-free diet most of the lipoproteins in rat intestinal lymph are α_2-lipoproteins (VLDL), which contain both the A and B apoproteins (63). The presence of malabsorption in abetalipoproteinemia indicates that synthesis of the B apoprotein is essential for the production of lymph chylomicrons and VLDL (35), whereas the normal fat absorption in Tangier disease suggests that synthesis of the A protein is not required (27). The B apoprotein is produced by the intestinal mucosal cell, but the source of the A apoprotein is uncertain; nor is it known whether lymph VLDL contain additional specific peptides analogous to those found in human-serum VLDL. When fat is absorbed, rat intestinal lymph contains a greater quantity of particles ($S_f > 1100$) that fail to migrate in paper or agarose-gel electrophoresis. Available data indicate that the intestinal mucosal cell assembles and releases VLDL and chylomicrons and that their triglyceride content depends on the dietary triglyceride load. It is not yet known whether dietary fat affects the content of peptides and other lipid components of intestinal VLDL and chylomicrons.

In the absence of dietary fat the extent of the intestinal contribution to the pool of serum VLDL triglycerides is unknown; estimates have varied from 10% (63) to 40% (64). The electrophoretic and immunochemical properties of VLDL released into the lymph are similar to those of VLDL discharged by the liver into the plasma (65), but plasma VLDL have more protein and less phospholipid than the VLDL initially secreted into the lymph (63). Compositional changes may occur as VLDL from either source circulate in the plasma. Such changes have been demonstrated *in vitro* during the incubation of $S_f > 400$ lipoproteins from rat lymph with rat serum (66).

Since chylomicron formation and fat absorption are discussed elsewhere in this volume, the remainder of this chapter focuses on lipoprotein synthesis in the liver.

B. Technical Problems in Studies of Lipoprotein Synthesis

Technical problems in the study of lipoprotein synthesis include the development of a sensitive and specific isolation procedure for newly synthesized lipoproteins, proof of the biosynthetic product, and dissociation of the individual steps in the overall process of lipoprotein synthesis. The following discussion focuses on the first two problems; the final one is treated in the next section (C).

The VLDL and LDL, but not the HDL, interact specifically with a variety of sulfated polysaccharides to form insoluble complexes. These polyanion-precipitation methods, which have been discussed in an excellent review (67), have been used in some studies of lipoprotein synthesis (52, 68). Such precipitation techniques are useful as preparative methods for the initial separation of lower density lipoproteins from serum since good agreement was found when the protein (69) and lipid content (70) of lipoproteins separated by flotation at *d* 1.063 g/ml were compared with those isolated by sulfated-polysaccharide precipitation. Moreover, workers in two different laboratories achieved comparable results when labeled $d < 1.063$ g/ml lipoproteins were separated by either heparin-divalent cation precipitation or by ultracentrifugal flotation, and the precipitated complex contained no labeled albumin (68). In our studies, however, labeled contaminants coprecipitated with VLDL and LDL when dextran sulfate–Ca^{2+} or sodium phosphotungstate was employed (52). Such results emphasize the need to test a particular precipitation technique before it is used to isolate labeled $d < 1.063$ g/ml lipoproteins. In addition, the reported interference by long-chain fatty acids with the formation of insoluble complexes (71) suggests that precipitation of VLDL and LDL with sulfated polysaccharides may be incomplete under certain conditions.

Preparative ultracentrifugation is the method used most commonly for isolating serum-lipoprotein subclasses. However, the criteria for the ultracentrifugal separation of serum lipoproteins may not apply to the isolation of lipoproteins newly made *in vitro*. Furthermore, the large centrifugal forces and the high salt concentration may cause structural changes. An altered form of HDL, with different electrophoretic, immunochemical, and ultracentrifugal behavior has been described (72). Thus the standard techniques for lipoprotein isolation are tedious, may yield products contaminated with other labeled peptides, and may produce molecular rearrangements that give rise to spurious heterogeneity.

Because of the unique affinity between an antibody and its antigen, immunoprecipitation of labeled serum lipoproteins by specific antiserums has proved to be a valuable isolation technique for studies of lipoprotein synthesis. Specific antiserums have been used to detect biosynthesis of rat LDL and HDL by perfused liver (50) and by hepatic ribosomes (56). Results obtained by immune precipitation of labeled VLDL and LDL released from isolated liver cells agreed closely with those obtained by ultracentrifugal flotation (52). Recently a radioimmunoassay method was developed to quantitate lipoprotein synthesis by rat-liver slices (73). Although immunoprecipitation techniques can separate HLD from LDL and from VLDL, the latter two lipoproteins cannot be distinguished from each other because they share a common antigen. Immunoprecipitation techniques for the assay of specific labeled proteins have been reviewed recently (74).

Another problem in the isolation of newly labeled lipoproteins is the requirement for added serum or lipoprotein carrier in most studies. Under such circumstances a highly labeled contaminant or an incomplete lipoprotein fragment may adsorb to the carrier lipoprotein. Thus a fall of 40 to 60% was found in the recovery of lipoproteins from ribosomes (56) and from isolated liver cells (52) when carrier was omitted. A carrier effect of serum may partly explain the fivefold stimulation of ^{14}C-leucine incorporation into lipoproteins released from rat-liver slices when serum replaced bicarbonate buffer as the incubation medium (51).

Finally in broken-cell preparations the separation of newly synthesized serum lipoproteins from the subcellular particles introduces further complications in the identification of the labeled product. Thus lipoprotein isolation may entail the opening of closed microsomal vesicles by sonication (55) or dissolution of ribosomes by lithium chloride (56). Such techniques may contaminate the product with labeled tissue lipoproteins or damage the serum lipoproteins and thus alter their physical characteristics.

C. Steps Involved in Lipoprotein Synthesis

The overall process of serum-lipoprotein production can be visualized as entailing synthesis of the lipid components of the lipoprotein, synthesis of the apolipoprotein (or apoglycolipoprotein), linkage of the apolipoprotein with lipid, and export of the completed molecule into the bloodstream. This process is diagramed schematically in Fig. 1. Trams and Brown (75), in a theoretical treatment of serum-lipoprotein synthesis, suggested several speculative schemes for this process.

By analogy with the synthesis of other proteins, and from direct demonstration of apolipoprotein synthesis in hepatic ribosomes (56), it seems reasonable to conclude that apolipoproteins are synthesized by ribosomes

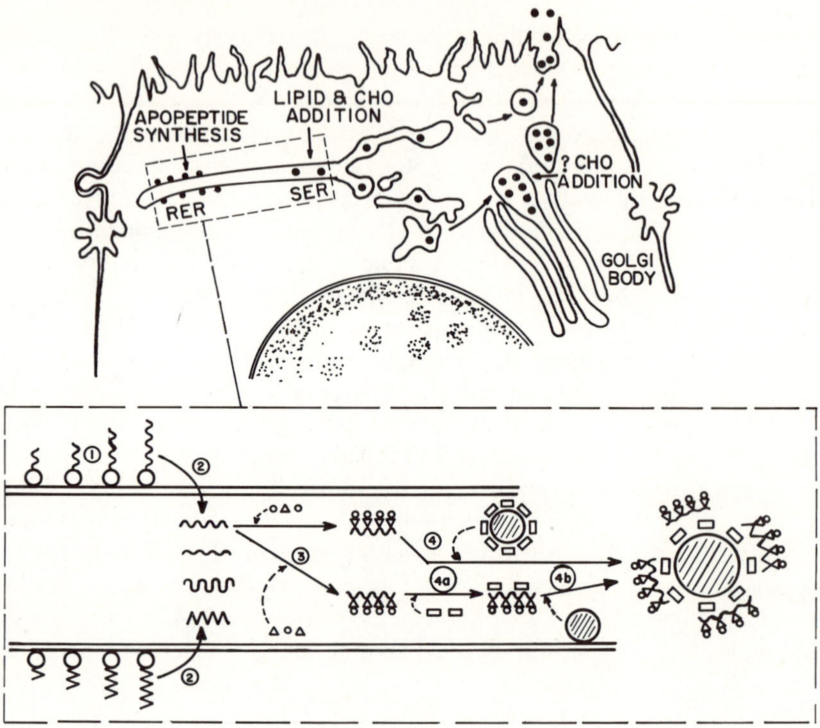

Fig. 1 Schematic diagram of VLDL synthesis. Apopeptides are synthesized on hepatic polysomes (step 1) and enter (step 2) the tubular lumen of the rough endoplasmic reticulum (RER). Carbohydrate (CHO) units are added (step 3) to form apoglycopeptides in the smooth endoplasmic reticulum (SER) and possibly the Golgi complex as well. The lipid may be coupled to the apoglycopeptide either in a single step (step 4) or in a staged process where phospholipids, and perhaps cholesterol, are added first (step 4*a*) and then the remaining lipids are added to complete the VLDL molecule (step 4*b*). The VLDL are stored in the Golgi complex. Secretory vesicles carry VLDL to the cell membrane where they are released into the space of Disse.

attached to the rough endoplasmic reticulum. As is the case with other serum proteins, the apolipoproteins probably pass into the channels of the endoplasmic reticulum. Carbohydrate attachment may occur while the apolipoprotein is bound to the ribosome, during passage through the endoplasmic reticulum, or in the Golgi apparatus. Coupling of the lipid and peptide portions may occur within the endoplasmic reticulum or the Golgi body. The newly synthesized lipoprotein is then secreted from the hepatocyte into the space of Disse. The lipid portion of the newly made lipoprotein differs from that bound to circulating lipoproteins since enzymatic modification and exchange of these lipids occurs during their circulation. These modifications are described in more detail in chapter 14 of this volume.

1. Lipid Components. The cholesterol component of serum lipoproteins is largely synthesized in the liver, although dietary cholesterol is removed by the liver from triglyceride-depleted chylomicrons (76). The fatty acids utilized for triglyceride and phospholipid synthesis are derived from de novo synthesis in the liver, dietary lipids transported on chylomicrons, and free fatty acids released from adipose tissue. The relative proportion of lipoprotein fatty acids derived from each of these sources varies with the species, with the time elapsed since the last meal, and with the composition of the diet.

In the postabsorptive state about 9 g/hr of fatty acids is released from the adipose stores of an adult man. Approximately one-third of these fatty acids are taken up by the liver (37), where they are mostly utilized as an energy source. Part of the remainder (about 0.5 g/hr) serves as the only source of phospholipid and triglyceride fatty acids for the serum lipoproteins synthesized during this time (8).

In the postprandial period dietary lipids and carbohydrates are the major sources of lipoprotein triglycerides. When the fat content of the diet is high, fatty acids are largely derived from the breakdown of chylomicrons. The feeding of fat has been shown to inhibit fatty acid synthesis and to increase cholesterol synthesis by the liver (77). Dietary carbohydrates are converted to fatty acids in both the liver and adipose tissue (78). In the rat and mouse adipose tissue plays a more important role than does the liver in the conversion of carbohydrates to fatty acids (79, 80). By contrast, in pigeon and man the liver is apparently the major site for de novo fatty acid synthesis (81–83).

2. Synthesis of Apolipoprotein. Net synthesis of serum lipoproteins by rat-liver slices and by perfused rat liver was demonstrated by Marsh and Whereat (50), who used specific antiserums to isolate the $d < 1.063$ g/ml and HDL fractions. Most other workers have utilized the incorporation of radioactive amino acids to measure the rate of lipoprotein production. Radding, Bragdon, and Steinberg (51) showed that labeled proteins with the ultracentrifugal characteristics of LDL and HDL were released during perfusion of rat liver with ^{14}C-leucine or incubation of rat-liver slices with labeled leucine. Autoradiography of peptide maps indicated that HDL peptide synthesized by liver slices was identical with the HDL peptide from rat serum (84). Evidence for the identity of labeled LDL with serum-LDL peptide was not conclusive. In these studies (51) and in later work by Haft et al. (85) amino acids were incorporated into LDL peptides at a faster rate than into HLD peptides. Recent work showed active synthesis and release of leucine-labeled VLDL and LDL by isolated rat-liver cells (52).

In studies on the synthesis of the peptide part of serum lipoproteins by isolated rat-liver microsomes, Marsh (55) observed that HDL were labeled more rapidly than LDL. He suggested that damage to LDL during microsomal disruption may explain the difference in labeling patterns between *in vivo* and *in vitro* studies. This difference may also be attributable to alteration of the endoplasmic reticulum during preparation of microsomes. Furthermore, studies with intact cells involved both synthesis and secretion of lipoproteins, whereas work with microsomes measured only the synthetic portion of this overall process. Although labeled lipoproteins were also released during a similar incubation of isolated mitochondria, these lipoproteins did not react with antibodies prepared against rat-serum lipoproteins (56). Serum-lipoprotein synthesis was also demonstrated with isolated ribosomes, in which equal incorporation of label was found in HDL and LDL peptides from solubilized ribosomes (56). Because ribosomes contain almost no lipid, these experiments clearly involved apolipoprotein synthesis. Tryptic peptides of apo-LDL had the same labeling pattern as LDL synthesized in slices, but the correlation was not as close in the case of apo-HDL. Since carrier lipoprotein was required for the ultracentrifugal isolation of immunologically reactive lipoprotein from ribosomes solubilized with lithium chloride, it is evident that the labeled product can combine in some fashion with the carrier.

3. Coupling of Apolipoprotein and Lipids. There is little data available on the mechanism for coupling of the lipid and protein moieties during the process of serum-lipoprotein formation. The accumulation of lipid droplets within the endoplasmic reticulum in fatty livers induced with orotic acid (86), which may result from defective coupling of lipids to peptide (87, 88), suggests that this organelle is a site for lipid–peptide assembly. The Golgi apparatus, a vesicular array usually isolated with the microsomal fraction and normally a continuation of the smooth endoplasmic reticulum, may also be a coupling site for carbohydrate or lipid. Jones, Ruderman, and Herrera (89) suggested that the Golgi complex is involved in the addition of the carbohydrate moiety to the peptide and thereby permits lipid addition. Complex carbohydrates and glycoproteins have been detected in the Golgi apparatus of rat-liver cells by electron-microscopy examination of histochemically stained sections (90).

The coupling or secretion mechanisms are probably the target sites for the inhibition of serum-lipoprotein production by specific toxic agents like carbon tetrachloride and phosphorus (91, 92). Such interference with the linking process has also been implicated in the causation of fatty liver by other agents, which are considered in detail later.

4. Secretion of Lipoproteins. Electron-microscopy and biochemical studies indicate that the Golgi apparatus has an important function in VLDL release. Such a secretory function for the hepatic Golgi is analogous to the role of this organelle in the formation of pancreatic zymogen granules preparatory to secretion (93). Large concentrations of osmiophilic particles with the size and dimensions of VLDL have been observed under the electron microscope in the Golgi cisternae and in the perfusate of rat livers during perfusion with media containing fatty acid (89, 94). Physiological studies have shown that these Golgi particles are present under conditions that lead to increased VLDL levels in plasma (95–97) and absent when VLDL synthesis or release is inhibited (95). Thus clusters of particles were prominent in secretory vesicles of the Golgi apparatus in rats given an acute, intoxicating dose of ethanol (97), in dogs infused with norepinephrine (96), and in rabbits injected for 4 to 6 days with cortisone (95). In each instance an increase in the number of particles was associated with elevated plasma levels of VLDL. The particles in cortisone-treated rabbits were larger than normal, as were the VLDL of plasma. In contrast, during the first 2 days of cortisone administration, when plasma-triglyceride levels fell, Golgi apparatus was scarce and contained few lipid particles (95). Mahley et al. (95) concluded that the disappearance of the Golgi apparatus or the presence of the Golgi apparatus without particles was indicative of a prolonged interruption of VLDL synthesis or release. Ten minutes after injection of radioactive palmitate or glycerol into rats, a technique that combined electron microscopy and radioautography indicated that the label was concentrated over the Golgi apparatus (98). The authors proposed that this label was present in newly synthesized lipoproteins.

The Golgi particles were further identified as VLDL or their precursors by biochemical studies on isolated Golgi apparatus. Golgi particles were separated by sonication followed by ultracentrifugation. The particles and VLDL formed lines of identity with antiserum against plasma VLDL. In addition the lipid and protein compositions of the Golgi particles were very similar to those of rat VLDL (99). Finally, the VLDL released from perfused liver and isolated Golgi particles contain the major apolipoproteins identified in delipidated rat-plasma VLDL (100). This finding suggests that the apolipoproteins are assembled in the liver before VLDL release rather than being added during circulation.

Newly synthesized serum lipoproteins are probably carried in secretory vesicles to the sinusoidal surface of the cell and there discharged into the space of Disse (98, 101). This proposal is supported by electron-microscopy findings that were interpreted as showing secretory vesicles in various stages of transport between the Golgi apparatus and the sinusoidal surface of the cell (101). Individual particles were readily identified in the space of Disse (101). The transport, but not synthesis, of rat-serum lipoproteins by liver slices was found to be dependent on the potassium-ion content of the slices (102).

In addition to the 300- to 800-Å lipid particles in the secretory vesicles of the Golgi apparatus, the liver may contain several other types of lipid deposits that turn over more slowly. Larger, membrane-bound lipid aggregates, called liposomes, accumulate in the livers of ethionine-treated rats. Liposomes have been identified by electron microscopy, isolated, and characterized chemically (103). These accumulations, which develop during experimental induction of fatty liver in rats, represent triglyceride-engorged dilatations of the ergastoplasm specialized for fatty acid esterification and possibly lipoprotein completion (103). They probably result from an imbalance between the rate of triglyceride synthesis and the rate of VLDL synthesis or export from the cell. Though they occur in small numbers in the livers of fasting rats, a striking increase is discernible in hepatic cells engaged in active fatty acid esterification or undergoing some types of fatty change. Liposomes appear in or near the Golgi apparatus when there is some inhibition of VLDL synthesis or release (94, 95). Fatty liver develops if this process is not reversed. Characteristic of fatty liver is the accumulation of larger lipid droplets that are not enclosed within a membrane. These droplets are isolated as "floating fat" from liver homogenates.

D. The Apolipoprotein Carrier Hypothesis

A series of studies by Eder and co-workers (85, 104–107) presented evidence of the existence in lipoprotein-free rat serum of an apolipoprotein that was capable of accepting a lipid cargo during its passage through the liver. When fatty livers from cholesterol-fed rats were perfused, they released triglyceride and cholesterol into the perfusion medium; the addition of $d > 1.21$ g/ml plasma proteins to the perfusion medium enhanced this release of lipids. Lipid secretion stopped after 2 hr, presumably because the lipid-acceptor capacity of the apolipoprotein was exceeded. The addition of fresh perfusion medium, which contained the plasma fraction of $d > 1.21$ g/ml, promoted a second release of lipid. The appearance of lipids in the perfusion fluid, almost exclusively as VLDL, and the incorporation of acceptor protein into VLDL exhibited a marked temperature dependence. When the $d > 1.21$ g/ml proteins were prelabeled *in vivo* with ^{14}C-amino acids and then perfused through the liver, the VLDL fraction in the perfusion medium achieved higher specific activity than the starting $d > 1.21$ g/ml proteins. This result suggests the presence of a precursor protein with a greater specific activity than the average of the entire fraction. An α_1-globulin fraction of the $d > 1.21$ g/ml infranatant was most active for promotion of lipid release. Since the incorporation of labeled $d > 1.21$ g/ml proteins into VLDL was unaffected by the presence of a large pool of unlabeled amino acids, the apolipoprotein did not break down to its constituent amino acids in the liver, but rather was incorporated directly into lipoprotein by combination with lipid. Moreover, puromycin did not diminish the appearance of labeled precursor protein in VLDL. During perfusion of livers with $d > 1.21$ g/ml proteins prelabeled with ^{14}C-glucosamine, lipoproteins in the perfusate became labeled, thereby suggesting that lipid-acceptor proteins are glycoproteins (105). Normal livers also incorporated labeled $d > 1.21$ g/ml proteins into lipoproteins, but net increase of VLDL levels occurred with fatty livers only (105).

The apolipoprotein hypothesis was strengthened by the results of Windmueller and Spaeth (108), who showed that livers with similar rates of fatty acid synthesis released more triglyceride, cholesterol, and newly formed fatty acid when the perfusion medium contained plasma. Ovalbumin, serum albumin, and fibrinogen failed to enhance lipid removal from the perfused liver. However, the apolipoprotein proposed by Eder may in fact be lipoproteins that are partially delipidated or otherwise changed during isolation.

The release of labeled lipid from liver slices, prepared from rats injected with ^{14}C-palmitate, was augmented by incubation in medium that contained serum (109, 110) or lipoprotein (109), but the enhancement was mainly in the phospholipid fraction. Kook and Rubinstein (110) noted that the increased label was present in $d < 1.063$ g/ml lipoproteins separated by flotation, but not in the lower density lipoproteins isolated by Ca^{2+}–heparin precipitation. The authors proposed that serum contains a lipoprotein capable of complexing with liver phospholipids. The resultant "hyperlipidated" lipoproteins can be separated by ultracentrifugal flotation, but do not precipitate with Ca^{2+}–herapin. However, phospholipid exchange between the prelabeled slices and serum may be partly responsible for these results. A $d > 1.21$ g/ml acceptor protein of serum enhanced ^{32}P-phospholipid release from liver slices (111). Since the phospholipid-acceptor protein decreased its density only to $1.063 < d < 1.21$ g/ml and did not increase phospholipid release into VLDL or LDL, it is not identical with the apolipoprotein postulated by Roheim et al. (104).

In rat livers perfused with fresh rat blood Buckley, Delahunty, and Rubinstein (112) found that lipid release was completely inhibited 2 hr after protein synthesis was stopped with puromycin. Similarly, *in vivo*, the secretion of labeled lipid from the liver ceased 1 hr after puromycin administration. They concluded that a circulating apolipoprotein, if it exists, plays a very limited role and is either readily saturated or has a very short half-life. Moreover, active protein synthesis is required for it to function.

Lees reported indirect evidence for the presence of apo-LDL in the plasma of patients with abetalipoproteinemia (113). Chemical modifications of native LDL from normal plasma rendered the molecule immunologically identical with a protein present in normal and abetalipoproteinemic plasma. This latter protein was characterized by immunoelectrophoresis as a lipid-free β-globulin and was presumed by Lees to be apo-LDL. However, Gotto and co-workers (114) detected no immunoreactivity between normal or abetalipoproteinemic plasma and antiserums to LDL, its chemical derivatives, or soluble apo-LDL.

At present the proposed model of a recycling apolipoprotein, synthesized by the liver and released into the serum or formed at extrahepatic sites by removal of lipid cargo, remains controversial. If such an acceptor protein does exist in rat or human serum, its quantitative importance in lipid transport is uncertain.

E. Control of Serum-Lipoprotein Synthesis

The fragmentary information about the sequential steps and mechanisms involved in serum lipoprotein synthesis makes it extremely difficult to unravel the factors that control this process in the liver. It is likely that hormones play an important part in the control of lipoprotein synthesis, but most studies on the effects of hormones have been done *in vivo*. Since it is difficult in such studies to distinguish between effects on serum-lipoprotein synthesis and those that alter lipid metabolism or lipoprotein catabolism, hormonal control is considered in Section III. Most available data are concerned with the influence of changes in hepatic lipogenesis or the quantity of lipid presented to the liver on the formation of serum lipoproteins. The discussion focuses on the factors that regulate the synthesis of lipoprotein peptide.

1. Cholesterol-Mediated Effects. Rat livers made fatty by feeding a high-cholesterol diet exhibited an enhanced release of cholesterol into the lower density lipoproteins during perfusion, but there was no stimulation of amino acid incorporation into VLDL or LDL protein (104). Perfusates from such fatty livers showed a net increase in LDL-bound cholesterol but no increase in LDL peptide (115). Despite its depression of cholesterol synthesis, cholesterol feeding stimulated the transfer of cholesterol and other lipids from perfused fatty livers (104, 107). The authors concluded that the formation of serum lipoproteins was independent of the rate of synthesis of its lipid constituents. Similarly the rate of lipoprotein production from ^{14}C-leucine in liver slices was not affected by prior stimulation of cholesterol synthesis *in vivo* with Triton WR-1339 or by inhibition of cholesterol synthesis by dietary cholesterol (84). Neither whole-body irradiation nor cholesterol feeding influenced the rate of ^{14}C-lysine incorporation into lipoproteins released by perfused rat livers, although both treatments altered the rate of hepatic cholesterol synthesis (85). When normal livers were perfused with blood from the cholesterol-fed animals, there was a considerable increase in ^{14}C-lysine incorporation into the $d < 1.063$ g/ml lipoproteins.

These studies suggest that the enhanced release of cholesterol in the presence of additional cellular cholesterol is not accomplished by an altered rate of apolipoprotein formation, but rather by an increased quantity of cholesterol carried by the individual lipoprotein molecules. Furthermore, a depressed rate of cholesterogenesis does not interfere with the formation of lipoprotein peptide. This last conclusion may not be true under all conditions, since liver slices, prepared from rats fed clofibrate, an antihyperlipemic drug, displayed a 70% fall in ^{14}C-acetate incorporation into cholesterol and a 50% inhibition in the secretion of labeled $d < 1.21$ g/ml lipoproteins (116). These drug-fed rats also had increased hepatic concentrations of protein, phospholipids and triglycerides, and an enhanced rate of hepatic triglyceride synthesis. It would be premature to conclude that the inhibition of cholesterol and lipoprotein synthesis were causally related in this study, though that remains a distinct possibility. The effect on lipoprotein labeling may have resulted from an independent action of clofibrate on some part of the endoplasmic reticulum or on the secretory mechanism of the liver cell.

Also receiving attention is the converse question: Do the serum lipoproteins influence cholesterol synthesis by the liver? A review by Dietschy and Wilson (34) concludes that the amount of cholesterol reaching the liver as chylomicrons controls the rate of hepatic cholesterol synthesis.

2. Fatty-Acid-Mediated Effects. There is good evidence that the presence of fatty acids in the perfusion medium stimulates the release of triglycerides by perfused liver. It is unclear whether this stimulation results from the output of additional lipoprotein molecules, an increased triglyceride load per molecule, or a combination of these processes.

In perfused livers from both normal rats and rats with alloxan-induced diabetes export of triglycerides was proportional to levels of free fatty acids in the perfusate (117, 118). However, both triglyceride synthesis and release were depressed in the diabetic animals (117, 118). Wilcox, Dishmon, and Heimberg (119) observed a reduction in the incorporation of labeled amino acids into all classes of serum lipoproteins and a decline in serum-triglyceride formation in perfused livers of rats with alloxan-induced diabetes. The former effect was refractory to insulin, whereas the latter was rectified by insulin administration. They concluded that the inhibition of triglyceride formation and the reduced synthesis of lipoprotein peptide were causally unrelated.

Wilcox, Fried, and Heimberg (120) also found no significant differences in the rates of lysine incorporation into VLDL or LDL when normal livers were perfused with normal rat serum or with serum that contained added palmitic acid. However, the serum alone may have contained sufficient levels of fatty acid to minimize the effect of added palmitate. These findings, nonetheless, raise some doubts concerning the importance of exogenous fatty acids and endogenous lipid production as determinants of the rapidity of lipoprotein-peptide formation.

Several studies indicate that stimulation of fatty acid synthesis by the liver enhances serum-lipoprotein production. Windmueller and Spaeth (108) confirmed previous reports showing that livers from fasted, refed rats synthesize fatty acids more actively than those from rats fed ad libitum. They also observed larger quantities of esterified fatty acids and cholesterol in the $d < 1.016$ g/ml fraction of the perfusate from fasted, refed rats than in the perfusate from control livers. They concluded that active fatty acid synthesis promoted the release of triglycerides and cholesterol, and that the rate of de novo fatty acid synthesis was an important determinant of the release of other lipids by the liver. β-lipoproteins were identified in the $d < 1.016$ g/ml fraction of both control and experimental groups, but the amount of peptide present and the rate of amino acid incorporation into lipoprotein peptide were not measured. In the fasted, refed rats the lipids of the $d < 1.016$ g/ml lipoproteins contained a disproportionate increase in the ratio of triglyceride and cholesterol to phospholipid.

These findings differ from those of Heimberg and co-workers (117, 121), who concluded that triglycerides, cholesterol, and phospholipids are released by rat livers into the $d < 1.006$ g/ml fraction of serum in constant molar ratios to one another. In isolated hepatocytes stimulation of lipid synthesis by the addition of a mixture of lipogenic cofactors resulted in enhanced VLDL and LDL synthesis and release (52). However, inhibition of lipid synthesis by addition of clofibrate *in vitro* failed to diminish the production of VLDL and LDL from ^{14}C-leucine. One possible explanation for this datum is that only the VLDL fraction is influenced by the rate of lipogenesis, whereas LDL peptides are synthesized at a rate independent of changes in lipid metabolism (52).

There is abundant evidence that free fatty acids stimulate the hepatic output of triglycerides by increasing the number and size of VLDL molecules formed. Thus presentation of an augmented input of free fatty acids to a perfused liver resulted in an accelerated rate of VLDL release into the perfusate (121). A similar effect was observed by Nestel and Steinberg (122), who reported that triglyceride secretion may be enhanced when free fatty acids are mobilized from fat depots. Conversely, the rate of hepatic triglyceride secretion may fall when free-fatty-acid mobilization is prevented (123, 124). Kay and Entenman (125) reported the release of chylomicronlike bodies of $d < 1.006$ g/ml by perfused livers of fed rats. This release did not occur in the livers of fasted rats.

To this evidence has been added the electron-microscopy data of Jones et al. (89, 126) and Hamilton et al. (94), who independently reported that the presence of unsaturated free fatty acids in the perfusion medium increased the size, number, and osmiophilia of electron-dense particles with the dimensions of VLDL (300–800 Å). These particles were observed as clusters in the Golgi cisternae, in the perfusate, and, to a lesser extent, in the smooth endoplasmic reticulum and the space of Disse. Puromycin markedly depressed the hepatic secretion of the electron-dense bodies into the $d < 1.006$ g/ml fraction during perfusion with an oleate-rich medium. In addition, puromycin blocked the appearance of ^{14}C-oleate in lipoprotein triglycerides in the perfusate but did not interfere with its incorporation into liver triglycerides (121). These data suggest that the transport of triglycerides into the perfusate requires the concurrent synthesis of lipoprotein peptide. Subsequently Ruderman and associates (127) discovered that perfusion of rat liver with a linoleate-rich medium resulted in a sharp rise in triglyceride release, a significant acceleration of net output of VLDL protein, and a stimulation of amino acid incorporation into the protein moiety of VLDL. They further reported that the rate of amino acid incorporation into $1.008 < d < 1.21$ protein was not affected by fatty acid concentration, but that the rate of synthesis of other perfusate and tissue proteins was lowered by the use of media enriched with fatty acids. Stimulation of triglyceride release also increased the number and size of osmiophilic particles in the perfusate. They concluded that the liver increases its delivery of triglycerides into the plasma primarily by the production of more lipoprotein molecules and suggested that the intracellular concentration of newly synthesized triglycerides may, in some specific way, alter the release and perhaps the synthesis of $d < 1.007$ g/ml lipoprotein peptide.

Kohout, Kohoutova, and Heimberg (128) have recently shown that the structure of the fatty acid perfused into the liver may also determine the rate of VLDL formation and secretion. Thus the release of triglycerides increased with the chain length of infused saturated fatty acids (C_6–C_{18}). Furthermore, triglyceride output fell as the number of double bonds in the C_{18} fatty acid was increased; more triglycerides were secreted with stearic acid than with linoleic or linolenic acid infusion. They concluded that the rate of VLDL-triglyceride secretion depends on the chain length, degree of unsaturation, and concentration of fatty acids in the perfusion medium and suggested that VLDL are probably secreted as a complete unit with constant molar ratios of cholesterol, phospholipids, and triglycerides.

In all probability free fatty acids mainly stimulate a parallel rise in the hepatic output of triglycerides and in de novo synthesis and release of VLDL peptide. However, individual lipoprotein molecules may be more heavily charged with additional triglycerides in some physiological situations. This does not exclude the possibility that increased lipoprotein release results from stabilization by triglycerides of an unstable lipoprotein peptide or peptide precursor in the liver. Nor does it preclude the possible participation of a circulating lipid-acceptor protein, as proposed by Eder et al. (105), although its quantitative significance in the physiological transport of lipids is probably small (112).

F. Fatty Liver

Intracellular deposition of lipid is a common response of the hepatic parenchymal cell to injury. The accumulated lipid is mainly triglyceride, even when the fatty liver results from the intake of a high-cholesterol diet by experimental animals. This stereotyped response suggests that unifying factors underlie the development of fatty livers from various causes and that different agents may affect the same mechanism, albeit in somewhat different ways.

In general, triglyceride buildup in the liver ensues when an imbalance exists between the rate at which fatty acids are made by, or brought to, the liver, and their rate of oxidation or export as lipoprotein triglycerides. The fatty changes induced by such agents as carbon tetrachloride, ethionine, white phosphorus, puromycin, and orotic acid all share a common feature. The deposition of triglycerides is preceded and accompanied by decreasing concentrations of serum lipids, especially triglycerides, and of serum lipoproteins, especially VLDL. Evidence from a number of laboratories (40–44, 54, 92, 129–133) indicates that many types of experimentally induced fatty livers result from a reduction in either the synthesis or release of serum lipoproteins, particularly VLDL. The hypothesis that depression of serum-lipoprotein production might form the basis for an increase in liver lipid concentrations was first proposed by Robinson and co-workers (40, 130), who also presented experimental evidence based on their studies with ethionine and carbon tetrachloride.

The pathogenesis of fatty liver is considered here primarily as it bears on the topic of serum-lipoprotein production. Types of fatty liver that can be reasonably attributed to inhibition of lipoprotein synthesis or release are covered in the first two parts of the following discussion. As indicated in the final section, however, a number of agents cause fatty liver without evident interference with lipoprotein production. Excellent reviews by Lombardi (129) and Recknagel (92) discuss the development of fatty liver in more detail.

1 Fatty Livers Associated with Depression of Hepatic Protein Synthesis. Impaired hepatic protein synthesis has been implicated as a basis for the fatty liver induced by ethionine (42, 131), carbon tetrachloride (43, 132), puromycin (42, 52), dimethylnitrosamine (44, 133), phosphorus (41, 134), and azaserine (135). Robinson and Harris (40) reported that liver slices prepared from ethionine-treated rats showed a diminished incorporation of leucine into the $d < 1.21$ g/ml lipoproteins released into the medium. They found that puromycin (42) or carbon tetrachloride (43) administration had the same effect. In these studies (41–43) development of fatty liver and diminished rates of protein synthesis were associated with decreased concentrations of all classes of serum lipids except fatty acids, which were mobilized under these conditions (136). Rat-liver-cell suspensions, prelabeled with ^{14}C-acetate or ^{14}C-palmitate, were unable to secrete labeled lipids when puromycin was added to the incubation medium, although lipid-labeled lipoproteins were released at a linear rate in the absence of puromycin (54).

Puromycin produced a similar inhibition of ^{14}C-leucine incorporation into VLDL and LDL released from isolated rat hepatocytes (52). An analogous effect was observed on the absorption of long-chain fatty acids in rats treated with puromycin (137), which inhibited chylomicron formation, suppressed the absorption of labeled lipid into the lacteals (137), and resulted in distention of the villous mucosal cells with lipids (46). In perfused livers from rats treated with carbon tetrachloride there was a reduction in the incorporation of lysine into all secreted lipoproteins (120) and in the output of cholesterol, phospholipids, and especially triglycerides (121).

The synthesis of serum proteins accounts for most of the active protein synthesis in the liver. Since the turnover rates of serum lipoproteins are much faster than those of most other serum proteins (138, 139), it might be concluded that hepatic accumulation of triglyceride is simply a consequence of the generalized impairment of protein synthesis in that organ. Support for this conclusion has been derived from ultrastructural evidence. After administration of carbon tetrachloride or ethionine to rats, electron microscopy showed detachment of ribosomes from the endoplasmic reticulum, polysomal disaggregation, and anomalous sedimentation characteristics of the ribosomes (92, 131, 140–142). As a result, numerous free ribosomes appeared in the cytoplasmic ground substance, and an increased number of lipid-containing droplets were seen in the smooth endoplasmic reticulum.

However, the dual effect of these agents on lipoprotein synthesis and hepatic triglyceride accumulation cannot be taken by itself as evidence that the lipid infiltration is caused by the inhibition of lipoprotein-peptide synthesis; and much evidence militates against this oversimplification. In the first place, actinomycin D markedly inhibits serum-lipoprotein synthesis in rats, both *in vivo* and in perfused liver (142), but does not produce fatty changes (143). Second, ethionine, carbon tetrachloride, and azaserine cause increases in plasma free fatty acids and may induce fatty liver through their effects on free-fatty-acid mobilization. In animals treated with carbon tetrachloride or azaserine injection of adenosine triphosphate (ATP) prevented the development of fatty liver without correcting the impairment of protein synthesis (135). Adenosine triphosphate also abolished the free-fatty-acid mobilization induced by the three hepatotoxic agents. Finally, in the case of carbon tetrachloride at least, peroxidative damage to the structural lipids of membranes, probably involving free radicals, occurs rather indiscriminately and involves membranous components besides the ergastoplasm, especially the mitochondria and lysosomes (92). Although decreased protein synthesis is a prominent feature of the liver damaged by carbon tetrachloride, Recknagel suggests that the coupling or release mechanisms may be the key targets that account for the rapid diminution in triglyceride secretion during carbon tetrachloride toxicity (92). He observed that inhibition of protein synthesis alone cannot explain the greatly disproportionate inhibition of VLDL labeling in comparison with that of the other serum proteins. But at the present time the available data appear to support the view that the inhibition of hepatic protein synthesis is an important contributing factor to the reduction of serum-lipid levels in ethionine-treated animals.

2. Fatty Livers with Normal Hepatic Protein Synthesis. In choline-deficient animals the synthesis of hepatic and plasma proteins is not impaired (129), and in orotic-acid-fed rats this synthesis is, if anything, increased (144, 145). However, as with the hepatotoxic agents, the fatty liver caused by dietary orotic acid (146, 147) or choline deficiency (148) shows a similar cytoarchitectural alteration of fine lipid droplets surrounded by a membrane in continuity with that of the endoplasmic reticulum. Presently available evidence in the case of the orotic acid and choline-deficient livers favors a defect in the coupling of lipid to lipoprotein peptide or in the mechanism for lipoprotein secretion. Fatty liver caused by each agent is considered individually.

In the orotic acid fatty liver, which was first reported by Standerfer and

Handler (149), plasma triglyceride, phospholipid, and cholesterol levels decline within the first 24 hr, and liver triglycerides begin to accumulate (150). Hepatic nucleotide metabolism is profoundly disturbed (151), and, in common with ethionine hepatotoxicity, intracellular ATP levels are depressed, but this is readily reversible by adenine administration (131, 152). Rubin and Pendleton (153) found that liver slices prepared from orotic-acid-fed rats exhibited a marked depression in their capacity to incorporate ^{14}C-leucine into β-lipoproteins. Since general protein synthesis in the liver slices was normal, they proposed that the defect in synthesis might be specific for the LDL peptide. Windmueller was unable to distinguish between a defect in LDL synthesis and one of LDL secretion in orotic acid fatty liver (150).

Roheim et al. (87, 88) confirmed the fact that orotic acid feeding did not depress the incorporation of ^{14}C-amino acids into tissue or plasma proteins by perfused livers. Yet, in agreement with the findings of Rubin and Pendleton, labeled VLDL were almost completely absent from the perfusate from orotic acid livers. Moreover, when an orotic acid fatty liver was perfused with labeled $d > 1.21$ g/ml proteins prepared from normal rat plasma, incorporation of radioactive high-density proteins into VLDL was markedly depressed. In contrast, when fatty livers from cholesterol-fed rats were perfused with labeled $d > 1.21$ g/ml plasma proteins from either normal or orotic-acid-fed rats, labeled VLDL rapidly appeared in the perfusate. Thus, according to these workers, the orotic-acid-fed animals did produce and release the apolipoprotein of LDL and VLDL, and some step subsequent to synthesis of the peptide was affected by the orotic acid intake.

Windmueller and Levy (60) demonstrated the complete, selective disappearance of β-lipoproteins from the bloodstream of rats fed orotic acid for 1 week. The concentration of HDL in the plasma was reduced by about 50%. The experimental design of this study does not permit a distinction between inhibited synthesis and an interruption of coupling or secretion. Analysis of thoracic-duct lymph from rats fed orotic acid suggested that the absorption of long-chain fatty acids and the formation of chylomicrons were unimpaired despite the lack of plasma β-lipoproteins and the development of hepatic steatosis (154). This finding is consistent with the fact that intestinal synthesis of β-lipoproteins is unimpaired in rats fed orotic acid (59). The difference between the liver and intestine in the sensitivity of β-lipoprotein synthesis to dietary orotic acid remains unexplained.

Lombardi, Ugazio, and Raick (155) reported that defective phospholipid synthesis in choline-deficient rats led to impaired utilization of dietary triglycerides by the liver. There was no inhibition of protein synthesis, but phospholipid levels in liver and serum were diminished. The plasma-phospholipid level decreased when the rats were on a choline-deficient diet for as little as 1 day, but the level of plasma triglycerides only fell after about 5 days on the deficient diet (156, 157). Contrary to earlier results (158), which indicated that development of fatty liver in choline-deficient rats preceded the reduction of plasma-triglyceride levels, Lombardi, Pani, and Schlunk (159) established that impaired triglyceride release occurred within 24 hr on a choline-deficient diet and accompanied the accumulation of liver triglycerides. This observation supports the possibility that the fatty liver of choline-deficient animals may, in part, result from a more gradual and subtle disturbance in triglyceride output. Since release of lipoproteins and other serum proteins was impaired despite normal protein synthesis, they suggested that altered phospholipid synthesis in subcellular membranes interfered with the conjugating or secretory mechanism of the liver cell. It should be emphasized that nearly all serum proteins are glycoproteins and that conjugation of carbohydrate to the protein moiety may be essential for secretion from the hepatocyte (39). In addition, they found an increased turnover of liver lecithins, as measured by the incorporation of ^{32}P-labeled inorganic phosphate. Meldolesi et al. (141), who had observed a similar enhancement of the incorporation of ^{32}P-labeled inorganic phosphate into microsomal phospholipids in carbon tetrachloride hepatotoxicity, proposed that this stimulation produced functionally abnormal membranes.

In a series of studies (157, 160–162), Mookerjea and co-workers developed evidence for a defect in the addition of carbohydrates to serum proteins in early choline deficiency. They found that added ^{14}C-glucosamine rapidly appeared in the protein moieties of various serum lipoproteins and in $d > 1.21$ g/ml proteins during perfusion of a normal rat liver. When livers obtained from 2-day choline-deficient rats were perfused with blood obtained from similarly treated rats, the appearance of protein-bound label in the perfusate was impaired. The incorporation of ^{14}C-glusosamine into VLDL, LDL, and $d > 1.21$ g/ml proteins was significantly reduced, whereas incorporation into HDL was unaffected. Triglyceride release by the choline-deficient liver was markedly inhibited but was corrected when blood from choline-fed animals was used to perfuse the liver. Livers from animals with early choline deficiency showed no deficiency in protein synthesis or fatty acid esterification.

On the basis of these findings Mookerjea et al. proposed the following sequence of events in early choline deficiency:

1. General impairment of glycoprotein synthesis in the hepatic smooth endoplasmic reticulum and a specific decrease in synthesis of plasma $d > 1.21$ g/ml α-globulins, corresponding to the lipid-acceptor protein of Eder.

2. Impairment of plasma VLDL and LDL glycolipoprotein formation and consequently a defect in triglyceride transport from the liver, leading to lipid accumulation in the parenchyma.

Hence fatty liver in choline deficiency may represent a postribosomal event and may result from alterations in carbohydrate addition in the membranes of the smooth endoplasmic reticulum.

3. Fatty Liver Associated with Increased Serum-Lipoprotein Production. Fatty liver may occur despite an enhanced release of lower density lipoproteins. Hypertriglyceridemia has been reported, for example, in cases of fatty liver due to ethanol intoxication (163, 164), and administration of catecholamines (165) or cortisone (166, 167) to experimental animals. Intracellular accumulation of lipid in the liver has accompanied hyperlipoproteinemia in nephrotic rats (168) and in the regenerating rat liver after partial hepatectomy (169).

The fatty liver resulting from acute administration of ethanol to well-nourished animals has been attributed to various causes by different investigators. These proposals have included increased hepatic lipogenesis, increased free-fatty-acid transport to the liver, inhibition of serum-lipoprotein synthesis or secretion, diversion of hepatic fatty acid esterification from phospholipids to triglyceride synthesis, and diminished hepatic oxidation of fatty acids (164). It has not been established that the fatty liver of ethanol intoxication is causally related to a change in the rate of serum-lipoprotein synthesis. However, hyperlipemia and triglyceride elevations in the plasma commonly appear at some point during the development of fatty liver (163, 164).

Baraona and Lieber (170) presented evidence that alcoholic hyperlipemia in rats is due, at least partially, to an increment in newly synthesized lipoproteins. Increased incorporation of ^{3}H-palmitate and ^{14}C-lysine into $d < 1.019$ g/ml serum lipoproteins occurred *in vivo* during ethanol-induced hyperlipemia. Administration of Triton had the same effect in ethanol-treated rats as it did in control rats in which ethanol was replaced isocalorically with carbohydrate. Hence Baraona and Lieber postulated that ethanol-induced hyperlipemia in rats is not caused by defective removal of lipids from the circulation. Furthermore, fat absorption and the clearance of injected chylomicrons were unchanged by ethanol feeding. The simultaneous production of fatty liver, hyperlipemia, and increased serum-lipoprotein synthesis provide evidence that in the rat the ethanol-induced fatty liver is probably not a result of defective lipoprotein production. Similar data were obtained in investigations of ethanol-induced lipemia in healthy volunteers and in subjects with fasting hypertriglyceridemia (171). The lipemic response to the ingestion of fat and ethanol was proportional to the initial fasting triglyceride level and was greater than the additive effects of either substance ingested alone. Elevated VLDL levels were responsible for the lipemia.

Fatty liver developed in dogs during the administration of intravenous norepinephrine over an 8-hr period (165). The principal cause of the fat accumulation was the lipolytic action of a norepinephrine-sensitive lipase in adipose tissue (172). Plasma free-fatty-acid levels rose promptly to 10 times control levels and remained elevated as long as the norepinephrine infusion was maintained; liver triglyceride content rose progressively together with plasma cholesterol and lipoprotein levels (77). However, in this study liver damage during prolonged anesthesia could not be dismissed as a contributing factor to the hepatic fat accumulation.

In cortisone-treated rabbits, coincident with the development of fatty liver and hyperlipemia, there was a dramatic increase in clusters of large particles in the secretory vesicles of the Golgi apparatus (95). On the basis of electron-microscope observations Mahley et al. suggested that the electron-translucent particles were large VLDL molecules (300–3000 Å) present within the Golgi vesicles and in the serum $d < 1.006$ g/ml fraction. Stenger and Confer (173) described similar "bodies" (300–1000 Å) in the cytoplasm of hepatocytes, the space of Disse, and the sinusoids of the liver after partial hepatectomy. Fex and Olivecrona (169) suggested that such "bodies" may result from accelerated VLDL synthesis by the liver after partial hepatectomy.

A sharp elevation in serum VLDL and LDL levels and a decline in serum HDL concentration were observed 24 hr after partial hepatectomy in rats undergoing liver regeneration (174). In addition, 22.5 hr postoperatively the incorporation of ^{14}C-leucine into all lipoprotein and protein fractions except HDL_2 was higher per gram of liver in partially hepatectomized rats than in normal or sham-operated controls (175). In another study (176) the hepatic uptake of labeled chylomicrons and the incorporation of labeled glycerol into liver lipids was much greater, 4 hr after operation, in partially hepatectomized rats than in laparotomized controls. Thus the regenerating liver may synthesize lipids, proteins, and lower density lipoproteins more rapidly than they can be cleared in extrahepatic tissues.

Rats made nephrotic by the administration of antikidney serum or the aminonucleoside of puromycin develop, in addition to hepatic lipid accumulation (168), hepatic hyperplasia, hypoalbuminemia, and marked increases in VLDL and LDL synthesis in perfused liver (177) and liver slices (84). The latter findings may explain the hyperlipemia in these animals. Though the largest increases occur in serum VLDL and LDL (178), the stimulation of serum-lipoprotein synthesis is probably not specific and could be explained by an overall acceleration of hepatic protein synthesis with no change in the relative rates of synthesis of individual liver proteins.

III. METABOLISM

A. Peptide and Lipid Turnover

Serum lipoproteins, like other serum proteins, are continuously degraded and replaced by newly synthesized, similar proteins. The body pool of each lipoprotein at any given time is determined by the balance between synthesis and degradation. In the steady state these two processes occur at identical rates, so that the concentration of each lipoprotein is maintained at a relatively stable level in the body fluids. It has long been recognized that serum proteins are synthesized and degraded as a unit, and presumably this is also true of each polypeptide of the serum lipoproteins. However, the various HDL and VLDL polypeptides may be degraded at different rates. For a general discussion of the turnover of plasma proteins the reader is referred to an excellent review (179).

However, there is also good evidence that the individual lipids of the lipoproteins turn over at different rates, which differ considerably from the turnover rate of the peptide portion of the molecule. It is therefore necessary to consider separately the turnover of the lipid and peptide moieties of the serum lipoproteins.

1. Peptide. Studies of lipoprotein-peptide turnover require the preparation of lipoprotein molecules with a suitable label on the peptide. An ideal label for such work would have the following properties:

1. The labeling process would not alter the biological properties of the protein.
2. The removal of the label would only occur when the lipoprotein was totally degraded.
3. The label would not be reutilized for the synthesis of new lipoproteins.

Label has been introduced by chemical modifications *in vitro,* such as with ^{131}I, or by the incorporation of a labeled amino acid during lipoprotein biosynthesis *in vivo.*

A variety of techniques are available for the addition of ^{131}I to serum lipoproteins (180–183). Mild conditions must be used to prevent damage to the lipoprotein, and the degree of labeling of the molecule should not exceed one atom of iodine per molecule. Even minimal damage to the lipoproteins, which may escape detection by electrophoresis or centrifugation, may result in more rapid catabolism of the labeled protein and a falsely low value for the half-life of the lipoprotein. The quality of the preparation can be assessed by infusion of the labeled lipoprotein into an animal. Extremely rapid catabolism indicates that the preparation is unsuitable for use in turnover studies.

The ^{131}I may also label the lipid portion of the lipoprotein and cause an erroneously low estimate of the lipoprotein half-life since the lipids are removed more rapidly than the peptide. The amount of label incorporated into the lipid portion of the labeled product should be determined. No significant error will result when the lipids contain only a few percent of the total label.

Biosynthetic labels are free from the problems outlined above. However, they have the disadvantage that labeled amino acids released during protein catabolism are continuously reutilized for the synthesis of new serum lipoproteins. Reutilization, which leads to spuriously high estimates of the half-life of the protein, is particularly great when turnover is measured in the same animal that has received the radioactive amino acid. Recycling can be diminished by following the turnover of the labeled lipoprotein in a second animal whose body pool of proteins is not labeled.

A potentially useful technique for determining the rate of plasma-lipoprotein synthesis was introduced by McFarlane (184). This method involves the injection of $Na_2{}^{14}CO_3$ as a precursor of ^{14}C-arginine, which is incorporated into proteins and degraded to urea. By measuring the radioactivity incorporated into lipoprotein and into urea, it is possible to calculate the mass of lipoprotein synthesized during the period of observation. This method is better than the other types of biosynthetic labels because there is little or no recycling of the label. To date this method has not been utilized in studies of lipoprotein synthesis.

After an intravenous injection of ^{131}I-labeled lipoprotein, radioactivity in plasma and urine is followed. The decline in plasma radioactivity results from equilibration of intravascular lipoproteins with those of the extravascular space and from catabolism of the labeled lipoproteins. The first process is generally completed within 3 to 4 days after injection, so that the subsequent decline in plasma radioactivity is a measure of the metabolic breakdown of the lipoprotein. Iodine released during the breakdown of the lipoprotein is excreted in the urine, and urinary radioactivity is another parameter that depends on the catabolic rate.

The rate of lipoprotein catabolism can be calculated from a plot of plasma radioactivity against time on semilogarithmic paper. After a period of rapid decline of plasma radioactivity, which results from equilibration with the extravascular space, this plot becomes a straight line. This line is extrapolated to zero time, and the half-life $T_{1/2}$ is calculated by determining the time that corresponds to half the ordinate of the intercept. The slope of the line measures the fractional turnover rate k. The half-life and fractional turnover rate are related in the following manner:

$$k = \frac{0.693}{T_{1/2}}$$

The fractional turnover rate can be calculated from the urinary excretion of radioactivity by the following relationship:

$$k = \frac{du/dt}{P}$$

where du/dt is the urinary radioactivity per 24 hr and P is the average plasma radioactivity over the 24-hr period.

Three relationships have been found between the turnover of plasma proteins and their concentration in plasma (179, 185). For one type of protein—for example, fibrinogen—k is independent of its concentration in plasma (186). The catabolism of a second group of proteins, including transferrin and haptoglobin, is inversely proportional to their plasma concentration (187, 188). In a third type of catabolism, found with albumin and γG-globulins, k is directly proportional to the plasma concentration (189–191). Since the catabolic rate for LDL was not dependent on LDL concentration in plasma (192), the turnover of this lipoprotein falls into the first pattern outlined above. Implicit in this result is the fact that the absolute turnover of LDL is directly proportional to LDL concentration in plasma.

Just as for other serum proteins, the organ (or organs) involved in serum-lipoprotein-peptide catabolism and the biochemical mechanisms involved in such peptide degradation are largely unknown. The liver and gastrointestinal tract are the two sites that have been suggested for the degradation of serum protein. The importance of the gastrointestinal tract in this process is the subject of considerable disagreement. Many workers believe that the liver is the more important catabolic organ, but firm evidence on this point is lacking (179).

The subcellular site for lipoprotein-peptide degradation is most likely the lysosome that contains the intracellular pool of proteolytic enzymes (193).

The first studies of the turnover rates of human-serum lipoproteins were carried out by Volwiler et al. (139), who used ^{35}S-cystine or ^{35}S-tagged whole plasma as biosynthetic precursors. In eight normal subjects the apparent LDL half-life ranged from 2.9 to 7.4 days. Probably because of isotopic reutilization, the LDL half-life reported in this study is considerably longer than that found by most later workers who utilized ^{131}I-LDL. In normal adults a half-life of 3.1 to 3.4 days was reported by Gitlin et al. (138) and of 3.0 days by Langer, Strober, and Levy (194). In the studies of Walton and co-workers (183, 195) the LDL half-life in six normal women (only one was premenopausal) was only 2.4 days. These authors concluded that females in general turn over LDL more rapidly than males do.

In these studies with ^{131}I-LDL the serum radioactivity was followed for a relatively short time. It was assumed that equilibration between intravascular and extravascular spaces was achieved rapidly and that the LDL half-life could be calculated from the decline in serum radioactivity over a period of 2 to 2.5 weeks. When Hurley and Scott (192, 196) extended to 6 weeks the period of observation of serum label after ^{131}I-LDL injection into two subjects, the curve of serum radioactivity did not reach a straight line until about the 26th day. These authors assumed that complete equilibration between intravascular and extravascular spaces was not achieved until this time. Using this longer period of observation, they calculated an LDL half-life of 6 to 8 days. They also found a more rapid fractional turnover rate in young women than in men or older women. These workers postulated that there are both rapidly and slowly exchangeable pools in the extravascular space, and that the studies that lasted less than 26 days would give LDL half-life values that were too short because part of the disappearance rate would represent continued equilibration between intravascular and extravascular space.

As a possible example of the delayed equilibration of tissues with intravascular LDL, there is a rather slow entry of labeled LDL peptide into the normal aortic wall in man (197) and dogs (198), into human thrombi (199), and into xanthomas (200) of patients with hypercholesteremia. Immunofluorescent studies showed an accumulation of LDL, but not HDL, in the extracellular lipid in the intima of atherosclerotic aorta. There was no evidence of intracellular LDL. Walton and Williamson concluded that LDL accumulation is largely responsible for the intimal lipid accumulations of atherosclerosis (201). The uptake of ^{131}I-LDL into aortic slices was greater in animals susceptible to atherosclerosis, such as rabbits and cockerels, than it was in the rat, which does not readily develop atherosclerotic lesions (202).

The turnover rate of ^{131}I-LDL has been determined in several pathological states. The turnover of LDL is apparently increased in nephrotic children (138), in patients with hyperthyroidism (183), and in patients with a variety of acute conditions, such as head injury, cerebrovascular accidents, rheumatoid arthritis, cancer, leukemia, and some infections (192). The

LDL half-life was increased in hypothyroidism (183) and was normal in a patient with abetalipoproteinemia (203). Patients with hyperlipemia had a normal fractional turnover rate but an increase in the absolute rate of LDL turnover (183, 200). In a group of four hypercholesteremic patients, whose LDL levels decreased on treatment with clofibrate, there was no change in the fractional catabolic rate, but the absolute turnover rate fell considerably because of the smaller pool of LDL. Since there was a proportionate fall in the extravascular pool of LDL, Scott et al. suggest that this reduction in LDL may have accounted for the gradual disappearance of xanthomas (196).

More recently Fredrickson's group (194, 204) reported that the fractional catabolic rate was slower in patients with familial hypercholesteremia (type II hyperlipoproteinemia) than it was in normal controls. Reduction of serum-cholesterol levels by dietary measures or by cholestyramine treatment increased the fractional catabolic rate. They also concluded that the rate of LDL synthesis in patients with hypercholesteremia was the same as in normal subjects and that reduction of serum-cholesterol levels did not affect the rate of synthesis. By analogy with the lipid-storage diseases in man, which have so far proved to be a consequence of abnormally slow catabolism rather than increased rates of synthesis (205), it is reasonable to propose, as Fredrickson et al. did, that type II hyperlipoproteinemia results from a defect in LDL degradation. However, it is difficult to understand how steady-state levels of serum LDL can be maintained with a normal rate of synthesis and a decreased catabolic rate.

In some patients hypercholesteremia may reflect a structural or compositional abnormality in the lower density lipoproteins that renders them relatively resistant to degradation. Thus in broad-β disease (type III hyperlipoproteinemia) lipoproteins with $d < 1.006$ g/ml are abnormally rich in cholesterol and poor in triglycerides, and exhibit decreased mobility in paper electrophoresis (206). In these subjects plasma chylomicrons collected after an overnight fast were also enriched in cholesterol, with a triglyceride-to-cholesterol ratio of < 3.0, whereas chylomicrons obtained at the peak of alimentary lipemia had a normal composition (207). These results suggest that chylomicrons, initially normal in composition, are gradually converted by lipolysis and cholesterol transfer to abnormal lipoproteins with a high cholesterol content. This compositional change may interfere with further lipoprotein-lipase activity and retard the removal of this lipoprotein.

A unique low-density lipoprotein (LP-X), with a characteristically high content of unesterified cholesterol and phospholipids, is found in the d 1.006 to 1.063 g/ml fraction of serum from patients with obstructive liver disease (208). This lipoprotein is immunochemically and electrophoretically distinct from the lipoproteins normally isolated in this density subfraction and is probably responsible for the increase in lipoproteins with *d* 1.006 to 1.063 g/ml and the decrease in HDL that accompanies biliary obstruction. This abnormal lipoprotein may be identical with Switzer's (209) "obstructive lipoprotein," whose amino acid composition and immunochemical properties differed from those of the A and B peptides of HDL and LDL, respectively. Seidel, Alaupovic, and Furman (208) have suggested that LP-X originates in the intestinal mucosa, where it participates in fat absorption and that its catabolism is inhibited by the elevated levels of circulating bile acids present in biliary obstructive disease. The LP-X or altered LP-X then accumulates in the *d* 1.006 to 1.063 g/ml fraction of plasma.

The catabolism of HDL in normal subjects has been studied by several groups who utilized ^{131}I-HDL. The average half-lives reported by these workers are 4 days in normal adult men and children (138), 3.5 days in three normal adult men and in one hypercholesteremic patient (20), and 4.3 days in two normal adults (210). When injected into a dog, canine HDL was removed at a similar rate; but human HDL had a half-life of only 2.6 days in the dog and 12 hr in the mouse (10). In normal subjects the half-life of the delipidated protein of HDL was very similar to that of intact HDL (20, 210). The half-time of either intact or delipidated HDL was much shorter (1.8 days) in two patients with hyperchylomicronemia and slightly shorter (2.6 days) in two patients with endogenous hypertriglyceridemia (20). Furman et al. suggest that the shortened half-life in these patients is due to their diminished pool of HDL. If this is the case, the turnover properties of HDL would differ from those of LDL, whose half-lives are not affected by their concentration in serum. It would be interesting to determine the turnover rate of infused HDL in patients with absent HDL, or Tangier disease (27), to find out whether the catabolic rate of HDL is normal in these patients, just as the turnover of LDL is normal in patients with abetalipoproteinemia (203).

The half-life of ^{131}I-VLDL injected into human subjects was 2 to 3 days (138), and part of the label subsequently was isolated from serum LDL. No label appeared in VLDL after injection of ^{131}I-LDL. The turnover of VLDL was slower in nephrotic patients.

The use of iodinated HDL and VLDL raises problems of interpretation since their various apoproteins are probably catabolized at different rates. To obtain maximal information from such studies, one should reisolate each serum-lipoprotein fraction and determine the radioactivity in each individual polypeptide instead of following the decline of total plasma label.

2. Lipid. About two-thirds of the serum lipids—cholesterol and phospholipids—probably function primarily as structural components of the serum lipoproteins. Other roles for these lipids, however, are suggested by the abnormalities found in the erythrocytes of patients who cannot synthesize β-lipoproteins (35, 47). The magnitude and rate of their turnover are relatively small. Moreover, their ready interchange with tissue lipids (28) makes it difficult to use tracer studies to determine their net turnover. Phospholipids are present in larger quantities than any other lipids in plasma, but they turn over at a rather slow rate. It has been estimated that the plasma phospholipid pool turns over in about 3 days in man (211).

The total daily turnover of cholesterol in man is slightly more than 1 g (212). Between 100 and 300 mg are absorbed from the diet (213), and about 900 mg are synthesized each day in a person of ideal body weight (214). Endogenous cholesterol synthesis increases with body weight (214), whereas dietary cholesterol inhibits cholesterol synthesis in the liver (34). Transported from the intestine largely as cholesteryl esters (215) associated with chylomicrons (216, 217), most of the absorbed cholesterol is removed from the circulation by the liver (76, 218). Since all tissues can synthesize cholesterol (219, 220), plasma-cholesterol transport from the liver is not required to meet the requirements of peripheral tissues. It is possible, however, that the adrenal, ovary, testis, and placenta may utilize circulating cholesterol in part as substrates for steroid-hormone synthesis (221, 222). Perhaps more significant is the postulated transport of cholesterol from sites of cell breakdown back to the liver, the only organ that can excrete cholesterol, either directly into the bile or after conversion into bile acids (25, 27).

After injection of radioactive acetate or mevalonate, equilibration between liver and plasma free cholesterol took place with a half-time of about 20 min in the dog (223) and 1 hr in man (224). The specific activity of plasma free cholesterol reached its peak about 3 hr after labeled precursor was injected in man (224, 225). Radioactivity appeared more slowly in plasma cholesteryl esters, which achieved their maximal specific activity after about 2 days (225, 226). Because of slow equilibration between the unesterified cholesterol of plasma and that of various tissues, the specific activity of plasma free cholesterol declined slowly for about 2 months after injection of label (227, 228). The rate of equilibration varied among different body tissues; complete equilibration required a month for some tissues and even longer for arteries (227, 228).

In the rat the catabolic rate of different cholesteryl esters was heterogeneous (229, 230). The half-time of monounsaturated esters, for example, was shorter than that of other cholesteryl esters. During perfusion of rat livers VLDL cholesteryl esters had a faster turnover rate than those of other lipoproteins (107). In contrast, all types of cholesteryl esters had similar fractional turnover rates in man (225, 229); and, after injection of ^{14}C-mevalonate, label appeared most rapidly in cholesteryl esters of HDL and least rapidly in those of VLDL (225).

The magnitude of free-fatty-acid and triglyceride transport far exceeds that of cholesterol and phospholipids. Despite their relatively low concentration in plasma, free fatty acids exceed all other lipid classes in their contribution to total fat transport. Over 200 g of fat may be transported daily as free fatty acids (37). Next in quantitative significance are triglycerides. Between 50 and 150 g of triglycerides is ingested and transported from the intestine each day as chylomicrons. In addition it has been estimated that about 50 g of VLDL triglycerides can be removed from the bloodstream daily (231).

Free fatty acids are the serum lipid component with the fastest turnover rate. The half-life of labeled free fatty acids in the bloodstream is shorter than 5 min (232) and may be less than 1 min (233). Somewhat less rapidly cleared from the circulation of man and animals are triglycerides. Their rate of removal is directly proportional to the size of the lipoprotein particle (231, 234, 235) and inversely related to the triglyceride concentration (236, 237). Thus fat emulsions are cleared faster than chylomicrons (234), and larger chylomicrons are removed more rapidly than smaller ones (235). The triglycerides of VLDL are cleared more slowly than those of chylomicrons (231), which have an average half-life of less than 15 min (237, 238). The calculated rate of removal of VLDL triglycerides, when present in normal concentrations in man, is about 2 g/hr (231). Because of the relatively slow turnover rate of VLDL triglycerides, endogenous hyperlipemia may readily occur whenever there is an increased rate of VLDL synthesis and release. The problem is accentuated by the decreased fractional clearance rate for triglycerides as their plasma levels rise (236, 237).

The steady-state rates of serum-triglyceride turnover have been determined by the use of two major methods. In the more widely used method a pulse of labeled precursor is injected, and the rate of disappearance of labeled triglycerides from the plasma is used to estimate the turnover rate (239). In the other method labeled free fatty acids are infused continuously, and the rate of accumulation of radioactivity in plasma triglycerides is measured. Simultaneous determination of the turnover rate of free fatty acids allows an estimate of the steady-state turnover rate of plasma triglycerides (240). Havel (241) pointed out that opposite conclusions were reached when these two methods were used to study endogenous hypertriglyceridemia in man. Application of the first method led one group to conclude that clearing mechanisms were normal and that lipemia was caused by increased triglyceride production (231). Workers who applied the second method maintained that an abnormality of removal was responsible for the lipemia since the production rate of triglycerides was not increased

(242). Baker (243) has reviewed the application of multicompartmental analysis and computer techniques to problems of lipid metabolism and has critically evaluated eight kinetic studies of hepatic triglyceride secretion.

A recent report by Redgrave (76) indicates that the metabolism of chylomicrons takes place in two discrete phases. Most of the triglycerides were removed in peripheral tissues to form a smaller, cholesterol-rich "remnant particle," which accumulated in the blood of functionally hepatectomized rats. When later injected into rats, the remnant particles were rapidly cleared by the liver. These findings are consistent with earlier work showing that the liver removed most of the cholesteryl esters from chylomicrons injected into the circulation (218). Prior hydrolysis was not needed for the hepatic uptake of cholesteryl esters, which were only fully split in the perfused rat liver during the 3 to 4 hr after uptake (244). Ten minutes after injection of doubly-labeled chylomicrons, 80% of the cholesteryl esters, but only 20% of the triglycerides, was in the liver (76). This result might be predicted from the low levels of lipoprotein-lipase activity in the liver (245), which in fact may contain an inhibitor of this enzyme (246). In contrast, lipoprotein-lipase activity is present (246) at the presumed major sites of chylomicron removal in adipose tissue (9–11), heart (12–16), and skeletal muscle (11).

The critical role of this enzyme in the metabolism of chylomicrons is illustrated by the persistence of chylomicronemia in untreated patients with type I hyperlipoproteinemia (32), who have an inherited deficiency of lipoprotein-lipase activity (247–250). Several reviews by Robinson (251–253) describe the properties of this enzyme and indicate its role in the removal of chylomicron triglycerides from the blood. A noteworthy advance in this area is a method for the purification of human-lipoprotein lipase from postheparin plasma (23). Significantly greater activation of triglyceride emulsions was obtained with HDL and chylomicrons than with LDL or VLDL.

The VLDL triglycerides are also removed in peripheral tissues by the action of lipoprotein lipase, but there has been considerable uncertainty concerning the end product of this action. Although early theories proposed that LDL was an intermediate in the breakdown of VLDL (254), it had been difficult to understand how triglyceride removal alone could transform VLDL into a residue that was similar to LDL in lipid and protein composition. Fredrickson and Gordon (232) reviewed the earlier evidence for the metabolic conversion of VLDL to lipoproteins with higher S_f-rates. With greater knowledge of the protein components of these two lipoproteins and elucidation of the function of LCAT, such an interconversion becomes even more plausible. The combined activity of lipoprotein lipase and LCAT could produce the required changes in lipid pattern. Release of

HDL and the apo-C peptides from VLDL during catabolism of its lipids would leave a residue with apo-B as the only protein component.

The results of various studies are consistent with conversion of VLDL to LDL. Several laboratories have demonstrated that serum levels of HDL and LDL vary reciprocally with VLDL concentration (19, 255). In addition, when labeled lysine was injected into the pig, incorporation reached a peak at 15 min in VLDL, but not until 3 hr in LDL (256). These findings are consistent with a precursor–product relationship between VLDL and LDL. Moreover, early work with injected ^{131}I-VLDL indicated possible conversion of VLDL to LDL (138). Finally, a study *in vitro* suggested that the action of lipoprotein lipase and LCAT converts VLDL to LDL (26).

B. Use of Nonionic Detergents to Study Serum-Lipoprotein Metabolism

In 1951 Kellner, Correll, and Ladd (257) reported that intravenous injection of certain surface-active agents produced a striking, sustained hyperlipemia in rabbits. Subsequently, the hyperlipemic effect of the nonionic detergent Triton was observed in mice (258), rats (259), and dogs (260). Intravenous administration of Triton to dogs resulted in sustained hyperlipemia with marked elevations of serum free fatty acids, VLDL, and LDL, but a reduction in HDL (260). Triton infusion into rats produced a thirtyfold increase in their serum levels of neutral fat during the first 24 hr, but Friedman and Byers (259) did not find any histopathological changes on postmortem examination. These workers suggested that the hyperlipemia was produced by a change in the properties of the serum lipoproteins. Similar conclusions were drawn by other workers (261, 262), who proposed that physical alterations of the serum lipoproteins produced resistance to the action of lipoprotein lipase. Moreover, treatment of canine-serum HDL, LDL, and chylomicrons with Triton *in vitro* caused changes in electrophoretic, ultracentrifugal, and other properties, preventing their utilization as substrates by lipoprotein lipase (263). A combination of hepatectomy and Triton administration, to retard the removal of triglycerides from the plasma, indicated that the liver was the major source of triglycerides in post-Triton hyperlipemia (264).

Triton's inhibitory effect on triglyceride removal from serum has been frequently employed to gain further understanding of triglyceride metabolism. If it is assumed that Triton inhibits triglyceride removal but has no effect on their secretion by the liver, its administration permits a distinction between hyperlipemias caused by hepatic overproduction of VLDL and those due to delayed removal from peripheral tissues. Thus Triton should enhance triglyceride accumulation resulting from VLDL overproduction, but it should have little or no effect on hyperlipemia caused by defective clearing of lipoproteins. Furthermore, Triton administration can be used to calculate the rate of hepatic triglyceride secretion, as described by Recknagel (92).

Such studies must be appraised with caution, however, because Triton also accelerates free-fatty-acid mobilization (265), stimulates hepatic cholesterol synthesis (266), has a detergent action on the membranes of the liver (267) and erythrocytes (263), and may have other, as yet undetermined, metabolic effects. Scanu and Page (265) postulated that the complexes that form *in vivo* between Triton and serum lipoproteins are preferentially removed by reticuloendothelial cells instead of by hepatic parenchymal cells; such an alteration of lipoprotein catabolism may affect the regulation of lipid production by the liver. Moreover, the results of Triton use vary with the dose and duration of administration (260) and perhaps with the species of animal. The various effects of Triton and its use as an experimental tool have been reviewed by Scanu (268).

C. Control of Lipoprotein Metabolism: Carbohydrates and Insulin

Since the recognition of carbohydrate-induced hypertriglyceridemia in man (269), increased attention has been focused on the effects of carbohydrate intake and serum insulin levels on the metabolism of lipids and lipoproteins. Comprehensive coverage of this topic is beyond the scope of this chapter, but further information is available in several reviews (31, 270–272).

There is general agreement that the concentration of serum triglycerides is readily increased in man by a carbohydrate-rich diet. The magnitude and duration of the increase are related to the quantity and type of carbohydrate (270, 273), age (274), sex (275), presence of obesity (276), and genetic factors (36, 272).

The type of dietary carbohydrate has been variously correlated with the triglyceride response. In most investigations (31, 273, 277) the effect of sucrose was greater than that of starch, though this observation was not universal (278, 279). Rats fed fructose had a greater rise in plasma-triglyceride levels than those given glucose (280), whereas the rate of L-α-glycerophosphate incorporation into hepatic triglycerides was similar with ingestion of either sugar (281). Nikkilä and Pelkonen (282) found enhanced endogenous hyperglyceridemia in man with fructose feeding, but Nestel, Carroll, and Havenstein (283) detected no clear-cut difference between fructose and glucose on the incorporation of labeled palmitate into serum triglycerides. Although the hyperglyceridemic response to sucrose has been attributed to its fructose moiety, striking stimulation of triglyceride turnover has been reported with diets in which glucose was the only sugar formed on complete hydrolysis (284). In addition, insulin responds to oral fructose at a much lower level than it does to an equal quantity of glucose (285). Regardless of the type of dietary carbohydrate, the incorporation of fatty acids into triglycerides first exhibited a rise and then a fall during carbohydrate induction of hypertriglyceridemia (283).

Although individual responses were quite variable, young women were far more resistant to high-carbohydrate diets than were men or postmenopausal women (275). Healthy young subjects did not readily develop hyperglyceridemia (286). The magnitude of serum insulin and triglyceride responses during ingestion of carbohydrate-rich diets has been significantly correlated with body weight (283), though one group (287) concluded that obesity was unimportant despite a positive relationship between insulin response and the degree of hypertriglyceridemia. In obese patients with carbohydrate-induced glyceridemia reduction to ideal body weight is often associated with a fall in serum-triglyceride levels (36), and the degree of carbohydrate-induced glyceridemia may be less marked (272).

Genetic factors have a major influence on the ease of carbohydrate induction. Patients with type III, IV, and V hyperlipoproteinemia exhibit an exaggerated response of serum triglycerides to dietary carbohydrate (36, 272). When compared with normal controls, 16 patients with type III or IV hyperlipoproteinemia, whose hyperglyceridemia was stabilized on a diet containing 60% carbohydrate, had a marked rise in serum insulin, without definite hyperglycemia, in response to oral sucrose and starch test meals (288). These findings suggest that insulin had a direct role in the production of hypertriglyceridemia in these patients, though it may simply indicate insulin resistance secondary to hyperlipemia.

In the postabsorptive state the level of serum triglycerides is the result of the influx of VLDL from the liver and the efflux of triglycerides from the serum. Dietary carbohydrates may produce hypertriglyceridemia by an effect on either or both of these processes; insulin undoubtedly plays a part in this response of serum lipids to carbohydrate intake. Several studies suggest that carbohydrates stimulate triglyceride release. In rats fed glucose for 48 hr the incorporation of ^{14}C-leucine into VLDL and LDL by liver slices was doubled and the serum concentrations of VLDL and LDL were elevated (289). After 4 wk of glucose supplementation, serum levels of VLDL were increased fourfold over those of control rats. These results suggest that diets rich in carbohydrates cause a synchronous stimulation of triglyceride and β-lipoprotein-peptide synthesis. Reaven et al. (284) also proposed that an increase in triglyceride production, as measured by the influx of ^{3}H-glycerol-labeled triglycerides into the plasma, is the primary factor in the development of endogenous hyperglyceridemia. Other investigators (240, 242, 290), however, were unable to demonstrate increased triglyceride secretion and maintain the view that reduced efflux of triglycerides from plasma is the basis of carbohydrate-induced hyperlipemia. In addition, Nestel et al. (283) suggested impaired triglyceride removal as a possible cause for the greater effectiveness of fructose in the production of glyceridemia.

The role of insulin in carbohydrate-induced hyperlipemia is obscure. In fact, peripheral resistance to insulin action, insulin deficiency, and insulin hypersecretion have each been postulated as the cause of carbohydrate-induced hyperlipemia. Peripheral resistance to insulin was proposed by several groups, who noted a diminished decline in blood glucose levels after intravenous administration of tolbutamide or insulin in such subjects (291–293). A causal role for impaired insulin secretion is suggested by the high frequency of abnormal glucose-tolerance curves and frank diabetes in patients with carbohydrate-induced hyperlipemia (36). Hyperinsulinism was proposed as a cause of hyperlipemia because some of these patients had a positive correlation between serum insulin levels and the rise in serum triglycerides in response to carbohydrate-rich diets (276, 283). In another study (272, 294), however, there was no consistent abnormality in insulin response during a glucose-tolerance test in subjects with any of the types of hyperlipemia. Although the insulin response was often low in patients with type IV hyperlipoproteinemia, many patients had normal insulin levels after oral administration of glucose. Hyperinsulinism was not a characteristic finding in any of the types of hyperlipoproteinemia and was not correlated with the extent of carbohydrate induction. Thus, although hyperinsulinism is common in obesity (295), and both obesity and glucose intolerance are frequently associated with hypertriglyceridemia, the enhanced response of serum triglycerides to carbohydrate intake may occur with elevated, normal, or diminished insulin levels.

Although its involvement in carbohydrate induction is uncertain, insulin can affect both the synthesis and removal of serum lipoproteins. No specific stimulatory effect of insulin has been demonstrated on lipoprotein-peptide formation, but hepatic triglyceride secretion is enhanced in man (296) and the rat (289) by glucose loading. In addition, VLDL-peptide formation is severely impaired in rats with alloxan-induced diabetes (119). It is not clear whether this reflects a general dependence of hepatic protein synthesis on insulin or a more specific action of this hormone on lipoprotein synthesis. Insulin may also increase triglyceride production because of its stimulatory effect on hepatic fatty acid synthesis. This action of insulin (31, 297–300) may be acute, through alteration of the concentration of metabolic intermediates in the liver, or chronic, by induction of the synthesis of acetyl-coenzyme A carboxylase and other enzymes. The esterification of palmitate in rat-liver slices was not changed by insulin (301).

Extrahepatic actions of insulin can affect serum-lipoprotein metabolism. The potent antilipolytic action of insulin on adipose tissue lowers serum free-fatty-acid levels (302). The resulting reduction in free-fatty-acid transport to the liver may diminish hepatic triglyceride synthesis and thus explain the fall in plasma-triglyceride levels during prolonged infusion of insulin in man (303). Insulin also enhances the removal of chylomicron and VLDL triglycerides since this hormone is required to maintain normal synthesis of lipoprotein lipase in adipose tissue (304, 305).

In brief, the level of circulating triglycerides and probably the rate of VLDL synthesis and disposal are modulated by carbohydrate intake and perhaps by insulin. Moreover, insulin may influence lipoprotein metabolism in a number of ways, but the relationship between insulin secretion or action and hyperglyceridemia remains unresolved.

D. Control of Lipoprotein Metabolism: Other Hormones

The fact that certain hormones have major effects on the metabolism of serum lipoproteins is evident from the many examples of hormonally induced alterations of serum lipid and lipoprotein levels in man and in experimental animals. Thus β-lipoproteins are often elevated in hypothyroidism (306–308); VLDL or chylomicron levels may be raised in patients with uncontrolled diabetes (36, 305). Increased estrogen levels, in pregnancy or during the use of oral contraceptives, may increase VLDL levels and thus produce hypertriglyceridemia (309–313), whereas treatment with progestational agents will return the serum-lipid pattern to normal in some patients with type V hyperlipoproteinemia (314). The level of LDL may be lowered by estrogens and raised by androgens; these sex hormones have the opposite effect on HDL concentrations, which are increased by estrogens and decreased by androgens (315). Reduction of serum LDL concentration is common in hyperthyroidism or during the treatment of hypothyroid patients with thyroid hormone (36). Several comprehensive reviews of this subject are available (268, 315, 316).

From presently available data it is difficult to decide whether these hormones regulate the provision of the lipid load or the apopeptide carrier, both required for lipoprotein synthesis, or the rate of lipid removal from the serum, or perhaps a combination of both. Some of these problems are illustrated by work on the incorporation of ^{35}S-methionine into the plasma β-lipoproteins of roosters (317). When injected prior to sacrifice, estrogen, epinephrine, cortisone, and thyroid hormones elevated the amount of radioactivity in isolated β-lipoproteins. Obviously such data do not de steps in lipoprotein metabolism that are affected by these hormon over, the observed effect of thyroid hormones on β-lipoprotein rad in the rooster is difficult to reconcile with its tendency to lower L cholesterol levels in man and other animals. Such difficulties in interpretation typify many of the experiments so far reported on hormonal modulation of lipoprotein synthesis and metabolism. Tissue preparations that are responsive to hormones *in vitro* would probably help to clarify these issues.

1. Catecholamines. In many species, including the dog, rat, and man, catecholamines activate adipose-tissue lipases and promote the release of free fatty acids both *in vivo* and *in vitro* (318). The large increase in serum-free-fatty-acid levels that follow epinephrine administration produces little or no change in serum-triglyceride levels in the rat (319) or dog (320, 321). However, catecholamine treatment in dogs did evoke a delayed increase in plasma levels of cholesterol, phospholipids, and lipoproteins with *d* 1.019 to 1.21 g/ml (165, 320). The response to catecholamines required normal function of the adrenal cortex (322).

One might conclude that the increase in serum lipid and lipoprotein levels is secondary to the stimulation of free-fatty-acid release by catecholamines, but the results of several studies cast doubt on this simple explanation. Concurrent administration of glucose or insulin prevented the release of free fatty acids, but not the delayed increase in serum cholesterol and phospholipids. Moreover, in rabbits a similar delayed increase in serum lipids, including triglycerides and lipoproteins, followed a single injection of epinephrine in oil (323), although catecholamines do not cause free-fatty-acid release in rabbits (324).

These studies suggest that the elevation of serum-lipoprotein levels was at least partially independent of free-fatty-acid mobilization. It is possible that some direct hepatic action of catecholamines stimulates lipoprotein synthesis or release. Thus it is not clear that the potent effect of catecholamines on adipose tissue is related to the increases in serum lipoproteins that follow the administration of these hormones.

2. Gonadal Hormones. Numerous investigations have demonstrated that gonadal steroids alter both the concentration and the composition of circulating lipoproteins. These effects vary with species, sex, age, and mode of administration.

In the frog (325) estrogen specifically induces hepatic synthesis of a serum lipophosphoprotein that is transported to the ovary for incorporation into yolk platelets. In lizards (326) the induction of plasma vitellin formation by estradiol is associated with increased free-fatty-acid release from the fat-bodies. Estrogen administration to fowl (327) causes hepatic production of plasma phosvitin and lipovitellin, proteins that are not ordinarily present in the circulation, and greatly increases the concentration of normally occurring low density lipoproteins. These effects in birds and lower vertebrates are associated with, and probably mediated by, the initial synthesis of a new RNA species (328) that is essential for the hepatic synthesis of yolk lipoprotein. These regulatory actions of estrogen on the hepatic biosynthesis of lipoproteins involved in vitellinogenesis may provide a useful experimental model for elucidation of the mechanism of hormonal control of serum-lipoprotein synthesis in mammals.

Present knowledge of the regulatory effects of gonadal hormones on serum-lipoprotein production in mammals is fragmentary. In rats estradiol elevates plasma-cholesterol and plasma-phospholipid concentrations, which gradually subside after several weeks (329). Androgen administration to rats lowers serum-cholesterol levels (330). In dogs, where HDL is the major circulating lipoprotein, androgens cause a decline in this fraction (331).

Considerable interest surrounds the effects of estrogens and androgens on serum-lipoprotein levels in man because of the widespread impression that estrogens protect against atherosclerosis by lowering serum-cholesterol levels. Scanu (268) and Furman et al. (315) have reviewed earlier studies indicating that women have higher concentrations of HDL, lower concentrations of LDL, and a lower ratio of cholesterol to phospholipids than do men of the same age.

In normolipemic subjects estrogens elevated the cholesterol and phospholipid content of the $d > 1.063$ g/ml lipoprotein fraction, but lowered the cholesterol-to-phospholipid and cholesterol-to-protein ratios (315). Thus estrogen administration increased the number of HDL molecules, each of which contained less cholesterol than was present in HDL prior to estrogen administration. Estrogen also caused a significant diminution in the cholesterol content of LDL and increases in the levels of serum triglycerides and VLDL.

During pregnancy or the administration of combination (estrogen and progesterone) oral contraceptives to premenopausal women, increases were found in serum triglycerides and VLDL (309–313). This response has been attributed to the estrogen component, which diminishes lipoprotein-lipase activity (312). In hyperlipemic individuals estrogens may diminish serum-cholesterol levels, mainly by a reduction in the cholesterol content of VLDL, with little change in serum-triglyceride levels (315).

The effects of androgen on VLDL and HDL were opposite to those of estrogen. Androgen administration to normal subjects reduced the lipid content of VLDL and HDL with consequent decreases in serum phospholipids and triglycerides, but this hormone had a variable effect on the cholesterol and phospholipids present in LDL (315). In some hyperlipemic subjects the effect of androgen on VLDL caused a profound reduction in serum triglycerides.

Although these hormones alter the cholesterol-to-protein and cholesterol-to-phospholipid ratios in α- and β-lipoproteins, the phospholipid-to-protein ratio remains constant. This finding is consistent with the concept of a basic, phospholipid-protein carrier unit for triglyceride transport.

In contrast to these easily demonstrable effects of estrogens and androgens, several studies indicated that progestational agents had little effect on the levels of serum cholesterol and triglycerides in either normal subjects or in those with moderately elevated concentrations of serum cholesterol (332–334). It was recently reported that progestational agents increase post-heparin lipoprotein-lipase activity and lower serum-triglyceride levels in some patients with type V hyperlipoproteinemia (314).

The response to estrogen and androgen may be due to modification of the synthesis or availability of hepatic messenger RNA, or to effects on hepatic lipid synthesis, lipoprotein catabolism, or free-fatty-acid mobilization. Elucidation of the mechanism of action of these hormones in lipoprotein metabolism may have far-reaching implications both for the therapy of hyperlipemia and for a better understanding of the influence of sex hormones on nonreproductive tissues.

3. Thyroid Hormone. Evidence from patients with thyroid deficiency or excess emphasizes the inverse relationship between the activity of the thyroid gland and circulating levels of LDL. Thus serum levels of LDL are consistently elevated in hypothyroid subjects (306–308), and VLDL concentrations may also increase when thyroid deficiency is prolonged; HDL levels are unchanged in such patients. Treatment with thyroid hormone usually restores the serum-lipoprotein pattern to normal (307). The levels of LDL and cholesterol are frequently low in hyperthyroidism (36). As already mentioned, LDL turnover is increased in hyperthyroidism and decreased in hypothyroidism (183).

Thyroid hormones exert a number of effects on lipid metabolism, but the mechanism of their action on lipoprotein metabolism is not established. Thyroxine influences cholesterol metabolism in rats in at least two different ways (335). It stimulates hepatic cholesterogenesis and the rate of cholesterol removal from plasma. Much evidence from *in vivo* experiments attests to a stimulation of cholesterol oxidation to bile acids by thyroxine. The effect on removal appears to be greater in most species, including man, since the net result of administration of this hormone is a reduction in serum-cholesterol levels.

Because of its cholesterol-decreasing action, D-thyroxine has been used in the therapy of type II hyperlipoproteinemia (336–338). Thyroid hormone also stimulates the release of free fatty acids from adipose tissue since the mean fasting free-fatty-acid level is elevated in hyperthyroid subjects and depressed in hypothyroid patients (339). No direct lipolytic effect has been demonstrated by adding thyroid hormone *in vitro*; however, it appears to potentiate the action of epinephrine or the sympathetic nervous system on adipose tissue (340). Finally postheparin lipolytic activity may be reduced in patients with hypothyroidism, who consequently have elevated levels of serum triglycerides (341).

4. Glucagon. The administration of glucagon to humans or laboratory animals lowers the concentrations of serum cholesterol and triglycerides (342–346). Conversely destruction or excision of the pancreatic α-cells, which produce this hormone, leads to hyperlipemia in experimental animals (347, 348).

Intravenous injection of glucagon 2.5 hr after the ingestion of a fatty meal produced a decline in serum-triglyceride levels within 30 min (342). Glucagon administration reduced serum cholesterol, phospholipids, and triglycerides in three patients with hypertriglyceridemia and lowered serum-cholesterol levels in three of five subjects with hypercholesteremia (344). Injections of glucagon also lowered serum-cholesterol levels in dogs (345) and both cholesterol and triglyceride concentrations in the rat (343, 346).

In rabbits (347), 24 hr after the destruction of the α-cells of the pancreatic islets by the intravenous administration of cobaltic chloride, a large elevation of plasma cholesterol occurred. Surgical removal of the portion of the dog pancreas that contains α-cells led to prominent hyperlipemia, which was abolished by intramuscular injections of glucagon (348). These experiments provide further evidence for the lipid-decreasing action of glucagon in mammals.

The mechanisms for the reduction of serum lipids by glucagon are unknown. Although glucagon stimulates the release of free fatty acids from adipose tissue in a number of species *in vitro* (349–353), glucagon administration *in vivo* may either increase (339, 344, 354) or decrease (339, 342, 346, 355) serum free fatty acids. The reduction in free-fatty-acid levels, which in turn may decrease hepatic production of serum lipoproteins, has been attributed to the hyperglycemic response (356), stimulation of the release of insulin (357), or increased free-fatty-acid oxidation by the liver (346).

Glucagon caused a decline in the release of cholesterol from the perfused rat liver (346). Moreover, it produced no alterations in the serum levels of cholesterol or triglycerides when injected into eviscerated, functionally hepatectomized rats. Accordingly, Gorman, Salter, and Penhos (346) suggested that this hormone directly altered lipid metabolism in the liver. This conclusion is supported by studies showing that glucagon inhibits fatty acid and cholesterol synthesis in rat and rabbit livers (358–360).

IV. SUMMARY

The synthesis and metabolism of plasma lipoproteins can best be summarized by an examination of the triglyceride transport of VLDL. Although the general picture outlined below is surely correct, it is clear that many details are unknown, and others are only hypotheses based on rather meager data. Furthermore, many conclusions are derived from experiments with rats and remain to be tested in man.

After their synthesis on hepatic polyribosomes, VLDL apopeptides enter the lumen of the endoplasmic reticulum. Carbohydrate and lipid moieties are added either as the polypeptide traverses the smooth endoplasmic reticulum or in the Golgi complex. From the Golgi complex, and possibly from the smooth endoplasmic reticulum as well, the completed VLDL are carried within secretory vesicles that move to, and fuse with, the cell membrane. The VLDL molecules are then extruded from the secretory vesicles into the space of Disse and enter the bloodstream.

The rate of VLDL production may be regulated by the rate of apopeptide synthesis or by the availability of cargo or structural lipids. The availability of these lipids depends on the relative rates of their synthesis and degradation in the liver, as well as the quantity of free fatty acids mobilized to the liver from adipose tissue. Each of these processes is modulated by hormonal influences. Thus, for example, thyroxine stimulates cholesterol catabolism, insulin enhances hepatic fatty acid synthesis, and many hormones affect the release of free fatty acids from adipose-tissue stores. Carbohydrate and fat ingestion also influence hepatic lipids, both directly and indirectly. Dietary glycerides directly increase the amount of triglyceride transported to the liver; dietary cholestrol inhibits hepatic cholesterol synthesis. Ingested carbohydrate is rapidly converted to lipid in the livers of certain patients (type III, IV, and V hyperlipoproteinemia) with consequent hypertriglyceridemia.

Little is known about the factors that direct the rate of apopeptide synthesis, although their production is probably stimulated by the presence of excessive lipid in the liver. The capacity of the hepatic cell for the synthesis of lipoprotein peptide may determine whether newly made triglycerides are incorporated into a cellular lipid droplet or exported into the plasma on

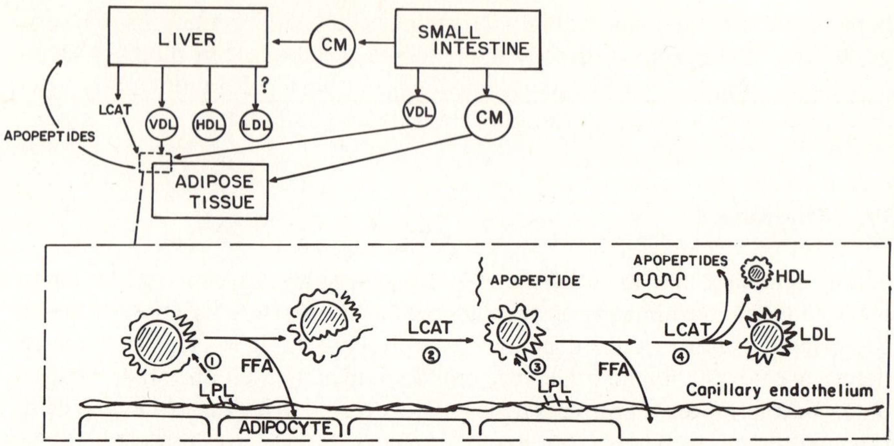

Fig. 2 Schematic diagram of lipoprotein metabolism. The VLDL are synthesized in the hepatocytes or cells of the intestinal mucosa. The triglycerides of VLDL are hydrolyzed to form free fatty acids (FFA) and glycerol by the action of lipoprotein lipase (LPL), which is bound to the inner surface of the capillary endothelium (step 1). Free fatty acids are taken up by the adipose-tissue cells. Triglyceride hydrolysis produces a perturbation of VLDL, which is attacked (step 2) by LCAT, synthetized in the liver, to release phospholipids and apopeptides and form cholesteryl esters. The triglycerides of the smaller VLDL are again split by LPL (step 3) and by LCAT (step 4), either sequentially or in concert. This causes further release of apopeptides and possibly lipid–apopeptide complexes of higher density. The LDL are the end products of VLDL metabolism. Apopeptides released from VLDL may return to the liver to be reutilized in the transport of an additional load of triglycerides. A similar scheme is postulated for the catabolism of chylomicrons.

VLDL. When production of lipoprotein carrier fails to keep pace with triglyceride formation, the resultant imbalance leads to the intracellular accumulation and coalescence of triglycerides. The end result is fatty liver.

A scheme for lipoprotein metabolism is shown in Fig. 2. The metabolism of plasma VLDL requires the action of two enzymes, lipoprotein lipase and LCAT. The former is probably bound to the capillary endothelium, where it splits VLDL triglycerides to free fatty acids and glycerol. The free fatty acids are stored in adipose tissue or used as an energy source in other tissues, such as skeletal muscle. Synthesized in the liver, LCAT promotes the removal of phospholipids and cholesterol, which have accumulated in excess on the surface of VLDL molecules during lipoprotein-lipase action. By repeated consecutive action or by a concerted attack of these two enzymes, the lipid moiety of VLDL is reduced in amount and altered in composition. Apopeptides, and perhaps polypeptide–lipid complexes, are also released from VLDL. As a result of these sequential modifications, VLDL are converted to LDL. The fate of the released apopeptides remains controversial. It has been suggested that these apoproteins may return to the liver to transport an additional load of lipids from that organ.

Various mechanisms have been proposed to account for abnormal accumulations of lipoproteins in plasma. These include an accelerated synthesis or diminished removal of the lipid or peptide portions of these molecules. Available data suggest that alcoholic hyperlipemia may be partly due to an increase in VLDL production. Much more commonly, however, the recognized defects result from reduced rates of lipoprotein-triglyceride lipolysis. Best understood are inherited deficiencies of lipoprotein lipase (type I hyperlipoproteinemia), which produce prolonged chylomicronemia whenever significant amounts of fat are ingested.

Lipoprotein-lipase activity is also under hormonal control. Insulin deficiency and estrogen administration diminish postheparin lipolytic activity; progestational agents, in contrast, increase the activity of this enzyme. Clearance of VLDL triglycerides is also slowed in patients with an inherited deficiency of LCAT (361, 362). Relatively less is known about the development of hyperlipoproteinemia as a consequence of abnormal degradation of the peptide portion of the lipoproteins. Recent studies, however, suggest that type II hyperlipoproteinemia results from a diminished rate of LDL peptide degradation. It seems likely that future research will uncover other hyperlipemic states that result from overproduction of serum lipoproteins or from a decreased capacity to catabolize the peptide portions of these molecules.

REFERENCES

1. Duff, G. L., *Arch. Pathol.* **20**, 81–123 (1935).
2. Steiner, A., and F. E. Kendall, *Arch. Pathol.* **42**, 433–444 (1946).
3. Reiser, R., M. F. Sorrels, and M. C. Williams, *Circulation Res.* **7**, 833–846 (1959).
4. Kannel, W. B., T. R. Dawber, G. T. Friedman, W. E. Glennon, and P. M. McNamara, *Ann. Intern. Med.* **61**, 888–899 (1964).
5. Albrink, M. J., *Arch. Intern. Med.* **109**, 345–359 (1952).
6. Stamler, J., D. M. Berkson, H. A. Lindberg, Y. Hall, W. Miller, L. Mojonnier, M. Levinson, D. B. Cohen, and Q. D. Young, *Med. Clin. N. Amer.* **50**, 229–254 (1966).
7. Heinle, R. A., R. I. Levy, D. S. Fredrickson, and R. Gorlin, *Amer. J. Cardiol.* **24**, 178–186 (1969).
8. Havel, R. J., *Metabolism* (*Clin. Exp.*) **10**, 1031–1034 (1961).
9. Markscheid, L., and E. Shafrir, *J. Lipid Res.* **6**, 247–257 (1965).
10. Moskowitz, M. S., and A. A. Moskowitz, *Science* **149**, 72–73 (1965).
11. Olivecrona, T., and P. Belfrage, *Biochim. Biophys. Acta* **98**, 81–93 (1965).

12. Delcher, H. K., M. Fried, and J. C. Shipp, *Biochim. Biophys. Acta* **106**, 10–18 (1965).
13. Crass, M. F., III, and H. C. Meng, *Biochim. Biophys. Acta* **125**, 106–117 (1966).
14. Scheuer, J., and R. E. Olson, *Amer. J. Physiol.* **212**, 301–307 (1967).
15. Enser, M. B., F. Kunz, J. Borensztajn, L. H. Opie, and D. S. Robinson, *Biochem. J.* **104**, 306–317 (1967).
16. Opie, L. H., *Amer. Heart J.* **77**, 100–122 (1969).
17. Schumaker, V. N., and G. H. Adams, *Annu. Rev. Biochem.* **38**, 113–136 (1969).
18. Schumaker, V. N., and G. H. Adams, *J. Theor. Biol.* **26**, 89–91 (1970).
19. Levy, R. I., R. S. Lees, and D. S. Fredrickson, *J. Clin. Invest.* **45**, 63–77 (1966).
20. Furman, R. H., S. S. Sanbar, P. Alaupovic, R. H. Bradford, and R. P. Howard, *J. Lab. Clin. Med.* **63**, 193–204 (1964).
21. Korn, E. D., *J. Biol. Chem.* **215**, 15–26 (1955).
22. Scanu, A., *J. Biol. Chem.* **242**, 711–719 (1967).
23. Fielding, C. J., *Biochim. Biophys. Acta* **206**, 109–117 (1970).
24. LaRosa, J. C., R. I. Levy, P. Herbert, S. E. Lux, and D. S. Fredrickson, *Circulation* **42**, III-6 (1970); Havel, R., V. Shore, B. Shore, and D. Bier, *Circulation* **42**, III-6 (1970).
25. Glomset, J. A., *J. Lipid Res.* **9**, 155–167 (1968).
26. Adams, G. H., and V. N. Schumaker, *Ann. N.Y. Acad. Sci.* **164**, 130–146 (1969).
27. Fredrickson, D. S., in *The Metabolic Basis of Inherited Disease*, 2nd ed., J. B. Stanbury, J. B. Wyngaarden, and D. S. Fredrickson, Eds., McGraw-Hill, New York, 1966, pp. 486–508.
28. Margolis, S., in *Structural and Functional Aspects of Lipoproteins in Living Systems,* E. Tria and A. M. Scanu, Eds., Academic Press, New York, 1969, pp. 369–424.
29. Marsh, J. B., in *Structural and Functional Aspects of Lipoproteins in Living Systems,* E. Tria and A. M. Scanu, Eds., Academic Press, New York, 1969, pp. 447–464.
30. Nestel, P. J., in *Newer Methods of Nutritional Biochemistry*, Vol. 3, A. A. Albanese, Ed., Academic Press, New York, 1967, pp. 243–302.
31. Nikkilä, E. A., *Adv. Lipid Res.* **7**, 63–134 (1969).
32. Robinson, D. S., in *Comprehensive Biochemistry*, Vol. 18, M. Florkin and E. H. Stotz, Eds., Elsevier, New York, 1970, pp. 51–116.
33. Nestel, P. J., *Adv. Lipid Res.* **8**, 1–39 (1970).
34. Dietschy, J. M., and J. D. Wilson, *New Engl. J. Med.* **282**, 1128–1138, 1179–1183, 1241–1249 (1970).
35. Farquhar, J. W., and P. Ways, in *The Metabolic Basis of Inherited Disease*, 2nd ed., J. B. Stanbury, J. B. Wyngaarden, and D. S. Fredrickson, Eds., McGraw-Hill, New York, 1966, pp. 509–522.
36. Fredrickson, D. S., R. I. Levy, and R. S. Lees, *New Engl. J. Med.* **276**, 34–42, 94–103, 148–156, 215–225, 273–281 (1967).
37. Havel, R. J., *Adv. Intern. Med.* **15**, 117–154 (1969).
38. Margolis, S., and R. G. Langdon, *J. Biol. Chem.* **241**, 469–476 (1966); Marsh, J. B., *Proc. Soc. Exp. Biol. Med.* **133**, 9–10 (1970).

39. Eylar, E. H., *J. Theor. Biol.* **10**, 89–113 (1966).
40. Robinson, D. S., and P. M. Harris, *Biochem. J.* **80**, 361–369 (1961).
41. Seakins, A., and D. S. Robinson, *Biochem. J.* **92**, 308–312 (1964).
42. Robinson, D. S., and A. Seakins, *Biochim. Biophys. Acta* **62**, 163–165 (1962).
43. Seakins, A., and D. S. Robinson, *Biochem. J.* **86**, 401–407 (1963).
44. Rees, K. R., and V. L. Shotlander, *Ann. N.Y. Acad. Sci.* **104**, 905–915 (1963).
45. Heimberg, M., I. Weinstein, and M. Kohout, *J. Biol. Chem.* **244**, 5131–5139 (1969); Van Harken, D. R., C. W. Dixon, and M. Heimberg, *J. Biol. Chem.* **244**, 2278–2285 (1969).
46. Sabesin, S. M., and K. J. Isselbacher, *Science* **147**, 1149–1151 (1965).
47. Isselbacher, K. J., R. Scheig, G. R. Plotkin, and J. B. Caulfield, *Medicine* **43**, 347–361 (1964).
48. Roheim, P. S., L. I. Gidez, and H. A. Eder, *J. Clin. Invest.* **45**, 297–300 (1966).
49. Faloona, G. R., B. N. Stewart, and M. Fried, *Arch. Biochem. Biophys.* **130**, 680–683 (1969).
50. Marsh, J. B., and A. F. Whereat, *J. Biol. Chem.* **234**, 3196–3200 (1959).
51. Radding, C. M., J. H. Bragdon, and D. Steinberg, *Biochim. Biophys. Acta* **30**, 443–444 (1958).
52. Capuzzi, D. M., Ph.D. thesis, Johns Hopkins University, Baltimore, 1969.
53. Capuzzi, D. M., and S. Margolis, *Clin. Res.* **17**, 42 (1969).
54. Daikuhara, Y., A. Ichihara, H. Tanioka, and Y. Takeda, *J. Biochem. (Tokyo)* **60**, 322–328 (1966).
55. Marsh, J. B., *J. Biol. Chem.* **238**, 1752–1756 (1963).
56. Bungenberg de Jong, J. J., and J. B. Marsh, *J. Biol. Chem.* **243**, 192–199 (1968).
57. Ockner, R. K., and A. L. Jones, *J. Lipid Res.* **11**, 284–292 (1970).
58. Jones, A. L., and R. K. Ockner, *J. Cell. Biol.* **43**, 62a (1969).
59. Windmueller, H. G., and R. I. Levy, *J. Biol. Chem.* **243**, 4878–4884 (1968).
60. Windmueller, H. G., and R. I. Levy, *J. Biol. Chem.* **242**, 2246–2254 (1967).
61. Isselbacher, K. J., and D. M. Budz, *Nature* **200**, 364–365 (1963).
62. Hatch, F. T., Y. Aso, L. M. Hagopian, and J. J. Rubenstein, *J. Biol. Chem.* **241**, 1655–1665 (1966).
63. Windmueller, H. G., F. T. Lindgren, W. J. Lossow, and R. I. Levy, *Biochim. Biophys. Acta* **202**, 507–516 (1970).
64. Ockner, R. K., F. B. Hughes, and K. J. Isselbacher, *J. Clin. Invest.* **48**, 2079–2088 (1969).
65. Windmueller, H. G., and R. I. Levy, *J. Biol. Chem.* **243**, 4878–4884 (1968).
66. Lossow, W. J., F. T. Lindgren, and L. C. Jensen, *Biochim. Biophys. Acta* **144**, 670–677 (1967).
67. Cornwell, D. G., and F. A. Kruger, *J. Lipid Res.* **2**, 110–134 (1961).
68. Buckley, J. T., T. J. Delahunty, and D. Rubinstein, *Can. J. Biochem.* **46**, 341–349 (1968); Eaton, R. P., and D. M. Kipnis, *Amer. J. Physiol.* **217**, 1153–1159 (1969).
69. Florsheim, W. H., and C. Gonzales, *Proc. Soc. Exp. Biol. Med.* **104**, 618–620 (1960).
70. Jordan, W. J., Jr., A. G. Faulkner, and E. C. Knoblock, *Anal. Biochem.* **14**, 91–94 (1966).
71. Cogan, V., and T. Nishida, *Biochim. Biophys. Acta* **187**, 444–446 (1969).
72. Levy, R. I., and D. S. Fredrickson, *J. Clin. Invest.* **44**, 426–441 (1965).

73. Eaton, R. P., and D. M. Kipnis, *J. Clin. Invest.* **48**, 1387–1396 (1969).
74. Sargent, J. R., in *Techniques in Protein Biosynthesis,* Vol. 1, P. N. Campbell and J. R. Sargent, Eds., Academic Press, New York, 1967, pp. 167–176.
75. Trams, E. G., and E. A. Brown, *J. Theor. Biol.* **12**, 311–326 (1966).
76. Redgrave, T. G., *J. Clin. Invest.* **49**, 465–471 (1970).
77. Bortz, W., *Biochim. Biophys. Acta* **137**, 533–539 (1967).
78. Favarger, P., in *Handbook of Physiology, Section 5: Adipose Tissue,* A. E. Renold and G. F. Cahill, Jr., Eds., American Physiological Society, Washington, D.C., 1965, pp. 19–23.
79. Favarger, P., and J. Gerlach, *Helv. Physiol. Pharmacol. Acta* **16**, 188–200 (1958); Patkin, J. K., and E. J. Masoro, *Can. J. Physiol. Pharmacol.* **42**, 101–107 (1964).
80. Jansen, G. R., M. E. Zanetti, and C. F. Hutchison, *Biochem. J.* **102**, 864–869 (1967).
81. Hirsch, J., and R. B. Goldrick, in *Handbook of Physiology, Section 5: Adipose Tissue,* A. E. Renold and G. F. Cahill, Jr., Eds., American Physiological Society, Washington, D.C., 1965, pp. 455–470.
82. Goodridge, A. G., and E. G. Ball, *Amer. J. Physiol.* **211**, 803–808 (1966).
83. Jeanrenaud, B., *Ergbn. Physiol.* **60**, 57–140 (1968).
84. Radding, C. M., and D. Steinberg, *J. Clin. Invest.* **39**, 1560–1569 (1960).
85. Haft, D. E., P. S. Roheim, A. White, and H. A. Eder, *J. Clin. Invest.* **41**, 842–849 (1962).
86. Rajalakshmi, S., W. R. Adams, and R. E. Handschumacher, *J. Cell Biol.* **41**, 625–636 (1969).
87. Roheim, P. S., S. Switzer, A. Girard, and H. A. Eder, *Biochem. Biophys. Res. Commun.* **20**, 416–421 (1965).
88. Roheim, P. S., S. Switzer, A. Girard, and H. A. Eder, *Lab. Invest.* **15**, 21–26 (1966).
89. Jones, A. L., N. B. Ruderman, and M. G. Herrera, *J. Lipid Res.* **8**, 429–446 (1967).
90. Rambourg, A., W. Hernandez, and C. P. Leblond, *J. Cell. Biol.* **40**, 395–414 (1969).
91. Reynolds, E. S., *J. Cell. Biol.* **19**, 139–157 (1963).
92. Recknagel, R. O., *Pharmacol. Rev.* **19**, 145–208 (1967).
93. Caro, L. G., *J. Biophys. Biochem. Cytol.* **10**, 37–45 (1961).
94. Hamilton, R. L., D. M. Regen, M. E. Gray, and V. S. Le Quire, *Lab. Invest.* **16**, 305–319 (1967).
95. Mahley, R. W., M. E. Gray, R. L. Hamilton, and V. S. Le Quire, *Lab. Invest.* **19**, 358–369 (1968).
96. Hamilton, R. L., and V. S. Le Quire, *Fed. Proc.* **26**, 575 (1967).
97. Stein, O., and Y. Stein, *Israel J. Med. Sci.* **1**, 378–388 (1965).
98. Stein, O., and Y. Stein, *J. Cell. Biol.* **33**, 319–339 (1967).
99. Mahley, R. W., R. L. Hamilton, and V. S. Le Quire, *J. Lipid Res.* **10**, 433–439 (1969).
100. Mahley, R. W., T. P. Bersot, V. S. Le Quire, R. I. Levy, H. G. Windmueller, and W. V. Brown, *Science* **168**, 380–382 (1970).
101. Parks, H. F., *Amer. J. Anat.* **120**, 253–280 (1967).
102. Judah, J. D., and M. R. Nicholls, *Biochem. J.* **116**, 663–669 (1970).
103. Schlunk, F. F., and B. Lombardi, *Lab. Invest.* **17**, 30–38 (1967).

104. Roheim, P. S., L. Miller, and H. A. Eder, *J. Biol. Chem.* **240**, 2994–3001 (1965).
105. Eder, H. A., P. S. Roheim, and S. Switzer, *Trans. Assoc. Amer. Physicians (Philadelphia)* **77**, 259–267 (1964).
106. Roheim, P. S., and H. A. Eder, *Circulation* **24**, 1101 (1961).
107. Roheim, P. S., D. E. Haft, L. I. Gidez, A. White, and H. A. Eder, *J. Clin. Invest.* **42**, 1277–1285 (1963).
108. Windmueller, H. G., and A. E. Spaeth, *Arch. Biochem. Biophys.* **122**, 362–369 (1967).
109. Hamosh, M., and B. Shapiro, *Amer. J. Physiol.* **201**, 1030–1034 (1961).
110. Kook, A. I., and D. Rubinstein, *Can. J. Biochem.* **47**, 65–69 (1969).
111. Kook, A. I., and D. Rubinstein, *Biochim. Biophys. Acta* **202**, 396–398 (1970).
112. Buckley, J. T., T. J. Delahunty, and D. Rubinstein, *Can. J. Biochem.* **46**, 341–349 (1968).
113. Lees, R. S., *J. Lipid Res.* **8**, 396–405 (1967).
114. Gotto, A. M., R. I. Levy, M. E. Birnbaumer, and D. S. Fredrickson, *Clin. Res.* **17**, 383 (1968).
115. Marsh, J. B., and F. Sherry, *Proc. Soc. Exp. Biol. Med.* **109**, 14–15 (1962).
116. Gould, R. G., E. A. Swyryd, D. Avoy, and B. Coan, *Progr. Biochem. Pharmacol.* **2**, 345–357 (1967).
117. Heimberg, M., A. Dunkerley, and T. O. Brown, *Biochim. Biophys. Acta* **125**, 252–264 (1966).
118. Van Harken, D. R., T. O. Brown, and M. Heimberg, *Lipids* **2**, 231–238 (1967).
119. Wilcox, H. G., G. Dishmon, and M. Heimberg, *J. Biol. Chem.* **243**, 666–675 (1968).
120. Wilcox, H. G., M. Fried, and M. Heimberg, *Biochim. Biophys. Acta* **106**, 598–602 (1965).
121. Heimberg, M., I. Weinstein, G. Dishmon, and M. Fried, *Amer. J. Physiol.* **209**, 1053–1060 (1965).
122. Nestel, P. J., and D. Steinberg, *J. Lipid Res.* **4**, 461–469 (1963).
123. Trout, D. L., *J. Pharmacol. Exp. Ther.* **152**, 529–534 (1966).
124. Carlson, L. A., and E. R. Nye, *Acta Med. Scand.* **179**, 453–461 (1966).
125. Kay, R. E., and C. Entenman, *J. Biol. Chem.* **236**, 1006–1012 (1961).
126. Jones, A. L., N. B. Ruderman, and M. G. Herrera, *Proc. Soc. Exp. Biol. Med.* **123**, 4–9 (1966).
127. Ruderman, N. B., K. C. Richards, V. Valles de Bourges, and A. L. Jones, *J. Lipid Res.* **9**, 613–619 (1968).
128. Kohout, M., B. Kohoutova, and M. Heimberg, *Biochim. Biophys. Acta* **210**, 177–179 (1970).
129. Lombardi, B., *Lab. Invest.* **15**, 1–20 (1966).
130. Robinson, D. S., and A. Seakins, *Biochem. J.* **82**, 9P (1961).
131. Farber, E., K. H. Shull, S. Villa-Trevino, B. Lombardi, and M. Thomas, *Nature* **203**, 34–40 (1964).
132. Recknagel, R. O., and B. Lombardi, *J. Biol. Chem.* **236**, 564–569 (1961).
133. Rees, K. R., and V. L. Shotlander, *Proc. Roy. Soc. (London)* **B157**, 515–535 (1963).
134. Smuckler, E. A., and E. A. Barker, *Fed. Proc.* **23**, 335 (1964).
135. Hyams, D. E., E. B. Taft, G. D. Drummey, and K. J. Isselbacher, *Lab. Invest.* **16**, 604–615 (1967).

136. Rees, K. R., and V. L. Shotlander, *Brit. J. Exp. Pathol.* **45**, 364–374 (1964).
137. Kayden, H. J., and M. Medick, *Biochim. Biophys. Acta* **176**, 37–43 (1969).
138. Gitlin, D., D. G. Cornwell, D. Nakasato, J. L. Oncley, W. L. Hughes, Jr., and C. A. Janeway, *J. Clin. Invest.* **37**, 172–184 (1958).
139. Volwiler, W., P. D. Goldsworthy, M. P. MacMartin, P. A. Wood, I. R. MacKay, and K. Fremont-Smith, *J. Clin. Invest.* **34**, 1126–1140 (1955).
140. Smuckler, E. A., O. A. Iseri, and E. P. Benditt, *J. Exp. Med.* **116**, 55–72 (1962).
141. Meldolesi, J., L. Vicenzi, P. Bassan, and M. T. Morini, *Lab. Invest.* **19**, 315–323 (1968).
142. Faloona, G. R., B. N. Stewart, and M. Fried, *Biochemistry* **7**, 720–725 (1968).
143. McLean, A. E. M., E. McLean, and J. D. Judah, *Int. Rev. Exp. Pathol.* **4**, 127–157 (1965).
144. Deamer, D. W., F. A. Kruger, and D. G. Cornwell, *Biochim. Biophys. Acta* **97**, 147–149 (1965).
145. Sidransky, H., E. Verney, and B. Lombardi, *J. Nutr.* **81**, 348–356 (1963).
146. Novikoff, A. B., P. S. Roheim, and N. Quintana, *Fed. Proc.* **23**, 126 (1964).
147. Novikoff, A. B., P. S. Roheim, and N. Quintana, *Lab. Invest.* **15**, 27–49 (1966).
148. Ashworth, C. T., E. Sanders, and N. Arnold, *Arch. Pathol.* **72**, 625–636 (1961).
149. Standerfer, S. B., and P. Handler, *Proc. Soc. Exp. Biol. Med.* **90**, 270–271 (1955).
150. Windmueller, H. G., *J. Biol. Chem.* **239**, 530–537 (1964).
151. Marchetti, M., P. Puddu, and C. M. Caldarera, *Biochem. J.* **92**, 46–51 (1964).
152. Handschumacher, R. E., W. A. Creasey, J. J. Jaffe, C. A. Pasternak, and L. Hankin, *Proc. Natl. Acad. Sci. U.S.* **46**, 178–186 (1960).
153. Rubin, R. J., and R. G. Pendleton, *Fed. Proc.* **23**, 126 (1964).
154. Kayden, H. J., M. I. Glassman, and M. Medick, *Biochim. Biophys. Acta* **176**, 44–47 (1969).
155. Lombardi, B., G. Ugazio, and A. N. Raick, *Amer. J. Physiol.* **210**, 31–36 (1966).
156. Haines, D. S. M., and S. Mookerjea, *Can. J. Biochem.* **43**, 507–520 (1965).
157. Mookerjea, S., *Can. J. Biochem.* **43**, 1733–1744 (1965).
158. Lombardi, B., and M. C. Schotz, *Proc. Soc. Exp. Biol. Med.* **112**, 400–401 (1963).
159. Lombardi, B., P. Pani, and F. F. Schlunk, *J. Lipid Res.* **9**, 437–446 (1968).
160. Mookerjea, S., *Can. J. Biochem.* **44**, 1064–1067 (1966).
161. Mookerjea, S., D. Jeng, and J. Black, *Can. J. Biochem.* **45**, 825–838 (1967).
162. Mookerjea, S., *Can. J. Biochem.* **47**, 125–133 (1969).
163. Isselbacher, K. J., and N. J. Greenberger, *New Engl. J. Med.* **270**, 351–356 (1964).
164. DiLuzio, N. R., *Lab. Invest.* **15**, 50–63 (1966).
165. Feigelson, E. B., W. W. Pfaff, A. Karmen, and D. Steinberg, *J. Clin. Invest.* **40**, 2171–2176 (1961).
166. Moran, T. J., *Arch. Pathol.* **73**, 300–312 (1962).
167. Hill, R. B., Jr., and W. A. Droke, *Proc. Soc. Exp. Biol. Med.* **114**, 766–769 (1963).
168. Hoak, J. C., W. E. Connor, M. L. Armstrong, and E. D. Warner, *Lab. Invest.* **19**, 370–375 (1968).
169. Fex, G., and T. Olivecrona, *Biochim. Biophys. Acta* **164**, 424–426 (1968).
170. Baraona, E., and C. S. Lieber, *J. Clin. Invest.* **49**, 769–778 (1970).
171. Wilson, D. E., P. H. Schreibman, A. C. Brewster, and R. A. Arky, *J. Lab. Clin. Med.* **75**, 264–274 (1970).

172. Steinberg, D., *Pharmacol. Rev.* **18**, 217–235 (1966).
173. Stenger, R. J., and D. B. Confer, *Exp. Mol. Pathol.* **5**, 455–474 (1966).
174. Narayan, K. A., G. E. S. Mary, and F. A. Kummerow, *Proc. Soc. Exp. Biol. Med.* **129**, 6–12 (1968).
175. Narayan, K. A., *Lipids* **5**, 156–158 (1970).
176. Olivecrona, T., and G. Fex, *Biochim. Biophys. Acta* **202**, 259–268 (1970).
177. Marsh, J. B., and D. L. Drabkin, *Metabolism (Clin. Exp.)* **9**, 946–955 (1960).
178. Sodhi, H. S., and N. Kalant, *Metabolism (Clin. Exp.)* **12**, 420–427 (1963).
179. Schultze, H. E., and J. F. Heremans, *Molecular Biology of Human Proteins*, Vol. 1, Elsevier, Amsterdam, 1966, pp. 450–517.
180. McFarlane, A. S., *Biochem. J.* **62**, 135–143 (1956).
181. McFarlane, A. S., *Nature* **182**, 53 (1958).
182. Hunter, W. M., and F. C. Greenwood, *Nature* **194**, 495–496 (1962).
183. Walton, K. W., P. J. Scott, P. Dykes, and J. Davis, *Clin. Sci.* (*London*) **29**, 217–238 (1965).
184. McFarlane, A. S., *Biochem. J.* **89**, 277–290 (1963).
185. Freeman, T., and A. H. Gordon, *Biblio. Haematol.* **23**, 1108–1115 (1965).
186. McFarlane, A. S., D. Todd, and S. Cromwell, *Clin. Sci.* (*London*) **26**, 415–420 (1964).
187. Cromwell, S., in *Protides of the Biological Fluids*, H. Peeters, Ed., Elsevier, Amsterdam, 1964, pp. 484–486.
188. Freeman, T., in *Protides of the Biological Fluids*, H. Peeters, Ed., Elsevier, Amsterdam, 1965, pp. 344–352.
189. Bennhold, H., and E. Kallee, *J. Clin. Invest.* **38**, 863–872 (1959).
190. Cohen, S., and J. D. L. Hanson, *Clin. Sci.* (*London*) **23**, 351–359 (1962).
191. Olhagen, B., G. Birke, L.-O. Plantin, and S. Ahlinder in *Protides of the Biological Fluids*, H. Peeters, Ed., Elsevier, Amsterdam, 1964, pp. 487–490.
192. Hurley, P. J., Ph.D. thesis, University of Otago, Auckland, New Zealand, 1968.
193. DeDuve, C., and R. Wattiaux, *Annu. Rev. Physiol.* **28**, 435–492 (1966).
194. Langer, T., W. Strober, and R. I. Levy, *J. Clin. Invest.* **48**, 49a (1969).
195. Walton, K. W., P. J. Scott, J. Verrier Jones, R. F. Fletcher, and T. Whitehead, *J. Atheroscler. Res.* **3**, 396–414 (1963).
196. Scott, P. J., and P. J. Hurley, *J. Atheroscler. Res.* **9**, 25–34 (1969).
197. Scott, P. J., and P. J. Hurley, *Israel J. Med. Sci.* **5**, 631–634 (1969).
198. Duncan, L. E., Jr., K. Buck, and A. Lynch, *Science* **142**, 972–973 (1963).
199. Scott, P. J., and P. J. Hurley, *J. Pathol.* **97**, 603–609 (1969).
200. Scott, P. J., and C. C. Winterbourn, *J. Atheroscler. Res.* **7**, 207–223 (1967).
201. Walton, K. W., and N. Williamson, *J. Atheroscler. Res.* **8**, 599–624 (1968).
202. Virag, S., T. Pozsonyi, R. Denes, and S. Gero, *J. Atheroscler. Res.* **8**, 859–860 (1968).
203. Lees, R. S., and E. H. Ahrens, Jr., *New Engl. J. Med.* **280**, 1261–1266 (1969).
204. Langer, T., R. I. Levy, and D. S. Fredrickson, *Circulation* **40**, III-14 (1969).
205. Brady, R. O., *Adv. Clin. Chem.* **11**, 1–19 (1968).
206. Hazzard, W. R., F. T. Lindgren, and E. L. Bierman, *Biochim. Biophys. Acta* **202**, 517–525 (1970).
207. Hazzard, W. R., D. Porte, Jr., and E. L. Bierman, *J. Clin. Invest.* **49**, 1853–1858 (1970).
208. Seidel, D., R. Alaupovic, and R. H. Furman, *J. Clin. Invest.* **48**, 1211–1223 (1969).

209. Switzer, S., *J. Clin. Invest.* **46**, 1855–1866 (1967).
210. Scanu, A., and W. L. Hughes, *J. Clin. Invest.* **41**, 1681–1689 (1962).
211. Moser, H. W., and K. Emerson, Jr., *J. Clin. Invest.* **34**, 1286–1296 (1955).
212. Bergström, S., *Fed. Proc.* **21** (Suppl. 11), 28–32 (1962); Danielsson, H., *Adv. Lipid Res.* **1**, 335–385 (1963).
213. Kaplan, J. A., G. E. Cox, and C. B. Taylor, *Arch. Pathol.* **76**, 359–368 (1963); Wilson, J. D., and C. A. Lindsey, Jr., *J. Clin. Invest.* **44**, 1805–1814 (1965); Grundy, S. M., and E. H. Ahrens, Jr., *J. Clin. Invest.* **45**, 1503–1515 (1966).
214. Nestel, P. J., H. M. Whyte, and D. S. Goodman, *J. Clin. Invest.* **48**, 982–991 (1969).
215. Byers, S. O., and M. Friedman, *Amer. J. Physiol.* **179**, 79–84 (1954); Fredrickson, D. S., D. L. McCollester, R. J. Havel, and K. Ono, in *Chemistry of Lipids as Related to Atherosclerosis*, I. H. Page, Ed., Thomas, Springfield, Ill., 1958, pp. 205–218.
216. Vahouny, G. V., and C. R. Treadwell, *Amer. J. Physiol.* **191**, 179–184 (1957).
217. Goodman, D. S., *Physiol. Rev.* **45**, 747–839 (1965).
218. Stein, O., Y. Stein, D. S. Goodman, and N. H. Fidge, *J. Cell. Biol.* **43**, 410–431 (1969).
219. Dietschy, J. M., and J. D. Wilson, *J. Clin. Invest.* **47**, 166–174 (1968).
220. Dietschy, J. M., and M. D. Siperstein, *J. Lipid Res.* **8**, 97–104 (1967).
221. Werbin, H., and I. L. Chaikoff, *Arch. Biochem. Biophys.* **93**, 476–482 (1961).
222. Hellig, H., D. Gattereau, Y. Lefebvre, and E. Botté, *J. Clin. Endocrinol.* **30**, 624–631 (1970).
223. Eckles, N. E., C. B. Taylor, D. J. Campbell, and R. G. Gould, *J. Lab. Clin. Med.* **46**, 359–371 (1955).
224. Gould, R. G., G. V. LeRoy, G. T. Okita, J. J. Kabara, P. Keegan, and D. M. Bergenstal, *J. Lab. Clin. Med.* **46**, 372–384 (1955).
225. Goodman, D. S., *J. Clin. Invest.* **43**, 2026–2036 (1964).
226. Hellman, L., R. S. Rosenfeld, and T. F. Gallagher, *J. Clin. Invest.* **33**, 142–149 (1954).
227. Field, H., Jr., L. Swell, P. E. Schools, Jr., and C. R. Treadwell, *Circulation* **22**, 547–558 (1960).
228. Chobanian, A. V., and W. Hollander, *J. Clin. Invest.* **41**, 1732–1737 (1962).
229. Goodman, D. S., and T. Shiratori, *Biochim. Biophys. Acta* **84**, 104–106 (1964).
230. Goodman, D. S., and T. Shiratori, *J. Lipid Res.* **5**, 578–586 (1964).
231. Reaven, G. M., D. B. Hill, R. C. Gross, and J. W. Farquhar, *J. Clin. Invest.* **44**, 1826–1833 (1965).
232. Fredrickson, D. S., and R. S. Gordon, Jr., *Physiol. Rev.* **38**, 585–630 (1958).
233. Baker, N., and M. C. Schotz, *J. Lipid Res.* **8**, 646–660 (1967).
234. Belfrage, P., B. Edgren, and T. Olivecrona, *Acta Physiol. Scand.* **62**, 344–351 (1964).
235. Quarfordt, H. S., and D. S. Goodman, *Biochim. Biophys. Acta* **116**, 382–385 (1966).
236. French, J. E., and B. Morris, *J. Physiol.* **138**, 326–339 (1957).
237. Nestel, P. J., *J. Clin. Invest.* **43**, 943–949 (1964).
238. Bates, M. W., *Amer. J. Physiol.* **212**, 662–668 (1967).
239. Farquhar, J. W., R. C. Gross, R. M. Wagner, and G. M. Reaven, *J. Lipid Res.* **6**, 119–134 (1965).
240. Ryan, W. G., and T. B. Schwartz, *Metabolism* (*Clin. Exp.*) **14**, 1243–1254 (1965).

241. Havel, R. J., in *Deuel Conference on Lipids, The Turnover of Lipids and Lipoproteins,* G. Cowgill, D. L. Estrich, and P. D. Wood, Eds., U.S. Government Printing Office, Washington, 1968, pp. 117–130.
242. Sailer, S., F. Sandhofer, and H. Braunsteiner, *Klin. Wochenschr.* **44**, 1032–1036 (1966).
243. Baker, N., *J. Lipid Res.* **10**, 1–24 (1969).
244. Quarfordt, S. H., and D. S. Goodman, *Biochim. Biophys. Acta* **176**, 863–872 (1969).
245. Felts, J. M., and P. A. Mayes, *Nature* **206**, 195–196 (1965).
246. Mayes, P. A., and J. M. Felts, *Biochem. J.* **108**, 483–487 (1968).
247. Havel, R. J., and R. S. Gordon, Jr., *J. Clin. Invest.* **39**, 1777–1790 (1960).
248. Fredrickson, D. S., K. Ono, and L. L. Davis, *J. Lipid Res.* **4**, 24–33 (1963).
249. Kuo, P., D. Bassett, A. D. George, and G. Carpenter, *Circulation Res.* **16**, 221–229 (1965).
250. Bradford, R. H., and R. H. Furman, *Biochim. Biophys. Acta* **164**, 172–184 (1968).
251. Robinson, D. S., *Adv. Lipid Res.* **1**, 133–182 (1963).
252. Robinson, D. S., in *Handbook of Physiology, Section 5: Adipose Tissue,* A. E. Renold and G. F. Cahill, Jr., Eds., American Physiological Society, Washington, D.C., 1965, pp. 295–300.
253. Robinson, D. S., in *Deuel Conference on Lipids, The Fate of Dietary Lipids,* G. Cowgill and L. W. Kinsell, Eds., U.S. Government Printing Office, Washington, D.C., 1967, pp. 166–194.
254. Lindgren, F. T., and A. V. Nichols, in *The Plasma Proteins,* Vol. 2, F. W. Putnam, Ed., Academic Press, New York, 1960, pp. 1–58.
255. Nichols, A. V., *Adv. Biol. Med. Phys.* **11**, 110–158 (1967).
256. Fried, M., H. G. Wilcox, G. R. Faloona, S. P. Eoff, M. S. Hoffman, and D. Zimmerman, *Comp. Biochem. Physiol.* **25**, 651–661 (1968).
257. Kellner, A., J. W. Correll, and A. T. Ladd, *J. Exp. Med.* **93**, 373–385 (1951).
258. Cornforth, J. W., P. D'Arcy Hart, R. J. W. Rees, and J. A. Stock, *Nature* **168**, 150–153 (1951).
259. Friedman, M., and S. O. Byers, *J. Exp. Med.* **97**, 117–130 (1953).
260. Scanu, A., P. Oriente, J. M. Szajewski, J. L. McCormack, and I. H. Page, *J. Exp. Med.* **114**, 279–294 (1961).
261. Brown, R. K., E. Boyle, and C. B. Anfinson, *J. Biol. Chem.* **204**, 423–434 (1953).
262. Schotz, M. C., A. Scanu, and I. H. Page, *Amer. J. Physiol.* **188**, 399–402 (1957).
263. Scanu, A., and P. Oriente, *J. Exp. Med.* **113**, 735–757 (1961).
264. Byers, S. O., and M. Friedman, *Amer. J. Physiol.* **198**, 629–631 (1960).
265. Scanu, A., and I. H. Page, *J. Clin. Invest.* **41**, 495–504 (1962).
266. Frantz, I. D., Jr., and B. T. Hinkelman, *J. Exp. Med.* **101**, 225–232 (1955).
267. Hunter, A. R., and A. Korner, *Biochem. J.* **100**, 73P (1966).
268. Scanu, A. M., *Adv. Lipid Res.* **3**, 63–138 (1965).
269. Ahrens, E. H., Jr., J. Hirsch, K. Oette, J. W. Farquhar, and Y. Stein, *Trans. Assoc. Amer. Physicians* (*Philadelphia*) **74**, 134–146 (1961).
270. MacDonald, I., *Adv. Lipid Res.* **4**, 39–67 (1966).
271. McGandy, R. B., D. M. Hegsted, and F. J. Stare, *New Engl. J. Med.* **277**, 417–419, 469–471 (1967).
272. Levy, R. I., and C. J. Glueck, *Arch. Intern. Med.* **123**, 220–228 (1969).
273. Kuo, P. T., *Trans. Assoc. Amer. Physicians* (*Philadelphia*) **78**, 97–116 (1965).

274. Schwartz, D., E. Patois, and J. L. Beaumont, *J. Atheroscler. Res.* **7**, 537–548 (1967).
275. MacDonald, I., *Amer. J. Clin. Nutr.* **18**, 369–372 (1966).
276. Bierman, E. L., and D. Porte, Jr., *Ann. Intern. Med.* **68**, 926–933 (1968).
277. Anderson, J. T., F. Grande, Y. Matsumoto, and A. Keys, *J. Nutr.* **79**, 349–359 (1963).
278. Lees, R. S., *Clin. Res.* **13**, 549 (1965).
279. Porte, D., Jr., E. L. Bierman, and J. D. Bagdade, *Proc. Soc. Exp. Biol. Med.* **123**, 814–816 (1966).
280. Nikkilä, E. A., and K. Ojala, *Life Sci.* **4**, 937–943 (1965).
281. Fallon, H. J., and E. L. Kemp, *J. Clin. Invest.* **47**, 712–719 (1968).
282. Nikkilä, E. A., and R. Pelkonen, *Proc. Soc. Exp. Biol. Med.* **123**, 91–94 (1966).
283. Nestel, P. J., K. F. Carroll, and N. Havenstein, *Metabolism (Clin. Exp.)* **19**, 1–18 (1970).
284. Reaven, G. M., R. L. Lerner, M. P. Stern, and J. W. Farquhar, *J. Clin. Invest.* **46**, 1756–1767 (1967).
285. Samols, E., and T. L. Dormandy, *Lancet* **i**, 478–479 (1963).
286. Anderson, J. T., *Amer. J. Clin. Nutr.* **20**, 168–175 (1967).
287. Farquhar, J. W., A. Frank, R. C. Gross, and G. M. Reaven, *J. Clin. Invest.* **45**, 1648–1656 (1966).
288. Kuo, P. T., and L. Y. Feng, *Metabolism (Clin. Exp.)* **19**, 372–380 (1970).
289. Eaton, R. P., and D. M. Kipnis, *Amer. J. Physiol.* **217**, 1153–1159 (1969).
290. Sailer, S., F. Sandhofer, and H. Braunsteiner, *Metabolism (Clin. Exp.)* **15**, 135–137 (1966).
291. Knittle, J. L., and E. H. Ahrens, Jr., *J. Clin. Invest.* **43**, 485–495 (1964).
292. Davidson, P. C., and M. J. Albrink, *Metabolism (Clin. Exp.)* **14**, 1059–1070 (1965).
293. Nestel, P. J., *Metabolism (Clin. Exp.)* **15**, 787–795 (1966).
294. Glueck, C. J., R. I. Levy, and D. S. Fredrickson, *Clin. Res.* **16**, 343 (1968).
295. Yalow, R. S., S. M. Glick, J. Roth, and S. A. Berson, *Ann. N.Y. Acad. Sci.* **131**, 357–373 (1965).
296. Schonfeld, G., *J. Lab. Clin. Med.* **75**, 206–211 (1970).
297. Haft, D. E., *Amer. J. Physiol.* **213**, 219–230 (1967).
298. Gellhorn, A., and W. Benjamin, *Biochim. Biophys. Acta* **84**, 167–175 (1964).
299. Kalkhoff, R. K., and D. M. Kipnis, *Diabetes* **15**, 443–450 (1966).
300. Myant, N. B., in *The Biological Basis of Medicine*, Vol. 2, E. E. Bittar and N. Bittar, Eds., Academic Press, London, 1968, pp. 151–191.
301. Rubenstein, B., and D. Rubenstein, *Can. J. Biochem.* **44**, 129–140 (1966).
302. Winegrad, A. I., in *Handbook of Physiology, Section 5: Adipose Tissue*, A. E. Renold and G. F. Cahill, Jr., Eds., American Physiological Society, Washington, D.C., 1965, pp. 319–329.
303. Jones, D. P., and R. A. Arky, *Metabolism (Clin. Exp.)* **14**, 1287 (1965).
304. Salaman, M. R., and D. S. Robinson, *Biochem. J.* **99**, 640–647 (1966).
305. Bagdade, J. D., D. Porte, Jr., and E. L. Bierman, *New Engl. J. Med.* **276**, 427–433 (1967).
306. Cornwell, D. G., F. A. Kruger, G. J. Hamwi, and J. B. Brown, *Amer. J. Clin. Nutr.* **9**, 24–40 (1961).
307. Olson, R. E., and J. W. Vester, *Physiol. Rev.* **40**, 677–733 (1960).
308. Furman, R. H., R. P. Howard, K. Lakshmi, and L. N. Norcia, *Amer. J. Clin. Nutr.* **9**, 73–102 (1961).

309. Pantelakis, S. N., A. S. Fosbrooke, J. K. Lloyd, and O. H. Wolff, *Diabetes* **13**, 153–160 (1964).
310. Aurell, M., K. Cramér, and G. Rybo, *Lancet* **i**, 291–293 (1966).
311. Wynn, V., J. Doar, and G. Mills, *Lancet* **ii**, 720–725 (1966).
312. Hazzard, W. R., M. J. Speiger, J. D. Bagdade, and E. L. Bierman, *New Engl. J. Med.* **280**, 471–474 (1969).
313. Sachs, B. A., L. Wolfman, and N. Herzig, *Obstet. Gynecol.* **34**, 530–535 (1969).
314. Glueck, C. J., W. V. Brown, R. I. Levy, H. Greten, and D. S. Fredrickson, *Lancet* **i**, 1290–1291 (1969).
315. Furman, R. H., P. Alaupovic, and R. P. Howard, *Progr. Biochem. Pharmacol.* **2**, 215–249 (1967).
316. Hess, R., *Adv. Lipid Res.* **2**, 295–445 (1964).
317. Florsheim, W. H., M. A. Faircloth, D. Graff, N. S. Austin, and S. M. Velcoff, *Metabolism* (*Clin. Exp.*) **12**, 598–607 (1963).
318. Wenke, M., *Adv. Lipid Res.* **4**, 69–105 (1966).
319. Shafrir, E., K. E. Sussman, and D. Steinberg, *J. Lipid Res.* **1**, 459–465 (1960).
320. Shafrir, E., K. E. Sussman, and D. Steinberg, *J. Lipid Res.* **1**, 109–117 (1959).
321. Carlson, L. A., S. O. Liljedahl, and C. Wirsén, *Acta Med. Scand.* **178**, 81–102 (1965).
322. Shafrir, E., and D. Steinberg, *J. Clin. Invest.* **39**, 310–319 (1960).
323. Dury, A., *Circulation Res.* **5**, 47–53 (1957).
324. Rudman, D., *J. Lipid Res.* **4**, 119–129 (1963).
325. Wallace, R. A., and D. W. Jared, *Develop. Biol.* **19**, 498–526 (1969).
326. Hahn, W. E., *Comp. Biochem. Physiol.* **23**, 83–93 (1967).
327. Schjeide, O. A., and M. Wilkens, *Nature* **201**, 42–44 (1964).
328. Hahn, W. E., R. B. Church, and A. Gorbman, *Endocrinology* **84**, 738–745 (1969).
329. Priest, R. E., M. T. Schroeder, R. Rasmussen, and R. W. Wissler, *Proc. Soc. Exp. Biol. Med.* **96**, 298–301 (1957).
330. Abell, L. L., E. H. Mosbach, and F. E. Kendall, *Circulation Res.* **10**, 846–850 (1962).
331. Mosbach, E. H., and L. L. Abell, *Circulation* **22**, 658–659 (1960).
332. Engelberg, H., and S. J. Glass, *Metabolism* (*Clin. Exp.*) **4**, 298–301 (1955).
333. Oliver, M. F., and G. S. Boyd, *Circulation* **13**, 82–91 (1956).
334. Svanborg, A., and O. Vikrot, *Acta Med. Scand.* **179**, 615–622 (1966).
335. Myant, N. B., in *Lipid Pharmacology*, R. Paoletti, Ed., Academic Press, New York, 1964, pp. 299–323.
336. Moyer, J. H., *Arch. Environ. Health* **14**, 337–347 (1957).
337. Strisower, E. H., G. Adamson, and B. Strisower, *Amer. J. Med.* **45**, 488–501 (1968).
338. Connor, W. E., *Med. Clin. N. Amer.* **52**, 1249–1260 (1968).
339. Levy, L. J., J. J. Adesman, and G. Spergel, *J. Clin. Endocrinol. Metab.* **30**, 372–379 (1970).
340. Steinberg, D., and M. Vaughan, in *Proceedings of the Fifth International Congress of Biochemistry,* Vol. 7, G. Popjak, Ed., Pergamon, New York, 1963, pp. 162–190.
341. Porte, D., D. D. O'Hara, and R. H. Williams, *Metabolism* (*Clin. Exp.*) **15**, 107–113 (1966).
342. Albrink, M. J., J. R. Fitzgerald, and E. B. Man, *Proc. Soc. Exp. Biol. Med.* **95**, 778–780 (1957).

343. Salter, J. M., *Amer. J. Clin. Nutr.* **8**, 535–539 (1960).
344. Amatuzio, D. S., F. Grande, and S. Wada, *Metabolism (Clin. Exp.)* **11**, 1240–1249 (1962).
345. Caren, R., and L. Corbo, *Metabolism (Clin. Exp.)* **9**, 938–945 (1960).
346. Gorman, C. K., J. M. Salter, and J. C. Penhos, *Metabolism (Clin. Exp.)* **16**, 1140–1157 (1967).
347. Caren, R., and L. Carbo, *J. Clin. Endocrinol. Metab.* **16**, 507–516 (1956).
348. Paloyan, E., and P. V. Harper, Jr., *Metabolism (Clin. Exp.)* **10**, 315–323 (1961).
349. Goodridge, A. G., and E. G. Ball, *Comp. Biochem. Physiol.* **16**, 367–381 (1965).
350. Carlson, L. A., S. O. Liljedahl, M. Verdy, and C. Wirsen, *Metabolism (Clin. Exp.)* **13**, 227–231 (1964).
351. Steinberg, D., E. Shafrir, and M. Vaughan, *Clin. Res.* **7**, 250 (1959).
352. Hagen, J. H., *J. Biol. Chem.* **236**, 1023–1027 (1961).
353. Sutherland, E. W., and G. A. Robison, *Diabetes* **18**, 797–819 (1969).
354. Lipsett, M. B., H. R. Engel, and D. M. Bergenstal, *J. Lab. Clin. Med.* **56**, 342–354 (1960).
355. Dreiling, D. A., E. L. Bierman, A. F. Debons, P. Elsbach, and I. L. Schwartz, *Metabolism (Clin. Exp.)* **11**, 572–578 (1962).
356. Sokal, J. E., *Amer. J. Med.* **41**, 331–341 (1966).
357. Grodsky, G. M., L. L. Bennett, D. F. Smith, and F. G. Schmid, *Metabolism (Clin. Exp.)* **16**, 222–233 (1967).
358. Haugaard, E. S., and W. C. Stadie, *J. Biol. Chem.* **200**, 753–757 (1953).
359. Haugaard, E. S., and N. Haugaard, *J. Biol. Chem.* **206**, 641–645 (1954).
360. Berthet, J., *Progr. Nucl. Energy Ser. VII Med. Sci.* **3**, 179–184 (1958).
361. Norum, K. R., and E. Gjone, *Scand. J. Clin. Lab. Invest.* **20**, 231–243 (1967).
362. Gjone, E., and K. R. Norum, *Acta Med. Scand.* **183**, 107–112 (1968).

Author Index

Numbers in brackets indicate the pages on which the complete references appear.

Subject Index